Diffusion-Weighted MR Imaging of the Brain, Head and Neck, and Spine

Toshio Moritani • Aristides A. Capizzano
Editors

Diffusion-Weighted MR Imaging of the Brain, Head and Neck, and Spine

Third Edition

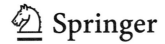

Editors
Toshio Moritani, MD, PhD
Professor of Radiology
Director of Clinical Neuroradiology Research
Division of Neuroradiology
University of Michigan
Ann Arbor, MI
USA

Aristides A. Capizzano, MD
Associate Professor of Radiology
Division of Neuroradiology
University of Michigan
Ann Arbor, MI
USA

ISBN 978-3-030-62119-3   ISBN 978-3-030-62120-9   (eBook)
https://doi.org/10.1007/978-3-030-62120-9

© Springer Nature Switzerland AG 2021, corrected publication 2021
This work is subject to copyright. All rights are reserved by the Publisher, whether the whole or part of the material is concerned, specifically the rights of translation, reprinting, reuse of illustrations, recitation, broadcasting, reproduction on microfilms or in any other physical way, and transmission or information storage and retrieval, electronic adaptation, computer software, or by similar or dissimilar methodology now known or hereafter developed.
The use of general descriptive names, registered names, trademarks, service marks, etc. in this publication does not imply, even in the absence of a specific statement, that such names are exempt from the relevant protective laws and regulations and therefore free for general use.
The publisher, the authors, and the editors are safe to assume that the advice and information in this book are believed to be true and accurate at the date of publication. Neither the publisher nor the authors or the editors give a warranty, expressed or implied, with respect to the material contained herein or for any errors or omissions that may have been made. The publisher remains neutral with regard to jurisdictional claims in published maps and institutional affiliations.

This Springer imprint is published by the registered company Springer Nature Switzerland AG
The registered company address is: Gewerbestrasse 11, 6330 Cham, Switzerland

To Lila, my mom, for being always there, to my wife, Nicoll, for her relentless patience and to Angela and Emma, source of my inspiration.

Aristides A. Capizzano

I dedicate this 3ʳᵈ edition to my father, Hideo Moritani, and my mother, Tomoko Moritani, who recently passed away from long fight against their illness.
I would like to thank my wife, Yumiko Moritani, for her strong support and editorial assistance with devotion.

Toshio Moritani

Preface to the 3rd edition

The routine application of diffusion-weighted imaging (DWI) in Neuroradiology has been expanded not only to the brain but also to head and neck, spine, and spinal cord. Accordingly, in addition to the cases presented in the 2nd edition of *"Diffusion-Weighted MR Imaging of the Brain"*, we have included head and neck and spine DWI cases in this 3rd edition; therefore, the title has been changed to *"Diffusion-Weighted MR Imaging of the Brain, Head and Neck, and Spine"*.

Remarkable progress has continuously been made in the field of diffusion imaging in the last 10 years, as exemplified by diffusion tensor imaging (DTI), fiber tractography, high b-value DWI, intravoxel incoherent motion (IVIM), diffusion kurtosis, Q-space imaging, and oscillating-gradient spin-echo (OGSE) diffusion. The emphasis of this 3rd edition, however, has remained in the clinical aspect of image interpretation, as has been the tradition in the two previous editions of this work. This is supported by the wealth of clinical cases presented, the vast majority from the authors' several year clinical experience at the Universities of Iowa and Michigan.

More recently, new technology and knowledge of genetics, epigenetics, and molecular biology of various neurologic and oncologic diseases have been rapidly progressing, even with faster pace than the progress of new imaging technologies. Numerous studies have been published especially in the last several years. The advancements of both molecular biology and cutting-edge imaging have greatly impacted on the diagnosis, management, and treatment of many diseases.

Without the same up-to-date background knowledge, it is sometimes hard for radiologists and clinicians to discuss diagnosis, management, and treatment. In this 3rd edition, we asked radiation oncologists, neurologists, clinicians, and neurosurgeons to contribute the essential most recent management and treatment for each chapter.

This 3rd edition consists of four parts. Part 1 (Chaps. 1, 2, 3, 4, 5, 6, and 7) was written by world experts in their respective fields, encompassing the following topics: basic and advanced physics of diffusion imaging (Chaps. 1 and 7), DWI and DTI anatomy (Chap. 2), pitfalls and artifacts (Chap. 3), diffusion kurtosis, Q-space imaging, glymphatic system and DTI (Chap. 4), intravoxel incoherent motion (IVIM) (Chap. 5), and functional MRI (Chap. 6).

Part 2 (Chaps. 8, 9, 10, 11, 12, 13, 14, 15, 16, 17, 18, 19, 20, 21, 22, and 23) was divided into imaging and treatment sections in each chapter. The authors of the treatment sections summarized the clinically important topics for interpreting the imaging findings. Each chapter presents correlations between many DW images and pathological tissues. Chapter 8 covered DWI of brain edema with relatively new underlying pathologic and pathophysiologic concepts such as intramyelinic edema, axonal swelling (beading), excitotoxic brain injury, cytokine cascade, and cortical spreading depression by using various illustrative cases. Chapter 9 (infarction) and Chap. 10 (hemorrhage) discussed the time course of signal abnormalities of infarction and hemorrhage with the background pathologies.

Chapter 11 (vasculitis/vasculopathy) was largely rewritten to update the latest advances in vascular diseases, including metabolic and inflammatory conditions, embolic diseases, coagulative and functional disorders. Chapter 12 (epilepsy) was substantially updated to include the last ILAE classifications of seizures and the epilepsies and expanded to review the imaging features of epileptogenic lesions including recently described entities such as amygdala enlargement and immune-mediated encephalitis. Chapter 13 (demyelinating disease) was updated to discuss neuromyelitis optica (NMO) spectrum disorders, anti-myelin oligodendrocyte glycoprotein (MOG) antibody-related demyelination and chronic lymphocytic inflammation with pontine perivascular enhancement responsive to steroids (CLIPPERS).

Chapter 14 (degenerative disease) was wholly rewritten to include discussion of the most prevalent neurodegenerative disorders such as Alzheimer's, Lewy body, Parkinson diseases, and frontotemporal lobar degeneration (FTLD) as well as neuronal intranuclear inclusion disease (NIID) and hereditary diffuse leukoencephalopathy with axonal spheroids (HDLS). Chapter 15 (toxic and metabolic disease) was updated to include more recently described metabolic conditions such as stroke-like migraine attacks after radiation therapy (SMART) syndrome.

We include new cases such as COVID-19 in Chap. 16 (infectious disease), traumatic optic neuropathy in Chap. 17 (trauma), various brain tumors based on the WHO 2016 classification in Chap. 18 (neoplasm), pediatric leukodystrophy and neoplasms in Chap. 19 (pediatrics), and various head and neck tumors and infections in Chap. 20 (head and neck).

This 3rd edition includes three new chapters of spine DWI: Chap. 21 (spine infection), Chap. 22 (spine neoplasm), and Chap. 23 (spinal cord lesion) with many DWI cases and discussion of management.

In Part 3 (Chaps. 24 and 25), experts of the field discuss the future of the DW imaging including oscillating-gradient spin-echo (OGSE) diffusion.

Part 4 (Chap. 26) lists important figures and imaging examples from each chapter, which should help the readers understand pathology, pathophysiology, and DWI cases visually.

We hope that this book, *"Diffusion-Weighted Imaging of the Brain, Head and Neck and Spine"*, will be useful for better understanding of the physics, anatomy, pathology, pathophysiology, and imaging characteristics of diseases in these anatomic fields, and a good companion to the Neuroradiologist in the reading room.

Ann Arbor, MI	Toshio Moritani
Ann Arbor, MI	Aristides A. Capizzano
August 2020	
March 2021	

Acknowledgements

We are sincerely grateful to all the authors and contributors to this book (see the list in authors and contributors section).

We wish to thank our Faculty colleagues, residents, fellows, MRI technologists, and other coworkers in the Departments of Radiology and allied Departments at the University of Michigan and the University of Iowa.

Our deepest gratitude goes to Ms Danielle Dobbs and Ms Sarah Abate, Media Division, Department of Radiology at the University of Michigan, for the beautiful illustrations.

We would like to especially thank Dr Ashok Srinivasan (Director, Neuroradiology, Department of Radiology, University of Michigan), Dr Thomas Chenevert (Professor, Department of Radiology, University of Michigan), Dr Vikas Glani (Chairman, Department of Radiology, University of Michigan), Dr N Reed Dunnick (Former Chairman, Department of Radiology, University of Michigan), Dr Colin P Derdeyn (Chairman, Department of Radiology, University of Iowa), Dr Joan E Maley (Director, Neuroradiology, Department of Radiology, University of Iowa), Dr Yutaka Sato (Director, Pediatric Radiology, Department of Radiology, University of Iowa), and Dr Yuji Numaguchi (Department of Radiology, St. Luke's International Hospital, Tokyo, Japan), who gave us encouragement and support.

Toshio Moritani
Aristides A. Capizzano
Ann Arbor, Michigan

Contents

Part I Principles of DW Imaging

1 **Basics of Diffusion Measurements by MRI** 3
Arun Venkataraman and Jianhui Zhong

2 **Diffusion-Weighted and Tensor Imaging of the Normal Brain** 11
Noriko Salamon and Toshio Moritani

3 **Pitfalls and Artifacts of Diffusion-Weighted Imaging** 29
Toshio Moritani, Akio Hiwatashi, and Jianhui Zhong

4 **Diffusion Tensor and Kurtosis** 43
Toshiaki Taoka

5 **Intravoxel Incoherent Motion Imaging** 67
Takashi Yoshiura

6 **Functional MRI and Diffusion Tensor Imaging** 77
Gaurang Shah

7 **Physics of Advanced Diffusion Imaging** 103
Arun Venkataraman and Jianhui Zhong

Part II Clinical Applications of DW Imaging

8 **Brain Edema** 113
Toshio Moritani

Badih Junior Daou, Gregory Palmateer, and Aditya S. Pandey

9 **Infarction** 155
John Kim, Toshio Moritani, Sven Ekholm, and Yoshimitsu Ohgiya

Julius Griauzde, and Neeraj Chaudhary

10 **Intracranial Hemorrhage** 187
Toshio Moritani, and Akio Hiwatashi

Sravanthi Koduri, Zachary Marcus Wilseck, Ankur Bhambri, and Aditya S. Pandey

11 Vasculopathy and Vasculitis...............217
Girish Bathla, Toshio Moritani, Patricia A. Kirby,
and Aristides A. Capizzano

Sadhana Murali, and Mollie McDermott

12 Epilepsy 275
Aristides A. Capizzano, and Toshio Moritani

Hiroto Kawasaki

13 Demyelinating Diseases 313
Aristides A. Capizzano, and Toshio Moritani

Andrew Romeo

14 Degenerative Diseases of the CNS...............353
Aristides A. Capizzano, and Toshio Moritani

Juana Nicoll Capizzano

15 Toxic and Metabolic Diseases...............391
Aristides A. Capizzano, and Toshio Moritani

Yang Mao-Draayer, Brian Chang, and Deema Fattal

16 Infectious Diseases 429
Toshio Moritani, Yoshiaki Ota, and Patricia A. Kirby

Eiyu Matsumoto

17 Trauma...............487
Vikas Jain, and Toshio Moritani

Hiroto Kawasaki

18 Brain Neoplasm...............521
Jayapalli Rajiv Bapuraj, Toshio Moritani, Shotaro Naganawa,
and Akio Hiwatashi

Christopher Becker, Yoshie Umemura, and Michelle M. Kim

19 Pediatrics 627
Lillian Lai, and Toshio Moritani

Satsuki Matsumoto, Mariko Sato, Jeremy D. Greenlee,
and John M. Buatti

20 Head and Neck 715
Jerry M. Kovoor, Jack Kademian, and Toshio Moritani

Molly Heft Neal, Andrew C. Birkeland, and Matthew E. Spector

Contents

21 Spine Infection 777
John Kim, Eiyu Matsumoto, and Toshio Moritani

22 Primary and Metastatic Spine Tumors 803
Patrick W. Hitchon, Shotaro Naganawa, John Kim,
Royce W. Woodroffe, Logan C. Helland, Mark C. Smith,
and Toshio Moritani

23 Spinal Cord Lesions 839
John Kim, Duy Q. Bui, Toshio Moritani,
Patrick W. Hitchon, Royce W. Woodroffe,
Jennifer L. Noeller, and Kirill V. Nourski

Part III Futures of Diffusion Imaging

**24 Future Directions for Diffusion Imaging
of the Brain and Spinal Cord** 877
Takayuki Obata, Jeff Kershaw, Akifumi Hagiwara,
and Shigeki Aoki

25 Diffusion Imaging of the Head and Neck in the Future 891
Ashok Srinivasan

Part IV How to use this book

26 How to Use This Book 903
Toshio Moritani and Per-Lennart A. Westesson

**Corrections to: Future Directions for Diffusion Imaging
of the Brain and Spinal Cord** C1

Editors and Contributors

Editors

Toshio Moritani, MD, PhD Professor of Radiology, Director of Clinical Neuroradiology Research, Division of Neuroradiology, University of Michigan, Ann Arbor, MI, USA

Aristides A. Capizzano, MD Associate Professor of Radiology, Department of Radiology, Division of Neuroradiology, University of Michigan, Ann Arbor, MI, USA

Authors

Shigeki Aoki, MD, PhD Professor and Chairman, Department of Radiology, Juntendo University, Tokyo, Japan

Jayapalli Rajiv Bapuraj, MBBS Associate Professor of Radiology, Division of Neuroradiology, University of Michigan, Ann Arbor, MI, USA

Girish Bathla, MBBS, MMeD, FRCR Clinical Assistant Professor of Radiology, Division of Neuroradiology, University of Iowa Hospitals & Clinics, Iowa City, IA, USA

Christopher Becker, MD Department of Neurology, University of Michigan, Ann Arbor, MI, USA

Ankur Bhambri, BS Department of Neurosurgery, University of Michigan, Ann Arbor, MI, USA

Andrew C. Birkeland, MD Assistant Professor of Otolaryngology Head and Neck Surgery, University of California Davis, Sacramento, CA, USA

John M. Buatti, MD Professor and Chair of Radiation Oncology, University of Iowa Hospitals and Clinics, Iowa City, IA, USA

Duy Q. Bui, MD Department of Radiology, University of Iowa Hospitals and Clinics, Iowa City, IA, USA

Aristides A. Capizzano, MD Associate Professor of Radiology, Division of Neuroradiology, University of Michigan, Ann Arbor, MI, USA

Juana Nicoll Capizzano, MD Assistant Professor of Family Medicine, University of Michigan, Ann Arbor, MI, USA

Brian Chang, MSCR University of Michigan Medical School, Ann Arbor, MI, USA

Neeraj Chaudhary, MD Associate Professor of Radiology, Neurosugery, Neurology, Division of Neuroradiology, University of Michigan, Ann Arbor, MI, USA

Badih Junior Daou, MD Department of Neurosurgery, University of Michigan, Ann Arbor, MI, USA

Sven Ekholm, MD, PhD Professor Emeritus, Department of Imaging Sciences, University of Rochester Medical Center, Rochester, NY, USA

Deema Fattal, MD Clinical Associate Professor of Neurology, University of Iowa Hospitals & Clinics, Iowa City, IA, USA

Jeremy D. Greenlee, MD Professor of Neurosurgery, University of Iowa Hospitals and Clinics, Iowa City, IA, USA

Julius Griauzde, MD Assistant Professor of Radiology, University of Michigan School of Medicine, Ann Arbor, MI, USA

Akifumi Hagiwara, MD, PhD Assistant Professor, Department of Radiology, Juntendo University, Tokyo, Japan

Molly Heft Neal, MD Department of Otolaryngology Head and Neck Surgery, University of Michigan, Ann Arbor, MI, USA

Logan C. Helland, MD Department of Neuroesurgery, University of Iowa Hospitals & Clinics, Iowa City, IA, USA

Patrick W. Hitchon, MD Professor of Neurosurgery, University of Iowa Carver College of Medicine, Iowa City, IA, USA

Akio Hiwatashi, MD, PhD Associate Professor, Department of Clinical Radiology, Kyushu University, Fukuoka, Japan

Vikas Jain, MD Associate Professor of Radiology, The MetroHealth System, Cleveland, OH, USA

Jack Kademian, DDS, MD Assistant Professor of Radiology, University of Iowa Hospitals & Clinics, Iowa City, IA, USA

Hiroto Kawasaki, MD, PhD Associate Professor of Neurosurgery, University of Iowa Hospitals & Clinics, Iowa City, IA, USA

Jeff Kershaw, PhD Senior Researcher, Applied MRI Research, National Institute of Radiological Sciences, QST, Chiba, Japan

John Kim, MD Assistant Professor of Radiology, Division of Neuroradiology, University of Michigan, Ann Arbor, MI, USA

Michelle M. Kim, MD Associate Professor of Radiation Oncology, University of Michigan, Ann Arbor, MI, USA

Patricia A. Kirby, MBBCh Professor Emerita of Pathology, University of Iowa Hospitals & Clinics, Iowa City, IA, USA

Sravanthi Koduri, MD Department of Neurosurgery, University of Michigan, Ann Arbor, MI, USA

Jerry M. Kovoor, MD Associate Professor of Clinical Radiology and Imaging Sciences, Indiana University School of Medicine, Indianapolis, IN, USA

Lillian Lai, MD Clinical Assistant Professor of Radiology, Children's Hospital Los Angeles, Los Angeles, CA, USA

Yang Mao-Draayer, MD, PhD Clinical Professor of Neurology, University of Michigan, Ann Arbor, MI, USA

Eiyu Matsumoto, MD Clinical Assistant Professor of Internal Medicine, University of Iowa Hospitals and Clinics, Iowa City, IA, USA

Satsuki Matsumoto, MD Clinical Assistant Professor of Pediatrics, University of Iowa Hospitals and Clinics, Iowa City, IA, USA

Mollie McDermott, MD Clinical Assistant Professor of Neurology, University of Michigan, Ann Arbor, MI, USA

Toshio Moritani, MD, PhD Professor of Radiology, Director of Clinical Neuroradiology Research, Division of Neuroradiology, University of Michigan, Ann Arbor, MI, USA

Sadhana Murali, MD Clinical Lecturer of Neurology, University of Michigan, Ann Arbor, MI, USA

Shotaro Naganawa, MD, PhD Department of Radiology, University of Michigan, Ann Arbor, MI, USA

Jennifer L. Noeller, ARNP Department of Neurosurgery, University of Iowa Hospitals and Clinics, Iowa City, IA, USA

Kirill V. Nourski, MD, PhD Associate Professor of Neurosurgery, University of Iowa Hospitals and Clinics, Iowa City, IA, USA

Takayuki Obata, MD, PhD Senior Researcher, Applied MRI Research, National Institute of Radiological Sciences, QST, Chiba, Japan

Yoshimitsu Ohgiya, MD, PhD Professor and Chairman, Department of Radiology, Showa University School of Medicine, Tokyo, Japan

Yoshiaki Ota, MD Department of Radiology, University of Michigan, Ann Arbor, MI, USA

Gregory Palmateer, BA University of Michigan, Ann Arbor, MI, USA

Aditya S. Pandey, MD Associate Professor of Neurological Surgery, Associate Professor of Otolaryngology of Head and Neck Surgery, University of Michigan, Ann Arbor, MI, USA

Andrew Romeo, MD Clinical Assistant Professor of Neurology, University of Michigan, Ann Arbor, MI, USA

Noriko Salamon, MD, PhD Professor of Radiology, Vice Chair of Academic Affairs, Chief of Diagnostic Neuroradiology, Director of Clinical Image Processing Laboratory, Department of Radiological Sciences, Ronald Reagan UCLA Medical Center, Los Angeles, CA, USA

Mariko Sato, MD, PhD Clinical Associate Professor of Pediatrics, University of Iowa Hospitals and Clinics, Iowa City, IA, USA

Gaurang Shah, MD, FACR Professor of Radiology, Director of Functional MRI, Division of Neuroradiology, University of Michigan, Ann Arbor, MI, USA

Mark C. Smith, MD Clinical Associate Professor of Radiation Oncology, University of Iowa Carver College of Medicine, Iowa City, IA, USA

Matthew E. Spector, MD Assistant Professor of Otolaryngology, Division of Head and Neck Surgery, University of Michigan, Ann Arbor, MI, USA

Ashok Srinivasan, MD Professor of Radiology, Director of Neuroradiology, University of Michigan, Ann Arbor, MI, USA

Toshiaki Taoka, MD, PhD Professor, Department of Radiology, Nagoya University, Nagoya, Japan

Yoshie Umemura, MD Clinical Assistant Professor of Neurology, University of Michigan, Ann Arbor MI, USA

Arun Venkataraman, BS Department of Imaging Sciences, University of Rochester Medical Center, Rochester, NY, USA

Per-Lennart A. Westesson, MD, DDS, PhD Professor of Imaging Sciences, University of Rochester Medical Center, Rochester, NY, USA

Zachary Marcus Wilseck, MD Department of Radiology, University of Michigan, Ann Arbor, MI, USA

Royce W. Woodroffe, MD Department of Neurosurgery, University of Iowa Carver College of Medicine, Iowa City, IA, USA

Takashi Yoshiura, MD, PhD Professor and Chairman, Department of Radiology, Kagoshima University, Kagoshima, Japan

Jianhui Zhong, PhD Professor of Imaging Sciences, University of Rochester Medical Center, Rochester, NY, USA

Contributors

Takashi Abe, MD Department of Radiology, Nagoya University, Nagoya, Japan

Noriko Aida, MD Department of Radiology, Kanagawa Children's Medical Center, Yokohama, Japan

Aaron Berg, MD Department of Radiology, Sanford Health, Sioux Falls, SD, USA

Felix Boucher, MD Department of Radiology, University of Michigan, Ann Arbor, MI, USA

Adam Bryant, MD Department of Radiology, University of Iowa Hospitals & Clinics, Iowa City, IA, USA

Sandra Camelo-Piragua, MD Department of Pathology, University of Michigan, Ann Arbor, MI, USA

Robert J. Casson, MD Ophthalmic Research Laboratories, Hanson Institute, The University of Adelaide, Adelaide, SA, Australia

Umar Shafique Chaudhary, MD Department of Radiology, University of Texas Medical Branch, Galveston, TX, USA

Kamani Chaula, RT Department of Radiology, University of Michigan, Ann Arbor, MI, USA

Thomas Chenevert, PhD Department of Radiology, University of Michigan, Ann Arbor, MI, USA

Ramon de Guzman, MD Department of Imaging Sciences, University of Rochester, Rochester, NY, USA

Joel Dennhardt, MD Department of Radiology, University of Iowa Hospitals & Clinics, Iowa City, IA, USA

Nancy A. Dudek, RT Department of Radiology, University of Michigan, Ann Arbor, MI, USA

Michaelangelo Fuortes, MD Department of Radiology, University of Iowa Hospitals & Clinics, Iowa City, IA, USA

Barbara Germin, MD Department of Pathology, University of Rochester, Rochester, NY, USA

Justin Guan, MD Department of Radiology, University of Iowa Hospitals & Clinics, Iowa City, IA, USA

Edip M. Gurol, MD Department of Neurology, Massachusetts General Hospital, Boston, MA, USA

Atsuhiko Handa, MD Department of Radiology, University of Iowa Hospitals & Clinics, Iowa City, IA, USA

Myles Horton, MD Section of Neurology, Department of Medicine, University of Manitoba, Winnipeg, Canada

Masahiro Ida, MD Department of Radiology, Mito Medical Center, Ibaraki, Japan

Karra A. Jones, MD Department of Pathology, University of Iowa Hospitals & Clinics, Iowa City, IA, USA

Jinsuh Kim, MD Department of Radiology, University of Alabama at Birmingham, Birmingham, AL, USA

Toshibumi Kinoshita, MD Department of Radiology, Akita Cerebrospinal and Cardiovascular Center, Akita, Japan

Takashi Kitanosono, MD Northfield International, INC, Honolulu, HI, USA

Nobuo Kobayashi, MD Department of Radiology, St. Luke's International Hospital, Tokyo, Japan

Ryo Kurokawa, MD Department of Radiology, University of Tokyo, Tokyo, Japan

Andrew Lee, MD Department of Ophthalmology, Blanton Eye Institute, Houston Methodist Hospital, Houston, TX, USA

Ho Kyu Lee, MD Department of Radiology, Jeju National University Hospital, Jeju, Republic of Korea

Michael Lee, MD Department of Radiology, University of Michigan, Ann Arbor, MI, USA

Vincet A. Magnotta, PhD Department of Radiology, University of Iowa Hospitals & Clinics, Iowa City, IA, USA

Joy Matsui, MD Department of Radiology, UT Southwestern Medical Center, Dallas, TX, USA

Mitsuru Matsuki, MD Department of Radiology, Kindai University, Osaka, Japan

Joel Morehouse, RT Department of Radiology, University of Michigan, Ann Arbor, MI, USA

Harushi Mori, MD Department of Radiology, Jichi Medical University, Tochigi, Japan

Minoru Morikawa, MD Department of Radiology, Nagasaki University, Nagasaki, Japan

Kristine M. Mosier, PhD Department of Radiology & Imaging Sciences, Indiana University, Indianapolis, IN, USA

Hisao Nakamura, MD Department of Radiology, St. Marianna University School of Medicine, Kawasaki, Japan

Jared W. Nelson, MD Department of Radiology, University of Iowa Hospitals & Clinics, Iowa City, IA, USA

Yuji Numaguchi, MD Department of Radiology, St. Luke's International Hospital, Tokyo, Japan

Hiroshi Oba, MD Department of Radiology, Teikyo University School of Medicine, Tokyo, Japan

Masaki Oka, MD Department of Radiology, Kikuna Memorial Hospital, Yokohama, Japan

Bruno Policeni, MD Department of Radiology, University of Iowa Hospitals & Clinics, Iowa City, IA, USA

James M. Powers, MD Department of Pathology and Laboratory Medicine, University of Rochester Medical, Center, Rochester, NY, USA

Michael Sacher, MD Department of Radiology, Mount Sinai Medical Center, New York, NY, USA

Sarabjit K. Saggu, MD Ophthalmic Research Laboratories, Hanson Institute, and The University of Adelaide, Adelaide, SA, Australia

Mio Sakai, MD Department of Radiology, Osaka International Cancer Institute, Osaka, Japan

Tomoaki Sasaki, MD Faculty of Health Sciences, Okayama University Medical School, Okayama, Japan

Takashi S. Sato, MD Department of Radiology, University of Iowa Hospitals & Clinics, Iowa City, IA, USA

Yutaka Sato, MD Department of Radiology, University of Iowa Hospitals & Clinics, Iowa City, IA, USA

R. Nuri Sener, MD Department of Radiology, Ege University Hospital, Izmir, Turkey

Umber Shafique, MBBS Department of Radiology, Indiana University, Indianapolis, IN, USA

Jay L. Starkey, MD Department of Diagnostic Radiology, Oregon Health & Science University, Portland, OR, USA

Sergei Syrbu, MD Department of Pathology, University of Iowa Hospitals & Clinics, Iowa City, IA, USA

Min D. Tang-Schomer, PhD Penn Center for Brain Injury and Repair and Department of Neurosurgery, University of Pennsylvania, Philadelphia, PA, USA

Keiko Toyoda, MD Department of Radiology, Jikei University School of Medicine, Tokyo, Japan

Ryutaro Ukisu, MD Department of Diagnostic Radiology, Kitasato University of School of Medicine, Tokyo, Japan

Hidetsuna Utsunomiya, MD Department of Radiology, Teikyo University School of Medicine, Tokyo, Japan

Matthew White, MD Department of Radiology, University of Nebraska Medical Center, Omaha, NE, USA

Kei Yamada, MD Department of Radiology, Kyoto Prefectural University of Medicine, Kyoto, Japan

Limin Yang, MD Department of Radiology, University of Iowa Hospitals & Clinics, Iowa City, IA, USA

Yan D. Zhang, MD Department of Radiology, University of Nebraska Medical Center, Omaha, NE, USA

Part I

Principles of DW Imaging

Basics of Diffusion Measurements by MRI

1

Arun Venkataraman and Jianhui Zhong

1.1 Diffusion: A Probabilistic Process

Diffusion in the context of diffusion-weighted imaging (DWI) refers to the probabilistic process of water movement over time. To better understand this process, we must first introduce the concept of a "random walk." To understand this process, we can picture a one-dimensional system with discrete time points. At each time point, one can move either left or right along this line, with equal probability to do either. If we plot the course of multiple "walkers" over time, we get a probability distribution resembling a normal distribution centered at the origin (Fig. 1.1). This process is the basis for movement of water, termed "Brownian motion," after the scientist who first described it [1, 2]. We can picture this movement by placing a drop of ink in a glass of water. The ink is initially concentrated where it initially hits the water, but over time it diffuses and becomes more diluted. If we discretized the time points (i.e., calculate how "diffuse" the ink is every second), we could get a measure of the "diffusivity" of the ink in the water by how quickly it spreads.

The quantification of this "diffusivity" of ink has interesting parallels in the realm of brain imaging. We can image that the diffusivity relies on the size of the container; the larger the container, the more distance can be traveled. Similarly, if we could inject "magic ink" into the brain tissue and follow its progress, we could infer details about the structure of brain tissue itself, as well as the changes occurring due to pathologic processes.

1.2 Diffusion Imaging in MR

The aforementioned "magic ink" is created in diffusion imaging by the application of specific magnetic field gradients [3]. When a patient enters the bore (central cavity) of the scanner, the large, static magnetic field (measured in Tesla) induces magnetic spins of protons (small magnets inside hydrogen nuclei) to align with the direction of the magnetic field. In addition, magnetic field gradients add a smaller, nonstatic magnetic field for a certain duration to "tag" different locations in the tissue of interest. This equates to dropping "magic ink" in a location that can be chosen. The application of another gradient after some time informs us about how much the spins have diffused in this time. This equates to taking a snapshot of the "magic ink" at a later time and

---

A. Venkataraman · J. Zhong (✉)
Department of Physics and Astronomy, Center for Advanced Brain Imaging and Neurophysiology, University of Rochester, Rochester, NY, USA

Department of Imaging Sciences, Center for Advanced Brain Imaging and Neurophysiology, University of Rochester, Rochester, NY, USA
e-mail: arun_venkataraman@urmc.rochester.edu; jianhui.zhong@rochester.edu

© Springer Nature Switzerland AG 2021
T. Moritani, A. A. Capizzano (eds.), *Diffusion-Weighted MR Imaging of the Brain, Head and Neck, and Spine*, https://doi.org/10.1007/978-3-030-62120-9_1

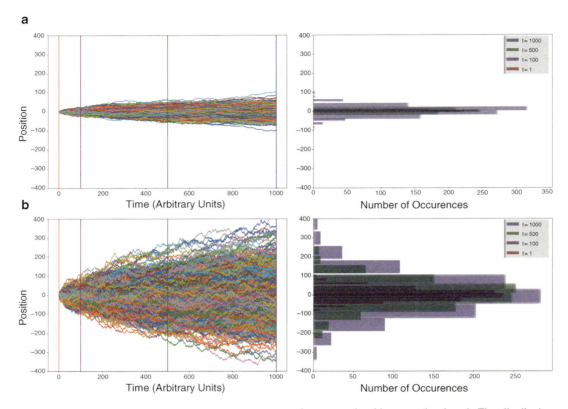

Fig. 1.1 Evolution of random walk over discretized time steps. (**a**) Shows a step size of one at each time point; the resulting trajectories (*left panel*) and histogram of position over time (*right panel*) are shown. (**b**) Same as (**a**), but with step size of five. Vertical bars on the left panel denote comparing to the initial snapshot to quantify how much the ink has diffused. However, the analogy of introducing "magic ink" to assess diffusivity ends here.

when respective histogram is plotted. The distribution widens over time, and as a function of step size, reflecting processes that influence "diffusivity." It is clear that a molecule represented by (**b**) would have a higher "diffusivity" that one represented by (**a**)

1.3 Diffusion Imaging of the Brain

The brain is composed of a multitude of structures, each with unique physical properties. Different tissues may, therefore, restrict motion of water to different degrees. Since water particles are performing a random walk at baseline, they will run into constituents of cells in different cellular compartments and will therefore spread at different rates when labeled with the magnetic field gradients. In addition, this motion need not be identical in different directions, based on the local cellular neighborhood. As explained later in the chapter, the overall tendencies of diffusion can be measured through metrics such as diffusion rate, diffusion coefficient, or diffusivity based on the unit used, and the asymmetry of diffusion can be measured using diffusion anisotropy, with a variety of parameters defined [4–7].

1.4 Principles of Magnetic Resonance Diffusion Imaging

The MRI sequence of diffusion studies can be classified into two portions: (1) Diffusion labeling, and (2) Image acquisition. This means that we need to apply diffusion magnetic field

1 Basics of Diffusion Measurements by MRI

gradients in addition to radiofrequency and gradient pulses used in conventional MRI imaging. A simplified version of the most commonly used pulse-gradient spin-echo (PGSE) pulse sequence for diffusion imaging is shown in Fig. 1.2.

During the diffusion labeling portion, a pair of field gradients are applied to perform "diffusion-encoding" (Fig. 1.2, shaded rectangles). Each gradient in this gradient pair lasts for a time, δ, with gradient magnitude, G (usually measured in mT/m). The gradient pairs are separated by time Δ. Note that the diffusion gradients can be applied in different spatial orientations, which is relevant to measurements of anisotropic diffusion as we will discuss later in the chapter. We can define the so-called diffusion-weighting factor, b, as

$$b = \gamma^2 G^2 \delta^2 \left(\Delta - \frac{\delta}{3} \right) \quad (1.1)$$

where γ is the gyromagnetic ratio of a proton (42.6 MHz/T). From Eq. (1.1), we can see that b, also called the b-factor, can be increased through increases in G, δ, Δ. A formal analysis tells us that the intensity of the signal can be calculated based on the b-factor, the relationship is given by

$$S = S_0 e^{-b \cdot \text{ADC}} \quad (1.2)$$

Here, ADC is the apparent diffusion coefficient and S_0 is the signal intensity when there is no diffusion gradient used. The apparent diffusion coefficient is so-named because it is an average measure of more complicated processes in the tissues, as discussed in the next section.

Equation (1.2) suggests that there is an exponential reduction in the measured signal, S, when diffusion-weighted gradients are applied; this can be understood with simple reasoning. The result of the diffusion gradients is a spatially varying magnetic field; as spins diffuse through this magnetic field, each spin is affected differently based on its location and trajectory. The net outcome is dephasing of the spins, when the spins are no longer aligned with the magnetic field. Since the signal is the summation of the small signals from individual spins, the dephasing caused by the gradient pulses leads to a drop in overall signal intensity. It is also evident that the longer the

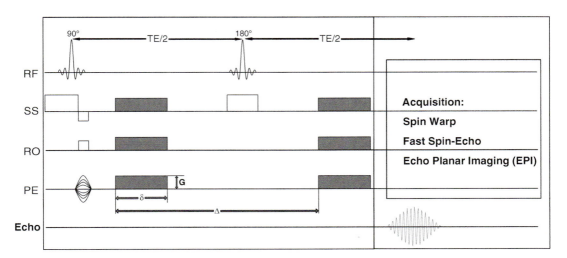

Fig. 1.2 Pulse sequence diagram for general diffusion imaging. *Blue* portion denotes the period of time corresponding to diffusion labeling; shaded rectangles are diffusion gradients. *Red* portion denotes image acquisition, which can be achieved with a variety of techniques (three examples given). *TE* echo time, *RF* radiofrequency, *SS* slice selection, *RO* readout, *PE* phase encoding

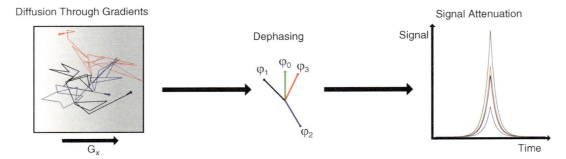

Fig. 1.3 Effects of gradients on diffusing spins. In the first panel, we see an example of three spins (*black*, *blue*, and *red*) diffusing randomly in a one-dimensional magnetic gradient (G_x). The result of motion is dephasing, shown in the second panel. In the final panel, we see that there is a reduction in measured signal resulting from any change in phase. Note that positive and negative phase changes equally attenuate signal. φ_0 represents phase without any diffusion gradients applied

diffusion proceeds, the more dephasing takes place and the lower the signal (Fig. 1.3).

1.5 Apparent Diffusion Coefficient

From Eq. (1.2), we can see that when a fixed b-factor is used, tissues with a higher ADC produce a lower signal intensity. Since brain cerebrospinal fluid (CSF) contains water that can move around relatively freely, it has a much higher ADC value than that of other brain tissues (either gray or white matter), which have diffusion restriction due to cellular structures. Therefore, in a diffusion-weighted (DW) image, one typically sees dark CSF space (due to pronounced dephasing) and brighter signal in the brain tissue (less dephasing). Equation (1.2) also tells us that if we collect a series of DW images with different *b* values, we can calculate ADC value for each volumetric pixel (voxel) and obtain a parametric map, referred to as an ADC map. The calculated ADC map would have voxel intensities reflecting the strength of diffusion in the pixels. Regions of CSF will, therefore, have higher intensity than other brain tissues, opposite of what is seen in the DW images. There are reasons the ADC map is advantageous to the DW image. One is the so-called T2 shine-through effect, which will be discussed in Chap. 2. It should also be noted that in Eq. (1.2), S_0 refers to the signal when no DW gradients are used. Figure 1.2 suggests that this is actually the same as would be obtained from a simple spin-echo sequence. In most clinical scanners, a long TE time (tens of milliseconds) is needed to accommodate the diffusion pulses, leading to T2 weighting of the S_0 image.

1.6 Diffusion Represents a Molecular Event

Despite resolution of MRI images on the order of a millimeter, the information provided by diffusion imaging reflects cellular or molecular events in much smaller scales. This is because the molecular diffusion process is highly influenced by these events. It can be shown that water spins diffuse about tens of micrometers during a typical MR imaging measurement time, which coincides with the dimension of typical cellular structures. If spins are relatively unrestricted by cellular structures during this time (as is the case in the CSF), the measured diffusion is "free" and "isotropic" (equal in all directions), and ADC is just the intrinsic molecular diffusion coefficient. On the other hand, when diffusing spins run into cellular constituents such as cell membranes, the value of ADC will be reduced when compared with the value in free space. Cellular diffusion events are represented schematically in Fig. 1.4.

1 Basics of Diffusion Measurements by MRI

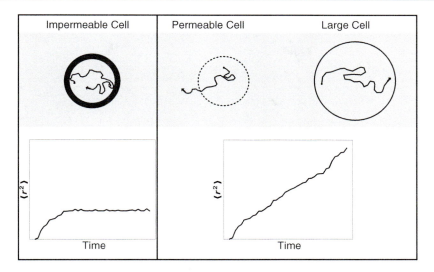

Fig. 1.4 Displacement profiles for different cell types. *Green* (*left*) panel depicts impermeable cell (*upper*) and corresponding mean displacement (<r^2>) graph (*lower*). The graph shows that water in an impermeable cell is hindered, seen by the plateau. *Blue* (*right*) panel depicts permeable and large cells, which have identical mean displacement graphs (*black line, lower panel*), compared to impermeable cell graph (*gray line, lower panel*). Diffusion barriers inside a permeable cell or in a cell much larger than mean displacement during diffusion (*blue panel*) show minimal diffusion barrier effects

For patients with neurologic abnormalities, which change the water distribution in various cellular compartments, or change the ability for water to pass through cell membranes, measured ADC values will be altered [4–7]. Therefore, MR diffusion measurement offers a unique opportunity to obtain information about morphology otherwise inaccessible to conventional MR imaging methods. A wide range of pathological conditions can be explored with water diffusion measurements, as described in later chapters. The measured ADC may also vary depending on the duration of the diffusion process, the direction in which diffusion is measured, and other factors. For diffusion in an anisotropic environment (brain white matter consisting of axons with myelin layers wrapped around them, making diffusion along the bundle much easier than through the bundle), diffusion becomes more complicated, and a complete description of the process relies on what is called tensor analysis [8, 9].

Diffusion tensor imaging (DTI) is an MRI sequence that is available on clinical scanners with diffusion sequences. Instead of monitoring the magnitude of water movement alone, DTI detects both the magnitude and directionality of water diffusion processes in three dimensions and allows the investigation of the microstructure of the CNS by measuring the diffusion properties of water protons in their microenvironment. It is expected that water molecules move less impeded along white matter bundles, than perpendicular to the bundles. The net effect is high directionality (high anisotropy) of movement in the white matter of the brain. In areas of high concentration of fluid (i.e., ventricles filled with CSF), there is little preferential directionality of movement (low anisotropy) and minimal hindrance to diffusion (high diffusivity); these scenarios are shown in Fig. 1.5. Here, we define fractional anisotropy (FA) and mean diffusivity (MD) in the context of DTI metrics used to measure microscopic motion of tissue water at each image voxel. In a DTI measurement, six or more DWI measurements are required; tensor eigenvalues ($\lambda_1, \lambda_2, \lambda_3$) and eigenvectors are derived from these measurements [8]. Maps of MD and FA can then be generated from the eigenvalues with the following relations:

Fig. 1.5 Illustration of diffusion and corresponding diffusion tensor and ellipsoid. *Upper row* illustrates the case with unrestricted diffusion, forming a spherical probability distribution. *Lower row* shows restricted diffusion, such as the case is in white matter. The diffusion ellipsoid is elongated along the direction of maximum diffusion. Note that the more elliptical the ellipsoid is, the higher the measured FA

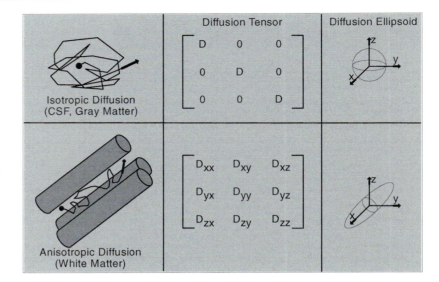

$$\mathrm{MD} = \frac{\lambda_1 + \lambda_2 + \lambda_3}{3} \tag{1.3}$$

$$\mathrm{FA} = \sqrt{\frac{2}{3}} \sqrt{\frac{(\lambda_1 - \mathrm{MD})^2 + (\lambda_2 - \mathrm{MD})^2 + (\lambda_3 - \mathrm{MD})^2}{\lambda_1^2 + \lambda_2^2 + \lambda_3^2}} \tag{1.4}$$

FA represents the anisotropy of the diffusion process, yielding values between 0 (perfectly isotropic diffusion) and 1 (completely anisotropic diffusion). MD represents overall strength of water mobility in different brain areas. A useful representation of DTI measurement results is given by a "color FA" map in which red, green, and blue colors are used to represent the orientation of the largest eigenvalue along left-right (LR), anterior-posterior (AP), and superior-inferior (SI) directions, respectively, while image intensity represents FA values in each voxel.

By following the main direction of water movement (the largest tensor eigenvalue) and its connection in adjacent voxels in the three-dimensional space, fiber tractography in white matter can be formed. We will discuss more advanced applications, and potentials of going beyond the tensor model in the final chapter. The overall impact of DTI is to increase the diagnostic ability of diffusion imaging in degenerative neurological diseases where damage to axon bundles or demyelination can be directly detected and visualized.

1.7 Requirements in Clinical Diffusion Imaging

In the clinical setting, certain requirements are imposed on diffusion studies. Imaging time is often limited to a few minutes for each scan (T1-W, T2-W, diffusion, and others). Multiple slices (15–20) are required to cover most of the brain. A good spatial resolution (~5 to 8 mm thick, 1 to 3 mm in plane) is required. A reasonably short TE (<100 ms) to reduce T2 decay and an adequate diffusion sensitivity (ADC ~ 0.2–1 × 10^{-3} mm²/s for brain tissues) are also needed. The most important requirement, however, is the almost complete elimination of sensitivity to subject motion during scanning. The best compromise so far in clinical diffusion imaging is the use of multidirectional (*x*, *y*, *z*), 2 *b*-factor (*b* = 0, *b* ~ 1/ADC = 1000) single-shot echo-planar imaging (EPI) technique. In addition, multiple *b* = 0 images can be acquired, usually with 6 diffusion-weighted images being acquired for every *b* = 0 image. A clinical scan may last around 5 min, and allow for the acquisition of up to 60 diffusion-weighted images. Sometimes, fluid attenuation with inversion recovery (FLAIR) is used to eliminate signal in the highly diffusive CSF space. Separation from relaxation effects (i.e., T2 shine-through) is achieved with calculation of ADC instead of just using DW. Elimination of anisotropic diffusion is achieved by averaging the diffusion measurements from three orthogonal directions.

1.8 Setting the *b* Value in Clinical DW Imaging

For the sake of standardization in the clinical setting, it is advisable to maintain the same *b* value for all examinations, making it easier to interpret images and become aware of the findings in various disease processes. The studies and discussions presented in this book are limited to DW imaging using *b* values of 0 and 1000 except in the case of advanced implementations of DW imaging (Chap. 7). An upper b-factor of around 1000 is available on most clinical scanners and DW imaging at these standard values has been shown to be a sensitive tool in detecting restricted diffusion (e.g., in acute ischemic lesions of the brain). DW imaging has become clinically important in many other disease processes, which will be discussed in this book.

1.9 Future Trends in Clinical Diffusion Imaging

Newer DW imaging techniques are using even higher *b* values: 8000 s/mm^2 and above. The advent of "Connectome" scanners (of which there are three in the world) allows for the creation of extremely large gradients in a small amount of time. These are currently being used to acquire extremely high-resolution (1.25 mm isotropic) DW images [10]. The increased *b* values may free up routine DW imaging from its most pressing problem, T2 shine-through. At high *b* values, more attention will be focused on the actual physiological basis of restricted and facilitated diffusion. Clearly, much of the advantage of increased *b* values may lie not with the diagnosis of lesions with restricted diffusion, especially acute infarcts, but with allowing a more complete understanding of more subtle or complicated pathologies.

The benefits of improved diffusion contrast at high *b* values can be seen in Eq. (1.2); an identical ADC with higher *b* value will give a lower signal. The overall effect is a higher sensitivity of the scan to motion. However, we can see this could be problematic in calculating the ADC. Because tissues are described by fast and slow components, the results of a two-point measurement will depend on the specific *b* values chosen. If the lower *b* value is set to 0 (T2-weighted image) and the upper value is allowed to vary, the ADC will vary as a function of the upper value. Specifically, one would expect the measured ADC to decrease as the upper *b* value increases.

Advances in acquisition hardware alongside RF coil development are now making it possible to collect data from multiple slices of the brain at once, a technique called simultaneous multislice (SMS) imaging [11]. In SMS imaging, a specialized pulse excited multiple slices within the same acquisition. In combination with multiple channels in the RF coils, imaging data of those slices are acquired. The so-called SMS factor tells us how many slices are being excited in one acquisition. In diffusion imaging, factors of up to four are used, resulting in an acquisition in one-fourth of the original time. It should be noted that there is a trade-off between SMS factor and signal to noise ratio (SNR); with increased SMS factors, SNR decreases. In addition, SMS is not as helpful in current clinical sequences, which are already fast. SMS, instead, is extremely useful in multi-shell acquisitions, which can last for up to 2 h without SMS. Further details about multi-shell acquisition and its advantages are discussed in Chap. 7.

References

1. Einstein A (1905) On the movement of small particles suspended in stationary liquids required by the molecularkinetic theory of heat. Ann. d. Phys 17. 549–560:1.

2. R. V.P.L.S (2009) XXVII. A brief account of microscopical observations made in the months of June, July and August 1827, on the particles contained in the pollen of plants; and on the general existence of active molecules in organic and inorganic bodies. Philosophical Mag Ser 2(21) (1828):161–173

3. Stejskal E, Tanner J (1965) Spin diffusion measurements: spin echoes in the presence of a time-dependent field gradient. J Chem Phys 42(1): 288–292

4. Bihan LD, Breton E, Lallemand D, Grenier P, Cabanis E, Laval-Jeantet M (1986) MR imaging of intravoxel incoherent motions: application to diffusion and perfusion in neurologic disorders. Radiology 161(2):401–407

5. Moseley M, Kucharczyk J, Mintorovitch J, Cohen Y, Kurhanewicz J, Derugin N, Asgari H, Norman D (1990) Diffusion-weighted MR imaging of acute stroke: correlation with T2-weighted and magnetic susceptibility-enhanced MR imaging in cats. AJNR Am J Neuroradiol 11(3): 423–429

6. Moonen CT, Pekar J, de Vleeschouwer MH, van Gelderen P, van Zijl PC, Despres D (1991) Restricted and anisotropic displacement of water in healthy cat brain and in stroke studied by NMR diffusion imaging. Magnet Reson Med 19(2):327–332

7. Zhong J, Petroff O, Prichard J, Gore J (1993) Changes in water diffusion and relaxation properties of rat cerebrum during status epilepticus. Magnet Reson Med 30(2):241–246

8. Basser PJ, Mattiello J, Lebihan D (1994). MR diffusion tensor spectroscopy and imaging. J Magnetic Reson Ser B 66(1):259–267

9. Bihan D, van Zijl P (2002) From the diffusion coefficient to the diffusion tensor. NMR Biomed. 15. 7–8:431–434

10. Essen DC, Ugurbil K, Auerbach E, Barch D, Behrens TEJ, Bucholz R, Chang A, Chen L, Corbetta M, Curtiss SW, Penna DS, Feinberg D, Glasser MF, Harel N, Heath AC, Larson-Prior L, Marcus D, Michalareas G, Moeller S, Oostenveld R, Petersen SE, Prior F, Schlaggar BL, Smith SM, Snyder AZ, Xu J, Yacoub E, Consortium W-M (2012) The Human Connectome Project: a data acquisition perspective. Neuroimage 62(4):2222–2231

11. Barth M, Breuer F, Koopmans PJ, Norris DG, Poser BA (2016) Simultaneous multislice (SMS) imaging techniques. Magnet Reson Med 75(1):63–81

Diffusion-Weighted and Tensor Imaging of the Normal Brain

2

Noriko Salamon and Toshio Moritani

2.1 Introduction

Diffusion-weighted images (DWI) are usually obtained in three orthogonal orientations using spin-echo type single-shot echo-planar imaging with b values around 0 and 1000 s/mm². These three planes are combined into isotropic DWI, and apparent diffusion coefficient (ADC) maps are calculated on a pixel-by-pixel basis (Fig. 2.1). To avoid misinterpretations, it is important to recognize the normal findings on DWI and ADC maps.

2.2 Adult Brain

2.2.1 Low Signal in Basal Ganglia

Isotropic DWI in adult brain often shows low signal intensity in the basal ganglia (Fig. 2.1). This low signal is caused by normal iron deposition. The hypointensity on DWI of these areas is essentially related to T2 contrast, which is also shown on b_0 images. ADC maps usually show the areas as isointense, but it can be hyper- or hypoin-

tense depending on the paramagnetic susceptibility artifact of iron deposition.

2.2.2 Diffusion-Weighted Imaging of Gray and White Matter

Gray matter on DWI is generally hyperintense when compared with white matter. ADC values of gray matter ($0.76 \pm 0.13 \times 10^{-3}$ mm²/s) and white matter ($0.77 \pm 0.18 \times 10^{-3}$ mm²/s) are, however, identical in the adult brain [1]. There are several reports about ADC increasing with age [2–8], but this increase is minimal and has been observed in all parts of the brain. It is usually more apparent in the white matter and lentiform nucleus than in the rest of the brain. Focal areas of DW hyperintensities are often seen in the posterior limbs of the internal capsule, corticospinal tract, cingulate gyrus, insula, medial lemniscus, and the decussation of the superior cerebellar peduncles (Figs. 2.1 and 2.2). These DW hyperintensities are caused by T2 contrast and represent normal findings without clinical significance. ADC maps are usually isointense in these areas [2].

2.2.3 Choroid Plexus

The choroid plexus occasionally shows prominent hyperintensity on DWI associated with mild elevation of ADC. In these situations the ADC is

N. Salamon
Department of Radiological Sciences, Ronald Reagan UCLA Medical Center, Los Angeles, CA, USA
e-mail: nsalamon@mednet.ucla.edu

T. Moritani (✉)
Division of Neuroradiology, University of Michigan, Ann Arbor, MI, USA
e-mail: tmoritan@med.umich.edu

© Springer Nature Switzerland AG 2021
T. Moritani, A. A. Capizzano (eds.), *Diffusion-Weighted MR Imaging of the Brain, Head and Neck, and Spine*, https://doi.org/10.1007/978-3-030-62120-9_2

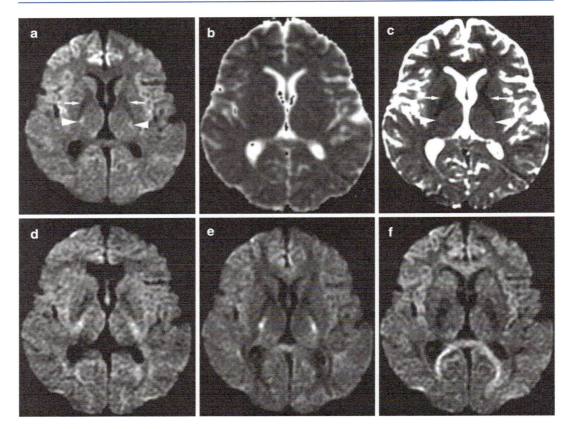

Fig. 2.1 Normal adult brain of a 40-year-old male without neurological deficits. (**a**) Isotropic DWI is obtained by combining b_0 image and three orthogonal unidirectional images (x, y, z axis). The bilateral globi pallidi have low signal on DWI as a result of physiological iron deposition (*arrows*). Corticospinal tracts have mildly high signal on DW image (*arrowheads*). *Gray* matter shows mildly high signal compared to *white* matter. These signal changes on isotropic DWI are normal and are caused by T2 contrast. (**b**) ADC map shows homogeneous ADC values in globi pallidi, corticospinal tracts, *gray* and *white* matter. (**c**) b_0 image shows low signal in globi pallidi (*arrows*), high signal in corticospinal tracts (*arrowheads*), and the gray-white matter contrast. (**d–f**) Diffusion weighting is applied in x axis (**d**), y axis (**e**), and z axis (**f**)

often higher than in white matter, but lower than in cerebrospinal fluid. The high DW signal is believed to represent gelatinous cystic changes of the choroid plexus, which can occur with age (Fig. 2.3) [9].

2.3 Pediatric Brain

2.3.1 Diffusion-Weighted Imaging and ADC of the Pediatric Brain

The normal brain of neonates and infants has significantly higher ADC values than the adult brain [10–15] (Fig. 2.4). ADC in neonates and infants varies markedly within different areas of the brain and is higher in white matter (1.13×10^{-3} mm²/s) than in gray matter (1.02×10^{-3} mm²/s) [13]. ADC at birth is higher in subcortical white matter (1.88×10^{-3} mm²/s) than in both the anterior (1.30×10^{-3} mm²/s) and posterior limbs of the internal capsule (1.09×10^{-3} mm²/s). It is also higher in cortex and the caudate nucleus (1.34×10^{-3} mm²/s) than in the thalamus and the lentiform nucleus (1.20×10^{-3} mm²/s) [15]. With the exception of the cerebrospinal fluid (CSF), there is a trend of decreasing ADC with increasing maturation in most areas of the pediatric brain. These ADC changes seem to reflect a combination of differ-

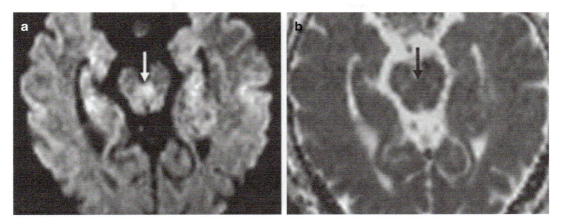

Fig. 2.2 (a) Decussation of the superior cerebellar peduncle has mildly high signal on DWI (*arrow*). (b) ADC map shows similar ADC values in the decussation of the superior cerebellar peduncle to those in cerebral peduncles (*arrow*)

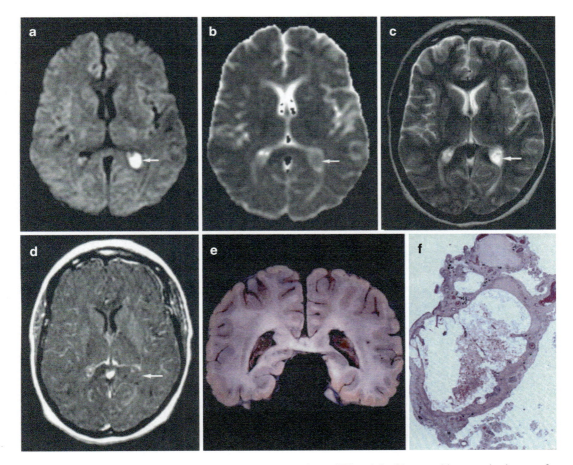

Fig. 2.3 Cystic changes in the choroid plexus. (a) DWI shows hyperintensity in cystic changes of the left choroid plexus (*arrow*). (b) ADC values of the cystic changes are lower than those of the CSF, which probably represent viscous gelatinous materials, but higher than those of brain parenchyma (*arrow*). (c) T2-weighted image shows the cystic changes as hyperintensity (*arrow*). (d) Gadolinium-enhanced T1-weighted image with magnetization transfer contrast reveals no enhancement in it (*arrow*). (e) Macropathology of choroid plexus cyst (another case). (f) Micropathology shows gelatinous content, foci of calcification with a thickened fibrous wall containing blood vessels. (Courtesy of Kinoshita T, MD, Research Institute for Brain and Blood Vessels Akita, Japan)

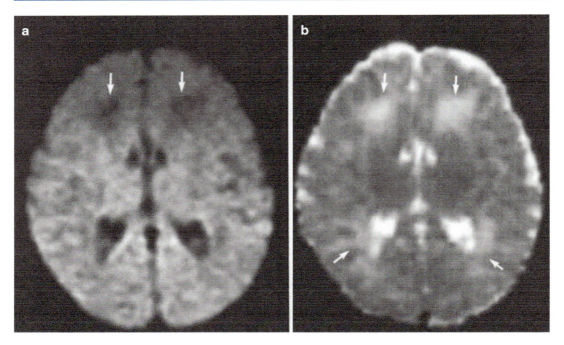

Fig. 2.4 Normal neonatal brain. (**a**) The appearance of the pediatric brain on DWI varies with age. In neonates it is normal to have low DW signal intensities in the frontal deep *white* matter (*arrows*). (**b**) ADC values of the corresponding areas are high in neonatal brain, especially in the *white* matter (*arrows*). These ADC changes seem to reflect a combination of factors, including a reduction of overall water content, cellular maturation, and *white* matter myelination

ent factors, including a reduction of overall water content, cellular maturation, and white matter myelination. In neonates and infants, ischemia is usually global and can therefore resemble the normal image with elevated DW signal and decreased ADC. White matter diseases can also be mimicked by the normal, age-related appearance of DWI and ADC. Out of necessity, the ADC values will therefore have to be age related for a correct interpretation of the DWI of the pediatric brains.

2.4 Diffusion Tensor Imaging and White Matter Anatomy

Diffusion tensor imaging (DTI) is available in many modern clinical scanners. A fractional anisotropy (FA) map represents the magnitude of the anisotropy of the diffusion process at each image voxel, yielding values between 0 (perfectly isotropic diffusion) and 1 (completely anisotropic diffusion) (Fig. 2.5). A color FA map represents the directionality of the anisotropy based on the orientation of the largest eigenvalue along left-right (red), anterior-posterior (green), and superior-inferior directions (blue) (Fig. 2.5).

A fiber tractography map is made by following the main direction of water movement (the largest tensor eigenvalue) and its connection in adjacent voxels in the three-dimensional space (Figs. 2.6, 2.7, 2.8, 2.9, 2.10, and 2.11). DTI with these maps has been used to investigate the microstructure of the CNS, and their clinical usefulness has been reported in the literature [16–18]. DTI can beautifully demonstrate white matter fiber tracts of the CNS in detail that is useful for understanding the anatomy.

White matter fiber tracts consist of myelinated fiber bundles, called the fasciculus. The white matter fibers are traditionally classified as follows: (1) association fibers that interconnect various cortical areas of the same hemisphere, (2) projection fibers that interconnect cortical areas with the thalami, brain stem, cerebellum, and spinal cord, and (3) commissural fibers that interconnect corresponding cortical areas of the two hemispheres [19–22]. However, the classification of the fiber bundles is complex and to date has remained unresolved [23–27].

2.4.1 Association Fibers

Short association fibers arch beneath the six layers of the cortex referred to as U-fibers or arcuate fibers. In long association fibers, the superior longitudinal fasciculus (SLF) is the largest bundle, connecting the frontal lobe cortex to the temporal and occipital lobe cortices (Fig. 2.6). The arcuate fasciculus (AF) is the part of the SLF that forms a curved shape and connects the Broca area

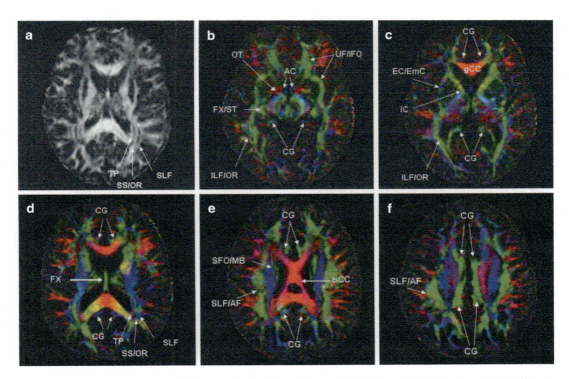

Fig. 2.5 (**a**) Fractional anisotropy (FA) map, (**b–f**) axial DTI color maps, (**g–i**) coronal DTI color maps, (**j–m**) sagittal DTI color maps, (**g–i**) coronal DTI color maps, (**j–m**) sagittal DTI color maps. DTI shows the *white* matter lateral to the posterior horn as three parts: the tapetum (TP), internal and external sagittal strata including optic radiation (SS/OR), and SLF. SLF/AF connects the frontal lobe to temporal and occipital lobes. SFO/MB is situated beneath the corpus callosum (CC) and medial to the corona radiata (CR). ILF connects temporal and occipital lobe cortices. The cingulum (CG) is situated on both sides of the midline on the surface of CC. The uncinate fasciculus (UF) connects the ventral and lateral frontal lobe with the anterior temporal lobe. EmC/EC is hard to be separately seen on DTI. *SLF* superior longitudinal fasciculus, *AF* arcuate fasciculus, *ILF* inferior longitudinal fasciculus, *CG* cingulum, *UF* uncinate fasciculus, *SFO* superior fronto-occipital fasciculus, *IFO* inferior fronto-occipital fasciculus, *EmC* extreme capsule, *EC* external capsule, *MB* subcallosal fasciculus of Muratoff, *IC* internal capsule, *CST* corticospinal tract, *OT* optic tract, *OR* optic radiation, *SS* sagittal stratum, *gCC* genu of corpus callosum, *bCC* body of corpus callosum, *sCC* splenium of corpus callosum, *TP* tapetum, *AC* anterior commissure, *FX* fornix, *ST* stria terminalis, *SCP* superior cerebellar peduncle, *MCP* middle cerebellar peduncle. (Courtesy of Kim J MD, The University of Iowa Hospitals and Clinics, USA, and White ML MD and Zhang Y MD, The University of Nebraska Medical Center, USA)

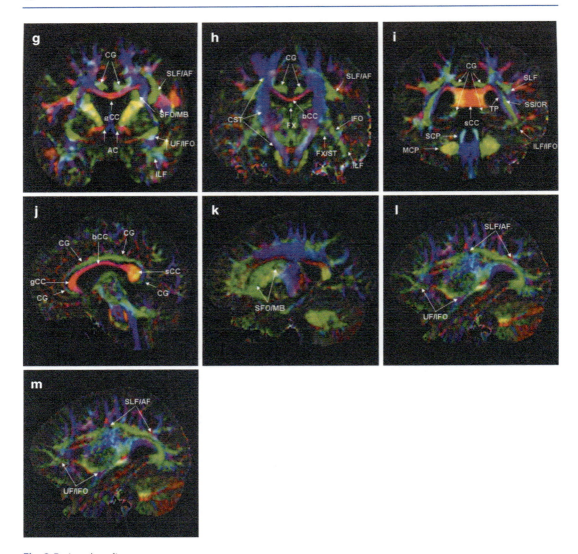

Fig. 2.5 (continued)

(motor area of speech) with the Wernicke area (language comprehension). The inferior longitudinal fasciculus (ILF) connects the temporal and occipital lobe cortices, which are concerned with visual perception, object identification, and recognition.

The cingulum (CG) is situated on both sides of the midline on the peripheral surface of the corpus callosum and courses within the cingulate gyrus that is concerned with behavior and regulation of emotional processing (Fig. 2.7). The cingulum bundle contains variable length fibers which connect the frontal and parietal lobes with the parahippocampal gyrus and adjacent temporal lobe cortex. The uncinate fasciculus (UF) connects the ventral and lateral frontal lobe cortex with the anterior temporal lobe cortex, which is concerned with memory integration (retrograde amnesia).

The existence of the superior or inferior fronto-occipital (occipitofrontal) fasciculus is controversial [23–27]. The superior fronto-occipital fasciculus (SFO) connects the frontal and parietal lobes. It is thought to be concerned with space perception. Ventrally its base rests on the subcallosal fasciculus of Muratoff (MB) [24, 26]. The

2 Diffusion-Weighted and Tensor Imaging of the Normal Brain

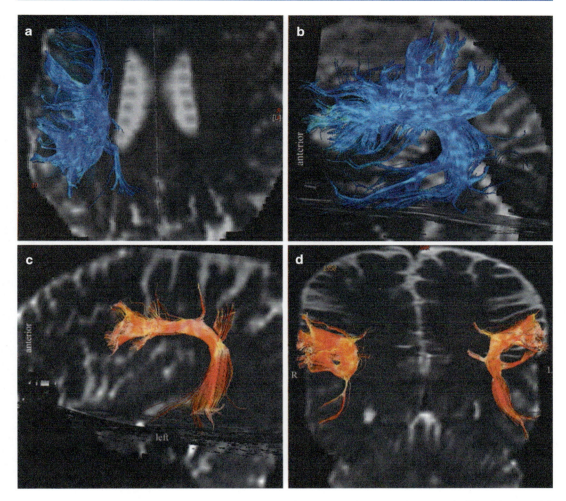

Fig. 2.6 (**a**, **b**) The superior longitudinal fasciculus (SLF) interconnects frontal lobe cortex to temporal and occipital lobe cortices. The inferior longitudinal fasciculus (ILF) connects temporal and occipital lobe cortices. (**c**) The arcuate fasciculus (AF) is the part of the SLF that forms a curved shape and connects the Wernicke area with Broca area. (**d**) There is asymmetry in right and left side of arcuate fasciculi (Courtesy of White ML MD and Zhang Y MD, The University of Nebraska Medical Center, USA)

SFO/MB is situated beneath the corpus callosum and medial to the corona radiata (Fig. 2.5). The SFO may not exist based on analyses using fiber dissection techniques [23]. The inferior fronto-occipital fasciculus (IFO) connects the frontal and temporo-occipital areas intermingled with the uncinate fasciculus antero-inferiorly, possibly concerned with auditory-visual association [24] (Fig. 2.7). The IFO may not exist based on analyses using isotope anterograde tract tracer in the macaque monkey [24–27].

The extreme capsules (EmC) contain association fibers parallel to the external capsule (EC), which are separated by a sheet of gray matter known as the claustrum.

Corticostriatal fibers interconnect the cortex with the striatum including the external capsule and the subcallosal fasciculus of Muratoff (MB) concerned with motor and cognitive–affective performance. The corticostriatal fibers are not exactly association fibers, based on the definition [25, 28].

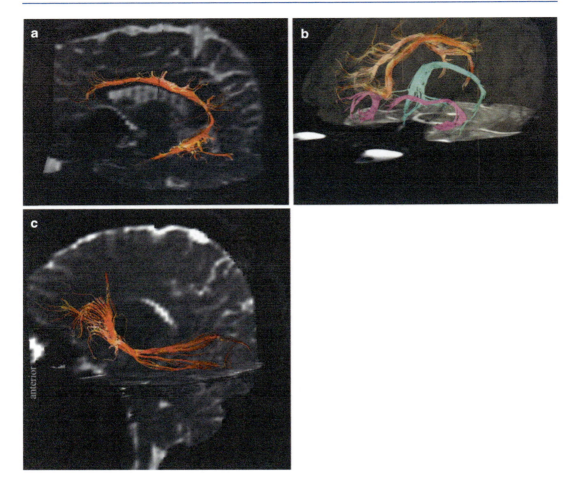

Fig. 2.7 (**a**) The cingulum bundle contains variable length fibers which connect frontal and parietal lobes with parahippocampal gyrus and adjacent temporal lobe cortex. (Courtesy of White ML, MD and Zhang Y MD, University of Nebraska Medical Center, USA). (**b**) The cingulum (*orange*) is situated on both sides of the midline on the peripheral surface of the corpus callosum and courses within the cingulate gyrus. The uncinate fasciculus (UF) (*pink*) connects the ventral and lateral frontal lobe cortex with the anterior temporal lobe cortex. The fornix (FX) (*light blue*) is also demonstrated. (Courtesy of Aoki S, MD, The University of Tokyo, Japan). (**c**) The inferior fronto-occipital fasciculus (IFO) connects frontal and temporo-occipital areas intermingled with the uncinate fasciculus antero-inferiorly. (Courtesy of White ML MD and Zhang Y MD, The University of Nebraska Medical Center, USA)

2.4.2 Projection Fibers

The corona radiata and internal capsule (IC) are composed of afferent and efferent fibers to and from the entire cerebral cortex. Efferent fibers in the internal capsule arise from the cortex and project to the brain stem and spinal cord and are categorized as corticothalamic, corticopontine, corticobulbar, and corticospinal tracts (Fig. 2.8) [29, 30]. The most posterior component of the posterior limb of the internal capsule contains fibers, connecting the lateral geniculate nucleus to the calcarine sulcus (geniculo-calcarine tract), also known as optic radiation (OR) (Fig. 2.9). The ventral bundle of the optic radiation passes anteriorly before making a sharp turn, known as the Meyer loop, and terminating in the inferior bank of the calcarine cortex. The temporal stem

2 Diffusion-Weighted and Tensor Imaging of the Normal Brain

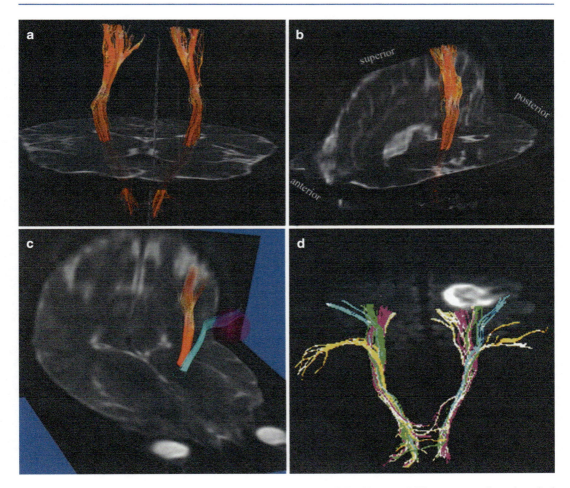

Fig. 2.8 (**a**, **b**) Anterior-posterior and oblique lateral views of the corticospinal tract. (Courtesy of White ML MD and Zhang Y MD, University of Nebraska Medical Center, USA). (**c**) The corticospinal tract (*orange*) and corticobulbar tract (*light blue*) are demonstrated. (Courtesy of Aoki S, MD, The University of Tokyo, Japan). (**d**) Multi-tensor DTI separates each corticospinal fiber projecting special areas: hand (green), tongue (*orange*), trunk (*purple*), face (blue), and lower extremity (*yellow*). (Courtesy of Yamada K MD, Kyoto Prefectural University of Medicine, Japan) (from [29])

is a critical landmark in temporal lobe surgery, which is crossed by the uncinate fasciculus, inferior fronto-occipital fasciculus, and Meyer's loop [24, 31]. The optic radiation is part of the sagittal stratum. The sagittal stratum not only conveys fibers from parietal, occipital, temporal, and cingulate regions to the thalamus and brain stem, but also conveys principally from the thalamus to the cortex. The thalamocortical (afferent) and corticothalamic (efferent) fibers are arrayed around the thalamus, termed thalamic radiations or peduncles (Fig. 2.10).

2.4.3 Commissural Fibers

The corpus callosum (CC) is a broad thick plate of dense myelinated fibers that reciprocally interconnect broad regions of the cortex (Fig. 2.11). The genu (gCC) contains fibers interconnecting rostral parts of the frontal lobes. Fibers from the remaining parts of the frontal lobe and the parietal lobe traverse the body of the corpus callosum (bCC). Fibers transversing the splenium relate regions of the temporal and occipital lobes. The tapetum comprises the

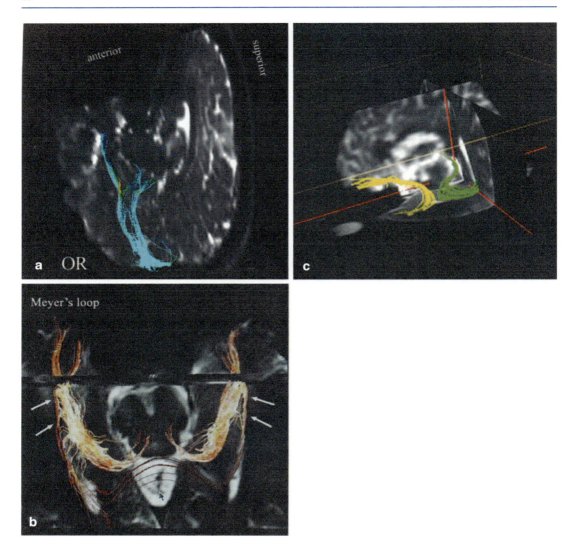

Fig. 2.9 (a) Optic radiations on the right (OR), (b) Meyer's loop (*arrows*). (Courtesy of White ML MD and Zhang Y MD, The University of Nebraska Medical Center, USA). (c) The relationship between the Meyer's loop (green) and the uncinate fasciculus. (Courtesy of Taoka T MD, Nara Medical University, Japan)

fibers in the splenium (sCC) which sweep inferiorly along the lateral margin of the posterior horn of the lateral ventricle. The white matter lateral to the posterior horn is divided into four layers: the tapetum, the internal and external sagittal strata, and the SLF [22, 32]. The anterior commissure (AC) is a small compact bundle that crosses the midline rostral to the columns of the fornix. The posterior commissure connects the right and left peritectal region. The hippocampal commissure joins the right and left hippocampi also known as the commissure of the fornix (FX). The fornix is the main efferent fiber system of the hippocampal formation, including both projection and commissural fibers, associated with antegrade amnesia. The stria terminalis is an efferent pathway from the amygdala, which arches along the medial border of the caudate nucleus and terminates in the hypothalamic nuclei lateral to the fornix. The stria terminalis is associated with the hypothalamus-pituitary-adrenal axis.

2 Diffusion-Weighted and Tensor Imaging of the Normal Brain

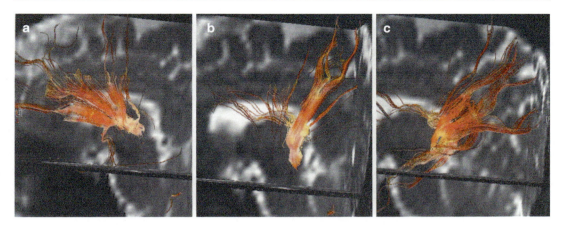

Fig. 2.10 Thalamic radiations (**a** anterior, **b** superior, **c** posterior) (Courtesy of White ML MD and Zhang Y MD, The University of Nebraska Medical Center, USA)

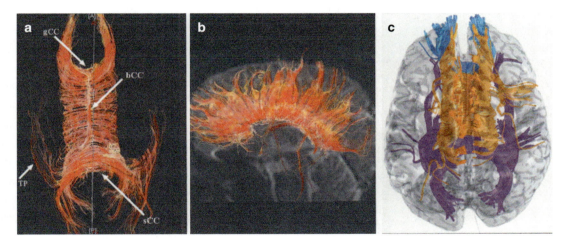

Fig. 2.11 (**a–c**)The corpus callosum is a broad thick plate of dense myelinated fibers that reciprocally interconnect broad regions of the cortex. The genu (gCC) contains fibers interconnecting rostral parts of the frontal lobes. Fibers from the remaining parts of the frontal lobe and the parietal lobe traverse the body of the corpus callosum (bCC). Fibers transversing the splenium relate regions of the temporal and occipital lobes. The tapetum (TP) is the extension into the hemisphere of the corpus callosum lying adjacent to the ventricular ependyma. (Courtesy of White ML MD and Zhang Y MD, The University of Nebraska Medical Center, USA)

2.4.4 Fibers of the Brain Stem and Cerebellum

The complex anatomy of the brain stem includes a large number of tracts, nuclei, commissures, and decussations (Fig. 2.12) [19, 33].

In the midbrain, the tegmentum and crus cerebri are separated by the substantia nigra. The crus cerebri consists of corticopontine, corticobulbar, and corticospinal fibers. The superior cerebellar peduncle (SCP) is seen on each side of the upper part of the fourth ventricle and decussates completely in the caudal midbrain tegmentum. The SCP is made up of predominantly efferent pathways arising from the cerebellar cortex and deep cerebellar nuclei to the thalamus and cerebral cortex but it also caries afferent pathways. It is associated with coordination of motor function. The ventral part of the pons consists of longitudinal descending fibers, pontine nuclei, and transverse pontine fibers projecting to the cerebellum. The dorsal tegmental portion contains

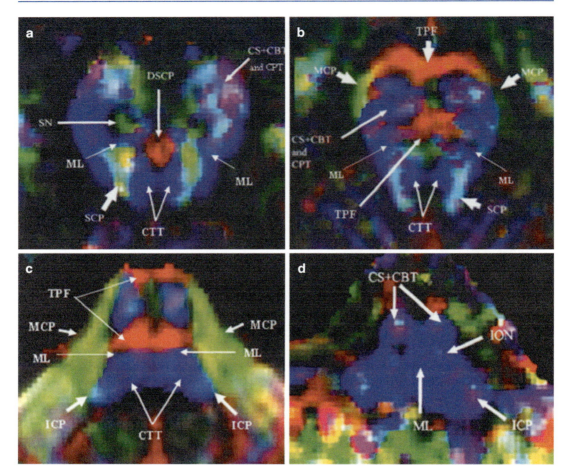

Fig. 2.12 (**a**) The midbrain: The crus cerebri consists of corticopontine, corticobulbar, and corticospinal fibers (CPT, CBT, CST). The tegmentum and crus cerebri are separated by the substantia nigra (SN). The superior cerebellar peduncle (SCP) and their decussation (DSCP, *round red spot*) are noted in the caudal midbrain tegmentum. The dorsal tegmental portion contains the central tegmental tract (CTT) and medial lemniscus (ML). The upper (**b**) and lower (**c**) pons: The ventral part of the pons contains CPT, CBT, CST, pontine nuclei, and transverse pontine fibers (TPF). The middle cerebellar peduncle (MCP) arises from pontine nuclei projecting to the cerebellar hemisphere. The inferior cerebellar peduncle is noted on each side of the lower part of the forth ventricle. (**d**) The medulla: The inferior olivary nuclei (ION), medullary pyramids (CST, CBT), medial lemniscus (ML), and ICP are demonstrated. (Courtesy of White ML MD and Zhang Y MD, The University of Nebraska Medical Center, USA)

the reticular formation, medial lemniscus, and cranial nerve nuclei. The medial lemniscus comprises large ascending fibers and terminates in the ventral posterolateral nucleus of the thalamus, which is concerned with sensation of touch, vibration, proprioception, and two-point discrimination.

The middle cerebellar peduncle (MCP) also known as the brachium pontis consists of predominantly afferent fibers arising from the pontine nuclei, and most of them decussate and terminate as mossy fibers projecting to the cerebellar hemisphere. The function of the MCP includes initiation, planning, and voluntary movement. The medulla contains the inferior olivary nuclei, cranial nerve nuclei, and decussation of the medullary pyramids and medial lemniscus.

The inferior cerebellar peduncle (ICP), seen on each side of the lower part of the fourth ventricle, connects the cerebellum and medulla

2 Diffusion-Weighted and Tensor Imaging of the Normal Brain

(Fig. 2.13). The ICP carries mostly afferent pathways from the spinal cord and conveys impulses from vestibular receptors, associated with balance coordination. The corpus medullare is a compact mass of cerebellar white matter imbedding four deep nuclei (dentate, fastigial, globose, and emboliform), continuous with the three cerebellar peduncles [34]. The corpus medullare splits in the roof of the fourth ventricle at an acute angle (fastigium) and forms the superior and inferior medullary vela.

2.4.5 Clinical Importance of White Matter Fiber Anatomy

White matter anatomy is a developing area in neuroimaging, and the structure and function of many white matter bundles are incompletely understood. Nevertheless, knowledge of white matter fiber tract anatomy can be clinically useful. The most common context in which white matter anatomy is clinically important is in preoperative planning, most often to avoid unneces-

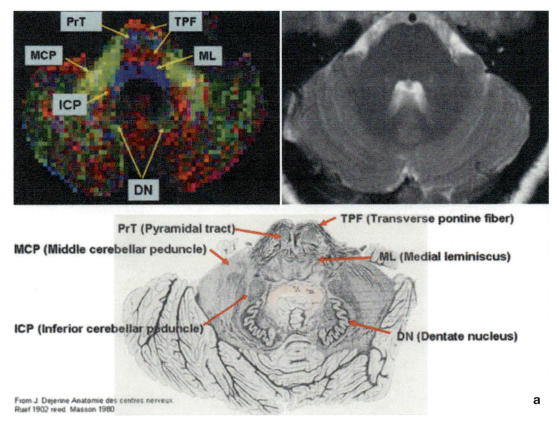

Fig. 2.13 a–c Axial (**a**), Coronal (**b**), and Sagittal (**c**) images. The ventral part of the pons consists of pyramidal tracts (PrT), pontine nuclei, and transverse pontine fibers (TPF) projecting to the cerebellum. The medial lemniscus (ML) is large ascending fibers and terminates in the ventral posterolateral nucleus of the thalamus. The middle cerebellar peduncle (MCP) consists of predominantly afferent fibers from TPF and most of them decussate and terminate as mossy fibers projecting to the cerebellar hemisphere. The inferior cerebellar peduncle (ICP), seen on each side of the lower part of the forth ventricle, connects the cerebellum and medulla. (**d–f**) Parasagittal images. The corpus medullare is a compact mass of cerebellar white matter imbedding 4 deep cerebellar nuclei (dentate, fastigial, globose, and emboliform), continuous with the three cerebellar peduncles. The superior cerebellar peduncle (SCP) is seen on each side of the upper part of the forth ventricle and decussates completely in the caudal midbrain tegmentum. (**g, h**) Fiber tractography. SCP is predominantly efferent pathways arising from cerebellar cortex and deep cerebellar nuclei to thalamus and cerebral cortex (*green*). Pyramidal tracts (*blue*) and middle cerebellar peduncles and transverse pontine fibers (*orange*) are demonstrated

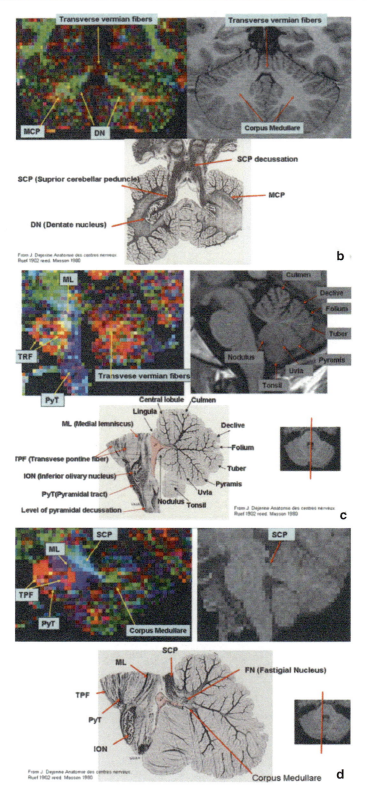

Fig. 2.13 (continued)

2 Diffusion-Weighted and Tensor Imaging of the Normal Brain 25

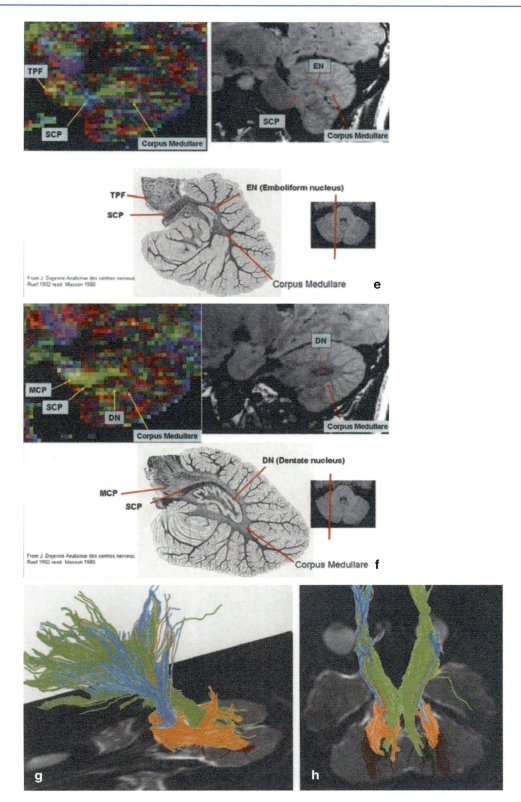

Fig. 2.13 (continued)

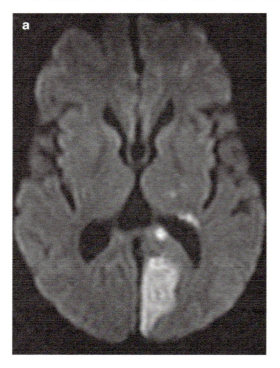 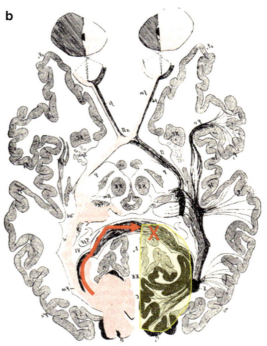

Fig. 2.14 A 45-year-old woman with pure alexia following left PCA territory infarction. (**a**) DWI demonstrates diffusion restriction in the left occipital lobe, left splenium of the corpus callosum, and left peritrigonal white matter. (**b**) The left occipital lobe infarction (*yellow*) and the lesion in the splenium of the corpus callosum (*red X*) disconnect the commissural fibers (*red arrow*) that connect the normal right occipital lobe (*pink*) to the visual-verbal association cortex in the left inferior parietal lobule. Therefore, the patient cannot read despite preserved ability to see letters and write

sary injury to projection fibers like the corticospinal tracts and optic radiations. Injuries to projection fibers are straightforward to understand and can result in devastating deficits in primary motor, sensory, and visual function. Injury to other white matter fibers is less straightforward to understand but can explain deficits in higher brain functions that result from association between cortical areas. These deficits, called disconnection syndromes, occur secondary to damage to one or more of the relevant cortical regions, the association white matter fibers connecting them, or both [35–37]. The prototypical disconnection syndrome is the conduction aphasia that results from injury to association fibers in the arcuate fasciculus that connect Broca's and Wernicke's areas. These patients have normal speech fluency and language comprehension but exhibit paraphasic speech and repetition deficits. Another classical disconnection syndrome is pure alexia without agraphia (i.e., the inability to read with preserved ability to see letters and write) that can occur with injury to the occipital lobe and splenium of the corpus callosum in the language dominant hemisphere (Fig. 2.14). These patients present with right hemianopsia and an inability to read even when written words are presented to the functioning visual field. The reading deficit is due to a disconnection in the white matter fibers connecting the normal right occipital lobe to the visual-verbal association cortex in the left inferior parietal lobule.

2.5 Conclusion

Knowledge of the DWI appearance of the normal adult and pediatric brain and variations is necessary to avoid misinterpretation. In children it is also important to match the findings with those of normal children of the same age. DTI and fiber tractography are useful for understanding the normal white matter fiber tract anatomy. White matter anatomy is a developing area in neuroimaging, and the structure and function of many white matter bundles are incompletely understood. Nevertheless, knowledge of white matter fiber tract anatomy can be clinically useful.

References

1. Yoshiura T, Wu O, Sorensen AG (1999) Advanced MR techniques: diffusion MR imaging, perfusion MR imaging, and spectroscopy. Neuroimaging Clin N Am 9:439–453
2. Asao C, Hirai T, Yoshimatsu S et al (2007) Human cerebral cortices: signal variation on diffusion-weighted MR imaging. Neuroradiology 50:205–211
3. Chun T, Filippi CG, Zimmerman RD, Ulug AM (2000) Diffusion changes in the aging human brain. Am J Neuroradiol 21:1078–1083
4. Engelter ST, Provenzale JM, Petrella JR, DeLong DM, MacFall JR (2000) The effect of aging on the apparent diffusion coefficient of normal-appearing white matter. Am J Roentgenol 175:425–430
5. Helenius J, Soinne L, Perkio J (2002) Diffusion-weighted MR imaging in normal human brains in various age groups. Am J Neuroradiol 23:194–199
6. Gideon P, Thomsen C, Henriksen O (1994) Increased self-diffusion of brain water in normal aging. J Magn Reson Imaging 4:185–188
7. Nusbaum AO, Tang CY, Buchsbaum MS, Wei TC, Atlas SW (2001) Regional and global changes in cerebral diffusion with normal aging. Am J Neuroradiol 22:136–142
8. Abe O, Aoki S, Hayashi N et al (2002) Normal aging in the central nervous system: quantitative MR diffusion-tensor analysis. Neurobiol Aging 23:433–441
9. Kinoshita T, Moritani T, Hiwatashi A et al (2005) Clinically silent choroid plexus cyst: evaluation by diffusion-weighted MRI. Neuroradiology 47:251–255
10. Sakuma H, Nomura Y, Takeda K et al (1991) Adult and neonatal human brain: diffusional anisotropy and myelination with diffusion-weighted MR imaging. Radiology 180:229–233
11. Morriss MC, Zimmerman RA, Bilaniuk LT, Hunter JV, Haselgrove JC (1999) Changes in brain water diffusion during childhood. Neuroradiology 41:929–934
12. Tanner SF, Ramenghi LA, Ridgway JP et al (2000) Quantitative comparison of intrabrain diffusion in adults and preterm and term neonates and infants. Am J Roentgenol 174:1643–1649
13. Neil JJ, Shiran SI, McKinstry RC et al (1998) Normal brain in human newborns: apparent diffusion coefficient and diffusion anisotropy measured by using diffusion tensor MR imaging. Radiology 209:57–66
14. Engelbrecht V, Scherer A, Rassek M, Witsack HJ, Modder U (2002) Diffusion-weighted MR imaging in the brain in children: findings in the normal brain and in the brain with white matter diseases. Radiology 222:410–418
15. Forbes KP, Pipe JG, Bird CR (2002) Changes in brain water diffusion during the 1st year of life. Radiology 222:405–409
16. Nucifora PGP, Verma R, Lee SK, Melhem ER (2007) Diffusion-tensor MR imaging and tractography: exploring brain microstructure and connectivity. Radiology 245:367–384
17. Assaf Y, Pasternak O (2008) Diffusion tensor imaging (DTI)-based white matter mapping in brain research: a review. J Mol Neurosci 34:51–61
18. Alexander AL, Lee JE, Lazar M, Field AS (2007) Diffusion tensor imaging of the brain. Neurotherapeutics 4:316–329
19. Jellison BJ, Field AS, Medow J, Lazar M, Salamat MS, Alexander AL (2004) Diffusion tensor imaging of cerebral white matter: a pictorial review of physics, fiber tract anatomy, and tumor imaging patterns. AJNR Am J Neuroradiol 25:356–369
20. Wakana S, Jiang H, Nagae-Poetscher LM, van Zijl PC, Mori S (2004) Fiber tract-based atlas of human white matter anatomy. Radiology 230:77–87
21. Mamata H, Mamata Y, Westin CF, Shenton ME, Kikinis R, Jolesz FA, Maier SE (2002) High-resolution line scan diffusion tensor MR imaging of white matter fiber tract anatomy. AJNR Am J Neuroradiol 23:67–75
22. Tamura H, Takahashi S, Kurihara N, Yamada S, Hatazawa J, Okudera T (2003) Practical visualization of internal structure of white matter for image interpretation: staining a spin-echo T2-weighted image with three echo-planar diffusion-weighted images. AJNR Am J Neuroradiol 24:401–409
23. Türe U, Yaşargil MG, Pait TG (1997 Jun) Is there a superior occipitofrontal fasciculus? A microsurgical anatomic study. Neurosurgery 40(6):1226–1232
24. Kier EL, Staib LH, Davis LM, Bronen RA (2004 May) MR imaging of the temporal stem: anatomic dissection tractography of the uncinate fasciculus, inferior occipitofrontal fasciculus, and Meyer's loop of the optic radiation. AJNR Am J Neuroradiol 25(5):677–691
25. Schmahmann JD, Pandya DN (2006) Fiber pathways of the brain. Oxford University Press, Oxford, NY
26. Schmahmann JD, Pandya DN, Wang R, Dai G, D'Arceuil HE, de Crespigny AJ, Wedeen VJ (2007) Association fibre pathways of the brain: parallel observations from diffusion spectrum imaging and autoradiography. Brain 130:630–653
27. Schmahmann JD, Pandya DN (2007) The complex history of the fronto-occipital fasciculus. J Hist Neurosci 16:362–377
28. Utsunomiya H, Nakamura Y (2007) MR features of the developing perianterior horn structure including subcallosal fasciculus in infants and children. Neuroradiology 49:947–954

29. Yamada K, Sakai K, Hoogenraad FG, Holthuizen R, Akazawa K, Ito H, Oouchi H, Matsushima S, Kubota T, Sasajima H, Mineura K, Nishimura T (2007) Multitensor tractography enables better depiction of motor pathways: initial clinical experience using diffusion-weighted MR imaging with standard b-value. AJNR Am J Neuroradiol 28:1668–1673
30. Aoki S, Iwata NK, Masutani Y et al (2005) Quantitative evaluation of the pyramidal tract segmented by diffusion tensor tractography: feasibility study in patients with amyotrophic lateral sclerosis. Radiat Med 23:195–199
31. Taoka T, Sakamoto M, Nakagawa H, Nakase H, Iwasaki S, Takayama K, Taoka K, Hoshida T, Sakaki T, Kichikawa K (2008) Diffusion tensor tractography of the Meyer loop in cases of temporal lobe resection for temporal lobe epilepsy: correlation between postsurgical visual field defect and anterior limit of Meyer loop on tractography. AJNR Am J Neuroradiol 29(7):1329–1334. [Epub ahead of print]
32. Kitajima M, Korogi Y, Takahashi M, Eto K (1996) MR signal intensity of the optic radiation. AJNR Am J Neuroradiol 17:1379–1383
33. Salamon N, Sicotte N, Alger J, Shattuck D, Perlman S, Sinha U, Schultze-Haakh H, Salamon G (2005) Analysis of the brain-stem white-matter tracts with diffusion tensor imaging. Neuroradiology 47:895–902
34. Salamon N, Sicotte N, Drain A, Frew A, Alger JR, Jen J, Perlman S, Salamon G (2007) White matter fiber tractography and color mapping of the normal human cerebellum with diffusion tensor imaging. J Neuroradiol 34:115–128
35. Catani M, Mesalum M (2008) What is a disconnection syndrome? Cortex 44:911–913
36. Catani M, ffytche D (2005) The rises and falls of disconnection syndromes. Brain 128:2224–2239
37. Catani M, Mesalum M (2008) The arcuate fasciculus and the disconnection theme in language and aphasia: history and current state. Cortex 44:953–961

Pitfalls and Artifacts of Diffusion-Weighted Imaging

3

Toshio Moritani, Akio Hiwatashi, and Jianhui Zhong

3.1 Introduction

There are many inherent artifacts and pitfalls in diffusion-weighted imaging (DWI) of the brain that are important to recognize to avoid misinterpretations.

3.2 Influence of ADC and T2 on the DW Appearance

DWI is inherently T2 weighted and changes in T2 signal characteristics will thus influence the appearance of DW independent of tissue diffusibility [1–16]. The effect of T2 prolongation, so-called "T2 shine-through," is well known. Less well known is the balance between apparent diffusion coefficient (ADC) and T2, sometimes called T2 washout. Also the effect of T2 shortening, or T2 blackout, and magnetic susceptibility effects will influence the DW appearance in many

T. Moritani (✉)
Division of Neuroradiology, Department of Radiology, University of Michigan, Ann Arbor, MI, USA
e-mail: tmoritan@med.umich.edu

A. Hiwatashi
Department of Clinical Radiology, Kyushu University, Fukuoka, Japan
e-mail: hiwatasi@radiol.med.kyushu-u.ac.jp

J. Zhong
University of Rochester Medical Center, Rochester, NY, USA
e-mail: jianhui.zhong@rochester.edu

situations. This chapter will illustrate and discuss the effects of T2 and ADC on DWI.

3.2.1 Concepts

The signal intensity (SI) on DWI is influenced by T2, ADC, the b-factor, the spin density (SD), and the echo time (TE), and is calculated as follows:

$$SI = SI_{b=0}e^{-b\mathrm{ADC}}$$

However,

$$SI_{b=0} = k\mathrm{SD}\left(1 - e^{-\mathrm{TR/T1}}\right)e^{-\mathrm{TE/T2}}$$

For TR $>>$ T1

$$SI = k\mathrm{SD}e^{-\mathrm{TE/T2}}e^{-b\mathrm{ADC}}$$

where k is a constant, TR is repetition time, and $SI_{b=0}$ is the signal intensity on the spin-echo echo-planar image (b_0 image) [1, 2, 5, 7, 8, 10, 12, 16].

To evaluate the tissue T2 and ADC, we should pay attention to the images discussed below as well as isotropic DWIs and b_0 images [3–5, 7, 8, 10, 11, 13–16].

3.2.2 Apparent Diffusion Coefficient Maps

To evaluate the diffusibility, ADC is calculated as:

$$ADC = -\ln\left(SI / SI_{b=0}\right) / b$$

© Springer Nature Switzerland AG 2021
T. Moritani, A. A. Capizzano (eds.), *Diffusion-Weighted MR Imaging of the Brain, Head and Neck, and Spine*, https://doi.org/10.1007/978-3-030-62120-9_3

Subsequently, increased ADC causes decreased SI on DWI, and decreased ADC causes increased SI on DWI [3–5, 7, 10, 15, 16].

3.2.3 Exponential Images

To remove the T2-weighted contrast, the DWI can be divided by the b_0 image to create an "exponential image" [4, 7, 10, 15].

The signal intensity (SIe_{Dwi}) on the exponential image is calculated as:

$$SIe_{DWI} = SI / SI_{b=0} = e^{-bADC}$$

Therefore, this image can eliminate the effect of T2. Contrary to ADC maps, hyperintensity on exponential DWI means decreased ADC, and hypointensity means increased ADC.

3.3 Clinical Conditions

3.3.1 T2 Shine-Through

This is a well-known phenomenon that causes hyperintensity on DWI by means of T2 prolongation [3–5, 7, 8, 10, 11, 15, 16]. If ADC is decreased at the same time, this can result in an accentuation of the hyperintensity on DWI (Figs. 3.1, 3.2, and 3.3).

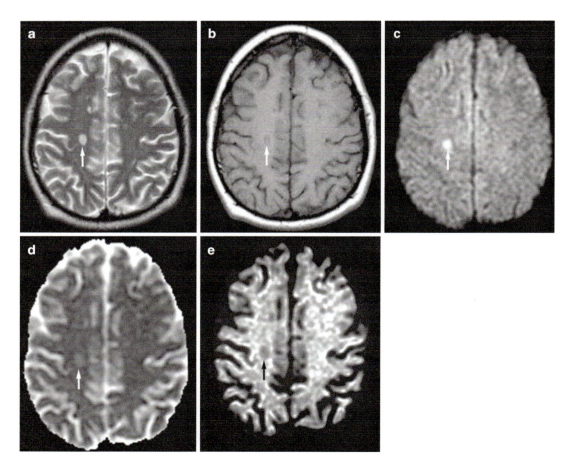

Fig. 3.1 T2 shine-through in a 35-year-old female patient with multiple sclerosis and weakness of the lower extremities. (**a**) T2-weighted image shows several hyperintense lesions, with the largest in the right frontal lobe (*arrow*). (**b**) On T1-weighted image the lesion was hypointense (*arrow*) and did not enhance with contrast (not shown). (**c**) On DWI the lesion is hyperintense (*arrow*). (**d**) ADC map also shows hyperintensity in the lesion (1.2 × 10⁻³ mm²/s; *arrow*). (**e**) Exponential image eliminates the T2 effect and shows the lesion to be hypointense (*arrow*). This confirms that the hyperintensity on DWI is due to a T2 shine-through effect

3 Pitfalls and Artifacts of Diffusion-Weighted Imaging

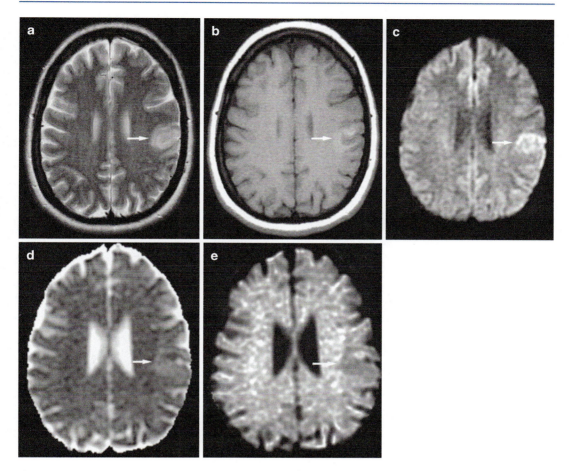

Fig. 3.2 T2 shine-through in a 45-year-old female patient with seizures caused by an anaplastic astrocytoma. (**a**) T2-weighted image shows a hyperintense lesion in the left frontal lobe (*arrow*). (**b**) On T1-weighted image the lesion is hypointense with a peripheral hyperintense area (*arrow*). The lesion did not enhance with contrast (not shown), (**c**) DWI shows hyperintensity (*arrow*). (**d**) ADC map also shows hyperintensity in the lesion (0.98–1.35 × 10^{-3} mm^2/s; *arrow*). (**e**) Exponential image eliminates the T2 effect and shows the lesion to be hypointense (*arrow*). This confirms that the hyperintensity on the DWI is due to a T2 shine-through effect

3.3.2 T2 Washout

This implies that isointensity on DWI is the result of a balance between hyperintensity on T2-weighted images and increased ADC [13, 14, 16]. This is often seen in vasogenic edema, where the combination of increased ADC and hyperintensity on T2-weighted images will result in isointensity on DWI (Fig. 3.4).

To the best of our knowledge there have been no systematic reports on pathological conditions with isointensity on DWI, caused by a balance of hypointensity on T2-weighted images and decreased ADC.

3.3.3 T2 Blackout

This indicates hypointensity on DWI caused by hypointensity on T2-weighted images and is typically seen in some hematomas [9, 16]. Paramagnetic susceptibility artifacts may occur in this situation (Figs. 3.5 and 3.6).

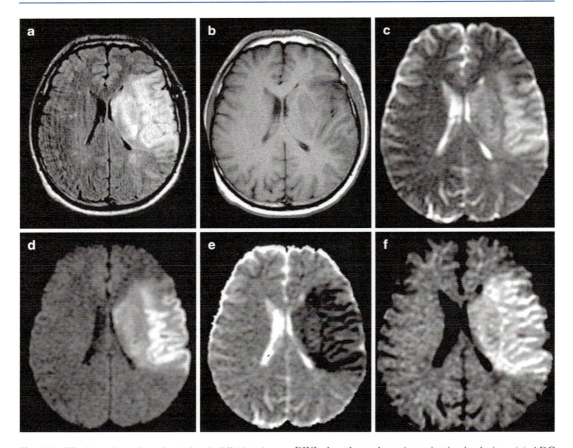

Fig. 3.3 T2 shine-through and restricted diffusion in a 56-year-old male patient with right-sided weakness due to acute infarction. MR imaging was obtained 24 h after the onset of symptoms. (**a**) FLAIR image shows a hyperintense lesion in the left middle cerebral artery territory. (**b**) On T1-weighted image the lesion is hypointense. (**c**) On T2-weighted image (b_0) the lesion is hyperintense. (**d**) DWI also shows hyperintensity in the lesion. (**e**) ADC map shows hypointensity in the lesion (0.27–0.45 × 10^{-3} mm^2/s). (**f**) On the exponential image, which eliminates the T2 effect, the lesion remains hyperintense. This confirms that the DW hyperintensity is due to both restricted diffusion and T2 prolongation

3.4 Artifacts

Numerous artifacts can be generated during the acquisition of DWI. There are five main artifacts of single-shot DW echo-planar imaging:

(1) Eddy current artifacts due to echo-planar imaging phase-encoding and readout gradients, and motion-probing gradient pulses for diffusion weighting.
(2) Susceptibility artifacts.
(3) N/2 ghosting artifacts.
(4) Chemical shift artifacts.
(5) Motion artifacts.

We will discuss each artifact separately.

3.4.1 Eddy Current Artifacts

Eddy currents are electrical currents induced in a conductor by a changing magnetic field. Eddy currents can occur in patients and in the MR scanner itself, including cables or wires,

3 Pitfalls and Artifacts of Diffusion-Weighted Imaging

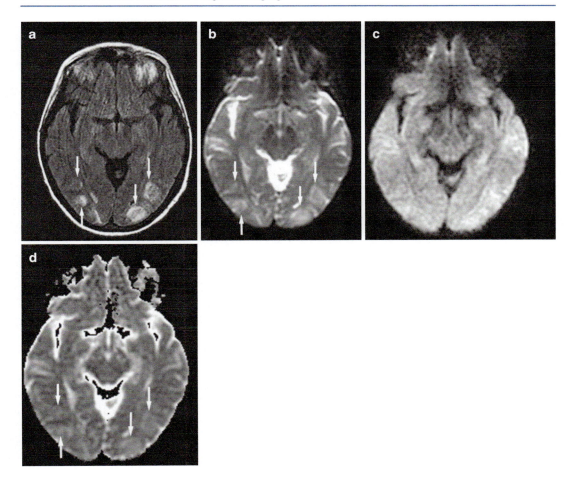

Fig. 3.4 T2 washout in a 45-year-old female patient with hypertension, seizures, and posterior reversible encephalopathy syndrome. (**a**) FLAIR image shows hyperintense lesions in the bilateral occipital lobe (*arrows*). (**b**) T2-weighted image (b_0) also shows hyperintensity of the lesions (*arrows*). (**c**) DWI shows mild hyperintensity in the lesions. (**d**) ADC map shows hyperintensity of the lesions ($1.18–1.38 \times 10^{-3}$ mm^2/s; *arrows*). With the strong T2 prolongation one would expect more hyperintensity on the DWI, but the T2 shine-through effect is reduced by the hyperintensity on the ADC, resulting in a balance between increased diffusibility and hyperintensity on the T2-weighted image (T2 washout)

gradient coils, cryoshields, and radiofrequency shields [17]. Eddy currents are particularly severe when gradients are turned on and off quickly, as in echo-planar imaging pulse sequences. Gradient waveforms are distorted due to eddy currents, which results in image artifacts, including spatial blurring and misregistration. In single-shot DW echo-planar imaging, eddy currents are due to both echo-planar imaging gradients and motion-probing gradients, which lead to image distortions (Fig. 3.7). Correction of image distortion is essential to calculate ADC values and especially to quantify anisotropy with diffusion tensor imaging.

Correction methods: (1) correction of distortion by using post-processing [18–21], (2) pre-emphasis or pre-compensation, purposely distorting the gradient driving currents [22, 23], (3) shielded gradients, redesigning the magnet to

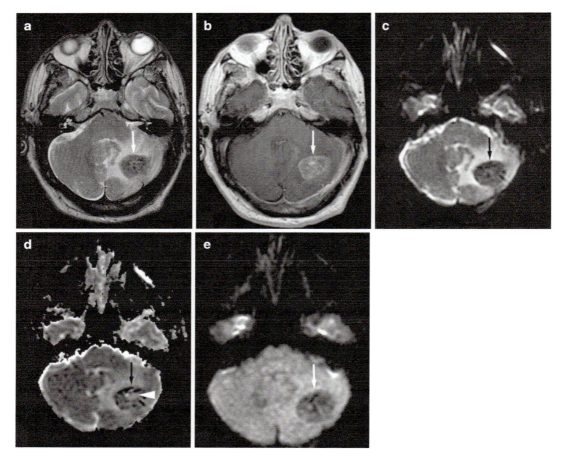

Fig. 3.5 T2 blackout in lung cancer metastasis in a 62-year-old male patient with adenocarcinoma of the lung. (**a**) T2-weighted image shows a hypointense mass (*arrow*) with surrounding edema in the left cerebellar hemisphere. (**b**) Gadolinium-enhanced T1-weighted image shows heterogeneous enhancement of the mass (*arrow*). (**c**) T2-weighted image (b_0) also shows hypointensity in the lesion with surrounding hyperintense edema (*arrow*), (**d**) ADC map shows central hyperintensity (1.63–2.35 × 10^{-3} mm^2/s; *arrowhead*) and peripheral hypointensity (1.13–1.38 × 10^{-3} mm^2/s; *arrow*) of the mass. There is also hyperintensity of the surrounding tissue, consistent with vasogenic edema. (**e**) DWI shows heterogeneous hypointensity of the mass (*arrow*) and isointensity of the surrounding edema. The DW hypointensity of the mass (*arrow*) is due to the increased diffusibility and the hypointensity on the T2-weighted image (T2 blackout). The isointensity in the surrounding edema is due to the balance between increased diffusibility and hyperintensity on the T2-weighted image (T2 washout)

incorporate shielding coils between the gradient coils and the main windings [24].

3.4.2 Susceptibility Artifacts

Single-shot echo-planar imaging is sensitive to susceptibility artifacts, especially frequency and phase errors due to paramagnetic susceptibility effects. These artifacts are seen near the skull base, especially near the air in paranasal sinuses and mastoid (Fig. 3.8). Susceptibility artifacts are more severe along the phase-encoding direction and phase encoding should thus be along the anterior-posterior direction for axial DW images. Coronal and sagittal DW images are helpful in detecting lesions in certain locations, such as the hippocampus and the brain stem, and to identify susceptibility artifacts (Fig. 3.9). Increased matrix size leads to elongation of the readout time, which causes even larger image distortions.

3 Pitfalls and Artifacts of Diffusion-Weighted Imaging

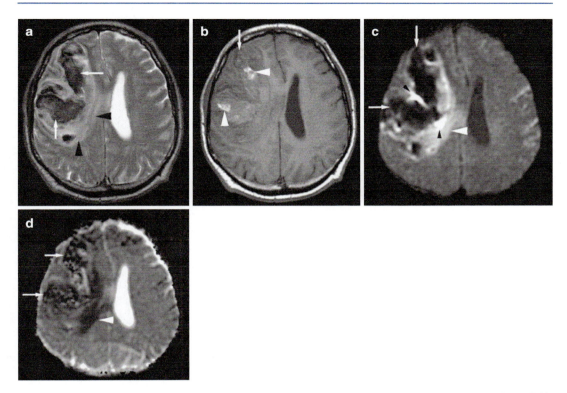

Fig. 3.6 T2 blackout from susceptibility artifacts in acute hemorrhage (deoxyhemoglobin and intracellular met-hemoglobin) in a 74-year-old man with left-sided weakness. MR imaging was obtained 24 h after the onset of symptoms. (**a**) T2-weighted image shows hypointense lesions in the right frontoparietal lobes (*arrows* deoxyhemoglobin and intracellular met-hemoglobin) with areas of surrounding hyperintensity consistent with edema (*arrowheads*). (**b**) T1-weighted image shows the heterogeneous lesion with hypointensity (*arrow* deoxyhemoglobin) and hyperintensity (*arrowheads* intracellular met-hemoglobin). (**c**) DWI shows hypointensity (*arrows* deoxyhemoglobin and intracellular met-hemoglobin) and hyperintensity in the region of edema (*arrowhead*). The surrounding hyperintense rims (*small arrowheads*) are due to magnetic susceptibility artifacts. (**d**) ADC could not be calculated accurately in the T2 "dark" hematoma due to magnetic susceptibility artifacts (*arrows*). The surrounding areas of hypointensity (*arrowhead*) probably correspond to cytotoxic edema surrounding the hematoma. This example shows how T2 hypointensity from susceptibility effects can produce a complex appearance in and around cerebral hemorrhage

Fig. 3.7 Misregistration due to eddy current artifact. a, b Misregistration artifact is noted in the occipital regions (*arrows*) on DWI (**a**) and the ADC map (**b**). Gradient waveforms are distorted due to eddy currents, which results in this misregistration

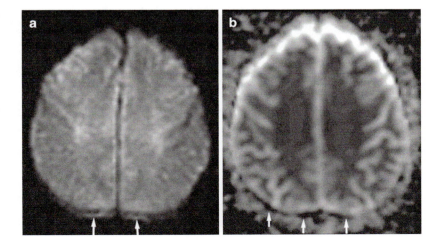

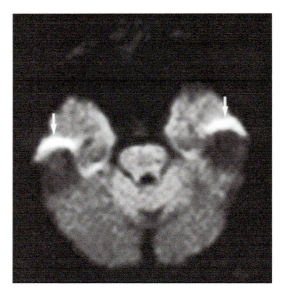

Fig. 3.8 Susceptibility artifact. Susceptibility artifacts are seen near the air content of the mastoids (*arrows*). This is generally prominent in echo-planar sequences

Correction methods: (1) multishot echo-planar imaging (to reduce the readout time, to enable high-resolution scanning) [25, 26], (2) line scan [27, 28], (3) single-shot fast spin echo (SSFSE) [29, 30], (4) periodically rotated overlapping parallel lines with enhanced reconstruction (PROPELLER) [31, 32], (5) sensitive encoding (SENSE)/array spatial and sensitivity-encoding technique (ASSET), undersampling of k-space which enables effective band width and shortens readout time, providing thin section and high-resolution matrix [33].

3.4.3 N/2 Ghosting Artifact (Nyquist Ghost)

The N/2 ghosting artifact occurs when there are differences between the even and odd lines of the k-space. Phase error is due to hardware imperfec-

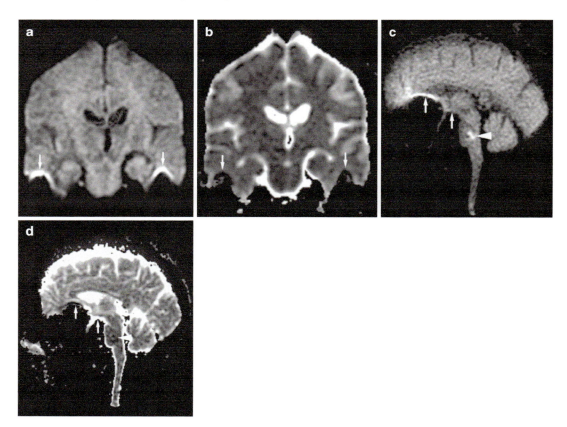

Fig. 3.9 Susceptibility artifact in coronal and sagittal plane DWIs. Coronal DWI (**a**) and the ADC map (**b**) are used to evaluate the hippocampus, but susceptibility artifacts distort the image near the mastoids. Sagittal DWI (**c**) and the ADC map (**d**) show a pontine infarct as hyperintense with decreased ADC (*arrowhead*). Susceptibility artifacts are caused by air in the ethmoid and sphenoid sinuses (*arrows*)

3 Pitfalls and Artifacts of Diffusion-Weighted Imaging

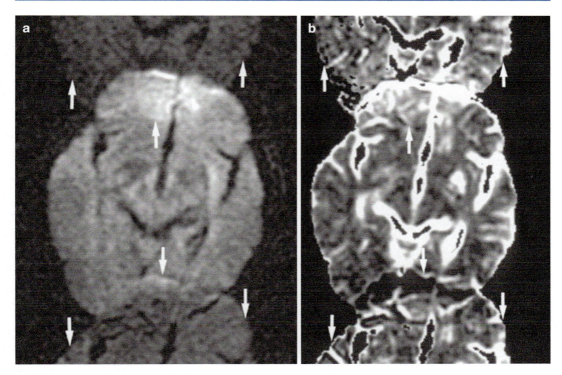

Fig. 3.10 N/2 ghosting artifact. (**a**) DWI shows N/2 ghosting artifacts (*arrows*), which are always shifted by half of the field of view in the phase-encoding direction. (**b**) On the ADC map severe N/2 ghosting artifacts are also seen (*arrows*)

tions (eddy currents, imperfect timing of even and odd echo, imperfect gradients, and magnetic field inhomogeneity), which can be produced by on-off switching during readout gradients. The ghosts in this artifact are always shifted by half of the field of view in the phase-encoding direction (Fig. 3.10). This ghost can produce severe artifacts when ADC maps are calculated.

Correction methods: (1) reduce eddy currents, (2) adjust gradients and magnetic field homogeneity, (3) high b-value, (4) fluid-attenuated inverse recovery (FLAIR) DWI (reduce cerebrospinal fluid signal) [33, 34].

3.4.4 Chemical Shift

In echo-planar DWI, chemical shift artifacts due to the different resonance frequencies in water and fat are produced along the phase-encoding direction, while they are along the frequency-encoding direction in conventional spin-echo type MR imaging. This artifact is more severe in echo-planar imaging than in conventional spin-echo type imaging. Effective fat suppression techniques, such as the chemical shift selective (CHESS) method and the spectral selective radio-frequency excitation method are necessary.

Correction methods: appropriate fat suppression techniques.

3.4.5 Motion Artifacts

The sources of motion artifacts include gross head motion, respiratory motions, cardiac-related pulsations, and patient bed vibration due to gradient pulses. Single-shot DW echo-planar imaging has relatively low sensitivity to patient motion, because each image is acquired in about 100–300 ms and the total acquisition time is less than 40 s. If one of the x, y, z or b_0 images is corrupted by motion artifacts during a scan, or if patient head motion occurs between scans, the isotropic DW images and the ADC maps will have these artifacts (Figs. 3.11 and 3.12). In those cases, unidirectional and b_0 images from the raw data of DWI can be free from the motion artifacts and

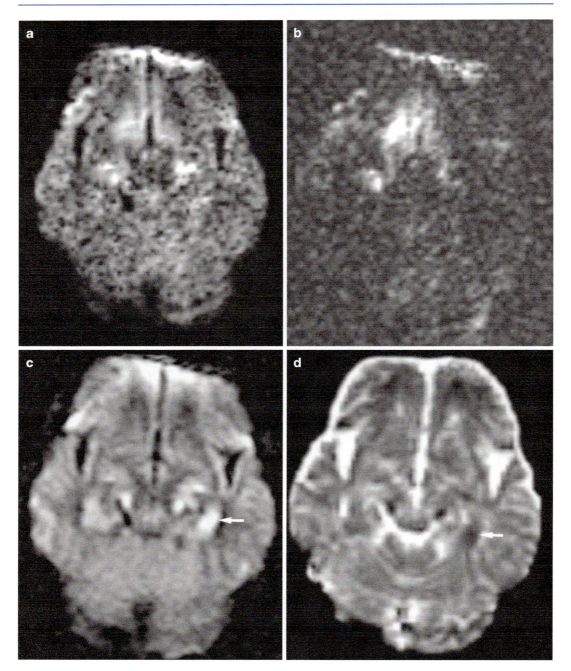

Fig. 3.11 Motion artifacts due to head motion during the scan of a patient with status epilepticus. (**a**) It is difficult to evaluate the DW image because of severe motion artifacts. (**b**) In the raw data of the DWI, the *x* axis image is corrupted by head motion during the scan. (**c**) The y axis image is free from the artifacts. This image shows a hyperintense lesion in the left hippocampus (*arrow*). (**d**) ADC map of *y* axis image also shows decreased ADC of the lesion (transferred to a workstation for image processing, using a home-made code, which is based on the numerical computation software)

3 Pitfalls and Artifacts of Diffusion-Weighted Imaging

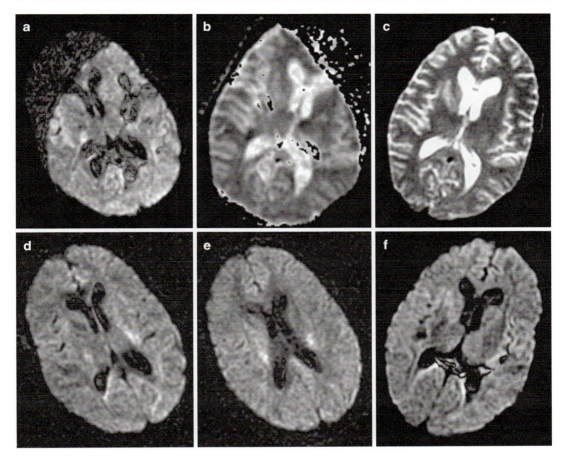

Fig. 3.12 Motion artifacts due to head motion between the scans. Chronic infarcts in the right basal ganglia. (**a**) DWI has motion artifacts due to head motion between the scans. This image is composed of overlapping b_0, x, y, and z axis images. (**b**) ADC map also shows severe motion artifacts. This map is composed of b_0, x, y, and z axis images. (**c**) b_0, (**d**) x axis, (**e**) y axis, (**f**) z axis. b_0 and unidirectional images are all free from the artifacts

remain diagnostically useful. Long (tens of ms) gradient pulses to reach sufficient diffusion weighting often increase sensitivity to motion.

Correction methods: (1) For a fixed b-factor, use high-gradient amplitude but reduce gradient pulse duration to minimize the sensitivity to motion, (2) post-processing to correct for phase error (navigator method) [35–37], (3) elimination of phase-encode step (line scan method, projection reconstruction), (4) minimize time for phase error accumulation (single-shot echo-planar imaging, hybrid method with multishot echo-planar imaging), (5) SSFSE, (6) PROPELLER [38], (7) SENSE.

3.5 Conclusion

DWI is inherently T2 weighted, and the interpretation of signal intensity on DW images requires a correlation between b_0 images, ADC maps, and exponential images to uncover the underlying pathophysiologic condition. It is also important to understand a variety of artifacts to avoid misinterpreting the DWIs. Understanding inherent artifacts and how to reduce the artifacts on DWI will improve the quality and accuracy of DW imaging.

References

1. Stejkal EO, Tanner J (1965) Spin diffusion measurements: spin echoes in the presence of a time-dependent field gradient. J Chemical Phys 42:288–292
2. LeBihan D, Breton E, Lallemand D, Grenier P, Cabanis E, Laval-Jeantet (1986) MR imaging of intravoxel incoherent motions: application to diffusion and perfusion in neurologic disorders. Radiology 161:401–407
3. Warach S, Gaa J, Siewert B, Wielopolski P, Edelman RR (1995) Acute human stroke studied by whole brain echo planar diffusion-weighted magnetic resonance imaging. Ann Neurol 37:231–241
4. Provenzale JM, Engelter ST, Petrella JR, Smith JS, MacFall JR (1999) Use of MR exponential diffusion-weighted images to eradicate T2 "shine-through" effect. AJR Am J Roentgenol 172:537–539
5. Burdette JH, Elster AD, Ricci PE (1999) Acute cerebral infarction: quantification of spin-density and T2 shine-through phenomena on diffusion-weighted MR images. Radiology 212:333–339
6. Coley SC, Porter DA, Calamante F, Chong WK, Connelly A (1999) Quantitative MR diffusion mapping and cyclosporine-induced neurotoxicity. AJNR Am J Neuroradiol 20:1507–1510
7. Schaefer PW, Grant PE, Gonzalez RG (2000) Diffusion-weighted MR imaging of the brain. Radiology 217:331–345
8. Field A (2001) Diffusion and perfusion imaging. In: Elster AD, Burdette JH (eds) Questions and answers in magnetic resonance imaging. Missouri, Mosby, St. Louis, pp 194–214
9. Maldjian JA, Listerud J, Moonis G, Siddiqi F (2001) Computing diffusion rates in T2-dark hematomas and areas of low T2 signal. AJNR Am J Neuroradiol 22:112–128
10. Engelter ST, Provenzale JM, Petrella JR, Alberts MJ, DeLong DM, MacFall JR (2001) Use of exponential diffusion imaging to determine the age of ischemic infarcts. J Neuroimaging 11:141–147
11. Chen S, Ikawa F, Kurisu K, Arita K, Takaba J, Kanou Y (2001) Quantitative MR evaluation of intracranial epidermoid tumors by fast fluid-attenuated inversion recovery imaging and echo-planar diffusion-weighted imaging. AJNR Am J Neuroradiol 22:1089–1096
12. Geijer B, Sundgren PC, Lindgren A, Brockstedt S, Stahlberg F, Holtas S (2001) The value of b required to avoid T2 shinethrough from old lacunar infarcts in diffusion-weighted imaging. Neuroradiology 43:511–517
13. Casey S (2001) "T2 washout": an explanation for normal diffusion-weighted images despite abnormal apparent diffusion coefficient maps. AJNR Am J Neuroradiol 22:1450–1451
14. Provenzale JM, Petrella JR, Cruz LC Jr, Wong JC, Engelter S, Barboriak DP (2001) Quantitative assessment of diffusion abnormalities in posterior reversible encephalopathy syndrome. AJNR Am J Neuroradiol 22:1455–1461
15. Eastwood JD, Engelter ST, MacFall JF, Delong DM, Provenzale JM (2003) Quantitative assessment of the time course of infarct signal intensity on diffusion-weighted images. AJNR Am J Neuroradiol 24:680–687
16. Hiwatashi A, Kinoshita T, Moritani T et al (2003) Hypointensity on diffusion-weighted MRI related to T2 shortening and susceptibility effects. AJR Am J Roentgenol 181(6):1705–1709
17. Elster AD, Burdette JH (2001) Scanner hardware. In: Elster AD, Burdette JH (eds) Questions and answers in magnetic resonance imaging. Missouri, Mosby, St. Louis, pp 54–71
18. Haselgrove JC, Moore JR (1996) Correction for distortion of echo-planar images used to calculate the apparent diffusion coefficient. Magn Reson Med 36:960–964
19. Horsfield MA (1999) Mapping eddy current induced fields for the correction of diffusion-weighted echo planar images. Magn Reson Imaging 17:1335–1345
20. Jezzard P, Barnett AS, Pierpaoli C (1998) Characterization of and correction for eddy current artifacts in echo planar diffusion imaging. Magn Reson Med 39:801–812
21. Calamante F, Porter DA, Gadian DG, Connelly A (1999) Correction for eddy current induced Bo shifts in diffusion-weighted echo-planar imaging. Magn Reson Med 41:95–102
22. Schmithorst VJ, Dardzinski BJ (2002) Automatic gradient preemphasis adjustment: a 15-minute journey to improved diffusion-weighted echo-planar imaging. Magn Reson Med 47:208–212
23. Papadakis NG, Martin KM, Pickard JD, Hall LD, Carpenter TA, Huang CL (2000) Gradient preemphasis calibration in diffusion-weighted echo-planar imaging. Magn Reson Med 44:616–624
24. Chapman BL (1999) Shielded gradients. And the general solution to the near field problem of electromagnet design. MAGMA 9:146–151
25. Robson MD, Anderson AW, Gore JC (1997) Diffusion-weighted multiple shot echo planar imaging of humans without navigation. Magn Reson Med 38:82–88
26. Brockstedt S, Moore JR, Thomsen C, Holtas S, Stahlberg F (2000) High-resolution diffusion imaging using phase-corrected segmented echo-planar imaging. Magn Reson Imaging 18:649–657
27. Maier SE, Gudbjartsson H, Patz S et al (1998) Line scan diffusion imaging: characterization in healthy subjects and stroke patients. AJR Am J Roentgenol 171:85–93
28. Robertson RL, Maier SE, Mulkern RV, Vajapayam S, Robson CD, Barnes PD (2000) MR line-scan diffusion imaging of the spinal cord in children. AJNR Am J Neuroradiol 21:1344–1348
29. Lovblad KO, Jakob PM, Chen Q et al (1998) Turbo spinecho diffusion-weighted MR of ischemic stroke. Am J Neuroradiol 19:201–208

30. Alsop DC (1997) Phase insensitive preparation of single-shot RARE: application to diffusion imaging in humans. Magn Reson Med 38:527–533
31. Forbes KP, Pipe JG, Karis JP, Farthing V, Heiserman JE (2003) Brain imaging in the unsedated pediatric patient: comparison of periodically rotated overlapping parallel lines with enhanced reconstruction and single-shot fast spin-echo sequences. AJNR Am J Neuroradiol 24:794–798
32. Bammer R, Keeling SL, Augustin M et al (2001) Improved diffusion-weighted single-shot echo-planar imaging (EPI) in stroke using sensitivity encoding (SENSE). Magn Reson Med 46:548–554
33. Porter DA, Calamante F, Gadian DG, Connelly A (1999) The effect of residual Nyquist ghost in quantitative echoplanar diffusion imaging. Magn Reson Med 42:385–392
34. Bastin ME (2001) On the use of the FLAIR technique to improve the correction of eddy current induced artefacts in MR diffusion tensor imaging. Magn Reson Imaging 19:937–950
35. Anderson AW, Gore JC (1994) Analysis and correction of motion artifacts in diffusion weighted imaging. Magn Reson Med 32:379–387
36. Ordidge RJ, Helpern JA, Zx Q, Knight RA, Nagesh V (1994) Correction of motional artifacts in diffusion-weighted MR images using navigator echoes. Magn Reson Imaging 12:455–460
37. Dietrich O, Heiland S, Benner T, Sartor K (2000) Reducing motion artefacts in diffusion-weighted MRI of the brain: efficacy of navigator echo correction and pulse triggering. Neuroradiology 42:85–91
38. Pipe JG (1999) Motion correction with PROPELLER MRI: application to head motion and free-breathing cardiac imaging. Magn Reson Med 42:963–969

Diffusion Tensor and Kurtosis

4

Toshiaki Taoka

4.1 Introduction

Diffusion of water is based on the principle that the water molecules show random motion. Water diffusion can provide unique information on the functional architecture of tissues, during their random displacements water molecules probe tissue structure at a microscopic scale [1, 2]. Since the introduction of imaging methods to visualize the diffusion phenomenon of the water molecule within tissue, this method has become one of the most important imaging techniques in clinical practice. In diffusion study on magnetic resonance imaging using motion proving gradient, signal decrease which is caused by molecular diffusion in the tissue provides information about tissue structure and physiological status. In this chapter, theoretical basis of diffusion tensor method and non-Gaussian diffusion technique including diffusion kurtosis imaging is discussed, and clinical or basic researches mainly using diffusion kurtosis imaging are introduced. In addition, the recently introduced concept of "glymphatic system" and the trial to evaluate the system using diffusion tensor method are also introduced.

4.1.1 Theoretical Considerations for Diffusion Tensor and Diffusion Kurtosis Imaging

4.1.1.1 Diffusion-Weighted Imaging

A method to observe in vivo diffusion phenomena using magnetic resonance techniques was first reported by Stajskal and Tanner in 1965 [3]. Subsequently, in 1986 LeBihan et al. applied diffusion techniques for the first time in MR imaging [1]. In this method, a pair of motion providing gradients (MPGs), which are gradient magnetic fields for detecting self-diffusion of water molecules, were applied with an inverted pulse of 180 degrees between them. The effects of the sequence cancel each other for stationary protons but cause additional dephasing in diffusing protons undergoing random motion which is proportional to the degree of movement. The commonly used index for the strength of the MPG is the b value, which is given by the formula $b = \gamma^2 G^2 \delta^2 (\Delta - \delta/3)$, where γ: gyromagnetic ratio, G: strength of the MPG, Δ: interval of the MPG, and δ: duration of the MPG. The unit of the b value is s/mm^2, and the reciprocal is thereby mm^2/s, which is the diffusion coefficient. For diffusion-weighted imaging of the brain, a b value of 1000 s/mm^2 is often used. On a diffusion-weighted image, tissues with high water diffusivity have low signal intensity and tissues with restricted diffusion have high signal intensity. In

T. Taoka (✉)
Department of Radiology, Nagoya University, Nagoya, Aichi, Japan
e-mail: ttaoka@med.nagoya-u.ac.jp

© Springer Nature Switzerland AG 2021
T. Moritani, A. A. Capizzano (eds.), *Diffusion-Weighted MR Imaging of the Brain, Head and Neck, and Spine*, https://doi.org/10.1007/978-3-030-62120-9_4

the method proposed by Stajskal and Tanner, the diffusion coefficient can be calculated from the slope of a graph of the logarithmic value of the signal acquired at different b-values. The values obtained by this method are called the apparent diffusion coefficient (ADC) and are different from the true tissue diffusion coefficients because they are influenced by phenomena other than pure diffusion, such as perfusion when measured in vivo.

Diffusion-weighted imaging plays a very important role in brain diagnoses particularly for acute infarctions and has become an essential tool for clinical practice. The most useful application of diffusion imaging in stroke has been supported by the finding that decreased diffusion can be used to detect brain ischemia at an early stage [4]. Although the underlying mechanisms for the decreased diffusion are not fully understood, cell swelling, changes in cell membrane permeability, decreased cytoplasmic streaming, and increased intracellular viscosity have been proposed [5–8]. Recently, a study of cerebral infarction using a very short diffusion time with oscillating gradient spin echo diffusion was reported. The findings indicated that a combination of neuronal beading and axonal swelling was the key structural changes leading to the reduced apparent diffusion coefficient after stroke [9]. This study indicates that alteration of the diffusion time is one method that may be applied to explore the microstructure of tissue; however there are alternative approaches that may also be used for this purpose.

4.1.1.2 Diffusion Tensor Imaging Based on a Gaussian Distribution

In neuronal tissue, the diffusion of water molecules is not uniform in all directions. Due to cell membranes and other tissue structures, the speed of diffusion varies depending on the direction, resulting in a state called anisotropic diffusion. In white matter of the brain, the diffusion in a direction perpendicular to the nerve fibers is more limited than along the axial direction of the fibers. The diffusion coefficient differs depending on the direction of motion probing gradient. Mathematically, scalars and

vectors are not sufficient to describe this phenomenon, and the application of a tensor is required. A tensor is a multidimensional array, where a rank 0 tensor is a scalar and a rank 1 tensor is a vector. When expressing diffusions in a three-dimensional space, a 3×3 matrix is used, and the diffusion tensor image (DTI) is acquired for this purpose. The diagonal components $\lambda 1$, $\lambda 2$, and $\lambda 3$ of the obtained diffusion tensor are called eigenvalues, and the eigenvectors of the eigenvalues coincide with the axes of the diffusion ellipsoid. In the white matter, the largest value of $\lambda 1$ is assumed to be the diffusion coefficient in the direction of fiber. The apparent diffusion coefficient (ADC) and fractional anisotropy (FA) value are often used as indices to evaluate the properties of this diffusion ellipsoid. For example, in tissue with dense fibers, the diffusivity in the direction perpendicular to the fiber is suppressed and thus the FA value is increased. In contrast, when the fiber structure is damaged as with degenerative diseases or other disorders, the diffusivity in the direction perpendicular to the fiber is increased and thus the FA value is reduced. So, by evaluating FA or ADC in the brain, the structural changes in tissue can be estimated [10].

Diffusion tensor tractography is a method to estimate white matter structural anatomy from diffusion tensor images [11–13]. In tractography, the direction of the principal axis of the eigenvector is assumed to coincide with the direction of the nerve fiber, and the direction of the principal axis for each voxel is traced to draw a virtual fiber. Although there are various algorithms, one type displays a virtual fiber path connecting a specified origin and endpoint, which is called the "deterministic model." This model is sufficient for gross anatomical information such as the anatomy of the pyramidal tract. However, in situations where more detailed spatial resolution is desired, or where there are many nerve fibers crossing, such as in the corona radiata, the resultant tracks obtained by the deterministic model may not be good enough. In these instances, a probabilistic model can be applied to obtain a more accurate depiction of the fiber tracts. This algorithm creates multiple tracts by taking into

4.1.1.3 Non-Gaussian Diffusion and Diffusion Kurtosis Imaging

A major assumption for conventional diffusion imaging is that "Diffusion has a Gaussian distribution." Diffusion tensor imaging using a Gaussian distribution model has been successful in evaluating anisotropic water diffusion in white matter, in which the diffusion is restricted by macromolecules, membranes, and myelin. Diffusion tensor imaging is based on a mathematical ellipsoid model. Thus, the principal direction of diffusion and the magnitude of diffusion along this direction can be calculated. Diffusion tensor tractography is an innovative application of the diffusion tensor method, which can delineate the neuronal fiber pathways. However, neuronal tissue has a highly heterogeneous structure and a Gaussian distribution is only applicable to free diffusion in fluid that is sufficiently large and uniform. Complicated structures exist in neuronal tissue, and the Gaussian distribution model does not truly represent the existence of a large number of compartments and nerve tracts, particularly in the central nervous system (CNS). Therefore, instead of a simple Gaussian distribution model, the application of probability distribution for a more detailed depiction of water molecule diffusion is necessary. To acquire probability distributions, dedicated model-free methods such as diffusion spectrum imaging have been introduced, which has high demand on scanner hardware and a long acquisition time [15, 16]. Another method to acquire a probability distribution is q-space imaging (QSI). QSI is performed by acquiring a large number of diffusion encodings and can provide a probability density function (PDF) of water molecules. In QSI, the diffusion phenomenon is not assumed to have a normal distribution. The information from fast diffusion to slow diffusion can be collected at various q values, and diffusion in each voxel can be expressed in the form of the PDF. The PDF in QSI is the distribution function of the distance traveled by the water

molecules and their probability. The q value represents the strength of the MPGs like a b value, and the definition is as follows. $q = \gamma/2\pi \ G\delta$ (where γ: gyromagnetic ratio, G: strength of the MPG, and δ: duration of the MPG). The unit of q is m^{-1}, that is, the spatial frequency, and the reciprocal is the distance of the water molecule movement. The shape of the PDF curvature is characterized by the mean displacement of the water molecule, which is calculated from the full width at half height and the probability for zero displacement, which is given by the height of the profile at zero displacement (Fig. 4.3).

Although QSI is theoretically superior to conventional Gaussian distribution analysis, one of the limitations is a long acquisition time due to the large number of sampling process. To further evaluate non-Gaussianity, the concept of kurtosis also can be applied. Diffusion kurtosis is a method to analyze the non-Gaussian distribution of water molecules within tissues [17, 18]. Kurtosis is a descriptor of the "Peakedness" relative to a Gaussian distribution of the probability distribution given by

$$K = \frac{1}{n}\sum_{i=1}^{n}\left(\frac{x_i - \overline{x}}{s_n}\right)^4$$

(where x: observed value and Sn: standard deviation). The higher the kurtosis, that is, the larger the deviation from the Gaussian distribution, the more the diffusion is restricted by the structure of the tissue and the structure of the cell. Therefore, the diversity of the diffusion distribution in the tissue is increased. Positive kurtosis means that distribution is more sharply peaked than Gaussian. The higher the diffusion kurtosis, the more the water molecule diffusion deviates from a Gaussian distribution, indicative of a more restricted diffusion environment. In other words, higher kurtosis means the distribution has a distinct peak near the mean and heavy tails, which is closely associated with diffusional heterogeneity [17, 19, 20]. Diffusion kurtosis can be calculated within a clinically feasible imaging time using a combination of more than three different MPG strengths with cumulant expansion [17]. Jensen et al. developed the method of cumulant expansion to obtain diffusion kurtosis, which was approximated by including a quadratic function [20]. In this method, a relatively low *b* value MPGs can be used to evaluate the non-Gaussian distribution diffusion. Diffusion kurtosis is sensitive to slow diffusional movement in a restricted environment, which may be mainly determined by microstructure. A diffusion kurtosis image (DKI) is reported to provide better characterization of both normal and pathological tissue and is less susceptible to free fluid contamination compared to the mean diffusivity or fractional anisotropy parameters provided by DTI [21]. Typical parameters in DKI include radial kurtosis (Krad), which is the diffusion kurtosis perpendicular to the principal diffusion tensor eigenvector, axial kurtosis (Kax), which is the diffusion kurtosis along the principal diffusion tensor eigenvector, and mean kurtosis (MK), which is a special mean of the diffusion kurtosis. These directional diffusion kurtosis parameters may provide detailed information regarding the tissue microstructure, thus improving the MR diffusion characterization of neural tissues. DKIs are reported to have a greater sensitivity to changes in myelination compared with conventional DTIs. In particular, both Krad and MK are reported to have stronger correlations with myelin content compared with diffusion tensor metrics [22] (Figs 4.1 and 4.2).

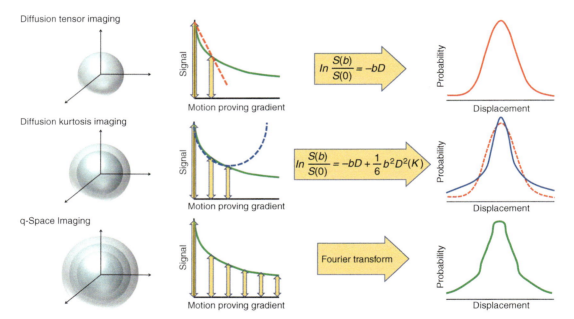

Fig. 4.1 The theory of diffusion tensor imaging, diffusion kurtosis imaging, and multi-shell diffusion imaging. A diffusion tensor image can be obtained by a set of multi-axes motion probing gradients (MPGs) in addition to no MPG for covering the special distribution of water diffusion. Since diffusion tensor imaging is based on the assumption that water diffusion obeys a Gaussian distribution, only a single set of b-values (calculated by the strength and duration of motion probing gradient) is required. Because the shape of the distribution is fixed to Gaussian, the logarithm of the diffusion-weighted signal intensity as a function of the MPG is fit to a following line:

$$\ln \frac{S(b)}{S(0)} = -bD.$$

(*S* signal intensity, *b* b value, *D* diffusivity). Kurtosis is a dimensionless statistical metric for quantifying the non-Gaussianity of an arbitrary probability distribution. To acquire a diffusion kurtosis image, at least two sets of MPGs in addition to no MPG is needed, because the following approximation can estimate both the diffusivity and kurtosis when the b values of the MPGs are sufficiently small:

$$\ln \frac{S(b)}{S(0)} = -bD + \frac{1}{6} b^2 D^2 (K).$$

(*K* kurtosis). With this approximation, one can estimate both D and K by fitting the diffusion-weighted signal intensity data with three or more MPGs while the logarithm of the signal intensity is fit to a parabola. Large kurtosis means a high peak and a fat tail in the probability distribution. Q-space imaging (QSI) is a method to measure the probability distribution of a detailed water molecule. The main principle in q-space analysis is that a Fourier transformation of the signal intensity with respect to the MPGs provides a probability density function (PDF). QSI is performed by the measurement of a large amount of diffusion encoding

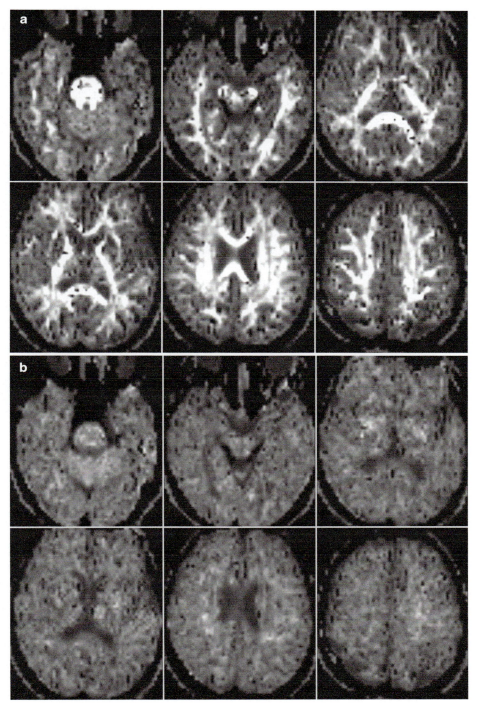

Fig. 4.2 Diffusion kurtosis images of the normal brain. (**a**) Radial kurtosis images, (**b**) axial kurtosis images, (**c**) mean kurtosis images. Radial kurtosis is the diffusion kurtosis perpendicular to the principal diffusion tensor eigenvector. On radial kurtosis images, white matter has a significantly higher value compared to gray matter. In white matter, myelin acts as a multiple barrier structure in the direction that is perpendicular to the fiber bundles. In contrast, on axial kurtosis images white matter shows lower value showing that barrier structure in the direction of fiber bundle is not dense

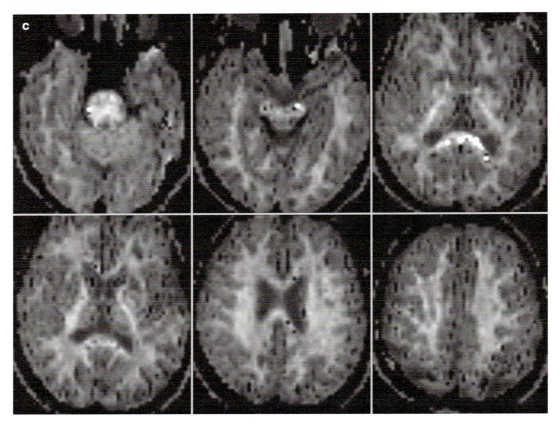

Fig. 4.2 (continued)

4.1.2 Studies Using Diffusion Kurtosis Imaging for Central Nervous System Diseases

4.1.2.1 Cerebrovascular Diseases

There are several reports on the application of DKI for ischemic stroke in human subjects [8, 20, 23, 24]. Jensen et al. reported that white matter infarction showed increased diffusion kurtosis with a strong fiber tract orientational dependence in their preliminary study. They showed a large increase in Kax in conjunction with a small increase in Krad. They speculated that it could be due to a large change in the intra-axonal diffusivity, which is possibly related to either axonal varicosities or alterations associated with the endoplasmic reticulum [8]. They also reported that the increased kurtosis in the ischemic lesion meant an increase in the complexity or heterogeneity of the water microenvironment in the tissue [17, 20]. Diffusion kurtosis imaging was also used to predict stroke outcome [24]. This study showed that the volume of an acute lesion on a kurtosis map was identical with the volume on the 1-month follow-up T2-weighted image (T2WI) for large (diameter ≥ 1 cm) lesions. For small (diameter <1 cm) lesions, the number of acute lesions on DKI was consistent with that found on follow-up T2WIs [24]. There is also a report of a longer time course of diffusion kurtosis changes after infarction in human subjects [23]. The study evaluated cases from 3 h to 122 days after onset and found that the diffusion kurtosis was highest immediately after the onset of infarction and decreased with time. Krad showed a pseudo-normalization earlier than the ADC, and the pseudo-normalization of Kax occurred slightly later than that of the ADC. The time course of the parameters differed by the location of the infarction. The pseudo-normalization for Krad/Kax occurred at 13.2/59.9 days for perforator infarctions, 33.1/40.6 days for white matter infarctions, 34.8/35.9 days for cortical infarctions, and 34.1/28.2 days after watershed infarctions [23] (Figs. 4.3, 4.4, and 4.5).

There are several reports of DKI in experimental models of cerebral infarction [25, 26]. Hui et al. investigated the time course of DKI in an experimental model of infarction in the rat brain. They found that MK increased in the hyperacute (0–2 h) and acute (24 hrs post-occlusion) phases after occlusion of middle cerebral artery, which was followed by renormalization or pseudo-normalization at days 1–2, and a decrease at day 7. The time course of diffusion kurtosis has also been evaluated in a transient cerebral artery occlusion model [27]. Adult male Wistar rats were subjected to 30 or 60 min of middle cerebral artery occlusion and imaged on a 7 T scanner. DKI was obtained before middle cerebral artery reperfusion and 3, 6, and 24 h after reperfusion. The study found that the relative FA and ADC values decreased at 3 h after MCA reperfusion and remained decreased through 24 h. The relative MK, Kax, and Krad values were increased at 3 h after MCA reperfusion, peaked at 6 h, and were slightly

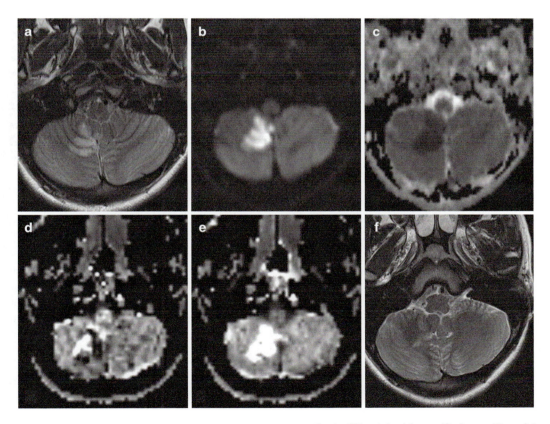

Fig. 4.3 Diffusion kurtosis image of early cerebral infarction. 18 years old female. Five days after the onset of cerebellar infarction due to vertebral artery dissection. A T2-weighted image (T2WI) (**a**) shows high signal intensity, the diffusion-weighted image (**b**) shows high signal intensity, and the ADC image (**c**) has lower values. At the same time, the radial (**d**) and axial (**e**) kurtosis images show increased kurtosis in the lesion. In particular, the axial kurtosis image has higher values. Sixteen days after onset. On the T2-weighted image (**f**), the swelling of the lesion has diminished and the high signal intensity of the diffusion-weighted image (**g**) has also decreased. The ADC image (**h**) shows pseudo-normalization at this time point. The radial kurtosis image (**i**) remains high and the axial kurtosis (**j**) indicates nearly pseudo-normalization. The changes over time of the diffusion kurtosis images including axial and radial kurtosis are different from the conventional T2 image or the diffusion tensor metrics

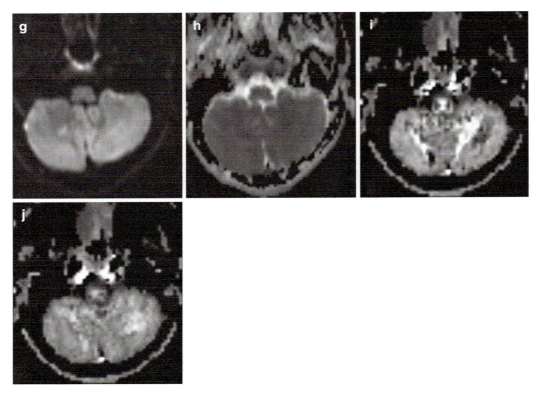

Fig. 4.3 (continued)

decreased at 24 h. In white matter, Kax showed larger changes than Krad. These results indicate that the diffusion kurtosis parameters show earlier pseudo-normalization than the ADC of the lesions. For white matter lesions, the increase in Kax was larger than that for Krad, suggesting that tissue changes after infarction mainly produce reduced diffusivity along the fiber tracts and lead to increased diffusion inhomogeneity [27].

4.1.2.2 Brain Tumors

The first report for the application of DKI in the diagnosis of brain tumors was published in 2010. The preliminary study of 34 patients with cerebral gliomas indicated that low-grade tumors are different from normal tissue, and higher-grade tumors demonstrate mean kurtosis values very similar to those of normal white matter. This phenomenon could be explained by the cellular differences between normal white matter versus low- and high-grade tumors. Normal white matter is highly organized and contains many barriers to diffusion such as the myelin sheath and tightly packed neuronal axons. In contrast, low-grade gliomas (LGGs) have low cellularity, large sized cells, and, usually, infiltrative growth; thus they contain fewer barriers to water diffusion. High-grade gliomas (HGGs) are characterized by high cellularity, more nuclear atypia, increased pleomorphism, and more vascular hyperplasia and necrosis. Thus the structural complexity is greater than in LGGs, but does not reach the complexity of normal white matter. These differences in tissue characteristics are reflected by the increasing MK of HGGs, which are somewhat similar to normal while matter [28]. A meta-analysis of 10 investigations involving 430 patients was published in 2017. The study assessed the diagnostic test accuracy and sources of heterogeneity for the discriminative potential of DKI to differentiate LGG, and indicated that the difference in MK between LGGs versus HGGs had high diagnostic accuracy with a z score equal to 5.86 ($P < 0.001$).

4 Diffusion Tensor and Kurtosis

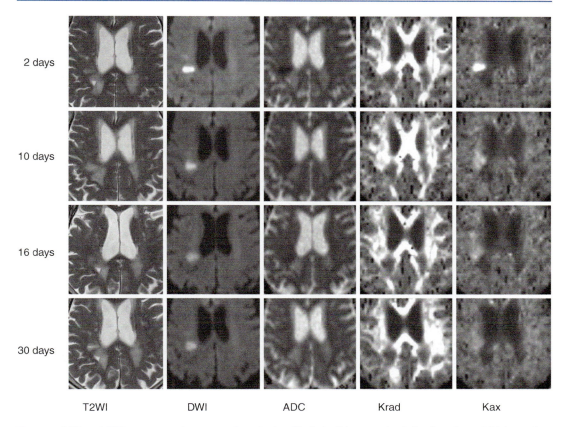

Fig. 4.4 DKI and DTI parameters in a case of cerebral infarction. MR images from a 76-year-old woman with a right corona radiata infarction. Images (T2WI, DWI, ADC, Krad, Kax) were acquired on days 2, 10, 16, and 30 after onset of infarction. On the T2WI, the lesion had uniform high signal intensity. The DWI demonstrated a prominent high-signal-intensity region, particularly on the image at day 2. The signal retained its high intensity even on the image at day 30. The ADC was low immediately after infarction, and became less obvious on the images at days 16 and 30. The white matter exhibited high Krad; in this case, the infarction showed higher values compared with the contralateral normal region. This elevation in Krad decreased soon after the infarction, and on the image at day 16, Krad was lower than in the normal region. The Kax values were similar in both white and gray matter, and the Kax images appeared homogeneous. The infarction lesion showed a very high Kax value compared with the normal region immediately after the onset of infarction, but this soon diminished to the negative value shown in the later images. Images from reference [23]

Furthermore, the study concluded that the heterogeneity was driven by the neuropathologic subtype as well as differences in DKI techniques [29] (Figs. 4.6 and 4.7).

A recent study which aimed to assess the diagnostic capabilities of DKI for grading glioma according to prognostic molecular characteristics suggested that mean kurtosis appears to be a promising in vivo biomarker for glioma. The study showed that the mean kurtosis was significantly lower in gliomas with the isocitrate-dehydrogenase (IDH1/2) mutation and the alpha-thalassemia/mental retardation syndrome X-linked (ATRX) loss of expression than in those with IDH1/2 wild type and ATRX maintained expression. Thus, MK may provide insight into the human glioma molecular profile with regard to IDH1/2 mutation status and ATRX expression [30].

There is also a study to discriminate metastatic brain tumor versus high-grade astrocytoma using diffusion kurtosis parameters including MK, Krad, and Kax, as well as diffusion tensor parameters including FA and MD values. The study indicated that the three diffusion kurtosis parameters in peritumoral edema were significantly higher in high-grade astrocytoma than metastatic brain tumors [31]. This difference in diffusion kurtosis parameters may reflect the tissue characteristics of peritumoral edema in high-grade astrocytoma, in which neoplastic cells may restrict diffusion in both the axial and radial directions. Assessment of malignant lymphoma is also a good application of diffusion kurtosis imaging. A study comparing diffusion kurtosis parameters between high-grade glioma and primary CNS lymphoma showed that primary CNS lymphoma had significantly higher mean kurtosis and axial kurtosis than high-grade gliomas. However, differences in diffusion parameters such as MD or FA were not significant [32]. In a study that examined DKI for the assessment of chemotherapy response in patients with cervical non-Hodgkin lymphoma, mean kurtosis was decreased significantly at follow-up of the responders compared to baseline images [33] (Fig. 4.8).

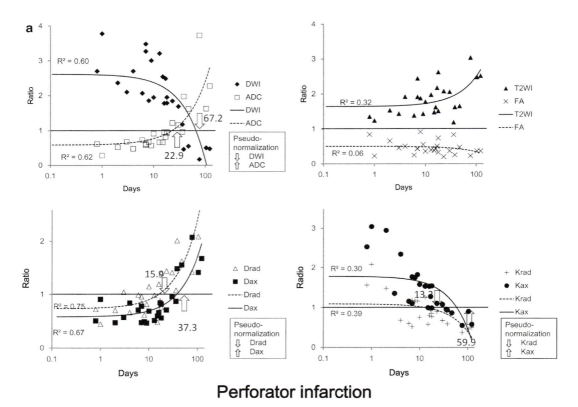

Perforator infarction

Fig. 4.5 Changes over time in DKI and DTI parameters of cerebral infarction. Plots of the ratios (lesion versus normal tissue) for each variable and duration after onset of the infarction. Linear regression lines are provided with their coefficient of determination (R^2). Because a logarithmic scale was used for the time axis, the first-order linear regression lines are drawn as exponential curves. (**a**) Perforator infarction group. (**b**) White matter territorial infarction group. (**c**) Cortical infarction group. (**d**) Watershed infarction group. For each variable (T2WI signal, DWI signal, ADC, FA, Drad: radial diffusivity, Dax: axial diffusivity, Krad, and Kax), the ratio of the value in the lesion compared with that in the contralateral normal tissue was plotted against time after infarction (days). The times at which pseudo-normalization occurred are indicated by arrows. In general, the T2WI showed increased signal intensity with time after infarction onset. The DWI signal tended to be higher immediately after onset and decreased with time after infarction onset. The ADC was lowest soon after onset and increased with time. Fractional anisotropy diminished throughout the observation period. Drad and Dax were lowest immediately after onset and increased with time; this increase was faster in Drad. Krad and Kax were highest immediately after onset and decreased with time. Images from reference [23]

4 Diffusion Tensor and Kurtosis

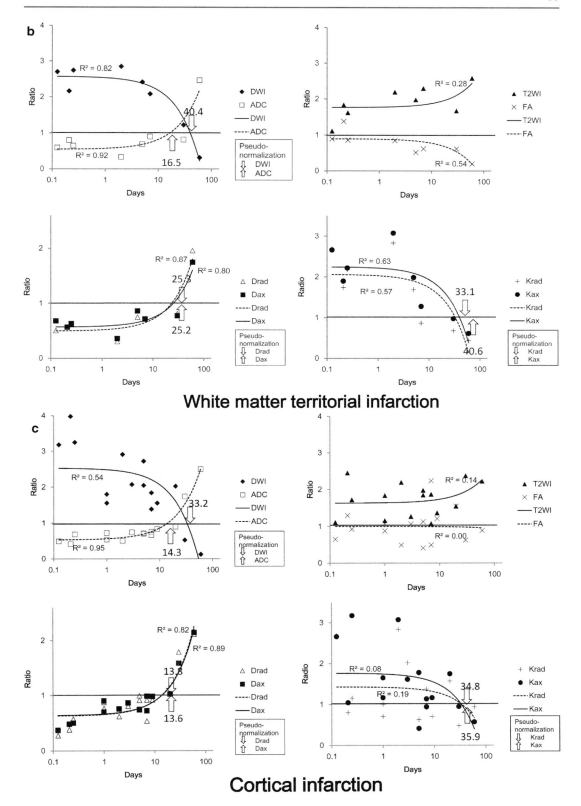

Fig. 4.5 (continued)

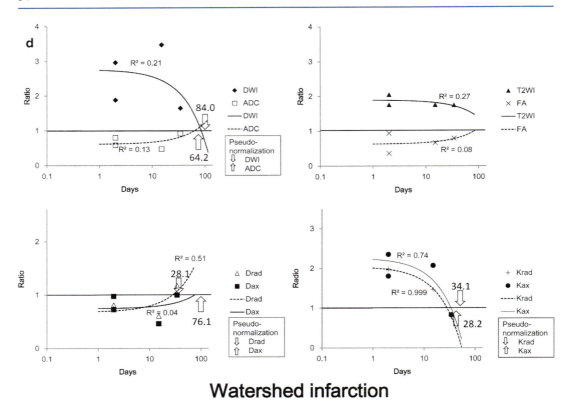

Fig. 4.5 (continued)

4.1.2.3 Demyelinating Diseases

Alterations in diffusion kurtosis parameters can detect tissue damage in multiple sclerosis (MS). In a study of DKI and DTI for normal appearing white matter in MS, significant differences in both FA and DK values were observed between control and MS groups. In addition, the differences in DK values between normal appearing white matter in MS and controls were more pronounced than those found with FA or ADC values [34]. Diffusion kurtosis can delineate changes in the optic pathway in MS cases. In a study of MS cases with unilateral and bilateral optic nerve damage, the bilaterally damaged group had significantly higher ADC and lower MK values relative to cases with unilateral damage or controls with no damage [35]. Another study evaluated the associations between diffusional kurtosis parameters in the corticospinal tract and disability in MS, which was quantified at the time of MR imaging using the Expanded Disability Status Scale. The study showed significant associations of Krad in the corticospinal tract with age, as well as the disability score during the baseline visit, suggesting that Krad in the corticospinal tract may have an association with neurologic disability in MS [36] (Figs. 4.9 and 4.10).

4.1.2.4 Neurodegenerative Diseases

Diffusion tensor imaging has been widely applied for the evaluation of Alzheimer's disease (AD) and other neurodegenerative diseases. In 2000, Rose et al. were the first to apply DTI to Alzheimer's disease [37]. Tract-based analysis permits the selective measurement of the white matter tracts. In tractography, the desired white matter tract is selected as a volume of interest and anisotropy or diffusivity are measured along the volume. In addition, Taoka et al. reported tract-based analysis of the uncinate fasciculus, which is part of limbic system circuitry in Alzheimer's disease cases [10].

4 Diffusion Tensor and Kurtosis

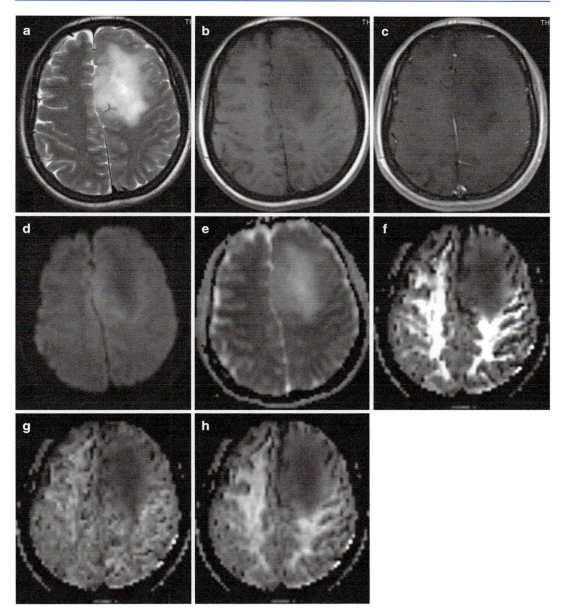

Fig. 4.6 A case of benign glioma. MR images of a 33-year-old woman suffering from convulsion. Surgery indicated a diffuse astrocytoma in the left frontal lobe. The T2-weighted image (**a**) shows diffuse high signal intensity and the T1-weighted image (**b**) shows low signal intensity. The contrast-enhanced image (**c**) does not show any enhancement in the lesion. The diffusion-weighted image (**d**) shows low signal intensity and the ADC image (**e**) has higher values. The radial (**f**), axial (**g**), and mean (**h**) kurtosis images show characteristic homogeneous lower values throughout the tumor

In a study investigating changes in brain microstructure by DKI and DTI parameters in AD and mild cognitive impairment (MCI) versus controls, Krad in the anterior corona radiata was the best individual discriminator of MCI from controls, and axial diffusivity in the hippocampus was the best discriminator of MCI from AD [38]. Another study used DKI to detect microstructural abnor-

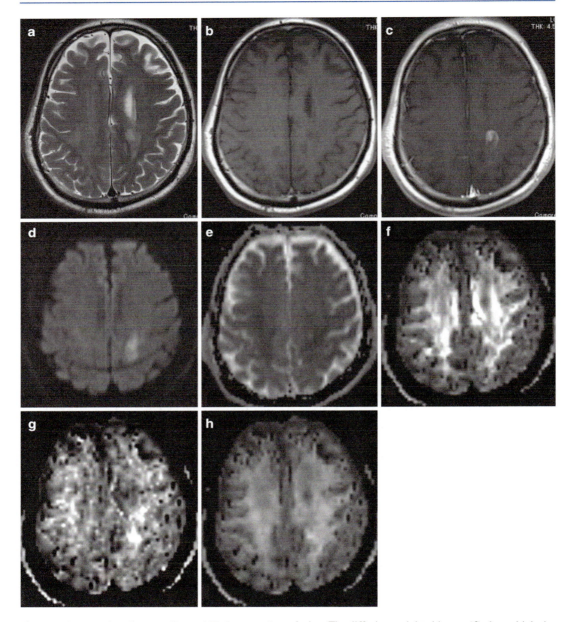

Fig. 4.7 A case of malignant glioma. MR images of a 74-year-old man suffering from weakness of the left lower extremity. Surgery indicated a glioblastoma in the left parietal lobe. The T2-weighted image (**a**) shows irregular high signal intensity, and the T1-weighted image (**b**) shows low signal intensity. The contrast-enhanced image (**c**) shows irregular but prominent enhancement of the lesion. The diffusion-weighted image (**d**) shows high signal intensity but the ADC image (**e**) shows small differences compared to the surrounding area. The radial (**f**), axial (**g**), and mean (**h**) kurtosis images show heterogeneous high values in the tumor. In particular, the axial kurtosis image showed high values compared to the surrounding tissue

malities of deep and cortical gray matter in AD. This study indicated that MK can complement conventional diffusion metrics to detect microstructural alterations, particularly in deep gray matter. They found that more regions in deep gray matter had DKI abnormalities than local volume loss in early MCI. Mean kurtosis exhibited the largest number of significant abnormalities

4 Diffusion Tensor and Kurtosis

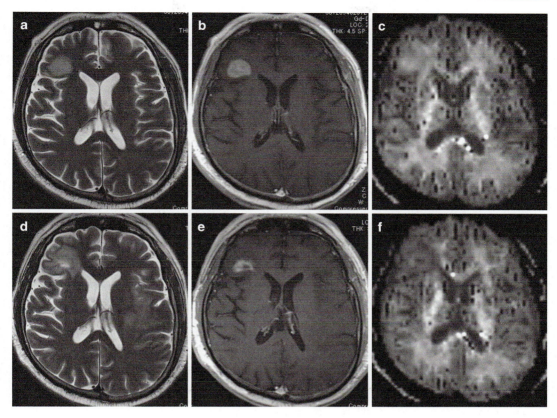

Fig. 4.8 A case of primary central nervous system lymphoma. MR images of a 49-year-old man suffering from convulsive attacks. Biopsy indicated a primary central nervous system lymphoma in the right frontal lobe. The pre-treatment T2-weighted image (**a**) shows homogenous slightly high signal intensity, and the contrast-enhanced image (**b**) shows homogeneous enhancement in the lesion. The mean kurtosis image (**c**) shows high values in the tumor. After treatment by high-dose methotrexate, the T2-weighted image (**d**) shows elevation of the signal intensity in the center of the tumor, and the contrast-enhanced image (**e**) indicates tumor volume loss, but still has prominent enhancement. The mean kurtosis image at post-treatment (**f**) shows a uniform decrease of the kurtosis in the tumor

among all DKI metrics. In more advanced AD, diffusional abnormalities were observed in fewer regions than atrophy. In gray matter, the abnormalities in cortical thickness were mainly in the medial and lateral temporal lobes [39].

4.1.2.5 Normal Brain Development and Developmental Abnormalities

Development is an important target for diffusion imaging. Although most studies of human brain development have used diffusion tensor imaging with an evaluation of FA or diffusivity metrics [40], recent studies have employed non-Gaussian methods for the evaluation of development and developmental abnormalities.

One study measured age-related microstructural changes in the developing human brain. The findings indicated that mean kurtosis detects significant microstructural changes consistent with known patterns of brain maturation compared to FA [41]. In the study, 90% of maximum FA was reached at 5 months, whereas 90% of maximum mean kurtosis occurred at 18 months for the external capsule, indicating that mean kurtosis detected continued microstructural changes in white matter past the FA plateau, accounting for more delayed isotropic changes.

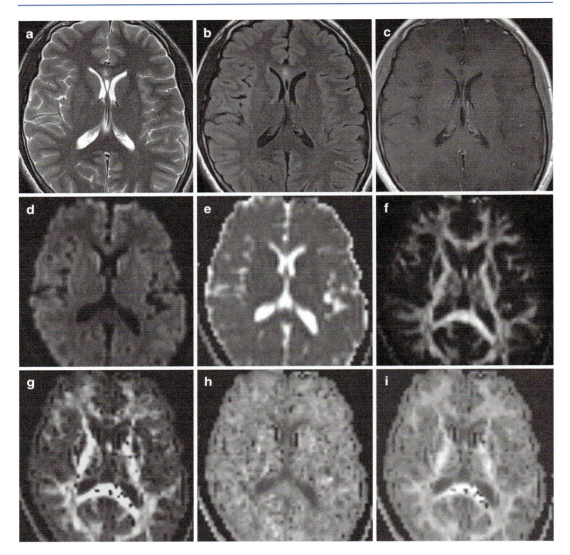

Fig. 4.9 A case of chronic lesion from multiple sclerosis. MR images of a 15-year-old man with multiple sclerosis. The T2-weighted image (**a**) shows a diffuse high signal intensity, and the T1-weighted image (**b**) shows low signal intensity in the midline of the genu of the corpus callosum. The contrast-enhanced image (**c**) does not show any enhancement of the lesion. The diffusion-weighted image (**d**) shows slightly high signal intensity; however the ADC image (**e**) shows equal value to the surrounding tissue indicating T2-shine through. The FA image (**f**) shows reduced FA in the lesion. The radial kurtosis image (**g**) shows obvious low values in the lesion; however, the axial kurtosis image (**h**) shows little difference, and the mean kurtosis image (**i**) seems to indicate intermediate values. These findings may indicate that the pathological change in the lesion is mainly due to the breakdown of myelin structure

Another study comparing diffusion tensor versus diffusion kurtosis imaging also indicated that DKI was more sensitive to developmental changes in local microstructure and environment, and was particularly powerful to unravel developmental differences in major association fibers, such as the cingulum and superior longitudinal fasciculus [42]. The study compared DTI and DKI between childhood (average age 10.3 years) and middle adult ages (average age 54.3 years) and showed that between-group differences in diffusion kurtosis metrics were more widespread

4 Diffusion Tensor and Kurtosis

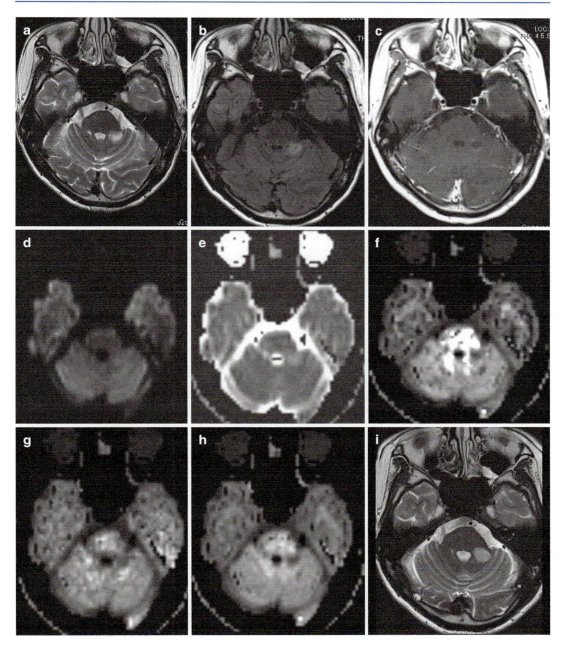

Fig. 4.10 A case of chronic lesion from multiple sclerosis at pre- and post-treatment. MR images of a 24-year-old man suffering from numbness and decreased grip in the left hand. Two sessions of steroid pulse therapy were applied under the diagnosis of multiple sclerosis. The pre-treatment T2-weighted (**a**) and FLAIR images (**b**) show high signal intensity in the left middle cerebellar peduncle. The contrast-enhanced image (**c**) shows a ring-like enhancement surrounding the lesion. The diffusion-weighted image (**d**) shows slightly high signal intensity, and the ADC image (**e**) shows high values indicating T2-shine through. While the radial (**f**) and mean (**h**) kurtosis images show low values in the lesion, the axial kurtosis image (**g**) shows a region with higher values at the edge of the lesion (*arrow*). The post-treatment T2-weighted image (**i**), FLAIR image (**j**), diffusion-weighted image (**k**), ADC image (**l**), radial (**m**) and mean (**o**) kurtosis images look very similar to the pre-treatment images. The post-treatment axial kurtosis image (**n**) indicates that the region with higher values at the edge of the lesion has disappeared

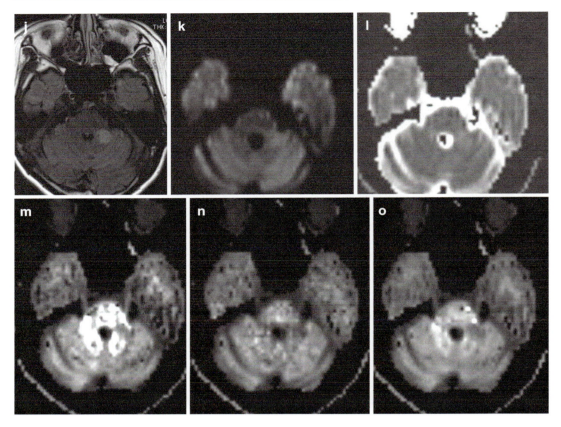

Fig. 4.10 (continued)

in comparison to diffusion tensor metrics for voxel-based analysis.

Diffusion kurtosis imaging has also been applied to developmental abnormalities. In a study of children with a clinical diagnosis of idiopathic generalized epilepsy and unilateral interictal epileptiform discharges, DKI was more sensitive for the detection of diffusion abnormalities in both white and gray matter compared to FA and diffusivity parameters [43]. The findings indicated a significant reduction in FA values in the left cerebrum white matter and increased MD in the left brainstem, particularly in the pons. In contrast, a significant reduction in MK was observed more extensively in both white matter and gray matter of the cerebrum including the contralateral hemisphere. In cases with congenital sensorineural hearing loss, significantly lower FA and MK values were found in 6 white matter regions. However, in 2 additional white matter regions and 2 gray matter regions, only MK was lower, with no appreciable change observed in FA values for patients over 3 years of age. In addition, in some gray matter regions of children with sensorineural hearing loss, there were significant changes in MK but no appreciable changes in FA values in the same areas. These results suggest that DKI is more sensitive to microstructural changes that occur in isotropic gray matter [44]. The author experienced a case of Pelizaeus-Merzbacher disease, in which no myelination pattern was observed on T1- and T2-weighted images. In this condition, the FA maps still had high values throughout the white matter, which may have been due to axonal structural elements. In contrast, the radial kurtosis image indicated higher kurtosis in the bilateral pyramidal tracts and in the corpus callosum, which may indicate that myelinic structure is present in these structures (Fig. 4.11).

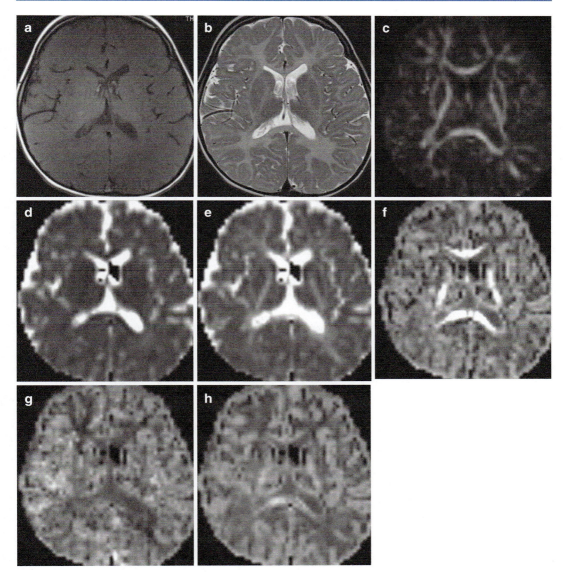

Fig. 4.11 A case of Pelizaeus-Merzbacher disease. MR images from a 2-year-old male with spastic paralysis and vertical nystagmus. Genetic diagnosis of Pelizaeus-Merzbacher disease was made. On both the T1-weighted (**a**) and the T2-weighted (**b**) images there is almost no signal, indicating normal myelination in the white matter including the pyramidal tracts. However, the FA image (**c**) has high values throughout the white matter, which may be due to the axonal structure of the white matter. The radial diffusivity (**d**) and axial diffusivity (**e**) images indicate that the diffusivity in the white matter is larger in the direction of the fiber bundles. On the radial kurtosis image (**f**) higher kurtosis can be observed in the bilateral pyramidal tracts and in the corpus callosum, which are not obvious on the axial (**g**) and mean (**h**) kurtosis images. This combination of results on the kurtosis images may indicate that the myelinic structure is present in the pyramidal tract and the corpus callosum

4.1.3 Glymphatic System and Diffusion Imaging

The glymphatic system is a recently discovered waste drainage system in the brain via the cerebrospinal fluid (CSF) along the perivascular spaces. This system promotes the elimination of soluble proteins including amyloid-β and metabolites, and also facilitates the distribution of glucose, lipids, amino acids, and neuromodulators [45, 46]. In this system, CSF and interstitial fluid (ISF) are known to interchange by the influx of

CSF along the loose fibrous matrix of the perivascular spaces. The CSF influx from the subarachnoid space into the deep peri-arterial space is driven by arterial pulsatile motion, slow motion of the vessels, respiratory motion, and CSF pressure. Subsequently, CSF is transported into the brain parenchyma via aquaporin-P4 (AQP4) water channels in astrocytic endfeet. CSF movement into the parenchyma drives convective ISF fluxes within the tissue toward the peri-venous spaces surrounding the deep veins and then, collected in the peri-venous space. From the peri-venous space, the fluid drains out of the brain toward the cervical lymphatic system [45, 47, 48] (Fig. 4.12).

A tracer study is an efficient method to visualize or evaluate this mass transportation system in vivo. The activity of the glymphatic system has been studied by intrathecally administered tracers in animal experiments. A tracer study permits the tracking of a substance and its interactions within the body through labeling of the substance in a manner that does not alter the substances original properties. Also for brain tissue, tracer studies have been used to simulate or trace substance transport in interstitial spaces [49]. However, the administration of tracers including gadolinium-based contrast agents (GBCAs) is invasive for human subjects, which is why the evaluation of the glymphatic system in humans is not well established.

Diffusion MR methods can also be applied to evaluate the dynamics of interstitial space. The tracer studies evaluate the behavior of the tracer though a time interval and require hours to follow the distribution of the tracer within the brain. In contrast, diffusion imaging provides information of the water molecule movement in tissue at the moment that the MPGs are applied. Therefore, a diffusion-based technique may provide very different information compared to a tracer study. Diffusion images including DTI can be acquired within several minutes and may have the potential to monitor the status of the glymphatic system over time. In addition, methods based on diffusion imaging are noninvasive compared to tracer studies which need intrathecal or intravenous injection of the tracers.

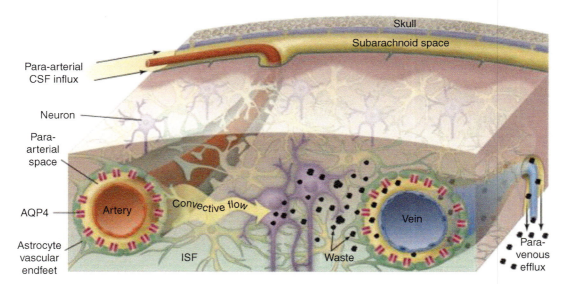

Fig. 4.12 Outline of the glymphatic system. Cerebrospinal fluid flows into the brain parenchyma via the perivascular space. From the perivascular space surrounding the artery, cerebrospinal fluid enters the interstitium of brain tissue via AQP4-controlled water channels, which are distributed in astrocytic endfeet constituting the outer wall of the perivascular space. Cerebrospinal fluid entering the interstitial fluid flows by convection, after washing waste proteins from the tissue. It then flows into the perivascular space around the vein and is discharged outside the brain. Images from reference [55]

Diffusion tensor image analysis along the perivascular space (DTI-ALPS) can evaluate diffusivity along the direction of the perivascular (peri-arterial and peri-venous) spaces compared with that of projection and association fibers on a slice at the level of the lateral ventricle body (Fig. 4.13). The medullary arteries and veins are the vessels of the brain parenchyma and are adjacent to the perivascular space, which is the major drainage pathway of the glymphatic system. At the level of the lateral ventricle body, the medullary veins run perpendicular to the ventricular wall [51, 52]. The perivascular space also runs in the same direction as the medullary veins, which is in the right-left direction (x-axis). In the plane of this region, projection fibers run in the head-

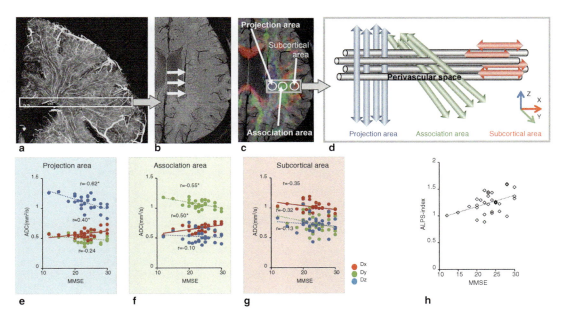

Fig. 4.13 The theory of diffusion tensor image analysis along the perivascular space (DTI-ALPS) and findings for Alzheimer's disease. (**a**) A roentgenogram of an injected coronal brain slice showing the parenchymal vessels that run horizontally on the slice (*white box*) at the level of the lateral ventricle body. (**b**) An axial susceptibility-weighted image (SWI) on the slice at the level of the lateral ventricle body indicates that the parenchymal vessels run laterally (x-axis). (**c**) A superimposed color display of the DTI on the SWI (**b**) indicating the distribution of the projection fibers (z-axis: *blue*), association fibers (y-axis: *green*), and subcortical fibers (x-axis: *red*). Three ROIs are placed in the region with the projection fibers (projection area), association fibers (association area), and subcortical fibers (subcortical area) to measure the diffusivities in the three directions (x, y, z). (**d**) A schematic indicating the relationship between the direction of the perivascular space (*gray cylinders*) and the directions of the fibers. Note that the direction of the perivascular space is perpendicular to both projection and association fibers. The correlation between directional diffusivity and MMSE scores. The correlation between MMSE and diffusivities for the three directions of the three areas (projection: (**e**), association: (**f**), subcortical: (**g**)) is indicated. The diffusivity of the x-axis is plotted as *red*, y-axis as *green*, and z-axis as *blue*. The regression lines are also shown in the same colors with the plots, accompanied by the values for the correlation coefficients. Statistically significant correlations are shown as asterisks. In the projection area (**e**), we found a significant positive correlation between the diffusivity along the perivascular space (x-axis) and MMSE score. In the association area (**f**), we found a significant positive correlation between the diffusivity along the perivascular space (x-axis) and MMSE score. However, there was a significant negative correlation between the diffusivity along the projection fibers (z-axis) in the projection area and MMSE score. There was also a significant negative correlation between the association fibers (y-axis) in the association area and MMSE score. These negative correlations may be explained by white matter degeneration in the projection or association fibers due to AD or MCI. (**h**) Correlation between the ALPS index and MMSE. Correlations between the MMSE and ALPS index, which is given by the following ratio, are shown.

ALPSindex = mean (Dxxproj, Dxxassoc)/
mean (Dyyproj, Dzzassoc).

There was a significant positive correlation ($r = 0.46$, $p = 0.0084$) between the ALPS index and MMSE score. Images from reference [50]

foot (z-axis) direction mainly adjacent to the lateral ventricle and the superior longitudinal fascicles (SLFs). In addition, the association fibers run in the anterior-posterior (y-axis) direction outside of the projection fibers. On the outside of the SLFs, the subcortical fibers run mainly in the right-left (y-axis) direction in the subcortical areas. Consequently, the perivascular space runs perpendicular to the projection fibers and the SLFs. This anatomical structure of the perivascular space and major fibers allows a nearly independent analysis of the diffusivity along the direction of perivascular spaces because the major fiber tracts do not run parallel to the perivascular space. When there are common changes of diffusivity in the right-left direction (x-axis) in both the projection and association fiber areas, the observed change could be due to an alteration of the diffusivity along the direction of the perivascular space. In a recent study to evaluate the activity of the glymphatic system in individual subjects, an ALPS score was calculated [50]. This score was provided by the ratio of two sets of diffusivity values, which are perpendicular to the dominant fibers in the tissue. It was hypothesized that the ratio of these values would represent the presence of water diffusion along the perivascular space, which should reflect the activity of the glymphatic system in an individual subject. If the ratio was close to 1, it meant that the water diffusion along the perivascular space was at a minimum, and alternatively, a larger ratio represented increased water diffusivity along the perivascular space. This study found that there was a significant positive correlation between the ALPS index and the MMSE scores. This result could indicate that the ALPS index may be used to evaluate the activity of the glymphatic system in individual subjects. Another investigation aimed to replicate the DTI-ALPS method in 36 patients with Alzheimer's disease and associated status (16 AD, 16 MCI, and 4 SMC). The study indicated significant correlations between the DTI-ALPS and the stratified Mini-Mental State Examination score [53]. This DTI-APLS method was also applied for the evaluation of glymphatic function in idiopathic normal pressure hydrocephalus (iNPH). Cekic et al.

reported that the ALPS index can distinguish reliably between iNPH, ventriculomegaly/pseudo-iNPH, and controls. In particular, the ALPS index performed better than both the Evans index and the callosal angle in distinguishing between pseudo-iNPH and iNPH [54].

4.2 Conclusion

Diffusion imaging is an indispensable tool for clinical practice of the nervous system today and is also a powerful tool for investigating the finer morphology of the brain. There have been technological advancements that allow more information to be obtained from fewer data sets, which result in reduced acquisition time. It is thought that technology considered currently to be at the forefront of research will be applied to a clinical setting in the relatively near future.

References

1. Le Bihan D, Breton E, Lallemand D, Grenier P, Cabanis E, Laval-Jeantet M (1986) MR imaging of intravoxel incoherent motions: application to diffusion and perfusion in neurologic disorders. Radiology 161(2):401–407
2. Le Bihan D (2014) Diffusion MRI: what water tells us about the brain. EMBO Mol Med 6(5):569–573
3. Stejskal EO, Tanner JE (1965) Spin diffusion measurements: spin echoes in the presence of a time-dependent field gradient. J Chem Phys 42:288–292
4. Le Bihan D, Turner R, Douek P, Patronas N (1992) Diffusion MR imaging: clinical applications. AJR Am J Roentgenol 159(3):591–599
5. Benveniste H, Hedlund LW, Johnson GA (1992) Mechanism of detection of acute cerebral ischemia in rats by diffusion-weighted magnetic resonance microscopy. Stroke 23(5):746–754
6. Lee JH, Springer CS Jr (2003) Effects of equilibrium exchange on diffusion-weighted NMR signals: the diffusigraphic "shutter-speed". Magn Reson Med 49(3):450–458
7. Dijkhuizen RM, de Graaf RA, Tulleken KA, Nicolay K (1999) Changes in the diffusion of water and intracellular metabolites after excitotoxic injury and global ischemia in neonatal rat brain. J Cereb Blood Flow Metab 19(3):341–349
8. Jensen JH, Falangola MF, Hu C et al (2011) Preliminary observations of increased diffusional kurtosis in human brain following recent cerebral infarction. NMR Biomed 24(5):452–457

9. Baron CA, Kate M, Gioia L et al (2015) Reduction of diffusion-weighted imaging contrast of acute ischemic stroke at short diffusion times. Stroke 46(8):2136–2141

10. Taoka T, Iwasaki S, Sakamoto M et al (2006) Diffusion anisotropy and diffusivity of white matter tracts within the temporal stem in Alzheimer disease: evaluation of the "tract of interest" by diffusion tensor tractography. AJNR Am J Neuroradiol 27(5):1040–1045

11. Melhem ER, Mori S, Mukundan G, Kraut MA, Pomper MG, van Zijl PC (2002) Diffusion tensor MR imaging of the brain and white matter tractography. AJR Am J Roentgenol 178(1):3–16

12. Ito R, Mori S, Melhem ER (2002) Diffusion tensor brain imaging and tractography. Neuroimaging Clin N Am 12(1):1–19

13. Taoka T, Hirabayashi H, Nakagawa H et al (2006) Displacement of the facial nerve course by vestibular schwannoma: preoperative visualization using diffusion tensor tractography. J Magn Reson Imaging 24(5):1005–1010

14. Habas C, Cabanis EA (2007) Anatomical parcellation of the brainstem and cerebellar white matter: a preliminary probabilistic tractography study at 3 T. Neuroradiology 49(10):849–863

15. Wedeen VJ, Wang RP, Schmahmann JD et al (2008) Diffusion spectrum magnetic resonance imaging (DSI) tractography of crossing fibers. NeuroImage 41(4):1267–1277

16. Reese TG, Benner T, Wang R, Feinberg DA, Wedeen VJ (2009) Halving imaging time of whole brain diffusion spectrum imaging and diffusion tractography using simultaneous image refocusing in EPI. J Magn Reson Imaging 29(3):517–522

17. Jensen JH, Helpern JA, Ramani A, Lu H, Kaczynski K (2005) Diffusional kurtosis imaging: the quantification of non-Gaussian water diffusion by means of magnetic resonance imaging. Magn Reson Med 53(6):1432–1440

18. Hori M, Fukunaga I, Masutani Y et al (2012) Visualizing non-Gaussian diffusion: clinical application of q-space imaging and diffusional kurtosis imaging of the brain and spine. Magn Reson Med Sci 11(4):221–233

19. Hui ES, Cheung MM, Qi L, Wu EX (2008) Towards better MR characterization of neural tissues using directional diffusion kurtosis analysis. NeuroImage 42(1):122–134

20. Jensen JH, Helpern JA (2010) MRI quantification of non-Gaussian water diffusion by kurtosis analysis. NMR Biomed 23(7):698–710

21. Hui ES, Cheung MM, Qi L, Wu EX (2008) Advanced MR diffusion characterization of neural tissue using directional diffusion kurtosis analysis. Conf Proc IEEE Eng Med Biol Soc 2008:3941–3944

22. Kelm ND, West KL, Carson RP, Gochberg DF, Ess KC, Does MD (2016) Evaluation of diffusion kurtosis imaging in ex vivo hypomyelinated mouse brains. NeuroImage 124(Pt A):612–626

23. Taoka T, Fujioka M, Sakamoto M et al (2014) Time course of axial and radial diffusion kurtosis of white matter infarctions: period of pseudonormalization. AJNR Am J Neuroradiol 35(8):1509–1514

24. Yin J, Sun H, Wang Z, Ni H, Shen W, Sun PZ (2018) Diffusion kurtosis imaging of acute infarction: comparison with routine diffusion and follow-up MR imaging. Radiology 287(2):651–657

25. Cheung JS, Wang E, Lo EH, Sun PZ (2012) Stratification of heterogeneous diffusion MRI ischemic lesion with kurtosis imaging: evaluation of mean diffusion and kurtosis MRI mismatch in an animal model of transient focal ischemia. Stroke 43(8):2252–2254

26. Hui ES, Fieremans E, Jensen JH et al (2012) Stroke assessment with diffusional kurtosis imaging. Stroke 43(11):2968–2973

27. Taoka T, Fujioka M, Kashiwagi Y et al (2016) Time course of diffusion kurtosis in cerebral infarctions of transient middle cerebral artery occlusion rat model. J Stroke Cerebrovasc Dis 25(3):610–617

28. Raab P, Hattingen E, Franz K, Zanella FE, Lanfermann H (2010) Cerebral gliomas: diffusional kurtosis imaging analysis of microstructural differences. Radiology 254(3):876–881

29. Figini M, Riva M, Graham M et al (2018) Prediction of Isocitrate dehydrogenase genotype in brain Gliomas with MRI: single-Shell versus multishell diffusion models. Radiology 289(3):788–796

30. Hempel JM, Bisdas S, Schittenhelm J et al (2017) In vivo molecular profiling of human glioma using diffusion kurtosis imaging. J Neuro-Oncol 131(1):93–101

31. Tan Y, Wang XC, Zhang H et al (2015) Differentiation of high-grade-astrocytomas from solitary-brain-metastases: comparing diffusion kurtosis imaging and diffusion tensor imaging. Eur J Radiol 84(12):2618–2624

32. Pang H, Ren Y, Dang X et al (2016) Diffusional kurtosis imaging for differentiating between high-grade glioma and primary central nervous system lymphoma. J Magn Reson Imaging 44(1):30–40

33. Wu R, Suo ST, Wu LM, Yao QY, Gong HX, Xu JR (2017) Assessment of chemotherapy response in non-Hodgkin lymphoma involving the neck utilizing diffusion kurtosis imaging: a preliminary study. Diagn Interv Radiol 23(3):245–249

34. Yoshida M, Hori M, Yokoyama K et al (2013) Diffusional kurtosis imaging of normal-appearing white matter in multiple sclerosis: preliminary clinical experience. Jpn J Radiol 31(1):50–55

35. Takemura MY, Hori M, Yokoyama K et al (2017) Alterations of the optic pathway between unilateral and bilateral optic nerve damage in multiple sclerosis as revealed by the combined use of advanced diffusion kurtosis imaging and visual evoked potentials. Magn Reson Imaging 39:24–30

36. Spampinato MV, Kocher MR, Jensen JH, Helpern JA, Collins HR, Hatch NU (2017) Diffusional kurtosis imaging of the corticospinal tract in multiple sclero-

sis: association with neurologic disability. AJNR Am J Neuroradiol 38(8):1494–1500

37. Rose SE, Chen F, Chalk JB et al (2000) Loss of connectivity in Alzheimer's disease: an evaluation of white matter tract integrity with colour coded MR diffusion tensor imaging. J Neurol Neurosurg Psychiatry 69(4):528–530

38. Falangola MF, Jensen JH, Tabesh A et al (2013) Non-Gaussian diffusion MRI assessment of brain microstructure in mild cognitive impairment and Alzheimer's disease. Magn Reson Imaging 31(6):840–846

39. Gong NJ, Chan CC, Leung LM, Wong CS, Dibb R, Liu C (2017) Differential microstructural and morphological abnormalities in mild cognitive impairment and Alzheimer's disease: evidence from cortical and deep gray matter. Hum Brain Mapp 38(5):2495–2508

40. Qiu A, Mori S, Miller MI (2015) Diffusion tensor imaging for understanding brain development in early life. Annu Rev Psychol 66:853–876

41. Paydar A, Fieremans E, Nwankwo JI et al (2014) Diffusional kurtosis imaging of the developing brain. AJNR Am J Neuroradiol 35(4):808–814

42. Grinberg F, Maximov II, Farrher E et al (2017) Diffusion kurtosis metrics as biomarkers of microstructural development: a comparative study of a group of children and a group of adults. NeuroImage 144(Pt A):12–22

43. Zhang Y, Gao Y, Zhou M, Wu J, Zee C, Wang D (2016) A diffusional kurtosis imaging study of idiopathic generalized epilepsy with unilateral interictal epileptiform discharges in children. J Neuroradiol 43(5):339–345

44. Zheng W, Wu C, Huang L, Wu R (2017) Diffusion kurtosis imaging of microstructural alterations in the brains of paediatric patients with congenital Sensorineural hearing loss. Sci Rep 7(1):1543

45. Iliff JJ, Wang M, Liao Y et al (2012) A paravascular pathway facilitates CSF flow through the brain parenchyma and the clearance of interstitial solutes, including amyloid beta. Sci Transl Med 4(147):147ra111

46. Iliff JJ, Lee H, Yu M et al (2013) Brain-wide pathway for waste clearance captured by contrast-enhanced MRI. J Clin Invest 123(3):1299–1309

47. Johnston M, Zakharov A, Papaiconomou C, Salmasi G, Armstrong D (2004) Evidence of connections between cerebrospinal fluid and nasal lymphatic vessels in humans, non-human primates and other mammalian species. Cerebrospinal Fluid Res 1(1):2

48. Murtha LA, Yang Q, Parsons MW et al (2014) Cerebrospinal fluid is drained primarily via the spinal canal and olfactory route in young and aged spontaneously hypertensive rats. Fluids Barriers CNS 11:12

49. Mardor Y, Rahav O, Zauberman Y et al (2005) Convection-enhanced drug delivery: increased efficacy and magnetic resonance image monitoring. Cancer Res 65(15):6858–6863

50. Taoka T, Masutani Y, Kawai H et al (2017) Evaluation of glymphatic system activity with the diffusion MR technique: diffusion tensor image analysis along the perivascular space (DTI-ALPS) in Alzheimer's disease cases. Jpn J Radiol 35(4):172–178

51. Okudera T, Huang YP, Fukusumi A, Nakamura Y, Hatazawa J, Uemura K (1999) Micro-angiographical studies of the medullary venous system of the cerebral hemisphere. Neuropathology 19(1):93–111

52. Taoka T, Fukusumi A, Miyasaka T, Kawai H (2017) … Structure of the medullary veins of the cerebral hemisphere and related disorders. …

53. Steward C, Venkatraman V, Lui E, et al. (2019) Reproducibility of the diffusion of the perivascular space in older adults with dementia. 27th International Society for Magnetic Resonance in Medicine. Montreal, p 3425

54. Cekic M, Yokota H, Ellingson B, Linetsk M, Salamon N (2018) Evaluation of the Glymphatic System with DTI in Idiopathic Normal Pressure Hydrocephalus. American Society of Neuroradiology Annual Meeting. Vancouver, p O-518

55. Nedergaard M (2013) Neuroscience. Garbage truck of the brain. Science 340(6140):1529–1530

Intravoxel Incoherent Motion Imaging

5

Takashi Yoshiura

5.1 Intravoxel Incoherent Motion Concept

Intravoxel incoherent motion (IVIM) was first proposed by Le Bihan [1, 2] and refers to the microscopic incoherent motion of water molecules within each imaging voxel during the observation that reduces the magnitude of the MR signal through phase dispersion of spins induced by molecular displacement under a magnetic field gradient. This includes both true molecular diffusion due to random Brownian motion and the pseudo-diffusion resulting from water flow through randomly oriented capillary segments (Fig. 5.1).

In the conventional model of diffusion, MR signal intensity under diffusion-weighted imaging (DWI) is described using a simple mono-exponential equation:

$$Sb / S0 = \exp(-bD)$$

where S0 and Sb represent signal intensities with b values of 0 and b respectively, and D is the apparent diffusion coefficient (ADC). In the IVIM model, signal intensity is instead described using a bi-exponential equation (Fig. 5.2):

T. Yoshiura (✉)
Department of Radiology, Graduate School of Medical and Dental Sciences, Kagoshima University, Kagoshima, Japan
e-mail: yoshiura@m3.kufm.kagoshima-u.ac.jp

$$Sb / S0 = f \exp(-bD^*) + (1 - f) \exp(-bD)$$

where S0 and Sb are signal intensities with b values of 0 and b, respectively, f is the volume fraction of the perfusion component, D^* is the pseudo-diffusion coefficient, and D is the true diffusion coefficient. It should be noted that D^* is distinctly larger than D. As a result, the relative contribution of the perfusion component is greater at lower b values, but is negligible at higher b values (Fig. 5.2).

The relationships between perfusion-related IVIM parameters and classical perfusion parameters have been documented [3]. Perfusion fraction f is proportional to cerebral blood volume (CBV), while pseudo-diffusion coefficient D^* is inversely proportional to the mean transit time (MTT). The product of f and D^* is thus proportional to cerebral blood flow (CBF).

$$f = \frac{CBV}{f_w}$$

$$D^* = L \cdot \frac{1}{6MTT}$$

$$f \cdot D^* = CBF \cdot L \cdot \frac{1}{6f_w}$$

where f_w is the fraction of MR visible water, L is the total capillary length, and l is the mean capillary segment length.

© Springer Nature Switzerland AG 2021
T. Moritani, A. A. Capizzano (eds.), *Diffusion-Weighted MR Imaging of the Brain, Head and Neck, and Spine*, https://doi.org/10.1007/978-3-030-62120-9_5

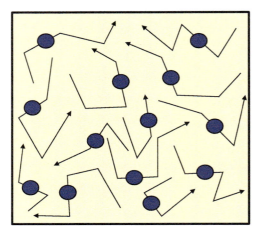
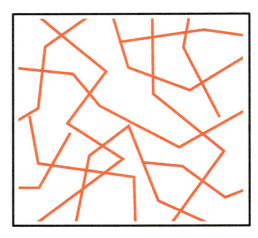

Fig. 5.1 Intravoxel incoherent motion (IVIM) refers to microscopic incoherent motion of water molecules within each imaging voxel that affects signal intensity on diffusion-weighted images. IVIM includes both true molecular diffusion due to random Brownian motion and pseudo-diffusion caused by capillary perfusion

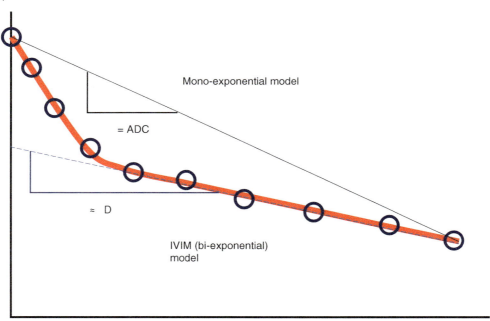

Fig. 5.2 Mono- and bi-exponential models of diffusion-weighted imaging. With the conventional mono-exponential diffusion model, the apparent diffusion coefficient (ADC) is calculated from signal intensities at two b values. In IVIM imaging, signal intensities at multiple b values are fitted to a bi-exponential function including both perfusion and true diffusion components. A steeper slope at low b values reflects the contribution of perfusion (D^*) in addition to the true diffusion (D). At higher b values, the contribution of perfusion components becomes negligible. Slope over high b values thus closely approximates the true diffusion coefficient D

5.2 IVIM Imaging

IVIM imaging provides a unique opportunity for the simultaneous evaluation of diffusion and capillary perfusion. IVIM does not require contrast administration for perfusion assessment. Moreover, IVIM perfusion assessment does not include tracer delivery, representing a potential advantage over tracer-based MR perfusion techniques such as the dynamic susceptibility contrast (DSC) technique and arterial spin labeling, as these techniques suffer from inherent issues of tracer bolus dispersion and elongated transit time. Furthermore, true diffusion coefficient D could offer a more accurate measure of tissue microstructure than conventional ADC because the contaminating effects of perfusion are eliminated.

IVIM parameters for each voxel can be obtained by fitting the bi-exponential model above to the measured signal intensities at a series of b values (Fig. 5.2). Accordingly, imaging is performed typically at 10–20 different b values ranging from 0 to 1000 s/mm^2. Figure 5.3 shows maps of IVIM-derived parameters (D, f, and D*) in a healthy sub-

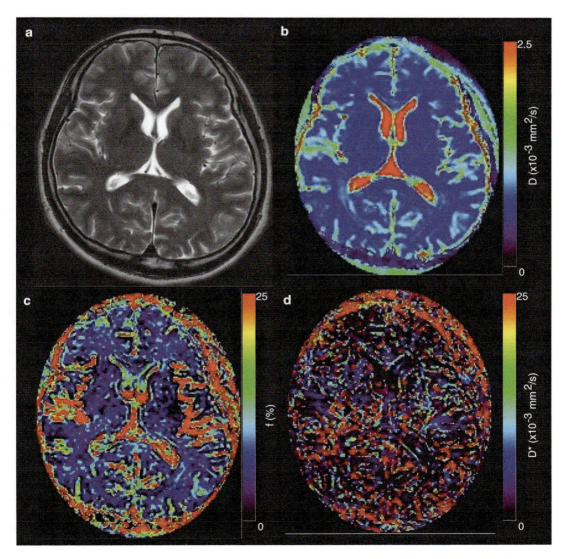

Fig. 5.3 (**a–d**) IVIM parametric brain maps of a healthy subject. T2-weighted image (**a**) and the corresponding maps of true diffusion coefficient D (**b**), perfusion fraction f (**c**), and pseudo-diffusion coefficient D* (**d**) are shown

ject. Notably, all other imaging parameters, i.e., echo time (TE) and diffusion time, should be kept constant while changing the b value. The optimal number and choice of b values for each organ have been subjects of debate, but no consensus has been reached for the brain. In most cases, motion probing gradients are applied in three orthogonal directions to obtain isotropic diffusion-weighted images at each b value.

IVIM imaging is most often based on single-shot echo planar (SSEP) DWI. SSEP-DWI is advantageous, with a short imaging time and high signal-to-noise ratio (SNR). However, SSEP-DWI suffers from image degradation due to magnetic field inhomogeneities, especially at the skull base and head and neck, limiting its utility in those areas. Several alternative approaches have been proposed to mitigate this issue. For example, non-EP-DWI methods such as shingle-shot turbo spin-echo DWI have been used for IVIM imaging [4, 5] (Fig. 5.4). Multi-shot EP-DWI could be alternative solution [6]. The

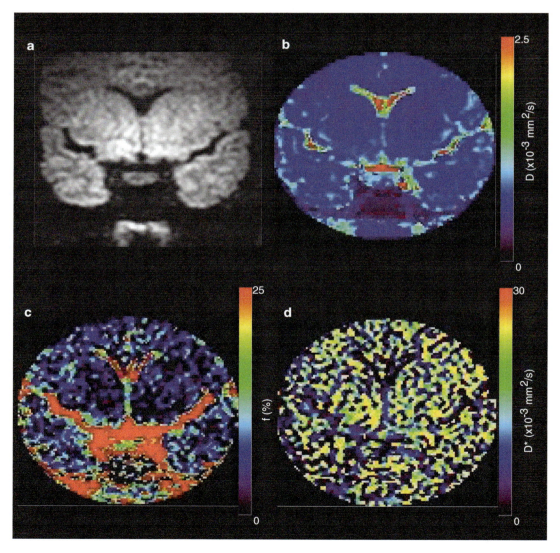

Fig. 5.4 (**a–d**) IVIM imaging based on single-shot turbo spin-echo acquisition. Isotropic diffusion-weighted image (b = 1000 s/mm^2) (**a**) and maps of D (**b**), f (**c**), and D* (**d**). Note the skull base structures including the pituitary gland are clearly visualized without distortion

5.3 Methods of IVIM Analysis

To obtain IVIM parameters for each voxel, signal intensities at different b values are fitted to the bi-exponential model above. A few different calculation methods have been proposed. The most straightforward method is fitting using all three parameters (f, D, and D^*) as variables. This method can, however, become unstable and is prone to fall into a local solution. The second method is a two-step approach in which D is first obtained by mono-exponential fitting using only data at higher b values (typically >200 s/mm^2); then f and D^* are obtained by fitting using all b values [7]. This method is popular because of its robustness. Finally, a third method uses only S0 and high-b-value data to obtain D and f. D^* is then calculated by bi-exponential fitting [8]. With this method, D and f could potentially be obtained without using low-b-value data, which may be susceptible to noise. One should be aware that these calculation methods can critically affect the estimates of IVIM parameters.

5.4 Neuroimaging Applications of IVIM Imaging

Despite the fact that IVIM was originally developed for the brain, neuroimaging applications have not been prevalent until recently.

5.4.1 Physiological Applications

As mentioned earlier, IVIM perfusion parameters (f and D^*) are closely related to classical perfusion parameters including CBV, CBF, and MTT. IVIM imaging allows noninvasive monitoring of physiological vascular responses to neuronal activation and CO_2 challenge. Federau et al. [9] demonstrated increases in f, D^* and f·D^* with increasing CO_2 concentrations during inhalation of carbogen (a mixture of O_2 and CO_2). Moreover, the same group reported increases in f, D^* and f·D^* during visual stimulation [10], suggesting the utility of IVIM imaging as a functional brain imaging tool.

5.4.2 IVIM Imaging of Brain Tumors

Diffusion and perfusion MR imaging have been widely used to characterize brain tumors. The ADC derived from DWI is considered to reflect tumor cell density and has been recognized as a useful imaging marker of proliferation. Angiogenesis is another important feature of a tumor. The tumor blood volume derived from perfusion MR imaging represents a marker for tumor vascularization. IVIM imaging has potential to evaluate these two key aspects of a tumor simultaneously without the need for a contrast agent.

DSC perfusion imaging is the current gold-standard imaging technique for evaluating tumor vascularity. IVIM perfusion fraction f has been directly compared to the tumor blood volume derived from DSC perfusion imaging in several types of tumors, demonstrating their close correlation [11]. Moreover, histopathological investigations have shown close agreement between perfusion fraction f and microvessel density in brain tumors [12].

5.4.3 IVIM Imaging of Gliomas

A few studies have reported the utility of IVIM in preoperative grading of diffuse gliomas. The most reproducible finding among these studies was an increased perfusion fraction (f) in high-grade gliomas (HGGs) compared to low-grade gliomas (LGGs) [13–15], which was attributable to the higher vascularity and tumor blood volume in HGGs. D was lower in HGGs than in LGGs, consistent with previous reports of ADC. As for another perfusion-related parameter, D^*, previous IVIM studies have shown inconsistent results [13–15]. In the majority of previous IVIM studies, D^* has been reported as a less reproducible index than D or f. Figures 5.5 and 5.6 show IVIM parametric maps of LGG and HGG.

IVIM has been reported to be useful in differentiating posttreatment effect and recurrence in glioma, as phenomena that are often difficult to distinguish by conventional imaging. Kim et al. [16] analyzed IVIM images of patients with glioma treated with concurrent chemoradiation after surgery. They found that perfusion fraction f was significantly higher in recurrence than in posttreatment effect, as was the CBV derived from DSC perfusion imaging. Furthermore, recent papers have shown that pretreatment IVIM perfusion parameters were predictive of survival in patients with glioma [17, 18].

5.4.4 Other Brain Tumors

Primary central nervous system lymphoma (PCNSL) is sometimes hard to distinguish from glioblastoma under conventional MR imaging, although the treatment strategies show critical differences. PCNSL has previously been charac-

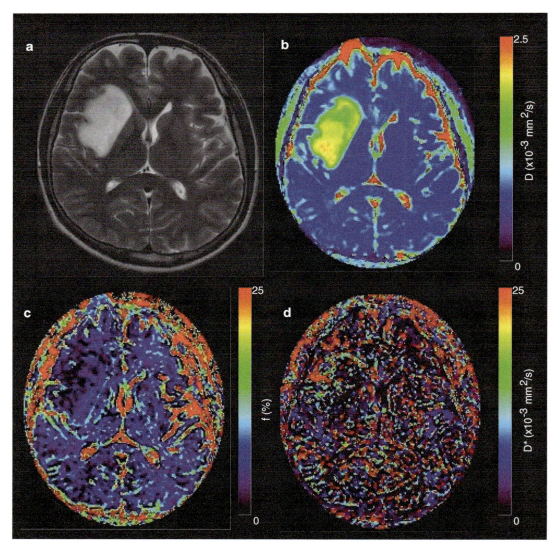

Fig. 5.5 (**a–d**) A male patient with diffuse astrocytoma (Grade II). The T2-weighted image (**a**) shows a homogeneously hyperintense mass in the right insula. IVIM imaging shows increased D (**b**) and decreased f (**c**), reflecting low cellularity and vascularity. The D* map (**d**) shows no specific findings

5 Intravoxel Incoherent Motion Imaging

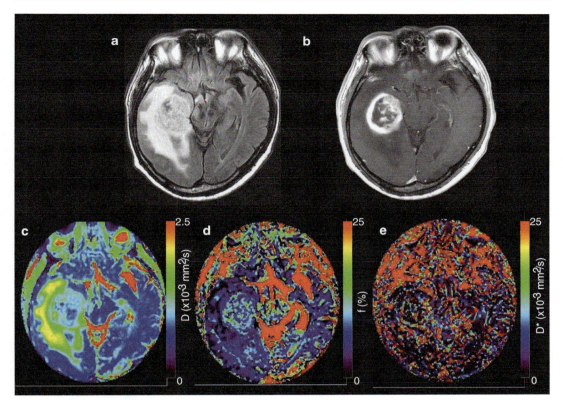

Fig. 5.6 (**a–d**) A male patient with glioblastoma (Grade IV). FLAIR image (**a**) shows an ill-defined mass in the right temporal lobe with extensive surrounding edema. A post-contrast T1-weighted image (**b**) shows heterogeneous enhancement in the mass. IVIM imaging shows heterogeneously lower D in the tumor (**c**), as compared with that in the diffuse astrocytoma in Fig. 5.5b. The tumor shows increased f, indicating hypervascularity (**d**). Focal areas of increased D^* are shown (**e**)

terized by lower DSC tumor blood volume compared to glioblastoma. Consistent with those results, some studies have shown that perfusion fraction f is useful in discriminating between the two tumors [19, 20].

As in the case of glioma, differentiation between treatment effect and tumor recurrence is often problematic in metastatic brain tumors treated with gamma knife radiosurgery. A previous study showed that the 90th percentiles of f and D^* histograms offered useful imaging markers for their discrimination [21].

5.4.5 Stroke and Brain Ischemia

Studies have shown the feasibility of IVIM assessment for acute brain infarction, where along with D, perfusion fraction f was signifi-cantly decreased in the infarcted area defined by reduced ADC compared to the contralateral normal brain parenchyma [22, 23]. Nevertheless, any additive clinical value of IVIM imaging in the management of acute stroke has not yet been elucidated.

A recent study showed that a decrease in the whole-brain perfusion fraction (f) and $f \cdot D^*$ was predictive for the development of delayed cerebral ischemia due to vasospasm in patients with ruptured cerebral aneurysm [24].

5.4.6 Head and Neck Lesions

IVIM has been used to characterize head and neck lesions. Sumi et al. [25] analyzed salivary gland tumors and reported that the combination of D and D^* allowed accurate discrimination among pleomorphic adenoma, malignant tumors, and Warthin tumor. That is, pleomorphic adenoma was characterized by high D and low D*, whereas malignant tumors showed intermediate D and D*, and Warthin tumor tended to have low D and high D*. The same authors have shown that the combination of D and the perfusion parameter (essentially f) helped characterize head and neck tumors including malignant lymphoma, squamous cell carcinoma (SCC) and schwannoma, as well as salivary gland tumors [26]. Fujima et al. [27] used IVIM along with diffusion kurtosis imaging (DKI) to predict outcomes after chemoradiation therapy in patients with nasal or sinonasal SCC. They reported that the 25th percentile of D was particularly useful in predicting local control.

5.5 Pitfalls and Technical Limitations

The most notorious technical issue in IVIM imaging is the high susceptibility to noise. A computer simulation in which SNR was controlled by adding Rician noise showed that low SNR seriously limited the accuracy and precision of the perfusion parameters (D* and f), particularly D*, while D was distinctly robust to the noise [28]. That report tells us that imaging with sufficient SNR is essential to obtain meaningful results. The effects of the cardiac and respiratory cycles on IVIM parametric measurement remain under investigation. Some evidence suggests that controlling those effects by gating will improve the reproducibility of IVIM measurement [29].

As shown above, the IVIM model is very simple and contains only three variables (D, D*, and f). This ignores differences in properties other than diffusivity of the perfusion and diffusion components such as longitudinal and transverse relaxivities. However, in reality, the two components can differ in terms of those properties. Estimated f and D* can therefore be influenced by the settings of TE. A previous IVIM study on normal prostate showed that f was strongly affected by the choice of TE in the central zone where T2 (of the diffusion component) is much

shorter than that of blood (i.e., the perfusion component), but not in the peripheral zone whose T2 is closer to blood T2 [30]. The TE dependence of f has also been reported for other organs, such as the pancreas [31]. Such effects should be considered when IVIM parameters of two tissues with very different T2s are compared, or when IVIM parameters obtained under different imaging conditions are compared.

The cerebrospinal fluid (CSF) is another factor that is not assumed in the bi-exponential model. This issue is most problematic in the cerebral cortex, where a substantial fraction of voxels is contaminated with CSF, especially when thick slices are used. In addition, even the deep brain parenchyma contains CSF that is characterized by free isotropic diffusion in locations such as perilesional edema and the perivascular space. The presence of CSF can lead to inaccurate estimation of the IVIM perfusion parameters. Attempts have been made to correct this CSF effect [32, 33].

References

1. Le Bihan D, Breton E, Lallemand D, Greiner P, Cabanis E, Laval-Jeantet M (1986) MR imaging of intravoxel incoherent motions: application to diffusion and perfusion in neurologic disorders. Radiology 161:401–407
2. Le Bihan D, Breton E, Lallemand D, Aubin ML, Vignaud J, Laval-Jeantet M (1988) Separation of diffusion and perfusion in intravoxel incoherent motion MR imaging. Radiology 168:497–505
3. Le Bihan TR (1992) The capillary network. A link between IVIM and classical perfusion. Magn Reason Med 27:171–178
4. Sakamoto J, Imaizumi A, Sasaki Y, Kamio T, Wakoh M, Oyani-Yamamoto M et al (2014) Comparison of accuracy of intravoxel incoherent motion and apparent diffusion coefficient techniques for predicting malignancy of head and neck tumors using half-Fourier single-shot turbo spin-echo diffusion-weighted imaging. Magn Reason Imaging 32:860–866
5. Kamimura K, Nakajo M, Fukukura Y, Iwanaga T, Saito T, Sasaki M et al (2016) Intravoxel incoherent motion in normal pituitary gland: initial study with turbo spin-echo diffusion-weighted imaging. AJNR Am J Neuroradiol 37:2328–2333
6. Lasbleiz J, Le Ster C, Guillin R, Saint-Jalmes H, Gamborota G (2018) Measurement of diffusion and perfusion in vertebral bone marrow using intravoxel

incoherent motion (IVIM) with multishot, readout-segmented (RESOLVE) echo-planar imaging. J Magn Reason Imaging. https://doi.org/10.1002/jmri.26270

7. Lucuani A, Vignaud A, Cavet M, Van Nhieu JT, Mallat A, Ruel L et al (2008) Liver cirrhosis: intravoxel incoherent motion MR imaging—pilot study. Radiology 249:891–899

8. Sigmund E, ViVier P-H, Sui D, Lamparello NA, Tantillo K, Mikheev A et al (2012) Intravoxel incoherent motion and diffusion-tensor imaging in renal tissue under hydration and furosemide flow challenges. Radiology 263:758–769

9. Federau C, Maeder P, O'Brien K, Browaeys P, Meuli R, Hagmann P (2012) Quantitative measurement of brain perfusion with intravoxel incoherent motion MR imaging. Radiology 265:874–881

10. Federau C, O'brien K, Birbaumer A, Meuli R, Hagmann P, Maeder P (2015) Functional mapping of the human visual cortex with intravoxel incoherent motion MRI. PLoS One. https://doi.org/10.1371/journal.pone.0117706

11. Federau C, O'Brien K, Meuli R, Hagmann P, Maeder P (2014) Measuring brain perfusion with intravoxel incoherent motion (IVIM): initial clinical experience. J Magn Reason Imaging 39:624–632

12. Togao O, Hiwatashi A, Yamashita K, Kikuchi K, Momosaka D, Yoshimoto K et al (2018) Measurement of the perfusion fraction in brain tumors with intravoxel incoherent motion MR imaging: validation with histopathological vascular density in meningiomas. Br J Radiol 91:20170912. https://doi.org/10.1259/bjr.20170912

13. Bisdas S, Koh TS, Order C, Braun C, Schottenhelm J, Ernemann U et al (2013) Intravoxel incoherent motion diffusion-weighted MR imaging of gliomas: feasibility of the method and initial results. Neuroradiology 55:1189–1196

14. Federau C, Meuli R, O'Brien K, Maeder P, Hagmann P (2014) Perfusion measurement in brain gliomas with intravoxel incoherent motion MRI. AJNR Am J Neuroradiol 35:256–262

15. Togao O, Hiwatashi A, Yamashita K, Kikuchi K, Mizoguchi M, Yoshimoto K et al (2016) Differentiation of high-grade and low-grade diffuse gliomas by intravoxel incoherent motion MR imaging. Neuro-Oncol 18:132–141

16. Kim HS, Suh CH, Kim N, Choi C-G, Kim SJ (2014) Histogram analysis of intravoxel incoherent motion for differentiating recurrent tumor from treatment effect in patients with glioblastoma: initial clinical experience. AJNR Am J Neuroradiol 35:490–497

17. Federau C, Cerny M, Roux M, Mosimann PJ, Maeder P, Meuli R et al (2017) IVIM perfusion fraction is prognostic for survival in brain glioma. Clin Neuroradiol 27:485–492

18. Puig J, Sanchez-Gonzalez J, Blasco G, Daunis-Estadella P, Federau C, Alberich-Bayarri A et al (2016) Intravoxel incoherent motion metrics as potential biomarkers for survival in glioblastoma. PLoS One 11:e0158887

19. Suh CH, Kim HS, Lee SS, Kim N, Yoon HM, Choi C-G et al (2014) Atypical imaging features of primary central nervous system lymphoma that mimics glioblastoma: utility of intravoxel incoherent motion MR imaging. Radiology 272:504–513

20. Yamashita K, Hiwatashi A, Togao O, Kikuchi K, Kitamura Y, Mizoguhi M et al (2016) Diagnostic utility of intravoxel incoherent motion MR imaging in differentiating primary central nervous system lymphoma from glioblastoma multiforme. J Magn Reason Imaging 44:1256–1261

21. Kim DY, Kim HS, Goh MJ, Choi CG, Kim SJ (2014) Utility of intravoxel incoherent motion MR imaging for distinguishing recurrent metastatic tumor from treatment effect following gamma knife radiosurgery: initial experience. AJNR Am J Neuroradiol 35:2082–2090

22. Federau C, Sumer S, Becce F, Maeder P, O'Brien K, Meuli R, Wintermark M (2014) Intravoxel incoherent motion perfusion imaging in acute stroke: initial clinical experience. Neuroradiology 56:629–635

23. Suo S, Cao M, Zhu W, Li L, Li J, Shen F et al (2016) Stroke assessment with intravoxel incoherent motion diffusion-weighted MRI. NMR Biomed 29:320–328

24. Heit J, Wintermark M, Martin BW, Zhu G, Marks MP, Zaharchuk G et al (2018) Reduced intravoxel incoherent motion microvascular perfusion predicts delayed cerebral ischemia and vasospasm after aneurysm rupture. Stroke 49:741–745. https://doi.org/10.1161/STROKEAHA.117.020395

25. Sumi M, Van Cauteren M, Sumi T, Obara M, Ichikawa Y, Nakamura T (2012) Salivary gland tumors: use of intravoxel incoherent motion MR imaging for assessment of diffusion and perfusion for the differentiation of benign from malignant tumors. Radiology 263:770–777

26. Sumi M, Nakamra T (2013) Head and neck tumors: assessment of perfusion-related parameters and diffusion coefficients based on the intravoxel incoherent motion model. AJNR Am J Neuroradiol 34:410–416

27. Fujima N, Yoshida D, Sakashita T, Homma A, Tsukahara A, Shimizu Y et al (2017) Prediction of the treatment outcome using intravoxel incoherent motion and diffusional kurtosis imaging in nasal or sinonasal squamous cell carcinoma patients. Eur Radiol 27:956–965

28. Wu W-C, Chen Y-F, Tseng H-M, Yang S-C, My P-C (2015) Caveats of measuring perfusion indexes using intravoxel incoherent motion magnetic resonance imaging in the human brain. Eur Radiol 25:2485–2492

29. Kang KM, Choi SH, Kim DE, Yun TJ, Kim J-H, Sohn C-H et al (2017) Application of cardiac gating to improve the reproducibility of intravoxel incoherent motion measurements in the head and neck. Magn Reson Med Sci 16:190–202

30. Feng Z, Min X, Wang L, Yan L, Li B, Ke Z et al (2018) Effects of echo time on IVIM quantification of the normal prostate. Sci Rep 8. https://doi.org/10.1038/s41598-018-19150-2

31. Lemke A, Laun FB, Simon D, Stieltjes B, Schad LR (2010) An in vivo verification of the intravoxel incoherent motion effect in diffusion-weighted imaging of the abdomen. Magn Reason Med 64:1580–1585
32. Federau C, O'Brien K (2015) Increased brain perfusion contrast with T2-prepared intravoxel incoherent motion (T2prep IVIM) MRI. NMR Biomed 28:9–16
33. Bisdas S, Klose U (2015) IVIM analysis of brain tumors: an investigation of the relaxation effects of CSF, blood, and tumor tissue on the estimated perfusion fraction. Magn Reason Mater Phys 28:377–383

Functional MRI and Diffusion Tensor Imaging

6

Gaurang Shah

6.1 Introduction

Magnetic resonance imaging (MRI) is more sensitive than computed tomography (CT) in detecting structural and functional abnormalities of the brain, providing superior structural resolution and tissue contrast. Modalities like positron emission tomography (PET), single-photon emission tomography (SPECT), magnetoencephalography (MEG), and functional magnetic resonance imaging (fMRI) inform us about functional aspect of the brain related to brain metabolism, receptor binding, cerebral blood flow, certain pathological molecular accumulations, and certain molecular changes. Diffusion tensor imaging (DTI) is an MRI method to delineate axonal tracts, utilizing a particular type of diffusion-weighted sequence that measures microstructural water diffusion properties within the brain.

6.2 Functional MRI

Functional magnetic resonance imaging (fMRI) implies any MRI technique that can measure local physiology of the brain and spine. However,

in a more specific sense, the term functional magnetic resonance imaging (fMRI) refers to the techniques that employ the blood Oxygenation Level Dependent (BOLD) MRI technique that was first observed by Ogawa et al. in 1990 to image rat brain [1, 2], which made MR signal to be more sensitive to local changes in the oxygenation of blood. They observed that a mouse brain image was uniform and exhibited less susceptibility when breathing 100% oxygen, as opposed to heterogeneous and with areas of parenchymal and vessel susceptibility when they breathed air with only 20% oxygen.

The human brain accounts for about 2% of the total body weight, but receives about 15% of the total cardiac output, with cerebral blood flow (CBF) of about 700 ml per minute. A neural activity of brain would require still increased amount of energy, namely glucose and oxygen. The increased metabolic requirement of the brain is generated by an array of complex tasks that the brain cells perform. Apart from basic cellular processes like chemical synthesis and chemical transport, the brain cells also perform neural signaling that requires generation of electrical activity with generation of action potential and release of neurotransmitters at synapses. Since the brain has no reserve store of oxygen or glucose, the increased neural activity results in almost instantly increased cerebral blood flow (CBF) and also increased cerebral blood volume (CBV).

G. Shah (✉)
Department of Radiology, University of Michigan, Ann Arbor, MI, USA
e-mail: gvshah@med.umich.edu

© Springer Nature Switzerland AG 2021
T. Moritani, A. A. Capizzano (eds.), *Diffusion-Weighted MR Imaging of the Brain, Head and Neck, and Spine*, https://doi.org/10.1007/978-3-030-62120-9_6

6.3 HRF and BOLD Imaging

A localized brain activity consumes increased oxygen that initially results in increased amount of deoxyhemoglobin and less availability of oxyhemoglobin. A neurovascular coupling occurs due to feedforward neural signaling to blood vessels through astrocytic activity. This activates a hemodynamic response function (HRF) within the brain; as a result, the capillaries and arterioles dilate (Fig. 6.1), resulting in increased CBF to supply more of oxygenated hemoglobin that results in increased local CBV containing increased amount of oxyhemoglobin than the resting stage, which overshoots the oxygen demand [3]. The increased CBF may be in part due to increased metabolic activities, but may also be due to increased secretion of glutamate neurotransmitter [4]. Oxyhemoglobin is diamagnetic, while deoxyhemoglobin is paramagnetic. This, in turn, the latter alters the local magnetic field. Initially, due to increased accumulation of deoxyhemoglobin, there is increased inhomogeneity (see initial deep in Fig. 6.2). However, due to HRF, there is increased amount of oxyhemoglobin within the activated brain parenchyma, resulting in diminished inhomogeneity [5].

These alterations in local magnetic field are best investigated by a gradient-echo pulse sequence, namely T2* weighted sequence that uses a single RF pulse with a flip angle for excitation, uses gradient pulse for refocusing the spin phase, and generates an echo. T2* at rest is a function of inherent T2 value of the tissue and local magnetic field. Local field inhomogeneity can be introduced by metal, blood products, air and also by altered composition of local blood volume. In activated state of the brain, T2* also reflects the inhomogeneity in local magnetic field introduced by increasing CBV that reflects increased amount

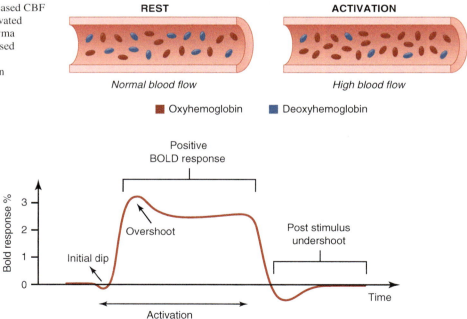

Fig. 6.1 Increased CBF within the activated brain parenchyma exhibits increased amount of oxyhemoglobin

Fig. 6.2 Hemodynamic response function (HRF). On functional activation, there is initial increase in local deoxyhemoglobin within the activated brain resulting in initial negative BOLD response. Feedforward neural signal involving blood vessels results in activation of hemodynamic response function, resulting in increased CBF, leading to increased amount of oxyhemoglobin that initially overshoots the tissue oxygen requirement. The BOLD response plummets on stopping the stimulus and results in momentary post-stimulus undershoot, before it normalizes

of oxyhemoglobin. A T2* signal is higher in intensity for diamagnetic tissues and lower for paramagnetic tissues. Hence, increased neuronal activities increases blood flow to the brain due to HRF and alters the local magnetic field inhomogeneity. This phenomenon is captured on MRI by T2* sequence and BOLD imaging, yielding valuable mapping of activated areas of the brain [6].

6.4 Regional Organization of Brain Systems

The anatomic organization of the brain in bilateral cerebral hemispheres, cerebellum, brainstem, central gray matter and white matter tracts belies an array of complex functional systems and subsystems that are distributed throughout the brain. All these areas are connected to each other structurally by white matter tracts and functionally by simultaneous and temporal activities. A deeper understanding and mapping of the location of the anatomic and structural distribution of these functional systems can be elicited by functional MRI [7].

6.4.1 Primary Sensorimotor Cortex

The primary motor cortex (PMC, M1, area 4) is situated within the precentral gyrus, in front of the central sulcus that separates the frontal lobe from the parietal lobe (Fig. 6.3). The precentral gyrus is the most posterior part of the frontal lobe and is the seat of motor movement function. The center of sensory reception is the postcentral gyrus, the very anterior part of the parietal lobe. The executive motor function of different body parts is located on PMC from superior medial to inferior lateral direction. The foot of the motor homunculus is located at the superior and medial most part of precentral sulcus, just over the interhemispheric fissure. The most characteristic representation of hand motor function is within the reverse omega-shaped region (Fig. 6.4) along the superior lateral part of precentral sulcus [8]. The inferior aspect of the central sulcus moves anteriorly as it courses inferiorly. The face and tongue

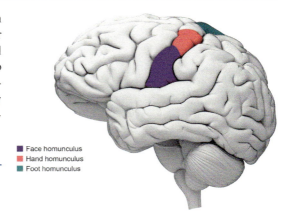

Fig. 6.3 Primary motor cortex (PMC). Precentral gyrus is the posterior most gyrus of the frontal lobe, situated anterior to the central sulcus. Executive function of motor activity is distributed throughout its course from superomedial to anteroinferior

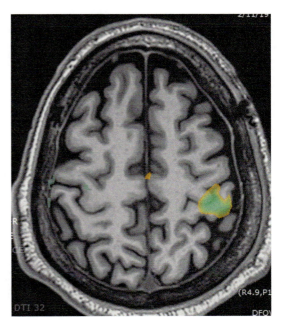

Fig. 6.4 Hand homunculus. (**a**) A reverse omega-shaped region along the superior and lateral part of the precentral sulcus represents executive hand motor function; (**b**) on the right finger tapping task, there is activation of the reverse omega-shaped region in the left precentral sulcus as well as adjoining, corresponding sensory cortex situated along the postcentral gyrus

of the motor homunculus is located along the lateral and inferior part of the PMC. This region is closely posterior to the Broca's area within the inferior frontal gyrus and separated by the Sylvain fissure from the superior temporal gyrus. Premotor cortex area (PMA, area 6) lies anterior to M1 with similar connections as PMC. It is primarily responsible for initiation and planning of motor movements. The primary sensory area along the postcentral gyrus is also organized from superior medial to inferior lateral just like the PMC. Together, these areas are referred to as primary sensory motor cortex [9].

fMRI is typically utilized to identify the 3 main motor areas of foot, hand, and face for neurosurgical motor mapping. A structural lesion can cause anatomic distortion of surface landmarks due to edema and mass effect, making identification of eloquent cortex difficult for the neurosurgeon. The very location of foot homunculus, in close association with superior sagittal sinus, makes its identification by direct intraoperative cortical stimulation very difficult.

6.4.2 Primary Language Areas

A complex network of frontal, parietal, and temporal regions make up the primary language areas. The receptive language area, also called Wernicke's area, is located along the posterior superior temporal gyrus, posterior superior temporal sulcus, and posterior middle temporal gyrus, also known as posterior Brodmann area 22 (Fig. 6.5). It is the primary location of receptive spoken and written language, speech perception, and phenological processing [10]. Additionally, the semantic meaning is also processed at angular gyrus and supramarginal gyrus [11].

The posterior inferior frontal gyrus, also known as pars orbitalis, adjacent pars opercularis, and pars triangularis is denoted as Brodmann areas 44 and 45. They make up the expressive language center generating words and spoken language and are knows as Broca's area (Fig. 6.6).

The lateral premotor cortex extends posterior and superior from Broca's area, anterior to the precentral gyrus, and is the primary location for written language [12]. Processing of complex semantic language and abstract ideas during language is located in the middle frontal gyrus, within dorsolateral prefrontal cortex, situated anterior and superior to Broca's area [13]. It is also known as Brodmann area 46.

Most of the population is left hemispheric dominant in language function. The total incidence of right-dominant or ambidextrous population is 5–6%. About 10% of left-handed population is right hemispheric dominant, while about 15%

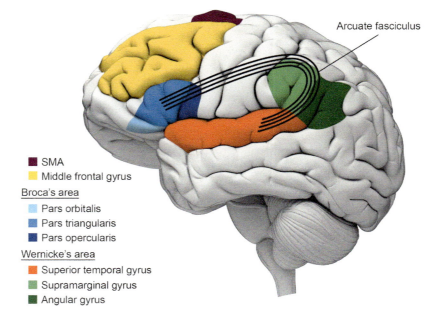

Fig. 6.5 Language areas. Wernicke's area represents comprehensive language function. It is situated at the posterior part of the superior temporal gyrus. The angular gyrus and supramarginal gyrus also participate in the activity. It is connected to the Broca's expressive language area by a fiber track called arcuate fasciculus. Middle frontal gyrus and supplemental motor area for language are ancillary language areas

6 Functional MRI and Diffusion Tensor Imaging

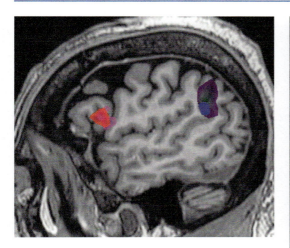

Fig. 6.6 Mapping language activation. Expressive language activation at Broca's area and comprehensive language activation seen at posterior part of superior temporal gyrus and angular gyrus

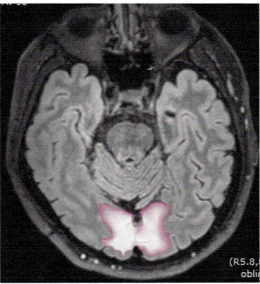

Fig. 6.7 Primary visual cortex. Bilateral medial and inferior occipital cortex along the calcarine sulcus receives, segments, and integrates visual information and sends it to other regions of the brain to analyze and utilize

of left-handed population has bilateral language representation [14, 15]. In 33% of patients with temporal lobe epilepsy, bilateral language distribution is seen. In case of slow growing neoplasm close to language areas, the phenomenon of crossed dominance is very common.

6.4.3 Primary Visual and Association Cortex

The primary visual cortex, area V1, lies along the calcarine fissure within the occipital lobes. The parieto-occipital sulcus forms its medial boundary, and the line connecting parieto-occipital sulcus and pre-occipital notch serves its lateral boundary, while the pre-occipital notch serves as its ventral margin. It comprises a part of lingual gyrus, cuneus, occipital pole, posterior part of fusiform gyrus, and superior, middle, and inferior occipital gyri. The primary visual cortex is responsible for the perception of margins, motion, and color.

Structurally it is connected to cingulum, temporal pole, lateral geniculate nucleus of thalamus, inferior frontal gyrus, orbito-frontal cortex, inferior and middle temporal gyrus, and parahippocampal gyrus. Functionally, it is connected to thalamus, fusiform gyrus, supplementary motor area (SMA), frontal eye fields, inferior frontal gyrus, and intraparietal sulcus. fMRI activation corresponds to a retinotopic distribution over the visual cortex (Fig. 6.7). fMRI mapping of eloquent visual cortex near a pathology is extremely useful for prognostication and risk assessment before a surgery or endovascular treatment [16].

6.4.4 Supplementary Motor Areas

The SMA is a secondary language area located in the superior frontal gyrus just medial to the superior frontal sulcus (Fig. 6.8). The anterior borders are ill-defined; however, the posterior border of the SMA is the foot motor region of the primary motor gyrus [17]. The anterior part of SMA is active on fMRI of language tasks. A more posterior portion is active during the fMRI of motor tasks [18–21].

The SMA is also organized along the anatomical regions, like in PMC. The three main motor areas of hand, foot, and face are sequentially mapped along the more posterior part of the SMA, called motor SMA [22, 23]. The SMA is broadly responsible for planning of motor activities and shows metabolic activity, which precedes activation of PMC [24, 25]. It is associated with voluntary movement, but also activates during passive tasks [26]. The SMA is associated with temporal planning and organization of motor movements before execution [25, 27]. SMA also plays a pivotal role in brain plasticity and cortical reorganizations, especially if the PMC is infiltrated by a tumor [28, 29]. Damage to SMA during brain tumor surgery increases the risk of patient morbidity and disability, which may or may not be transient [30–33].

6.5 Paradigms and Design

fMRI can be performed by either an event-related design or a block design [34]. In an event-related paradigm, discrete events of short duration are performed in varying orders with varying timings. An event-related paradigm can detect detailed transient changes in hemodynamic response, documenting temporal BOLD signal changes [35]. Now, a single event results in change in BOLD response by only 3–5% and hence has limited statistical power (Fig. 6.2). A patient task can be followed by rest, but the study requires multiple repetitions and increased study time to compensate for lower detection power and can lead to diminished patient compliance [36, 37].

In a block design, the same stimulus is presented sequentially, alternating with periods of rest [38]. Then the task-related acquisitions and resting-state acquisitions are averaged for signal, creating increased statistical power and significant activations. A typical boxcar design would have the patient performing the same task (e.g., finger tapping) for 10–15 seconds, followed by 10–15 seconds of lack of activity (Fig. 6.9). This cycle would be repeated 5–6 times and can last for 5 to 6 minutes [39, 40].

The brain mapping achieved by performance of fMRI depends on precise execution of different tasks to elicit a specific functional activation [38]. Most commonly utilized paradigms for

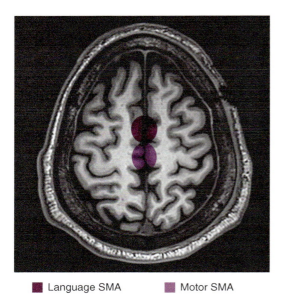

Fig. 6.8 Supplementary motor area (SMA). Posterior one third of superior frontal gyrus represents SMA. It is responsible for planning of complex movements. Language SMA is the anterior most part, just in front of the motor SMA, which is just anterior to activated feet homunculus

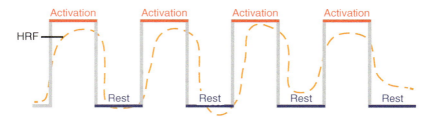

Fig. 6.9 Boxcar design of fMRI paradigm. The experimental "activation" stimuli for motor or language functions result in positive hemodynamic response function (HRF) with increased BOLD response at the corresponding area of the brain. Any areas that are used in a lower level "rest condition" are statistically subtracted out from the "activation condition"

mapping of the motor area are foot tapping or toe wriggle, finger tapping, lip smacking, or tongue motion.

Motor foot localization is achieved with repetitive flexion and extension of the toes, but without moving the ankles. Finger tapping paradigm is performed by the patients tapping their fingers while in the scanner (Fig. 6.10). It is important to avoid movement of the arms or shoulders. During the lip smacking paradigm, the patient is asked to purse the lips during the activation phase. In tongue motion paradigm, patients keep their teeth closed and rotate their tongue against the back of their teeth or along the palate.

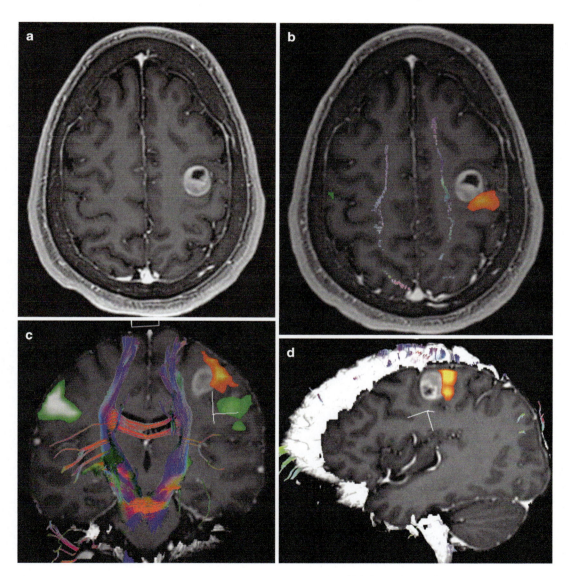

Fig. 6.10 CNS lymphoma infiltrating hand homunculus. (**a**) Intensely enhancing, well-defined mass at high convexity left frontal lobe also shows diffusion restriction and hypointense T2 signal; (**b**) right finger tapping paradigm results in activation of sensorimotor hand homunculus, which is partially infiltrated by the mass; (**c**) right finger tapping task activates hand homunculus of left PMC (*orange*), which is partially infiltrated by the mass. Lip smacking task activates bilateral face homunculus (*green*), situated at the lower part of bilateral PMC. The bilateral corticospinal tracts are unaffected; (**d**) 3-D sagittal orientation exhibits a more anterior, intensely enhancing focal mass, infiltrating the anterior part of activated hand homunculus of left sensory motor cortex

Close to 95% of right-handed people show left-sided hemispheric localization, while 6–15% of left-handed people show right-sided localization [41]. However, an atypical language lateralization is possible in patients with lesions in the left cerebral hemisphere [42–44]. The presence of brain tumor is also known to alter language lateralization [45]. Patients with intractable seizures have demonstrated reorganization of language circuits [46, 47].

The Wada test is an invasive endovascular method that is considered the gold standard for language localization [48, 49]. It also requires many human and material resources and is expensive to perform. Investigating laterality of language function with fMRI is noninvasive, relatively quick, and utilizes far less resources (Fig. 6.11). It has become very popular and is the mainstay of presurgical functional mapping of brain. For fMRI mapping of language laterality, at least 2–3 language tasks are performed. Silent word generation, verb generation, sentence completion, and picture naming are some of the language paradigms that are eminently suitable to boxcar design [50]. Performance of language fMRI tasks with boxcar design is found to have a high degree of congruence with Wada test to determine language laterality [51–53].

6.6 Functional Mapping in Brain Tumor Surgery

It is well known that infiltrating primary malignant brain tumor like glioma extend much beyond what is detected by structural brain MRI [54]. Surgical resection of brain tumor beyond the margins perceived on FLAIR, T2-weighted, or post-contrast brain MRI delays the malignant transformation of lower grade tumor and improves the true extent of tumor resection [55]. The primary goal of brain surgery for malignant masses is to maximize the extent of resection and minimize morbidity, since surgery-induced neu-

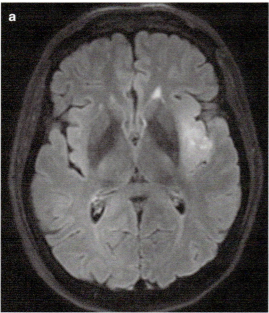
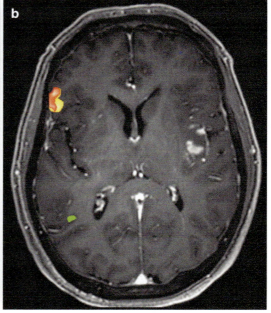

Fig. 6.11 Language laterality in the left-handed man with left insular GBM. (**a**) An infiltrating hyperintense FLAIR signal mass at left insular and subinsular region; (**b**) significant activation at the expected location of right-sided Broca's area on silent word generation and verb generation tasks without evidence for secondary activation on the left side, which may or may not be due to uncoupling of hemodynamic response function due to adjacent left insular mass

rological deficits result in lower quality of life and shortened survival [56]. fMRI allows identification of eloquent cortex to prevent damage during surgical removal [40] (Fig. 6.12). Better extent of tumor resection results in better patient outcome for both the low- and high-grade glioma [57–60]. Presurgical sensory motor mapping by fMRI accurately identifies the location of sensory and motor cortex [61]. This is especially useful when the normal sulcal and gyral pattern is distorted due to mass effect and brain edema and normal anatomic landmarks are not identified [62] (Fig. 6.13). Presurgical brain mapping with fMRI data allows for gross total resection of

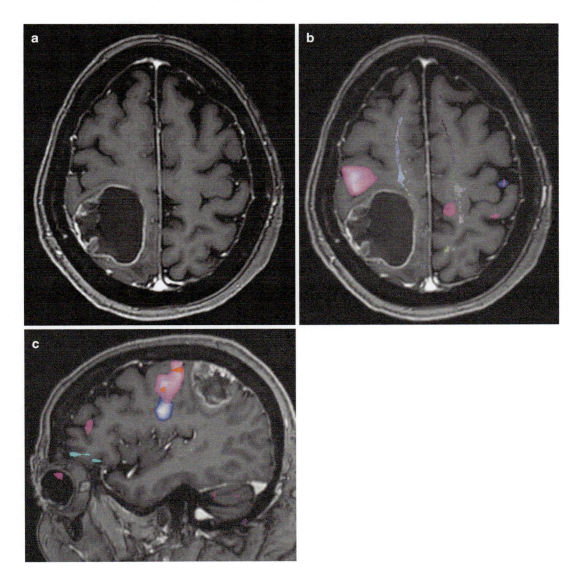

Fig. 6.12 Mapping of right PMC in a patient with right high convexity frontoparietal, peripherally enhancing malignant glioma. (**a**) A peripherally enhancing, hypointense T1 signal mass at high convexity right frontoparietal region with anatomic distortion and indistinct right central sulcus; (**b**, **c**) Left finger tapping (*pink*) and lip smacking (*blue*) tasks exhibit anterior displacement of right primary motor cortex with activated right hand homunculus and face homunculus (*blue*) seen anterior and inferior to the heterogeneous, ring-enhancing right frontoparietal mass

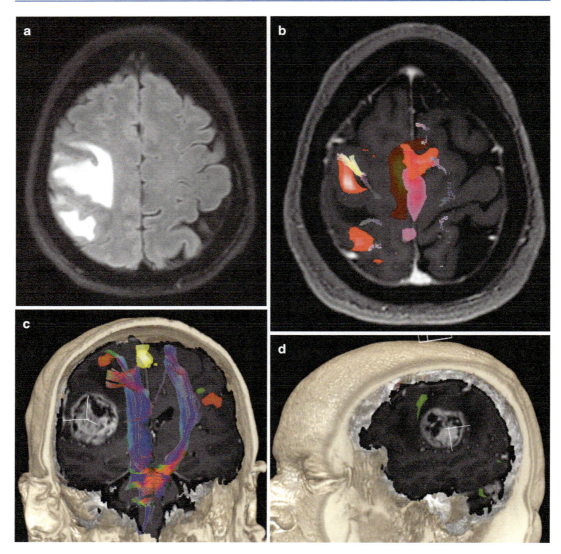

Fig. 6.13 Right frontal opercular GBM with large perilesional edema infiltrating primary motor cortex. (**a**) FLAIR-weighted axial imaging shows a large amount of edema blurring the normal sulcal and gyral landmarks; (**b**) the perilesional edema cleaves the right sensory motor cortex. The right corticospinal tracts terminates at hand motor area, which is displaced anteriorly. Motor SMA is seen in the midline; (**c**) 3-D coronal image shows intact but medially deviated right corticospinal tract, terminating at the homunculus; (**d**) 3-D sagittal imaging shows presence of hand homunculus anterior to the opercular tumor

brain tumors without postsurgical deficits [63]. Presurgical sensory motor fMRI is also known to change treatment options, allowing surgeons to operate on tumors previously deemed unresectable [64] and increasing confidence levels in further treatment planning. fMRI also helps avoid further studies including Wada imaging [51] and minimizes resources [49]. It also alters surgical planning and intraoperative brain cortical mapping strategies [51]. There is a high congruence in results of intraoperative cortical mapping and fMRI, which is also available in patients who are not amenable to the intraoperative procedure [65]. fMRI can also predict outcome of language functionality following epilepsy surgery. Presurgical contralateral language recruitment is

6.7 Pearls and Pitfalls of Interpretation

Some of the artifacts specific to fMRI include motion-related artifacts, susceptibility artifacts, and perfusion-related BOLD signal modulation [67]. The motion-related artifacts can appear as a halo around the brain due to nodding movement of the head while performing a motor paradigm, or may be due to linear motion of the head. Most statistical analysis software can correct some of the motion-related artifacts, although the nodding artifacts are difficult to remove. Previous surgery with possible metallic staples, titanium plates, or even suture material with trace metal can give rise to enhanced susceptibility on source T2* images. Dental work or air interface at skull base or hyperpneumatized sinuses can also result in significant distortion and lack of registration of BOLD activation [26]. Residual blood products in surgical cavity or underneath the craniotomy site can also cause significant diminution in BOLD signal or blooming susceptibility artifact. BOLD imaging coregistered with anatomic sequences can sometimes give rise to false negative interpretation.

Malignant brain tumors are associated with neovascularity with dilation of blood vessels supplying the tumor that results in increased perfusion parameters with elevated CBV and CBF. Conversely, an avidly enhancing mass-like lesion on follow-up study may represent a recurrent mass, in which case, it will exhibit increased perfusion parameters, or pseudo-progression, in which case the perfusion image may show hypo or normal perfusion (Fig. 6.14). In a high-grade malignant brain tumor, there is loss of autoregulation of blood vessels, with lack of the expected increased vascularity on performing functional paradigm, diminishing the BOLD effect [68]. This false negative phenomenon is known as uncoupling of HRF (Fig. 6.15). It can also be seen on restoration of normal perfusion in brain surrounding the tumor once it is surgically resected [69]. When a mass infiltrates PMC, the false negative BOLD signal on motor paradigm is associated with ipsilateral motor weakness and paresis [70]. By the same token, the BOLD signal is larger in low-grade gliomas and smaller in high-grade gliomas, which are associated with neovascularity and hyperperfusion [71]. The false negative BOLD signal is inversely proportionate to the distance between the eloquent cortex and the tumor and is reported to normalize at the distance of 3.1 cm [72].

6.8 Diffusion Tensor Imaging

The functional connectivity of different parts of the brain is measured by BOLD fMRI during task performance or even in resting state [73]. However, the structural connectivity of brain by white matter tracts can be best studied by diffusion tensor imaging (DTI) [74].

The principle of anisotropic diffusion is employed to generate white matter fiber tract trajectories in the brain and spinal cord; made possible with the advent of faster, more powerful gradients, and utilizing single-shot diffusion-weighted echoplanar imaging (DW-EPI) sequences with higher SNR and reduced motion artifacts [75]. DTI measures diffusion characteristics of water to differentiate local microstructural features and delineates axonal tracts within the white matter of brain [76]. In isotropic diffusion, the magnitudes of diffusion quantify equally in all directions. However, the white matter tracts are composed of axons that contain microtubules and neurofilaments, contain a cell membrane, and are covered by a myelin sheath that is longitudinally oriented. Hence the water molecules move more freely parallel to the long axis of the axons [77]. This phenomenon is known as anisotropic diffusion (Fig. 6.16).

Diffusion-weighted images are obtained at three different angles, and the corresponding eigenvalues are fitted into a diffusion tensor model, which can be visualized in three dimensions as an ellipsoid and represented as a matrix [78]. The anisotropy of white matter tracts is higher than other brain parenchyma. Because of

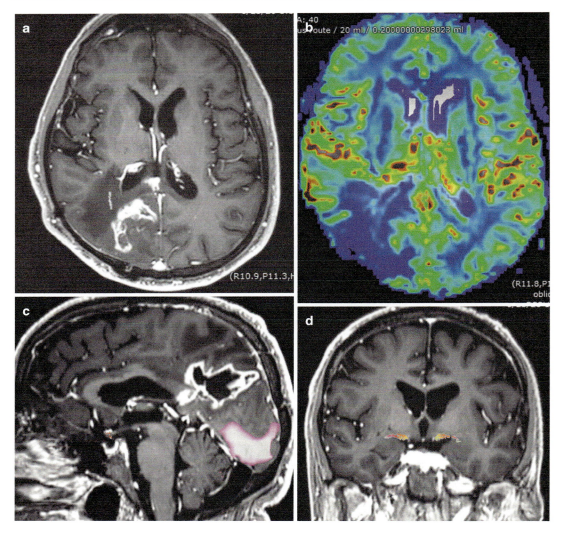

Fig. 6.14 Intensely and peripherally enhancing right parietal lesion, concerning for a recurrent GBM. (**a**) Axial post-contrast T1-weighted images exhibit intense patchy post-contrast enhancement with perilesional edema. Terminal right optic radiation seen within perilesional edema; (**b**) diminished perfusion in this area favors the possibility of pseudo-progression, which was confirmed on biopsy; (**c**) the activated primary visual cortex appears to be posterior to the lesion; (**d**) bilateral optic tracts, which can be traced onto optic radiations

this difference, it is possible to mathematically calculate a matrix called fractional anisotropy (FA) [79, 80]. The FA value ranges from 0 to 1, with 1 being a perfectly linear anisotropic diffusion and 0 being an isotropic diffusion lacking any directionality [81]. FA values reflect axonal density and high degree of myelination, but can also be influenced by axonal diameter and membrane permeability [82, 83]. Mean diffusivity (MD) represents the rate of diffusion averaged in all directions, axial diffusivity (AD) denotes rate of diffusivity parallel to white matter tracts, while radial diffusivity (RD) describes diffusivity perpendicular to the tracts; their exact significance with relation to information about axonal density and myelination is still uncertain [84].

The relative directional information of white matter tracts, based on three components of diffusion vector, can be displayed in color-coded voxels of DTI imaging by fractional anisotropy (FA) maps. Each voxel is coded with a color

6 Functional MRI and Diffusion Tensor Imaging

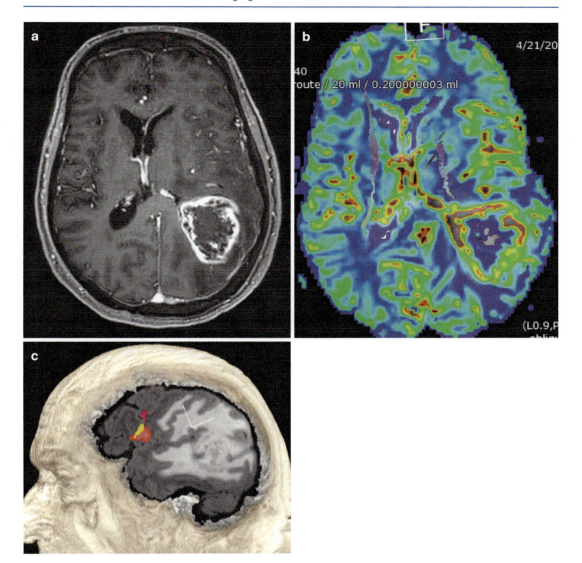

Fig. 6.15 Uncoupling of hemodynamic response function. (**a**) Post-contrast T1 axial images exhibit peripherally enhancing large left temporoparietal mass with perilesional edema; (**b**) hyperperfusion seen along the irregular peripheral wall of the mass; (**c**) 3-D parasagittal FLAIR weighted image shows activation of Broca's expressive language area. Complete lack of activation at the left superior temporal gyrus, angular gyrus, or supramarginal gyrus, likely related to uncoupling of hemodynamic response function

according to the eigenvector with the greatest eigenvalue. Green represents the anterior-posterior axis, red represents the transverse axis, while blue represents the cranio-caudal direction. The intensity of the color is a function of the magnitude of the FA value [85]. This allows visualization of global white matter tracts along with conventional MR imaging technique.

6.9 White Matter Tracts

White matter fiber tracts consist of bundles of myelinated fibers called fasciculi. They are classified in four groups: a group of brainstem white matter tracts and three in cerebral hemispheres called the projection fibers, the association fibers, and the commissural fiber tracts [86–88].

ISOTROPIC DIFFUSION | ANISOTROPIC DIFFUSION

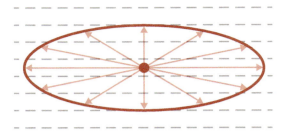

Fig. 6.16 Water diffusion in brain tissue. Isotropic diffusion is equal in all directions, mostly taking place in liquids, with the self-diffusion coefficient (D) of the same magnitude in all directions. An anisotropic diffusion is not equal in all directions and depends on the composition of the matrix. D is calculated by eigenvalue decomposition of multiple, at least six gradients in different directions

6.9.1 Projection Fibers

The projection fibers are divided into 2 classes. The thalamic radiations contain the cortical thalamic/thalamic cortical fibers and the long corticofugal fibers including the corticopontine, corticoreticular, corticobulbar, and corticospinal tracts. The thalamic radiations include the anterior, the superior, and the posterior thalamic radiations [89]. The posterior thalamic radiations include the optic radiation that connects the lateral geniculate nucleus and the occipital lobe. They all penetrate the anterior or posterior limb of internal capsule: between the thalamus and the putamen or the caudate head and the putamen. While ascending they fan out to form the corona radiata (Fig. 6.17). The internal capsule also contains long corticofugal pathways, descending towards the brainstem and include cortical pontine tracts, which can be further differentiated into frontal, parietal, occipital, and temporal pontine tracts. From the pontine nuclei, they project into the contralateral cerebellar hemisphere through the middle cerebellar peduncle, forming the prominent cortico-ponto-cerebellar pathway. The DTI-based reconstruction of corticopontine tracts cannot be differentiated from corticoreticular and corticobulbar tracts. The corticospinal tracts passing through the middle portion of cerebral peduncle predominantly contain projections from precentral gyrus (primary motor cortex); however some of the somatosensory and parietal cortical fibers are also included within this bundle [90].

6.9.2 Association Fibers

The association fibers connect different areas of cerebral cortex and are divided into short association fibers and long association fibers [91]. The short association fibers include those connecting adjacent gyri, called the U-fibers. The long association fibers connect the different lobes of the cerebral hemispheres and are some of the prominent fiber tracts. These include the superior longitudinal fasciculus (slf), inferior longitudinal fasciculus (ilf), superior frontal occipital fasciculus (sfo), inferior frontal occipital fasciculus (ifo), and uncinate fasciculus (unc). Cingulum (cg), fornix (fx), and stria terminalis (st) are major association fibers connecting the limbic system (Fig. 6.17).

Superior longitudinal fasciculus is a long tract along the superior lateral side of the putamen, connecting the frontal, the parietal, temporal, and occipital lobes, and also forms a large arcuate fasciculus, connecting the Broca's area and the Wernicke's area [92]. The inferior longitudinal fasciculus connects the occipital and temporal lobes, and the inferior frontal occipital fasciculus connects the frontal and occipital lobes. The superior frontal occipital fasciculus is seen along the superior edge of the anterior limb of the internal capsule and projects into the frontal lobe [93].

The cingulum extends underneath the cingulate gyrus, along its entire length, and collects axons from the cingulate gyrus in a large C-shaped trajectory. The fornix contains both the afferent and efferent connections between the hypothalamus and the hippocampus. The smaller C shape of fornix anteriorly contains the column, the body, and the posterior crus, which projects into bilateral hippocampi.

6.9.3 Commissural Fibers

The corpus callosum, anterior commissure, posterior commissure, and hippocampal commissure make for the commissural fibers. Corpus callo-

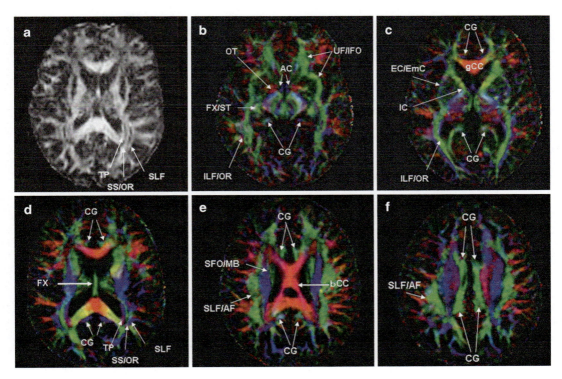

Fig. 6.17 Cerebral white matter tracts. (**a**) Fractional anisotropy (FA) map, (**b–f**) axial DTI color maps, (**g–i**) coronal DTI color maps, (**j–m**) sagittal DTI color maps, (**g–i**) coronal DTI color maps, (**j–m**) sagittal DTI color maps. DTI shows the white matter lateral to the posterior horn as three parts: the tapetum (TP), internal and external sagittal strata including optic radiation (SS/OR), and SLF. SLF/AF connects the frontal lobe to temporal and occipital lobes. SFO/MB is situated beneath the corpus callosum (CC) and medial to the corona radiata (CR). ILF connects temporal and occipital lobe cortices. The cingulum (CG) is situated on both sides of the midline on the surface of CC. The uncinate fasciculus (UF) connects the ventral and lateral frontal lobe with the anterior temporal lobe. EmC/EC is hard to be separately seen on DTI. SLF superior longitudinal fasciculus, AF arcuate fasciculus, ILF inferior longitudinal fasciculus, CG cingulum, UF uncinate fasciculus, SFO superior fronto-occipital fasciculus, IFO inferior fronto-occipital fasciculus, EmC extreme capsule, EC external capsule, MB subcallosal fasciculus of Muratoff, IC internal capsule, CST corticospinal tract, OT optic tract, OR optic radiation, SS sagittal stratum, gCC genu of corpus callosum, bCC body of corpus callosum, sCC splenium of corpus callosum, TP tapetum, AC anterior commissure, FX fornix, ST stria terminalis, SCP superior cerebellar peduncle, MCP middle cerebellar peduncle

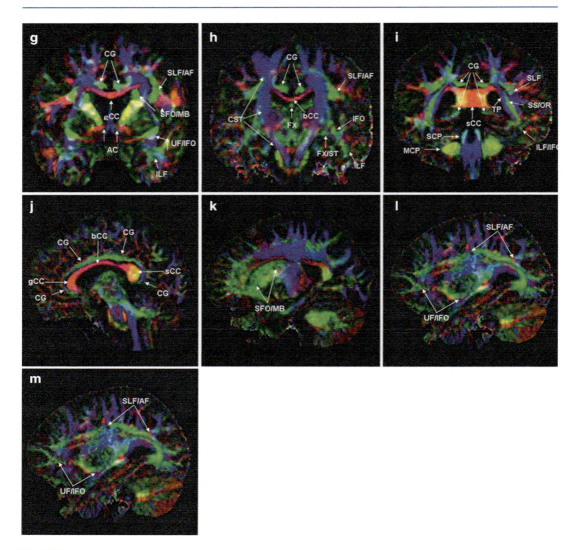

Fig. 6.17 (continued)

sum is the largest fiber bundle in the human brain and is predominantly symmetrical with mirror image sites [94]. The fibers course through the genu of corpus callosum (gCC), connecting the anterior part of frontal lobes. The body of corpus callosum (bCC) connects the remaining part of the frontal lobe and parietal lobes (Fig. 6.17). The splenium of corpus callosum (sCC) connects the temporal and occipital lobes. The anterior commissure (AC) is a tiny structure that is seen anterior to the column of the fornix. The posterior commissure (PC) is seen just above the tectal plate and connects the bilateral peritectal regions.

The hippocampal commissure is also known as the psalterium and connects the bilateral hippocampi between the fornices. The fornix contains both the projection and commissural fibers and is the main outflow tract of hippocampus.

6.9.4 Fibers of Brainstem and Cerebellum

There are 5 major white matter tracts within the brainstem: the superior cerebellar peduncles, the middle cerebellar peduncles, the inferior cerebellar peduncles, the corticospinal tracts, and the medial lemniscus [95].

The corticospinal tract (CST) is a descending pathway originating from the primary motor cortex. It passes through the cerebral peduncles and courses inferiorly through the pons and medulla [96]. The medial lemniscus (ml) is an ascending sensory pathway. It decussates at the ventral medulla and ascends into the dorsal pons and midbrain and then disperses. It cannot be traced any further. The superior cerebellar peduncle (scp) is the efferent pathway from dentate nucleus of cerebellum and extends into thalamus. The middle cerebellar peduncle (mcp) contains afferent pontocerebellar tracts, extending from the pons to cerebellum (Fig. 6.18). The inferior cerebellar peduncle includes both afferent and the efferent connections to the cerebellum. It originates in the dorsal medulla, traverses the pons, and branches within the cerebellar hemispheres.

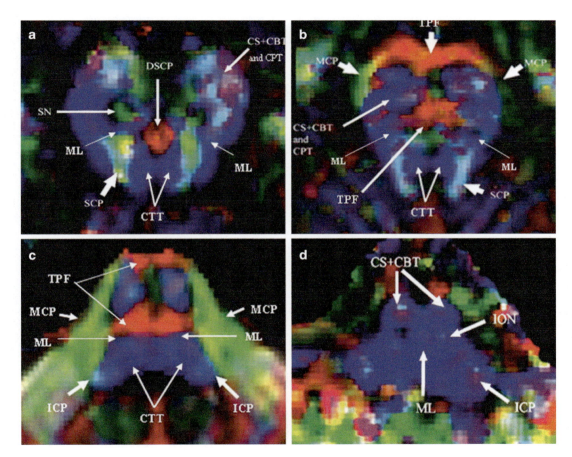

Fig. 6.18 Brainstem and cerebellar white matter tracts. (**a**) The midbrain: The crus cerebri consists of corticopontine, corticobulbar and corticospinal fibers (CPT, CBT, CST). The tegmentum and crus cerebri are separated by the substantia nigra (SN). The superior cerebellar peduncle (SCP) and their decussation (DSCP, round red spot) are noted in the caudal midbrain tegmentum. The dorsal tegmental portion contains the central tegmental tract (CTT) and medial lemniscus (ML). (**b, c**) The upper (**b**) and lower (**c**) pons: The ventral part of the pons contains CPT, CBT, CST, pontine nuclei, and transverse pontine fibers (TPF). The middle cerebellar peduncle (MCP) arises from pontine nuclei projecting to the cerebellar hemisphere. The inferior cerebellar peduncle is noted on each side of the lower part of the forth ventricle. (**d**) The medulla: The inferior olivary nuclei (ION), medullary pyramids (CST, CBT), medial lemniscus (ML), and ICP are demonstrated. (Courtesy of White ML, MD and Zhang Y MD, The University of Nebraska Medical Center, USA, and Courtesy of Salamon N MD, The University of California, Los Angeles, USA)

6.10 Diffusion Fiber Tracking

DTI sequence needs a minimum of 6 directional gradients. However, with advancement in MR imaging techniques, up to 128 direction gradients are applied sequentially during activation of diffusion tensor imaging (Fig. 6.19). From this DTI data, a diffusion fiber tracking or diffusion tractography can be obtained [75, 92, 97–101]. This allows three-dimensional (3-D) mapping of individual white matter fiber tracts within the brain, based on the directionality information that is derived from the FA values [102].

Numerous DTI tractography algorithms have been utilized, the two most common being the deterministic and the probabilistic tractography [98–100]. The probabilistic method estimates and displays the uncertainty in propagation between the two points. However, the deterministic approach uses the best estimate of the major eigenvector to propagate the fiber tracts and follows the primary eigenvector from the voxel to voxel in three dimensions. At the edge of the voxel, the direction of fiber trajectory changes to match the closest eigenvector in the next voxel [98, 103–106]. This makes it possible to reconstitute the entire pathway of the fiber tract coursing through the brain (Fig. 6.20). The possibility of crossing fibers, noise, or image artifacts can confuse the algorithm [106, 107]. However, there is potential to distinguish between the white matter tracts running in the same bundle [88, 92, 101], increasing the specificity of critical spatial relationships [108].

6.11 Presurgical Brain Mapping with DTI

A unique, patient-specific neurosurgical plan can be created by presurgical mapping from functional imaging and DTI data. This can establish spatial relationships between a brain mass or other lesion and the eloquent cortex and eloquent white matter tracts [109], reducing the morbidity and surgical complication. There is a high congruence between DTI fiber tracking and intraoperative subcortical mapping with decreased

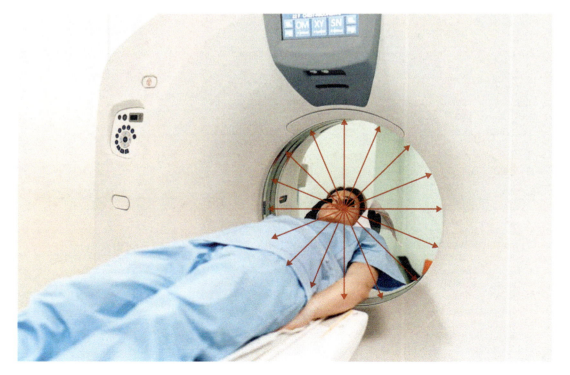

Fig. 6.19 Acquisition of diffusion tensor imaging. Within MRI machine, at least six and up to 128 gradients in different directions are applied sequentially to the brain

6 Functional MRI and Diffusion Tensor Imaging

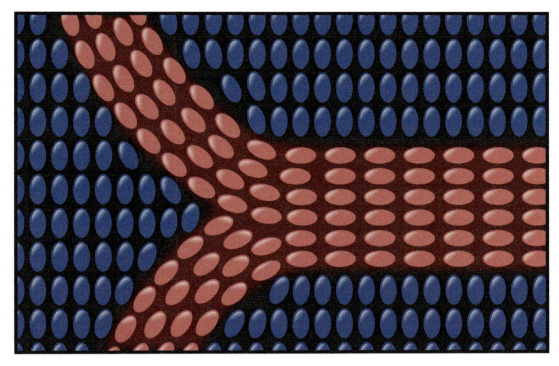

Fig. 6.20 Diffusion tractography. The vector information in each voxel can be exploited by different pixel connection techniques. Seeding a pixel with a ROI, propagation and termination by a probabilistic or deterministic algorithm like Fiber Assignment by Continuous Tracking (FACT) defines specific anatomic fiber tracks

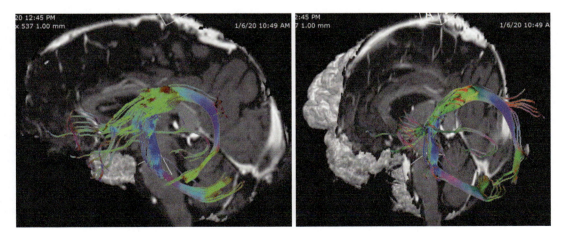

Fig. 6.21 Arcuate fasciculus. An association fiber tract connecting the Broca's expressive language area at inferior frontal lobe to Wernicke's comprehensive language center at posterior part of superior temporal gyrus

duration of surgery, patient fatigue, and intraoperative seizures [110]. DTI was also able to identify the eloquent primary motor cortex without the aid of functional imaging in patients with brain neoplasm and anatomic distortion [111].

The classic theory for language is based on anatomic location of Wernicke's area and Broca's area and their interconnection by arcuate fasciculus (Fig. 6.21). The current dual-stream hypothesis of language includes the sensorimotor features of dorsal stream and the speech comprehension of ventral stream. The uncinate fasciculus connects the inferior longitudinal fasciculus to the inferior frontal area and appears to be one of the main tracts on the ventral stream [112, 113]. Fiber tractography can define the course of arcuate fasciculus and inform the neurosurgeon about its precise course and whether they are displaced or infiltrated (Fig. 6.22).

Atypical language lateralization is seen in patients with epilepsy and left-handed people [46, 47]. As a result, further assessment with DTI and a precise location of language susceptibility and its relationship with an epileptogenic or mass lesion is very important [114, 115]. Wada test is considered gold standard for language lateralization; however, it remains an invasive, expansive, and unpleasant experience for the patients [116] and can result in complications in 10.9% of the cases, such as encephalopathy (7.2%), seizures (1.2%), stroke (0.6%), or carotid artery dissection [117]. A large number of studies have established a correlation between DTI and fMRI that helps to define language lateralization through DTI [118, 119]. A recent analysis of 10 patients with temporal lobe of epilepsy found that FA, volume, and number of fibers of the arcuate fasciculus were greater, and the volume and length of fibers of uncinate fasciculus were higher in the dominant hemisphere [120]. An analysis of arcuate fasciculus and other tract bundles by DTI can help determine language dominance in patients [116, 121].

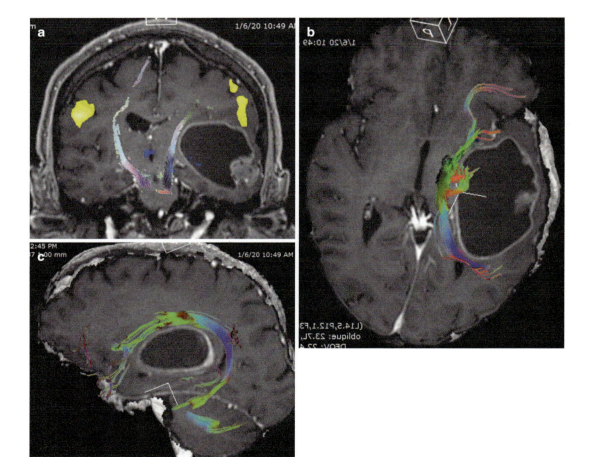

Fig. 6.22 Left temporal GBM. (**a**) Marked medial deviation of left corticospinal tract without infiltration by the tumor; (**b**) medial displacement of left arcuate fasciculus by the irregular ring-enhancing mass without infiltration; (**c**) an intact arcuate fasciculus wraps around the left fronto-temporal mass

While conventional MRI with newer techniques helps diagnose a brain mass or epilepsy focus, presurgical evaluation of fMRI and DTI further defines eloquent cortex and white matter tracts and defines the extent of tumor resection. It also gives valuable prognostic information and helps identify infiltration of vital white matter structures (Fig. 6.23). Diffusion imaging techniques like high angular diffusion imaging (HARDI), diffusion spectral imaging, and diffusion kurtosis imaging are promising and can help resolve conundrums like crossing tracts [122–125]. Increasing compatibility of fMRI and DTI software with neuronavigation systems and increased intraoperative availability has increased the utility of these techniques, allowing the neurosurgeons to achieve maximal cytoreduction and reduce surgical time, while limiting morbidity and complications. By providing the accurate and detailed information about the spatial relationships of various vital brain structures, fMRI and DTI are soon becoming the standard of care for neurosurgical procedures.

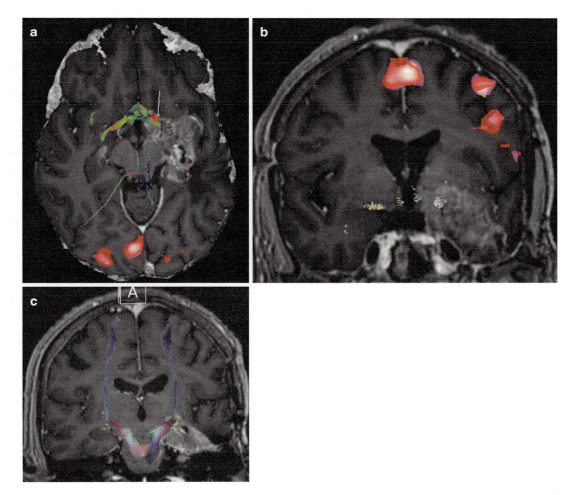

Fig. 6.23 Fiber tracking in recurrent anaplastic glioneural tumor. (**a**) The left optic tract on the way to lateral geniculate nucleus is infiltrated by enhancing left frontotemporal recurrent tumor mass; (**b**) left optic tract is infiltrated by enhancing recurrent mass; (**c**) the left corticospinal tract is infiltrated by enhancing left frontal temporal mass

References

1. Ogawa S, Lee TM, Nayak AS, Glynn P (1990) Oxygenation-sensitive contrast in magnetic resonance image of rodent brain at high magnetic fields. Magn Reson Med 14(1):68–78
2. Ogawa S, Lee TM, Kay AR, Tank DW (1990) Brain magnetic resonance imaging with contrast dependent on blood oxygenation. Proc Natl Acad Sci USA 87(24):9868–9872
3. Buxton RB, Uludag K, Dubowitz DJ, Liu TT (2004) Modeling the hemodynamic response to brain activation. NeuroImage 23(Suppl 1):S220–S233
4. Logothetis NK, Pauls J, Augath M, Trinath T, Oeltermann A (2001) Neurophysiological investigation of the basis of the fMRI signal. Nature 412(6843):150–157
5. Logothetis NK, Wandell BA (2004) Interpreting the BOLD signal. Annu Rev Physiol 66:735–769
6. Raichle ME, Mintun MA (2006) Brain work and brain imaging. Annu Rev Neurosci 29:449–476
7. Hampson M, Peterson BS, Skudlarski P, Gatenby JC, Gore JC (2002) Detection of functional connectivity using temporal correlations in MR images. Hum Brain Mapp 15(4):247–262
8. Stippich C, Blatow M, Durst A, Dreyhaupt J, Sartor K (2007) Global activation of primary motor cortex during voluntary movements in man. NeuroImage 34(3):1227–1237
9. Tieleman A, Deblaere K, Van Roost D, Van Damme O, Achten E (2009) Preoperative fMRI in tumour surgery. Eur Radiol 19(10):2523–2534
10. Price CJ (2010) The anatomy of language: a review of 100 fMRI studies published in 2009. Ann N Y Acad Sci 1191:62–88
11. Binder JR, Desai RH, Graves WW, Conant LL (2009) Where is the semantic system? A critical review and meta-analysis of 120 functional neuroimaging studies. Cereb Cortex 19(12):2767–2796
12. Price CJ (2000) The anatomy of language: contributions from functional neuroimaging. J Anat 197(Pt 3):335–359
13. Friederici AD (2011) The brain basis of language processing: from structure to function. Physiol Rev 91(4):1357–1392
14. Szaflarski JP, Binder JR, Possing ET, McKiernan KA, Ward BD, Hammeke TA (2002) Language lateralization in left-handed and ambidextrous people: fMRI data. Neurology 59(2):238–244
15. Binder JR, Frost JA, Hammeke TA, Cox RW, Rao SM, Prieto T (1997) Human brain language areas identified by functional magnetic resonance imaging. J Neurosci 17(1):353–362
16. DeYoe EA, Carman GJ, Bandettini P, Glickman S, Wieser J, Cox R et al (1996) Mapping striate and extrastriate visual areas in human cerebral cortex. Proc Natl Acad Sci USA 93(6):2382–2386
17. Dassonville P, Lewis SM, Zhu XH, Ugurbil K, Kim SG, Ashe J (1998) Effects of movement predictability on cortical motor activation. Neurosci Res 32(1):65–74
18. Fried I, Katz A, McCarthy G, Sass KJ, Williamson P, Spencer SS et al (1991) Functional organization of human supplementary motor cortex studied by electrical stimulation. J Neurosci 11(11):3656–3666
19. Matsuzaka Y, Aizawa H, Tanji J (1992) A motor area rostral to the supplementary motor area (presupplementary motor area) in the monkey: neuronal activity during a learned motor task. J Neurophysiol 68(3):653–662
20. Mitz AR, Wise SP (1987) The somatotopic organization of the supplementary motor area: intracortical microstimulation mapping. J Neurosci 7(4):1010–1021
21. Arienzo D, Babiloni C, Ferretti A, Caulo M, Del Gratta C, Tartaro A et al (2006) Somatotopy of anterior cingulate cortex (ACC) and supplementary motor area (SMA) for electric stimulation of the median and tibial nerves: an fMRI study. NeuroImage 33(2):700–705
22. Rijntjes M, Dettmers C, Buchel C, Kiebel S, Frackowiak RS, Weiller C (1999) A blueprint for movement: functional and anatomical representations in the human motor system. J Neurosci 19(18):8043–8048
23. Chainay H, Krainik A, Tanguy ML, Gerardin E, Le Bihan D, Lehericy S (2004) Foot, face and hand representation in the human supplementary motor area. Neuroreport 15(5):765–769
24. Tanji J, Kurata K (1982) Comparison of movement-related activity in two cortical motor areas of primates. J Neurophysiol 48(3):633–653
25. Nachev P, Kennard C, Husain M (2008) Functional role of the supplementary and pre-supplementary motor areas. Nat Rev Neurosci 9(11):856–869
26. Tharin S, Golby A (2007) Functional brain mapping and its applications to neurosurgery. Neurosurgery 60(4 Suppl 2):185–201; discussion-2
27. Tanji J, Shima K (1994) Role for supplementary motor area cells in planning several movements ahead. Nature 371(6496):413–416
28. Peck KK, Bradbury M, Psaty EL, Brennan NP, Holodny AI (2009) Joint activation of the supplementary motor area and presupplementary motor area during simultaneous motor and language functional MRI. Neuroreport 20(5):487–491
29. Peck KK, Bradbury MS, Hou BL, Brennan NP, Holodny AI (2009) The role of the Supplementary Motor Area (SMA) in the execution of primary motor activities in brain tumor patients: functional MRI detection of time-resolved differences in the hemodynamic response. Med Sci Monit 15(4):MT55–MT62
30. Bannur U, Rajshekhar V (2000) Post operative supplementary motor area syndrome: clinical features and outcome. Br J Neurosurg 14(3):204–210
31. Fontaine D, Capelle L, Duffau H (2002) Somatotopy of the supplementary motor area: evidence from correlation of the extent of surgical resection with the

clinical patterns of deficit. Neurosurgery 50(2):297–303; discussion-5

32. Krainik A, Lehericy S, Duffau H, Capelle L, Chainay H, Cornu P et al (2003) Postoperative speech disorder after medial frontal surgery: role of the supplementary motor area. Neurology 60(4):587–594

33. Zentner J, Hufnagel A, Pechstein U, Wolf HK, Schramm J (1996) Functional results after resective procedures involving the supplementary motor area. J Neurosurg 85(4):542–549

34. Petersen SE, Dubis JW (2012) The mixed block/event-related design. NeuroImage 62(2):1177–1184

35. Birn RM, Cox RW, Bandettini PA (2002) Detection versus estimation in event-related fMRI: choosing the optimal stimulus timing. NeuroImage 15(1):252–264

36. Liu TT (2012) The development of event-related fMRI designs. NeuroImage 62(2):1157–1162

37. Friston KJ, Zarahn E, Josephs O, Henson RN, Dale AM (1999) Stochastic designs in event-related fMRI. NeuroImage 10(5):607–619

38. Amaro E Jr, Barker GJ (2006) Study design in fMRI: basic principles. Brain Cogn 60(3):220–232

39. Zarahn E, Aguirre G, D'Esposito M (1997) A trial-based experimental design for fMRI. NeuroImage 6(2):122–138

40. Kim PE, Singh M (2003) Functional magnetic resonance imaging for brain mapping in neurosurgery. Neurosurg Focus 15(1):E1

41. Lurito JT, Dzemidzic M (2001) Determination of cerebral hemisphere language dominance with functional magnetic resonance imaging. Neuroimaging Clin N Am 11(2):355–363

42. Woods RP, Dodrill CB, Ojemann GA (1988) Brain injury, handedness, and speech lateralization in a series of amobarbital studies. Ann Neurol 23(5):510–518

43. Kurthen M, Helmstaedter C, Linke DB, Hufnagel A, Elger CE, Schramm J (1994) Quantitative and qualitative evaluation of patterns of cerebral language dominance. An amobarbital study. Brain Lang 46(4):536–564

44. Staudt M, Lidzba K, Grodd W, Wildgruber D, Erb M, Krageloh-Mann I (2002) Right-hemispheric organization of language following early left-sided brain lesions: functional MRI topography. NeuroImage 16(4):954–967

45. Partovi S, Jacobi B, Rapps N, Zipp L, Karimi S, Rengier F et al (2012) Clinical standardized fMRI reveals altered language lateralization in patients with brain tumor. AJNR Am J Neuroradiol 33(11):2151–2157

46. Rodrigo S, Oppenheim C, Chassoux F, Hodel J, de Vanssay A, Baudoin-Chial S et al (2008) Language lateralization in temporal lobe epilepsy using functional MRI and probabilistic tractography. Epilepsia 49(8):1367–1376

47. Thivard L, Hombrouck J, du Montcel ST, Delmaire C, Cohen L, Samson S et al (2005) Productive and perceptive language reorganization in temporal lobe epilepsy. NeuroImage 24(3):841–851

48. Woermann FG, Jokeit H, Luerding R, Freitag H, Schulz R, Guertler S et al (2003) Language lateralization by Wada test and fMRI in 100 patients with epilepsy. Neurology 61(5):699–701

49. Medina LS, Aguirre E, Bernal B, Altman NR (2004) Functional MR imaging versus Wada test for evaluation of language lateralization: cost analysis. Radiology 230(1):49–54

50. Caulo M, Esposito R, Mantini D, Briganti C, Sestieri C, Mattei PA et al (2011) Comparison of hypothesis- and a novel hybrid data/hypothesis-driven method of functional MR imaging analysis in patients with brain gliomas. AJNR Am J Neuroradiol 32(6):1056–1064

51. Medina LS, Bernal B, Dunoyer C, Cervantes L, Rodriguez M, Pacheco E et al (2005) Seizure disorders: functional MR imaging for diagnostic evaluation and surgical treatment–prospective study. Radiology 236(1):247–253

52. Jones SE, Mahmoud SY, Phillips MD (2011) A practical clinical method to quantify language lateralization in fMRI using whole-brain analysis. NeuroImage 54(4):2937–2949

53. Dym RJ, Burns J, Freeman K, Lipton ML (2011) Is functional MR imaging assessment of hemispheric language dominance as good as the Wada test?: a meta-analysis. Radiology 261(2):446–455

54. Kelly PJ, Daumas-Duport C, Kispert DB, Kall BA, Scheithauer BW, Illig JJ (1987) Imaging-based stereotaxic serial biopsies in untreated intracranial glial neoplasms. J Neurosurg 66(6):865–874

55. Yordanova YN, Moritz-Gasser S, Duffau H (2011) Awake surgery for WHO Grade II gliomas within "noneloquent" areas in the left dominant hemisphere: toward a "supratotal" resection. Clinical article. J Neurosurg 115(2):232–239

56. Verburg N, de Witt Hamer PC (2020) State-of-the-art imaging for glioma surgery. Neurosurg Rev. https://doi.org/10.1007/s10143-020-01337-9. Epub ahead of print. PMID: 32607869

57. Smith JS, Chang EF, Lamborn KR, Chang SM, Prados MD, Cha S et al (2008) Role of extent of resection in the long-term outcome of low-grade hemispheric gliomas. J Clin Oncol 26(8):1338–1345

58. Lacroix M, Abi-Said D, Fourney DR, Gokaslan ZL, Shi W, DeMonte F et al (2001) A multivariate analysis of 416 patients with glioblastoma multiforme: prognosis, extent of resection, and survival. J Neurosurg 95(2):190–198

59. Capelle L, Fontaine D, Mandonnet E, Taillandier L, Golmard JL, Bauchet L et al (2013) Spontaneous and therapeutic prognostic factors in adult hemispheric World Health Organization Grade II gliomas: a series of 1097 cases: clinical article. J Neurosurg 118(6):1157–1168

60. Sanai N, Polley MY, McDermott MW, Parsa AT, Berger MS (2011) An extent of resection threshold

for newly diagnosed glioblastomas. J Neurosurg 115(1):3–8

61. Pujol J, Torres L, Deus J, Cardoner N, Pifarre J, Capdevila A et al (1999) Functional magnetic resonance imaging study of frontal lobe activation during word generation in obsessive-compulsive disorder. Biol Psychiatry 45(7):891–897

62. Bittar RG, Olivier A, Sadikot AF, Andermann F, Pike GB, Reutens DC (1999) Presurgical motor and somatosensory cortex mapping with functional magnetic resonance imaging and positron emission tomography. J Neurosurg 91(6):915–921

63. Wilkinson ID, Romanowski CA, Jellinek DA, Morris J, Griffiths PD (2003) Motor functional MRI for pre-operative and intraoperative neurosurgical guidance. Br J Radiol 76(902):98–103

64. Petrella JR, Shah LM, Harris KM, Friedman AH, George TM, Sampson JH et al (2006) Preoperative functional MR imaging localization of language and motor areas: effect on therapeutic decision making in patients with potentially resectable brain tumors. Radiology 240(3):793–802

65. Roessler K, Donat M, Lanzenberger R, Novak K, Geissler A, Gartus A et al (2005) Evaluation of pre-operative high magnetic field motor functional MRI (3 Tesla) in glioma patients by navigated electro-cortical stimulation and postoperative outcome. J Neurol Neurosurg Psychiatry 76(8):1152–1157

66. Foesleitner O, Sigl B, Schmidbauer V, Nenning KH, Pataraia E, Bartha-Doering L et al (2020) Language network reorganization before and after temporal lobe epilepsy surgery. J Neurosurg 1–9. https://doi.org/10.3171/2020.4.JNS193401. Epub ahead of print. PMID: 32619977

67. Krings T, Topper R, Willmes K, Reinges MH, Gilsbach JM, Thron A (2002) Activation in primary and secondary motor areas in patients with CNS neoplasms and weakness. Neurology 58(3):381–390

68. Holodny AI, Schulder M, Liu WC, Maldjian JA, Kalnin AJ (1999) Decreased BOLD functional MR activation of the motor and sensory cortices adjacent to a glioblastoma multiforme: implications for image-guided neurosurgery. AJNR Am J Neuroradiol 20(4):609–612

69. Roux FE, Boulanouar K, Ibarrola D, Tremoulet M, Chollet F, Berry I (2000) Functional MRI and intra-operative brain mapping to evaluate brain plasticity in patients with brain tumours and hemiparesis. J Neurol Neurosurg Psychiatry 69(4):453–463

70. Krings T, Reinges MH, Erberich S, Kemeny S, Rohde V, Spetzger U et al (2001) Functional MRI for presurgical planning: problems, artefacts, and solution strategies. J Neurol Neurosurg Psychiatry 70(6):749–760

71. Ludemann L, Forschler A, Grieger W, Zimmer C (2006) BOLD signal in the motor cortex shows a correlation with the blood volume of brain tumors. J Magn Reson Imaging 23(4):435–443

72. Hou BL, Bradbury M, Peck KK, Petrovich NM, Gutin PH, Holodny AI (2006) Effect of brain tumor neovasculature defined by rCBV on BOLD fMRI activation volume in the primary motor cortex. NeuroImage 32(2):489–497

73. Biswal B, Yetkin FZ, Haughton VM, Hyde JS (1995) Functional connectivity in the motor cortex of resting human brain using echo-planar MRI. Magn Reson Med 34(4):537–541

74. Basser PJ, Mattiello J, LeBihan D (1994) Estimation of the effective self-diffusion tensor from the NMR spin echo. J Magn Reson B 103(3):247–254

75. Basser PJ, Pajevic S, Pierpaoli C, Duda J, Aldroubi A (2000) In vivo fiber tractography using DT-MRI data. Magn Reson Med 44(4):625–632

76. Mori S, Zhang J (2006) Principles of diffusion tensor imaging and its applications to basic neuroscience research. Neuron 51(5):527–539

77. Beaulieu C, Allen PS (1994) Determinants of anisotropic water diffusion in nerves. Magn Reson Med 31(4):394–400

78. Mukherjee P, Berman JI, Chung SW, Hess CP, Henry RG (2008) Diffusion tensor MR imaging and fiber tractography: theoretic underpinnings. AJNR Am J Neuroradiol 29(4):632–641

79. Beaulieu C (2002) The basis of anisotropic water diffusion in the nervous system—a technical review. NMR Biomed 15(7–8):435–455

80. Basser PJ, Pierpaoli C (1996) Microstructural and physiological features of tissues elucidated by quantitative-diffusion-tensor MRI. J Magn Reson B 111(3):209–219

81. Pierpaoli C, Basser PJ (1996) Toward a quantitative assessment of diffusion anisotropy. Magn Reson Med 36(6):893–906

82. Ulug AM, van Zijl PC (1999) Orientation-independent diffusion imaging without tensor diagonalization: anisotropy definitions based on physical attributes of the diffusion ellipsoid. J Magn Reson Imaging 9(6):804–813

83. Jones DK, Knosche TR, Turner R (2013) White matter integrity, fiber count, and other fallacies: the do's and don'ts of diffusion MRI. NeuroImage 73:239–254

84. Wheeler-Kingshott CA, Cercignani M (2009) About "axial" and "radial" diffusivities. Magn Reson Med 61(5):1255–1260

85. Pajevic S, Pierpaoli C (1999) Color schemes to represent the orientation of anisotropic tissues from diffusion tensor data: application to white matter fiber tract mapping in the human brain. Magn Reson Med 42(3):526–540

86. Wakana S, Jiang H, Nagae-Poetscher LM, van Zijl PC, Mori S (2004) Fiber tract-based atlas of human white matter anatomy. Radiology 230(1):77–87

87. Mori S, van Zijl PC (2002) Fiber tracking: principles and strategies—a technical review. NMR Biomed 15(7–8):468–480

88. Jellison BJ, Field AS, Medow J, Lazar M, Salamat MS, Alexander AL (2004) Diffusion tensor imaging

of cerebral white matter: a pictorial review of physics, fiber tract anatomy, and tumor imaging patterns. AJNR Am J Neuroradiol 25(3):356–369

89. Poupon C, Clark CA, Frouin V, Regis J, Bloch I, Le Bihan D et al (2000) Regularization of diffusion-based direction maps for the tracking of brain white matter fascicles. NeuroImage 12(2):184–195

90. Lori NF, Akbudak E, Shimony JS, Cull TS, Snyder AZ, Guillory RK et al (2002) Diffusion tensor fiber tracking of human brain connectivity: acquisition methods, reliability analysis and biological results. NMR Biomed 15(7–8):494–515

91. Makris N, Worth AJ, Sorensen AG, Papadimitriou GM, Wu O, Reese TG et al (1997) Morphometry of in vivo human white matter association pathways with diffusion-weighted magnetic resonance imaging. Ann Neurol 42(6):951–962

92. Mori S, Kaufmann WE, Davatzikos C, Stieltjes B, Amodei L, Fredericksen K et al (2002) Imaging cortical association tracts in the human brain using diffusion-tensor-based axonal tracking. Magn Reson Med 47(2):215–223

93. Schmahmann JD, Pandya DN, Wang R, Dai G, D'Arceuil HE, de Crespigny AJ et al (2007) Association fibre pathways of the brain: parallel observations from diffusion spectrum imaging and autoradiography. Brain 130(Pt 3):630–653

94. Jones DK, Simmons A, Williams SC, Horsfield MA (1999) Non-invasive assessment of axonal fiber connectivity in the human brain via diffusion tensor MRI. Magn Reson Med 42(1):37–41

95. Stieltjes B, Kaufmann WE, van Zijl PC, Fredericksen K, Pearlson GD, Solaiyappan M et al (2001) Diffusion tensor imaging and axonal tracking in the human brainstem. NeuroImage 14(3):723–735

96. Wakana S, Caprihan A, Panzenboeck MM, Fallon JH, Perry M, Gollub RL et al (2007) Reproducibility of quantitative tractography methods applied to cerebral white matter. NeuroImage 36(3):630–644

97. Mori S, Crain BJ, Chacko VP, van Zijl PC (1999) Three-dimensional tracking of axonal projections in the brain by magnetic resonance imaging. Ann Neurol 45(2):265–269

98. Conturo TE, Lori NF, Cull TS, Akbudak E, Snyder AZ, Shimony JS et al (1999) Tracking neuronal fiber pathways in the living human brain. Proc Natl Acad Sci USA 96(18):10422–10427

99. Lazar M, Alexander AL (2005) Bootstrap white matter tractography (BOOT-TRAC). NeuroImage 24(2):524–532

100. Parker GJ, Haroon HA, Wheeler-Kingshott CA (2003) A framework for a streamline-based probabilistic index of connectivity (PICo) using a structural interpretation of MRI diffusion measurements. J Magn Reson Imaging 18(2):242–254

101. Catani M, Howard RJ, Pajevic S, Jones DK (2002) Virtual in vivo interactive dissection of white matter fasciculi in the human brain. NeuroImage 17(1):77–94

102. Ulmer JL, Klein AP, Mueller WM, DeYoe EA, Mark LP (2014) Preoperative diffusion tensor imaging: improving neurosurgical outcomes in brain tumor patients. Neuroimaging Clin N Am 24(4):599–617

103. Basser PJ, Jones DK (2002) Diffusion-tensor MRI: theory, experimental design and data analysis—a technical review. NMR Biomed 15(7–8):456–467

104. Mori S, Barker PB (1999) Diffusion magnetic resonance imaging: its principle and applications. Anat Rec 257(3):102–109

105. Behrens TE, Woolrich MW, Jenkinson M, Johansen-Berg H, Nunes RG, Clare S et al (2003) Characterization and propagation of uncertainty in diffusion-weighted MR imaging. Magn Reson Med 50(5):1077–1088

106. Hess CP, Mukherjee P (2007) Visualizing white matter pathways in the living human brain: diffusion tensor imaging and beyond. Neuroimaging Clin N Am 17(4):407–426, vii

107. Anderson AW (2001) Theoretical analysis of the effects of noise on diffusion tensor imaging. Magn Reson Med 46(6):1174–1188

108. Han BS, Hong JH, Hong C, Yeo SS, Lee D, Cho HK et al (2010) Location of the corticospinal tract at the corona radiata in human brain. Brain Res 1326:75–80

109. Berman J (2009) Diffusion MR tractography as a tool for surgical planning. Magn Reson Imaging Clin N Am 17(2):205–214

110. Bello L, Gambini A, Castellano A, Carrabba G, Acerbi F, Fava E et al (2008) Motor and language DTI Fiber Tracking combined with intraoperative subcortical mapping for surgical removal of gliomas. NeuroImage 39(1):369–382

111. Berman JI, Berger MS, Chung SW, Nagarajan SS, Henry RG (2007) Accuracy of diffusion tensor magnetic resonance imaging tractography assessed using intraoperative subcortical stimulation mapping and magnetic source imaging. J Neurosurg 107(3):488–494

112. Chang EF, Raygor KP, Berger MS (2015) Contemporary model of language organization: an overview for neurosurgeons. J Neurosurg 122(2):250–261

113. Kim CH, Chung CK, Koo BB, Lee JM, Kim JS, Lee SK (2011) Changes in language pathways in patients with temporal lobe epilepsy: diffusion tensor imaging analysis of the uncinate and arcuate fasciculi. World Neurosurg 75(3–4):509–516

114. Garcia-Pallero MA, Hodaie M, Zhong J, Manzanares-Soler R, Navas M, Pastor J et al (2019) Prediction of laterality in temporal lobe epilepsy using white matter diffusion metrics. World Neurosurg 128:e700–e7e8

115. Garcia-Pallero MA, Torres CV, Manzanares-Soler R, Camara E, Sola RG (2016) The role of diffusion

tensor imaging in the pre-surgical study of temporal lobe epilepsy. Rev Neurol 63(12):537–542

116. Ellmore TM, Beauchamp MS, Breier JI, Slater JD, Kalamangalam GP, O'Neill TJ et al (2010) Temporal lobe white matter asymmetry and language laterality in epilepsy patients. NeuroImage 49(3):2033–2044

117. Loddenkemper T, Morris HH, Moddel G (2008) Complications during the Wada test. Epilepsy Behav 13(3):551–553

118. Silva G, Citterio A (2017) Hemispheric asymmetries in dorsal language pathway white-matter tracts: a magnetic resonance imaging tractography and functional magnetic resonance imaging study. Neuroradiol J 30(5):470–476

119. Vassal F, Schneider F, Boutet C, Jean B, Sontheimer A, Lemaire JJ (2016) Combined DTI tractography and functional MRI study of the language connectome in healthy volunteers: extensive mapping of white matter fascicles and cortical activations. PLoS One 11(3):e0152614

120. Delgado-Fernandez J, Garcia-Pallero MA, Manzanares-Soler R, Martin-Plasencia P, Blasco G, Frade-Porto N et al (2020) Language hemispheric dominance analyzed with magnetic resonance DTI: correlation with the Wada test. J Neurosurg 1–8. https://doi.org/10.3171/2020.4.JNS20456. Epub ahead of print. PMID: 32707542

121. Matsumoto R, Okada T, Mikuni N, Mitsueda-Ono T, Taki J, Sawamoto N et al (2008) Hemispheric asymmetry of the arcuate fasciculus: a preliminary diffusion tensor tractography study in patients with unilateral language dominance defined by Wada test. J Neurol 255(11):1703–1711

122. Frank LR (2002) Characterization of anisotropy in high angular resolution diffusion-weighted MRI. Magn Reson Med 47(6):1083–1099

123. Wedeen VJ, Hagmann P, Tseng WY, Reese TG, Weisskoff RM (2005) Mapping complex tissue architecture with diffusion spectrum magnetic resonance imaging. Magn Reson Med 54(6):1377–1386

124. Leclercq D, Duffau H, Delmaire C, Capelle L, Gatignol P, Ducros M et al (2010) Comparison of diffusion tensor imaging tractography of language tracts and intraoperative subcortical stimulations. J Neurosurg 112(3):503–511

125. Wu EX, Cheung MM (2010) MR diffusion kurtosis imaging for neural tissue characterization. NMR Biomed 23(7):836–848

Physics of Advanced Diffusion Imaging

7

Arun Venkataraman and Jianhui Zhong

Abbreviations

CHARMED	Composite hindered and restricted model of diffusion
DKI	Diffusion kurtosis imaging
dMRI	Diffusion MRI
dODF	Diffusion orientation distribution function
DSI	Diffusion spectrum imaging
HARDI	High angular resolution diffusion imaging
HCP	Human connectome project
NODDI	Neurite orientation dispersion and density imaging
QBI	Q ball imaging
QSI	Q-space imaging
SMS	Simultaneous multislice

A. Venkataraman · J. Zhong (✉)
Department of Physics and Astronomy, Center for Advanced Brain Imaging and Neurophysiology, University of Rochester, Rochester, NY, USA

Department of Imaging Sciences, Center for Advanced Brain Imaging and Neurophysiology, University of Rochester, Rochester, NY, USA
e-mail: arun_venkataraman@urmc.rochester.edu; jianhui.zhong@rochester.edu

7.1 Pitfalls of the Diffusion Tensor Model

Advances in MRI hardware have allowed for much faster and stronger magnetic field gradients, leading to a decrease in time of acquisition, allowing for utilization of multiple and high b-value imaging. The resulting images are more sensitive to the diffusion process and have shown that the diffusion tensor model does not describe all diffusion phenomena in the brain. In Chap. 1, the diffusion tensor was described as a matrix, from which the principal directions of diffusion could be derived (Fig. 1.5). The tensor itself was fit on the assumption of a single exponential decay model (Chap. 1, Eq. 1.2), derived from the assumption of Gaussian diffusion. As we will see, these assumptions are faulty in certain situations and can lead us to false outcomes based on data derived from the tensor model, such as FA maps.

The diffusion tensor introduced in Chap. 1, as mentioned, has an underlying assumption of Gaussian diffusion, i.e., the probability of a particle traveling some distance has a normal distribution. This relationship is given in Eq. (7.1).

$$P(\vec{r},t) = \left(4\pi\ddot{D}t\right)^{-3/2} e^{-\vec{r}\cdot\vec{r}/4\ddot{D}t}, \qquad (7.1)$$

where $\ddot{D}$ is the diffusion tensor, t is the diffusion time (from Fig. 1.2), and $\vec{r}$ is the displacement vector. We can immediately see that this model is

---

© Springer Nature Switzerland AG 2021
T. Moritani, A. A. Capizzano (eds.), *Diffusion-Weighted MR Imaging of the Brain, Head and Neck, and Spine*, https://doi.org/10.1007/978-3-030-62120-9_7

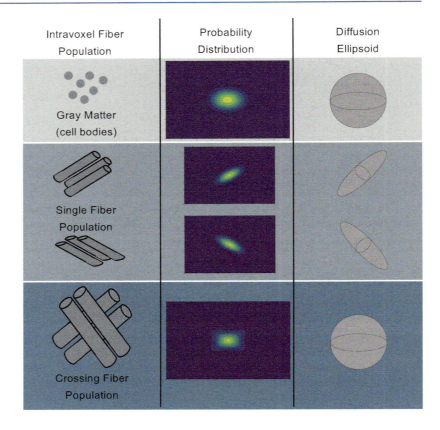

Fig. 7.1 DTI reconstruction of different intravoxel fiber populations. Left panel describes dominant fiber population in an arbitrary voxel. Center panel describes the resulting probability distribution of diffusion in two dimensions. Right panel describes the diffusion ellipsoid based on tensor model reconstructed from data. Note that gray matter and crossing fiber population have identical ellipsoids

a problem if a voxel of interest contains more than one fiber population (Fig. 7.1).

The main effect of crossing fibers is a blurring of the diffusion tensor, leading to a picture of more isotropic diffusion. The diffusion tensor, due to the assumption of a single orientation in a voxel, cannot uniquely describe a voxel containing multiple fibers. It is then important to ask how such a situation should be modeled. In the next section, we will address the physical basis of signals from voxels with crossing fibers, and will lead into modern innovations in diffusion MRI (dMRI) that allow for the estimation of these more complex situations.

7.2 Diffusion Signal of Crossing Fibers

Crossing fibers have become more of a concern as more quantitative dMRI scans are used. Even with increased spatial resolution in dMRI; with up to 90% of voxels potentially contain crossing fibers [1]. The main pitfall of the diffusion tensor model is the assumption of a normal distribution (Eq. 7.1). We can picture a system such as that shown in the bottom panel of Fig. 7.1, where a voxel contains crossing fibers. From a naïve understanding of probability dsitributions, and since the crossing fibers are independent of each other, the signal from this voxel should be the sum of two normal distributions, with Eq. (7.1) added to itself with corresponding changes to the displacement vector and diffusion tensor. This is where the diffusion tensor model falls short, since it can only account for one tensor and vector per voxel. It has been shown in literature that the diffusion tensor model does a poor job modeling brain fibers in certain situations. In order to accurately model crossing fiber voxels, it is essential that the model go beyond the assumption of a single normal distribution, or potentially beyond the formulation of the classical diffusion probability. In the next sections,

7.3 Modifications to the Single Exponential Decay Assumption

One of the earliest models applied past the tensor model is called the bi-exponential model [2]. An early observation of the diffusion model is that the data was decaying faster than expected from a single exponential decay (Chap. 1, Eq. 1.2). It was then proposed that perhaps the signal is a result of a bi-exponential decay function, essentially the sum of two decaying exponentials with different diffusion coefficients. In essence, this is modeling a system with two "pools" of Gaussian diffusion, with different diffusion rates for each pool. From modeling the data, it turned out that one of the pools was "fast" and the other was "slow," as defined by their diffusion coefficients. However, this model fell short, as the pools contradicted what was known about the population distribution of cellular components.

After the bi-exponential model was proposed, another model was introduced, this time to better explain the heterogeneity of the tissue being imaged [3]. This model was termed the "stretched-exponential" model, where a stretching exponent, γ, was used to quantify the nature of the tissue that spins diffused through. This proved to be effective in certain pathologies such as gliomas, where there are changes in tissue structure and, therefore, heterogeneity. This model, though, does not take into account the tensorial nature of diffusion, i.e., there is no modeling of the directionality of the exponent, so the exponent itself is dependent on the b-vectors.

One of the most popular non-Gaussian techniques is called Diffusion Kurtosis Imaging (DKI) [4], as discussed in an earlier chapter. Similar to the two previous models, DKI attempts to modify the assumption of a simple exponential decay. In this model, the signal is expanded as a series in terms of the b-value (Eq. 7.2).

$$\log\left[S(b)\right] = \log\left[S(0)\right] - b\bar{D} + \frac{1}{6}b^2\bar{D}^2\bar{K}, \quad (7.2)$$

where the original equation (Chap. 1, Eq. 1.2) did not address the final term. This term includes a new variable, the kurtosis tensor, $\bar{K}$. Kurtosis, in this context, measures how far from a Gaussian distribution the signal is, noting that when $K = 0$, we recover the original diffusion tensor model. Here, $\bar{K}$ is a 15-component tensor, meaning that we need to measure at least 15 diffusion directions in order to determine the full tensor. In addition, the number of b-values that have to be applied is still debated and must be less than 3000 s/mm^2 due to assumptions of the series expansion in Eq. (7.2). The reconstructed data is presented alongside DTI data, with Mean Kurtosis (MK) maps giving contest to MD maps of DTI.

7.4 Biophysical Compartment Models

In dMRI, a single voxel represents a cube of brain tissue with side length on the order of 2 mm. Within this voxel, there is a diverse population of cells in addition to neurons, containing thousands of cells and tissue components. In addition, there are regions of intra- and extracellular spaces. Notice, in the previously described models, the issue of cellular compartment was not addressed; if spins inside and outside a cell diffuse differently, the fraction of spins in each comparment will influence the overall signal.

The first methodology used to address the biophysical compartments is called the ball-and-stick model [5, 6]. This model splits each voxel into an infinitely anisotropic component, the "stick," for each fiber orientation, and an isotropic component, the "ball," to describe the extracellular space (Fig. 7.2). This is also the first model discussed that explicitly allows for multiple fiber orientations in one voxel, which is a major pitfall of DTI.

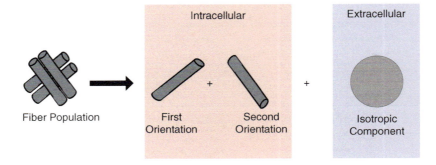

Fig. 7.2 Illustration of ball-and-stick model representation of voxel containing crossing fibers

The signal at each voxel has to now be fit to a model with more unknowns, as the fraction of the voxel containing each component has to be calculated, as well as the number of fiber orientations. Computational techniques have been created to estimate the number of fibers at each orientation, which is much more difficult than assessing the fraction of voxel belonging to each compartment. The ball-and-stick method was found to detect white matter regions of complex fiber architecture that DTI missed, as is expected with the addition of multiple fiber orientations.

At the same time as the ball-and-stick model, the composite hindered and restricted model of diffusion (CHARMED) was developed [7]. CHARMED proposes the same two components, but models them in a different way. The intracellular compartment is now termed as the "restricted" compartment; the diffusion is broken down into two components, diffusion along the fiber and diffusion perpendicular to the fiber. The extracellular compartment is now termed the "hindered" compartment and is modeled using the diffusion tensor model. In addition, the hindered compartment includes effects from glia as a result of the formulation. Therefore, the idea of intra- and extracellular compartments is left behind. It should be noted that CHARMED requires a large range of b-values, with up to ten b-values used ranging from 0 to 10,000 s/mm^2, and leads to a long scan time, making it less frequently used for *in vivo* scanning. Nevertheless, literature has suggested that CHARMED provides better angular resolution of fiber orientations that is more robust to noise compared to diffusion tensor methods [8].

The problem of long scan times in these compartment models has limited their implementation in clinical and research practice. Therefore, a new methodology that can assess cellular compartments in a short acquisition time is extremely desirable. In order to solve this problem, Neurite Orientation Dispersion and Density Imaging (NODDI) was introduced. Neurite is a term for the collective structure of axons and dendrites. NODDI was initially created because models such as ball-and-stick and CHARMED fail to address the effect of the dispersion of axonal orientation due to bending and fanning of fiber bundles throughout the brain. NODDI explicitly defines three compartments: intracellular, extracellular, and CSF compartments, each with unique diffusion characteristics. The intracellular compartment is the space bounded by neurites, which can be modeled as a set of sticks. The extracellular compartment is the space around the neurites, composed of glial cells and, in the gray matter, cell bodies. Here, diffusion is modeled as an anisotropic Gaussian, as it is not restricted. The CSF compartment is modeled as an isotropic Gaussian, as spins can diffuse equally in all directions. The overall representation of tissues in NODDI is shown in Fig. 7.3.

NODDI, as the name implies, mainly measures neurite orientation dispersion (OD) and neurite density. The OD is a measure of how many orientations the neurites take in each voxel. It is high when neuronal projections are equally

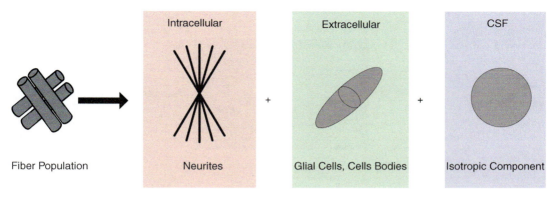

Fig. 7.3 Schematic of NODDI model. Intracellular diffusion is now modeled as neurites modeled as sticks, with extracellular representation as a tensor model with anisotropic diffusion allowed. The model also addresses CSF diffusion as isotropic

distributed in all directions, and low in the case of neurites that are linear. The neurite density is an estimate of how many neuronal projections exist in a voxel.

NODDI is one of the most popular compartment models due to its accuracy, and its model allows for accurate predictions with the use of only two non-zero b-values. In addition, literature has shown that these b-values can be low, still within the realm of clinical scanning, with 30 vectors with a b-value of 700 s/mm^2 and 60 vectors with a b-value of 2000 s/mm^2 [9]. Scanning with b-value 1000 s/mm^2, such as that used in current clinical sequences, has shown good estimates of OD, but it seems that neurite density is only properly modeled in a multi-shell sequence.

7.5 Q-Space Imaging Approaches

In order to discuss Q-space imaging (QSI), we must introduce the diffusion wavevector, $\vec{q}$ (Eq. 7.3).

$$\vec{q} = \frac{\gamma \delta \vec{g}}{2\pi}, \qquad (7.3)$$

where γ is the gyromagnetic ratio, introduced in Chap. 1, δ is the length of the diffusion pulse (Fig. 1.2), and $\vec{g}$ is the b-vector. Q-space is similar to k-space, in that it signifies a Fourier relationship with another variable. K-space is the space defining the Fourier transform of the position variable, and similarly, q-space is the space defining the Fourier transform of the displacement, or the change in position over the diffusion time. The terms single-shell and multi-shell now begin to make sense, as, in q-space, vectors with the same magnitude over different directions form the surface of a sphere. We are then sampling q-space over these shells at radii defined by the b-values. QSI, unlike other diffusion sequences, requires high sampling of q-space on a cartesian grid (called Diffusion Spectrum Imaging, DSI), which is time-intensive, and requires a large range of gradients. The upside of QSI is that it is a model-free method to estimate the "ensemble average propagator" (EAP) (Fig. 7.4). The EAP is the probability density function of diffusion displacement, which, in DTI, for example, is estimated as a Gaussian. The limitations discussed, however, make QSI impractical in most settings; however, adaptations of QSI methods have allowed for faster imaging by exploiting physical properties of diffusion. We will discuss Q-ball imaging (QBI) below.

We will first introduce the High Angular Resolution Diffusion Imaging (HARDI), which governs the underlying image acquisition of QBI. HARDI samples q-space over a

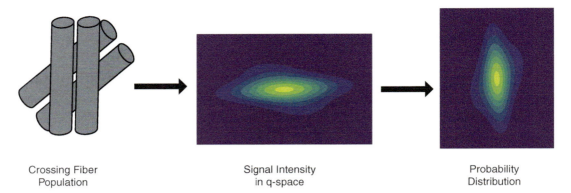

Fig. 7.4 Estimation of EAP using QSI. The signal in q-space is acquired from the scanner; a Fourier transform then gives the estimate of the EAP. Note that the peaks of the EAP correspond to fiber directions. The probability distribution can also be called the Orientation Distribution Function (ODF)

sphere at a high b-value, usually around 3000 s/mm^2; however, research on the b-value and number of b-vectors needed is ongoing. The spherical acquisition allows the sequence to be less time-consuming than QSI. However, since we are no longer sampling on a cartesian grid, the Fourier relationship cannot be directly reconstructed. QBI utilizes the HARDI acquisition protocol, in order to reconstruct the Fourier relationship; QBI exploits the Funk-Radon Transform, which is discussed elsewhere [10]. QBI provides an estimate of the diffusion orientation distribution function (dODF), which describes the angular distribution of diffusion in each voxel, but does not give any information about the radial direction. In addition, by looking at the peaks of the dODF, fiber orientations can be extracted and used for tractography algorithms to generate a tract map of the brain.

7.6 Summary of Advanced Diffusion Protocols

In this chapter, we have discussed three major classes of non-Gaussian diffusion imaging: (1) Models with changes to the exponential model, (2) Biophysical compartment models, and (3) Q-space imaging (model-free imaging). A summary of the discussed models and their main features is given in Fig. 7.5.

7.7 Future Development of Advanced Diffusion Studies

Many of the techniques discussed are now feasible due to technical implementations such as Simultaneous Multislice (SMS) sequences, which allow multiple slices of brain tissue to be imaged at once. These advances have allowed for shortening of the repetition time (TR) and are essential to developing methodologies and models [11]. An example of this is the Human Connectome Project (HCP), a multi-site study which uses the so-called Connectom scanners, which are able to increase gradient strength substantially. The application of SMS and other acceleration factors allows for a high-resolution DSI scan in less than 5 minutes [12]. Although technical advances also potentially introduce new sources of error, for example, SMS carries a risk of leakage artifact, in which signals from slices being acquired at the same time may influence each other. Methods to correct for this phenomenon are already being implemented [13]. In addition, machine learning has been used in the design of faster acquisition sequences and post-processing with heavily undersampled dMRI data [14–17], which further speed up dMRI scans. Overall, the future of advanced dMRI techniques is trending towards higher spatial and temporal resolution with clinical implementation not far behind.

Class	Range of b-values (s/mm^2)	Assumptions	Metrics	Measurement Time
Altered Exponential Model				
Bi-exponential model	2,000 - 10,000	Diffusion can be expressed as sum of two exponentials	Fast and slow diffusion coefficients (D_1, D_2) and volume fractions(f_1, f_2)	20-30 minutes
Stretched-exponential model	500 - 6,500	Diffusion can be expressed as an exponential with a stretching factor, γ	Stretching Factor, γ	20-30 minutes
DKI	Up to 2,000	Non-Gaussian nature of diffusion can be captured by kurtosis	Mean Kurtosis, Apparent Kurotsis	5-10 minutes
Biophysical Compartment Model				
Ball-and-stick model	1,000 - 2,000	Two compartments: Intracellular with restricted diffusion, Extracellular with isotropic diffusion	Fiber Orientation (used for tractography)	5-10 minutes
CHARMED	Up to 10,000	Two compartments: Intracellular with restricted diffusion (parallel and perpendicular), Extracellular with hindered diffusion	Fiber Orientation, Microstructural Parameters, Compartmental diffusion coefficients	20-40 minutes
NODDI	Up to 2,000	Three compartments: Intracellular with restricted diffusion, extracellular with hindered diffusion, CSF with isotropic diffusion	Neurite Density, Orientation Dispersion	20-30 minutes
QSI				
DSI	Up to 12,000	No assumptions	Orientation Distribution Function (ODF)	40-60 minutes
QBI	Above 2,000 (still being investigated)	No assumptions	Diffusion Orientation Distribution Function (dODF)	10-30 minutes

Fig. 7.5 Summary of discussed advanced diffusion imaging techniques along with information about measurements and representative measurement time

References

1. Jeurissen B, Leemans A, Tournier J, Jones D, Sijbers J (2010) Estimating the number of fiber orientations in diffusion MRI voxels: a constrained spherical deconvolution study. ISMRM. p. 573
2. Niendorf T, Dijkhuizen RM, Norris DG, van Campagne M, Nicolay K (1996) Biexponential diffusion attenuation in various states of brain tissue: implications for diffusion-weighted imaging. Magn Reson Med 36:847–857
3. Bennett KM et al (2003) Characterization of continuously distributed cortical water diffusion rates with a stretched-exponential model. Magn Reson Med 50:727–734
4. Jensen JH, Helpern JA, Ramani A, Lu H, Kaczynski K (2005) Diffusional kurtosis imaging: The quantification of non-Gaussian water diffusion by means of magnetic resonance imaging. Magn Reson Med 53:1432–1440
5. Behrens TEJ et al (2003) Characterization and propagation of uncertainty in diffusion-weighted MR imaging. Magn Reson Med 50:1077–1088
6. Behrens TEJ, Berg JH, Jbabdi S, Rushworth MFS, Woolrich MW (2007) Probabilistic diffusion tractography with multiple fibre orientations: what can we gain? NeuroImage 34:144–155
7. Assaf Y, Freidlin RZ, Rohde GK, Basser PJ (2004) New modeling and experimental framework to characterize hindered and restricted water diffusion in brain white matter. Magn Reson Med 52:965–978
8. Assaf Y, Basser PJ (2005) Composite hindered and restricted model of diffusion (CHARMED) MR imaging of the human brain. NeuroImage 27:48–58
9. Zhang H, Schneider T, Wheeler-Kingshott CA, Alexander DC (2012) NODDI: practical in vivo neurite orientation dispersion and density imaging of the human brain. NeuroImage 61:1000–1016
10. Tuch DS (2004) Q-ball imaging. Magn Reson Med 52:1358–1372
11. Feinberg DA, Setsompop K (2013) Ultra-fast MRI of the human brain with simultaneous multi-slice imaging. J Magn Reson 229:90–100
12. Setsompop K et al (2013) Pushing the limits of in vivo diffusion MRI for the Human Connectome Project. NeuroImage 80:220–233
13. Cauley SF et al (2014) Interslice leakage artifact reduction technique for simultaneous multislice acquisitions. Magn Reson Med 72(1):93–102
14. Gao Z (2017) HEp-2 Cell Image Classification with Deep Convolutional Neural Networks. IEEE J Biomed Health Inform 21(2):416–428
15. Rumelhart DE, Hinton GE, Williams RJ (1986) Learning representations by back-propagating errors. Nature 323(6088):533–536
16. Gong T, He H, Li Z, Lin Z, Tong Q, Li C, Sun Y, Yu F, Zhong J (2018) Efficient reconstruction of diffusion kurtosis imaging based on a hierarchical convolutional neural network. ISMRM. 71398–71411
17. Gong T, He H, Lin Z, Li Z, Tong Q, Sun Y, Yu F, Zhong J (2018) Direct and fast learning of fiber orientation distribution function for tractography. ISMRM 46(7):3101–3116

Part II

Clinical Applications of DW Imaging

Brain Edema

8

Toshio Moritani

Badih Junior Daou, Gregory Palmateer, and Aditya S. Pandey

8.1 Characterization and Classification of Brain Edema

Brain edema is defined as an accumulation of excess fluid in cells or in the extracellular space. Brain edema can be classified as cytotoxic (cellular), vasogenic [1], or interstitial. Cytotoxic and vasogenic edema often coexist in pathological conditions such as infarction, hypoxic ischemic encephalopathy, toxic metabolic encephalopathy, encephalitis, trauma, and demyelinating disease. The edema may primarily be either vasogenic or cytotoxic, but as the process evolves over time, the injury can lead to a combination of cellular swelling and vascular damage. Interstitial edema occurs with hydrocephalus, water intoxication, or plasma hyposmolarity [2].

Conventional MR imaging does not always allow distinction between the different forms of edema. However, diffusion-weighted imaging (DWI), which is based on the microscopic movement of water molecules in brain tissue, can differentiate cytotoxic edema from vasogenic or interstitial edema [3].

8.2 Cytotoxic or Cellular Edema

Cytotoxic or cellular edema is defined as an abnormal uptake of fluid in the cytoplasm due to abnormal cellular osmoregulation. Cytotoxic edema is the premorbid cellular process, otherwise known as cellular edema, oncotic cell swelling, or oncosis, whereby extracellular Na^+ and other cations enter into neurons and astrocytes through several different cation channels and accumulate intracellularly, in part due to failure of energy-dependent mechanisms [2].

Recent experimental evidence shows several nonselective cation channels that have been implicated in cytotoxic edema: (1) acid-sensing ion channel, (2) SUR1-regulated NC_{Ca-ATP} channel, (3) TRP channel, (4) NKCC channel, (5) Aquaporin (AQP) channel, and (6) N-methyl-D-aspartate (NMDA) receptor channel [2]. Acid-sensing ion channel may be responsible for acidosis-mediated, glutamate receptor-independent neuronal injury. Depletion of ATP triggers NC_{Ca-ATP} channel opening. NKCC channel mediates the movement of Na^+ and/or K^+ with Cl^-. AQP4 channel is predominantly expressed in astrocytic foot processes surrounding blood vessels and ependymocytes. It is implicated in the formation of either cytotoxic or vasogenic edema [4].

T. Moritani (✉)
Division of Neuroradiology, Department of Radiology, University of Michigan, Ann Arbor, MI, USA
e-mail: tmoritan@med.umich.edu

B. J. Daou
Department of Neurosurgery, University of Michigan, Ann Arbor, MI, USA
e-mail: bdaou@umich.edu

G. Palmateer · A. S. Pandey
University of Michigan, Ann Arbor, MI, USA
e-mail: gpalmate@umich.edu; adityap@umich.edu

© Springer Nature Switzerland AG 2021
T. Moritani, A. A. Capizzano (eds.), *Diffusion-Weighted MR Imaging of the Brain, Head and Neck, and Spine*, https://doi.org/10.1007/978-3-030-62120-9_8

Cytotoxic/cellular edema may accompany various processes that damage cells, such as ischemic stroke, status epilepticus, cortical spreading depression, trauma, toxic metabolic disease, encephalitis, demyelination, and even the early phase of neurodegeneration.

Classification of the involved cell types may explain the pathophysiology and different prognosis of these conditions. CNS is composed of neuroglial units including 100 billion neurons, 1 trillion glia, and 100–500 trillion synapses. The gray and white matters are mainly composed of neurons, glial cells, axons, and myelin sheaths (Fig. 8.1). Oligodendrocytes are glial cells producing myelin sheaths in the CNS. Myelin sheath is continuous with the perikaryon of oligodendrocyte. One oligodendrocyte has approximately 40–50 branches of myelin sheath. Astrocyte end-feet support and regulate myelinated fibers at the node of Ranvier.

In the gray matter, cytotoxic edema occurs mainly in neurons and glial cells (astrocytes, oligodendrocytes) (Fig. 8.2). In the white matter,

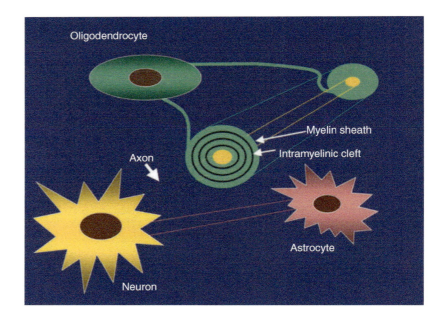

Fig. 8.1 Normal brain tissue is mainly composed of neurons, glial cells (astrocytes or oligodendrocytes), axons, and myelin sheaths surrounded by an extracellular space

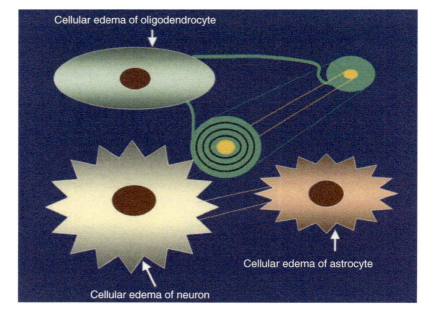

Fig. 8.2 Cytotoxic edema occurs in neurons and glial cells (astrocytes and oligodendrocytes). These cells are vulnerable to ischemia. As cells increase in size, there is a shift of water from extracellular to intracellular compartments, which can occur without a net gain in water (compared with Fig. 8.1). Cytotoxic edema results in increased intracellular space and decreased extracellular space, which may cause a decrease in ADC

however, the edema occurs in glial cells, axons (axonal swelling) (Fig. 8.3), and myelin sheaths (intramyelinic edema) (Fig. 8.4), either selectively or with the combination depending on the underlying disease or the severity of the disease [5]. Ultrastructural appearance of cellular edema after NMDA injection shows swelling of the intracellular organelles such as mitochondrion and endoplasmic reticulum (ER) as well as some scattered ribosomes in the cytoplasm (Fig. 8.5). In intramyelinic edema, trapped water mainly accumulates between the intraperiod lines of the myelin sheath, widened potential space of the extracellular space rather than the cytoplasm. It may be inappropriate to continue to label this phenomenon cytotoxic [6].

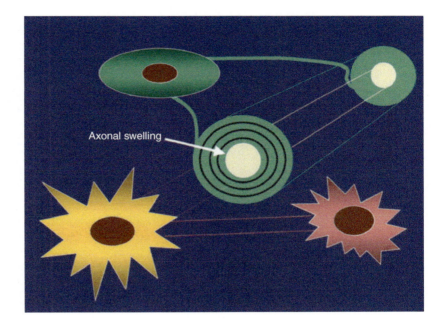

Fig. 8.3 Cytotoxic edema can occur in axons

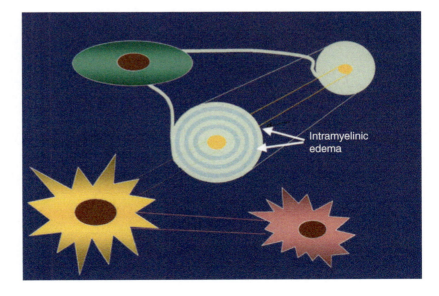

Fig. 8.4 Cytotoxic edema can occur in myelin sheaths in which edema is found in either the myelin sheath itself or in the intramyelinic cleft

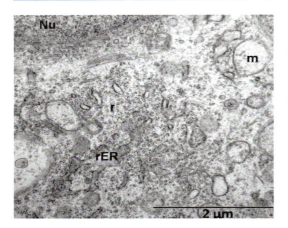

Fig. 8.5 Ultrastructural appearance of cellular edema after NMDA injection shows swelling of the intracellular organelles such as mitochondrion (m) and endoplasmic reticulum (ER) as well as some scattered ribosomes (r) in the cytoplasm. Courtesy of Saggu S, MD, and Casson R, MD (from [51])

8.3 Pathophysiology of Cytotoxic Edema

8.3.1 Energy Failure

In ischemia or hypoxia, cytotoxic edema is mainly caused by energy failure [7]. The insult initiates substrate depletion, which leads to a decrease in intracellular ATP used for oxidative phosphorylation, and a failure of the sodium–potassium pump (Fig. 8.6) [8]. This will cause an influx of sodium and calcium into the cells, subsequently increasing the osmotic gradient and the transport of water into the cells, resulting in cellular swelling, mainly seen in the neurons and astrocytes (Fig. 8.7). Moreover, in an attempt to produce ATP, the cells switch from oxidative phosphorylation to anaerobic glycolysis, resulting in intracellular lactate formation. This will further increase the osmotic gradient across the cell membrane, which exacerbates the cytotoxic edema. Pathologically, injured neurons shrink and become eosinophilic due to increased density of damaged mitochondria. Astrocytes swelling (Alzheimer type II cells) is seen as a response to metabolic insults. The damaged neurons disintegrate and are removed by macrophages. With time, cortical atrophy and gliosis develop.

Energy failure is not the only mechanism responsible for the cytotoxic edema [7]. The insult such as ischemia and seizure initiates substrate depletion in the organelles via secondary messengers (calcium) which leads to a decrease in intracellular ATP, depending on the severity of mitochondrial dysfunction. Severe mitochondrial dysfunction results in pan-necrosis, moderate dysfunction in selective necrosis, and mild or no dysfunction in apoptosis/gliosis or reversible lesion respectively (Fig. 8.6). Membrane transporters can be triggered or inhibited by a range of excitatory neurotransmitters, such as glutamate and aspartate, but also other agents such as cytokines, acidosis, and free radicals [9]. Any cell, including neuron, glia, axon, myelin sheath, and endothelial cells, can be a target of these toxic substances. Neuropathologic examination shows that the acutely reactive astrocytes have swollen cytoplasm and neurophil, consistent with cytotoxic edema [10]. Reactive astrocytes play a significant role in cellular and tissue repair by detoxifying various noxious substances (such as glutamate, free radicals, ammonia, and metals).

8.3.2 Excitotoxic Brain Injury

Excitotoxic brain injury plays an important role in cellular damage in various diseases, and it is the final common pathway resulting in brain injury from any seemingly unrelated diseases [7]. Glutamate, aspartate, and glycine are the dominant excitatory amino acids (EAAs) and the primary neurotransmitters in about one-half of all the synapses in the brain [4]. Among them, glutamate is the most important and responsible for many neurologic functions including cognition, memory, movement, and sensation. In normal brain tissues, concentration of glutamate in the cytoplasm is 10 mmol and only 5 μmol in the extracellular space. High concentration of glutamate in the synaptic and extracellular space is one of the important mechanisms associated with cytotoxic edema of various diseases, including infarction, hypoxic ischemic encephalopathy, status epilepticus, and traumatic brain injury such as diffuse axonal injury, contusion, and abused head injury [11]. In acute excitotoxic injury, increased extracellular glutamate results from an

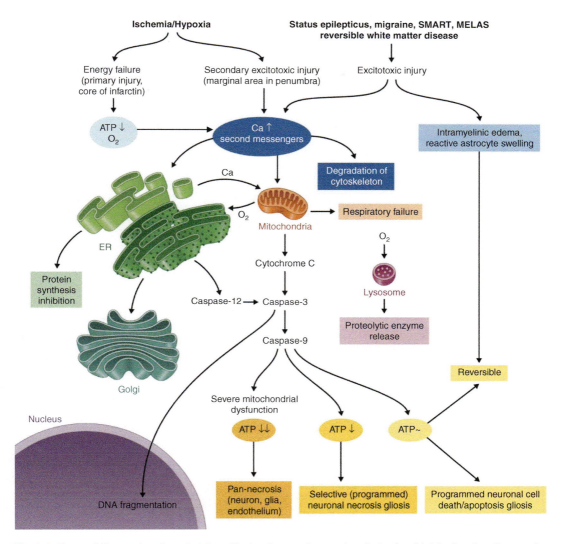

Fig. 8.6 Energy failure and excitotoxic injury. The insult such as ischemia and seizure initiates substrate depletion in the organelles via secondary messengers (calcium) which leads to a decrease in intracellular ATP depending on the severity of mitochondrial dysfunction. Severe mitochondrial dysfunction results in pan-necrosis, moderate dysfunction in selective necrosis, and mild or no dysfunction in apoptosis/gliosis or reversible lesion respectively

increased release/leakage of glutamate or a decreased reuptake (Figs. 8.8 and 8.9) [5].

NMDA receptors are located in the cell membrane of the neurons, glial cells, myelin sheaths, and endothelial cells. Glutamate is released from the presynaptic terminal into the synaptic cleft. The glutamate binding to NMDA receptors allows entry of Ca^{2+} into the postsynaptic neuron, which results in necrotic cell death or apoptosis. Apoptosis is defined as a programmed cell death and is histologically characterized by fragmentation of DNA in the nucleus of the cell. Activation of NMDA receptors also triggers a significant increase in intracellular Na^+ and Cl^-. The glutamate binding to non-NMDA receptors (AMPA receptors and kainic receptors) allows entry of Na^+ into the postsynaptic neuron, resulting in cytotoxic edema. Reuptake of extracellular glutamate takes place at the presynaptic terminals and in adjacent glial cells, which causes cytotoxic edema (acute phase of reactive astrocytosis). Excessive extracellular glutamate depolar-

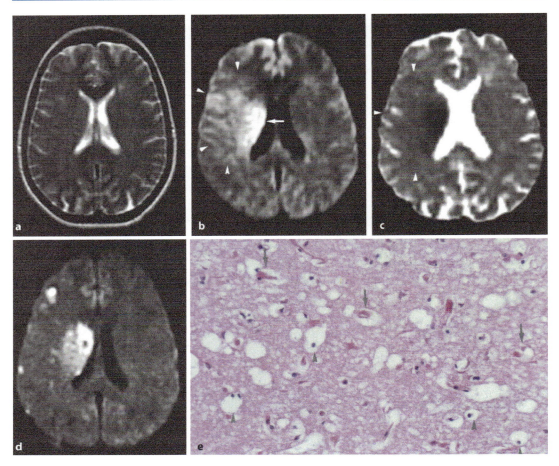

Fig. 8.7 (a–e) Hyperacute cerebral infarction (3 h after onset) in a 39-year-old woman with decreased consciousness. Her neurologic functions improved after intra-arterial thrombolytic therapy. (**a**) T2-weighted image appears normal. (**b**) DWI shows a hyperintense lesion in the right corona radiata (arrow) and a slightly hyperintense lesion in the right middle cerebral artery (MCA) territory, which may correspond to ischemic penumbra (arrowheads). (**c**) ADC map shows a definite decrease in ADC in the corona radiata and slightly decreased ADC in the right MCA territory (arrowheads). (**d**) On DWI after fibrinolytic therapy (3 days after onset), the hyperintense lesion in the cortical area is largely resolved, with remaining small, peripheral infarcts. Early cytotoxic edema with slightly decreased ADC does not always result in infarction. (**e**) Another case. Pathology of cytotoxic edema in the cortex in an acute stroke shows shrunken eosinophilic neurons which are anoxic (arrows) and swollen glial cells (arrowheads) (hematoxylin–eosin stain, original magnification ×200)

izes injured adjacent glial cells or neurons and in turn causes release or leakage of glutamate.

Excitotoxic injury is self-propagating through neuron-glial cell units, and transaxonal or transsynaptic routes along the white matter fiber tracts [5], also known as secondary neuronal degeneration. It can also propagate to other locations through synaptic connections between the various white matter tracts, corpus callosum, superficial and deep gray matter, which is called "Excitatory Circuits" (Figs. 8.10, 8.11, and 8.12).

Excitotoxic injury can also occur likely related to the functional failure of the glutamate receptor in Creutzfeldt–Jakob disease (CJD) [12] (Fig. 8.13, see Chap. 9, Figs. 9.13, 9.14, and 9.15), autoantibodies to the NMDA receptor in anti-NMDA antibody receptor encephalitis (see Chap. 12, Fig. 12.25) and Rasmussen encephalitis [13] (see Chap. 12, Fig. 12.23), or the presence of structurally similar substances to glutamate at the receptor sites such as hydroxyglutarate or glutarate in some metabolic diseases [7].

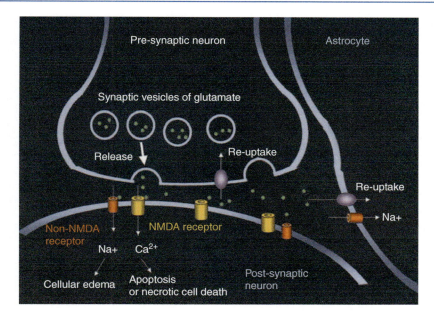

Fig. 8.8 Excitotoxic mechanisms in the neuron and astrocyte. In the neuron, glutamate is released from the presynaptic terminal into the synaptic cleft. The glutamate binding to NMDA receptors allows entry of Ca2+ into the postsynaptic neuron, which can result in necrotic cell death or apoptosis. The glutamate binding to non-NMDA receptors allows entry of Na+ into the postsynaptic neuron, resulting in cytotoxic edema of the neuron. Reuptake of extracellular glutamate takes place at the presynaptic terminals and in adjacent astrocytes. Similar mechanisms also cause cytotoxic edema in the astrocyte

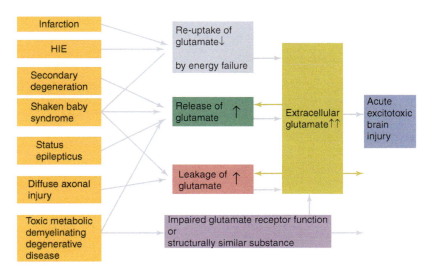

Fig. 8.9 Acute excitotoxic brain injury in various diseases. Various diseases are associated with acute excitotoxic brain injury. The mechanisms are classified into: (1) decreased reuptake, (2) increased release, (3) leakage due to disruption of axonal membranes, (4) others, including impaired glutamate receptor function or substances structurally similar to glutamate. There are various combinations of mechanisms according to each disease process. There are two positive feedback loops (yellow arrow): (1) increased extracellular glutamate depolarizes adjacent neurons that release intracellular glutamate; (2) neuronal injury causes leakage of glutamate. This mechanism is self-propagating via neuron-glial cell units and via transaxonal or transsynaptic routes along the fiber tracts. (From [5])

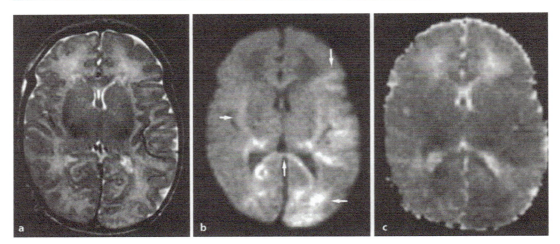

Fig. 8.10 (**a–c**) A 2-day-old term girl with hypoxic ischemic encephalopathy due to perinatal hypoxia–ischemia event. (**a**) T2-weighted image appears normal. (**b**) DWI shows hyperintense lesions in the temporo-occipital gray and white matter including the corpus callosum (*arrows*). Low intensity in bilateral frontal deep white matter (*arrowheads*) is a normal finding in a patient of this age. (**c**) ADC map shows these lesions as decreased ADC representing cytotoxic edema. Increased ADC in the frontal deep white matter is also a normal finding in a patient of this age. These ischemic lesions are more clearly seen on DWI than on the ADC map because DWI depicts subtle T2 contrast abnormalities (T2 shine-through effect) in addition to the contrast of diffusion restriction of these lesions

Glutamate also directly modulates vascular permeability [14]. Glutamate enhances calcium influx and NO levels within or adjacent to microvascular structures, leading to increased vascular permeability through activation of NMDA receptor. High extracellular concentration of glutamate is potentially related to blood–brain barrier (BBB) breakdown and vasogenic edema.

Glutamate receptor-mediated excitatory neurotransmission plays a key role in neural development, differentiation, and synaptic plasticity [15]. During brain development (perinatal, early infant), the pediatric brain is more vulnerable to the excitotoxic injury than the adult brain. The pediatric brain during the first 2 years of life has abundant EAA (such as glutamate) receptors. There is overexpression of EAA receptors related to synaptogenesis. NMDA receptors dominate in the immature brain. GABA receptors are excitatory in early infants whereas inhibitory in adults. However, non-NMDA receptors (AMPA receptors and kainic receptors) predominate during maturation. Pediatric secondary degeneration tends to be more widely distributed via Wallerian and trans-synaptic degenerations and therefore presents earlier when compared to adults (Figs. 8.10, 8.11, and 8.12). With shaken baby syndrome, glutamate levels in the CSF are extremely high (see Chap. 19, Figs. 19.14, 19.15, and 19.16) [16]. In experimental acute subdural hematomas in shaken infant rat brain, glutamate increases more than seven times over baseline levels [17].

8.3.3 Cytokinopathy/Cytokine Storm and Excitotoxic Mechanisms (Fig. 8.14)

Cytokines are a group of proteins for inter-cell communication and biological protection. The cytokines from different cells upregulate or downregulate each other constituting the "Cytokine Networks" or "Cytokine Cascades." Many of these cell-cytokine relationships include feedback loops that are exponentially amplified resulting in so-called "Cytokine Storm" [18]. Cytokine storm and cytokinopathy have been reported to be related to a variety of diseases and syndromes including COVID-19 (see Chap. 16, Figs. 16.5 and 16.51).

Tumor necrosis factor-α (TNF-α), interleukin 1 (IL-1), and IL-6 are especially important in

8 Brain Edema

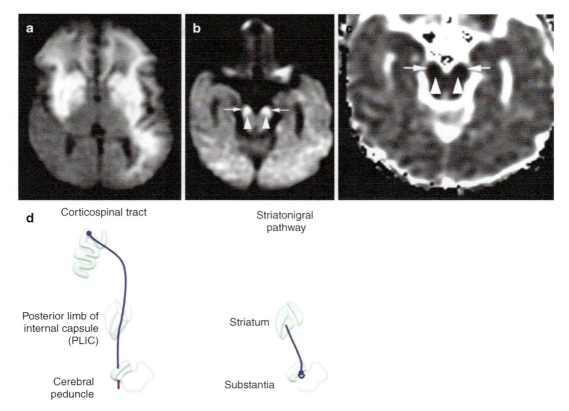

Fig. 8.11 (a–d) Bilateral pre-Wallerian and transsynaptic degeneration in a 10-day-old baby with hypoxic ischemic encephalopathy. (a, b) DWI shows hypoxic ischemic encephalopathy involving bilateral fronto-parietal lobes and basal ganglia as well as pre-Wallerian degeneration along the corticospinal tracts (arrows) and substantia nigra (arrowheads) bilaterally via striatonigral pathway associated with decreased ADC (c), which comprise "Excitotoxic Circuits." (d) Striatonigral pathway is fiber connections originating in the striatum projecting over the substantia nigra. Courtesy of Dr. Atsuhiko Handa and Dr. Jay Starkey. Loss of inhibitory GABAergic output from the ischemic lesion can induce postsynaptic long-term potentiation or a continuous excitatory state in the substantia nigra, resulting in neuronal swelling

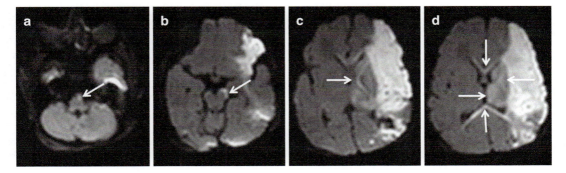

Fig. 8.12 (a–d) Pre-Wallerian and transsynaptic degeneration in a 6-day-old full-term baby with acute infarction in the left middle cerebral artery territory. (a, b) DWI shows acute infarcts involving the left middle cerebral artery territory with pre-Wallerian degeneration along the left corticospinal tract (arrows), and anterior and posterior corpus callosum (arrows). (c, d) Mild diffusion hyperintensities in the left basal ganglia and thalamus (arrows) are likely due to transsynaptic degeneration via striatocortical and thalamocortical connections, which comprise "Excitotoxic Circuits"

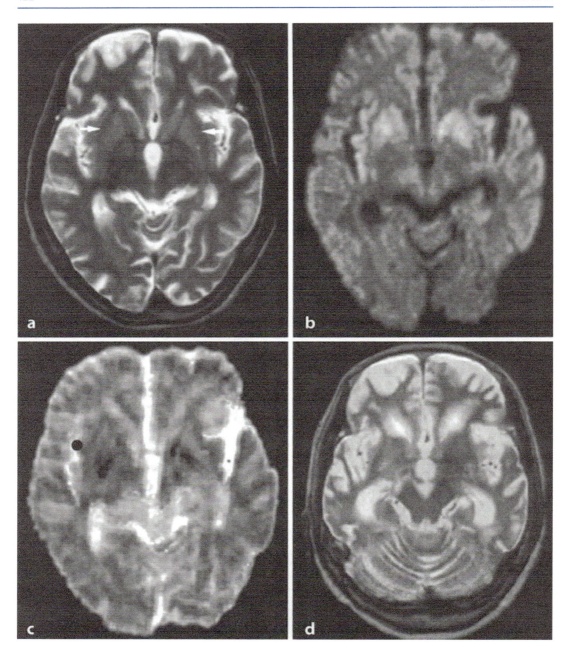

Fig. 8.13 (**a–d**) Creutzfeldt–Jakob disease in a 72-year-old woman with progressive dementia. (**a**) T2-weighted image demonstrates mildly increased signal bilaterally in the caudate nuclei and putamina (*arrows*). (**b**) DWI clearly demonstrates bilateral, symmetrical increase in signal intensity in the caudate nuclei and putamina. (**c**) ADC map shows these lesions as decreased ADC. (**d**) Four-month follow-up MR imaging shows prominent brain atrophy

CNS pathology. These cytokines modulate ion currents through neuronal membrane in glia and neurons and modify synthesis of neurotransmitters. Astrocytes and oligodendrocytes secrete cytokines and regulate homeostasis of glutamate.

With CNS infection and inflammation, monocytes are activated, migrate into the brain tissue, and become macrophages. The macrophages are activated and release IL-1 and IL-6 into the extracellular matrix [19]. T cell lymphocytes are

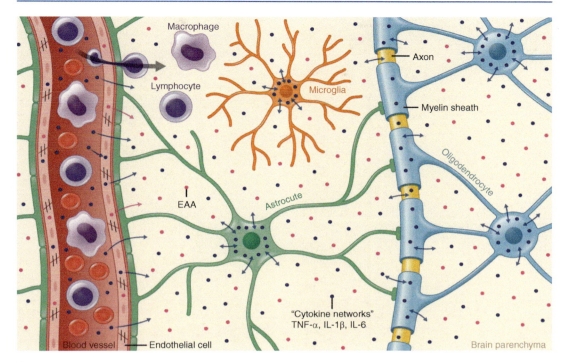

Fig. 8.14 With CNS infection and inflammation, monocytes are activated, migrate into the brain tissue, and become macrophages. The macrophages are activated and release IL-1 and IL-6 into the extracellular matrix. T cell lymphocytes are recruited and affect the endothelial cells leading to BBB breakdown. Microglia subsequently become activated and produce more cytokines. IL-1β induces synthesis of TNF-α and inhibits glutamate reuptake by astrocytes and increases glutamate release, thus increasing extracellular glutamate which results in cytotoxic edema

recruited and affect the endothelial cells leading to BBB breakdown. Microglia subsequently become activated and produce more cytokines. IL-1β induces synthesis of TNF-α and inhibits glutamate reuptake by astrocytes and increases glutamate release, thus increasing extracellular glutamate which results in cytotoxic edema (Figs. 8.8 and 8.14).

Mild encephalitis/encephalopathy with a reversible splenial lesion (MERS), or cytotoxic lesions of the corpus callosum (CLOCCs) have been reported in influenza, rotavirus (Fig. 8.15), and Epstein-Barr virus, measles encephalopathy, Salmonella, herpes 6, mumps, varicella-zoster, adenovirus, legionnaires, and hemolytic uremic syndrome [19, 20, 21]. Markedly elevated IL-6 in CSF and serum has been reported in MERS. Elevated IL-6 level suggests that remote activation of intracerebral immune response through the immune-neuroendocrine pathway plays an important role in the pathophysiology. CLOCCs occur in epileptic patients with or without medication (Fig. 8.16). A number of irregularities in cytokine production have been found in epileptic patients [22]. Antiepileptic medication such as phenytoin, vigabatrin, carbamazepine, and valproic acid can influence the production of pro-inflammatory and pro-convulsive cytokines. Excitatory synaptic cortico-cortical connections are mediated by the corpus callosum. 200–350 million nerve fibers are connected through the corpus callosum in humans. The corpus callosum, especially the splenium, has higher density of cytokine, EAA, toxin, and drug receptors than other brain areas [23], which presumably induces more cytotoxic edema.

Increased various cytokines in the CSF are observed as an inflammatory response to infection in bacterial or viral meningoencephalitis. Some of these virus and bacterial infections are associated with acute necrotizing encephalopa-

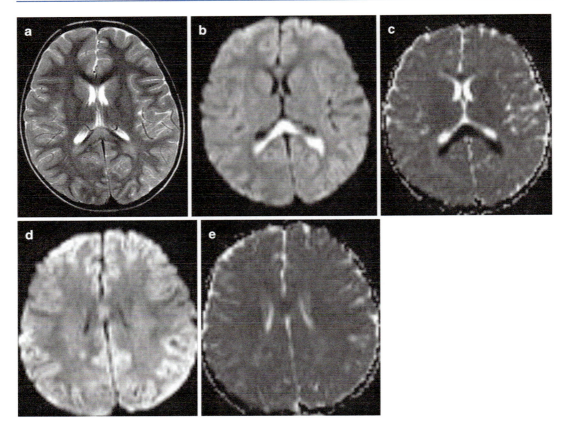

Fig. 8.15 (**a–e**) Symmetric corpus callosum lesions in acute encephalopathy with rotavirus gastroenteritis. 5-years-old male. T2-weighted image and DWI with ADC maps show splenial lesions extending in posterior deep white matter bilaterally and in the anterior corpus callosum (**a–c**) through the callosal body (**d, e**) which are completely resolved at 4-day follow-up MRI

thy (ANE) (Fig. 8.17), hemorrhagic shock and encephalopathy syndrome, Reye syndrome, and hemophagocytic lymphohistiocytosis (HLH) (see Chap. 16, Fig. 16.9), which are characterized by hypercytokinemia and cytokine storm. Toxin-mediated immune activation can cause endothelial injury and edema in sepsis-associated encephalopathy and hemolytic uremic syndrome (see Chap. 11, Fig. 11.24).

In cerebral malaria, essentially 2 types of mechanism causing brain parenchymal lesions are suggested: (1) Capillaries blockage causes ischemia and (2) Cerebral toxicity by cytokine. Pathologically, infected RBC, platelet, and leukocyte sequestration adhesive to the endothelium are observed within microvessels [24]. Activated macrophage and lymphocytes migrate into the Virchow-Robin space. CD8 T lymphocyte mediates to damage the microvascular endothelium causing leakage of pro-inflammatory cytokines (TNF-α, lymphotoxin-α, interferon-γ) and increased BBB permeability to cytokines. These cytokines activate microglia and astrocytes producing more cytokines resulting in extensive cytotoxic edema (see Chap. 16, Fig. 16.32).

8.4 Diffusion-Weighted Imaging and Cytotoxic Edema

Cytotoxic edema characteristically shows hyperintensity on DWI associated with decreased apparent diffusion coefficient (ADC). The precise mechanisms underlying the reduction in

8 Brain Edema

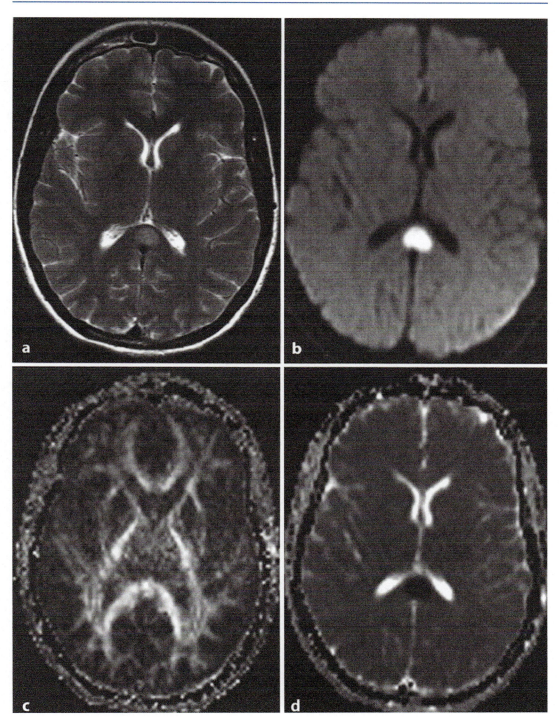

Fig. 8.16 (**a–d**) A reversible focal lesion of the splenium of the corpus callosum in a 26-year-old woman. (**a**) T2-weighted image shows a hyperintense lesion in the splenium of the corpus callosum. (**b**) DWI shows this lesion as hyperintense. (**c**) This lesion has decreased ADC, representing cytotoxic edema, presumably intramyelinic edema which is usually completely reversible. (**d**) FA is relatively preserved

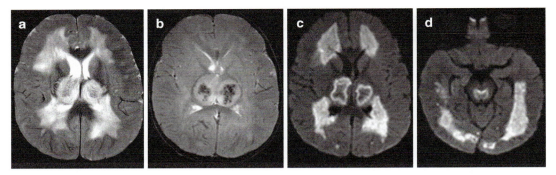

Fig. 8.17 (**a–d**) Acute necrotizing encephalopathy (ANE) with parainfluenza virus infection. A 13-month-old male presented with unresponsiveness after viral upper respiratory infection. T2-weighted image (**a**) and SWI (**b**) and DWI (**c, d**) show extensive symmetric lesions involving bilateral thalami, brainstem, and deep white matter with microhemorrhage and necrosis. The pathogenesis of ANE is thought to be overproduction of cytokines, so-called cytokine storm

ADC are not well understood. The most common explanation is a shift of extracellular water to the intracellular space. There must be a reduction in diffusivity of water molecules in the intracellular space which may be explained by the large number of intracellular organelles, which may act as obstacles for diffusion.

There are two things that prevent water molecule movement in the biological tissues: (1) Membranous structures and (2) Macromolecules (Fig. 8.18). Membranous geometric deformation of the cell membrane, axonal membrane, myelin sheath, or intracellular organelle's membrane is one of the important causes of the water molecule diffusion restriction. Neurite beading has recently been proposed as a mechanism for the diffusion changes after ischemic stroke with some ex vivo evidence. This has been studied using complex geometric models of non-uniformed swollen neurites (i.e., beading) and oscillating gradient spin-echo (OGSE) diffusion MRI (see Chap. 26) [25–27]. Normally, the intracellular space composes 80% and extracellular space 20% of the total brain volume. If pure cytotoxic/cellular edema occurs, the volume of the intracellular space is increased to 95% of the brain volume, while the extracellular space is decreased to 5%. The decrease in water ADC arises largely from the changes in the intracellular space based on Cs 133 NMR study with global CNS ischemia in rat brain [28]. However, the observed 40% reduction of ADC cannot be explained by an increase in intracellular water alone, even if all extracellular fluid went intracellular [29]. A recent study suggests that a decrease in the energy-dependent intracellular circulation, cytoplasmic streaming, or axoplasmic flow is too slow (less than 1 μm/s) to affect the ADC values [30].

The macromolecules are another cause of water molecule diffusion restriction, which is called viscosity. Diffusion coefficient and viscosity have the negative correlation based on Stokes-Einstein's formula which was originated from Albert Einstein's PhD thesis [31].

$$D = kT / 6\pi r \times \eta$$

where D: diffusion coefficient, k: constant, T: temperature, r: radius of macromolecule, η: viscosity.

A decrease in intracellular ADC could also be due to an increase in cytoplasmic viscosity from a swelling of intracellular organelles [32]. Neoplasms, epidermoids, hemorrhages, abscesses, and coagulative necrosis also result in a decrease in ADC. The mechanisms underlying the reduction in ADC in those lesions are also not well understood, but can be related to membranous barrier/deformation (edema, epidermoid), macromol-

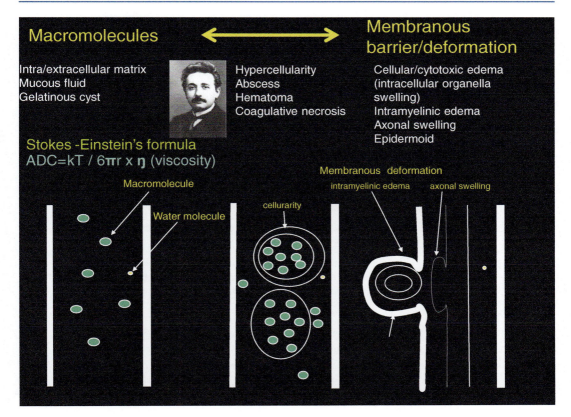

Fig. 8.18 Water molecule diffusion is restricted by "macromolecules" and "membranous barrier/deformation." Water molecule diffusion restriction by macromolecules is so-called viscosity. Diffusion coefficient and viscosity have the negative correlation based on Stokes-Einstein's formula which was originated from Albert Einstein's PhD thesis. Many of the biological and pathological tissues are consistent of the combination of macromolecules and membranous structures

ecules (mucous, hyperviscosity), or a combination of both (hypercellularity, abscess, hematoma, coagulative necrosis) [33, 34] (Fig. 8.18).

8.4.1 Conditions that Cause Cytotoxic Edema, and Reversibility

8.4.1.1 Cytotoxic Edema of Neurons and Glial Cells

Cytotoxic edema of neurons and glial cells usually accompany infarction (Figs. 8.7 and 8.12) [35–38], hypoxic ischemic encephalopathy (Figs. 8.9, 8.10, and 8.11) [39, 40], traumatic brain injury (Fig. 8.19, see Chap. 17, Figs. 17.1, 17.2, 17.3, 17.4, 17.5, 17.6, 17.7, and 17.8) [41, 42], hepatic encephalopathy (see Chap. 15, Fig. 15.21), Wernicke encephalopathy (see Chap. 15, Figs. 15.19 and 15.20), status epilepticus (Figs. 8.20 and 8.21) [11, 43, 44], migraine (Fig. 8.22) [45, 46], stroke-like migraine attacks after radiation therapy (SMART) syndrome (Fig. 8.23), metabolic encephalopathy such as mitochondrial encephalopathy, lactic acidosis, stroke-like episodes (MELAS) (Fig. 8.24), infectious or autoimmune mediated encephalitis [47], CJD (Fig. 8.12, see Chap. 14, Figs. 14.13, 14.14, and 14.15), and other neurodegenerative diseases such as neuronal intranuclear inclusion disease (see Chap. 14, Fig. 14.16) [48, 49].

Neurons and glial cells are the cells most vulnerable to ischemia and hypoxia; however, if the ischemia is severe, axons and myelin sheaths are

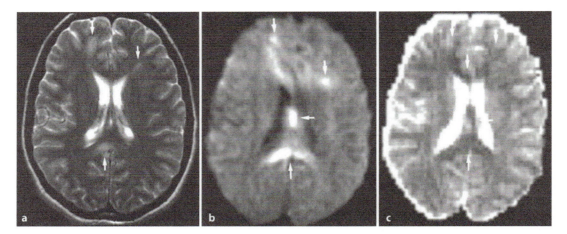

Fig. 8.19 (a–c) Diffuse axonal injury in an 18-year-old female patient 48 h after motor vehicle accident. (**a**) T2-weighted image shows mildly hyperintense lesions in the corpus callosum and the white matter of bilateral frontal lobes (arrows). (**b**) DWI demonstrates diffuse axonal injury as high signal intensity, representing cytotoxic edema (arrows). (**c**) ADC map shows decreased ADC lesions in the anterior to posterior corpus callosum and the frontal deep white matter (arrows)

also affected [7]. Astrocytes are more prone to pathological swelling than neurons, because they are involved in the clearance of K+ and glutamate [2]. Expression of high levels of the water channel AQP4 in astrocytes is also important. These differences among cell types for cytotoxic edema can explain the different time courses of diffusion abnormalities between gray and white matter in cerebral infarction and hypoxic ischemic encephalopathy [25, 50]. Recent studies have shown that the receptors related to excitotoxic mechanisms are widely distributed in the brain, not only in the gray matter (neurons and astrocytes) but also in the white matter (astrocytes, oligodendrocytes, myelin sheaths, and possibly in axons) [51, 52].

In arterial infarction, the area of cytotoxic edema on DWI seems to be irreversibly damaged tissue, resulting in coagulative or liquefactive necrosis. However, the area of decreased ADC in the ischemic penumbra can be reversible after intra-arterial or intravenous fibrinolytic therapy or even spontaneously (Fig. 8.7). In transient ischemic attack and venous infarction, an initially abnormal signal on DWI has occasionally been reversed, partially or completely, on follow-up MR images.

In hyperammonemic hepatic encephalopathy (see Chap. 15, Fig. 15.21), extracellular glutamine accumulation causes selective astrocyte swelling. Ammonia is normally detoxified in the liver and extrahepatic tissues by conversion to urea and glutamine. In the brain, glutamine synthesis is largely confined to astrocytes [53]. Brain edema in hyperammonemic hepatic encephalopathy shows diffusion restriction which is potentially reversible if it is not severe and treated earlier.

In Wernicke encephalopathy (see Chap. 15, Figs. 15.19 and 15.20), thiamine deficiency reduces Krebs cycle and pentose phosphate pathway efficiency [54]. Intracellular accumulation of glutamate from transamination of alpha-ketoglutarate limits the function of ATP-dependent cellular pumps, inducing failure to maintain cellular electrolyte homeostasis. Glutamate is consequently discharged in the extracellular space causing cytotoxic edema of glial cells and neurons. The edema is potentially reversible after immediate thiamine administration.

8.4.1.2 Cytotoxic Edema and Cortical Spreading Depolarization/Depression

There are several conditions related to cortical spreading depolarization/depression, including status epilepticus (Figs. 8.19 and 8.20, see Chap. 12, Fig. 12.19), acute encephalopathy with biphasic seizures and late reduced diffusion (AESD) (see Chap. 12, Fig. 12.21), migraine (Fig. 8.21),

8 Brain Edema

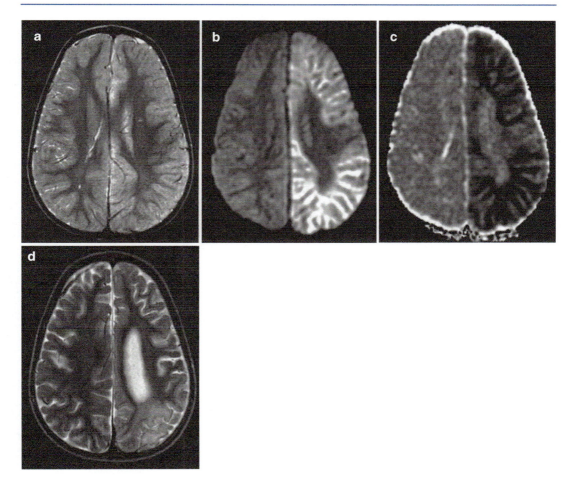

Fig. 8.20 (**a–d**) Status epilepticus in a 2-year-old girl 24 h after onset. (**a**) T2-weighted image shows diffuse cortical hyperintensity in the entire left hemisphere cortex. (**b**) DWI shows diffuse hyperintensity mainly in the gray matter of the left hemisphere. (**c**) ADC map shows decreased ADC of these lesions. (**d**) Diffuse brain atrophy and hyperintense lesions in the left hemisphere are seen on a 5-month follow-up T2-weighted image

SMART syndrome (Fig. 8.22), and possibly with MELAS (Fig. 8.23). Cortical spreading depolarization is a self-propagating wave of abruptly developing, near-complete breakdown of transmembrane ion gradients in neurons and astrocytes that spreads through contiguous cerebral gray matter [55]. The lesion does not correspond to the vascular territory. Spreading depression is a consequence of spreading depolarization.

In status epilepticus, cytotoxic edema is thought to be primarily located in neurons of the cortex but may extend into the subcortical white matter likely via excitotoxic mechanisms. Intramyelinic edema can also be seen in the underlying subcortical white matter in status epilepticus (see Chap. 12, Fig. 12.19d). It is often partially or completely reversible because the edema is likely due to pure excitotoxic injury without an energy failure. However, if severe, they may result in selective necrosis followed by brain atrophy or gliosis [11, 46]. A cytotoxic edema of reactive astrocytes in the acute phase can be responsible for the reversible signal abnormalities [11]. In status epilepticus, the hippocampus is often involved (70%), particularly CA1 and CA4 which have high density of NMDA receptors. Pulvinar involvement is also common (26%) which has rich reciprocal axonal connections to the temporal lobe and plays a role in seizure propagation and generalization [56].

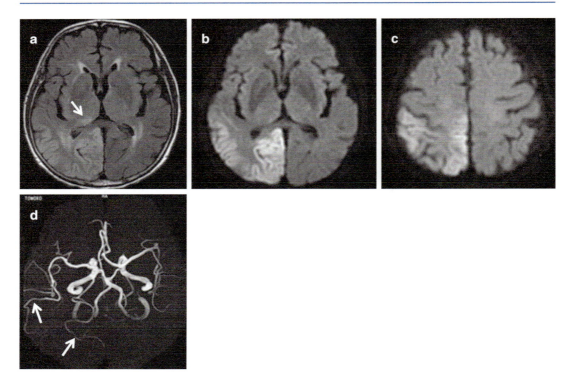

Fig. 8.21 (**a–d**) Status epilepticus with Lance-Adams syndrome. An 81-year-old female who developed status epilepticus several months after the treatment of CO_2 narcosis. Hyperintense FLAIR (**a**), and DWI (**b** and **c**) signal lesions are noted in the right parietal and occipital lobe, and pulvina of the right thalamus. Right pulvinar lesion shows no diffusion restriction likely representing a vasogenic edema (arrow). MRA (**d**) shows dilated right middle and posterior cerebral artery branches (arrows), compared to the left side. The cause of Lance-Adams syndrome is thought to be functional or microscopic abnormalities which later leads to status epilepticus. Prophylactic anti-epileptic medication is very important to avoid status epilepticus

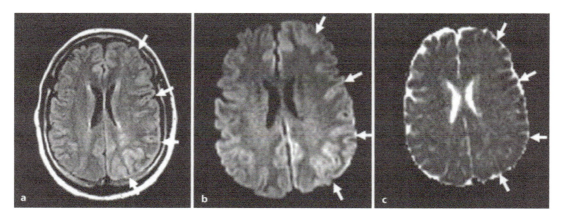

Fig. 8.22 (**a–c**) Migraine in a 37-year-old woman. (**a**) FLAIR image shows diffuse mild cortical hyperintensity in the left hemisphere (*arrows*). (**b**) DWI shows slightly increased intensity in the cortex (*arrows*). (**c**) ADC map shows decreased ADC of the lesions (*arrows*)

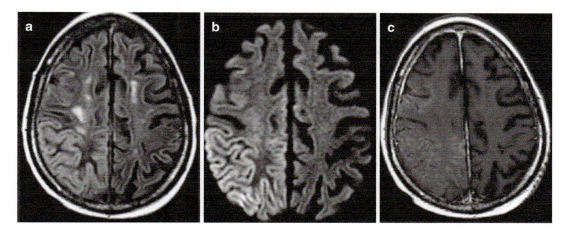

Fig. 8.23 (a–c) SMART syndrome. A 50-year-old man who presents with subacute onset of left-sided weakness, dysphagia, dysarthria, and possible seizure activity. There is a history of pineal teratoma status post whole brain radiation 20 years ago. FLAIR (a) and DWI (b) show hyperintensity along the right fronto-parietal cortices with enhancement on postcontrast-T1-weighted image (c)

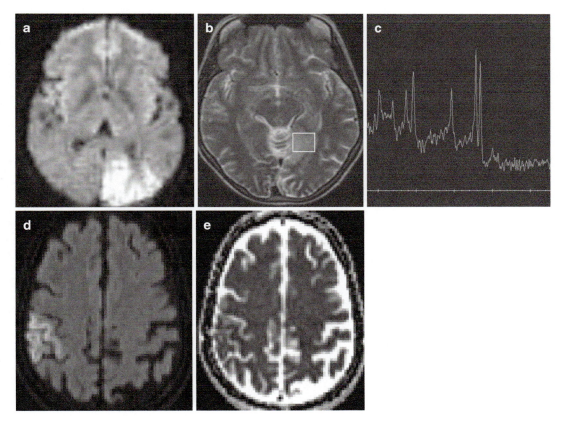

Fig. 8.24 (a–e) MELAS. A 24-year-old woman with a stroke-like symptom. (a) DWI and T2-weighted image (b) show hyperintense lesion in the left occipital and temporal lobes mimicking cortical diffusion restriction seen in status epilepticus. However, MR spectroscopy reveals the classic doublet lactate peak (c). (d, e) Three years later, DWI (d) shows the diffusion hyperintense lesion with mildly decreased ADC (e) which is now seen in the right parietal lobe

In MELAS, neuronal hyperexcitability and cortical spreading play an important role in lesion distribution and reversibility [57, 58]. Energy imbalance between energy requirement and availability of ATP due to oxidative phosphorylation defect in the susceptible neuron, which may cause cortical necrosis. SMART syndrome is a rare delayed complication of brain irradiation. The pathogenesis may be closer to migraine or epilepsy [59]. Radiation-induced mitochondrial dysfunction is one of the suggested pathogeneses of SMART syndrome.

8.4.1.3 Axonal Swelling

Axonal swelling with neurite beading has recently been proposed as a mechanism for the diffusion changes after ischemic stroke [25]. Axonal swelling also accompanies traumatic (diffuse) axonal injury which is usually irreversible (Fig. 8.19, see Chap. 17). Axonal injury represents mechanical breaking of the axonal cytoskeleton and microtubules, transport interruption and accumulation of transported materials with proteolysis, and axonal swelling which is called "axonal bulb/beads" or "retraction ball" [60, 61] (Fig. 8.25). Other possible mechanism of cytotoxic edema is axonal disruption at the node of Ranvier, leading to leakage of glutamate into the extracellular space producing swelling of the surrounding axons and myelin sheaths (Fig. 8.26). Diffusion-tensor imaging (DTI) may be useful in assessing patients with traumatic brain injury, although it remains unclear what neuropathological substrates are for changes on DTI (see Chap. 17, Fig. 17.18).

In acute stroke, decreased ADC in the white matter is thought to be mainly related to axonal beading and swelling based on Monte-Carlo simulations using OGSE diffusion [25].

Secondary neuronal degeneration occurs in the CNS after many primary events including various acute and chronic diseases. The early phase of Wallerian degeneration (pre-Wallerian

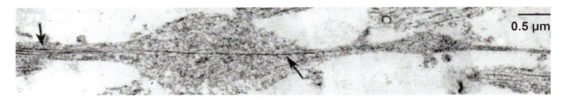

Fig. 8.25 Electron microscopy of axonal swelling. Microtubule breakage and varicose axonal swellings after dynamic stretch injury of axons. Transmission electron microscopy shows a solitary intact microtubule traversing a large swelling (arrow) whereas multiple microtubules can be observed in the adjacent non-swollen region from which it emerged (arrow). Courtesy of Tang-Schomer M PhD. (From [60])

Fig. 8.26 One of the mechanisms of cytotoxic edema in traumatic axonal injury is due to axonal disruption at the node of Ranvier, leading to leakage glutamate into the extracellular space, which causes swelling in the surrounding myelin sheath and astrocyte (excitotoxic mechanisms)

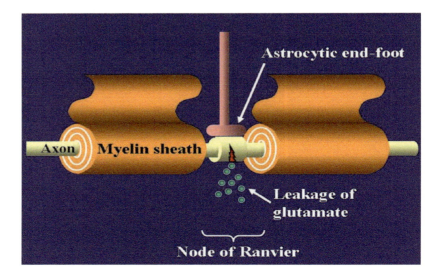

degeneration) pathologically demonstrates axonal spheroid formation (swelling) and surrounding intramyelinic edema, both of which cause diffusion restriction (Figs. 8.11, 8.12, 8.27 and 8.28) [51, 62]. Wallerian-type degeneration can occur in the corpus callosum and middle cerebellar peduncles (Fig. 8.12) [63]. Transsynaptic (transneuronal) degeneration is another specific type of injury which can occur in variable locations in the CNS (Fig. 8.11). Restriction of diffusion in the striatum and/or thalamus is likely due to transsynaptic degeneration via the striatocortical and/or thalamocortical connections (Fig. 8.12) [64].

In CJD, spongiform degeneration, actually representing cellular edema in early phase, is noted in the axons, dendrites, and astrocytes, which causes diffusion restriction (Fig. 8.13). CJD will eventually develop into prominent brain atrophy. One of the key physiological roles of prion protein may be regulation of NMDA receptor activity, leading to chronic "cytodegeneration" of elements in both gray and white matter regions of the CNS [12].

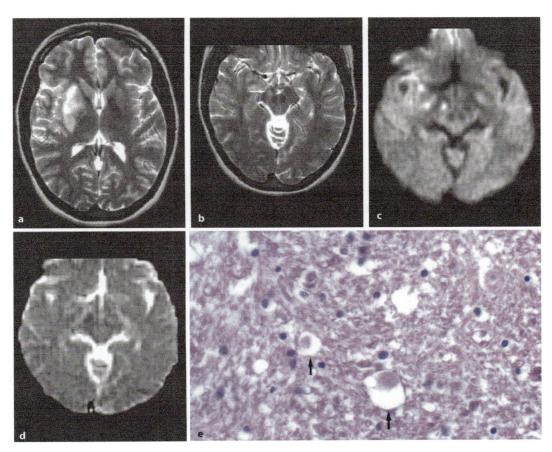

Fig. 8.27 (a–e) An early phase of Wallerian degeneration in a 20-year-old woman with subacute infarction (72 h after onset). (a) T2-weighted image shows a hyperintense lesion involving the right basal ganglia, the posterior limb of the internal capsule and corona radiata, representing a subacute infarct. (b) T2-weighted image shows a hyperintense lesion along the ipsilateral corticospinal tract (arrow) and substantia nigra (arrowheads) in the cerebral peduncle, which represents Wallerian and transneuronal degeneration secondary to the infarction in the right basal ganglia and corona radiata. (c, d) DW image shows a hyperintense spot in the right cerebral peduncle associated with decreased ADC, which may represent axonal swelling in the early phase of Wallerian and transneuronal degeneration. (e) Another case of the early phase of Wallerian degeneration. Histopathology shows axonal swelling as an enlarged axon in the corticospinal tract in the brain stem (arrows) (hematoxylin–eosin stain, original magnification ×200)

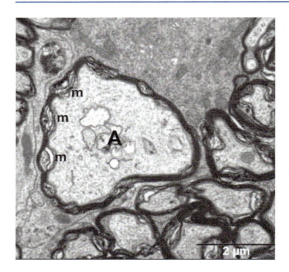

Fig. 8.28 Electron microscopy of axonal swelling. Ultrastructural appearances of axonal swellings after NMDA injection. Electron microscopy shows swollen axons (A) with abnormal collection of altered tubulovesicular structures and surrounding multilayered myelin sheath (m). Courtesy of Saggu S, MD, and Casson R, MD (from [51])

8.4.1.4 Intramyelinic Edema

Intramyelinic edema is one of the plausible explanations of complete or nearly complete reversibility of diffusion restricted edema in various diseases. Intramyelinic edema can occur in an acute cytotoxic plaque of multiple sclerosis (Fig. 8.29) [65], acute disseminated encephalomyelitis (see Chap. 13, Fig. 13.14), vigabatrin-associated vacuolar myelinopathy (Fig. 8.30), spectrum of reversible splenial lesion of corpus callosum (Figs. 8.15 and 8.16), metronidazole-induced encephalopathy (see Chap. 15, Fig. 15.7), drug-induced encephalopathy (see Chap. 15, Figs. 15.2, 15.3, 15.5, and 15.6), delayed post-anoxic leukoencephalopathy (see Chap. 15, Fig. 15.11), chemotherapy-induced leukoencephalopathy (Figs. 15.2 and 15.3), osmotic myelinolysis (see Chap. 15, Fig. 15.16) [67], metabolic and toxic leukoencephalopathies (phenylketonuria, maple syrup urine disease, Canavan disease, metachromatic leukodystrophy etc.) (Fig. 8.31, see Chap. 19, Figs. 19.85 and 19.88), and X-linked dominant Charcot Marie Tooth neuropathy [68–70] (see Chap. 19, Fig. 19.49).

Myelin sheath is composed of the inner and outer membranes: the cell processes of oligodendrocyte (Fig. 8.32) [71]. Fusion of the inner membranes forms the major dense line made by the part of the cytoplasm (intracellular space), line to line 12 nm. Fusion of the outer membrane forms the minor dense line (intraperiod or interperiod line, intramyelinic cleft) which is potentially the "extracellular space (ECS)." Intramyelinic edema predominantly occurs within the intramyelinic cleft, potential ECS but not continuous with ECS of the brain, and the BBB remains intact. Intramyelinic edema may occur in the intracellular space (major dense line) if the insult is more severe [72]. The edema even in the "closed" extracellular space in the myelin sheath can cause restricted diffusion probably related to the geometric distortion of the membranous structures. Complete reversibility of intramyelinic edema appears to be related to the edema in the intramyelinic cleft. Myelin sheath is one of the targets of the excitotoxic amino acids such as a glutamate.

In an immunohistochemical study, acute multiple sclerosis plaques showed high glutamate concentration in close proximity to axonal damage that may cause intramyelinic edema [73]. In vigabatrin-associated vacuolar myelinopathy, electron microscopy demonstrates splitting myelin at minor dense (intraperiod) line, which is a potential ECS (Fig. 8.30) [66]. Vigabatrin (antiepileptic drug) increases GABA concentration and inadvertently leads to excitotoxicity to the myelin sheath in infants. Function and predominant distribution of the excitatory and inhibitory receptors evolve along brain maturation. A focal lesion in the splenium of the corpus callosum in epileptic patients or those with encephalitis/encephalopathy is often completely reversible (Fig. 8.15 and 8.16) [74–76]. The explanation for this complete reversibility of the lesion is probably the intramyelinic edema where the edema is often primarily located in the intramyelinic cleft (minor dense or interperiod line), which is a potential ECS [5]. However, in a recent OGSE DWI study with Monte Carlo simulation, axonal swelling is a suggested cause of diffusion restriction of the splenial lesion [77].

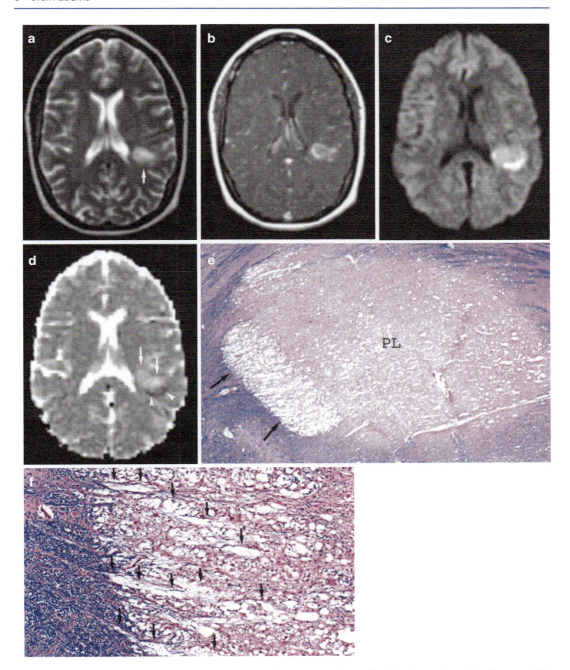

Fig. 8.29 (**a–f**) Multiple sclerosis in a 36-year-old woman with subacute onset of progressive aphasia. (**a**) T2-weighted image shows a hyperintense lesion in the periventricular white matter (*arrow*). (**b**) Gadolinium T1-weighted image with magnetization transfer contrast shows rim enhancement of this lesion. (**c**) DWI shows a combination of moderately hyperintense and significantly hyperintense lesions. (**d**) On ADC, the moderately hyperintense lesion on DWI has an increased ADC, which may represent demyelination (*arrows*), while the markedly hyperintense lesion on the DWI, with decreased ADC, may represent intramyelinic edema (*arrowheads*). (**e**) Another case. Histopathology shows that intramyelinic edema (*arrows*) is located in the periphery of a plaque (*PL*) (Luxol fast blue PAS stain, original magnification ×40). (**f**) Magnification of (**e**). Intramyelinic edema is seen along the myelin sheaths (*arrows*) (Luxol fast blue PAS stain, original magnification ×200). (From [43])

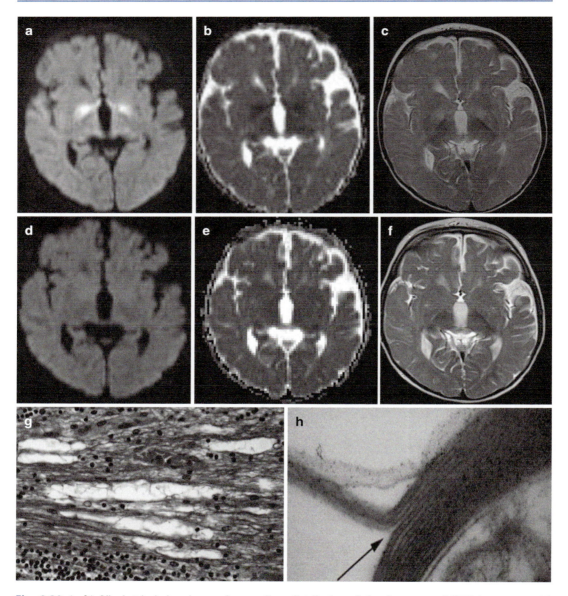

Fig. 8.30 (**a–h**) Vigabatrin-induced vacuolar myelinopathy. A 9 month-old boy with seizures. DWI (**a**), ADC map (**b**), and T2-weighted image (**c**) show symmetric high signal and diffusion restriction in the globi pallidi and thalami bilaterally. 3-month follow-up MRI (**d–f**) demonstrates complete reversibility of the lesions. The distribution of the lesions corresponds to distribution of abundant areas of GABA receptors. (**g**) In a different case from [66], light micrograph shows vacuoles 25 to 50 mm diameter in white matter. (**h**) Electron microscopy demonstrates splitting myelin at minor dense (intraperiod) line, which is a potential extracellular space. Courtesy of Horton M, MD, and Del Bigio MR, MD

8 Brain Edema 137

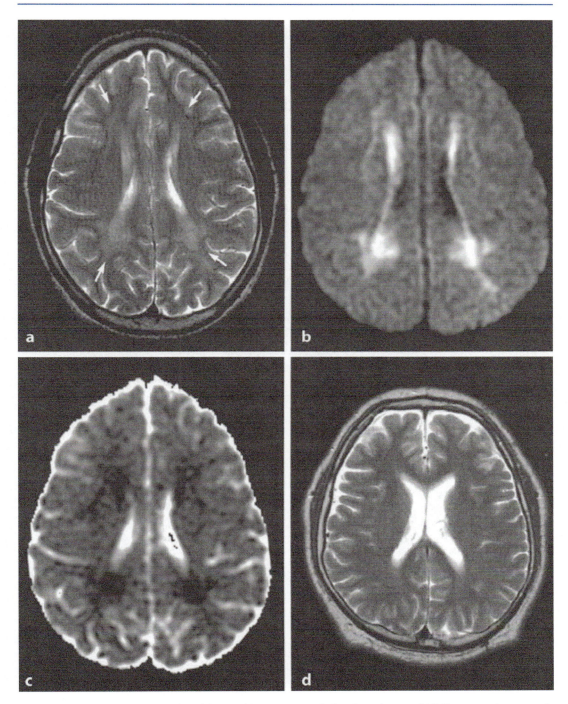

Fig. 8.31 (**a–d**) Phenylketonuria in a 36-year-old man. (**a**) T2-weighted image shows hyperintense lesions in the periventricular white matter (*arrows*). (**b**) DW image shows these lesions as hyperintense. (**c**) These hyperintense lesions have decreased ADC, representing cytotoxic edema, presumably intramyelinic edema. (**d**) Three-month follow-up MR imaging shows complete resolution of these lesions with clinical improvement

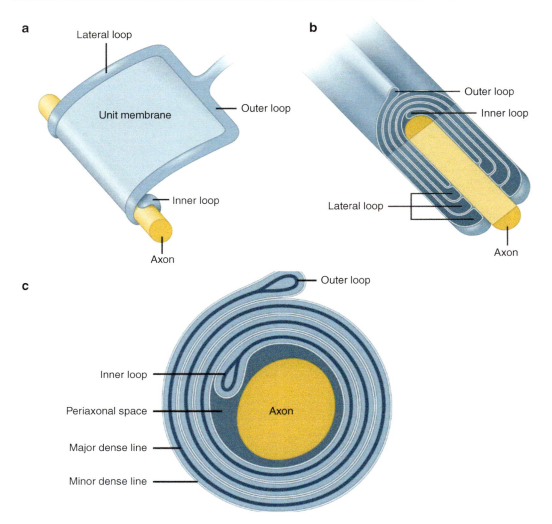

Fig. 8.32 (**a–c**) Myelin sheath is composed of the inner and outer membranes and loops: the cell processes of oligodendrocyte (**a, b**). Fusion of the inner membranes forms the major dense line made by the part of the cytoplasm (intracellular space). Fusion of the outer membrane forms the minor dense line (intraperiod line) which is potentially the "extracellular space (ECS)" (**c**). Intramyelinic edema predominantly occurs within the intramyelinic cleft (minor dense line), which is potential ECS but not continuous with ECS of the brain. Intramyelinic edema may occur in the intracellular space (major dense line) if the insult is more severe. The edema in the "closed" extracellular space in the myelin sheath can cause restricted diffusion likely related to the geometric distortion of membranous structures. (modified from [71, 72])

8.5 Vasogenic or Interstitial Edema

Vasogenic edema is characterized by dysfunction of the blood–brain barrier (BBB) or abnormal tumor endothelial tight junction—blood tumor barrier (BTB), allowing an abnormal passage of proteins, electrolytes, and water into the extracellular compartments [4]. Fluid leaving the capillaries enlarges the extracellular space, predominantly in the white matter. Brain tumor cells secrete vasogenic endothelial growth factor (VEGF) causing the formation of microvessels with lack of tight junction, allowing vasogenic edema. AQP4 plays an important role in brain tumor edema. Brain tumor-associated AQP4 expression is seen not only in the foot process but throughout the entire astrocyte cell membrane [4].

8 Brain Edema

Osmotic and hydrostatic gradients will also cause interstitial edema, increasing the extracellular space as water shifts from blood vessels and/or ventricles. Intracellular components are relatively preserved (Fig. 8.33), although some swelling of myelin sheaths and astrogliosis may be seen histologically [7]. Glutamate also directly modulates vascular permeability [14]. High extracellular concentration of glutamate is potentially related to blood–brain barrier (BBB) breakdown and vasogenic edema.

Fifteen to 30% of brain volume is the extracellular space, which is composed of extracellular matrix containing macromolecules such as proteoglycans (lectican, tenascin), hyaluronic acid, and free water. The function of the extracellular matrix is (1) cell adhesion, (2) short/long distance communication of neuronal-glial units by neurotransmitters, ions, and carrier proteins, (3) trophic effect, and (4) resistance to non-neuronal tumor invasion [78].

Pathological specimen of vasogenic edema shows leakage of plasma from the vessel and diffuse expansion of the extracellular space in the white matter (Fig. 8.34). In vasogenic and interstitial edema, electron microscopy has shown an increase of extracellular spaces in white matter amounting to 1000 nm, versus 60 nm in normal white matter [79]. These enlarged extracellular spaces, with free water, may be the dominant source for the total brain water signal, resulting in increased ADC.

8.5.1 Conditions that Cause Vasogenic Edema

Vasogenic edema is related to multiple pathological conditions. It typically occurs in the vicinity of brain tumors, intracerebral hematomas,

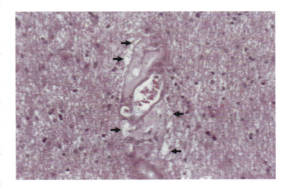

Fig. 8.34 Vasogenic edema, as shown on this tissue stain of a trauma case (arrows), is the result of plasma leakage through the blood vessel walls. The increase in extracellular space osmolarity will result in a marked increase in extracellular water, i.e., vasogenic edema (hematoxylin–eosin stain, original magnification ×200)

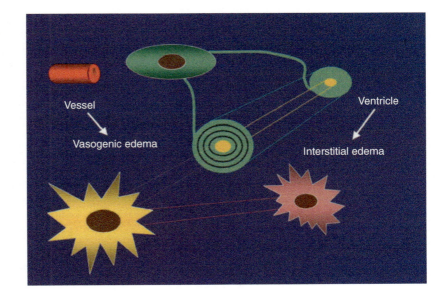

Fig. 8.33 Vasogenic or interstitial edema. There is enlarged extracellular space as water shifts from the blood vessels and/or ventricles. Intracellular compartments are relatively preserved

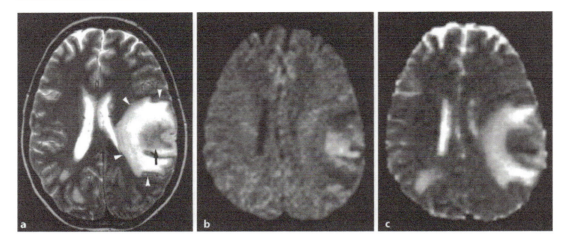

Fig. 8.35 (**a–c**) Cerebral toxoplasmosis and vasogenic edema in an 18-year-old female patient with headache. (**a**) T2-weighted image shows central necrosis as slightly hyperintense (arrow) and peripheral vasogenic edema as very hyperintense in the left hemisphere (arrowheads). Multiple lesions of toxoplasmosis are also seen in the right occipital and left periventricular areas. (**b**) DWI reveals vasogenic edema as hypointense, while the central necrosis shows hyperintensity on DWI. (**c**) ADC map shows increased ADC from the vasogenic edema. Decreased ADC of the central necrosis is probably due to hyperviscosity of the coagulative necrosis

infarctions, vasculitis (see Chap. 11, Figs. 11.2 and 11.3), abscesses/encephalitis (Fig. 8.35), contusions, posterior reversible encephalopathy syndrome (PRES) (Fig. 8.36), and hyperperfusion syndrome (Fig. 8.37) [80]. Venous ischemia at first shows a vasogenic edema due to venous congestion and a breakdown of BBB (see Chap. 9, Figs. 9.7 and 9.8). Progressive venous ischemia results in reduced capillary perfusion pressure which can lead to cytotoxic edema (see Chap. 9, Fig. 9.8) [81].

DWI shows low signal intensity, isointensity or slightly increased intensity, depending on T2 contrast, and an increase in ADC that reflects free water in the enlarged extracellular space (Figs. 8.35, 8.36 and 8.37).

8.6 Diffusion Tensor Imaging and Edema

Diffusion tensor imaging (DTI) measures the translation of extracellular water in the white matter tracts by directional evaluation of the water diffusivity (diffusion anisotropy) [82]. Fractional anisotropy (FA), a parameter derived from DTI computations, is sensitive for detecting extracellular edema (vasogenic and interstitial edema) in the white matter tracts. DTI shows decreased FA in the area of vasogenic edema (Fig. 8.36) and interstitial edema (Fig. 8.38) while FA is preserved or increased in pure cytotoxic edema (Fig. 8.39) [83]. In cytotoxic edema, increased tortuosity of the extracellular space and movement of water into the more restricted environment of the intracellular space may cause increased FA.

8.7 Conclusion

8.7.1 Cytotoxic or Cellular Edema

Cytotoxic or cellular edema is hyperintense on DWI and associated with decreased ADC. It can occur in neurons, glial cells, axons (axonal swelling), and myelin sheaths (intramyelinic edema). Excitotoxic brain injury plays an important role in cytotoxic edema, and it is the final common pathway in any seemingly unrelated diseases. Cytotoxic edema may be present not only in infarction/ischemia and trauma, but also in status epilepticus, the acute phase of multiple sclerosis, toxic or metabolic leukoen-

8 Brain Edema

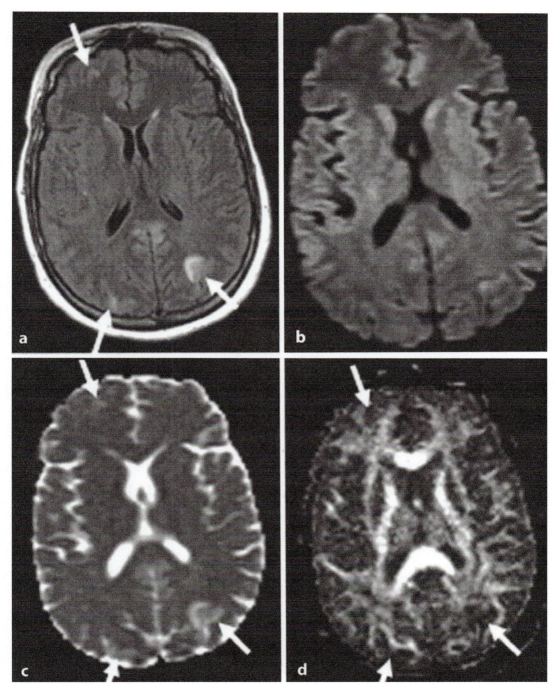

Fig. 8.36 (**a–d**) Posterior reversible encephalopathy syndrome (PRES) in a 42-year-old-woman with hypertension after liver transplant. (**a**) FLAIR image shows multiple hyperintense lesions in the right frontal and bilateral parieto-occipital areas (arrows). (**b**) DWI reveals these lesions as isointense. (**c**) ADC map shows increased ADC consistent with the vasogenic edema seen in PRES (arrows). (**d**) FA map shows decreased FA in the area of the subcortical vasogenic edema (arrows)

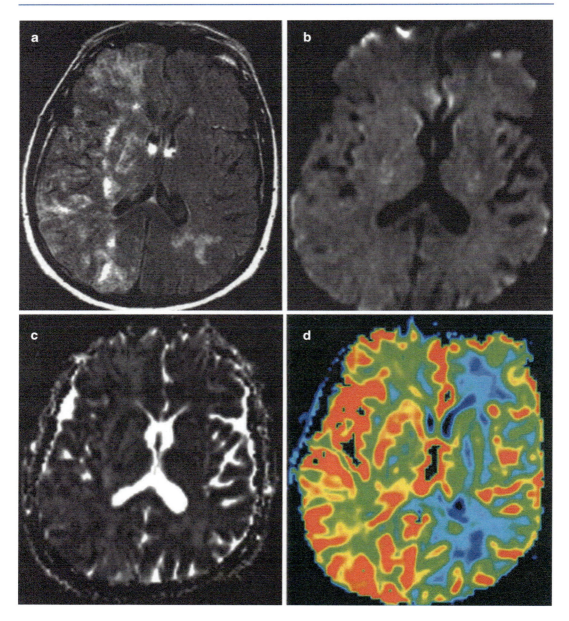

Fig. 8.37 (**a–d**) Hyperperfusion syndrome in a 72-year-old man after carotid endoatherectomy. (**a**) FLAIR image shows diffuse hyperintensity in the entire right hemisphere. (**b**) DWI reveals these areas as isointense. (**c**) ADC map shows increased ADC consistent with vasogenic edema. (**d**) Perfusion-weighted image (rCBV) shows increased cerebral blood volume in the entire right hemisphere

cephalopathy, osmotic myelinolysis, encephalitis, and presumably in the early phase of transneuronal or Wallerian degeneration and Creutzfeldt–Jakob disease. The differential diagnosis for hyperintense DWI also includes tumor, abscess, and hemorrhage, conditions that also may have decreased ADC. The decreased ADC in these latter conditions may be due to hypercellularity and/or hyperviscosity rather than the cytotoxic edema.

8 Brain Edema

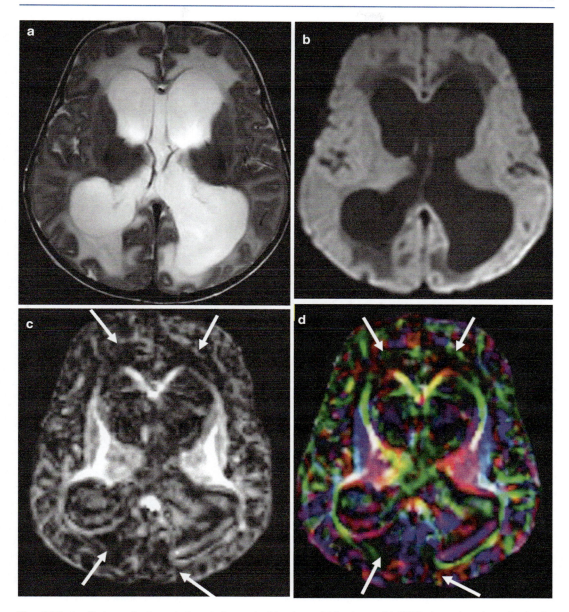

Fig. 8.38 (a–d) Acute hydrocephalus. A 3-month-old girl with posterior fossa mass (atypical teratoid/rhabdoid tumor). (**a**) T2-weighted image shows hydrocephalus and diffuse periventricular hyperintensity consistent with interstitial edema. (**b**) DWI shows hypointensity in the periventricular interstitial edema with decreased FA on FA map (arrows) (**c**) and decreased directional anisotropy on color map (arrows) (**d**)

8.7.2 Vasogenic Edema

Vasogenic edema has a variable appearance on DWI, with increased ADC. It is reversible but occasionally associated with cytotoxic edema, which usually is not reversible. DWI and ADC maps are useful for understanding MR images of various diseases with cytotoxic and/or vasogenic edema. These images are more sensitive than conventional MR imaging to determine the extent of edema in both gray and white matter.

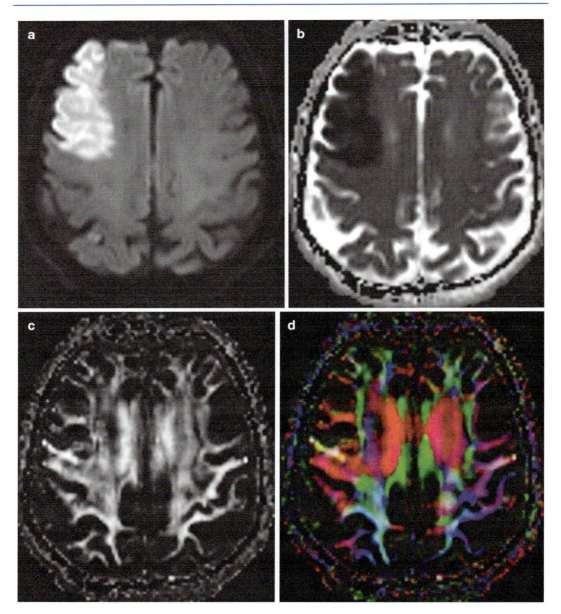

Fig. 8.39 (**a–d**) Acute cerebral infarction. A 70-year-old male with history of hypertension, hyperlipidemia, and atrial fibrillation who presented with left-sided weakness and difficulty following commands. DWI (**a**) and ADC map (**b**) show diffusion restriction in the anterior/superior right middle cerebral artery distribution cardioembolic stroke. FA and directional anisotropy are preserved in the area of the acute infarction on FA map (**c**) and color map (**d**). (Courtesy of Dr. Girish Bathla)

8.8 Brain Edema—Treatment

Badih J. Daou, Gregory Palmateer, and Aditya S. Pandey

8.8.1 Introduction

Cerebral edema is a process defined by a pathologic increase in the amount of total brain water with a resultant increase in brain volume [84]. There are three intracranial compartments consisting of brain tissue, blood, and cerebrospinal fluid (CSF); therefore, the accumulation of extracellular fluid can result in expansion of brain volume and resultant elevation of intracranial pressure [85], leading to mass effect and impairment of brain and cranial nerve functions. Cerebral edema can arise from multiple causes such as stroke, brain tumors, and traumatic brain injury. The amount of brain edema is variable, ranging from a small focal area of edema that may be asymptomatic in certain locations but can occasionally be associated with severe consequences, and can be fatal, if left untreated. The pathophysiological mechanisms underlying the formation of cerebral edema are complex [86]. In this chapter, we will discuss the etiology of brain edema, mechanisms of formation, as well as the medical and surgical treatment options and possible future therapeutic targets.

8.8.2 Types of Cerebral Edema and Diagnosis

Two main types of cerebral edema can be distinguished based on the underlying mechanisms: vasogenic and cytotoxic [87–89]. Vasogenic edema results from a disruption of the blood–brain barrier (BBB), leading to increased permeability and extravasation of fluid from the intravascular to the extracellular space [90]. In vasogenic edema, endothelial tight junctions are disrupted by the underlying injury resulting in inflammation, oxidative stress, and the release of vascular permeability factors by activated glial cells. The extravasated fluid accumulates outside the cells and leads to an increase in the brain volume [90]. In contrast, cytotoxic edema is characterized by an increased water content within the intracellular space and is due to intracellular ATP depletion, failure of ionic pumps, and disruption of the osmotic pressure gradient and ion balance that normally maintain cellular homeostasis, without disruption of the BBB [91]. This leads to an abnormal entry of extracellular fluid into cells and swelling of brain cells.

Cerebral edema can be further viewed as focal or diffuse edema. Focal edema accompanies a brain lesion and causes tissue shifts whereas diffuse edema affects the whole brain and is seen with more generalized etiologies [89].

8.8.3 Mechanisms of Cerebral Edema by Pathology

8.8.3.1 Tumor-Associated Edema

Cerebral edema associated with brain tumors is common and occurs in malignant primary brain tumors, metastatic tumors, as well as aggressive benign tumors (Fig. 8.40) [92, 93]. Tumor-associated edema is considered vasogenic in origin [94]. Edema formation is associated with a primary disturbance at the level of the microvasculature and BBB with leakage of plasma fluid and proteins across the vessel wall into the parenchyma [95]. One of the mostly described pathways leading to edema in brain tumors is the upregulation of VEGF [96]. Brain tumors including gliomas, meningiomas, and metastatic tumors have upregulation of VEGF which stimulates fenestrations in the brain endothelium and degeneration of the basement membrane [93, 97, 98].

8.8.3.2 Stroke-Associated Edema

Cerebral edema in ischemic stroke can be divided into three phases: (1) cytotoxic with swelling of the astrocytes and neuronal dendrites impacting cellular ionic gradients with entry of ions into cells, followed by water, with resultant cellular swelling [99, 100], (2) ionic with alterations to the ionic gradients of endothelial cells, including transcapillary flux of Na^+ with tissue swelling and early transient leakage of the BBB [101], and (3) vasogenic that further increases the water content of the tissue (Fig. 8.41) [102].

8.8.3.3 Intracranial Hemorrhage-Associated Edema

Intracranial hemorrhage (ICH)-associated edema or peri-hematomal edema develops in response to multiple processes including clot retraction and hydrostatic pressure changes, thrombin formation, erythrocyte lysis and hemoglobin toxicity,

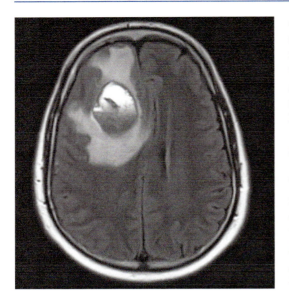

Fig. 8.40 Brain MRI, T2 FLAIR sequence, axial cut, demonstrates a right frontal lobe mass with surrounding T2 hyperintense signal consistent with vasogenic edema, with significant mass effect and an associated leftward midline shift of 6 mm

complement activation, plasma protein leakage, and disruption of the BBB [103]. Cerebral edema is also thought to occur in three phases with initial vasogenic edema, followed by inflammation and thrombin activation resulting in cytotoxic edema, and followed by erythrocyte lysis and hemoglobin toxicity [103].

8.8.3.4 Traumatic Brain Injury-Related Edema

The pathogenesis of traumatic brain injury (TBI) is complex and multifactorial [104]. Historically, edema following TBI was primarily thought to be vasogenic in nature; however, more recent studies have proven that there is a mix between vasogenic and cytotoxic edema [105–107]. Vascular injury and BBB disruption following TBI result in extravasation of fluid from the intravascular into the extracellular space and development of vasogenic edema. Afterwards, the decrease in cerebral blood flow reduces the delivery of oxygen and glucose to the brain, thereby leading to a

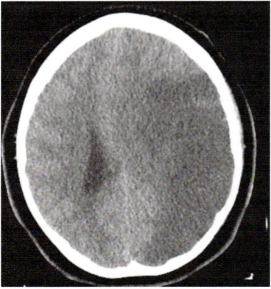 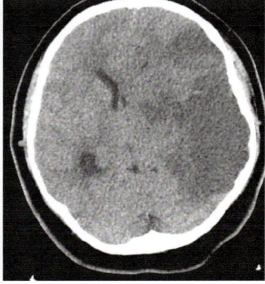

Fig. 8.41 Non-contrast head CT, axial cuts, demonstrates a large left MCA territory infarct with significant hypoattenuation of the left frontal parietal and temporal lobes consistent with a malignant infarct and edema, with associated midline shift of 12 mm and subfalcine herniation, left uncal herniation, and effacement of the left lateral ventricle and basal cisterns

drop of ATP production with sodium accumulation within the cells and resultant cytotoxic edema [104].

8.8.4 Diagnosis and Clinical Monitoring of Cerebral Edema

Diagnosing cerebral edema is directly related to methods used to evaluate the primary condition resulting in edema. A combination of history and physical examination, imaging, and often more invasive methods including intracranial pressure (ICP) monitoring are used. Localized cerebral edema can cause focal weakness, cranial nerve deficits, visual disturbances, and sensory changes. More diffuse cerebral edema may result in headaches, nausea, vomiting, confusion, mental status changes, lethargy, and seizures. While some patients do not show specific clinical symptoms for brain edema, other cases may have a more severe or malignant presentation. Cushing's triad (bradycardia, hypertension, and respiratory depression) suggests resultant elevated ICPs. Abnormal movements of the eyes and/or pupillary dilatation and unresponsiveness to light suggest a resultant herniation syndrome (transtentorial, uncal, or subfalcine). Furthermore, in acute pathologies, cerebral edema often peaks at the third or fourth day after the initial injury and can result in clinical worsening around that time.

Computed tomography (CT) of the head is often the first imaging tool used for evaluation. Cerebral edema resulting from a focal pathology will show up as an area of hypodensity surrounding a brain lesion (e.g., tumor, hemorrhage, abscess). This could result in significant mass effect, compression, and displacement of adjacent structures and midline shift. The degree of edema is highly variable, and even varies in the same patient at different timelines. Edema from a diffuse process can be demonstrated as diffuse effacement of the basal cisterns, ventricles and CSF containing spaces, and loss of gray-white matter differentiation.

Magnetic resonance imaging (MRI) of the brain is more sensitive in identifying cerebral edema and further demonstrates the above listed findings. Edema is represented on MRI by areas of T2-weighted hyperintensity, hyperintense areas on fluid-attenuated inversion recovery (FLAIR) sequences (most sensitive sequence), and low signal on T1-weighted sequences. Furthermore, these areas do not enhance with contrast and do not restrict diffusion.

The indication for invasive ICP monitoring is based on concomitant assessment of clinical and imaging findings [108]. ICP monitoring can be accomplished through a burr hole and placement of an epidural, subarachnoid, intraparenchymal, or intraventricular catheter. Intraventricular catheters are often preferred when possible, as it provides a way to measure ICP and also to drain cerebrospinal fluid (CSF) to reduce the ICP.

Noninvasive tonometry to measure the intraocular pressure represents an indirect way to evaluate for cerebral edema and elevated ICPs, if papilledema is demonstrated.

8.8.5 Medical Management of Cerebral Edema

8.8.5.1 General Measures
A. Head of bed elevation

Elevating the head of the bed to 30 degrees in patients with notable cerebral edema can assist in decreasing CSF hydrostatic pressure and facilitate venous blood drainage and can assist with reduction of ICP [109, 110]. Also the head should be kept neutral, to decrease jugular vein compression.

B. Analgesia and sedation

Analgesia and sedation should be considered in patients with severe cerebral edema with signs or symptoms of elevated ICP [111]. Opioids, benzodiazepines, and propofol are the most commonly used agents for sedation. Pharmacologic neuromuscular paralysis is reserved for severe cases refractory to other ICP lowering measures [112].

C. Ventilation

Hypoxia and hypercapnia act as cerebral vasodilators and lead to increased cerebral blood volume and ICP elevations. Intubation and mechanical ventilation are indicated if ventilation or oxygenation is insufficient in patients with cerebral edema, with the use of rapid-sequence intubation protocols [113]. Hyperventilation can be used as an initial measure to lower the ICP by reducing PCO2 and cerebral vasoconstriction [114]. This strategy should be used temporarily due to the risk of cerebral ischemia with continued hyperventilation [115].

D. Fluid and Sodium managements

Hypotonic fluids should be minimized or avoided in patients with cerebral edema as they can lower the serum osmolality and possibly worsen the edema. Fluid balance should be maintained within the euvolemia zone. Osmotic therapy with mannitol or hypertonic saline would be recommended for brain edema especially with high ICPs [116–120]. A standard mannitol bolus would be 1 g/kg of 20% mannitol. Volume depletion represents the main complication of mannitol administration [121]. Serum osmolality is typically monitored and should be maintained at less than 320 mOsm/L (number above which the risk of renal failure increases). Hypertonic saline concentration ranges from 1.8% to 23.4%. Three percent hypertonic saline is the most utilized concentration and requires a central line for administration (while 1.8% can be initiated at first if no central line is present); 23.4% is often reserved for patients with cerebral edema and signs of high ICP or brain herniation [122]. The excess volume from hypertonic saline can exacerbate congestive heart failure in patients with preexistent cardiac dysfunction. There is some data favoring hypertonic saline over mannitol in TBI; however, no definite advantage has been found [120].

8.8.5.2 Tumor-Related Edema
A. Steroids

Corticosteroids are the most commonly used medications in managing tumor-related edema

[93, 123, 124]. Dexamethasone is the most widely utilized drug. Steroids are associated with neurological and radiological improvement in edema [125]. The duration of treatment with steroids, and taper regimens vary widely and depend on the degree of edema, patient characteristics, and type of tumor. However, given the systemic effect and toxicity of steroids, patients with cerebral edema should be continuously monitored and the steroids should be tapered to off or to a lower maintenance dose, if and when possible.

B. Antiangiogenic agents

Brain tumor-associated edema is associated with VEGF expression, which increases vascular permeability and disruption of the BBB [126]. Bevacizumab (Avastin) is a recombinant human monoclonal antibody that works on inhibiting VEGF. It is FDA approved for the treatment of recurrent glioblastomas and may prolong progression-free survival, partly because of a reduction in vasogenic edema and its sequelae [127].

8.8.5.3 Stroke-Related Edema
Besides optimization of hemodynamics and temperature, avoiding hyperglycemia and applying general measures to control swelling, there are limited specific medical strategies to reduce cerebral edema following an ischemic stroke. Steroids do not have any benefit in stroke-related edema and their use is not recommended [128].

8.8.5.4 Traumatic Brain Injury-Related Edema
A. Blood Pressure and Cerebral Perfusion Pressure

Cerebral perfusion pressure (CPP) which equals mean arterial pressure–ICP is routinely monitored in TBI. CPP could be jeopardized in TBI if the injury results in high ICPs and especially if accompanied by hypotension. A low CPP would compromise CBF in this population that can have impaired cerebral autoregulation and causes impaired brain tissue oxygenation [129]. CPP should be maintained between 50 and 70 mm Hg in patients with significant cerebral edema and TBI [130].

B. Hypothermia and Barbiturates

Although these strategies can be applied to the management of cerebral edema and elevated ICPs from multiple causes, they have been studied mostly in TBI and represent tools used for cases refractory to other treatment measures. Multiple trials have studied the effect of hypothermia in TBI with inconsistent results and variations in the duration of cooling and target temperature [131]. Hypothermia has been shown to reduce ICPs, but its effect on clinical outcomes is questionable [132]. Pentobarbital reduces the cerebral metabolic activity and has a role in controlling edema and high ICPs, but barbiturates have not been shown to improve clinical outcomes [133].

8.8.6 Surgical Management of Cerebral Edema

8.8.6.1 Tumor-Related Edema

Surgical resection of the tumor is the ultimate method to treat peri-tumoral edema as it eliminates the tissue releasing factors and cytokines [134]. Although complete tumor resection would be ideal and leads to better outcomes and reduction of edema, certain eloquent locations may make complete resection risky or non-feasible; therefore the goal should be a maximal safe resection.

Cerebral edema associated with tumors may persist or worsen immediately following surgical resection due to brain irritation. This is also sometimes seen with brain biopsies. A steroid course following surgical resection is typically recommended. Some tumors may be amenable to stereotactic radiosurgery which can also cause treatment-associated cerebral edema and radionecrosis [135].

8.8.6.2 Stroke-Related Edema

Decompressive hemicraniectomy is the main treatment strategy for malignant ischemic cerebral edema [136–138]. Patients who undergo this procedure are those who develop increasing cerebral edema despite best medical measures, have a large hemispheric infarction, and experience neurological worsening in the first few days after the index event [139]. This is more likely to be encountered in younger patients who have a "full brain." The evidence is strongest for patients <60 years of age. Treatment should still be considered in older patients and individualized on a case-to-case basis [140]. Furthermore, there is strong evidence for a suboccipital decompressive craniectomy (± resection of necrotic cerebellar tissue) in patients with large cerebellar infarcts [141].

8.8.6.3 Traumatic Brain Injury-Associated Edema

Decompression surgery, with a wide hemicraniectomy or bifrontal craniectomy (Kjellberg procedure), is indicated for patients with refractory intracranial hypertension and edema following TBI [142]. The DECRA trial that included 155 patients who underwent a bifrontal decompressive craniectomy for TBI patients reported a higher rate of unfavorable outcomes in the surgical group than those receiving standard of care and a similar morality rate at 6 months [143]. This trial was thought to have several design flaws. The RescueICP trial, published in 2016, enrolled 408 patients with severe TBI and refractory ICPs to either undergo a craniectomy or continue with standard medical treatment and reported a significant reduction in morality (22.7% vs 48.5%) as well a reduction in unfavorable outcome at 6 months (26.9% vs 48.9%) and 12 months (30.4% vs 52%) after trauma, though there were also significantly more patients in a vegetative status (6.2% vs 1.7%) after surgery [142].

8.8.7 Future of Edema Management

Due to the complexity of cerebral edema formation and lack of experimental tools to investigate the cellular and molecular pathways for a long time, the options available for treatment are few. As our understanding of the pathogenesis has increased, and with the advent of newer imaging techniques and genetic and molecular tools, research pertaining to cerebral edema has expanded significantly. Molecular targets that are currently being investigated include myosin light chain kinase [144], matrix metalloproteinases [145], peroxisome proliferator-activated receptor [146], VEGF receptor [147], Substance P [148],

AQP-4 [149], vasopressin receptor [150], and the SUR1-TRPM4 channel [151]. More research efforts are required moving forward to identify targets that can be translated into clinical practice.

8.8.8 Summary of Cerebral Edema Treatment

Treatment section: Cerebral edema is associated with multiple neurological conditions including brain tumors, stroke, and traumatic brain injury. It can result in elevation of intracranial pressure and impairment of brain and cranial nerve functions. The severity of edema and associated symptoms is highly variable. Two main types of cerebral edema can be distinguished based on the underlying mechanisms: vasogenic and cytotoxic. A combination of history, physical examination, imaging, and occasionally invasive intracranial pressure monitoring is used to evaluate cerebral edema. General measures to manage cerebral edema include head of bed elevation, analgesia and sedation, and osmotic therapy with mannitol or hypertonic saline. Steroids are the mainstay of medical treatment of tumor-related edema whereas surgical tumor resection is the ultimate method to treat peri-tumoral edema. Decompressive hemicraniectomy is the main treatment strategy for malignant ischemic cerebral edema. A hemicraniectomy or bifrontal craniectomy is indicated in patients with refractory intracranial hypertension and edema following traumatic brain injury. Several genetic and molecular targets are currently being evaluated to treat cerebral edema and more research efforts are required to identify targets that can be translated into clinical practice.

References

1. Milhorat TH (1992) Classification of the cerebral edemas with reference to hydrocephalus and pseudotumor cerebri. Childs Nerv Syst 8(6):301–306
2. Liang D et al (2007) Cytotoxic edema: mechanisms of pathological cell swelling. Neurosurg Focus 22(5):E2
3. Ebisu T et al (1993) Discrimination between different types of white matter edema with diffusion-weighted MR imaging. J Magn Reson Imaging 3(6):863–868
4. Papadopoulos MC et al (2004) Molecular mechanisms of brain tumor edema. Neuroscience 129(4):1011–1020
5. Moritani T et al (2005) Diffusion-weighted imaging of acute excitotoxic brain injury. AJNR Am J Neuroradiol 26(2):216–228
6. Rosenblum WI (2007) Cytotoxic edema: monitoring its magnitude and contribution to brain swelling. J Neuropathol Exp Neurol 66(9):771–778
7. Ironside J, Pickard J (2002) Raised intracranial pressure, oedema and hydrocephalus. In: Graham D, Lantos P (eds) Greenfield's neuropathology. Arnold, London, pp 193–231
8. Hayashi T, Abe K (2004) Ischemic neuronal cell death and organellae damage. Neurol Res 26(8):827–834
9. Lipton SA, Rosenberg PA (1994) Excitatory amino acids as a final common pathway for neurologic disorders. N Engl J Med 330(9):613–622
10. Chan S et al (1996) Reversible signal abnormalities in the hippocampus and neocortex after prolonged seizures. AJNR Am J Neuroradiol 17(9):1725–1731
11. Mark LP et al (2001) Pictorial review of glutamate excitotoxicity: fundamental concepts for neuroimaging. AJNR Am J Neuroradiol 22(10):1813–1824
12. Zamponi GW, Stys PK (2009) Role of prions in neuroprotection and neurodegeneration: a mechanism involving glutamate receptors? Prion 3(4):187–189
13. Fukuyama T et al (2015) Semi-quantitative analyses of antibodies to N-methyl-d-aspartate type glutamate receptor subunits (GluN2B & GluN1) in the clinical course of Rasmussen syndrome. Epilepsy Res 113:34–43
14. Vazana U et al (2016) Glutamate-mediated blood-brain barrier opening: implications for neuroprotection and drug delivery. J Neurosci 36(29):7727–7739
15. Wang Y, Qin ZH (2010) Molecular and cellular mechanisms of excitotoxic neuronal death. Apoptosis 15(11):1382–1402
16. Pu Y et al (2000) Increased detectability of alpha brain glutamate/glutamine in neonatal hypoxic-ischemic encephalopathy. AJNR Am J Neuroradiol 21(1):203–212
17. Ruppel RA et al (2001) Excitatory amino acid concentrations in ventricular cerebrospinal fluid after severe traumatic brain injury in infants and children: the role of child abuse. J Pediatr 138(1):18–25
18. Tisoncik JR et al (2012) Into the eye of the cytokine storm. Microbiol Mol Biol Rev 76(1):16–32
19. Starkey J et al (2017) Cytotoxic lesions of the corpus callosum that show restricted diffusion: mechanisms, causes, and manifestations. Radiographics 37(2):562–576
20. Takanashi J et al (2006) Widening spectrum of a reversible splenial lesion with transiently reduced diffusion. AJNR Am J Neuroradiol 27(4):836–838
21. Takanashi J et al (2010) Differences in the time course of splenial and white matter lesions in clinically mild encephalitis/encephalopathy with

21. a reversible splenial lesion (MERS). J Neurol Sci 292(1–2):24–27
22. Mlodzikowska-Albrecht J, Steinborn B, Zarowski M (2007) Cytokines, epilepsy and epileptic drugs—is there a mutual influence? Pharmacol Rep 59(2):129–138
23. Domercq M, Matute C (1999) Expression of glutamate transporters in the adult bovine corpus callosum. Brain Res Mol Brain Res 67(2):296–302
24. Hunt NH et al (2006) Immunopathogenesis of cerebral malaria. Int J Parasitol 36(5):569–582
25. Baron CA et al (2015) Reduction of diffusion-weighted imaging contrast of acute ischemic stroke at short diffusion times. Stroke 46(8):2136–2141
26. Landman BA et al (2010) Complex geometric models of diffusion and relaxation in healthy and damaged white matter. NMR Biomed 23(2):152–162
27. Portnoy S et al (2013) Oscillating and pulsed gradient diffusion magnetic resonance microscopy over an extended b-value range: implications for the characterization of tissue microstructure. Magn Reson Med 69(4):1131–1145
28. Goodman JA, Ackerman JJ, Neil JJ (2008) Cs + ADC in rat brain decreases markedly at death. Magn Reson Med 59(1):65–72
29. Duong TQ et al (1998) Evaluation of extra- and intracellular apparent diffusion in normal and globally ischemic rat brain via 19F NMR. Magn Reson Med 40(1):1–13
30. Mussel M, Inzelberg L, Nevo U (2017) Insignificance of active flow for neural diffusion weighted imaging: a negative result. Magn Reson Med 78(2):746–753
31. Einstein A (1956) A new determination of molecular dimensions. In: Furth R (ed) Investigations on the theory of the Brownian movement. Dover Publications, INC, New York, pp 37–62
32. van der Toorn A et al (1996) Dynamic changes in water ADC, energy metabolism, extracellular space volume, and tortuosity in neonatal rat brain during global ischemia. Magn Reson Med 36(1):52–60
33. Tien RD et al (1994) MR imaging of high-grade cerebral gliomas: value of diffusion-weighted echo-planar pulse sequences. AJR Am J Roentgenol 162(3):671–677
34. Desprechins B et al (1999) Use of diffusion-weighted MR imaging in differential diagnosis between intracerebral necrotic tumors and cerebral abscesses. AJNR Am J Neuroradiol 20(7):1252–1257
35. Desmond PM et al (2001) The value of apparent diffusion coefficient maps in early cerebral ischemia. AJNR Am J Neuroradiol 22(7):1260–1267
36. Burdette JH et al (1998) Cerebral infarction: time course of signal intensity changes on diffusion-weighted MR images. AJR Am J Roentgenol 171(3):791–795
37. Kamal AK, Segal AZ, Ulug AM (2002) Quantitative diffusion-weighted MR imaging in transient ischemic attacks. AJNR Am J Neuroradiol 23(9):1533–1538
38. Forbes KP, Pipe JG, Heiserman JE (2001) Evidence for cytotoxic edema in the pathogenesis of cerebral venous infarction. AJNR Am J Neuroradiol 22(3):450–455
39. Arbelaez A, Castillo M, Mukherji SK (1999) Diffusion-weighted MR imaging of global cerebral anoxia. AJNR Am J Neuroradiol 20(6):999–1007
40. Wolf RL et al (2001) Quantitative apparent diffusion coefficient measurements in term neonates for early detection of hypoxic-ischemic brain injury: initial experience. Radiology 218(3):825–833
41. Barzo P et al (1997) Contribution of vasogenic and cellular edema to traumatic brain swelling measured by diffusion-weighted imaging. J Neurosurg 87(6):900–907
42. Liu AY et al (1999) Traumatic brain injury: diffusion-weighted MR imaging findings. AJNR Am J Neuroradiol 20(9):1636–1641
43. Kim JA et al (2001) Transient MR signal changes in patients with generalized tonicoclonic seizure or status epilepticus: periictal diffusion-weighted imaging. AJNR Am J Neuroradiol 22(6):1149–1160
44. Men S et al (2000) Selective neuronal necrosis associated with status epilepticus: MR findings. AJNR Am J Neuroradiol 21(10):1837–1840
45. Butteriss DJ, Ramesh V, Birchall D (2003) Serial MRI in a case of familial hemiplegic migraine. Neuroradiology 45(5):300–303
46. Liang Y, Scott TF (2007) Migrainous infarction with appearance of laminar necrosis on MRI. Clin Neurol Neurosurg 109(7):592–596
47. Tsuchiya K et al (1999) Diffusion-weighted MR imaging of encephalitis. AJR Am J Roentgenol 173(4):1097–1099
48. Demaerel P et al (1997) Diffusion-weighted magnetic resonance imaging in Creutzfeldt-Jakob disease. Lancet 349(9055):847–848
49. Bahn MM, Parchi P (1999) Abnormal diffusion-weighted magnetic resonance images in Creutzfeldt-Jakob disease. Arch Neurol 56(5):577–583
50. Kuroiwa T et al (1999) Different apparent diffusion coefficient: water content correlations of gray and white matter during early ischemia. Stroke 29(4):859–865
51. Saggu SK et al (2010) Wallerian-like axonal degeneration in the optic nerve after excitotoxic retinal insult: an ultrastructural study. BMC Neurosci 11:97
52. Hassel B et al (2003) Glutamate transport, glutamine synthetase and phosphate-activated glutaminase in rat CNS white matter. A quantitative study. J Neurochem 87(1):230–237
53. Brusilow SW et al (2010) Astrocyte glutamine synthetase: importance in hyperammonemic syndromes and potential target for therapy. Neurotherapeutics 7(4):452–470
54. Manzo G et al (2014) MR imaging findings in alcoholic and nonalcoholic acute Wernicke's encephalopathy: a review. Biomed Res Int 2014:503596
55. Hartings JA et al (2017) The continuum of spreading depolarizations in acute cortical lesion development:

examining Leao's legacy. J Cereb Blood Flow Metab 37(5):1571–1594

56. Chatzikonstantinou A et al (2011) Features of acute DWI abnormalities related to status epilepticus. Epilepsy Res 97(1–2):45–51

57. Iizuka T et al (2002) Neuronal hyperexcitability in stroke-like episodes of MELAS syndrome. Neurology 59(6):816–824

58. Sakai S et al (2018) Association between stroke-like episodes and neuronal hyperexcitability in MELAS with m.3243A>G: a case report. eNeurologicalSci 12:39–41

59. Zheng Q et al (2015) Stroke-like migraine attacks after radiation therapy syndrome. Chin Med J 128(15):2097–2101

60. Tang-Schomer MD et al (2012) Partial interruption of axonal transport due to microtubule breakage accounts for the formation of periodic varicosities after traumatic axonal injury. Exp Neurol 233(1):364–372

61. Johnson VE, Stewart W, Smith DH (2013) Axonal pathology in traumatic brain injury. Exp Neurol 246:35–43

62. Beirowski B et al (2010) Mechanisms of axonal spheroid formation in central nervous system Wallerian degeneration. J Neuropathol Exp Neurol 69(5):455–472

63. O'uchi T (1998) Wallarian degeneration of the pontocerebellar tracts after pontine hemorrhage. Int J Neuroradiol 4:171–177

64. Kamiya K et al (2013) Postoperative transient reduced diffusion in the ipsilateral striatum and thalamus. AJNR Am J Neuroradiol 34(3):524–532

65. Tievsky AL, Ptak T, Farkas J (1999) Investigation of apparent diffusion coefficient and diffusion tensor anisotropy in acute and chronic multiple sclerosis lesions. AJNR Am J Neuroradiol 20(8):1491–1499

66. Horton M, Rafay M, Del Bigio MR (2009) Pathological evidence of vacuolar myelinopathy in a child following vigabatrin administration. J Child Neurol 24(12):1543–1546

67. Cramer SC et al (2001) Decreased diffusion in central pontine myelinolysis. AJNR Am J Neuroradiol 22(8):1476–1479

68. Matsumoto S et al (1995) Carmofur-induced leukoencephalopathy: MRI. Neuroradiology 37(8): 649–652

69. Phillips MD et al (2001) Diffusion-weighted imaging of white matter abnormalities in patients with phenylketonuria. AJNR Am J Neuroradiol 22(8):1583–1586

70. Sener RN (2002) Metachromatic leukodystrophy: diffusion MR imaging findings. AJNR Am J Neuroradiol 23(8):1424–1426

71. Hirano A (2005) The role of electron microscopy in neuropathology. Acta Neuropathol 109(1):115–123

72. Hirano A, Zimmerman HM, Levine S (1968) Intramyelinic and extracellular spaces in triethyltin intoxication. J Neuropathol Exp Neurol 27(4):571–580

73. Werner P, Pitt D, Raine CS (2001) Multiple sclerosis: altered glutamate homeostasis in lesions correlates with oligodendrocyte and axonal damage. Ann Neurol 50(2):169–180

74. Maeda M et al (2003) Transient splenial lesion of the corpus callosum associated with antiepileptic drugs: evaluation by diffusion-weighted MR imaging. Eur Radiol 13(8):1902–1906

75. Tada H et al (2004) Clinically mild encephalitis/encephalopathy with a reversible splenial lesion. Neurology 63(10):1854–1858

76. Maeda M et al (2006) Reversible splenial lesion with restricted diffusion in a wide spectrum of diseases and conditions. J Neuroradiol 33(4):229–236

77. Maekawa T, Kamiya K, Murata K, Feiweier T, Hori M, Aoki S (2020) Time-dependent Diffusion in Transient Splenial Lesion: Comparison between Oscillating-Gradient Spin-echo Measurements and Monte-Carlo Simulation. Magn Reson Med Sci. https://doi.org/10.2463/mrms.bc.2020-0046. Epub ahead of print. PMID: 32611990

78. Ruoslahti E (1996) Brain extracellular matrix. Glycobiology 6(5):489–492

79. Gonatas NK, Zimmerman HM, Levine S (1963) Ultrastructure of inflammation with edema in the rat brain. Am J Pathol 42:455–469

80. Mukherjee P, McKinstry RC (2001) Reversible posterior leukoencephalopathy syndrome: evaluation with diffusion-tensor MR imaging. Radiology 219(3):756–765

81. Keller E et al (1999) Diffusion- and perfusion-weighted magnetic resonance imaging in deep cerebral venous thrombosis. Stroke 30(5):1144–1146

82. Basser PJ, Pierpaoli C (1996) Microstructural and physiological features of tissues elucidated by quantitative-diffusion-tensor MRI. J Magn Reson B 111(3):209–219

83. Green HA et al (2002) Increased anisotropy in acute stroke: a possible explanation. Stroke 33(6):1517–1521

84. Fishman RA (1975) Brain edema. N Engl J Med 293(14):706–711

85. Neff S, Subramaniam RP (1996) Monro-Kellie doctrine. J Neurosurg 85(6):1195

86. Stokum JA, Gerzanich V, Simard JM (2016) Molecular pathophysiology of cerebral edema. J Cereb Blood Flow Metab 36(3):513–538

87. Marmarou A (2007) A review of progress in understanding the pathophysiology and treatment of brain edema. Neurosurg Focus 22(5):E1

88. Klatzo I (1987) Pathophysiological aspects of brain edema. Acta Neuropathol 72(3):236–239

89. Rabinstein AA (2006) Treatment of cerebral edema. Neurologist 12(2):59–73

90. Michinaga S, Koyama Y (2015) Pathogenesis of brain edema and investigation into anti-edema drugs. Int J Mol Sci 16(5):9949–9975

91. Rungta RL, Choi HB, Tyson JR et al (2015) The cellular mechanisms of neuronal swelling underlying cytotoxic edema. Cell 161(3):610–621

92. Papadopoulos MC, Saadoun S, Binder DK, Manley GT, Krishna S, Verkman AS (2004) Molecular mechanisms of brain tumor edema. Neuroscience 129(4):1011–1020

93. Esquenazi Y, Lo VP, Lee K (2017) Critical care management of cerebral edema in brain tumors. J Intensive Care Med 32(1):15–24

94. Bruce JN, Criscuolo GR, Merrill MJ, Moquin RR, Blacklock JB, Oldfield EH (1987) Vascular permeability induced by protein product of malignant brain tumors: inhibition by dexamethasone. J Neurosurg 67(6):880–884

95. Criscuolo GR (1993) The genesis of peritumoral vasogenic brain edema and tumor cysts: a hypothetical role for tumor-derived vascular permeability factor. Yale J Biol Med 66(4):277–314

96. Goldman CK, Bharara S, Palmer CA et al (1997) Brain edema in meningiomas is associated with increased vascular endothelial growth factor expression. Neurosurgery 40(6):1269–1277

97. Gorman AM, Hirt UA, Orrenius S, Ceccatelli S (2000) Dexamethasone pre-treatment interferes with apoptotic death in glioma cells. Neuroscience 96(2):417–425

98. Kalkanis SN, Carroll RS, Zhang J, Zamani AA, Black PM (1996) Correlation of vascular endothelial growth factor messenger RNA expression with peritumoral vasogenic cerebral edema in meningiomas. J Neurosurg 85(6):1095–1101

99. Kimelberg HK (2004) Volume activated anion channel and astrocytic cellular edema in traumatic brain injury and stroke. Adv Exp Med Biol 559:157–167

100. Pantoni L, Garcia JH, Gutierrez JA (1996) Cerebral white matter is highly vulnerable to ischemia. Stroke 27(9):1641–1646; discussion 1647

101. Simard JM, Kent TA, Chen M, Tarasov KV, Gerzanich V (2007) Brain oedema in focal ischaemia: molecular pathophysiology and theoretical implications. Lancet Neurol 6(3):258–268

102. Vella J, Zammit C, Di Giovanni G, Muscat R, Valentino M (2015) The central role of aquaporins in the pathophysiology of ischemic stroke. Front Cell Neurosci 9:108

103. Zheng H, Chen C, Zhang J, Hu Z (2016) Mechanism and therapy of brain edema after Intracerebral hemorrhage. Cerebrovasc Dis 42(3–4):155–169

104. Winkler EA, Minter D, Yue JK, Manley GT (2016) Cerebral edema in traumatic brain injury: pathophysiology and prospective therapeutic targets. Neurosurg Clin N Am 27(4):473–488

105. Beaumont A, Fatouros P, Gennarelli T, Corwin F, Marmarou A (2006) Bolus tracer delivery measured by MRI confirms edema without blood-brain barrier permeability in diffuse traumatic brain injury. Acta Neurochir Suppl 96:171–174

106. Marmarou A (2003) Pathophysiology of traumatic brain edema: current concepts. Acta Neurochir Suppl 86:7–10

107. Marmarou A, Signoretti S, Fatouros PP, Portella G, Aygok GA, Bullock MR (2006) Predominance of cellular edema in traumatic brain swelling in patients with severe head injuries. J Neurosurg 104(5): 720–730

108. Bratton SL, Chestnut RM, Ghajar J et al (2007) Guidelines for the management of severe traumatic brain injury. VI. Indications for intracranial pressure monitoring. J Neurotrauma 24(Suppl 1):S37–S44

109. Magnaes B (1976) Body position and cerebrospinal fluid pressure. Part 1: clinical studies on the effect of rapid postural changes. J Neurosurg 44(6):687–697

110. Durward QJ, Amacher AL, Del Maestro RF, Sibbald WJ (1983) Cerebral and cardiovascular responses to changes in head elevation in patients with intracranial hypertension. J Neurosurg 59(6):938–944

111. Oddo M, Crippa IA, Mehta S et al (2016) Optimizing sedation in patients with acute brain injury. Crit Care 20(1):128

112. Juul N, Morris GF, Marshall SB, Marshall LF (2000) Neuromuscular blocking agents in neurointensive care. Acta Neurochir Suppl 76:467–470

113. Kramer N, Lebowitz D, Walsh M, Ganti L (2018) Rapid sequence intubation in traumatic brain-injured adults. Cureus 10(4):e2530

114. Stocchetti N, Maas AI, Chieregato A, van der Plas AA (2005) Hyperventilation in head injury: a review. Chest 127(5):1812–1827

115. Muizelaar JP, Marmarou A, Ward JD et al (1991) Adverse effects of prolonged hyperventilation in patients with severe head injury: a randomized clinical trial. J Neurosurg 75(5):731–739

116. Hinson HE, Stein D, Sheth KN (2013) Hypertonic saline and mannitol therapy in critical care neurology. J Intensive Care Med 28(1):3–11

117. Battison C, Andrews PJ, Graham C, Petty T (2005) Randomized, controlled trial on the effect of a 20% mannitol solution and a 7.5% saline/6% dextran solution on increased intracranial pressure after brain injury. Crit Care Med 33(1):196–202; discussion 257–198

118. Berger-Pelleiter E, Emond M, Lauzier F, Shields JF, Turgeon AF (2016) Hypertonic saline in severe traumatic brain injury: a systematic review and meta-analysis of randomized controlled trials. CJEM 18(2):112–120

119. Burgess S, Abu-Laban RB, Slavik RS, Vu EN, Zed PJ (2016) A systematic review of randomized controlled trials comparing hypertonic sodium solutions and mannitol for traumatic brain injury: implications for emergency department management. Ann Pharmacother 50(4):291–300

120. Li M, Chen T, Chen SD, Cai J, Hu YH (2015) Comparison of equimolar doses of mannitol and hypertonic saline for the treatment of elevated intracranial pressure after traumatic brain injury: a systematic review and meta-analysis. Medicine (Baltimore) 94(17):e736

121. Manninen PH, Lam AM, Gelb AW, Brown SC (1987) The effect of high-dose mannitol on serum and urine electrolytes and osmolality in neurosurgical patients. Can J Anaesth 34(5):442–446

122. Kerwin AJ, Schinco MA, Tepas JJ 3rd, Renfro WH, Vitarbo EA, Muehlberger M (2009) The use of 23.4% hypertonic saline for the management of elevated intracranial pressure in patients with severe traumatic brain injury: a pilot study. J Trauma 67(2):277–282

123. Galicich JH, French LA, Melby JC (1961) Use of dexamethasone in treatment of cerebral edema associated with brain tumors. J Lancet 81:46–53

124. Ryken TC, McDermott M, Robinson PD et al (2010) The role of steroids in the management of brain metastases: a systematic review and evidence-based clinical practice guideline. J Neuro-Oncol 96(1):103–114

125. Vecht CJ, Hovestadt A, Verbiest HB, van Vliet JJ, van Putten WL (1994) Dose-effect relationship of dexamethasone on Karnofsky performance in metastatic brain tumors: a randomized study of doses of 4, 8, and 16 mg per day. Neurology 44(4): 675–680

126. Berkman RA, Merrill MJ, Reinhold WC et al (1993) Expression of the vascular permeability factor/vascular endothelial growth factor gene in central nervous system neoplasms. J Clin Invest 91(1): 153–159

127. Ellingson BM, Cloughesy TF, Lai A et al (2012) Quantification of edema reduction using differential quantitative T2 (DQT2) relaxometry mapping in recurrent glioblastoma treated with bevacizumab. J Neuro-Oncol 106(1):111–119

128. Poungvarin N (2004) Steroids have no role in stroke therapy. Stroke 35(1):229–230

129. Needham E, McFadyen C, Newcombe V, Synnot AJ, Czosnyka M, Menon D (2017) Cerebral perfusion pressure targets individualized to pressure-reactivity index in moderate to severe traumatic brain injury: a systematic review. J Neurotrauma 34(5):963–970

130. Prabhakar H, Sandhu K, Bhagat H, Durga P, Chawla R (2014) Current concepts of optimal cerebral perfusion pressure in traumatic brain injury. J Anaesthesiol Clin Pharmacol 30(3):318–327

131. Sadaka F, Veremakis C (2012) Therapeutic hypothermia for the management of intracranial hypertension in severe traumatic brain injury: a systematic review. Brain Inj 26(7–8):899–908

132. Lewis SR, Evans DJ, Butler AR, Schofield-Robinson OJ, Alderson P (2017) Hypothermia for traumatic brain injury. Cochrane Database Syst Rev 9:Cd001048

133. Roberts I, Sydenham E (2012) Barbiturates for acute traumatic brain injury. Cochrane Database Syst Rev 12:Cd000033

134. Stummer W, Reulen HJ, Meinel T et al (2008) Extent of resection and survival in glioblastoma multiforme: identification of and adjustment for bias. Neurosurgery 62(3):564–576; discussion 564–576

135. Harat M, Lebioda A, Lasota J, Makarewicz R (2017) Evaluation of brain edema formation defined by MRI after LINAC-based stereotactic radiosurgery. Radiol Oncol 51(2):137–141

136. Alexander P, Heels-Ansdell D, Siemieniuk R et al (2016) Hemicraniectomy versus medical treatment with large MCA infarct: a review and meta-analysis. BMJ Open 6(11):e014390

137. Geurts M, van der Worp HB, Kappelle LJ, Amelink GJ, Algra A, Hofmeijer J (2013) Surgical decompression for space-occupying cerebral infarction:

outcomes at 3 years in the randomized HAMLET trial. Stroke 44(9):2506–2508

138. Juttler E, Schwab S, Schmiedek P et al (2007) Decompressive surgery for the treatment of malignant infarction of the middle cerebral artery (DESTINY): a randomized, controlled trial. Stroke 38(9):2518–2525

139. Frank JI, Schumm LP, Wroblewski K et al (2014) Hemicraniectomy and durotomy upon deterioration from infarction-related swelling trial: randomized pilot clinical trial. Stroke 45(3):781–787

140. Vahedi K, Hofmeijer J, Juettler E et al (2007) Early decompressive surgery in malignant infarction of the middle cerebral artery: a pooled analysis of three randomised controlled trials. Lancet Neurol 6(3):215–222

141. Wijdicks EF, Sheth KN, Carter BS et al (2014) Recommendations for the management of cerebral and cerebellar infarction with swelling: a statement for healthcare professionals from the American Heart Association/American Stroke Association. Stroke 45(4):1222–1238

142. Hutchinson PJ, Kolias AG, Timofeev IS et al (2016) Trial of decompressive craniectomy for traumatic intracranial hypertension. N Engl J Med 375(12):1119–1130

143. Cooper DJ, Rosenfeld JV, Murray L et al (2011) Decompressive craniectomy in diffuse traumatic brain injury. N Engl J Med 364(16):1493–1502

144. Luh C, Kuhlmann CR, Ackermann B et al (2010) Inhibition of myosin light chain kinase reduces brain edema formation after traumatic brain injury. J Neurochem 112(4):1015–1025

145. Rosenberg GA (2002) Matrix metalloproteinases in neuroinflammation. Glia 39(3):279–291

146. Stahel PF, Smith WR, Bruchis J, Rabb CH (2008) Peroxisome proliferator-activated receptors: "key" regulators of neuroinflammation after traumatic brain injury. PPAR Res 2008:538141

147. van Bruggen N, Thibodeaux H, Palmer JT et al (1999) VEGF antagonism reduces edema formation and tissue damage after ischemia/reperfusion injury in the mouse brain. J Clin Invest 104(11):1613–1620

148. Donkin JJ, Nimmo AJ, Cernak I, Blumbergs PC, Vink R (2009) Substance P is associated with the development of brain edema and functional deficits after traumatic brain injury. J Cereb Blood Flow Metab 29(8):1388–1398

149. Yao X, Uchida K, Papadopoulos MC, Zador Z, Manley GT, Verkman AS (2015) Mildly reduced brain swelling and improved neurological outcome in Aquaporin-4 knockout mice following controlled cortical impact brain injury. J Neurotrauma 32(19):1458–1464

150. Ameli PA, Ameli NJ, Gubernick DM et al (2014) Role of vasopressin and its antagonism in stroke related edema. J Neurosci Res 92(9):1091–1099

151. Simard JM, Chen M, Tarasov KV et al (2006) Newly expressed SUR1-regulated NC(Ca-ATP) channel mediates cerebral edema after ischemic stroke. Nat Med 12(4):433–440

Infarction

9

John Kim, Toshio Moritani, Sven Ekholm,
and Yoshimitsu Ohgiya

Julius Griauzde, and Neeraj Chaudhary

9.1 Introduction

Stroke is the *fifth* leading cause of death in the USA with 142,142 deaths in the year 2016, and one of the most common causes of disability among adult Americans [1]. Until recently these patients were mainly imaged with computed tomography (CT) to establish if the cause of stroke was ischemic or hemorrhagic. With further advances and widespread availability of CT and magnetic resonance imaging (MRI), both modalities play a major role in the diagnosis and treatment of stroke.

J. Kim (✉) · T. Moritani · N. Chaudhary
Division of Neuroradiology, University of Michigan,
Ann Arbor, MI, USA
e-mail: johannk@med.umich.edu;
tmoritan@med.umich.edu; neerajc@med.umich.edu

S. Ekholm
Department of Imaging Sciences, University of
Rochester Medical Center, Rochester, NY, USA
e-mail: sven.ekholm@gu.se

Y. Ohgiya
Department of Radiology, Showa University School
of Medicine, Tokyo, Japan
e-mail: ohgiya@med.showa-u.ac.jp

J. Griauzde
University of Michigan School of Medicine,
Ann Arbor, MI, USA
e-mail: jgriauz@umich.edu

The National Institute for Neurological Disease and Stroke Trial demonstrated clinical benefit for intravenous thrombolytic drug therapy (e.g., IV-tPA) for many years [2]. In recent years, new landmark randomized clinical trials published in 2015 and 2018 (MR CLEAN, ESCAPE, EXTEND-IA, and SWIFT PRIME, DAWN, DEFUSE-3) have shown the superior benefit of endovascular thrombectomy with IV-tPA for ischemic strokes within 24 h of onset [3–7]. (Please see the Sect. 9.18 in the latter part of this chapter for more detailed discussion.) Many patients are triaged based on CT perfusion, CT angiography, and MR findings for treatment decisions.

Due to continuous research and improvements in endovascular techniques and technology, the future of treatment of ischemic strokes appears bright with improved patient outcomes.

9.1.1 Diffusion-Weighted Imaging (DWI)

CT and conventional MR imaging have sensitivities below 50% with regard to detection of infarcts in the hyperacute stage, within 6 h [8]. In recent years, DWI has been proven as the most sensitive MR imaging technique to diagnose hyperacute cerebral infarction, with a sensitivity

---

© Springer Nature Switzerland AG 2021
T. Moritani, A. A. Capizzano (eds.), *Diffusion-Weighted MR Imaging of the Brain, Head and Neck, and Spine*, https://doi.org/10.1007/978-3-030-62120-9_9

of 88%–100% and a specificity of 86%–100% [9–12]. The detection of acute ischemic lesions is based on alterations in motion of water molecules [13, 14].

DWI techniques employ echo-planar sequences that are highly resistant to patient motion. DWI of the brain can usually be accomplished in less than 2 min. Other methods of diffusion imaging include multi-shot echo-planar, single-shot fast spin-echo techniques, line scan DW MR imaging, and spiral DW MR imaging [15, 16].

The ischemic event results in restricted diffusion of the affected tissue, which can be seen as early as 30 min after ictus [14]. A few rare cases of false-negative DWI have been reported [17, 18]. These infarcts were seen on perfusion-weighted images and later on DW images [17, 18].

9.2 Diffusion-Weighted Imaging and Pathophysiology of Cerebral Infarction

The abnormal imaging finding of cerebral and cerebellar infarctions is an area of hyperintensity on DWI of the involved vascular territory. This hyperintensity is presumed to be caused by cytotoxic edema as a result of cessation of ATP production [19]. Under normal circumstances, ATP maintains the Na^+/K^+ pump activity and other intracellular energy-related processes. When the Na^+/K^+ pump is not functioning properly, an inability to remove excess water from the cells develops, resulting in intracellular edema [20]. With cellular swelling, there is a reduction in the volume of extracellular space. A decrease in the diffusion of low-molecular-weight tracer molecules has been demonstrated in animal models [21, 22], which suggests that the increased tortuosity of extracellular space pathways contributes to restricted diffusion in acute ischemia. The outcome of this on DW imaging is restriction of water diffusion, which results in a signal increase on DWI and a decrease in diffusion shown as a reduced apparent diffusion coefficient [23]. These findings in acute stroke usually represent irreversible damage of brain tissue, or infarction [24, 25].

9.3 Apparent Diffusion Coefficient (ADC)

The actual diffusion coefficient cannot be measured by using DW imaging for a number of reasons [14]. When measuring molecular motion with DW imaging, the diffusion coefficient obtained from orthogonal DW images in all three planes is called the ADC. The ADC is used to determine whether the signal abnormality on DWI is caused by restricted diffusion or a T2 shine-through effect [26], as seen in subacute–chronic infarctions. ADC represents the degree of diffusivity of water molecules and aids in detecting subtle fluid changes in the hyperacute–acute stages of ischemic stroke. Reduced diffusion is seen as an area of low signal intensity on ADC maps.

9.3.1 Explanation for Restricted Diffusion

Several mechanisms have been proposed to explain the restricted diffusion in ischemia. These include cellular necrosis, shift of fluid from extra- to intracellular spaces causing a reduction in size and increase in tortuosity of the extracellular space, but there is also rather strong evidence that at least parts of these findings relate to a reduction in intracellular diffusion [27].

Regions of decreased or restricted diffusion are best seen on DWI, while ADC maps will verify the findings by eliminating the T2 shine-through effect as a cause of the increased signal intensity on DWI [14]. DWI and ADC can also show changes in diffusion that vary for the different stages of a stroke [28], and they can possibly distinguish between multiple strokes over time versus a single, progressive stroke by determining the time course of a cerebral infarction.

In animal models of ischemia, an ADC threshold for reversibility has been demonstrated [29, 30]. In humans, ADC values may also be of help in the future to assist in selecting patients with salvageable tissue within an ischemic penumbra for thrombolysis.

In older patients it is not uncommon to detect older lesions with prolonged T2 that are indistinguishable from acute lesions using conventional

9 Infarction

MR imaging. Acute infarctions are hyperintense on DWI and hypointense on the ADC map, whereas chronic foci are usually isointense on DWI and hyperintense on ADC maps [31].

Intermediate ADC values are noted in the ischemic penumbra, indicating tissue at risk of infarction [32]. An approach that is used more often to select patients who may benefit from thrombolysis is by comparing DWI and perfusion MR imaging to look for hypoperfused but not diffusion-restricted regions. The mismatch between DWI and perfusion demonstrates affected tissue that is still salvageable and not yet infarcted: the penumbra.

9.4 Time Course of Infarction

Infarctions may be classified as hyperacute (less than 6 h from time of onset of symptoms), acute (6 h to 3 days), subacute (3 days to 3 weeks), or chronic (3 weeks to 3 months), each having its characteristic signal abnormalities (Table 9.1).

9.4.1 Hyperacute (<6 h)

One of the main clinical applications of DW imaging is to detect a hyperacute cerebral infarction. This information is critical, particularly in cases of territorial thromboembolic infarction, as thrombolytic therapy can be started within the golden period of 3 h from onset of symptoms. Such treatment can result in early reperfusion and reduce the extension of the infarction [23, 33]. Diffusion restriction with reduced ADC has been observed as early as 30 min after the onset of ischemia, at a time when T2-weighted images still show a normal appearance. The DW signal intensity is increased during the hyperacute stage (<6 h) (Fig. 9.1). DW signal intensity changes are

Table 9.1 Time course of thromboembolic infarction of the middle cerebral artery [33]

	<6 h	3 days	7 days	30 days
T2	Isointense	Bright	Bright	Bright
DW imaging	Bright	Very bright	Bright	Isointense
ADC	Dark	Very dark	Dark to Isointense	Bright

generally considered to be permanent (and therefore reflect infarction) in clinical studies. However, some cases could be reversed with prompt treatment [34].

9.4.2 Acute (6 h to 3 Days)

Almost all acute (6 h to 3 days) stroke patients examined within 24 h of onset of symptoms show abnormal signal intensity on DW imaging [35]. At this stage the infarctions show a further increase in DW signal intensity and also a lower ADC than in the hyperacute stage (Fig. 9.2). The ADC continues to decrease and is most reduced at 8–32 h, remaining markedly reduced for 3–5 days. In most patients, a secondary increase in the size of the DW imaging abnormality was seen within 1 week [36].

9.4.3 Subacute (3 Days to 3 Weeks)

As the infarct continues to evolve into the subacute stage (3 days to 3 weeks), there is pseudo-normalization of the ADC, most likely attributed to a combination of (a) persistence of cytotoxic edema, and (b) development of vasogenic edema and cell membrane disruption, which results in increased amounts of extracellular water. The hyperintensity on DW imaging usually decreases within 1–2 weeks [37], but is still slightly hyperintense, while ADC is usually normalized within 10 days [26, 38]. This time gap is thought to result from T2 shine-through effects on DW imaging in the late subacute infarction (Fig. 9.3).

9.4.4 Chronic (3 Weeks to 3 Months)

In the chronic stage (3 weeks to 3 months) of infarction, there is a more or less complete necrosis of the cells, and at this stage there is an increase in ADC with a bright signal on the ADC map. On T2-weighted images the infarction is seen as a bright signal and this, in combination with the increased ADC, will result in a decrease in the signal on DW imaging; the gliosis in the infarction is isointense with surrounding tissue (Fig. 9.4).

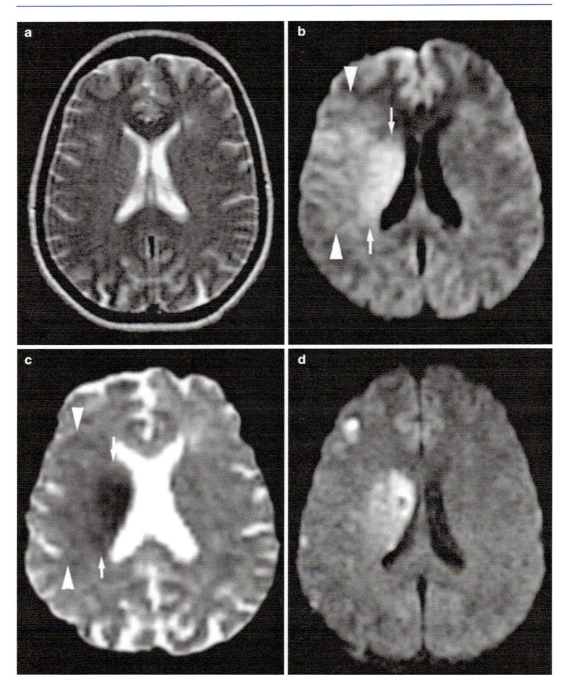

Fig. 9.1 (**a**–**d**) Hyperacute infarction (2 h after onset) in a 39-year-old woman with decreased consciousness. The symptoms improved after intra-arterial fibrinolytic therapy. (**a**) T2-weighted image appears normal. (**b**) DW image shows a hyperintense lesion in the right corona radiata (*arrows*) and a slightly hyperintense lesion in the right middle cerebral artery (MCA) territory (*arrowheads*). (**c**) ADC map shows decreased ADC in the corona radiata (*arrows*) and slightly decreased ADC in the cortical area of the MCA territory (*arrowheads*). (**d**) On DW image after fibrinolytic therapy (3 days after onset), the hyperintense lesion in the cortical area mostly resolved with peripheral small infarcts. Early cytotoxic edema with mild decreased ADC does not always result in infarction after treatment

9 Infarction

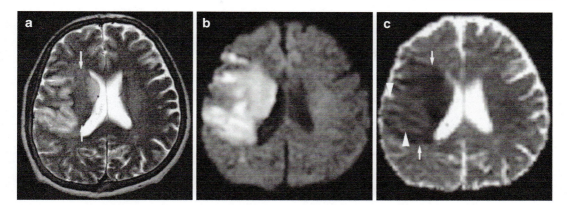

Fig. 9.2 (**a–c**) Acute infarction (24 h after onset) in a 56-year-old man with left hemiparesis. (**a**) T2-weighted image shows hyperintense lesions preferentially involving the right posterior frontal cortex and the right caudate region, sparing the right corona radiata (*arrows*). This finding is consistent with a relatively greater involvement of gray matter in the early infarction. (**b**) DW image shows the entire right MCA territory as hyperintense. (**c**) Decreased ADC is seen in the right MCA territory (*arrows*). However, some cortical lesions seem to be isointense or have a slightly increased ADC (*arrowheads*). This may reflect relative vulnerability for brain tissue. Hyperintensity on DW image of these cortical lesions is due to a T2 shine-through effect. DW images and ADC maps are more sensitive than conventional MR imaging for showing both gray and white matter involvement. ADC maps precisely reflect diffusion restrictions of the lesion within the gray and white matter

9.5 Diffusion-Weighted Imaging and ADC Characteristics of Gray and White Matter Ischemia

Diffusion-weighted imaging and ADC maps are more sensitive than conventional MR imaging in demonstrating both gray and white matter ischemia (Figs. 9.1, 9.2, and 9.3). Changes in ADC values in acute infarctions seem to be different for gray matter and white matter. Thus, there is a more prominent decrease in ADC in white matter than in gray matter. This decrease also remains for a longer period than in gray matter (Figs. 9.2 and 9.3). One of the explanations for these phenomena is that necrosis may be completed earlier in gray matter infarctions than in white matter infarctions. Another explanation is that the prominent and prolonged decrease in ADC in white matter may reflect cytotoxic edema in different cell types, such as myelin sheaths, axons, and glial cells [27, 28, 38].

Fiebach et al. observed a decrease in the relative ADC up to 3 days after the stroke and an increase in relative ADC from the third to the tenth day [28]. The relative ADC increased slightly faster in gray matter than in white, which may be due to the variability between these two tissue types at any stage in the ischemic process, which leads to an altered diffusion. The observed diffusion contrast in gray and white matter could be caused by differences in the mismatch between blood supply and metabolic demand, the type and/or severity of the histopathologic response to ischemic injury (vulnerability) or mechanisms by which histopathologic changes lead to altered diffusion [39]. Regarding the histopathologic response, gray matter has traditionally been considered to be more vulnerable than white matter to early ischemia. More recent findings in experimental models of stroke have demonstrated that ischemic damage to white matter occurs earlier and with greater severity than previously appreciated [40]. However, if this is true for humans as well is to our knowledge not yet established.

9.6 Reversibility and Treatment

Reversible ADC is rare but can be found in cases of transient ischemic attack in which imaging was performed within 4 h, venous infarction,

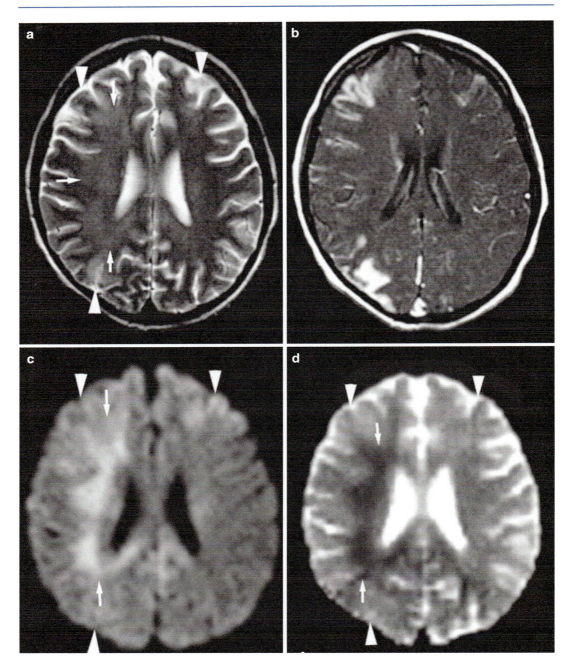

Fig. 9.3 (**a–d**) Subacute infarction (10 days after onset) in a 19-year-old woman with loss of consciousness due to cerebral embolism after cardiac surgery for endocarditis. (**a**) T2-weighted image shows hyperintense lesions in the gray (*arrowheads*) and white matter (*arrows*) in the right hemisphere and left frontal region. (**b**) Gadolinium T1-weighted image with magnetization transfer contrast shows gyral enhancement in the cortical lesions, representing subacute infarcts. (**c**) DW image also shows hyperintense lesions in the right deep white matter (*arrows*), and gray matter of both frontal and right parieto-occipital regions (*arrowheads*). (**d**) The ADC map shows decreased ADC in the right deep white matter lesion (*arrows*), and normal or slightly increased ADC in the gray matter lesions (*arrowheads*). The prolonged decreased ADC in the white matter may reflect edema of myelin sheaths or axons

9 Infarction

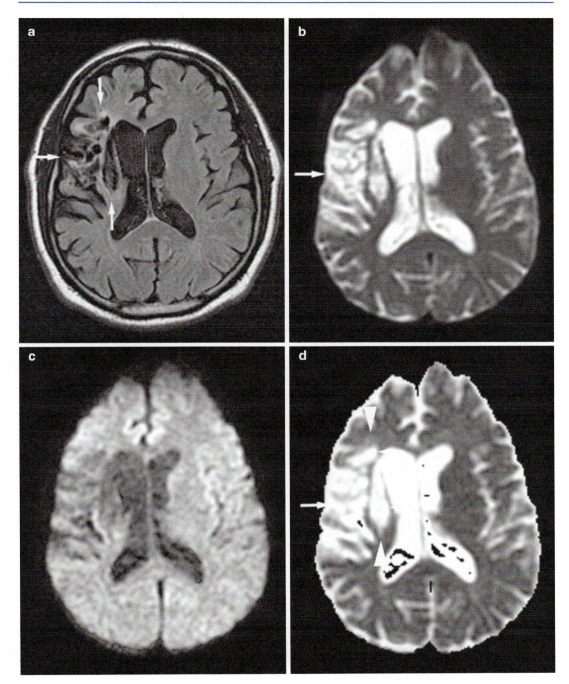

Fig. 9.4 (a–d) Chronic infarction (10 months after onset) in a 54-year-old man with numbness and weakness of the left lower extremity. (a) Fluid-attenuated inversion recovery (FLAIR) image shows chronic infarction in the right MCA territory as a cystic lesion with low signal intensity (cystic necrosis) and peripheral mild hyperintensity (gliosis) with atrophy (*arrows*). (b) b0 image shows the hyperintense cystic lesion (*arrow*). (c) DW image shows chronic infarction as hypointense cystic areas, and iso- or slightly hyperintense areas representing gliosis. (d) The ADC map shows marked increased ADC in the cystic necrosis (*arrow*), and slightly increased ADC in the gliotic periphery of the lesion (*arrowheads*)

hemiplegic migraine, and transient global amnesia. In these rare clinical settings, ischemia does not progress to complete necrosis but a minor subclinical, irreversible injury cannot be ruled out [27].

Clinically, the area of cytotoxic edema with bright DW signal seems to be irreversibly damaged resulting in permanent infarction. In early cerebral ischemia, mildly decreased ADC in the ischemic penumbra is indicative of viable tissue, but hypoperfused tissue at risk of infarction [41]. After intra-arterial or intravenous fibrinolytic therapy, or spontaneous lysis of a clot, abnormal signal in such areas is occasionally reversed, partially or completely (Figs. 9.4 and 9.5).

ADC normalization is not a rare event in acute stroke after thrombolytic therapy [42]. ADC normalization occurred predominantly in the basal ganglia and white matter after thrombolytic therapy in patients with more distal vessel occlusions. Early reperfusion is a prerequisite for ADC normalization. Tissue prone to ADC normalization is characterized by less severe initial ADC decreases.

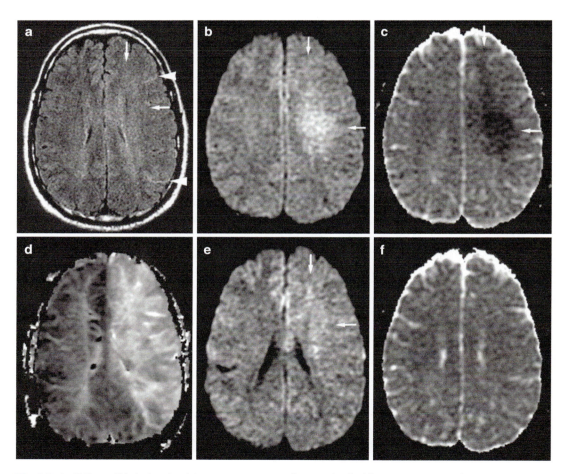

Fig. 9.5 (**a–f**) Reversible ischemia with cytotoxic edema (2 h from onset) in a 39-year-old man with left internal carotid artery dissection, presenting with right-sided weakness. (**a**) FLAIR image shows a subtle hyperintensity in the left frontoparietal white matter (*arrows*), and linear hyperintensity representing slow flow in the peripheral arteries (*arrowheads*). (**b, c**) DW image (**b**) shows a hyperintense lesion with decreased ADC (**c**) in the left frontoparietal white matter, representing cytotoxic edema (*arrows*). (**d**) Perfusion-weighted image shows increase in mean transit time of the entire left ACA and MCA territories. (**e**) Follow-up DW image 2 days later shows only a very subtle hyperintensity in the left frontal white matter (*arrows*). (**f**) ADC was normalized, which is in accordance with clinical improvement. Early ischemia with cytotoxic edema may have spontaneously resolved

9.7 Watershed Infarction

Watershed infarction may develop between two major vascular territories or within a single territory in the supraganglionic white matter, a border zone of the superficial and deep penetrating arterioles (Fig. 9.6). As mentioned above, thrombolytic therapy within the first 3 h from acute onset of symptoms can be effective to limit the size of the infarct under those circumstances. This is, however, not the case in watershed infarctions, as the basic etiology for these lesions is a significant reduction in perfusion secondary to an overall decrease in cerebral blood flow with subsequent poor perfusion pressure distally [33, 43].

There is a difference in the evolution time of ADC between watershed and thromboembolic infarction, the latter having an earlier normalization (Table 9.2). However, T2 signal intensity is the same for both types of infarction. The reason for this difference most likely lies in the different pathophysiologic features and cerebral perfusion of the two stroke subtypes. It is important to note that strokes with different pathogenetic, hemodynamic mechanisms may have different evolution in the ADC courses as well [33].

In fact, perfusion-weighted MR imaging demonstrated differences between territorial infarction and watershed infarction in the temporal changes of both relative cerebral blood volumes

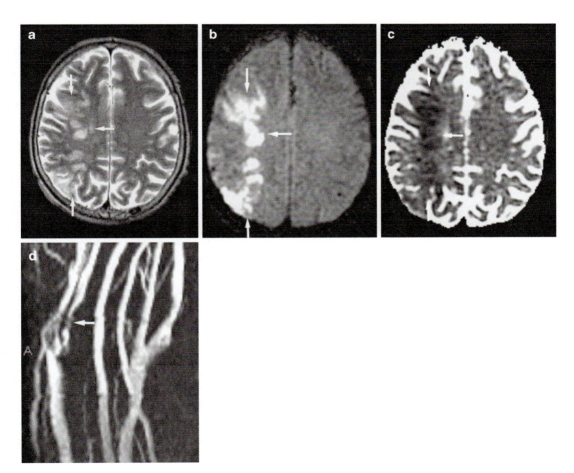

Fig. 9.6 (**a–d**) Watershed infarction. A 66-year-old man presented with stroke and seizure. (**a**) T2-weighted image shows multiple hyperintense lesions in the right frontoparietal area (*arrows*). (**b, c**) DW image shows these lesions as very hyperintense with decreased ADC, representing acute infarcts in the watershed area between anterior and middle cerebral arteries (*arrows*). (**d**) MR angiography shows a stenosis of the right internal carotid artery (*arrow*)

Table 9.2 Time course of watershed infarction of middle cerebral arterial territory [33]

	3 days	7 days	14 days	30 days
T2	Bright	Bright	Bright	Bright
DW imaging	Bright	Bright	Bright	Bright
ADC	Dark	Dark	Dark	Less dark

[43]. Patients with territorial infarction showed a progressively increasing pattern in relative cerebral blood volume from initial low values to peak high values at an early chronic stage. On the other hand, patients with watershed infarction showed consistently high relative cerebral blood volume throughout all stages.

9.8 Perfusion Versus Diffusion Imaging

MR perfusion-weighted (PW) imaging may be more sensitive than DW imaging in the detection of a hyperacute cerebral infarction, but it currently entails extensive post-processing to create interpretable perfusion maps (Figs. 9.5 and 9.6). Moreover, MR perfusion determines the degree of blood flow reduction at the level of the cerebral microvasculature, but it will not tell if a hypoperfused area represents an area of infarction or severe hypoperfusion. Perfusion MR can, however, be matched with the infarcted area on DW images and can demonstrate the area of hypoperfusion outside the infarction—the so-called penumbra. This is the area where neural tissue is at risk for infarction if perfusion is not re-established and ischemic penumbra is assumed to be salvageable by means of thrombolysis.

Many acute ischemic stroke patients arrive after the 4.5-h time window for recombinant tissue plasminogen activator administration. Intravenous desmoteplase administered 3–9 h after acute ischemic stroke in patients selected with perfusion/diffusion mismatch is associated with a higher rate of reperfusion and a better clinical outcome compared with placebo [44]. A wider time-to-treatment window may be achievable in patients selected by PW and DW imaging.

In fact, recent randomized clinical trials have used mostly CT perfusion and some MR to guide treatment and management of patients. In the DEFUSE 3 trial, CT perfusion was used to randomly assign patients to either endovascular thrombectomy versus medical therapy groups in an extended time-to-treatment window of up to 16 h [45]. The benefit of CT perfusion is its widespread availability and speed of acquisition. With the use of an automated image post-processing software, quantitative perfusion maps can be quickly created for patient triage and management. For the DEFUSE 3 and many other trials, the patients were eligible if the initial infarct volume (ischemic core) was less than 70 mL (as defined by a cerebral blood flow of <30% of normal), the ratio of volume of ischemic tissue to initial infarct volume was 1.8 or more, and an absolute volume of potentially reversible ischemia (penumbra) was 15 mL or more [45].

Initially developed for non-contrast CT imaging, the Alberta Stroke Program Early Computed Tomography Score (ASPECTS) can be used in both MR DW and CT PW imaging to assess the extent of acute ischemic stroke [46–48]. Originally the threshold of ASPECTS ≤7 was used to identify patients at high risk for intracerebral hemorrhage and poor clinical outcome [49]. The new recent clinical trials and American Heart Association have shown an ASPECTS ≥6 threshold to be useful criteria for endovascular thrombectomy.

9.9 Venous Infarction

Cerebral venous sinus thrombosis accounts for only a small percentage of cerebral infarctions in general. Because of its nonspecific presentation, cerebral venous sinus thrombosis can be difficult to diagnose. In about 50% of cases, cerebral venous sinus thrombosis results in cerebral venous infarction. This usually presents as a hemorrhagic infarction or focal edema in regions that are not typical for an arterial vascular distribution, usually occurring within the white matter or at the gray–white matter junction (Fig. 9.7).

9 Infarction

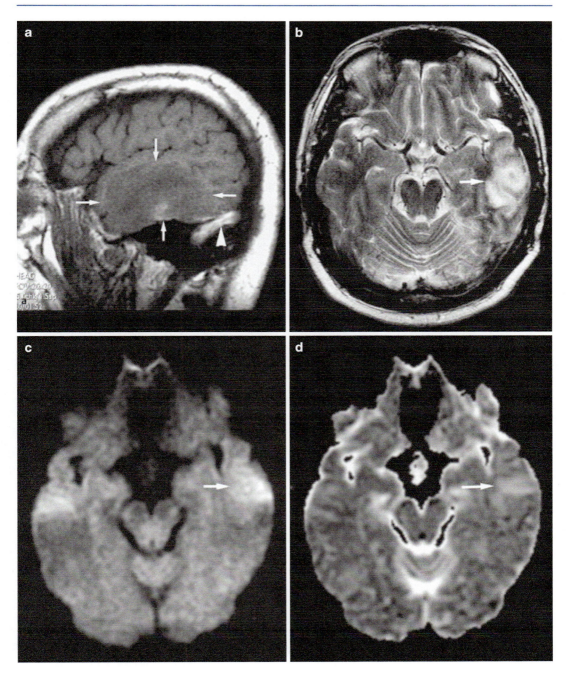

Fig. 9.7 (a–d) Venous infarction in a 57-year-old man with dysarthria. (**a**) Sagittal T1-weighted image shows a large area of hypointensity in the left temporal lobe (*arrows*) with a small area (hemorrhage). The hyperintensity in the left transverse sinus represents sinus thrombosis (*arrowhead*). (**b**) T2-weighted image shows a hyperintense lesion in the left temporal lobe (*arrow*). (**c**) DW image reveals this lesion as mildly hyperintense. (**d**) ADC is increased, representing vasogenic edema. On DW image, the lesion is overlapped with diamagnetic susceptibility artifacts from air in the mastoid cells

9.9.1 Predisposing Factors

There are several predisposing factors for thrombus formation within the cerebral venous sinuses. These include pregnancy, infection, extrinsic compression or local invasion by tumor, dehydration, oral contraceptives, hypercoagulable state, trauma, and drug abuse. It may also be idiopathic. Thrombus initially forms within the venous sinuses, eventually extending to the veins draining into the sinuses, leading to infarction.

9.9.2 Pathophysiology and Imaging

The pathophysiological mechanisms that lead to cerebral venous infarction are unclear. It has been postulated that: (1) retrograde venous pressure may cause breakdown of the blood–brain barrier, with leakage of fluid (vasogenic edema) and hemorrhage into the extracellular space, or (2) retrograde venous pressure may cause a decrease in cerebral blood flow, causing tissue damage similar to that seen in arterial infarctions. Restricted water diffusion suggesting cytotoxic edema is found in patients with acute cerebral venous infarction [50, 51]. However, areas without diminishment in ADC may primarily represent vasogenic edema from venous hypertension [52] (Figs. 9.7 and 9.8). Complete or nearly complete resolution of edema in patients with cerebral venous thrombosis and diminished ADC values has also been reported [53].

Gradient echo T2* and susceptibility-weighted images are very useful in the detection of acute- to subacute-phase thrombi which are hypointense (deoxy- or intracellular methemoglobin), especially before T1-weighted images show high signal in the subacute-phase thrombi (Fig. 9.8). DW imaging shows subacute-phase thrombi as high signal with decreased ADC (Fig. 9.9). Diffusion restriction of the thrombi may be predictive of a low rate of recanalization [54].

Preferred imaging modalities when suspecting cerebral venous sinus thrombosis are conventional MR imaging including gradient echo T2* or susceptibility-weighted images combined with MR venography.

9.10 Small Vessel (Lacunar) Infarcts

These are small infarcts measuring approximately 5–15 mm, usually seen in the basal ganglia, internal capsule, thalamus, pons, and corona radiata. They account for about 20% of all infarctions and are secondary to an embolus, thrombus, or atheromatous lesion within long, single, penetrating end arterioles.

These infarcts show increased signal in DW imaging with low ADC values (Fig. 9.10). However, unlike the usual time course of cerebral infarctions, they may show a prolonged increase in DW imaging signal and decrease in ADC values, sometimes seen beyond 60 days after onset of symptoms [55, 56].

Differential diagnoses include widened perivascular spaces (Virchow–Robin spaces) and subependymal myelin pallor.

9.11 Brain Stem and Cerebellar Infarcts

Cerebellar infarction is caused by occlusion of one of the major posterior circulation branches, which include the superior cerebellar, the anterior and posterior inferior cerebellar arteries, and the basilar artery. The posterior inferior cerebellar artery (PICA) supplies the postero-inferior portions of the cerebellum and is the most commonly obstructed cerebellar artery. The size of the infarct is important because a large infarct may cause a significant mass effect on the fourth ventricle and lead to hydrocephalus as well as brain stem compression. PICA infarctions can also result in the so-called lateral medullary (Wallenberg) syndrome, manifested by ipsilateral Horner's syndrome, ataxia, dysphagia, vertigo, nystagmus, hiccups and contralateral numbness, diminished

9 Infarction

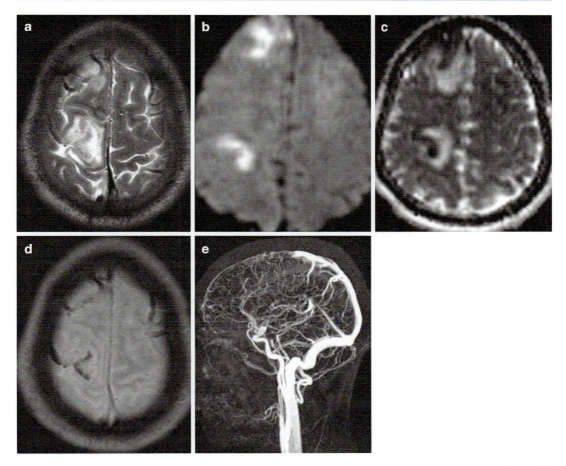

Fig. 9.8 (a–e) Acute-phase thrombosis with venous infarcts. A 23-year-old man with hypercoagulative state. (**a**) T2-weighted image shows hyperintense lesions in the right frontal lobe. It is difficult to detect the thrombi in the superior sagittal sinus and cortical veins. (**b, c**) DW image demonstrates hyperintense lesions with decreased ADC (cytotoxic edema) and surrounding increased ADC (vasogenic edema) consistent with venous infarcts. (**d**) On GRE hypointense thrombi in an arborizing fashion are clearly noted in the cortical veins in the bilateral frontal lobes. (**e**) Dynamic contrast 3D MR venogram shows nonvisualization of the anterior 2/3 of the superior sagittal sinus and the cortical veins

pain and temperature sensation. The brain stem and cerebellar infarcts behave similar to cerebral infarcts on DW imaging and ADC maps (Fig. 9.11).

Substantial image distortions are observed in the areas close to the base of the skull, which include areas in the posterior fossa. Some MR imaging techniques such as parallel MR imaging with SENSE and PROPELLER diffusion-weighted MR imaging reduce the susceptibility effect and image distortions. These techniques may improve detection of brain stem and cerebellar infarcts [57, 58].

9.12 Atypical Infarcts

9.12.1 Anterior Choroidal Artery

The anterior choroidal artery arises from the distal internal carotid artery just inferior to the carotid terminus. It courses laterally to the optic tract and then posterolaterally through the choroidal fissure to the posterior limb of the internal capsule. Infarcts of the anterior choroidal artery typically involve the posterior limb of the internal capsule, medial globus pallidus, and lateral

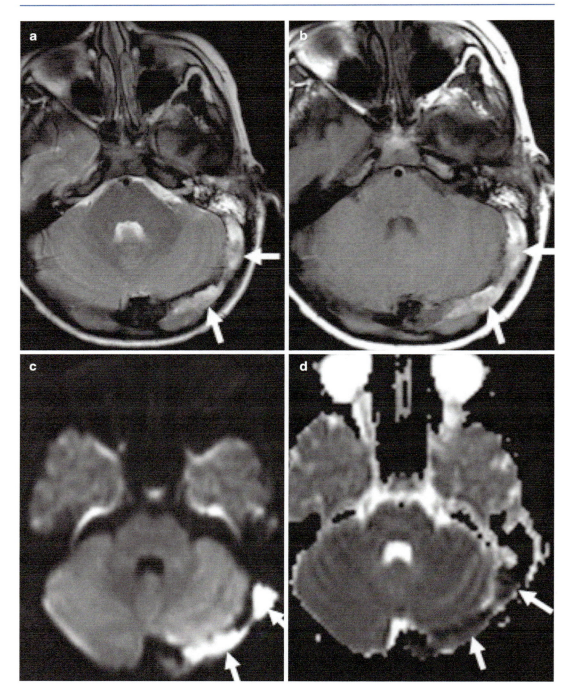

Fig. 9.9 (**a–d**) Subacute to chronic-phase thrombosis in the left jugular vein, transverse and sigmoid sinuses after decompression surgery for high jugular bulb in a 7-year-old boy. (**a, b**) T2- and T1-weighted images show subacute-phase thrombi (*arrows*) in the left transverse and sigmoid sinuses extending from the left jugular bulb as hyperintense. (**c, d**) DW image shows the subacute thrombi (*arrows*) as hyperintense with decreased ADC

9 Infarction

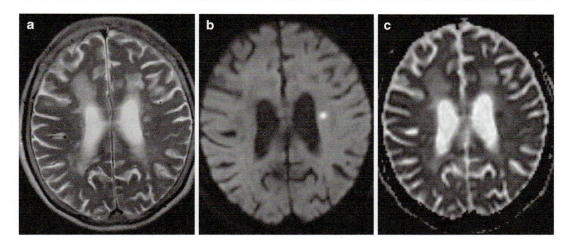

Fig. 9.10 (**a–c**) Small vessel infarction in a 74-year-old woman. (**a**) T2-weighted image shows periventricular hyperintensities; however, it is difficult to detect acute small infarction. (**b**) DW image clearly shows a small hyperintensity spot in the left white matter. (**c**) ADC is decreased, representing the acute phase of small vessel infarction

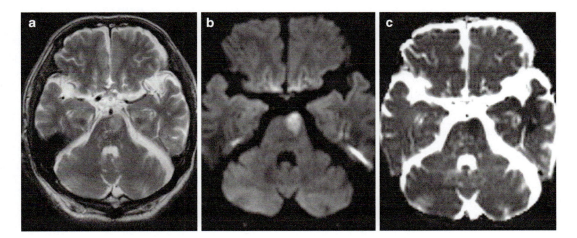

Fig. 9.11 (**a–c**) Brain stem infarction in an 85-year-old man with slurred speech and gait difficulties. (**a**) T2-weighted image shows a hyperintense lesion in the left side of the pons. (**b**) DW image clearly shows a hyperintense lesion. (**c**) The ADC is decreased, representing acute infarction

geniculate body of the thalamus (Fig. 9.12). Clinical presentation usually is a classic triad of hemianopia, hemiplegia, and hemisensory loss.

9.12.2 Subcallosal Artery

The subcallosal artery is the largest of the perforating branches of the anterior communicating artery. It branches posteriorly and superiorly to supply the bilateral anterior cingulate gyri, paraterminal gyrus, fornix, genu of the corpus callosum, and the anterior commissure. It is an uncommon location for infarct and is commonly related to surgical or endovascular treatment of anterior communicating artery aneurysms [59]. Patients with these infarcts present with antegrade amnesia with occasional confabulatory features, making it difficult to distinguish from Wernicke-Korsakoff encephalopathy. However, the classic imaging features are shown in Fig. 9.13.

9.12.3 Recurrent Artery of Heubner

The recurrent artery of Heubner is the largest of the medial lenticulostriate arteries, which arise from the anterior cerebral artery just distal to the anterior communicating artery. The caudate head, anterior limb of the internal capsule, and ventral globus pallidus are involved with these infarcts. Patients with these infarcts may present with pure contralateral motor hemiparesis (Fig. 9.14).

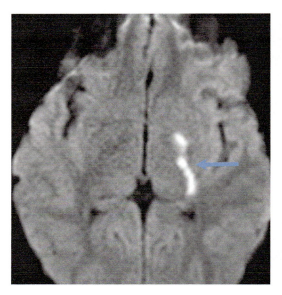

Fig. 9.12 Restricted diffusion of the left posterior limb of the internal capsule and left globus pallidus

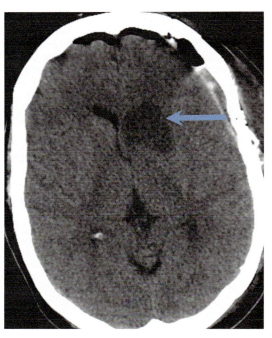

Fig. 9.14 Recurrent artery of Heubner infarct. There is hypoattenuation of the left caudate, anterior limb of internal capsule, and anterior putamen

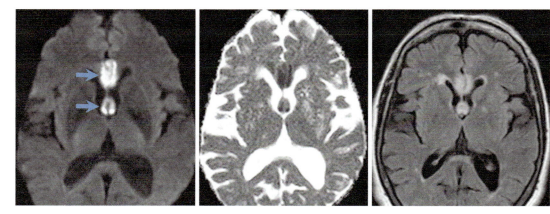

Fig. 9.13 A 74-year-old female with history of hypertension and pre-diabetes presented with altered mental status and cognitive decline. Diffusion-weighted imaging demonstrates restricted diffusion of the bilateral anterior cingulate gyri, genu of the corpus callosum, and bilateral fornices (arrows). ADC map shows corresponding low ADC values with T2 prolongation on FLAIR

9.12.4 Artery of Percheron

The artery of Percheron is an uncommon anatomic variant where a single unilateral artery arises from the posterior cerebral artery supplies the bilateral paramedian thalamus with variable midbrain supply (Fig. 9.15). The clinical presentation is variable but may include altered mental status, coma, hypersomnolence, aphasia/dysarthria, amnesia, ocular movement disorders, and pupillary abnormalities.

9.12.5 Transient Global Amnesia

Transient global amnesia (TGA) refers to sudden onset of antegrade amnesia that general resolves within 24 h. Patients may be disoriented to time and space with repetitive questioning. Common causes or triggers may include strenuous physical activity, sexual intercourse, trauma, conventional angiography, or acute emotional distress. TGA tends to occur in middle or late age adults (>50 years). Diffusion-weighted imaging for these patients often shows a small focus of restricted diffusion in the hippocampus (Fig. 9.16). The etiology of TGA is unclear or multifactorial. Vascular factors such as arterial ischemia, venous congestion, hyperlipidemia, and ischemic heart disease may play a role [60, 61]. Due to the focal restricted diffusion in the hippocampus and occurrence in patients with vascular risk factors, it is likely a tiny focal infarct off the posterior cerebral artery branch that is responsible for TGA.

9.12.6 Corpus Callosum Infarcts

Isolated corpus callosum infarction due to pericallosal artery disease is rare, but can present as an alien hand syndrome. These patients fail to recognize the ownership of one hand when placed in certain positions or situations [62]. Patients

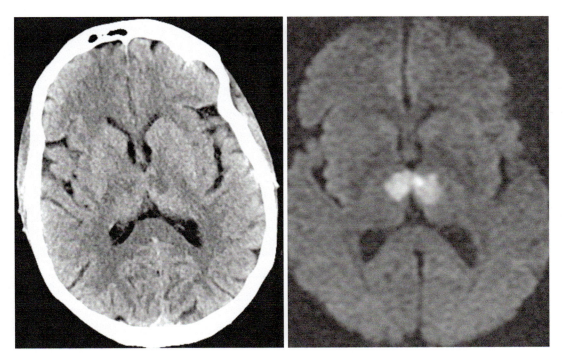

Fig. 9.15 The bilateral anterior thalami demonstrate hypoattenuation on CT and restricted diffusion on diffusion-weighted imaging

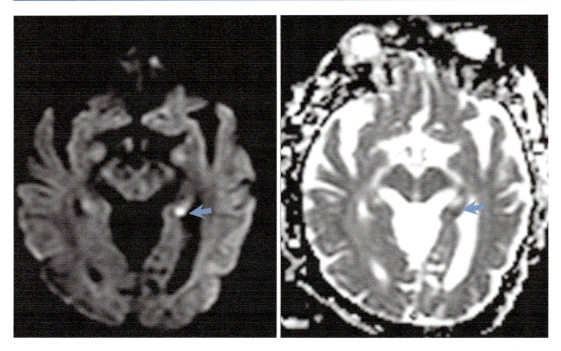

Fig. 9.16 Transient Global Amnesia. A 70-year-old male with history of hypertension and type 2 diabetes presented with episode of amnesia after having sexual intercourse following the use of sildenafil. Focal restricted diffusion in the left posterior hippocampus, which is usually supplied by the left posterior cerebral artery

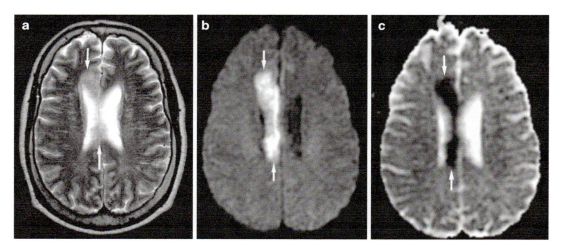

Fig. 9.17 (**a**–**c**) Corpus callosum infarction in a 64-year-old man with left-sided weakness. (**a**) T2-weighted image shows a hyperintense lesion in the anterior part and body of the corpus callosum extending into right frontal white matter (*arrows*). (**b**) DW image clearly shows this lesion as hyperintense (*arrows*). (**c**) ADC is decreased, representing acute infarction (*arrows*)

with corpus callosum infarcts can present with a variety of clinical signs and symptoms, which further complicates the diagnosis [63]. These lesions are readily detected by DW imaging and have signal characteristics similar to cerebral infarcts (Fig. 9.17).

9 Infarction

9.13 Stroke Mimickers

There is a long list of conditions that mimic the symptoms of an acute ischemic stroke. The most common ones include intracranial hemorrhage, migraines, seizures, functional and metabolic disorders, and also vasogenic edema syndromes. It is important to visualize and verify that an ischemic lesion is indeed the cause of the clinical symptoms before therapy is initiated, as these non-ischemic stroke mimickers should not be treated with thrombolysis and such therapy could actually be harmful. Moreover, in older patients it is not uncommon to detect older lesions with prolonged T2 that are indistinguishable from acute lesions using conventional MR imaging.

9.13.1 Hemiplegic Migraine

Hemiplegic migraine is a rare subtype which presents with severe headache attack that causes unilateral motor, sensory, or verbal weakness. Its prevalence is at around 1 in 10,000 with age of onset around 12 to 17 years of age. Like other migraine subtypes, it is more common in females. The attacks with auras may include visual field defects, numbness, paresthesias, motor weakness, aphasia, lethargy, and seizures. More severe attacks may mimic strokes or encephalopathy as patients may present with neurologic deficits and/or altered mental status.

Brain imaging is usually normal by CT or conventional MRI. However, a few patients may show unilateral hypo-/hyperperfusion, cortical edema, and/or high susceptibility of prominent cortical cerebral veins (Fig. 9.18).

9.13.2 Stroke-like Migraine Attacks after Radiation Therapy (SMART) Syndrome

Stroke-like migraine attacks after radiation therapy (SMART) syndrome is a rare complication occurring in patients with a history of brain irradiation 1–35 years prior. The syndrome typically occurs on average approximately 15–20 years after administration of high doses of radiation (>5000 centiGray). SMART syndrome is characterized by stroke-like symptoms, seizures, and migraines that often resolve spontaneously. Characteristic findings on MRI include transient unilateral cortical enhancement and high cortical T2 and FLAIR hyperintensity. Although a majority of cases are reversible (55%), some patients may present with irreversible superimposed infarcts (27%) (Fig. 9.19) [64].

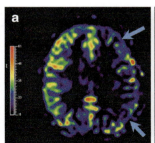 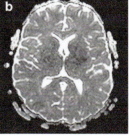 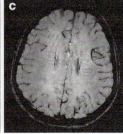 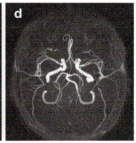

Fig. 9.18 (**a–d**) Young 13-year-old male presented with headache, right-sided facial droop, right upper weakness, and difficulty speaking. (**a**) The left hemisphere shows subtle but abnormally decreased cerebral blood flow or hypoperfusion (arrows) on pseudo-continuous arterial spin labeling (pCASL). (**b**) ADC map and DWI (not shown) are normal. (**c**) The left cortical veins are more prominent when compared to the right on susceptibility weighted imaging. (**d**) Time-of-flight MR angiogram of the circle of Willis showed slightly decreased overall flow-related enhancement of the left MCA vessels

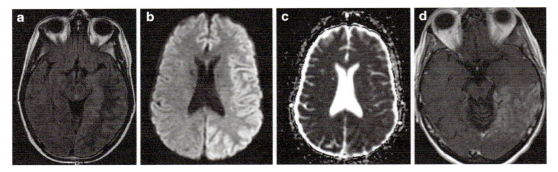

Fig. 9.19 (a–d) Remote history of metastatic melanoma and whole brain radiation therapy. (a) Subtle left temporal lobe gyriform edema on T2 FLAIR. (b, c) DWI shows increased signal in left cerebral hemisphere with minimal low ADC abnormality. (d) Gyriform left temporal lobe enhancement

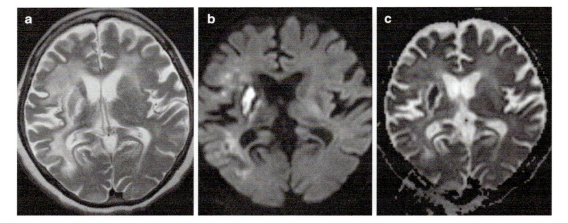

Fig. 9.20 (a–c) Hemorrhagic infarction in a 78-year-old woman with cardiogenic embolic-type acute infarction. (a) T2-weighted image shows a hyperintense area in the right white matter and hypointense lesions in right basal ganglia. (b) DW image shows hyperintense lesions in right basal ganglia, representing acute hemorrhagic infarction. (c) ADC is decreased with an area of hypointensity

9.14 Hemorrhagic Infarcts

About 40–50% of all stroke patients develop hemorrhagic transformation of their infarcts (Figs. 9.20 and 9.21). This usually occurs during the first week after onset of symptoms. The cause may be a spontaneous lysis of an embolus, which took place at a time when endothelial cells of the vessel had also been damaged by the ischemia, thus resulting in a breakthrough hemorrhage into the infarcted region. The incidence of hemorrhage is increased with use of thrombolytic therapy, as well as in the presence of certain clinical conditions, such as hypertension, embolic etiology, use of anticoagulant therapy, and increasing stroke severity.

Studies have shown that neuroimaging can predict which lesions are prone to progress into a hemorrhagic infarction [65]. Thus, ischemic lesions with a significantly greater percentage of low ADC values have a higher risk for hemorrhagic transformation than lesions with a smaller proportion of low ADC [65].

The most feared complication of tissue plasminogen activator therapy for acute stroke patients is symptomatic intracerebral hemorrhage. Patients with large baseline DW image lesion volumes who achieve early reperfusion

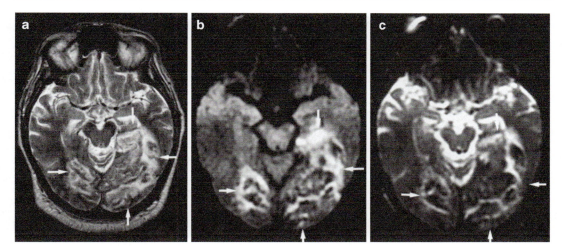

Fig. 9.21 (a–c) Hemorrhagic infarction in a 64-year-old man with mental status change. (**a**) T2-weighted image shows mixed hyper- and hypointense lesions in bilateral occipital lobes (*arrows*). (**b**) DW image shows these lesions as mixed hyper-, hypo-, and isointense, representing acute hemorrhagic infarction (*arrows*). (**c**) ADC is decreased with areas of DWI hyperintensity (*arrows*)

appear to be at greatest risk of symptomatic intracerebral hemorrhage after tissue plasminogen activator therapy [66].

9.15 Diffusion Tensor Imaging

The success of DW imaging is rooted in the concept that during their random diffusion-driven displacements, molecules probe the tissue structure. As diffusion is a three-dimensional process, molecular mobility in tissues may be anisotropic. With diffusion tensor (DT) imaging, diffusion anisotropy effects can be extracted, providing more details on tissue microstructure [37].

Both reduced [37, 67] and normal-to-elevated [68, 69] anisotropy have been reported in acute infarcts less than 24 h after the onset of symptoms. Some have proposed that increased diffusion anisotropy indicates continued structural integrity and tissue salvageability [68] and that increased anisotropic diffusion occurs as a result of fluid shift from the extracellular space to the intracellular space without membrane rupture [68]. Decreased diffusion anisotropy may signify the loss of cellular integrity with irreversible cellular injury.

Fiber tractography (FT) is a new method that can demonstrate the orientation and integrity of white matter fibers in vivo [70–72]; however, its

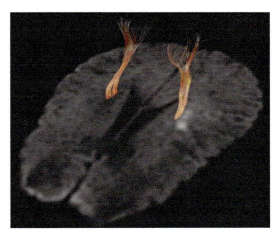

Fig. 9.22 An acute infarct in the left corona radiata in a 51-year-old woman. A 3D tractography superimposed on an axial isotropic DW image (from left anterosuperior viewpoint). An acute infarct is shown in the left corona radiata. The corticospinal tract (*orange lines*) of the affected cerebral hemisphere appears to be just medial to, but not to run through, the infarct. (Courtesy of Aoki S MD, University of Tokyo, Japan)

clinical application is still under investigation. In stroke, FT may improve our understanding of the symptom progression and predict functional recovery [73–75] (Figs. 9.22 and 9.23).

Kunimatsu et al. used FT to show the corticospinal tract in patients with acute or early subacute ischemic stroke involving the posterior

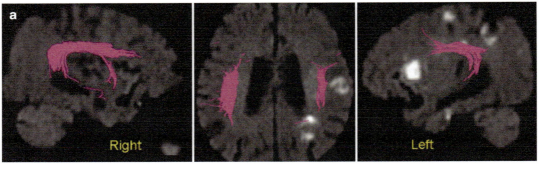

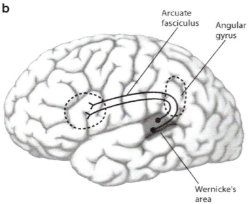

Fig. 9.23 (**a, b**) Acute left MCA infarcts in an 85-year-old woman with motor aphasia. (**a**) Sagittal and axial DW images superimposed with fiber tractography show the relationship between infarcts and the arcuate fasciculus. (**b**) The arcuate fasciculus forms a curved shape along the angular gyrus and connects the Wernicke area with the Broca area. (Courtesy of Yamada K MD, Kyoto Prefectural University of Medicine, Japan)

limb of the internal capsule or corona radiata and to assess involvement of the tract [73]. Infarcts and the tract were shown simultaneously, providing information on their spatial relationships. In five of the eight patients, three-dimensional fiber tract maps showed the corticospinal tract in close proximity to the infarct but not passing through it. All these patients recovered well, with maximum improvement from the lowest score on manual muscle testing (MMT) up to the full score through rehabilitation. In the other three patients the corticospinal tract was shown running through the infarct; reduction in MMT did not improve favorably or last longer, other than in one patient. Three-dimensional white matter tractography can show spatial relationships between the corticospinal tract and an infarct. The authors concluded that FT might be helpful in prognosis of gross motor function.

9.16 High-*b*-Value Diffusion-Weighted Imaging

The *b*-values applied in the stroke diffusion studies were usually in the range of 800–1500 s/mm². This range of *b*-values is considered reasonable based on contrast-to-noise ratio (CNR) estimates at gradient strengths of clinical MR instruments. MR technology has allowed higher *b*-values in recent years [76].

High-*b*-value DW imaging using a clinical MR imaging system has been applied and its clinical benefit has been discussed in the diagnosis of cerebral infarction. The initial application of DW imaging with high *b*-values of 2500–3000 s/mm² for acute or subacute infarction provided no apparent diagnostic advantages compared with those of usual images of $b = 1000$ s/mm² [77, 78].

However, the amount of diffusion weighting increases as the b-value increases [79]. Therefore, higher b-value DW imaging would be more advantageous in the diagnosis of hyperacute ischemic lesions in which mild diffusion changes can be present within the lesions than in the diagnosis of acute or subacute lesions. DW imaging at $b = 2000$ s/mm^2 was better than that at $b = 1000$ s/mm^2 for the detection and estimation of the extent of ischemia in patients with hyperacute ischemic stroke [80]. Toyoda et al. suggested that the size of the final infarction or irreversible cytotoxic edema was more predictable on high-b-value DW images than on the usual $b = 1000$ DW images (Fig. 9.24) [81].

9.17 Thin-Section Diffusion-Weighted Imaging

Conventional DW imaging uses 5–8-mm sections with a field of view of 20–40 cm and a matrix of 128–256, which produces in-plane resolution of $1–2 \times 1–2$ mm. Therefore, the in-plane resolution of DW imaging is higher than the section thickness. When a lesion is smaller than the section thickness and when it occupies only part of a voxel, the contrast relative to background tissue depends on both the signal intensity from the lesion and the proportion of the voxel that it occupies. Small, low-contrast lesions occupying only part of a voxel may go undetected. This phenomenon is known as partial volume effect [82, 83]. Nakamura et al. concluded that thin-section DW imaging with a 3-mm section thickness increased lesion conspicuity and improved the accuracy of stroke subtype diagnosis when comparing conventional 5-mm section DW imaging [84].

9.18 Treatment of Ischemic Stroke

Julius Griauzde and Neeraj Chaudhary

Intravenous tissue plasminogen activator (IV-tPA) has been the mainstay of ischemic stroke therapy for many years. Patients are deemed eligible for tPA if they are older than 18 years of age, have a measurable neurologic deficit, and have onset of symptoms within 3 h. The time window is expanded to 4.5 h in patients <80 years old and those whose stroke involves less than 1/3 of the affected middle cerebral artery territory. A complete discussion of contraindications to tPA is beyond the scope of this section, and is available via the American Heart Association's guidelines [85]. Key *imaging* exclusion criteria include CT demonstrating multilobar infarct, evidence of intracranial hemorrhage on CT, and presence of an intra-axial neoplasm. Patients with large intracranial aneurysms (<10 mm) and arteriovenous malformations may also be excluded.

In 2015, four landmark randomized control trials were published which placed mechanical thrombectomy at the forefront of the treatment of ischemic stroke. These trials (MR CLEAN, ESCAPE, EXTEND-IA, and SWIFT PRIME) demonstrated that mechanical thrombectomy in addition to IV-tPA was superior to IV-tPA alone in appropriately selected patients with large vessel occlusion ischemic stroke (internal carotid artery, middle cerebral artery) [86–89]. Patients in the thrombectomy groups were shown to have a significant increase in their chance of good neurologic outcomes at 90-day follow-up (Table 9.3). The outcomes of these trials led to broadly accepted guidelines for mechanical thrombectomy including ischemic stroke symptom onset within 6 h, Alberta stroke program early CT (ASPECT) score >6, and a national institute of health stroke scale (NIHSS) of ≥ 6.

More recently, two trials (DAWN and DEFUSE-3) were published which established treatment algorithms for late presenting anterior circulation large vessel ischemic stroke patients (6–24 h since last known neurologically normal) [90, 91]. These trials vastly expanded the role of perfusion imaging in treatment decisions of mechanical thrombectomy, with imaging criteria for inclusion in the DEFUSE 3 trial including <70 cc core infarct, a penumbra:core

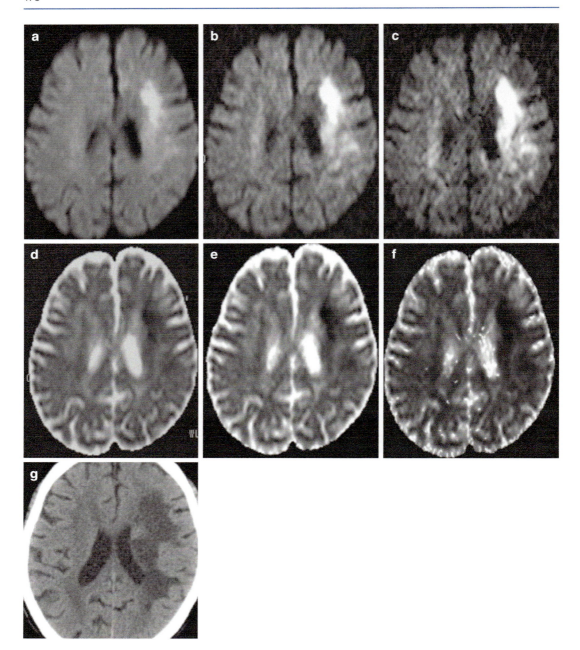

Fig. 9.24 (**a–g**) A cardiogenic embolic-type acute infarct in the left corona radiata in an 87-year-old woman. (**a**) $b = 1000$ isotropic DW image, (**b**) $b = 2000$ isotropic DW image, (**c**) $b = 3000$ isotropic DW image, (**d**) $b = 1000$ ADC map, (**e**) $b = 2000$ ADC map, (**f**) $b = 3000$ ADC map at the same level. (**g**) Follow-up CT. On the isotropic DW images (**a–c**) and ADC map (**d–f**), the area of restricted diffusion became more distinct and more extensive with increasing b-value. The area of the final infarct (**g**) was partly included in the site of decreased diffusion on the $b = 3000$ DW image. Such a change was hardly indicated on the $b = 1000$ DW images or ADC map. (Courtesy of Toyoda K MD, Kameda Medical Center, Japan)

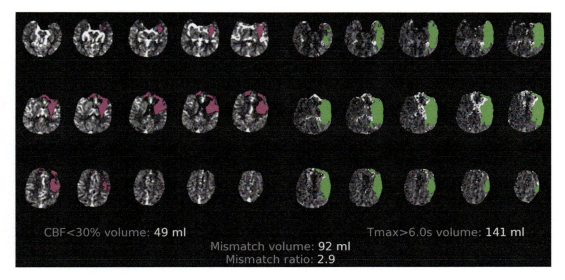

Fig. 9.25 Example of a patient with left MCA occlusion who underwent endovascular thrombectomy based on CT perfusion scan and use of automated image post-processing software. There is a small region of severely reduced cerebral blood flow (<30% of that in normal tissue), which represents early infarct (ischemic core), of 49 mL (pink) and a region of perfusion delay of more than 6 s, which represents hypoperfused tissue, of 141 mL (green). The penumbra:core mismatch ratio is 2.9

Table 9.3 Mechanical thrombectomy trial outcomes (thrombectomy + IV-tPA vs IV-tPA alone)

	MR CLEAN	ESCAPE	EXTEND-IA	SWIFT PRIME
% with good neurologic outcome	33% vs 19% $P < 0.05$	53% vs 29% $P < 0.001$	71% vs 40% $P < 0.01$	60% vs 35% $P < 0.001$
% with symptomatic hemorrhagic conversion	8% vs 6% Difference not significant	4% vs 3% Difference not significant	11% vs 15% Difference not significant	0% vs 3% Difference not significant

mismatch ratio of 1.8 or greater, and a mismatch volume of >15 cc (Fig. 9.25). Mechanical thrombectomy in posterior circulation stroke patients with large vessel occlusion remains a topic of some debate, but indications are largely extrapolated from anterior circulation trials and treatment windows are often extended to 24 h, given the dire outcome of posterior circulation stroke in untreated patients. Recently the WAKE-UP trial has been published utilizing MRI diffusion and FLAIR imaging to assess onset of ischemia in patients with unknown onset time of neurologic symptoms. Patients without FLAIR signal changes corresponding to areas of restricted diffusion were assumed to have had onset within 4.5 h, making them eligible for IV-tPA administration (Fig. 9.26) [92].

9.18.1 Procedural Details and Considerations

Mechanical thrombectomy is performed utilizing either stent retrievers, aspiration catheters, or both. Balloon guide catheters are sometimes used in the more proximal vasculature to arrest forward flow within the involved vascular distribution, decreasing the risk of distal embolization. At our institution, a combined approach is often utilized employing both a stent retriever and an aspiration catheter (termed the SOLUMBRA technique) [93]. Once a stable position is achieved in the ipsilateral cervical ICA with a guide catheter, intracranial catheterization is performed with an intermediate suction catheter and a microcatheter advanced over a microwire. The

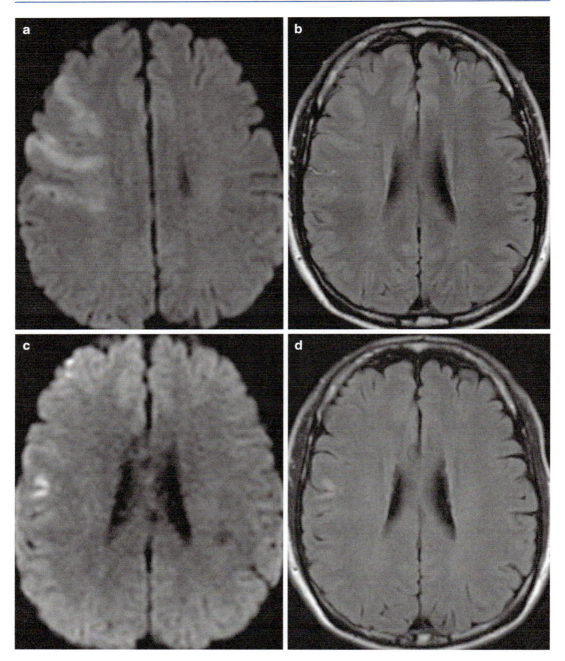

Fig. 9.26 (**a** and **b**) Diffusion and FLAIR MR images in a patient presenting within 4 h of symptom onset demonstrating abnormal diffusion hyperintensity in the right frontal region without corresponding FLAIR hyperintensity. (**c** and **d**) Follow-up images after IV-tPA and endovascular therapy showing near complete resolution of diffusion hyperintensities. The patient made a complete neurologic recovery

intermediate suction catheter is left proximal to the occlusive thrombus and connected to a mechanical suction device (Fig. 9.27). The microcatheter and microwire are advanced beyond the occlusive thrombus and a stent retriever device is deployed from distal to proximal across the occlusive thrombus (Fig. 9.27). Initially, recommendations were for

9 Infarction

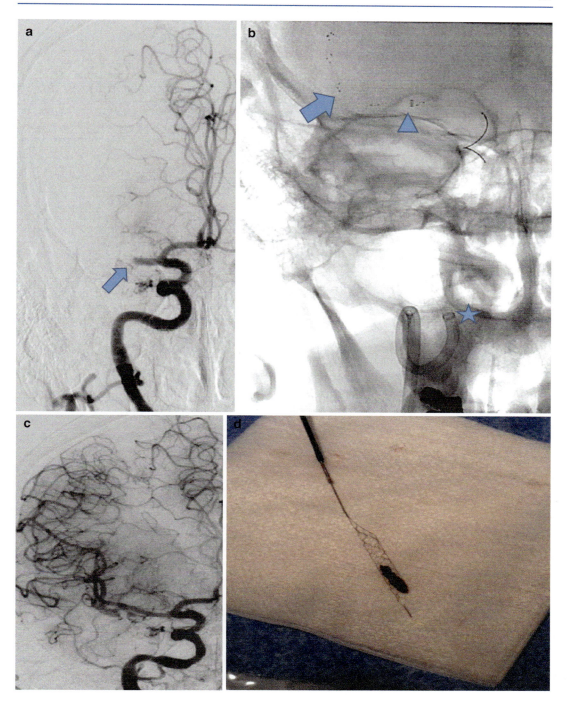

Fig. 9.27 (a) AP digital subtraction angiographic image with injection of the right internal carotid artery demonstrating abrupt cutoff of the M1 portion of the right middle cerebral artery (arrow). (b) Single shot fluoroscopic image demonstrating deployed stent retriever across the occlusion (arrow), the intermediate suction catheter just proximal to the site of occlusion (arrowhead), and the guide catheter within the tortuous right internal carotid artery (star). (c) Post-thrombectomy AP digital subtraction angiographic image with injection of the right internal carotid artery demonstrating recanalization of the right middle cerebral artery with complete filling of all distal branches (TICI3). (d) Picture of the stent retriever and removed embolus ex vivo

the stent retriever device to be left open for 5 min prior to removal. More recently, authors have advocated for a longer stent retriever dwell time (up to 8 min) to allow for improved expansion of the stent and incorporation of the thrombus within the tines of the stent [94]. Following the dwell time, the stent retriever and suction catheter are removed in tandem, often with manual negative aspiration applied to the guide catheter. Mechanical thrombectomy is often repeated until all proximal thrombus is removed. Subsequent attempts at thrombectomy must be performed judiciously as studies have shown that clot compaction occurs with each attempt, decreasing the chances of recanalization and increasing the chances of vessel injury [95].

Vessel recanalization is reported based on the thrombolysis in cerebral infarction score (TICI score) as follows: 0—No perfusion, 1—penetration with minimal perfusion, 2a—partial perfusion filling less than 50% of the distal branches, 2b—partial perfusion with filling of >50% of the distal branches, 3—full perfusion with filling of all distal branches [96]. Patients in whom TICI2b or 3 recanalization is achieved have been shown to have better outcomes than those with less robust recanalization [97]. Dual energy CT is performed on post procedure day 1, to evaluate for hemorrhagic conversion, which would alter subsequent clinical management.

References

1. Xu JQ, Murphy SL, Kochanek KD, Bastian B, Arias E (2018) Deaths: Final data for 2016. National Vital Statistics Reports. National Center for Health Statistics: Hyattsville, MD
2. National Institute of Neurological, D. and P.A.S.S.G. Stroke rt (1995) Tissue plasminogen activator for acute ischemic stroke. N Engl J Med 333(24):1581–1587
3. Berkhemer OA et al (2015) A randomized trial of intraarterial treatment for acute ischemic stroke. N Engl J Med 372(1):11–20
4. Campbell BC et al (2015) Endovascular therapy for ischemic stroke with perfusion-imaging selection. N Engl J Med 372(11):1009–1018
5. Goyal M et al (2016) Endovascular thrombectomy after large-vessel ischaemic stroke: a meta-analysis

of individual patient data from five randomised trials. Lancet 387(10029):1723–1731
6. Saver JL et al (2015) Stent-retriever thrombectomy after intravenous t-PA vs. t-PA alone in stroke. N Engl J Med 372(24):2285–2295
7. Goyal M et al (2015) Randomized assessment of rapid endovascular treatment of ischemic stroke. N Engl J Med 372(11):1019–1030
8. Mohr JP et al (1995) Magnetic resonance versus computed tomographic imaging in acute stroke. Stroke 26(5):807–812
9. Moseley ME et al (1990) Diffusion-weighted MR imaging of acute stroke: correlation with T2-weighted and magnetic susceptibility-enhanced MR imaging in cats. AJNR Am J Neuroradiol 11(3):423–429
10. Marks MP et al (1996) Acute and chronic stroke: navigated spin-echo diffusion-weighted MR imaging. Radiology 199(2):403–408
11. Gonzalez RG et al (1999) Diffusion-weighted MR imaging: diagnostic accuracy in patients imaged within 6 hours of stroke symptom onset. Radiology 210(1):155–162
12. Lovblad KO et al (1998) Clinical experience with diffusion-weighted MR in patients with acute stroke. AJNR Am J Neuroradiol 19(6):1061–1066
13. Chien, D et al (1992) MR diffusion imaging of cerebral infarction in humans. AJNR Am J Neuroradiol 13(4):1097–1102; discussion 1103–5
14. Schaefer PW, Grant PE, Gonzalez RG (2000) Diffusion-weighted MR imaging of the brain. Radiology 217(2):331–345
15. Gudbjartsson H et al (1996) Line scan diffusion imaging. Magn Reson Med 36(4):509–519
16. de Crespigny AJ et al (1995) Navigated diffusion imaging of normal and ischemic human brain. Magn Reson Med 33(5):720–728
17. Lefkowitz D et al (1999) Hyperacute ischemic stroke missed by diffusion-weighted imaging. AJNR Am J Neuroradiol 20(10):1871–1875
18. Wang PY et al (1999) Diffusion-negative stroke: a report of two cases. AJNR Am J Neuroradiol 20(10):1876–1880
19. Benveniste H, Hedlund LW, Johnson GA (1992) Mechanism of detection of acute cerebral ischemia in rats by diffusion-weighted magnetic resonance microscopy. Stroke 23(5):746–754
20. Mintorovitch J et al (1994) Diffusion-weighted magnetic resonance imaging of acute focal cerebral ischemia: comparison of signal intensity with changes in brain water and Na+,K(+)-ATPase activity. J Cereb Blood Flow Metab 14(2):332–336
21. Sykova E et al (1994) Extracellular volume fraction and diffusion characteristics during progressive ischemia and terminal anoxia in the spinal cord of the rat. J Cereb Blood Flow Metab 14(2):301–311
22. Niendorf T et al (1996) Biexponential diffusion attenuation in various states of brain tissue: implications for diffusion-weighted imaging. Magn Reson Med 36(6):847–857

23. Provenzale JM, Sorensen AG (1999) Diffusion-weighted MR imaging in acute stroke: theoretic considerations and clinical applications. AJR Am J Roentgenol 173(6):1459–1467
24. Keller E et al (1999) Diffusion- and perfusion-weighted magnetic resonance imaging in deep cerebral venous thrombosis. Stroke 30(5):1144–1146
25. Busza AL et al (1992) Diffusion-weighted imaging studies of cerebral ischemia in gerbils. Potential relevance to energy failure. Stroke 23(11):1602–1612
26. Burdette JH, Elster AD, Ricci PE (1999) Acute cerebral infarction: quantification of spin-density and T2 shine-through phenomena on diffusion-weighted MR images. Radiology 212(2):333–339
27. Grant PE et al (2001) Frequency and clinical context of decreased apparent diffusion coefficient reversal in the human brain. Radiology 221(1):43–50
28. Fiebach JB et al (2002) Serial analysis of the apparent diffusion coefficient time course in human stroke. Neuroradiology 44(4):294–298
29. Hasegawa Y et al (1994) MRI diffusion mapping of reversible and irreversible ischemic injury in focal brain ischemia. Neurology 44(8):1484–1490
30. Dardzinski BJ et al (1993) Apparent diffusion coefficient mapping of experimental focal cerebral ischemia using diffusion-weighted echo-planar imaging. Magn Reson Med 30(3):318–325
31. Singer MB et al (1998) Diffusion-weighted MRI in acute subcortical infarction. Stroke 29(1):133–136
32. Desmond PM et al (2001) The value of apparent diffusion coefficient maps in early cerebral ischemia. AJNR Am J Neuroradiol 22(7):1260–1267
33. Huang IJ et al (2001) Time course of cerebral infarction in the middle cerebral arterial territory: deep watershed versus territorial subtypes on diffusion-weighted MR images. Radiology 221(1):35–42
34. Kidwell CS et al (2000) Thrombolytic reversal of acute human cerebral ischemic injury shown by diffusion/perfusion magnetic resonance imaging. Ann Neurol 47(4):462–469
35. Burdette JH et al (1998) Cerebral infarction: time course of signal intensity changes on diffusion-weighted MR images. AJR Am J Roentgenol 171(3):791–795
36. Provenzale JM et al (2003) Assessment of the patient with hyperacute stroke: imaging and therapy. Radiology 229(2):347–359
37. Mukherjee P et al (2000) Differences between gray matter and white matter water diffusion in stroke: diffusion-tensor MR imaging in 12 patients. Radiology 215(1):211–220
38. Krueger K et al (2000) Late resolution of diffusion-weighted MRI changes in a patient with prolonged reversible ischemic neurological deficit after thrombolytic therapy. Stroke 31(11):2715–2718
39. Fitzek C et al (1998) Differentiation of recent and old cerebral infarcts by diffusion-weighted MRI. Neuroradiology 40(12):778–782
40. Pantoni L, Garcia JH, Gutierrez JA (1996) Cerebral white matter is highly vulnerable to ischemia. Stroke 27(9):1641–1646; discussion 1647
41. Kuroiwa T et al (1998) Different apparent diffusion coefficient: water content correlations of gray and white matter during early ischemia. Stroke 29(4):859–865
42. Fiehler J et al (2004) Predictors of apparent diffusion coefficient normalization in stroke patients. Stroke 35(2):514–519
43. Caplan LR et al (1997) Should thrombolytic therapy be the first-line treatment for acute ischemic stroke? Thrombolysis--not a panacea for ischemic stroke. N Engl J Med 337(18):1309–1310; discussion 1313
44. Hacke W et al (2005) The Desmoteplase in Acute Ischemic Stroke Trial (DIAS): a phase II MRI-based 9-hour window acute stroke thrombolysis trial with intravenous desmoteplase. Stroke 36(1):66–73
45. Albers GW et al (2018) Thrombectomy for stroke at 6 to 16 hours with selection by perfusion imaging. N Engl J Med 378(8):708–718
46. Barber PA et al (2005) Imaging of the brain in acute ischaemic stroke: comparison of computed tomography and magnetic resonance diffusion-weighted imaging. J Neurol Neurosurg Psychiatry 76(11):1528–1533
47. Mitomi M et al (2014) Comparison of CT and DWI findings in ischemic stroke patients within 3 hours of onset. J Stroke Cerebrovasc Dis 23(1):37–42
48. Aviv RI et al (2007) Alberta stroke program early CT scoring of CT perfusion in early stroke visualization and assessment. AJNR Am J Neuroradiol 28(10):1975–1980
49. Barber PA et al (2000) Validity and reliability of a quantitative computed tomography score in predicting outcome of hyperacute stroke before thrombolytic therapy. ASPECTS Study Group. Alberta Stroke Programme Early CT Score. Lancet 355(9216):1670–1674
50. Yoshikawa T et al (2002) Diffusion-weighted magnetic resonance imaging of dural sinus thrombosis. Neuroradiology 44(6):481–488
51. Forbes KP, Pipe JG, Heiserman JE (2001) Evidence for cytotoxic edema in the pathogenesis of cerebral venous infarction. AJNR Am J Neuroradiol 22(3):450–455
52. Leach JL et al (2006) Imaging of cerebral venous thrombosis: current techniques, spectrum of findings, and diagnostic pitfalls. Radiographics 26 Suppl 1:S19–S41; discussion S42–3
53. Ducreux D et al (2001) Diffusion-weighted imaging patterns of brain damage associated with cerebral venous thrombosis. AJNR Am J Neuroradiol 22(2):261–268
54. Favrole P et al (2004) Diffusion-weighted imaging of intravascular clots in cerebral venous thrombosis. Stroke 35(1):99–103
55. Geijer B et al (2001) Persistent high signal on diffusion-weighted MRI in the late stages of small

cortical and lacunar ischaemic lesions. Neuroradiology 43(2):115–122

56. Noguchi K et al (1998) Diffusion-weighted echo-planar MRI of lacunar infarcts. Neuroradiology 40(7):448–451

57. Kuhl CK et al (2005) Sensitivity encoding for diffusion-weighted MR imaging at 3.0 T: intraindividual comparative study. Radiology 234(2):517–526

58. Forbes KP et al (2002) Improved image quality and detection of acute cerebral infarction with PROPELLER diffusion-weighted MR imaging. Radiology 225(2):551–555

59. Pardina-Vilella L et al (2018) The goblet sign in the amnestic syndrome of the subcallosal artery infarct. Neurol Sci 39(8):1463–1465

60. Jang JW et al (2014) Different risk factor profiles between transient global amnesia and transient ischemic attack: a large case-control study. Eur Neurol 71(1–2):19–24

61. Zhang Z, Liu Z, Peng D (2019) Transient global amnesia secondary to atherosclerotic stenosis of accessory posterior cerebral artery. J Stroke Cerebrovasc Dis 28:e22–e23

62. Suwanwela NC, Leelacheavasit N (2002) Isolated corpus callosal infarction secondary to pericallosal artery disease presenting as alien hand syndrome. J Neurol Neurosurg Psychiatry 72(4):533–536

63. Riedy G, Melhem ER (2003) Acute infarct of the corpus callosum: appearance on diffusion-weighted MR imaging and MR spectroscopy. J Magn Reson Imaging 18(2):255–259

64. Black DF, Morris JM, Lindell EP et al (2013) Stroke-Like Migraine Attacks after Radiation Therapy (SMART) Syndrome Is Not Always Completely Reversible: A Case Series. AJNR Am J Neuroradiol. https://doi.org/10.3174/ajnr.A3602

65. Tong DC et al (2000) Relationship between apparent diffusion coefficient and subsequent hemorrhagic transformation following acute ischemic stroke. Stroke 31(10):2378–2384

66. Lansberg MG et al (2007) Risk factors of symptomatic intracerebral hemorrhage after tPA therapy for acute stroke. Stroke 38(8):2275–2278

67. Sorensen AG et al (1999) Human acute cerebral ischemia: detection of changes in water diffusion anisotropy by using MR imaging. Radiology 212(3):785–792

68. Yang Q et al (1999) Serial study of apparent diffusion coefficient and anisotropy in patients with acute stroke. Stroke 30(11):2382–2390

69. Ozsunar Y et al (2004) Evolution of water diffusion and anisotropy in hyperacute stroke: significant correlation between fractional anisotropy and T2. AJNR Am J Neuroradiol 25(5):699–705

70. Le Bihan D et al (2001) Diffusion tensor imaging: concepts and applications. J Magn Reson Imaging 13(4):534–546

71. Stieltjes B et al (2001) Diffusion tensor imaging and axonal tracking in the human brainstem. NeuroImage 14(3):723–735

72. Lee SK et al (2005) Diffusion-tensor MR imaging and fiber tractography: a new method of describing aberrant fiber connections in developmental CNS anomalies. Radiographics 25(1):53–65; discussion 66–8

73. Kunimatsu A et al (2003) Three-dimensional white matter tractography by diffusion tensor imaging in ischaemic stroke involving the corticospinal tract. Neuroradiology 45(8):532–535

74. Yamada K et al (2004) Stroke patients' evolving symptoms assessed by tractography. J Magn Reson Imaging 20(6):923–929

75. Konishi J et al (2005) MR tractography for the evaluation of functional recovery from lenticulostriate infarcts. Neurology 64(1):108–113

76. Yoshiura T et al (2001) Highly diffusion-sensitized MRI of brain: dissociation of gray and white matter. Magn Reson Med 45(5):734–740

77. Meyer JR et al (2000) High-b-value diffusion-weighted MR imaging of suspected brain infarction. AJNR Am J Neuroradiol 21(10):1821–1829

78. Burdette JH, Elster AD (2002) Diffusion-weighted imaging of cerebral infarctions: are higher B values better? J Comput Assist Tomogr 26(4):622–627

79. Stejskal EO, Tanner JE (1965) Spin diffusion measurements: spin echoes in the presence of a time-dependent field gradient. J Chem Phys 42:288–292

80. Kim HJ et al (2005) High-b-value diffusion-weighted MR imaging of hyperacute ischemic stroke at 1.5T. AJNR Am J Neuroradiol 26(2):208–215

81. Toyoda K et al (2007) Usefulness of high-b-value diffusion-weighted imaging in acute cerebral infarction. Eur Radiol 17(5):1212–1220

82. Molyneux PD et al (1998) The effect of section thickness on MR lesion detection and quantification in multiple sclerosis. AJNR Am J Neuroradiol 19(9):1715–1720

83. Bradley WG, Glenn BJ (1987) The effect of variation in slice thickness and interslice gap on MR lesion detection. AJNR Am J Neuroradiol 8(6):1057–1062

84. Nakamura H et al (2005) Effect of thin-section diffusion-weighted MR imaging on stroke diagnosis. AJNR Am J Neuroradiol 26(3):560–565

85. Powers WJ, Rabinstein AA, Ackerson T et al (2018) 2018 guidelines for the early management of patients with acute ischemic stroke: a guideline for healthcare professionals from the American Heart Association/American Stroke Association. Stroke 49(3):e46–e110

86. Berkhemer OA, Fransen PS, Beumer D et al (2015) A randomized trial of intraarterial treatment for acute ischemic stroke. N Engl J Med 372(1):11–20

87. Campbell BC, Mitchell PJ, Kleinig TJ et al (2015) Endovascular therapy for ischemic stroke with perfusion-imaging selection. N Engl J Med 372(11):1009–1018

88. Goyal M, Demchuk AM, Menon BK et al (2015) Randomized assessment of rapid endovascular treatment of ischemic stroke. N Engl J Med 372(11):1019–1030

89. Saver JL, Goyal M, Bonafe A et al (2015) Stent-retriever thrombectomy after intravenous t-PA vs. t-PA alone in stroke. N Engl J Med 372(24):2285–2295

90. Albers GW, Marks MP, Kemp S et al (2018) Thrombectomy for stroke at 6 to 16 hours with selection by perfusion imaging. N Engl J Med 378(8):708–718
91. Nogueira RG, Jadhav AP, Haussen DC et al (2018) Thrombectomy 6 to 24 hours after stroke with a mismatch between deficit and infarct. N Engl J Med 378(1):11–21
92. Thomalla G, Simonsen CZ, Boutitie F et al (2018) MRI-guided thrombolysis for stroke with unknown time of onset. N Engl J Med 379(7):611–622
93. Humphries W, Hoit D, Doss VT et al (2015) Distal aspiration with retrievable stent assisted thrombectomy for the treatment of acute ischemic stroke. J Neurointerv Surg 7(2):90–94
94. Kannath SK, Rajan JE, Sylaja PN et al (2018) Dwell time of stentriever influences complete revascular-ization and first-pass TICI 3 revascularization in acute large vessel occlusive stroke. World Neurosurg 110:169–173
95. Baek JH, Kim BM, Heo JH et al (2018) Number of Stent retriever passes associated with futile recanalization in acute stroke. Stroke 49(9):2088–2095
96. Zaidat OO, Yoo AJ, Khatri P et al (2013) Recommendations on angiographic revascularization grading standards for acute ischemic stroke: a consensus statement. Stroke 44(9):2650–2663
97. Goyal M, Menon BK, van Zwam WH et al (2016) Endovascular thrombectomy after large-vessel ischaemic stroke: a meta-analysis of individual patient data from five randomised trials. Lancet 387(10029):1723–1731

Intracranial Hemorrhage

10

Toshio Moritani, and Akio Hiwatashi

Sravanthi Koduri, Zachary Marcus Wilseck, Ankur Bhambri, and Aditya S. Pandey

10.1 Introduction

Intracranial hemorrhages are often characterized according to their location, such as intraparenchymal, subarachnoid, subdural, epidural, and intraventricular hemorrhages. The etiology of these hemorrhages includes a variety of heterogeneous conditions, such as trauma, hypertension, infarction, infection, neoplasm, vascular malformations, vasculitis, vasculopathy, coagulopathy, and drugs. This chapter will describe diffusion-weighted (DW) imaging characteristics of intracranial hemorrhages in relation to their location and evolutionary stage.

T. Moritani (✉)
Division of Neuroradiology, Department of Radiology, Clinical Neuroradiology Research, University of Michigan, Ann Arbor, MI, USA
e-mail: tmoritan@med.umich.edu

A. Hiwatashi
Department of Clinical Radiology, Kyushu University, Fukuoka, Japan

S. Koduri · A. Bhambri
Department of Neurosurgery, University of Michigan, Ann Arbor, MI, USA
e-mail: skoduri@umich.edu; abhambri@umich.edu

Z. M. Wilseck
Department of Radiology, University of Michigan, Ann Arbor, MI, USA
e-mail: zwilseck@umich.edu

A. S. Pandey
University of Michigan, Ann Arbor, MI, USA
e-mail: adityap@umich.edu

10.2 Intraparenchymal Hemorrhages: Appearance and Evolution (Fig. 10.1 and Tables 10.1 and 10.2)

The classic pattern for the temporal evolution of intracerebral hematomas on MR images at 1.5 T is well known [1–37]. However, actual evolution of hematoma is thought to be more complex. The change in signal intensity over time depends on many factors, such as the oxygenation state of hemoglobin, the status of red blood cell membranes, hematocrit, proteins, and clot formation [1–33, 36, 37]. Among these, the evolution of hemoglobin and the red cell membrane integrity are the most important [1–22, 24, 27, 29, 30, 32, 33]. The transition of oxy-hemoglobin to deoxy-hemoglobin (deoxyHb) and thereafter to met-hemoglobin (metHb) depends primarily upon the oxygen tension in the vicinity of the lesion as well as inside the hematoma itself. Therefore, the determination of the age of a hemorrhage is often inaccurate because of the variations between individual patients.

In the hyperacute phase of hemorrhage, oxy-hemoglobin (oxyHb) will dominate initially (Fig. 10.1). However, transformation into deoxyHb with deoxygenation will soon take place and deoxyHb will dominate after several hours to few days—the acute phase of hematoma. Within a few days to a week, deoxyHb will transform to metHb with oxidative denaturation—the early subacute phase of hematoma. The rate of this oxidation to

© Springer Nature Switzerland AG 2021
T. Moritani, A. A. Capizzano (eds.), *Diffusion-Weighted MR Imaging of the Brain, Head and Neck, and Spine*, https://doi.org/10.1007/978-3-030-62120-9_10

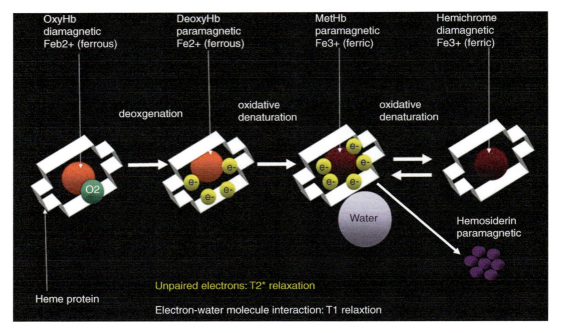

Fig. 10.1 OxyHb (diamagnetic, ferrous heme iron with oxygen molecule) predominates in the circulation and hyperacute hemorrhage. OxyHb is transformed into deoxyHb (paramagnetic, ferrous heme iron with 4 unpaired electrons) with deoxygenation after a few to several hours following hemorrhage, which dominates in acute hematoma. Within a few days to a week, deoxyHb will transform to metHb (paramagnetic, ferric heme iron with 5 unpaired electrons and a water molecule) with oxidative denaturation, which dominates in early subacute hematoma. Unpaired electrons cause T2* relaxation. Electron–water molecule interaction causes T1 relaxation. When the red cell membranes start to rupture, metHb will be found in the extracellular fluid space, which takes place about two weeks to a few months (late subacute to early chronic hematoma). In the chronic stage, there is continuous phagocytation of the breakdown products of hemoglobin by macrophages, resulting in hemosiderin and ferritin deposition in the periphery of the hematoma, which starts about one month following hemorrhage. On the other hand, the center of the chronic hematoma is a proteinaceous viscous solution that may contain "hemichrome" (diamagnetic, ferric heme) which is transformed and interchangeable from extracellular metHb with continued oxidative denaturation after a few to several months

Table 10.1 Time course of intraparenchymal hematomas

	Hyperacute	Acute	Early subacute	Late subacute	Chronic
T2	Hyper	Dark	Dark	Bright	Bright with dark rim
T1	Hypo/iso	Hypo/iso	Bright	Bright	Hypo
DW	Bright	Dark	Dark	Bright	Hyper-hypo
ADC	Dark	NAC	NAC	Dark	Increase/NAC

NAC no accurate calculation

metHb will depend on the oxygen tension in the tissue, which may further complicate the temporal pattern of expected signal changes.

Initially, metHb will be found within intact red blood cells in the early subacute stage, but when the red cell membranes start to rupture, metHb will be found in the extracellular fluid space, which takes place about two weeks to a few months following hemorrhage—the late subacute to early chronic phase of hematoma.

In the chronic stage, there is continuous phagocytation of the breakdown products of hemoglobin by macrophages, resulting in hemosiderin and ferritin deposition in the periphery of the hematoma, which starts about one month following hemorrhage. On the other hand, the center of the chronic hematoma is still proteinaceous viscous solution that contains "hemichrome" which is transformed from extracellular metHb with continued oxidative denaturation, seen after

Table 10.2 Time course of intraparenchymal hematomas (schematic more in detail)

	Hyperacute (oxyHb)	Acute (deoxyHb)	Early subacute (metHb)	Late subacute (extracellular metHb)	Early chronic (hemichrome/hemosiderin rim)	Late chronic (hemosiderin rim/deposition)
T1	Iso	Iso	Bright	Bright	Isocenter with dark rim	Dark center with dark rim to dark
T2	Iso	Dark	Dark	Bright	Isocenter with dark rim	Bright center with dark rim to dark
DWI	Bright	Dark	Dark	Bright	Bright center with dark rim	Dark center with dark rim to dark
ADC	Dark	NAC	NAC	Dark	Dark center with NAC rim	Bright center with NAC rim to NAC

NAC: no accurate calculation

a few months in the late chronic phase [38]. The chronic hematoma is resorbed over time, leading to less viscous solution and cavity collapse. However, the accumulation of the hemosiderin and ferritin within the phagocytic cells will remain for years or maybe indefinitely, as a marker of an old hemorrhage.

10.2.1 Hyperacute Hematoma

In the early stage of a hyperacute hematoma (Figs. 10.2 and 10.3), oxygenated hemoglobin within intact red blood cells is dominant. OxyHb is a diamagnetic substance and will, as such, generate an opposing magnetic field that reduces the applied

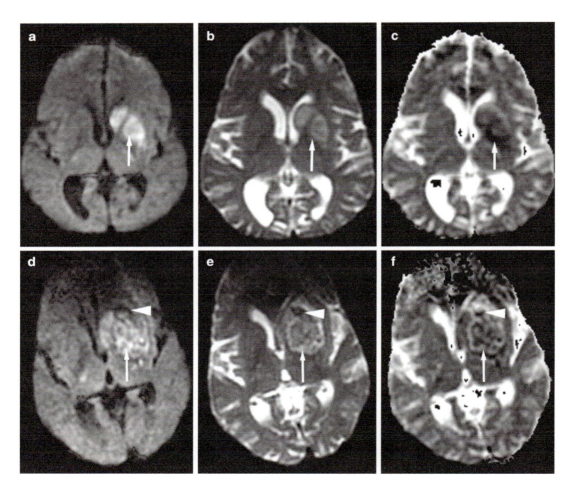

Fig. 10.2 (**a**–**f**) Acute infarction with hyperacute hemorrhage (oxyHb/deoxyHb). A 72-year-old woman suffered from a right-sided weakness. MR imaging 30 hours after the onset of symptoms (**a**–**c**) showed a lesion in the right basal ganglia (arrow) that is hyperintense on DW (**a**) and b$_0$ images (**b**). On the ADC map (**c**) the lesion is hypointense (arrow), indicating that this is a non-hemorrhagic acute infarction. During the end of the MR scanning, 30.5 hours after the onset of symptoms (**d**–**f**), the patient suddenly lost consciousness. The study was repeated, showing the increased size of the basal ganglia lesion. On the DW image (**d**) there is now a heterogeneous hyperintensity (arrow), consistent with oxy-hemoglobin. The b$_0$ image (**e**) also shows the lesion as heterogeneous, hyperintense (arrow), supporting oxy-hemoglobin. Note the new regions of hypointensity around the lesion (arrowhead), indicating deoxyHb (**d**–**f**). The ADC map (**f**) shows the lesions as heterogeneously hypointense, consistent with oxyHb (arrow). However, it is difficult to calculate the ADC due to the presence of paramagnetic deoxyHb (arrowhead)

10 Intracranial Hemorrhage

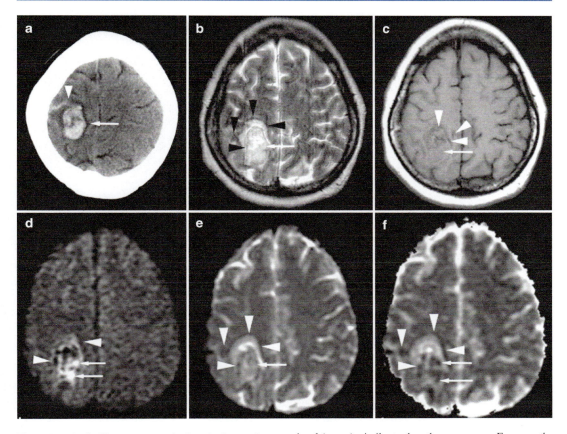

Fig. 10.3 (**a–f**) Hyperacute and chronic hemorrhage (oxyHb/deoxyHb, metHb, and hemosiderin/ferritin). A 40-year-old woman developed an acute left-sided weakness. A non-enhanced CT scan 6 hours after the onset of symptoms (**a**) shows a hyperdense lesion (arrow) in the right frontoparietal region associated with a small amount of subarachnoid hemorrhage (arrowhead). MR imaging 12 hours after the onset of symptoms (**b–h**) shows a heterogeneous lesion with areas of central hyperintensity on the T2-weighted image (**b**) (arrow; oxyHb) with a peripheral hypointensity from the susceptibility influence of paramagnetic material (arrowheads; deoxyHb). The T1-weighted image (**c**) shows the lesion as heterogeneous with areas of isointensity (arrow; oxyHb) and hypointensity (arrowheads; deoxyHb). Both the DW (**d**) and b_0 images (**e**) show the lesion as heterogeneous with areas of hyperintensity (arrows; oxyHb) and hypointensity (arrowheads; deoxyHb). The hypointensity is more prominent on these sequences than on the T2-weighted image (**b**). The ADC map (**f**) has a similar appearance of a heterogeneous lesion with areas of hypointensity (arrows; oxyHb and arrowheads; deoxyHb). As usual, when there is a strong susceptibility influence, it is difficult to calculate ADC (**g–n**) The coronal GRE image (**g**) and the GRE–echoplanar image (**h**) are more sensitive in depicting the susceptibility effect from deoxy-hemoglobin (arrowheads). The diamagnetic oxyHb will, as expected, show an isointense signal (arrow), similar to the other sequences. Four months after the onset of symptoms (**i–n**), the patient had a new MR examination. On a T2-weighted image (**i**), the lesion is still heterogeneous, but there are now areas of hyperintensity (extracellular metHb; arrow) and hypointensity (arrowheads; hemosiderin/ferritin). The T1-weighted image (**j**) shows the heterogeneous lesion with areas of hyperintensity (arrow; extracellular metHb) and hypointensity (hemosiderin/ferritin). The DW image (**k**) shows the lesion as hypointense overall and the same is seen on the b_0 image (**l**), but this "T2-weighted" image has a small hyperintense zone in the center of the hematoma, probably due to extracellular metHb (arrow). The hypointensity (arrowheads) on the b_0 image (**l**) is more pronounced than on the conventional T2-weighted image (**i**), demonstrating the higher sensitivity to susceptibility with this imaging sequence. The susceptibility effect will make it difficult to calculate ADC accurately, but the ADC map (**m**) will demonstrate the susceptibility from hemosiderin/ferritin as peripheral hypointense areas (arrowheads). In the center there are hyperintense areas (arrow), probably containing extracellular metHb. The hypointensity on the DW image (**k**) is probably a combined effect of T2 shortening, magnetic susceptibility, and increased diffusivity. A marked peripheral hypointensity from hemosiderin/ferritin will also be seen when a GRE technique (**n**) is used (arrowheads)

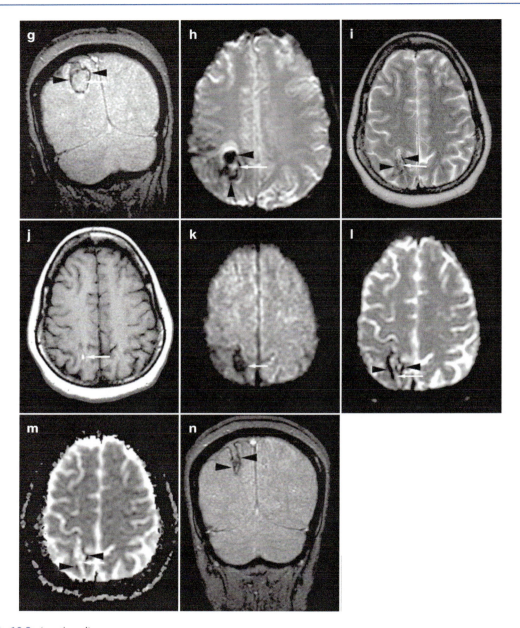

Fig 10.3 (continued)

magnetic field, as in most normal tissues in the body. Since there are no unpaired electrons in the iron of oxygenated hemoglobin, both longitudinal and transverse relaxation will be created by the so-called proton–proton, dipole–dipole interactions. At this stage, hematomas will have shorter relaxation times than water due to their protein content and will be slightly hypo- or isointense when compared with brain parenchyma on T1-weighted images. On T2-weighted images, oxyHb will be seen as a slightly hyperintense region because of the high water content [7, 11, 33].

Results of DW imaging of hematomas at this stage have not been well characterized. In our experience, however, a hyperacute intraparenchymal hemorrhage is hyperintense on DW images,

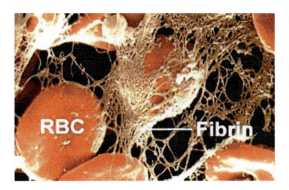

Fig. 10.4 Changes in concentration of red blood cells (RBC) and fibrin formation cause high viscosity and shrinkage of extracellular space

with a decreased apparent diffusion coefficient (ADC) (Tables 10.1 and 10.2). This is in accordance with observations of other authors [27, 32]. The causes for the decreased ADC are high viscosity and shrinkage of extracellular space due to clot retraction with fibrin and changes in the concentration of hemoglobin [19, 22, 27] (Fig. 10.4).

10.2.2 Acute Hematoma

Following hemorrhage there is normally a gradual oxygen desaturation of hemoglobin transforming oxyHb into deoxyHb (Fig. 10.4) [7, 11, 19, 33]. The loss of oxygen will change the binding geometry of iron from a six-ligand system to a five-ligand system, leaving four unpaired electrons and making it paramagnetic. When exposed to a magnetic field, paramagnetic substances will enhance the applied field locally. This will influence image contrast by means of so-called magnetic susceptibility-induced relaxation, which only effects transverse relaxation (T2* effect). The susceptibility effects create local field inhomogeneities, with a rapid loss of transverse magnetization of protons within this region resulting in signal loss on T2-weighted images. DeoxyHb will therefore demonstrate a marked hypointensity on T2-weighted images. Besides the concentration of deoxyHb, red blood cell concentration and/or clot formation may also contribute to this T2 hypointensity. Since this is an effect of magnetic susceptibility, gradient-echo (GRE) images will be more sensitive than DW- and T2-weighted images for the detection of acute as well as chronic hematomas [19, 25, 26, 31]. The T1 relaxivity effect is related to dipole–dipole relaxation, in this case the dipoles of water and unpaired electrons of the paramagnetic center. This would normally result in a shortening of relaxation time; however, the molecular configuration of deoxy-hemoglobin will act as a shield for such a close approach of water molecules to the unpaired electrons of the paramagnetic, ferrous iron. The acute hematoma containing deoxy-hemoglobin will thus show an iso- to hypointense signal on T1-weighted images, similar to oxyHb [5, 22, 33].

DW images of an acute hematoma show a marked hypointensity [27–30, 32], caused by the magnetic field inhomogeneity created by the paramagnetic deoxyHb. Although the ADC has been reported to be decreased, accurate calculations are often difficult [27–29, 32, 35].

10.2.3 Early Subacute Hematoma

In the early stage of the subacute hematoma (Figs. 10.3 and 10.5), there is a decline in the energy state of the red blood cell and hemoglobin is oxidized to metHb [3, 7, 11, 22, 33]. In metHb the iron is still bound to the heme moiety within the globin protein, but it is now in the ferric state with five unpaired electrons. This transformation normally starts in the periphery of the hemorrhage and gradually evolves to the center. In the transition to met-hemoglobin, conformational changes will take place in the molecule and water protons will now have access to the unpaired electrons of iron in metHb, creating a proton–electron, dipole–dipole interaction. Dipolar relaxation enhancement will then take place, making metHb appear hyperintense on T1-weighted images. MetHb, as a paramagnetic substance, will induce magnetic susceptibility relaxation affecting the transverse relaxation (T2* effect), which results in a marked hypointensity on T2-weighted images.

On DWI, intracellular metHb shows hypointensity due to these paramagnetic susceptibility effects and ADC measurements are not reliable due to the susceptibility effects [27–29, 32].

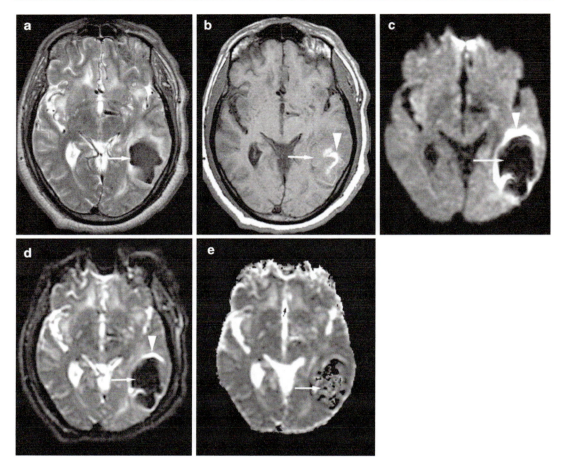

Fig. 10.5 (**a–e**) Acute to early subacute hemorrhage (deoxyHb and intracellular metHb). A 49-year-old man with headache and aphasia was referred for MR imaging 24 hours after the onset of symptoms. This study shows a left temporal lobe lesion that is hypointense on the T2-weighted image (**a**) (arrow; deoxyHb and intracellular metHb) with surrounding edema. On the T1-weighted image (**b**) the lesion is heterogeneous with areas of hypointensity (arrow; deoxyHb) and hyperintensity (arrowhead; intracellular metHb). The DW image (**c**) demonstrates hypointensity (arrow; deoxyHb and intracellular metHb). The surrounding hyperintense rim (arrowhead) represents magnetic susceptibility artifact and perihematomal injury. This peripheral artifact is also seen around the hypointensity (arrow) created by deoxyHb and intracellular metHb on the b_0 image (**d**). ADC cannot be calculated accurately, which is easy to understand when looking at the extremely heterogeneous lesion depicted on the ADC map (**e**)

10.2.4 Late Subacute Hematomas

The decline in energy state of the red blood cell will eventually damage the integrity of the red cell membrane, releasing the intracellular content to the extracellular fluid space (Figs. 10.3 and 10.6). Subsequently, there will be a dilution of the paramagnetic metHb in extracellular fluid, reducing the susceptibility effect of metHb [7, 11, 22, 33] (Fig. 10.7). The signal intensity on T2-weighted images will thus relate to the water content, creating a hyperintense signal on T2-weighted images. Extracellular metHb will, however, still have high signal intensity on T1-weighted images created by the same proton–electron, dipole–dipole relaxation as described in early subacute hematomas [5–7, 22].

It has been reported that late subacute hematomas are hyperintense on DW imaging [27, 28]. The ADC value for late subacute hematoma is

10 Intracranial Hemorrhage

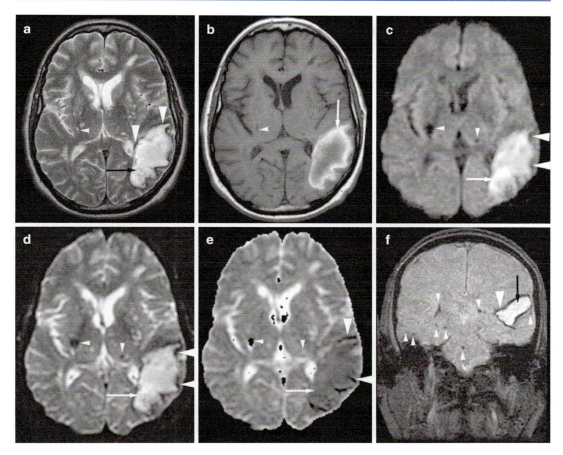

Fig. 10.6 (a–f) Late subacute-chronic hemorrhage (extracellular metHb, hemichrome, and hemosiderin/ferritin). A 52-year-old man with a history of chronic hypertension complained of headache and aphasia. MR examination 2 months after the onset of symptoms shows a left temporal lobe lesion that is hyperintense on the T2-weighted image (a) (arrow; extracellular metHb) and surrounded by a hypointense rim (arrowheads; hemosiderin/ferritin). Another hypointense lesion is visualized in the right basal ganglia (small arrowhead; hemosiderin/ferritin), compatible with chronic hemorrhage secondary to hypertension. The T1-weighted image (b) shows the temporal lobe lesion as peripheral hyperintensity (arrow; extracellular metHb) and central isointensity (hemichrome). The lesion in the right basal ganglia is also hypointense on this sequence (small arrowhead; hemosiderin/ferritin). On the DWI (c) the temporal lobe lesion is hyperintense (arrow; extracellular metHb and hemichrome) with a hypointense rim (arrowheads; hemosiderin/ferritin). The basal ganglia lesion remains hypointense, but the signal void is more extensive than on the conventional T2-weighted image (a), since spin-echo type EPI does not compensate for signal loss due to local magnetic field inhomogeneities and is thus more sensitive than regular spin-echo imaging. This increased susceptibility sensitivity revealed a second, old hemorrhagic lesion in the left thalamus (small arrowhead; hemosiderin/ferritin). The b_0 image (d) also shows the hyperintense lesion (arrow; extracellular metHb) with the hypointense rim (arrowheads; hemosiderin/ferritin) as well as the older lesions in the basal ganglia and thalamus (small arrowheads; hemosiderin/ferritin). On the ADC map (e) the temporal lesion is hypointense (arrow; extracellular metHb and hemichrome) with a hypointense rim (arrowheads; hemosiderin/ferritin). The other lesions are also visualized (small arrowheads); however, ADC cannot be calculated. Finally, the coronal GRE image (f) shows the temporal lesion as hyperintense (arrow; extracellular metHb with a hypointense rim) (arrowhead; hemosiderin/ferritin). The GRE sequence is the most sensitive and shows multiple small hypointense lesions (old hemorrhagic breakdown products) in the cerebral hemispheres and in the pons (small arrowheads; hemosiderin/ferritin)

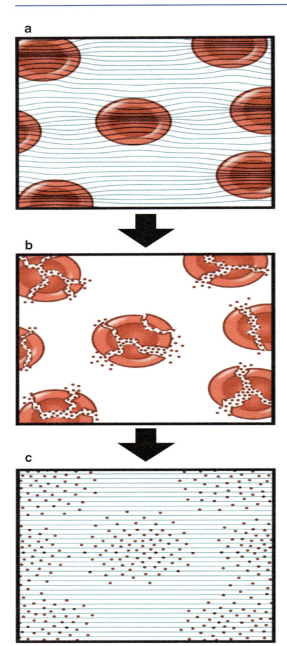

Fig. 10.7 (a-c) After hemorrage, intracellular paramagnetic deoxyHb followed by metHb cause magnetic field distortion in acute to early subacute phase (**a**). Decrease in the energy state damages the integrity of the RBC membrane, releasing the intracellular content to the extracellular space (**b**). With lysis of RBCs, metHb becomes uniformly dispersed throughout the hematoma cavity in late subacute to early chronic phase (**c**)

controversial. Ebisu et al. [23] reported decreased ADC in hematomas of hemorrhagic infarctions, whereas Atlas et al. reported ADC values higher than normal white matter in late subacute hematomas and suggested this was due to increased diffusivity [27]. Decreased ADC in late subacute hematomas is thought to be due to the high viscosity [32]. It is important to differentiate late subacute hematomas from abscesses since both can show hyperintensity on DWI and decreased ADC. Late subacute hematomas are hyperintense on T1-weighted images but abscesses are usually hypointense.

10.2.5 Chronic Hematomas

Over time, metHb will be resorbed or degraded and the effect on T1 high signal will be reduced (Figs. 10.3 and 10.5). The high water content in the chronic stage will result in prolonged T1 as well as T2 relaxation. From the start of the hemorrhage there is a continuous phagocytation of heme proteins. Ferritin and hemosiderin, the final breakdown products of hemoglobin, will remain within the phagocytic cells, which accumulate in the periphery of the hematoma, where they may remain indefinitely as a marker of an old hemorrhage [17, 33, 36, 37]. Ferritin and hemosiderin within these cells will have no access to water protons and thus there are no relaxivity effects. Magnetic susceptibility is the only factor influencing the signal, creating a marked signal loss on T2-weighted images. As mentioned earlier, the magnetic susceptibility effects are most prominent on T2*-weighted images.

DW images can show hyperintensity in early chronic hematomas which contains diamagnetic heme protein called "hemichrome" [28, 32, 38]. However, DW images can show hypointensity in late chronic hematomas depending on the viscosity. The ADC value has been reported to be increased, but decreased in early chronic hematomas due to the high viscosity of hemichrome-contained fluid. Differentiation between early chronic hematomas and abscesses on MR imaging is difficult because both can

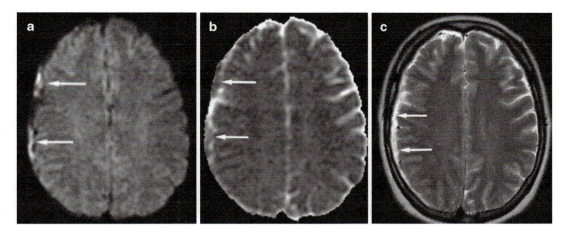

Fig. 10.8 (**a–c**) Perihematomal edema and injury. A 61-year-old man presented with headache. (**a**) T2-weighted image shows an acute hematoma as hypointense and the surrounding edema as hyperintense. (**b**) DW image shows the hematoma as mixed intense (arrows) and show the edema as hyper- or isointense (arrowheads). (**c**) The ADC map shows most of the edema as increased ADC, which represents vasogenic edema (arrows). However, there is a peripheral decreased ADC rim that probably represents perihematomal injury (arrowheads)

show hyperintensity on DW images and iso- or hypointensity on T1-weighted images. The presence of the hemosiderin rim may be the only clue for the differential diagnosis on the imaging. Measurement of the ADC is not always accurate due to magnetic susceptibility artifacts from the surrounding deposition of ferritin and hemosiderin [27–29, 32, 35].

10.2.6 Perihematomal Edema and Injury

Morbidity and mortality are associated with hematoma enlargement and the development of perihematomal edema. Serum protein penetration from the clot into the surrounding white matter and blood-brain barrier breakdown have been proposed as mechanisms leading to edema formation in the extracellular compartment (vasogenic edema). There is a significant direct relationship between ADC elevation in the edema and the volume of hematoma [39].

A rim of decreased ADC (perihematomal diffusion restriction) outside the hematoma is commonly observed in the hyperacute or acute phase. Mechanisms proposed as contributing factors to the perihematomal injury include ischemia resulting from mechanical compression and cytotoxic edema, or neurotoxicity resulting from breakdown products of blood, inflammation, or excitotoxic brain injury (Figs. 10.5 and 10.8) [40, 41]. Perihematomal diffusion restriction (cytotoxic edema) in hyperacute phase can be transient without short-term clinical impact [42, 43]. However, perihematomal diffusion restriction in the subacute phase may represent irreversible damage related to poor clinical outcome [44].

10.3 Subarachnoid Hemorrhage

Computed tomography (CT) is still essential in the diagnosis of acute subarachnoid hemorrhages, as the sensitivity and usefulness of MR imaging is controversial [4, 5, 9, 33, 45–50]. Fluid-attenuated inversion recovery (FLAIR) imaging has a high sensitivity for subarachnoid hemorrhage [51–54]. However, the specificity is low because there are several other causes for the appearance of subarachnoid hemorrhage on FLAIR imaging, such as high proton concentration, mass effect, vascular disease, contrast medium, and use of specific intravenous anesthetic agents [55–58].

It is often difficult to detect subarachnoid hemorrhage on DW images [32, 59]. Lin et al. detected subarachnoid hemorrhage in two of four cases on GRE imaging, but it could not be detected on b_0 images [30]. Wiesmann et al.

reported that proton density and FLAIR images could detect subarachnoid hemorrhage, but T2-weighted and DW images could not [59].

However, DW images may be useful to visualize parenchymal injuries secondary to subarachnoid hemorrhage. Ischemic changes, probably related to subarachnoid hemorrhage, have shown hyperintensity on DW images in both clinical and animal studies [60–65]. This finding depends on the timing of imaging and the severity of injury (Fig. 10.9).

10.4 Subdural and Epidural Hematoma

Subdural and epidural hematomas (Fig. 10.10) are well demonstrated on T1- and T2-weighted images. In the acute and subacute stages, the evolution of signal intensity generally follows the one of intraparenchymal hematomas with a slower rate because of higher oxygen tension in the subdural or epidural space. In the chronic stage, MR images often show hyperintensity of the hematoma, which may be iso- to hypodense on CT [66–72].

DW imaging findings of subdural and epidural hematomas have not been well described. Lin et al. reported that all three lesions could be detected on b_0 images, but GRE images were better at detecting lesions [30]. One of the benefits of DW imaging is for the detection of underlying or associated parenchymal lesions [73, 74]. Mixed signal intensity on DW imaging in chronic subdural hematomas may be related to postoperative treatment failure or complications [75].

10.5 Intraventricular Hemorrhage

Intraventricular hemorrhages (Figs. 10.9 and 10.11) are well demonstrated on FLAIR, T1-, T2-, and proton density-weighted images [61, 76–78]. FLAIR has been reported to have the highest sensitivity for detection of intraventricular hematomas [77]. DW images can demonstrate intraventricular hemorrhages, but in general the GRE images have a higher sensitivity [30].

10.6 Intratumoral Hemorrhage

Many primary brain tumors and metastases can bleed [33, 79–84]. The signal intensity of intratumoral hemorrhage (Fig. 10.12) tends to be more complex and its evolution tends to be delayed when compared with non-neoplastic hemorrhages [33, 84]. DW and b_0 images are useful to detect the hemorrhage in tumors [30].

10.7 Hemorrhage Related to Vascular Malformation

Vascular malformations can also cause intracranial hemorrhages (Fig. 10.13). Cavernous angioma is a vascular malformation that contains blood cavities surrounded by a single layer of endothelium [85–89]. MR imaging findings are well known and characterized as a central reticulated core with a peripheral rim of hypointensity due to the deposition of hemosiderin [85, 88, 89]. DW and b_0 images are useful for detecting hemorrhages related to vascular malformations.

10.8 Hemorrhage Related to Trauma (See Also Chap. 17)

Trauma is one of the most common causes of intracranial hemorrhages in younger patients (Fig. 10.14). Recently, head trauma has been increasing in the elderly patients because of increased elderly populations with or without dementia. Falls to the ground from standing or heights are the most common causes, since both motor and physiological functions are degraded. Subdural, contusional, and intracerebral hematomas are more common in the elderly than the young (Fig. 10.15). MR imaging is valuable in detecting intracranial injuries. DW and b_0 images and an ADC map can be more sensitive than conventional MR images to detect whether the abnormality includes diffuse axonal injury [90].

10 Intracranial Hemorrhage

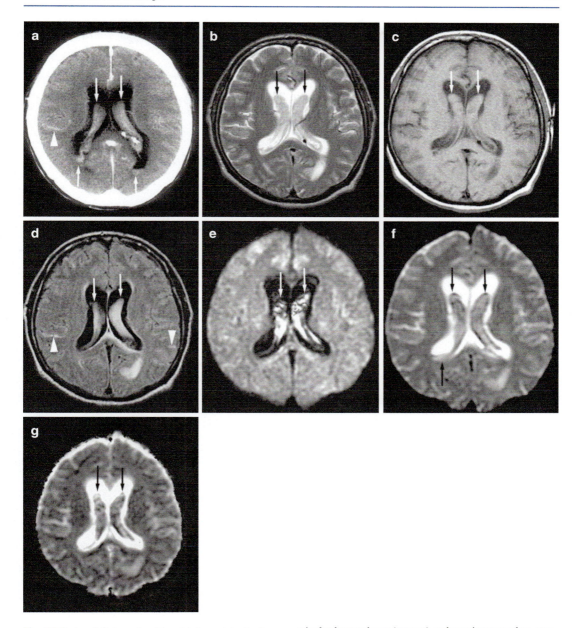

Fig. 10.9 (**a–g**) Subarachnoid and intraventricular hemorrhage due to arteriovenous malformation (intracellular met-hemoglobin). A 48-year-old woman presented with acute onset of severe headache had a CT scan 24 hours after the onset of symptoms (**a**), which shows diffuse subarachnoid (arrowhead) and intraventricular hemorrhage (arrows). Forty-eight hours after the onset of symptoms (**b–g**) she underwent MR imaging. On this examination the T2-weighted image (**b**) showed intraventricular hemorrhage (arrows), which is hypointense when compared with the cerebrospinal fluid. The diffuse subarachnoid hemorrhage cannot be visualized on the T2-weighted image. The T1-weighted image (**c**) shows the intraventricular hemorrhage (arrows) as hyperintense when compared with cerebrospinal fluid, but neither sequence can visualize the subarachnoid hemorrhage. The FLAIR image (**d**), however, shows both the subarachnoid (arrowheads) and intraventricular hemorrhage (arrows). The subarachnoid hemorrhage cannot be visualized on the DW image (**e**), but the intraventricular hemorrhage (arrows) can easily be seen as hyperintense when compared with cerebrospinal fluid and brain parenchyma. As expected, the subarachnoid hemorrhage cannot be demonstrated on either b_0 image (**f**) or ADC maps (**g**), but both sequences will depict the intraventricular hematoma as hypointense (arrows)

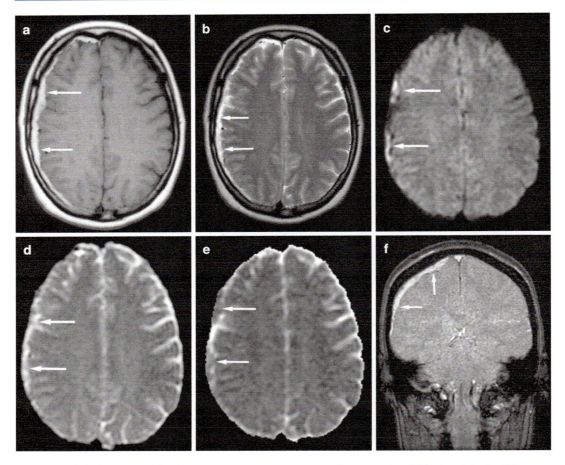

Fig. 10.10 (**a–f**) Subacute subdural hematoma (extracellular met-hemoglobin). A 49-year-old woman with headache following head trauma had an MR examination 2 weeks after the trauma, which shows right subdural hematoma as a hyperintense lesion (arrows) on the T1-weighted (**a**) and T2-weighted (**b**) images. The lesion was hyperintense on the DW (**c**) and the b_0 (**d**) images (arrows). On the ADC map (**e**) there are hypointense lesions (arrows), which correspond to the hyperintense lesions on the DW image (**c**). The coronal GRE image (**f**) shows the subdural hematoma to be hyperintense (arrows)

10.9 Conclusions

Diffusion-weighted imaging is often of limited value for diagnosis and staging of intracranial hemorrhages because accurate ADC measurements are only possible in the hyperacute stage, which contains diamagnetic oxy-hemoglobin, and in the late subacute phase, which contains extracellular met-hemoglobin, whose paramagnetic susceptibility artifacts are diminished by the dilution of extracellular fluid. CT and routine MR imaging continue to be the mainstay in diagnosing and characterizing intracranial hemorrhages. A thorough understanding of DW imaging characteristics is important, however, in order to avoid misinterpretations and inaccurate conclusions.

10.10 Treatment of Intracranial Hemorrhage

Sravanthi Koduri, Zachary Marcus Wilseck, Ankur Bhambri and Aditya S. Pandey

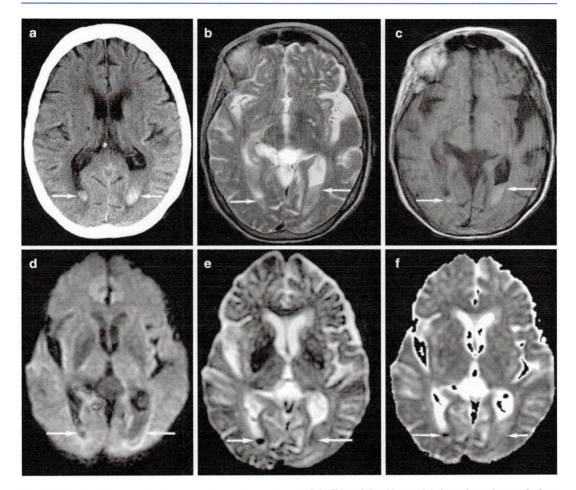

Fig. 10.11 (a–f) Intraventricular hemorrhage (intracellular met-hemoglobin). A 78-year-old woman with headache after thrombolytic therapy for femoral artery occlusion had a scan 6 hours after surgery (a). This shows intraventricular hemorrhage in the bilateral lateral ventricles (arrows). Three days after surgery (b–f), the T2-weighted image (b) shows hypointense lesions in the bilateral lateral ventricles with fluid-fluid levels (arrows) and the T1-weighted image (c) shows hyperintense lesions in the same distributions (arrows). The DW image (d) shows hypointense lesions (arrows) with surrounding hyperintensities. These are ascribed to magnetic susceptibility artifacts. The b_0 image (e) also shows hypointense lesions (arrows). These hypointensities are more prominent than on the T2-weighted images (b). The ADC map (f) shows hypointense lesions (arrows)

10.10.1 Introduction

Intracranial hemorrhage encompasses four main types of hemorrhage: epidural hemorrhage (EDH), subdural hemorrhage (SDH), subarachnoid hemorrhage (SAH), and intraparenchymal hemorrhage (IPH), which can be visualized in Figs. 10.16, 10.17, and 10.18. The epidemiology, pathophysiology, diagnosis, prognosis, and outcomes vary depending on the type of hemorrhage.

10.10.2 Extra-axial Hemorrhage (Epidural and Subdural Hematoma)

10.10.2.1 Epidemiology

Extra-axial hemorrhage primarily includes epidural and subdural hematomas. Epidural hemorrhages occur in 2% of all traumatic brain injury but account for up to 15% of all fatal head traumas [91]. Epidural hematomas are associated with an overlying skull fracture 85–95% of the

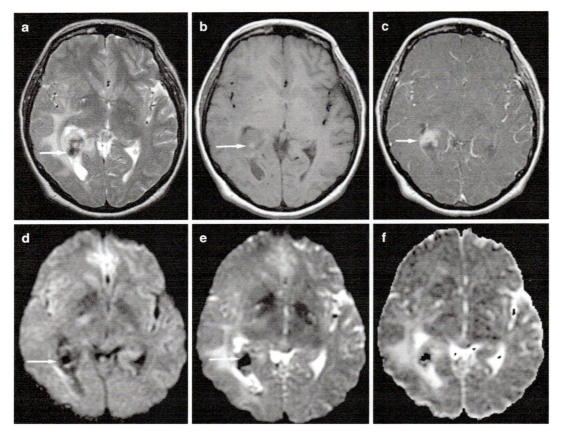

Fig. 10.12 (**a–f**) Hemorrhagic tumor. The T2-weighted MR image (**a**) in a 54-year-old woman with glioblastoma shows a mass lesion with heterogeneous intensity near the right lateral ventricle. The irregular hypointensities centrally in the lesion (arrow) indicate hemorrhage. The T1-weighted image (**b**) shows the heterogeneous hypointense to isointense mass, with a central area of higher signal intensity consistent with hemorrhage (arrow). The gadolinium-enhanced T1-weighted image (**c**) shows heterogeneous enhancement (arrow). On the DW image (**d**) the hemorrhage is heterogeneously hypointense (arrow). The b_0 image (**e**) shows the hemorrhage to be more hypointense (arrow) than on the T2-weighted image (**a**). The ADC (**f**) cannot be calculated due to magnetic susceptibility artifacts

time leading to a tear in the middle meningeal arterial branches. Subdural hemorrhages have a slightly higher frequency of up to 25% of traumatic brain injury patients and tend to be associated with more severe trauma [92]. In the elderly population, however, subdural hematomas (both acute and chronic) are found with reports of minimal trauma [93]. Both epidural and subdural hemorrhages tend to be more predominant within the male population. However, whereas epidural hematomas occur within young adults, subdural hemorrhages are more frequent with increasing age [94]. There are other causes of EDHs and SDH aside from trauma and these include coagulation abnormalities, vascular malformations, and hemorrhagic tumors [95–97].

10.10.2.2 Pathophysiology

Epidural hematomas occur when blood fills in the potential space between the inner table of the calvarium and the dura. This hemorrhage is most frequently secondary to arterial bleeding, with the middle meningeal artery being the most common offender, though venous bleeding has been shown to be the cause in 10% of instances [98, 99]. Subdural hematomas occur when blood fills

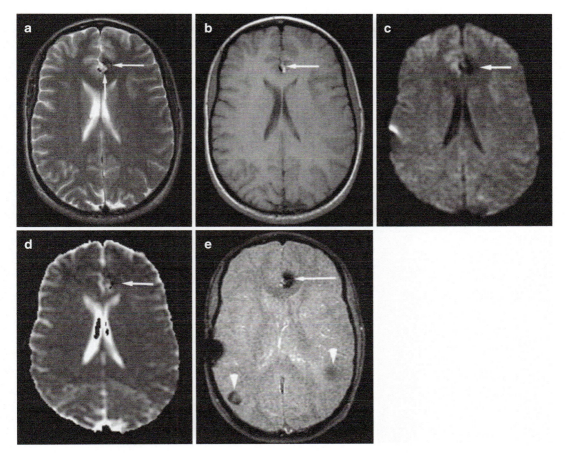

Fig. 10.13 (**a–e**) Multiple cavernous malformations. The T2-weighted image (**a**) in a 30-year-old woman with seizures shows a hyperintense lesion in the left frontal lobe with a surrounding hypointense rim (arrows). This is a characteristic finding for a cavernous angioma. The lesion is hyperintense on the T1-weighted image (**b**) (arrow) and hypointense on the DW image (**c**) (arrow). The ADC map (**d**) shows heterogeneous intensity and the GRE image (**e**) shows marked hypointensity in the left frontal lobe (arrow). The hypointensities in the right and left temporo-occipital region (arrowheads) suggest multiple cavernous malformations

the potential space between the dura and the arachnoid. SDHs tend to be secondary to tearing of the bridging veins, which are straight bridges between the cortical surface of the brain and the superior sagittal sinus [100]. Given the brain atrophy seen in the elderly, the subdural space enlarges, which increases the stretch on bridging veins thus increasing the probability of a tear with minimal trauma.

10.10.2.3 Clinical Presentation

The clinical presentation for these patients varies greatly from asymptomatic to severe neurologic deficit. Patients with either type of hemorrhage may present with headaches, nausea, vomiting, focal neurologic deficit, seizures, and coma [101, 102]. Patients found to have EDH frequently report a history of a blunt trauma and have a classic presentation of a lucid interval following the trauma. This is usually described as loss of consciousness at the time of trauma, followed by a nearly normal interval that then quickly leads into a deteriorating level of consciousness. Though this is the classic presentation, this history is described in less than 20% of patients [103]. EDHs in the posterior fossa are rare but the patient usually presents as conscious and neurologically intact until he/she suddenly loses con-

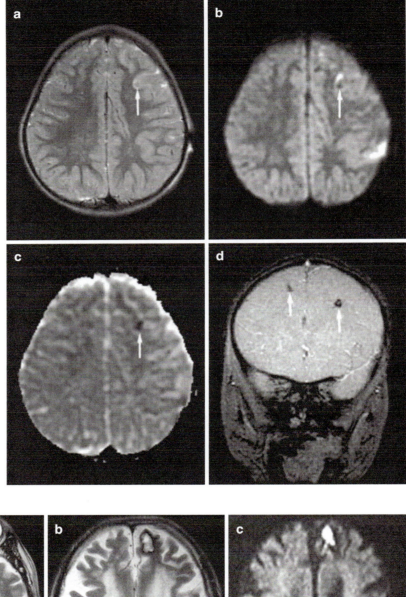

Fig. 10.14 (a–d) Trauma with hemorrhagic diffuse axonal injury. T2-weighted image of a 2-year-old girl 12 hours after a motor vehicle accident shows (**a**) a hyperintense lesion in the left frontal lobe (arrow). The corresponding area on the DW image (**b**) is hypointense with surrounding hyperintensity (arrow). The ADC map (**c**) shows hypointensity (arrow). The coronal GRE (**d**) image shows hypointense lesions in the bilateral frontal lobes (arrows)

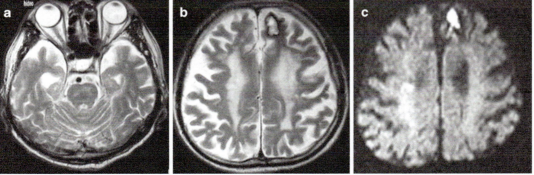

Fig. 10.15 (a–c) Trauma with hemorrhagic contusion. T2-weighted images of an 84 year-old man after fall show bilatral temporal lobe atrophy consistent with Alzheimer type dementia (a), and a hyperintense lesion in the left frontal lobe and diffuse white matter changes consistent with chronic ishemic small vessel disease (**b**). The corresponding area on the DW image (**c**) is hypointense with surrounding hyperintensity

10 Intracranial Hemorrhage

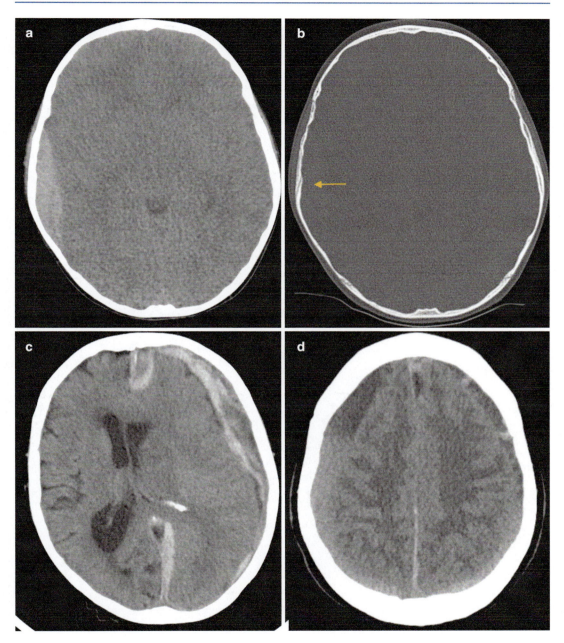

Fig. 10.16 Extra-axial hemorrhage. (**a**) Right-sided epidural hematoma, (**b**) right-sided non-displaced temporal bone fracture, (**c**) acute left-sided holo-hemispheric subdural hemorrhage, (**d**) acute on chronic bilateral subdural hemorrhages depicting hypodense chronic component and hyperdense acute component

sciousness, becomes apneic, and dies [104, 105]. Subdural hematomas do not have a classic presentation but present with any of the generalized or focal symptoms described above.

10.10.2.4 Diagnosis
Prior to evaluating for an intracranial pathology, the first and foremost consideration should be for airway, breathing, and the circulatory system.

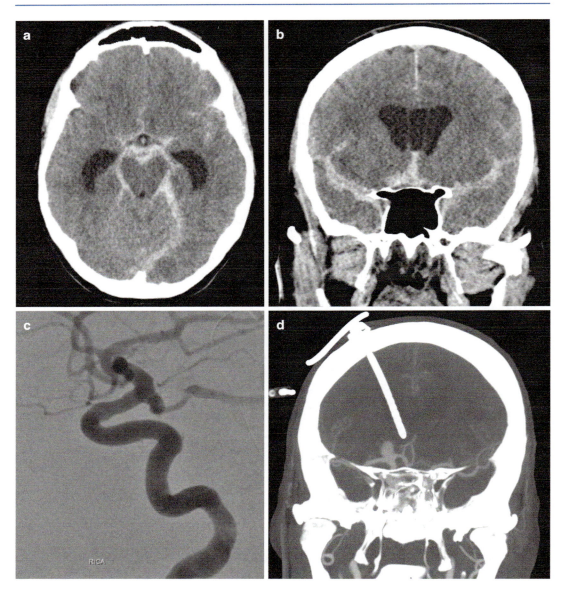

Fig. 10.17 Subarachnoid hemorrhage. (**a**) Subarachnoid hemorrhage within the perimesencephalic cisterns, (**b**) subarachnoid hemorrhage throughout bilateral Sylvian fissures, (**c**) digital subtraction angiography showing a right posterior communicating artery aneurysm, (**d**) CT angiography depicting a right internal carotid artery bifurcation aneurysm

Following cardiopulmonary stabilization, a neurologic exam should be obtained to determine the extent and laterality of the pathology. While this process is occurring, the patient's medication (particularly with respect to antiplatelet and anticoagulant medications) should be reconciled and laboratory studies completed to evaluate for any coagulation abnormalities. The most frequent next step is to have the patient undergo computed tomography (CT) scan of the head. In the setting of trauma, if there is concern for loss of consciousness, presence of severe mechanism of injury or any neurologic deficit, then the patient must undergo CT of the head [106].

10 Intracranial Hemorrhage

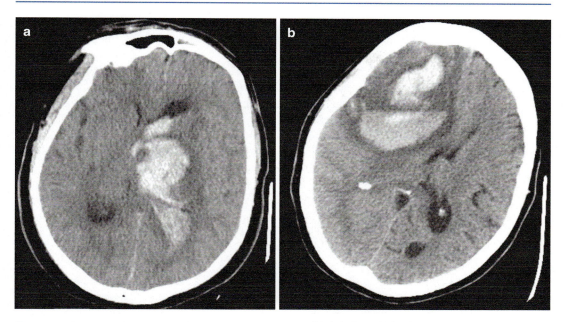

Fig. 10.18 Intraparenchymal hemorrhage. (**a**) Left basal ganglia hemorrhage with intraventricular extension and left to right midline shift due to likely hypertensive etiology, (**b**) right frontal lobar hemorrhage likely secondary to cerebral amyloid angiopathy

In the presence of a large compressive extra-axial hematoma, patients frequently present with symptoms of elevated intracranial pressure, which include decreased level of consciousness, severe headache, nausea, and vomiting. These generalized symptoms are associated with lateralizing signs such as contralateral hemiparesis as well as ipsilateral pupillary asymmetry, such as a fixed and dilated pupil [107]. In critically injured patients, the presentation can often be one of uncal herniation, which may include vital abnormalities such as bradycardia and hypertension, known as Cushing's reflex [108].

10.10.2.5 Imaging

Based on presentation, the most frequently imaging modality utilized is computed tomography. Non-contrast CT of the head is able to differentiate acute, subacute, and chronic hemorrhage in relation to brain parenchyma. Acute intracranial hemorrhage has an increased density compared to brain parenchyma, whereas subacute tends to be isodense and chronic hemorrhage tends to be hypodense compared to brain parenchyma (Fig. 10.16). There are a few distinguishing characteristics between epidural and subdural hematoma on imaging. Epidural hematomas tend to be lens shaped, hemispheric, and since they are outside the dura, they are confined by calvarial suture lines. EDHs can sometimes have a "swirl sign," which is indicative of an active hemorrhage [109]. Subdural hematomas have a crescentic shape and frequently are holo-hemispheric since they are not confined by suture lines.

Epidural hematomas are thought to originate from trauma to the middle meningeal artery, which is a branch of the external carotid artery. Subdural hematomas are thought to present due to tearing of bridging cortical veins. Neither of these vessels are well visualized on CT angiography so this imaging modality is not a routine part of the evaluation process in patients presenting with EDH or SDH specifically secondary to trauma.

10.10.2.6 Acute Management

When there is concern for a herniation syndrome, acute management involves temporizing the patient until definitive management, likely surgical, can be pursued. These temporizing measures are similar to those involved with treatment of acutely elevated intracranial pressure and involve securing the airway, elevating the head of bed, hyperventilating, and administering mannitol or hypertonic saline [110]. If a patient is on anticoagulant or antiplatelet medications, then administration of reversal agents should be completed at this time. Prophylactic platelet transfusion is not warranted unless the patient is to be taken to the operating room or has increase in size of hemorrhage on follow-up imaging.

10.10.2.7 Surgical Management

From the time of presentation, the primary decision that needs to be made is regarding whether or not the patient needs surgical intervention. With both epidural and subdural hematomas, there are specific guidelines towards surgical management. In these settings, patients should be temporized while on the way to the Operating Room as the definitive treatment is surgical evacuation.

Based on the most recent Brain Trauma Foundation guidelines for surgical management of acute epidural hematomas, an EDH measuring greater than 30 cm^3 should be evacuated regardless of the patient's clinical examination. If the patient has a EDH less than 30 cm^3, less than 1.5 cm in thickness, less than 5 mm of midline shift, and a GCS greater than 8, then these hemorrhages can be managed with serial CT scans to monitor for evolution with the next scan planned for 6–8 hours after the original. Any sign of expansion of hemorrhage or deteriorating neurologic exam is an indication for emergent surgical evacuation. It is strongly recommended that patients who are candidate for surgical evacuation undergo surgical evacuation as soon as possible. At this time, there is no consensus on the best surgical approach, though a craniotomy does lead to the most complete hematoma evacuation [111].

A subdural hemorrhage patient is a candidate for surgical intervention if the SDH is greater than 1 cm in thickness and causes more than 5 mm of midline shift, regardless of the patient's neurologic exam. If a patient has GCS < 9, then he/she should undergo surgical intervention regardless of SDH size if GCS decreased by more than 2 points from time of trauma to hospital admission, or if the patient has a fixed and dilated pupil or if ICP is greater than 20 mmHg [112]. Surgical treatment for acute SDHs involves craniotomy with/without bone flap removal/duraplasty [113] while treatment of chronic SDHs can be accomplished with burr holes [114].

Regardless of whether the patient undergoes surgical intervention, the patient should undergo intracranial pressure monitoring with an intracranial pressure monitor or external ventricular drain if he/she has GCS less than 9 and has intracranial pathology on CT scan.

10.10.2.8 Medical Management

In addition to surgical management, medical management plays a significant role in prognosis. Majority of these patients are admitted to an Intensive Care Unit for frequent neurologic checks. Regardless of whether the patient underwent surgical decompression, there can be significant cerebral edema secondary to the primary hemorrhage and thus the patient requires close neurological evaluation [110]. Such edema and associated intracranial hypertension must be closely monitored and treated with hyperosmolar and hypertonic therapy to ensure no further secondary injury takes place [115].

10.10.2.9 Prognosis

EDHs have been associated with a mortality rate of up to 15% and a rate of disability among survivors of 20% [103]. The patients with the most optimal prognosis include those with an early diagnosis and treatment. Prognosis for both EDH and SDH worsens with delay in diagnosis/treatment, pupillary abnormalities, poor GCS on arrival, elevated ICP post-surgically as well as other concomitant intracranial injuries on imaging [116].

10.10.3 Subarachnoid Hemorrhage

10.10.3.1 Epidemiology

Subarachnoid hemorrhage has an incidence of 3–5% of all hemorrhagic strokes with a subtle predominance in women over men [117, 118].

There are several modifiable risk factors for aSAH, which include hypertension, smoking, and sympathomimetic drug use. Non-modifiable risk factors include prior history of SAH, family history of SAH, autosomal dominant polycystic kidney disease (ADPKD), and Ehlers-Danlos syndrome [118, 119]. It is frequently divided either into traumatic and nontraumatic SAH or aneurysmal and non-aneurysmal SAH. The overall incidence of SAH increases as patients age, making it quite rare in the pediatric population.

10.10.3.2 Pathophysiology

Aneurysmal subarachnoid hemorrhage occurs due to the rupture of an intracranial aneurysm that leads to blood leaking into the subarachnoid space. Non-aneurysmal SAH is the presence of SAH without an identifiable aneurysm. The most frequent cause of non-aneurysmal SAH is trauma due to rupture of cortical vessels during sudden acceleration changes [120]. In addition, perimesencephalic hemorrhage is presence of SAH within the posterior fossa cisterns and thought to be related to venous bleeding as cerebral angiography is always negative. Aside from aneurysms and trauma, subarachnoid hemorrhage is noted with vascular malformations and antiplatelet/anticoagulant use.

10.10.3.3 Clinical Presentation

The classic presentation for patients with aneurysmal SAH is a sudden, severe headache that is frequently described as "the worst headache of life." Patients may also present with nausea, vomiting, dizziness, photophobia, seizures, loss of consciousness, altered mental status, and focal neurologic deficits. A small fraction of patients present with a sentinel headache but no other signs or symptoms of SAH and as a result, are misdiagnosed [121]. This population of patients are at high risk of a life-threatening hemorrhage in the next few hours to days given that the sentinel bleed may represent aneurysmal growth or hemorrhage within the wall of the aneurysm [122].

10.10.3.4 Diagnosis

Following initial cardiopulmonary stabilization, neurologic exam, and laboratory evaluation, patients presenting with sudden severe headache, neurologic deficit, or any other symptoms concerning for SAH should be evaluated with a CT head. If CT is positive for subarachnoid hemorrhage, then the next step of the diagnostic process is to obtain vascular imaging to evaluate for the presence of an intracranial aneurysm.

If there is a high index of suspicion for SAH based on the patient's clinical presentation and CT shows no evidence of hemorrhage, a lumbar puncture (LP) is the next best step to rule out xanthochromia [123, 124]. If a LP is performed within 6 hours of symptom onset, it may be false negative as there is insufficient time for the development of xanthochromia. Furthermore, results can be clouded with a traumatic tap; however, this can be mitigated with CSF collection in four consecutive tubes and RBC count measured in tube 1 and 4 to ensure that there is an appropriate decrease. Once the diagnosis of SAH is established, the presence of an aneurysm is determined based on CT angiography, MR angiography, or formal diagnostic angiography. The gold standard for intracranial vascular imaging is with cervico-cerebral digital subtraction angiography [125, 126].

10.10.3.5 Imaging

Initial imaging evaluation in subarachnoid hemorrhage involves a CT head. It is important to remember that the sensitivity of head CT findings decreases with time from onset of symptoms with less than 60% sensitivity at 7 days [127]. The classic imaging characteristics were the presence of hyperdensity within the basal cisterns, interhemispheric, and Sylvian fissures (Fig. 10.17). It is important to keep in mind that if the patient was administered contrast, the contrast can create a false positive hyperdensity within the subarachnoid space; however, this can be subtracted with a dual energy CT scan. If a patient presents with subarachnoid hemorrhage on CT but no significant history of trauma, then vascular imaging should be obtained to rule out an aneurysmal origin. Imaging should also be evaluated for the presence of hydrocephalus and other foci of hemorrhage.

If vessel imaging is negative for an aneurysm, the patient should also undergo MRI brain and cervical spine to evaluate for potential cervical AVM/AVs as well as the possibility of hemorrhagic tumors. To complete the evaluation, patients with angio-negative SAH should undergo repeat vessel imaging at 7–10 days following initial assessment given that thrombosed aneurysms may recanalize with time [127]. Angio-negative SAH can sometimes be further subclassified into perimesencephalic hemorrhage, which is when the hemorrhage is primarily concentrated within the perimesencephalic cisterns.

10.10.3.6 Acute Management

The initial acute management involves stabilization of the patient and evaluation of the patient's current intracranial pressure. If the patient has a poor neurologic exam or concern for hydrocephalus on imaging, an external ventricular drain (EVD) is placed for cerebrospinal fluid (CSF) diversion and intracranial pressure (ICP) monitoring. More rarely, a lumbar drain is inserted in lieu of an EVD based on surgeon and site preference. The patient should be monitored with frequent neurologic checks immediately after presentation. Furthermore, due to the risk of rebleeding, which is highest within the first 6 hours of presentation [128], it is paramount to control blood pressure and prevent rapid spikes in the systolic blood pressure with current guidelines recommending SBP less than 160 [128, 129]. This is frequently achieved with the use of an arterial line and intravenous antihypertensive medications to allow for continuous titration.

10.10.3.7 Surgical Management

If the patient is diagnosed with aneurysmal subarachnoid hemorrhage on angiography, the patient will need surgical treatment, either via microsurgical or endovascular approaches, to secure the intracranial aneurysm. The publication of the International Subarachnoid Aneurysm Trial (ISAT) showed that patients treated with endovascular coiling had a higher rate of disability-free survival at one-year posthemorrhage compared to patients who underwent microsurgical clipping [130, 131]. As a result, the trends of aneurysm treatment have greatly shifted towards favoring endovascular

coiling. However, endovascular coiling does have a higher risk of incomplete occlusion and aneurysm recurrence when compared to microsurgical clipping so routine follow-up vascular imaging is essential [132].

In addition to securing the aneurysm, patients may also develop chronic hydrocephalus and require permanent CSF diversion with the placement of a ventriculoperitoneal shunt. Patients who have an unsuccessful EVD wean require placement of a VPS.

10.10.3.8 Medical Management

Patients presenting with aSAH are routinely admitted to the Intensive Care Unit for a minimum of 14 days due to the potential for many medical and neurologic complications in the ensuing days. The medical complications include cardiac (Takotsubo cardiomyopathy), pulmonary (Acute Respiratory Distress Syndrome), alterations in fluid balance/electrolytes, and infections. Neurologic complications include hydrocephalus, delayed cerebral ischemia, and seizures.

Of these, delayed cerebral ischemia, which is defined as a new neurologic deficit that cannot be explained by any other cause, is the leading cause of morbidity in patients who survive the initial insult. Therefore, DCI is a diagnosis of exclusion. DCI occurs from day 3 to 14 following aneurysm rupture and has an association with increased thickness of SAH/IVH, as seen with the Fisher scale [133]. At this time, the only options for DCI prophylaxis are nimodipine and maintenance of euvolemia [129, 133]. Patients are monitored closely in the ICU for deterioration with frequent neurologic examination, transcranial Dopplers (TCDs), and blood pressure management. TCDs allow for the assessment of the velocity in major intracranial vessels and are a noninvasive way of determining the severity of arterial vasospasm. Unfortunately, TCDs are dependent on the person performing them and can be unreliable. If there is concern for DCI, then next steps include vessel imaging, either with CT angiogram/perfusion or digital subtraction angiography (DSA), which is the gold standard. These imaging techniques allow for the visualization of arterial narrowing while DSA also provides a mechanism of treatment, via the injection of intra-arterial verapamil vs milrinone. In addition to endovascular treatment, patients with symptomatic DCI have elevated mean arterial pressure goals via the use of vasopressors to allow for improved cerebral perfusion [129, 134].

10.10.3.9 Prognosis

Morbidity and mortality following aneurysmal subarachnoid hemorrhage is high with about a 35% rate of 30-day mortality and 30–35% of survivors reporting permanent disability [135, 136]. Traumatic and perimesencephalic subarachnoid hemorrhage have a better prognosis than patients with aSAH. There are several scales utilized for prognostication such as the Hunt Hess scale and Functional Recovery Expected after Subarachnoid Hemorrhage (FRESH) that aim to determine cognitive outcome and quality of life based on initial clinical presentation [137]. However, all these scales should be used with some caution.

10.10.4 Intraparenchymal Hemorrhage

10.10.4.1 Epidemiology/ Pathophysiology

The final category of intracranial hemorrhage is intraparenchymal hemorrhage (IPH), which is any hemorrhage within the brain parenchyma. Spontaneous IPH accounts for about 20% of all stroke and has a significant predominance within the elderly and a slight predominance among the male and African American population [138]. Intraparenchymal hemorrhage has many causes, the two most common of which are hypertension and cerebral amyloid angiography (most common cause of recurrent lobar hemorrhages) [139–141]. Other causes include trauma, infection, tumor, vasculitis, coagulopathy, venous hypertension, Moya-moya, sickle cell disease, eclampsia, etc.

10.10.4.2 Clinical Presentation/ Diagnosis/Imaging

Patients frequently present with acute onset of neurologic deficit and some present with the previously discussed symptoms of elevated intracranial pressure, including headache, nausea, vomiting, and decreased level of consciousness. The diagnosis of intraparenchymal hemorrhage is arrived at based on imaging, where a CT head shows hyperdensity within the brain parenchyma (Fig. 10.18). This is frequently followed by additional imaging, including a CT angiogram and MRI of the brain, to evaluate for vascular malformations or an underlying space-occupying lesion [22]. CT angiogram may have a "spot sign," which is an area of contrast enhancement that indicates likely acute, ongoing hemorrhage [142, 143]. Intraparenchymal hemorrhage most frequently occurs in the basal ganglia and the lobar regions with less frequent sites being the cerebellum, brainstem, and thalamus [144].

10.10.4.3 Surgical Management

Following acute management with cardiopulmonary stabilization, a thorough neurologic examination, and laboratory evaluation, a decision regarding whether the patient is a candidate for surgical intervention is made. There are no strict criteria at this time regarding indications for hematoma evacuation and surgery continues to remain controversial [145]. However, some indications for lobar hemorrhages include the presence of significant midline shift or a large compressive hematoma that comes to the cortical surface [146]. Patients presenting with posterior fossa hemorrhages tend to present more frequently in extremis and require emergent surgical intervention. There have been recent clinical trials with catheter-based delivery of clot busters that have showed promise but are not part of the standard of care at this time [147]. Surgical evacuation of the hematoma can be detrimental in certain situations if the hemorrhage is within the deep structures. In such a situation, a craniectomy may be a better option as it would reduce the intracranial pressure without causing further parenchymal damage; however, the role of surgical evacuation post ICH is currently being studied with numerous minimally invasive techniques.

10.10.4.4 Medical Management

Regardless of whether the patient undergoes surgical intervention, he/she will require frequent neurologic checks and close blood pressure monitoring with likely admission to an ICU [148, 149]. Patient should undergo repeat imaging at 6–8 hours to ensure stability of the hemorrhage as well as stroke prevention measures such as lipid panel monitoring and glycemic control [150]. If any anticoagulant or antiplatelet agents were on board, these should be reversed with the appropriate reversal agent prior to any surgical intervention.

10.10.4.5 Prognosis

Long-term prognosis is dependent on the size and location of hemorrhage, age of the patient, and neurologic exam at presentation, as well as patient-related comorbidities. Outcomes range from brain death to complete recovery. This population of patients has a 30-day mortality rate of 40–45% signifying the critical nature of ICH [151].

10.10.5 Summary

Intracranial hemorrhage can be divided into four major categories including epidural hemorrhage, subdural hemorrhage, subarachnoid hemorrhage, and intraparenchymal/intraventricular hemorrhage. Risk factors and pathophysiology of each subtype of hemorrhage vary but there are numerous similarities in terms of clinical presentation and acute management secondary to intracranial hypertension. Patients frequently present with any combination of headaches, nausea, vomiting, altered level of consciousness, seizures, and neurologic deficit. The acute management for all intracranial hemorrhage is cardiopulmonary stabilization, followed by complete laboratory and imaging evaluation. Due to the efficiency of computed tomography (CT), initial imaging is routinely a CT head, followed by vessel imaging (MR angiography, CT angiography, or cervico-cerebral angiography), and MRI as appropriate. Surgical intervention including ventriculostomy placement for hydrocephalus and intracranial hypertension management, endovascular or microsurgical management of intracranial vascular sites, and craniotomy-based ICH evacuation all play a significant role in the management of all of the previously described intracranial hemorrhage types. Majority of the patients presenting with intracranial hemorrhage require close neurological and blood pressure monitoring and thus frequently managed in an intensive care unit setting. Regardless of the subtype of hemorrhage, prognosis continues to remain relatively poor with significant morbidity and mortality.

References

1. Thulborn KR et al (1982) Oxygenation dependence of the transverse relaxation time of water protons in whole blood at high field. Biochim Biophys Acta 714(2):265–270
2. Fullerton GD, Potter JL, Dornbluth NC (1982) NMR relaxation of protons in tissues and other macromolecular water solutions. Magn Reson Imaging 1(4):209–226
3. Sipponen JT, Sepponen RE, Sivula A (1983) Nuclear magnetic resonance (NMR) imaging of intracerebral hemorrhage in the acute and resolving phases. J Comput Assist Tomogr 7(6):954–959
4. DeLaPaz RL et al (1984) NMR imaging of intracranial hemorrhage. J Comput Assist Tomogr 8(4):599–607
5. Bradley WG Jr (1985) and P.G. Schmidt, Effect of methemoglobin formation on the MR appearance of subarachnoid hemorrhage. Radiology 156(1):99–103
6. Gomori JM et al (1985) High-field MR imaging of superficial siderosis of the central nervous system. J Comput Assist Tomogr 9(5):972–975
7. Gomori JM et al (1985) Intracranial hematomas: imaging by high-field MR. Radiology 157(1):87–93
8. Sipponen JT et al (1985) Intracranial hematomas studied by MR imaging at 0.17 and 0.02 T. J Comput Assist Tomogr 9(4):698–704
9. Grossman RI et al (1986) Importance of oxygenation in the appearance of acute subarachnoid hemorrhage on high field magnetic resonance imaging. Acta Radiol Suppl 369:56–58
10. Di Chiro G et al (1986) Sequential MR studies of intracerebral hematomas in monkeys. AJNR Am J Neuroradiol 7(2):193–199
11. Gomori JM et al (1987) NMR relaxation times of blood: dependence on field strength, oxidation state, and cell integrity. J Comput Assist Tomogr 11(4):684–690
12. Zimmerman RD et al (1988) Acute intracranial hemorrhage: intensity changes on sequential MR scans at 0.5 T. AJR Am J Roentgenol 150(3):651–661
13. Hayman LA et al (1988) T2 effect of hemoglobin concentration: assessment with in vitro MR spectroscopy. Radiology 168(2):489–491

14. Brooks RA, Di Chiro G, Patronas N (1989) MR imaging of cerebral hematomas at different field strengths: theory and applications. J Comput Assist Tomogr 13(2):194–206
15. Hayman LA et al (1989) MR imaging of hyperacute intracranial hemorrhage in the cat. AJNR Am J Neuroradiol 10(4):681–686
16. Hayman LA et al (1989) Effect of clot formation and retraction on spin-echo MR images of blood: an in vitro study. AJNR Am J Neuroradiol 10(6):1155–1158
17. Hardy PA, Kucharczyk W, Henkelman RM (1990) Cause of signal loss in MR images of old hemorrhagic lesions. Radiology 174(2):549–555
18. Bryant RG et al (1990) Magnetic relaxation in blood and blood clots. Magn Reson Med 13(1):133–144
19. Clark RA et al (1990) Acute hematomas: effects of deoxygenation, hematocrit, and fibrin-clot formation and retraction on T2 shortening. Radiology 175(1):201–206
20. Thulborn KR et al (1990) The role of ferritin and hemosiderin in the MR appearance of cerebral hemorrhage: a histopathologic biochemical study in rats. AJNR Am J Neuroradiol 11(2):291–297
21. Bizzi A et al (1990) Role of iron and ferritin in MR imaging of the brain: a study in primates at different field strengths. Radiology 177(1):59–65
22. Bradley WG Jr (1993) MR appearance of hemorrhage in the brain. Radiology 189(1):15–26
23. Ebisu T et al (1997) Hemorrhagic and nonhemorrhagic stroke: diagnosis with diffusion-weighted and T2-weighted echo-planar MR imaging. Radiology 203(3):823–828
24. Atlas SW, Thulborn KR (1998) MR detection of hyperacute parenchymal hemorrhage of the brain. AJNR Am J Neuroradiol 19(8):1471–1477
25. Liang L et al (1999) Detection of intracranial hemorrhage with susceptibility-weighted MR sequences. AJNR Am J Neuroradiol 20(8):1527–1534
26. Kinoshita T et al (2000) Assessment of lacunar hemorrhage associated with hypertensive stroke by echo-planar gradient-echo T2*-weighted MRI. Stroke 31(7):1646–1650
27. Atlas SW et al (2000) Diffusion measurements in intracranial hematomas: implications for MR imaging of acute stroke. AJNR Am J Neuroradiol 21(7):1190–1194
28. Schaefer PW, Grant PE, Gonzalez RG (2000) Diffusion-weighted MR imaging of the brain. Radiology 217(2):331–345
29. Maldjian JA et al (2001) Computing diffusion rates in T2-dark hematomas and areas of low T2 signal. AJNR Am J Neuroradiol 22(1):112–118
30. Lin DD et al (2001) Detection of intracranial hemorrhage: comparison between gradient-echo images and b(0) images obtained from diffusion-weighted echo-planar sequences. AJNR Am J Neuroradiol 22(7):1275–1281
31. Hermier M et al (2001) MRI of acute post-ischemic cerebral hemorrhage in stroke patients: diagnosis with T2*-weighted gradient-echo sequences. Neuroradiology 43(10):809–815
32. Kang BK et al (2001) Diffusion-weighted MR imaging of intracerebral hemorrhage. Korean J Radiol 2(4):183–191
33. Atlas SW, Thulborn KR (2002) Intracranial hemorrhage. In: Atlas SW (ed) Magnetic resonance imaging of the brain and spine. Lippincott Williams & Wilkins, Philadelphia, pp 773–832
34. Latour LL et al (1994) Time-dependent diffusion of water in a biological model system. Proc Natl Acad Sci U S A 91(4):1229–1233
35. Does MD, Zhong J, Gore JC (1999) In vivo measurement of ADC change due to intravascular susceptibility variation. Magn Reson Med 41(2):236–240
36. Harrison PM et al (1967) Ferric oxyhydroxide core of ferritin. Nature 216(5121):1188–1190
37. Munro HN, Linder MC (1978) Ferritin: structure, biosynthesis, and role in iron metabolism. Physiol Rev 58(2):317–396
38. Bradley WG (1999) Hemorrhage. In: Stark DD, Bradley WG (eds) Magnetic resonance imaging. Mosby, St. Louis, pp 1329–1346
39. Carhuapoma JR et al (2002) Human brain hemorrhage: quantification of perihematoma edema by use of diffusion-weighted MR imaging. AJNR Am J Neuroradiol 23(8):1322–1326
40. Kidwell CS et al (2001) Diffusion-perfusion MR evaluation of perihematomal injury in hyperacute intracerebral hemorrhage. Neurology 57(9):1611–1617
41. Forbes KP, Pipe JG, Heiserman JE (2003) Diffusion-weighted imaging provides support for secondary neuronal damage from intraparenchymal hematoma. Neuroradiology 45(6):363–367
42. Stosser S et al (2016) Perihematomal diffusion restriction in intracerebral hemorrhage depends on hematoma volume, but does not predict outcome. Cerebrovasc Dis 42(3–4):280–287
43. Schneider T et al (2017) Perihematomal diffusion restriction as a common finding in large intracerebral hemorrhages in the hyperacute phase. PLoS One 12(9):e0184518
44. Fainardi E et al (2013) Temporal changes in perihematomal apparent diffusion coefficient values during the transition from acute to subacute phases in patients with spontaneous intracerebral hemorrhage. Neuroradiology 55(2):145–156
45. Chakeres DW, Bryan RN (1986) Acute subarachnoid hemorrhage: in vitro comparison of magnetic resonance and computed tomography. AJNR Am J Neuroradiol 7(2):223–228
46. Jenkins A et al (1988) Magnetic resonance imaging of acute subarachnoid hemorrhage. J Neurosurg 68(5):731–736
47. Satoh S, Kadoya S (1988) Magnetic resonance imaging of subarachnoid hemorrhage. Neuroradiology 30(5):361–366
48. Atlas SW (1993) MR imaging is highly sensitive for acute subarachnoid hemorrhage ... not! Radiology 186(2):319–322; discussion 323
49. Ogawa T et al (1993) Subarachnoid hemorrhage: evaluation with MR imaging. Radiology 186(2):345–351

50. Griffiths PD et al (2001) Multimodality MR imaging depiction of hemodynamic changes and cerebral ischemia in subarachnoid hemorrhage. AJNR Am J Neuroradiol 22(9):1690–1697
51. Noguchi K et al (1994) MR of acute subarachnoid hemorrhage: a preliminary report of fluid-attenuated inversion-recovery pulse sequences. AJNR Am J Neuroradiol 15(10):1940–1943
52. Noguchi K et al (1995) Acute subarachnoid hemorrhage: MR imaging with fluid-attenuated inversion recovery pulse sequences. Radiology 196(3):773–777
53. Noguchi K et al (1997) Subacute and chronic subarachnoid hemorrhage: diagnosis with fluid-attenuated inversion-recovery MR imaging. Radiology 203(1):257–262
54. Noguchi K et al (2000) Comparison of fluid-attenuated inversion-recovery MR imaging with CT in a simulated model of acute subarachnoid hemorrhage. AJNR Am J Neuroradiol 21(5):923–927
55. Melhem ER, Jara H, Eustace S (1997) Fluid-attenuated inversion recovery MR imaging: identification of protein concentration thresholds for CSF hyperintensity. AJR Am J Roentgenol 169(3):859–862
56. Singer MB, Atlas SW, Drayer BP (1998) Subarachnoid space disease: diagnosis with fluid-attenuated inversion-recovery MR imaging and comparison with gadolinium-enhanced spin-echo MR imaging—blinded reader study. Radiology 208(2):417–422
57. Dechambre SD et al (2000) High signal in cerebrospinal fluid mimicking subarachnoid haemorrhage on FLAIR following acute stroke and intravenous contrast medium. Neuroradiology 42(8):608–611
58. Taoka T et al (2001) Sulcal hyperintensity on fluid-attenuated inversion recovery MR images in patients without apparent cerebrospinal fluid abnormality. AJR Am J Roentgenol 176(2):519–524
59. Wiesmann M et al (2002) Detection of hyperacute subarachnoid hemorrhage of the brain by using magnetic resonance imaging. J Neurosurg 96(4):684–689
60. Busch E et al (1998) Diffusion MR imaging during acute subarachnoid hemorrhage in rats. Stroke 29(10):2155–2161
61. Rordorf G et al (1999) Diffusion- and perfusion-weighted imaging in vasospasm after subarachnoid hemorrhage. Stroke 30(3):599–605
62. Domingo Z et al (2000) Diffusion weighted imaging and magnetic resonance spectroscopy in a low flow ischaemia model due to endothelin induced vasospasm. NMR Biomed 13(3):154–162
63. Condette-Auliac S et al (2001) Vasospasm after subarachnoid hemorrhage: interest in diffusion-weighted MR imaging. Stroke 32(8):1818–1824
64. Hadeishi H et al (2002) Diffusion-weighted magnetic resonance imaging in patients with subarachnoid hemorrhage. Neurosurgery 50(4):741–747; discussion 747-8
65. Leclerc X et al (2002) Symptomatic vasospasm after subarachnoid haemorrhage: assessment of brain damage by diffusion and perfusion-weighted MRI and single-photon emission computed tomography. Neuroradiology 44(7):610–616
66. Fobben ES et al (1989) MR characteristics of subdural hematomas and hygromas at 1.5 T. AJR Am J Roentgenol 153(3):589–595
67. Ebisu T et al (1989) Nonacute subdural hematoma: fundamental interpretation of MR images based on biochemical and in vitro MR analysis. Radiology 171(2):449–453
68. Wilms G et al (1992) Isodense subdural haematomas on CT:MRI findings. Neuroradiology 34(6):497–499
69. Ashikaga R, Araki Y, Ishida O (1997) MRI of head injury using FLAIR. Neuroradiology 39(4):239–242
70. Williams VL, Hogg JP (2000) Magnetic resonance imaging of chronic subdural hematoma. Neurosurg Clin N Am 11(3):491–498
71. Tsui EY et al (2000) Rapid spontaneous resolution and redistribution of acute subdural hematoma in a patient with chronic alcoholism: a case report. Eur J Radiol 36(1):53–57
72. Lee Y et al (2001) MR imaging of shaken baby syndrome manifested as chronic subdural hematoma. Korean J Radiol 2(3):171–174
73. Biousse V et al (2002) Diffusion-weighted magnetic resonance imaging in Shaken Baby Syndrome. Am J Ophthalmol 133(2):249–255
74. Mesiwala AH, Goodkin R (2002) Reversible ischemia detected by diffusion-weighted magnetic resonance imaging. Case illustration. J Neurosurg 97(1):230
75. Lee SH et al (2018) The potential of diffusion-weighted magnetic resonance imaging for predicting the outcomes of chronic subdural hematomas. J Korean Neurosurg Soc 61(1):97–104
76. Bakshi R et al (1999) MRI in cerebral intraventricular hemorrhage: analysis of 50 consecutive cases. Neuroradiology 41(6):401–409
77. Bakshi R et al (1999) Fluid-attenuated inversion-recovery MR imaging in acute and subacute cerebral intraventricular hemorrhage. AJNR Am J Neuroradiol 20(4):629–636
78. Nakai Y et al (2002) Fatal cerebral infarction after intraventricular hemorrhage in a pregnant patient with moyamoya disease. J Clin Neurosci 9(4):456–458
79. Scott M (1975) Spontaneous intracerebral hematoma caused by cerebral neoplasms. Report of eight verified cases. J Neurosurg 42(3):338–342
80. Mandybur TI (1977) Intracranial hemorrhage caused by metastatic tumors. Neurology 27(7):650–655
81. Little JR et al (1979) Brain hemorrhage from intracranial tumor. Stroke 10(3):283–288
82. Zimmerman RA, Bilaniuk LT (1980) Computed tomography of acute intratumoral hemorrhage. Radiology 135(2):355–359
83. Leeds NE, Elkin CM, Zimmerman RD (1984) Gliomas of the brain. Semin Roentgenol 19(1):27–43

84. Atlas SW et al (1987) Hemorrhagic intracranial malignant neoplasms: spin-echo MR imaging. Radiology 164(1):71–77

85. Brunereau L et al (2000) Familial form of intracranial cavernous angioma: MR imaging findings in 51 families. French Society of Neurosurgery. Radiology 214(1):209–216

86. Tagle P et al (1986) Intracranial cavernous angioma: presentation and management. J Neurosurg 64(5):720–723

87. Zabramski JM et al (1994) The natural history of familial cavernous malformations: results of an ongoing study. J Neurosurg 80(3):422–432

88. Gomori JM et al (1986) Occult cerebral vascular malformations: high-field MR imaging. Radiology 158(3):707–713

89. Sigal R et al (1990) Occult cerebrovascular malformations: follow-up with MR imaging. Radiology 176(3):815–819

90. Liu AY et al (1999) Traumatic brain injury: diffusion-weighted MR imaging findings. AJNR Am J Neuroradiol 20(9):1636–1641

91. Fernandez-Abinader JA et al (2017) Traumatic brain injury profile of an elderly population in Puerto Rico. P R Health Sci J 36(4):237–239

92. Kotwica Z, Brzezinski J (1993) Acute subdural haematoma in adults: an analysis of outcome in comatose patients. Acta Neurochir 121(3–4):95–99

93. Roh D, Reznik M, Claassen J (2017) Chronic subdural medical management. Neurosurg Clin N Am 28(2):211–217

94. Kronsbein K et al (2020) Updating the risk profile of fatal head trauma: an autopsy study with focus on age- and sex-dependent differences. Int J Legal Med 134(1):295–307

95. Neeley OJ et al (2020) Tumoral mimics of subdural hematomas: case report and review of diagnostic and management strategies in primary B-cell lymphoma of the subdural space. World Neurosurg 133:49–54

96. Ruschel LG et al (2016) Spontaneous intracranial epidural hematoma during rivaroxaban treatment. Rev Assoc Med Bras (1992) 62(8):721–724

97. Chen CY et al (2012) Intracranial hemorrhage in adult patients with hematological malignancies. BMC Med 10:97

98. Chmielewski P, Skrzat J, Walocha J (2013) Clinical importance of the middle meningeal artery. Folia Med Cracov 53(1):41–46

99. Lee S et al (2018) The pathogenesis of delayed epidural hematoma after posterior fossa surgery. J Clin Neurosci 47:223–227

100. Rambaud C (2015) Bridging veins and autopsy findings in abusive head trauma. Pediatr Radiol 45(8):1126–1131

101. Gottesman RF, Komotar R, Hillis AE (2003) Neurologic aspects of traumatic brain injury. Int Rev Psychiatry 15(4):302–309

102. Araki T, Yokota H, Morita A (2017) Pediatric traumatic brain injury: characteristic features, diagnosis, and management. Neurol Med Chir (Tokyo) 57(2):82–93

103. Heiskanen O (1975) Epidural hematoma. Surg Neurol 4(1):23–26

104. Chaoguo Y et al (2019) Traumatic posterior fossa epidural hematomas in children: experience with 48 cases and a review of the literature. J Korean Neurosurg Soc 62(2):225–231

105. Winter RC (2015) Posterior fossa epidural hematoma. Pediatr Emerg Care 31(11):808–809

106. Rincon S, Gupta R, Ptak T (2016) Imaging of head trauma. Handb Clin Neurol 135:447–477

107. Maramattom BV, Wijdicks EF (2005) Uncal herniation. Arch Neurol 62(12):1932–1935

108. Dinallo S, Waseem M (2020) Cushing reflex. StatPearls, Treasure Island (FL)

109. Al-Nakshabandi NA (2001) The swirl sign. Radiology 218(2):433

110. Freeman WD (2015) Management of intracranial pressure. Continuum (Minneap Minn) 21(5 Neurocritical Care):1299–1323

111. Carney N et al (2017) Guidelines for the management of severe traumatic brain injury, fourth edition. Neurosurgery 80(1):6–15

112. Grandhi R et al (2014) Surgical management of traumatic brain injury: a review of guidelines, pathophysiology, neurophysiology, outcomes, and controversies. J Neurosurg Sci 58(4):249–259

113. Servadei F, Compagnone C, Sahuquillo J (2007) The role of surgery in traumatic brain injury. Curr Opin Crit Care 13(2):163–168

114. D'oria S, Dibenedetto M, Squillante E, Delvecchio C, Zizza F, Somma C, Godano U. Chronic subdural hematomas: single versus double burr holes. J Neurosurg Sci. 2020;64(2):216–18.

115. Chen H, Song Z, Dennis JA (2019) Hypertonic saline versus other intracranial pressure-lowering agents for people with acute traumatic brain injury. Cochrane Database Syst Rev 12:CD010904

116. Servadei F (1997) Prognostic factors in severely head injured adult patients with epidural haematoma's. Acta Neurochir 139(4):273–278

117. Go AS et al (2014) Heart disease and stroke statistics—2014 update: a report from the American Heart Association. Circulation 129(3):e28–e292

118. Macdonald RL, Schweizer TA (2017) Spontaneous subarachnoid haemorrhage. Lancet 389(10069):655–666

119. Greving JP et al (2014) Development of the PHASES score for prediction of risk of rupture of intracranial aneurysms: a pooled analysis of six prospective cohort studies. Lancet Neurol 13(1):59–66

120. Graff-Radford J et al (2016) Distinguishing clinical and radiological features of non-traumatic convexal subarachnoid hemorrhage. Eur J Neurol 23(5):839–846

121. Edlow JA, Malek AM, Ogilvy CS (2008) Aneurysmal subarachnoid hemorrhage: update for emergency physicians. J Emerg Med 34(3):237–251

122. Linn FH et al (1994) Prospective study of sentinel headache in aneurysmal subarachnoid haemorrhage. Lancet 344(8922):590–593

123. Suarez JI, Tarr RW, Selman WR (2006) Aneurysmal subarachnoid hemorrhage. N Engl J Med 354(4):387–396
124. Nagy K et al (2013) Cerebrospinal fluid analyses for the diagnosis of subarachnoid haemorrhage and experience from a Swedish study. What method is preferable when diagnosing a subarachnoid haemorrhage? Clin Chem Lab Med 51(11):2073–2086
125. McKinney AM et al (2008) Detection of aneurysms by 64-section multidetector CT angiography in patients acutely suspected of having an intracranial aneurysm and comparison with digital subtraction and 3D rotational angiography. AJNR Am J Neuroradiol 29(3):594–602
126. Donmez H et al (2011) Comparison of 16-row multislice CT angiography with conventional angiography for detection and evaluation of intracranial aneurysms. Eur J Radiol 80(2):455–461
127. de Oliveira Manoel AL et al (2014) Aneurysmal subarachnoid haemorrhage from a neuroimaging perspective. Crit Care 18(6):557
128. Tang C, Zhang TS, Zhou LF (2014) Risk factors for rebleeding of aneurysmal subarachnoid hemorrhage: a meta-analysis. PLoS One 9(6):e99536
129. Diringer MN et al (2011) Critical care management of patients following aneurysmal subarachnoid hemorrhage: recommendations from the Neurocritical Care Society's multidisciplinary consensus conference. Neurocrit Care 15(2):211–240
130. Molyneux A et al (2002) International Subarachnoid Aneurysm Trial (ISAT) of neurosurgical clipping versus endovascular coiling in 2143 patients with ruptured intracranial aneurysms: a randomized trial. J Stroke Cerebrovasc Dis 11(6):304–314
131. Molyneux AJ et al (2005) International subarachnoid aneurysm trial (ISAT) of neurosurgical clipping versus endovascular coiling in 2143 patients with ruptured intracranial aneurysms: a randomised comparison of effects on survival, dependency, seizures, rebleeding, subgroups, and aneurysm occlusion. Lancet 366(9488):809–817
132. Molyneux AJ et al (2015) The durability of endovascular coiling versus neurosurgical clipping of ruptured cerebral aneurysms: 18 year follow-up of the UK cohort of the International Subarachnoid Aneurysm Trial (ISAT). Lancet 385(9969):691–697
133. Macdonald RL (2014) Delayed neurological deterioration after subarachnoid haemorrhage. Nat Rev Neurol 10(1):44–58
134. Connolly ES Jr et al (2012) Guidelines for the management of aneurysmal subarachnoid hemorrhage: a guideline for healthcare professionals from the American Heart Association/American Stroke Association. Stroke 43(6):1711–1737
135. Lovelock CE, Rinkel GJ, Rothwell PM (2010) Time trends in outcome of subarachnoid hemorrhage: population-based study and systematic review. Neurology 74(19):1494–1501
136. Nieuwkamp DJ et al (2009) Changes in case fatality of aneurysmal subarachnoid haemorrhage over time, according to age, sex, and region: a meta-analysis. Lancet Neurol 8(7):635–642
137. Witsch J et al (2016) Prognostication of long-term outcomes after subarachnoid hemorrhage: the FRESH score. Ann Neurol 80(1):46–58
138. Gross BA, Jankowitz BT, Friedlander RM (2019) Cerebral intraparenchymal hemorrhage: a review. JAMA 321(13):1295–1303
139. Woo D et al (2004) Effect of untreated hypertension on hemorrhagic stroke. Stroke 35(7):1703–1708
140. Finelli PF, Kessimian N, Bernstein PW (1984) Cerebral amyloid angiopathy manifesting as recurrent intracerebral hemorrhage. Arch Neurol 41(3):330–333
141. Ritter MA et al (2005) Role of cerebral amyloid angiopathy in intracerebral hemorrhage in hypertensive patients. Neurology 64(7):1233–1237
142. Wada R et al (2007) CT angiography "spot sign" predicts hematoma expansion in acute intracerebral hemorrhage. Stroke 38(4):1257–1262
143. Demchuk AM et al (2012) Prediction of haematoma growth and outcome in patients with intracerebral haemorrhage using the CT-angiography spot sign (PREDICT): a prospective observational study. Lancet Neurol 11(4):307–314
144. Aguilar MI, Brott TG (2011) Update in intracerebral hemorrhage. Neurohospitalist 1(3):148–159
145. Mendelow AD et al (2013) Early surgery versus initial conservative treatment in patients with spontaneous supratentorial lobar intracerebral haematomas (STICH II): a randomised trial. Lancet 382(9890):397–408
146. Auer LM et al (1989) Endoscopic surgery versus medical treatment for spontaneous intracerebral hematoma: a randomized study. J Neurosurg 70(4):530–535
147. Ziai WC et al (2019) A randomized 500-subject open-label phase 3 clinical trial of minimally invasive surgery plus alteplase in intracerebral hemorrhage evacuation (MISTIE III). Int J Stroke 14(5):548–554
148. Honner SK et al (2011) Emergency department control of blood pressure in intracerebral hemorrhage. J Emerg Med 41(4):355–361
149. Qureshi AI et al (2010) Effect of systolic blood pressure reduction on hematoma expansion, perihematomal edema, and 3-month outcome among patients with intracerebral hemorrhage: results from the antihypertensive treatment of acute cerebral hemorrhage study. Arch Neurol 67(5):570–576
150. Biffi A et al (2011) Statin use and outcome after intracerebral hemorrhage: case-control study and meta-analysis. Neurology 76(18):1581–1588
151. Castellanos M et al (2005) Predictors of good outcome in medium to large spontaneous supratentorial intracerebral haemorrhages. J Neurol Neurosurg Psychiatry 76(5):691–695

Vasculopathy and Vasculitis

11

Girish Bathla, Toshio Moritani,
Patricia A. Kirby, and Aristides A. Capizzano

Sadhana Murali, and Mollie McDermott

11.1 Definition

Vasculopathy is a general term used to describe any disease affecting blood vessels [1]. It includes vascular abnormalities caused by degenerative, metabolic and inflammatory conditions, embolic diseases, coagulative disorders, and functional disorders such as posterior reversible encephalopathy syndrome. The etiology of vasculopathy is generally unknown, and the condition is frequently not pathologically proven. Vasculitis, on the other hand, is a more specific term and is defined as inflammation of the wall of a blood vessel [2]. However, the term vasculopathy is also used for "vasculitis" that has not been pathologically established.

G. Bathla (✉)
Division of Neuroradiology, University of Iowa
Hospitals & Clinics, Iowa City, IA, USA
e-mail: girish-bathla@uiowa.edu

T. Moritani · A. A. Capizzano
Division of Neuroradiology, University of Michigan,
Ann Arbor, MI, USA
e-mail: tmoritan@med.umich.edu;
capizzan@med.umich.edu

P. A. Kirby
University of Iowa Hospitals & Clinics,
Iowa City, IA, USA
e-mail: patricia-kirby@uiowa.edu

S. Murali · M. McDermott
University of Michigan, Ann Arbor, MI, USA
e-mail: msadhana@umich.edu; mcdermom@umich.edu

11.2 Clinical Presentation

Vasculitis and vasculopathy of the central nervous system (CNS) often have similar clinical and radiological characteristics. Both result in ischemia, which can be reversible or develop into infarction. The reversibility of a lesion is related to the size and location of vessels involved and the severity of ischemia. Diffusion-weighted (DW) imaging has been useful in the early detection of cytotoxic edema in hyperacute or acute infarctions and can distinguish cytotoxic edema from vasogenic edema and chronic infarctions [3]. Some specific types of vasculitis or vasculopathy demonstrate primarily vasogenic edema [4–8].

11.3 Role of Imaging

Digital subtraction catheter angiography and brain biopsy are the diagnostic foundations in establishing the diagnosis of CNS vasculitis (CNSV). However, the sensitivity and specificity of cerebral angiography in pathologically proven cases of primary angiitis of the central nervous system (PACNS) can be as low as 27 and 30%, respectively [9]. Because. while large/medium vessel PACNS can show angiographic abnormalities, small vessel PACNS usually has more severe encephalopathic symptoms with unrevealing angiographic findings. Similarly, neural

© Springer Nature Switzerland AG 2021
T. Moritani, A. A. Capizzano (eds.), *Diffusion-Weighted MR Imaging of the Brain, Head and Neck, and Spine*, https://doi.org/10.1007/978-3-030-62120-9_11

tissue biopsy also suffers from low sensitivity and may be false-negative in up to 25% of cases autopsy-proven cases [9]. Brain biopsy is still considered the most reliable diagnostic method even though it lacks sensitivity, nondiagnostic in up to 50% of the cases, with invasive procedures. CTA and MRA on the other hand can adequately document proximal vascular involvement but may not be reliable for more distal vascular involvement. Another limitation of all these modalities is that they predominantly evaluate the lumen of the vessel without any direct information about the vessel wall.

Advances in MRI techniques have allowed direct visualization of the vessel wall. Even though the visualization of the smaller vessels is beyond the resolution currently afforded by vessel wall imaging (VWI), the more proximal vessels, which are often involved, can be imaged with reasonable accuracy [10]. More recently, smaller case series have also demonstrated the utility of VWI for selecting biopsy site and monitoring response to therapy. The use of 7 T magnets may further expand the scope of VWI in future, given the higher signal-to-noise ratio.

Besides the evaluation of the vessel wall itself, MRI can often provide useful secondary information such as the presence of strokes and hemorrhages. Cerebral ischemia, which may result in focal infarction, is the major neurological manifestation of CNS vasculitis. Multifocal and multiphasic ischemia are some of the characteristic sequelae of CNS vasculitis. DW imaging can differentiate the phases of cerebral infarction as hyperacute, acute, subacute, or chronic. Additionally, DW imaging can be useful to differentiate an acute or subacute infarction from vasogenic edema, the latter being more common with arteriolar, capillary, or venular involvement. This is important both for choice of treatment and to predict the long-term prognosis. Diffuse increase in water diffusion in the normal-appearing brain with CNS vasculitis is also observed [11]. Even though the diagnostic and prognostic significance of this finding is unclear, it may imply a much more widespread involvement of the brain parenchyma at a microscopic level as is also seen on autopsy.

Parenchymal or subarachnoid hemorrhage may also be seen with CNSV. The widespread use of SWI has led to a greater recognition of microhemorrhages and venous involvement in CNSV [12, 13]. The improved detection of microhemorrhages with SWI is likely to increase the overall sensitivity of MRI in detection of underlying parenchymal abnormalities in CNSV, and an SWI sequence should ideally be performed in suspected CNSV. Overall, even though the imaging findings are often nonspecific, brain MRI is abnormal in more than 90% of patients with PACNS [14]. In fact, a normal brain MRI and CSF analysis has a high negative predictive value for CNS vasculitis.

11.4 Treatment

Vasculitis and vasculopathy of the CNS caused by an abnormal immune reaction are often treated with immunosuppressant agents. In the absence of prospective trials, the guidelines are primarily based on review of retrospective data and expert consensus. For PACNS, glucocorticoids are used as first-line therapy, and may be combined with cyclophosphamide or other biologics in more severe cases [15]. For secondary vasculitis involving the CNS, the underlying cause also needs to be concurrently addressed. Overall, the treatment response and patient outcomes seem to be related to the size of the involved vessels, with small cortical and leptomeningeal involvement associated with a more benign course and larger vessel involvement associated with a less favorable course [16]. Prompt characterization of the nature of CNS vasculitis and vasculopathy, by imaging and/or biopsy, is thus necessary to institute appropriate management.

11.5 Vasculitis of the CNS

The term vasculitis encompasses a heterogeneous group of multisystemic disorders characterized pathologically by inflammation and necrosis of the blood vessel wall. The clinical manifestations can be quite heterogeneous and include headache, transient ischemic attacks (TIAs), altered mental status, seizures, cranial nerve palsies, and localized neurologic deficits.

The 2012 Revised Chapel Hill Consensus Conference (CHCC) described various vasculitides in the context of (a) size of the involved vessels, and (b) associated pathologic lesions (Fig. 11.1) [17]. It is important to note here that CHCC only addresses etiologies which are not secondary to vessel wall invasion by infectious pathogens. Also, even though the different vasculitides are primarily defined on the basis of size of vessel involved, the vasculitis in all three major categories can affect vessel of any caliber.

Within the CNS, the vasculitis may be primary when it is restricted to the CNS, or secondary when it is associated with systemic disorders. What follows is a broad overview of the different vasculitides involving the brain along with a discussion of the pertinent pathophysiology and imaging.

11.5.1 Primary Angiitis of the Central Nervous System

Primary angitis (angiitis) of the central nervous system (PACNS) is a noninfectious granulomatous angiitis, pathologically characterized by infiltration of the vessel walls with lymphocytes, histiocytes, and/or multinucleated giant cells, with a variable degree of fibrinoid necrosis [18]. Under the revised CHCC classification, PACNS is categorized under single organ vasculitis [17]. PACNS is usually seen in middle-aged individuals (mean age 50 years) and is twice as common in men. In general, patients younger than 30 years and older than 70 years are rarely affected [14]. A potential caveat here is occurrence of PACNS in association with amyloid angiopathy which has been reported in older patients [19, 20]. Headaches and cognitive impairment are the most common symptoms and end to be indolently progressive. Spinal cord involvement is

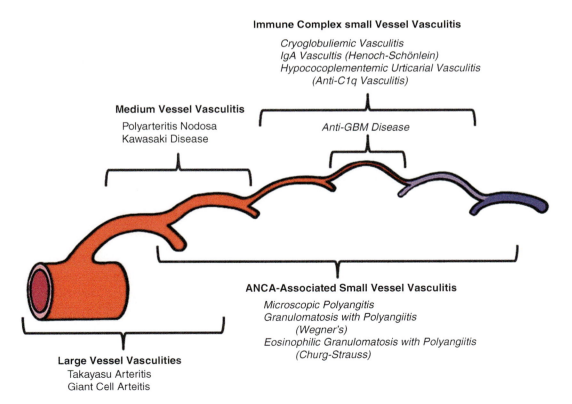

Fig. 11.1 Classification of CNS vasculitis. (Modified from [17])

seen in about 5% and most frequently affects the thoracic cord [21].

The pathogenesis is probably related to T-cell-mediated inflammation. PACNS tends to affect small- to medium-sized vessels of the brain parenchyma and meninges but can affect vessels of any size. Over the years, multiple subsets of PACNS have been described and may differ in terms of prognosis and management. These include angiography-negative variant, PACNS with prominent leptomeningeal enhancement, rapidly progressive PACNS, PACNS with intra-cranial hemorrhage, and PACNS associated with cerebral amyloid angiopathy [21].

Angiography may show a "string-of-beads" appearance, which is usually seen in PACNS involving medium-sized arteries, but it has a false-negative rate of 20–30% [22]. Microaneurysms are rare. Brain and meningeal biopsies are diagnostic in only 50–72% of patients with PACNS. Magnetic resonance imaging findings in PACNS are highly variable, ranging from multi-phasic cerebral infarction, vasogenic edema, and gliosis to hemorrhage and leptomeningeal enhancement [23, 24]. Infarcts may be seen in about 50% of cases. When present, these may be bilateral, involve different vascular territories and show temporal distribution. DW imaging is useful in differentiating an acute or subacute infarction from reversible vasogenic edema (Figs. 11.2 and 11.3), and can demonstrate multiphasic infarctions (Fig. 11.4). Mass-like lesions may be seen in about 15% of cases. Both subarachnoid and intra-parenchymal hemorrhages have been reported and may be seen in 10% of cases. Similarly, leptomeningeal enhancement is seen in 10–15% of cases and may suggest a more favorable prognosis [14, 21]. High-resolution VWI may show segmental areas of concentric wall thickening and enhancement although the sensitivity and specificity of this technique need to be validated [10, 21].

Prompt diagnosis is important as PACNS is often fatal if not treated with aggressive immuno-suppression [26]. PACNS involving small vessels tends to be responsive to immunosuppressive drugs, but often there is relapse. PACNS involv-ing medium-sized vessels tend to have isolated episodes with paucity of relapses [27].

11.5.2 Giant Cell (Temporal) Arteritis

GCA is the most common type of systemic vas-culitis in adults and is characterized by panarteri-tis of medium- to large-sized arterial vessels [28]. This falls under the large vessel vasculitis cate-gory in the revised CHCC classification. The American College of Rheumatology developed the following criteria for the classification of GCA: (1) age at disease onset >50 years, (2) new onset of headache, (3) tenderness of the temporal artery on palpation or decreased pulsation, (4) erythrocyte sedimentation ratio >50 mm/h, and (5) temporal artery biopsy showing vasculitis with multinucleated giant cells. In the traditional format classification, a minimum of three criteria are required for diagnosis, and provide a sensitiv-ity of 93.5% and specificity of 91.2% of the diag-nosis. Another classification tree along similar lines uses six criteria. These include all the above criteria except elevated ESR and additional vari-ables of scalp tenderness and claudication of the jaw or tongue on deglutition. These are margin-ally more sensitive but less specific than the tradi-tional criteria [29].

Giant cell arteritis is probably a T-cell-mediated vasculitis, and it can affect medium to large arteries. The superficial temporal, vertebral, and ophthalmic arteries are more commonly involved than the internal carotid arteries. Involvement of the intracranial arteries was con-sidered rare but has been observed more fre-quently with the use of VWI [30]. Other less common sites of involvement include axillary artery, aorta, coronary, and mesenteric vessels (Fig. 11.5) [32, 33]. Abrupt and irreversible visual loss is the most dramatic complication of giant cell arteritis, while TIA and stroke are rare (7%), but when present most often involve the vertebrobasilar territory.

On imaging, "halo sign" around the vessel wall has been described with ultrasound imaging. A recent meta-analysis showed a sensitivity and

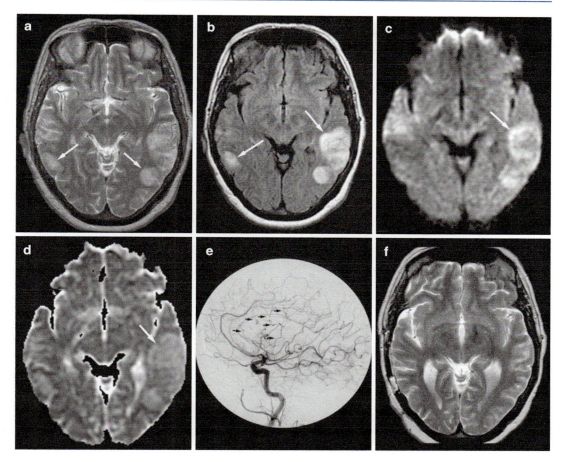

Fig. 11.2 Primary angiitis of central nervous system (proven by biopsy) in a 60-year-old woman with dizziness and speech difficulties. (**a**) T2-weighted image shows hyperintense lesions in the bilateral tempo-occipital cortices (*arrows*). (**b**) FLAIR image shows hyperintense lesions in the bilateral tempo-occipital cortices (*arrows*). (**c**) DW image shows slightly high signal in the lesions (*arrow*) with increased ADC (**d**), mainly representing vasogenic edema (*arrow*). (**e**) DSA shows multiple focal stenoses of distal branches of left middle cerebral arteries (*arrows*). (**f**) 2-month follow-up T2-weighted image shows no infarction in the bilateral tempo-occipital areas. (From [25])

specificity of 68 and 81%, respectively [28]. Recent studies using high-resolution VWI have shown a sensitivity and specificity of 89 and 75% in patients with biopsy-proved GCA [34]. Even though the role of DW imaging in diagnosing GCA of scalp vessel remains unexplored, a recent study highlighted the usefulness of DWI in a patient with aortic involvement [35]. On VWI, the involved vessels may show segmental wall thickening and enhancement which may involve the peri-adventitial tissue in severe cases. Intracranially, ischemic infarcts have been reported in 3–15% of cases [30]. Steroids are effective, and giant cell arteritis is usually self-limited and rarely fatal.

11.5.3 Takayasu's Arteritis (Aortitis Syndrome)

Takayasu's arteritis (Fig. 11.6) is a primary arteritis of unknown cause but probably also related to T-cell-mediated inflammation. Takayasu's arteritis again falls under the large vessel

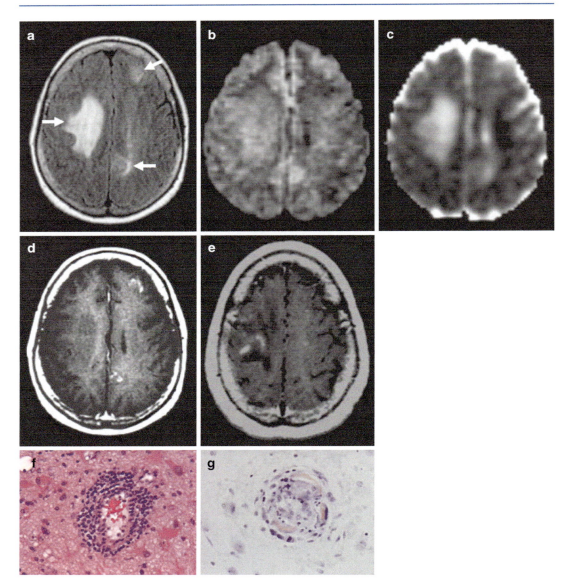

Fig. 11.3 Primary angiitis of the central nervous system associated with amyloid angiopathy (proven by biopsy) in a 56-year-old woman. (**a**) FLAIR image shows multiple hyperintense lesions in the bilateral frontoparietal areas (*arrows*). (**b**) DW image shows slightly increased signal with increased ADC (**c**), representing vasogenic edema. (**d**, **e**) Postcontrast T1weighted image shows prominent leptomeningeal enhancement in these lesions. (**f**) Pathology shows lymphocytic infiltration in the wall of the small artery. (**g**) Congo *red* stain reveals amyloid deposition (*orange*) and granulomatous inflammation in a vessel wall

vasculitis category of the revised CHCC and commonly affects large vessels including the aorta and its major branches to the arms and the head. It is more commonly seen in Asia and usually affects young women in the second and third decades of life [36, 37]. Pulseless upper extremities and hypertension are the common clues to suggest the diagnosis. Most patients are treated with steroids alone to reduce the inflammation. The prognosis is relatively good, and 90% of patients are still alive after 10 years. TIA or stroke is rare but can occasionally occur in severe

11 Vasculopathy and Vasculitis

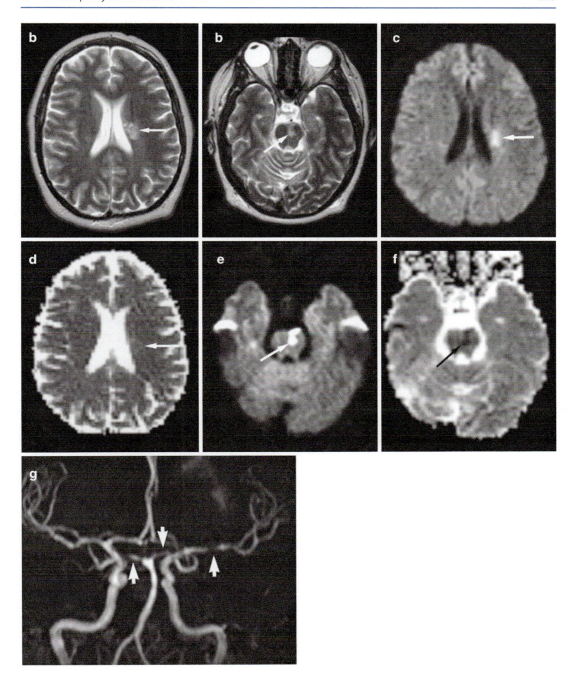

Fig. 11.4 Primary angiitis of central nervous system (proven by biopsy) in a 35-year-old woman with right hemiparesis. (**a, b**) T2-weighted image shows hyperintense lesions in the left corona radiata (*arrow*) and left side of the pons (*arrow*). (**c**) DW image shows slightly increased signal in the left corona radiata, indicating subacute infarction. (**d**) ADC map shows slightly increased ADC in this lesion (*arrow*). (**e**) DW image simultaneously shows very high signal in the left side of the pons, indicating acute infarction (*arrow*). (**f**) ADC map shows decreased ADC in this lesion (*arrow*). (**g**) MR angiography shows stenosis in the left middle cerebral and posterior cerebral arteries (*arrows*). (From [25]). (**h, i**) Digital subtraction angiography (DSA) confirms the stenosis in the left middle cerebral (*arrow*) and posterior cerebral arteries, consistent with PACNS involving medium-sized arteries (*arrows*). (**j**) Pathological specimen by meningeal biopsy shows infiltration of the vessel wall with lymphocytes, multinucleated giant cells, and intramural granulomatous inflammation (*arrows*). (From [25])

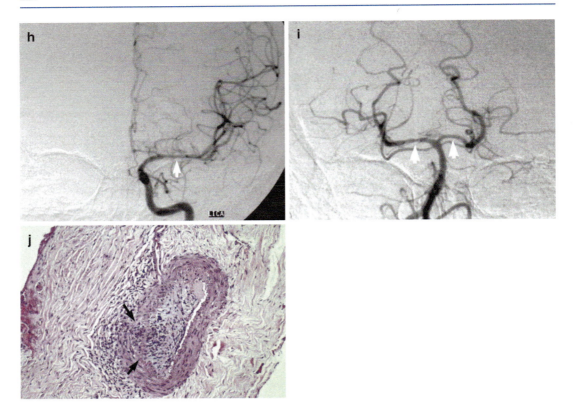

Fig. 11.4 (continued)

cases with significant stenosis of arteries supplying the CNS (Fig. 11.6). Additionally, patients may have intra-cranial aneurysms or show changes of reversible cerebral vasoconstriction syndrome [38].

11.5.4 Polyarteritis Nodosa

Polyarteritis nodosa often involves medium-sized arteries and is characterized by panmural necrotizing vasculitis [37]. The criteria of the American College of Rheumatology for the diagnosis of polyarteritis nodosa include at least three of the following: (1) weight loss >4 kg, (2) livedo reticularis, (3) testicular pain or tenderness, (4) myalgias, weakness, or leg tenderness, (5) mono or polyneuropathy, (6) hypertension, (7) elevated blood creatinine or blood urea nitrogen, (8) hepatitis B antigen or antibodies in the serum, (9) aneurysm or occlusion of the visceral arteries, and (10) granulocytes in small- or medium-sized arteries on vessel wall biopsy. Neurologic abnormalities occur in 10% of cases and is usually characterized by aneurysms and vascular stenoses [39]. Ischemic stroke can result from vasculitis, severe hypertension, or embolism secondary to cardiac involvement [40]. The treatment usually requires both cytotoxic agents and steroids.

11.5.5 Eosinophilic Granulomatosis with Polyangiitis (Churg-Strauss Syndrome)

This is an antineutrophil cytoplasmic autoantibody-mediated vasculitis, defined by at least four of the following: (1) asthma, (2) history of allergy, (3) eosinophilia (>10%), (4) mono- or polyneuropathy, (5) migratory or transitory pulmonary infiltrates, and (6) sinusitis. Under the revised CHCC classification,

11 Vasculopathy and Vasculitis

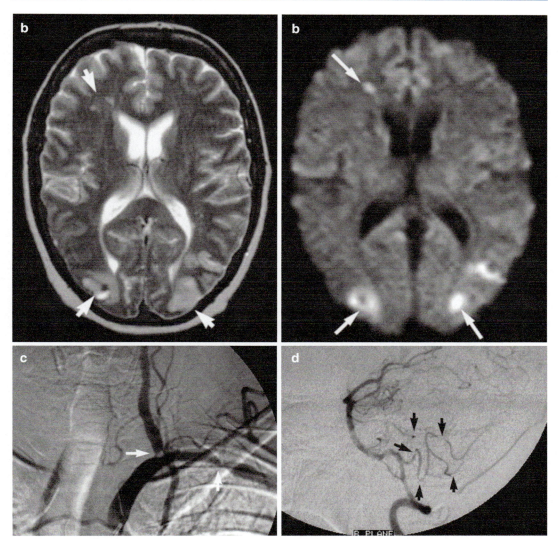

Fig. 11.5 Giant cell arteritis (proven by biopsy) in a 48-year-old woman with visual loss. (**a**) T2-weighted image shows hyperintense lesions in the bilateral parieto-occipital cortices and right frontal deep white matter (*arrows*). (**b**) DW image shows these lesions as high signal intensity, representing acute infarcts (*arrows*). (**c**) DSA of the left subclavian artery shows stenoses of the left vertebral and subclavian arteries (*arrows*). (**d**) DSA of the left vertebral artery shows extensive multifocal arterial stenoses (*arrows*). (From [31])

this is grouped under the small vessel vasculitis category. A biopsy of affected organs, including small arteries, arterioles, or venules shows a vasculitis with extravascular eosinophils, which confirms the diagnosis. Involvement of the peripheral nervous system is common and may present as mononeuritis multiplex. CNS involvement occurs in up to 10% of cases and may manifest as macro- and micro-infarctions and hemorrhages as well as subarachnoid hemorrhages (Figure 11.7) [39, 41–43]. Steroids usually stabilize this condition, but treatment with cyclophosphamide may be required. A normal angiogram does not exclude this form of vasculitis, as affected vessels are often smaller than the resolution of angiography.

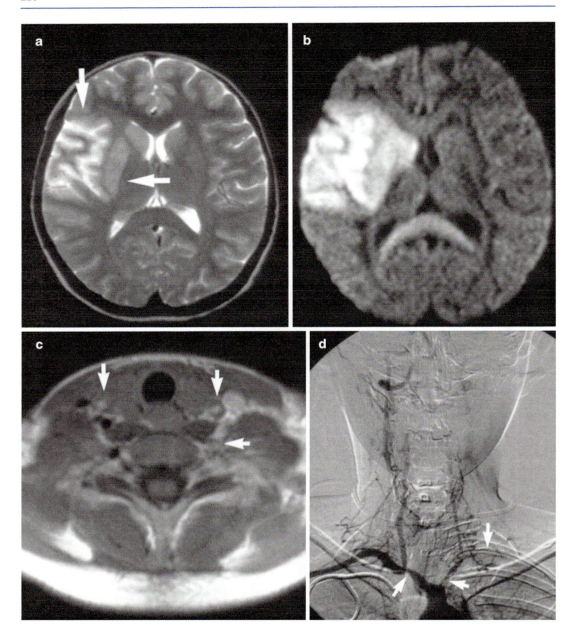

Fig. 11.6 Takayasu's arteritis in an 18-year-old woman with left hemiparesis. (**a**) T2-weighted image shows a hyperintense lesion in the right basal ganglia and temporal lobe (*arrows*). (**b**) DW image shows a very high signal lesion, indicating an acute infarct. (**c**) T1-weighted axial image shows occlusion of internal carotid arteries bilaterally and the left vertebral artery, with thickening of the wall and thrombosis (*arrows*). (**d**) DSA shows occlusion of both carotid arteries, and stenosis of the brachiocephalic and left subclavian arteries (*arrows*)

11.5.6 Other Small Vessel Vasculitis

The incidence of neurological symptoms in granulomatosis with polyangiitis (Wegener's granulomatosis) varies from 11 to 54%, but cerebral or meningeal involvement is uncommon, occurring in 2–8% of cases (Fig. 11.8) [44]. Involvement of the CNS in other forms of small vessel vasculitis (microscopic polyangitis, Henoch–Schönlein purpura, essential cryoglobulinemia, and hyper-

11 Vasculopathy and Vasculitis

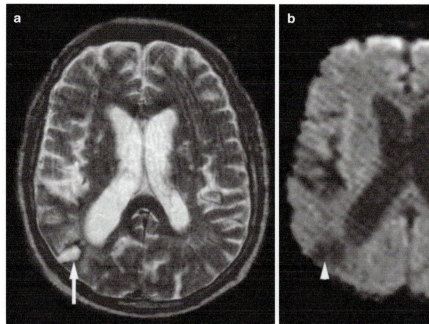

Fig. 11.7 Churg–Strauss disease in a 65-year-old man with seizures. (a) T2-weighted image shows multiple hyperintense lesions in both corona radiata and right parieto-occipital area, the latter with a hemosiderin rim, representing old hemorrhage (*arrow*). (b) DW image shows a hyperintense lesion (*arrow*) in the left corona radiata, representing an acute infarct. An old hemorrhage shows hypointensity (*arrowhead*) on DW image. MR angiography and DSA revealed no abnormalities (not shown). (From [25])

sensitivity vasculitis) is rare. In the case of Henoch–Schönlein purpura, MR imaging can show reversibility of lesions [7].

11.5.7 Variable Vessel Vasculitis

Under the revised CHCC classification, this category includes Bechet's disease and Cogan's syndrome [17]. Both these entities can affect vessels of any size and type (including capillaries and veins).

11.5.7.1 Bechet's Disease

Behçet's disease is a multisystem vasculitis of unknown origin. It is most common in Middle Eastern and Mediterranean countries. CNS involvement has been described in up to 30% of cases and is rare in the absence of mucocutaneous lesions and ocular symptoms [37, 42]. CNS involvement can be broadly classified into parenchymal (80%) and non-parenchymal (20%) groups. The former includes parenchymal lesions, meningoencephalitis, and cranial nerve involvement, while the latter includes sinus thrombosis, arterial occlusions, and aneurysms. Lesions more commonly involve the diencephalic structures, brainstem, and basal ganglia in the acute phase. During the recovery phase, new lesions may be seen in the periventricular white matter. The chronic phase is characterized by atrophy of the brainstem and posterior fossa structures. Overall, solitary lesions are more common in the acute phase, while the involvement in the chronic phase is more widespread [45]. The parenchymal distribution of lesions in Behçet's disease, especially at the mesodiencephalic junction (46%), supports small vessel vasculitis involving both the arterial and venous system, mainly venules. Occasionally, these lesions are reversible on MR images that mainly represent vasogenic edema. This is why DW imaging is useful in distinguishing them from infarction (Fig. 11.9). The treatment is usually a combination of cytotoxic agents and steroids. In other types of collagen diseases, such as scleroderma or rheumatoid arthritis, involvement of the CNS is very rare.

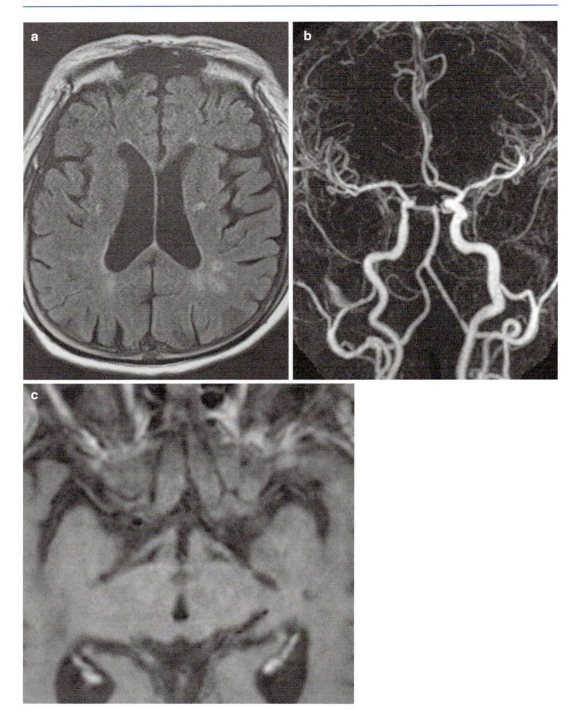

Fig. 11.8 Granulomatosis with polyangiitis. Axial FLAIR image (**a**) reveals small bilateral infarcts involving the PVWM, more on the left side. MIP image of the contrast enhanced MRA (**b**) reveals mild focal narrowing of the left proximal M1 segment. Magnified post contrast axial MPR image of the VWI study (**c**) reveals circumferential thickening and enhancement of the MCA vessels bilaterally, consistent with vasculitis.

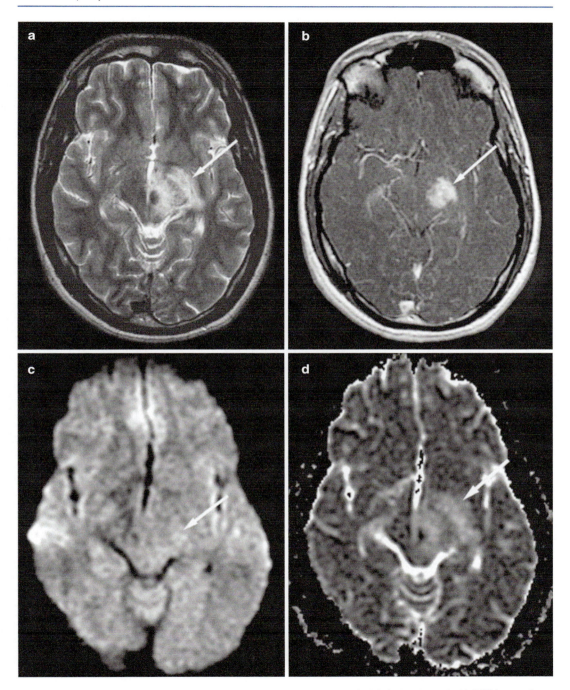

Fig. 11.9 Neuro-Behçet's disease in a 24-year-old man. (**a**) T2-weighted image shows a hyperintense lesion in the left midbrain extending into the left temporal lobe, with enlargement of the left cerebral peduncle (*arrow*). (**b**) Gadolinium-enhanced T1-weighted image shows enhancement in this lesion (*arrow*). (**c**) DW image shows a hyperintense lesion with increased signal intensity in the left cerebral peduncle, probably representing vasogenic edema (*arrow*). (**d**) ADC map shows increased ADC in this lesion (*arrow*). (From [46])

11.5.7.2 Cogan Syndrome

Common presentations of Cogan syndrome include ocular inflammatory lesions and inner ear disease. Even though the primary ocular vascular inflammatory target are the small vessels of the anterior globe, aortitis, aortic aneurysms, and aortic and/or mitral valvulitis may also occur [17]. Within the CNS, imaging findings may include infarcts, meningoencephalitis, venous sinus thrombosis, and enhancement of the membranous labyrinth [37].

11.5.8 Infectious Vasculitis

Infections can cause vasculitis both by direct invasion of the vessel walls and by an immune-mediated response to the pathogens. Bacterial, fungal, and some viral infections (e.g., herpes virus) result in a vasculitis. Vessel wall involvement may or may not result in subsequent infarction (Fig. 11.10) [2, 47]. Concurrent fever, leukocytosis, and ongoing or recent infection are important clues while considering infectious vas-

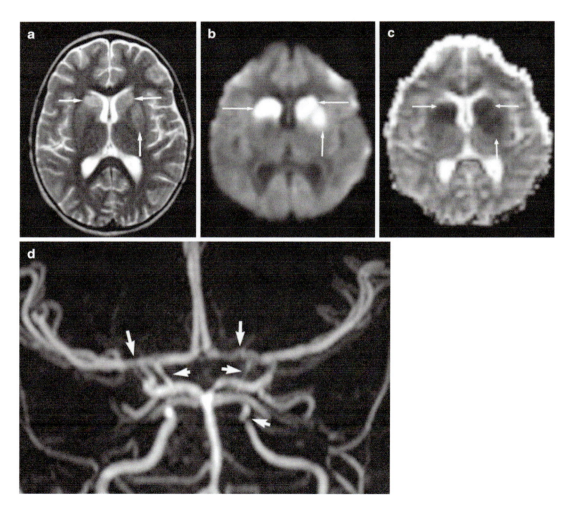

Fig. 11.10 Pneumococcal meningitis and vasculitis in a 4-year-old girl with high fever. (**a**) T2-weighted image reveals hyperintense lesions in bilateral basal ganglia (*arrows*). (**b**) OW Image shows these lesions as very hyperintense, representing acute or subacute infarcts caused by infectious vasculitis (*arrows*). (**c**) ADC demonstrates low signal, confirming acute or subacute infarcts (*arrows*). (**d**) MR angiography shows stenosis of internal carotid arteries, right middle cerebral and left anterior cerebral arteries (*arrows*)

culitis. Vasculitis and cerebral infarcts may be seen in 5–15% of adults with bacterial meningitis [39]. Globally, tuberculous meningitis is the most common cause of chronic meningitis and may have associated infarcts in about 40% of cases. Vasculitis with aseptic meningitis is probably related to an immunologic reaction, which can show reversible lesions. Aspergillus infiltrates and destroys the internal elastic lamina of major cerebral arteries, which results in infarction, abscess formation, and hemorrhage [48] (Fig. 11.11). Infection of the infarcted tissue may be aggressive, and direct extension into the surrounding brain may progress quickly.

11.5.9 Drug-Induced Vasculitis, Including Illicit Drugs

Some drugs, such as chemotherapeutic agents (e.g., sulfonamide, thiouracil) and illicit drugs (e.g., cocaine), can cause vasculitis [49]. Stroke can occur soon after administration of illicit drugs by an intravenous, oral, or nasal route. Cocaine, heroin, amphetamine, and other sympathomimetic drugs are most commonly implicated. The diagnosis of "vasculitis" depends on the pathological findings, not on the angiographic findings, which are usually nonspecific and may simply indicate vasospasm induced by these drugs.

Cocaine use has emerged as an important cause of cerebrovascular events in young adults and often involves medium-sized arteries [39, 50]. Vasculitic changes can be present on angiography, but the significance of these changes has been debated. However, both biopsy-proven vasculitis and wall enhancement on VWI have been reported in cocaine users [51, 52]. MR angiography may reveal irregularity of the intracerebral vessels, and DW imaging is useful for the detection of acute ischemic changes (Fig. 11.12).

11.5.10 Vasculitis Associated with Systemic Diseases

This category includes CNS vasculitis secondary to systemic lupus erythematosus (SLE), antiphospholipid antibody (ALPA) syndrome, Sjogren syndrome, rheumatoid arthritis, scleroderma, and sarcoidosis. In most cases, findings likely reflect a combination of thrombotic vasculopathies and (a smaller component of) immune-complex-mediated vasculitis [42].

SLE is distinctly more common in women and involves the CNS (neuropsychiatric SLE) in 14–75% of cases. On imaging, sub-cortical and parenchymal white matter lesions are seen in about 60–86% of patients and are the most common MRI finding. This is followed by parenchymal atrophy which is seen in about 43% of patients [37]. Overall, abnormal MRI findings are more common in those with associated APLA syndrome as compared to those with only SLE and no APLA syndrome (73 vs. 53%) (Fig. 11.13). Additionally, SLE patients with APLA syndrome are more likely to have both large territorial and lacunar infarcts, borderzone infarcts, basal ganglia lesions, and stenotic arterial lesions [53]. Intracranial hemorrhages, including parenchymal, subarachnoid, and subdural hemorrhages, may also be seen.

In Sjogren syndrome, CNS involvement is reported in 25–30% of cases, but it has been reported in up to 60% in some studies [37, 54]. Imaging manifestations include white and grey matter lesions, infarctions, and microhemorrhages as well as arterial stenoses. Posterior fossa and spinal cord involvement are considered rare. More recently, isolated case reports have described large vessel wall involvement in Sjogren syndrome cases presenting with cerebral infarcts [55].

Cerebral vasculitis in rheumatoid arthritis is rare but may be seen in about 1–8% of patients. Vasculitis in such cases is often accompanied by prominent extra-articular manifestations but little joint involvement [56]. Angiographic changes of vasculitis/vasculopathy may also be seen in patients with scleroderma (progressive systemic sclerosis). These are overall rare but tend to involve medium-sized arteries when present. Parenchymal hemorrhages and prominent vascular calcifications may also be seen [37, 39].

The exact incidence of vasculitis in sarcoidosis remains unclear. Although it was previously considered rare, data from autopsy studies and recent larger retrospective studies have shown

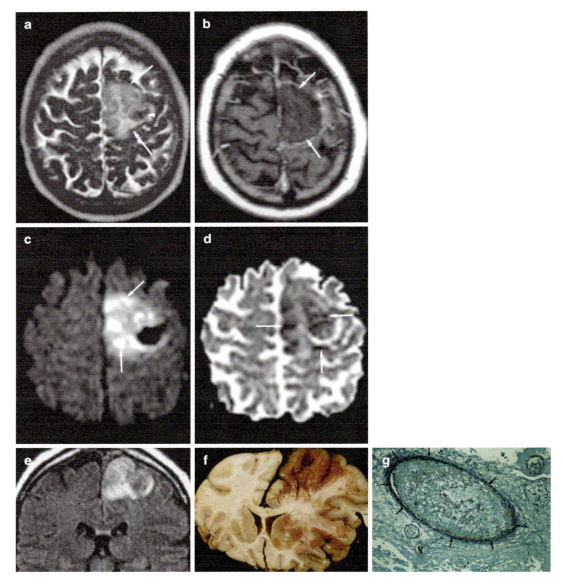

Fig. 11.11 Disseminated aspergillosis in a 48-year-old woman presenting with altered mental status and a history of acute lymphoblastic leukemia, post recent bone marrow transplant. (**a**) T2-weighted image shows a round high signal intensity lesion (*arrow*) at the corticomedullary junction in the medial left frontal lobe. A hypointense spot in this lesion represents a hemorrhagic component (*arrow head*). (**b**) Gadolinium-enhanced T1-weighted image reveals no enhancement within this lesion (*arrows*). (**c**) DW image shows this lesion containing areas of very high signal intensity (*arrows*), indicating a vasculitis-mediated acute septic infarction. (**d**) ADC shows heterogeneous decreased signal (*arrows*) in the lesion, confirming a conglomerate of acute septic infarctions. (**e**) Coronal FLAIR image shows a hyperintense mass in the left frontal lobe. (**f**) Gross specimen reveals a hemorrhagic necrotic lesion in the left frontal lobe. (**g**) Methenamine *Silver* stain shows numerous aspergillus hyphae involving the wall of the small artery (*arrows*). (From [25])

11 Vasculopathy and Vasculitis

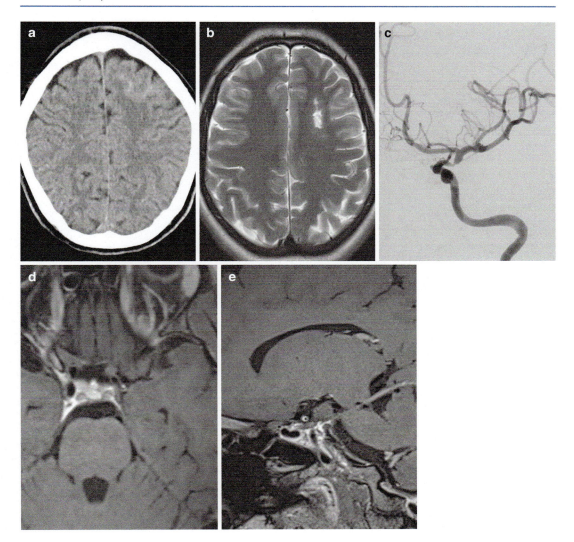

Fig. 11.12 Cocaine-induced vasculitis/vasculopathy. Axial CT image (**a**) in a young patient shows focal subarachnoid hemorrhage over left frontal convexity. Axial T2WI (**b**) also shows a chronic infarct in left centrum semiovale. DSA image (**c**) of left ICA injection shows a short segment of significant vascular stenosis involving the ICA. Axial MPR (**d**) and sagittal post contrast (**e**) images reveal circumferential, segmental vessel wall thickening, and enhancement

that it may be higher, perhaps in the range of 10–20% at initial presentation [12]. Most of these cases pertain to involvement of small vessels and often present with micro-infarcts, especially in the distribution of the perforator vessels. The routine use of SWI has further highlighted the role of sarcoid phlebitis, which appears to be more often associated with parenchymal micro-hemorrhages (Fig. 11.14) [12, 57]. Overall, large vessel vasculitis is probably the rarest, but may be seen with VWI [58].

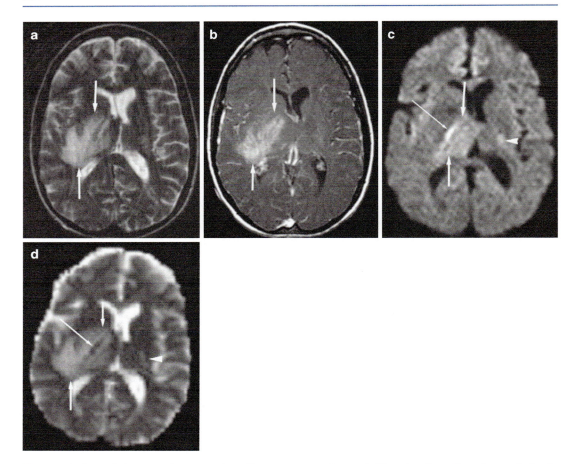

Fig. 11.13 Systemic lupus erythematosus in a 39-year-old woman with recurrent episodes of stroke, who presented with fever and disturbance of consciousness. (**a**) T2-weighted image shows hyperintense lesions in the right thalamus, internal capsule, putamen, subcortical white matter, and the left internal capsule (*arrows*). (**b**) Gadolinium-enhanced T1-weighted image reveals marked enhancement of the lesion on the right side, suggesting blood–brain barrier breakdown (*arrows*). (**c**) DW image shows a slightly hyperintense lesion in the right thalamus, but an isointense lesion in the right putamen and white matter (*arrows*). There is a linear hyperintense lesion in the right internal capsule (*long thin arrow*). A subtle hyperintense lesion in the left internal capsule is also seen (*arrowhead*). (**d**) The ADC map shows increased ADC of the lesion on the right side (*short thick arrows*), representing vasogenic edema. Increased ADC of the lesion in the left internal capsule (*arrowhead*) represents an old infarct. Decreased ADC is seen in the lesion in the right internal capsule (*long thin arrow*), presumably representing acute microinfarcts. (From [5])

11.6 Vasculopathy of the CNS

Vasculopathy is caused by a wide variety of underlying conditions such as degenerative, metabolic, inflammatory, embolic, coagulative, and functional disorders [1]. This presentation focuses on vasculopathies that mimic vasculitis but have no inflammation in the wall of the blood vessel (Fig. 11.15).

11.6.1 Moyamoya Disease

Moyamoya disease (MMD) is a rare, non-inflammatory vasculopathy of the intracranial vessels of unknown cause, which is found predominantly in East Asia, but it is also being increasingly recognized in Caucasian population, owing to increased recognition of disease [60]. The term moyamoya syndrome is used in cases

11 Vasculopathy and Vasculitis 235

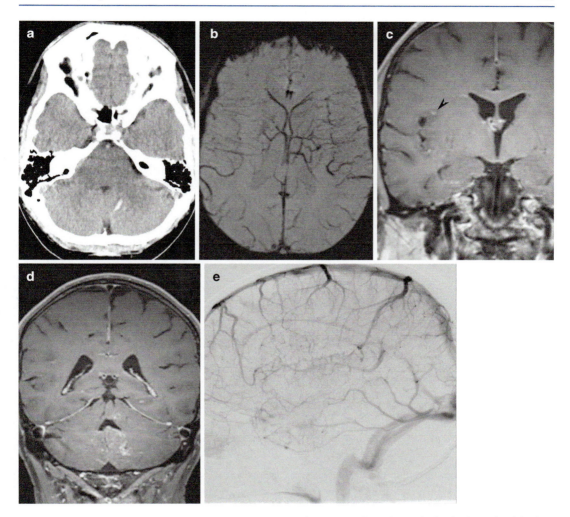

Fig. 11.14 Axial NCCT image (**a**) shows a small left vermian hemorrhage. Axial MIP SWI image (**b**) shows multiple dilated and irregular medullary veins, and few cortical veins, worse on the left side (**b**). Magnified coronal MPR post-contrast VWI images at the level of third ventricle (**c**) and vermis (**d**) reveal circumferential wall enhancement along the cortical vein (arrowhead in **c**) as well as patchy leptomeningeal and perivascular enhancement in the posterior fossa (**d**). Venous phase DSA image (**e**) from left ICA injection again reveals tortuous medullary veins

with an identifiable underlying etiology (sickle cell anemia, Down syndrome, atherosclerotic disease, etc.) [39]. MMD has a bimodal age presentation, the first in childhood (first decade) and the second in adults (fourth decade). Endothelial thickening, the main pathological finding, leads to chronic progressive arterial stenosis of the circle of Willis. Presentation with ischemic strokes are more common in the pediatric age group, while adults may present with ischemic or hemorrhagic strokes. In contrast to the Asian population however, presentation with hemorrhagic stroke is much lower in north American adults [39, 61]. The stenosis or occlusion of the terminal ICA is commonly bilateral although the involvement may be asymmetric or occasionally unilateral. Involvement of the proximal posterior cerebral arteries may be seen in up to 25% of patients with MMD [39]. These result in significant impairment of the cerebrovascular reserve

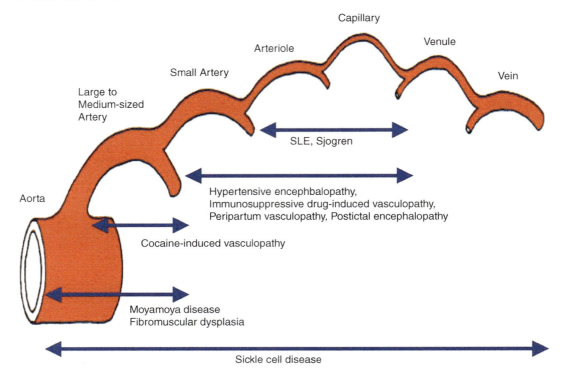

Fig. 11.15 Spectrum of CNS vasculopathy. (Modified from [59])

and compensatory development of tortuous collateral networks. Cerebral microbleeds may be seen in up to 46% of patients and are more common in those with hemorrhagic onset-type MMD [62]. DW imaging is useful in evaluating cerebral ischemia in Moyamoya disease (Fig. 11.16) [63]. Additional well-described imaging findings in MMD include "puff of smoke" sign on DSA and Ivy sign on FLAIR images.

11.6.2 Sickle Cell Disease (SCD)

Up to 25% if patients with SCD may develop neurological complications, often with evidence of territorial infarcts, silent ischemia, or hemorrhage on imaging [65]. The risk of stroke is greatest during thrombotic crises and during the first 15 years of life [66]. Vasculopathy is the hallmark of SCD and occurs secondary to non-inflammatory intimal hyperplasia. Both large and small vessels may be involved although terminal ICA and proximal ACA/MCA are typically affected. These result in increased ischemic susceptibility of the borderzone vascular distributions, resulting in more common and severe involvement. Additionally, infarcts may also occur secondary to thromboembolism [65, 67]. Approximately 75% of strokes are the result of an occlusion of the large arteries at the base of the brain. If progression is associated with neurologic dysfunction, strong consideration should be given to place the patient on a long-term transfusion program. DW imaging is useful in detecting active ischemic changes and in differentiating them from chronic ischemic changes (Fig. 11.17) [64].

11.7 Posterior Reversible Encephalopathy Syndrome

Posterior reversible encephalopathy syndrome (PRES) is a remarkably heterogeneous group of disorders, related to hypertensive encephalopathy, severe preeclampsia/eclamp-

Fig. 11.16 Probable Moyamoya disease in a 7-year-old girl with left hemiparesis. (**a**) T2-weighted an image shows lesions with mildly increased signal in the right basal ganglia and parieto-occipital cortex (*arrows*). (**b**) DW image clearly shows these lesions as high signal intensity, representing acute infarcts (*arrows*). (**c**) MR angiography shows occlusion of the right middle cerebral artery, and stenosis of the right internal carotid artery (*arrows*) and bilateral posterior cerebral arteries (*arrowheads*)

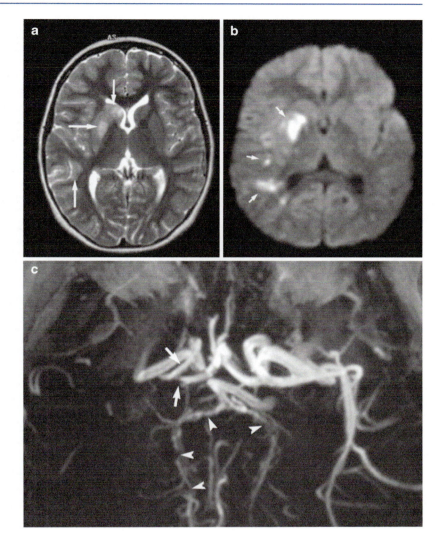

sia, immunosuppressive drug or interferon neurotoxicity, uremia, and thrombotic thrombocytopenic purpura [68]. Many synonyms of PRES have been reported includes reversible posterior leukoencephalopathy syndrome (RPLS), posterior leukoencephalopathy syndrome, or occipital parietal encephalopathy. However, PRES can also involve the frontal lobes, basal ganglia, brain stem, and cerebellum. In addition, the posterior reversible encephalopathy syndrome may not be entirely reversible as infarction and hemorrhage may develop.

The clinical symptoms are headache, altered mental status, seizures, and visual loss. The exact pathophysiology remains unclear, with some authors attributing changes to systemic hypertension, while others proposing widespread endothelial dysfunction from systemic conditions as the inciting event [69]. The pathophysiology is related to dysfunction of a cerebrovascular autoregulatory system. Generally, brain perfusion is maintained by the autoregulatory system of the small arteries and arterioles that have myogenic and neurogenic components. Since the vertebrobasilar system and the posterior cerebral arteries are sparsely innervated by sympathetic nerves, posterior brain regions are more susceptible to a breakthrough of the autoregulation in case of a sudden elevation of the systemic blood pressure.

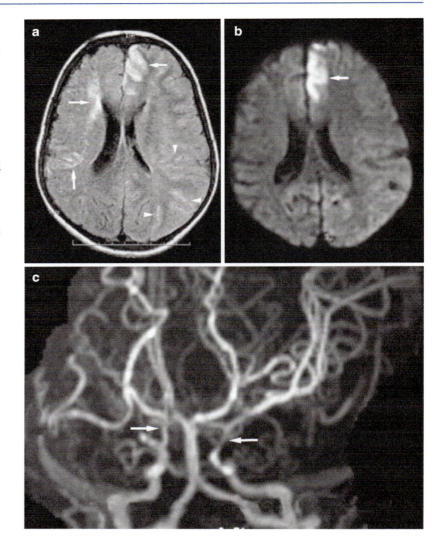

Fig. 11.17 Sickle cell disease. 3-year-old boy presented with right side weakness as a recurrent stroke. He has been non-compliant to transfusion therapy. (**a**) FLAIR image shows multiple hyperintense lesions in the left frontal and right frontotemporal regions (*arrows*). FLAIR image also shows multiple curvilinear hyperintensities along the peripheral vessels that probably reflects the slow flow in the collateral circulation (*arrow heads*). (**b**) DW image shows the left frontal lesion as very hyperintense representing an acute infarct (*arrow*). (**c**) MR angiography shows bilateral stenoses of internal carotid, and middle and anterior cerebral arteries (*arrows*). (From [64])

The primary cause of hypertensive encephalopathy is thought to be fluid extravasation through the interstitium, resulting from overdistension of distal small cerebral vessels (breakthrough of autoregulation) causing vasogenic edema. Ischemic processes can be triggered by the vasospasm of the cerebral arteriole in response to a severe increase in blood pressure (overregulation), which occasionally results in infarction. Hypertensive encephalopathy is a clinical syndrome in which morphological and clinical phenomena are not correlated to each other. However, plasma proteins and fibrin are deposited in the walls of small arteries (the so-called hypertensive vasculopathy). This process leads to destruction of smooth muscle cells (fibrinoid necrosis).

Any endothelial damages attenuate the myogenic response of the autoregulatory system. Endothelial dysfunction due to circulating endothelial toxins or antibodies against the endothelium has been suggested to be the primary cause of preeclampsia/eclampsia.

Regardless, the imaging manifestation are characterized predominantly by cortical and subcortical involvement predominantly in the occipital and parietal regions, followed by the frontal and inferior temporal lobe regions (Fig. 11.18). Involvement of the basal ganglia and brainstem is less common but may be seen. Some authors

11 Vasculopathy and Vasculitis

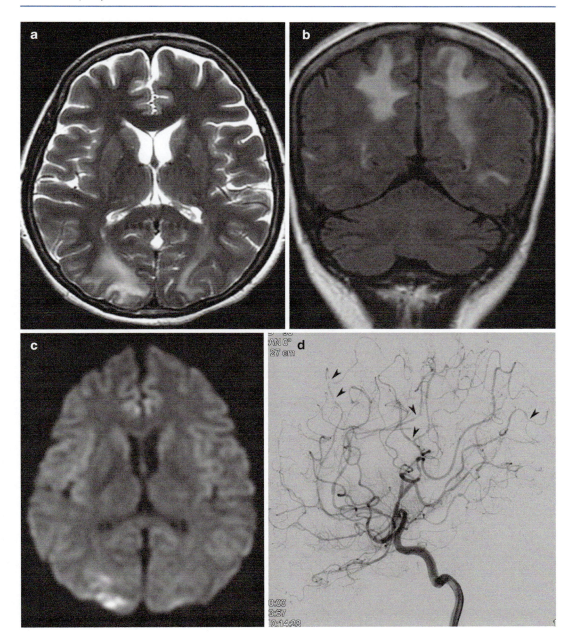

Fig. 11.18 PRES. 55-year-old man with hypertension. Axial T2WI (**a**) and coronal FLAIR (**b**) images reveal symmetrical areas of T2 prolongation involving the bilateral parieto-occipital regions. Axial DWI (**c**) shows a small focus of cytotoxic edema in the right occipital region. DSA (**d**) of the right ICA reveals multiple areas of vasoconstriction involving the distal ACA and MCA vessels (*arrowheads*)

have previously categorized the imaging manifestations into four patterns, each seen in about 20–30% of cases. The diagnostic and prognostic significance of these patterns however remains to be further defined. Intracranial hemorrhage and infarction may be seen in about 10–30% of cases. These tend to be more common in patients with preeclampsia/eclampsia (Fig. 11.19).

Hemorrhage is also more common in patients receiving anticoagulation or those post allogenic

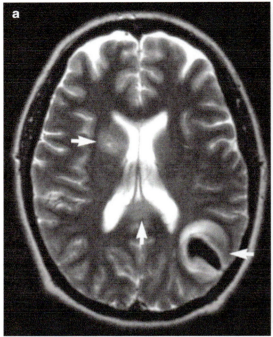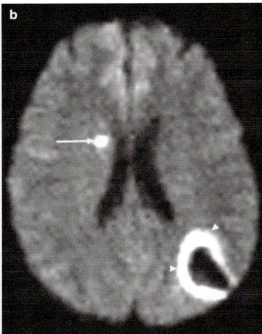

Fig. 11.19 Eclampsia in a 30-year-old woman with seizures. (**a**) T2-weighted image shows high signal intensity lesions in the right corona radiata, posterior corpus callosum, and left parieto-occipital region (*arrows*). The lesion in the left parieto-occipital region has a central, very low signal intensity, representing hemorrhage. (**b**) On DW image, a small infarct in the right corona radiata (*arrow*) and a hemorrhagic infarct in the left parieto-occipital region (*arrowheads*) are shown as hyperintense associated with decreased ADC (not shown). The lesion in the posterior corpus callosum represents vasogenic edema

marrow transplantation. Diffusion abnormalities in PRES tend to be punctate and interspersed with areas of vasogenic edema. Occasionally, patients may show gyral patterns of restricted diffusion and parenchymal atrophy on follow-up [31]. Angiographic findings reported in PRES include focal areas of vasoconstriction and dilatation as well as vessel pruning and reduced capillary blush [70].

Cyclosporine, tacrolimus (FK506), and interferon-α are effective immunosuppressive agents for the treatment of cerebral autoregulation. Neurotoxicity usually coexists with hypertensive crisis; however, it also occurs in normotensive individuals. These drugs have profound effects directly on the endothelium and cause release of potent vasoconstrictors such as endothelin. Disruption of the blood–brain barrier with possible focal loss of vascular autoregulation causes extravasation of fluid, which leads to vasogenic edema. MRI shows signal changes within the cortex and subcortical white matter in the occipital, posterior, temporal, parietal, and frontal lobes (Fig. 11.20). Non-transplant patients or those with total body irradiation develop white matter lesions, whereas those conditioned with chemotherapy develop mixed cortical and white matter lesions [71].

11.7.1 Reversible Cerebral Vasoconstriction Syndrome (RCVS)

RCVS refers to a clinical and radiological syndrome characterized by severe thunderclap headache and diffuse cerebral arterial vasoconstriction that typically resolves spontaneously within

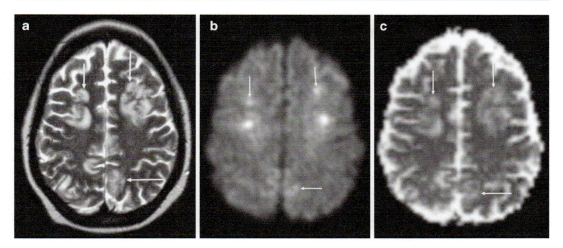

Fig. 11.20 Tacrolimus neurotoxicity in a 42-year-old woman with confusion after liver transplantation. (**a**) T2-weighted image shows high signal intensity lesions in the bilateral fronto-parieto-occipital subcortical white matter (*arrows*). (**b**) On DW image, these lesions show slightly hyperintense or isointense signal intensity (*arrows*). (**c**) ADC map shows increased ADC, which with hyperintense lesions (*arrows*) on DW image indicates T2 shine-through effect. These lesions had resolved on follow-up MR imaging (not shown)

3 months [72, 73]. Overall, RCVS is the second most common cause of thunderclap headache; the most common cause of isolated convexity subarachnoid hemorrhage in patients younger than 60 years as well as the commonest reason for recurrent severe secondary headaches [74].

RCVS is more common in women with peak incidence around 42 years (range 10–76). The exact incidence is unclear but is considered to be higher than initially reported. RCVS has been associated with multiple conditions, prominent among them being migraine, vasoactive agents (both therapeutic and recreational drugs), pregnancy/post-partum, catecholamine-secreting tumors, auto-immune diseases, and vascular abnormalities such as vascular dissections and aneurysms [72, 74]. PRES also demonstrates a significant overlap with RCVS, both in terms of disease associations and imaging findings. In fact, some authors believe that the two entities represent a continuum and share a common underlying pathophysiology.

On DSA, the vascular caliber abnormalities can affect the anterior and posterior circulation and are often bilateral and diffuse. These abnormalities may affect different vascular segments over time and may rarely involve extra-cranial vertebral and carotid vessels. Additionally, up to one-third of patients may have normal imaging at presentation and repeat imaging at approximately 2 weeks may help secure the diagnosis [72–74]. VWI imaging has shown promise in differentiation RCVS from vasculitis, with the former showing predominantly wall thickening with none or minimal post contrast enhancement [52, 72].

Complications of RCVS include convexity SAH which occurs in one-third of patients, parenchymal hemorrhage (6–20%), and ischemic complications which may occur in up to 40% of patients and often involve watershed distributions (Fig. 11.21) [74].

11.7.2 CADASIL and CARASIL

CADASIL stands for cerebral autosomal dominant arteriopathy with subcortical infarcts and leukoencephalopathy [75, 76]. Currently, CADASIL is considered the most common hereditary vascular dementia and occurs secondary to mutations of the NOTCH3 gene on chromosome 19. Common clinical manifestations include migraine with (20–40%) or without aura, TIA/ischemic strokes (85%), cognitive decline, and psychiatric manifestations [75, 77].

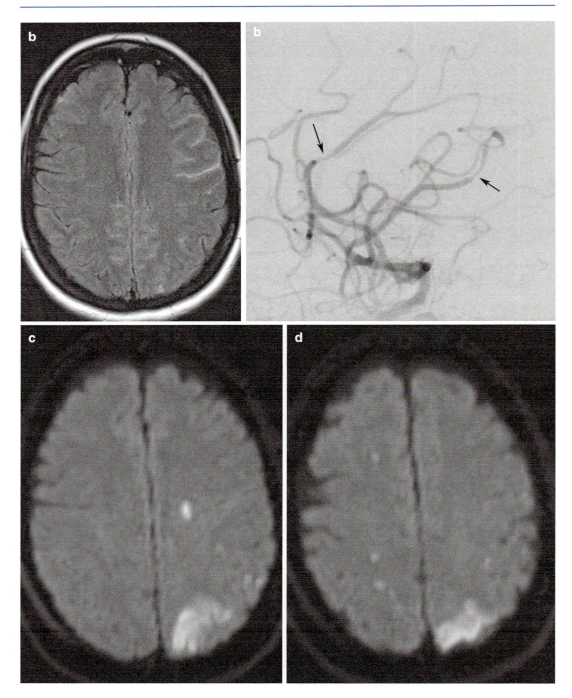

Fig. 11.21 RCVS. Axial FLAIR image (**a**) in a young patient who presented with thunderclap headache shows focal non-suppression of CSF over bilateral cerebral convexities (worse on left) corresponding to SAH on the NCCT (not shown). DSA (**b**) of ICA injection in the early arterial phase shows focal areas of luminal narrowing in the ACA (*long arrow*) and MCA (*short arrow*) distribution. Axial DWI images (**c, d**) obtained at day 6 show interval development of multiple acute infarcts in a watershed distribution, largest in the left parietal region

Abnormal MRI findings may be seen in virtually all patients by the age of 35 years. On imaging, foci of T2 prolongation involving the anterior temporal lobes and external capsule are common and considered virtually pathognomonic (Fig. 11.22). Patients often have patchy PVWM leukoaraiosis. The white matter lesions may be seen in the presymptomatic stage, even in patients younger than 20 years. Additionally, patients may show lacunar infarcts which are often subcortical may occasionally be multiple. Microhemorrhages may be seen in a third to one-half of patients and predominantly involve the cortex, subcortical WM, striatum, and brainstem. Larger intracerebral bleeds have also been reported [75–77]. A few studies have also shown underlying large vessel involvement, which is seen in up to one-fourth of patients and may be more common in the Asian population [76, 78].

CARASIL on the other hand is an autosomal recessive arteriopathy that is considerably rare. Important clinical differences from CADASIL include more severe memory dysfunction, earlier onset of strokes, premature diffuse baldness, and low back pain secondary to spondylosis. MRI findings of white matter changes and lacunar infarcts are often similar to CADASIL [75].

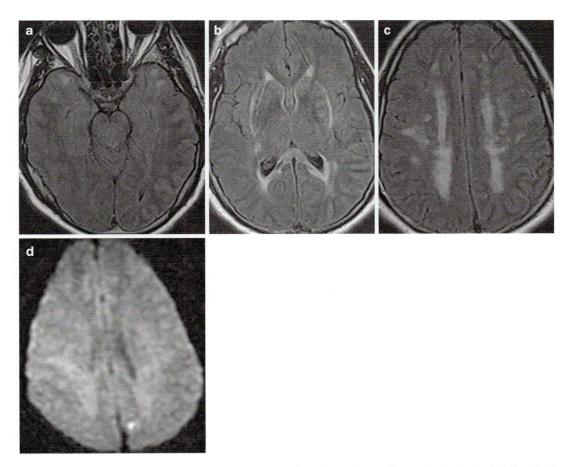

Fig. 11.22 CADASIL in a 34-year-old male with a history of complicated migraines. Axial FLAIR images (**a**–**c**) demonstrate multiple bilateral areas of T2 prolongation involving bilateral anterior temporal lobes (**a**), external capsules (**b**), and PVWM (**c**). Axial DWI obtained 1 year later shows a focus of lacunar infarction in the left parietal region (**d**). (Image courtesy of Dr. Suyash Mohan, Perelman school of Medicine, University of Pennsylvania, PA)

11.7.3 Susac Syndrome

Susac syndrome is a rare, presumably autoimmune disease which involves the smaller arterial vessels in the brain, retina, and inner ear. Clinically, the triad of encephalopathy, sensorineural hearing loss, and occlusion of the retinal artery branch are considered pathognomonic but is only seen in about 13% of the patients [79, 80]. Other common associated symptoms include headache, focal neurological deficits, tinnitus, and vertigo. Susac syndrome typically involves younger women between 20 and 40 years (range 7–70 years) and shows mild female predilection (F:M: 3:1) [79]. The basic histologic feature is microinfarctions. On imaging, the most characteristic feature is involvement of the corpus callosum and presence of brain infarctions (Fig. 11.23). The corpus callosal lesions are often described as central, small-to-large round white matter lesions ("snowballs") or linear lesions ("spokes"). Even though the involvement of corpus callosum is most common, the cortex, periventricular white matter, deep grey matter, cerebellum, and brainstem may also be involved. During the chronic phase, these lesions may appear as "punched out" holes on the T1WI. Multiple acute infarcts, again more frequently involving the corpus callosum, may also be seen. Similarly, DTI studies may show underlying widespread white matter injury. Both scattered parenchymal and leptomeningeal enhancement have been reported [79, 81, 82]. The disease may have a self-limited course, but patients usually have residual cognitive and visual/hearing disability.

11.7.4 Uremic Encephalopathy and Uremic Hemolytic Syndrome

Uremic encephalopathy is the name given to a brain syndrome that occurs in patients with renal failure. The pathogenesis is unknown, but it has been hypothesized that it may be caused by various toxins associated with uremia (elevated parathyroid hormone level, hypercalcemia, and other metabolic abnormalities) [83]. MR imaging usually shows reversible bilateral symmetric white matter lesions. The lesions predominantly involve the basal ganglia but may occasionally affect the cortex. Lesions are often T2 hyperintense and expansile (lentiform fork sign). These tend to be bilateral and often symmetrical. Occasionally, lesions may show true restricted diffusion (Fig. 11.24). Lesions often improve/resolve with hemodialysis [84].

Hemolytic uremic syndrome is defined as a multiorgan disease characterized by the triad of microangiopathic hemolytic anemia, thrombocytopenia, and uremia. CNS complications are commonly seen (20–50%) [85]. Hemolytic uremic syndrome caused by 0–157 *Escherichia coli* enterocolitis can potentially result in fatal CNS complications in infants and children. MR imaging sometimes shows irreversible lesions in the basal ganglia or cortex, representing infarction or cortical laminar necrosis. DW imaging can show these lesions as hyperintense with decreased ADC (Fig. 11.25). Imaging manifestations in adults on the other hand more frequently involves the pons and often does not show hemorrhage or contrast enhancement [86].

11.7.5 Thrombotic Thrombocytopenic Purpura

Thrombotic thrombocytopenic purpura is a multisystem vasculopathy characterized by microangiopathic hemolytic anemia, thrombocytopenia, renal involvement, fluctuating neurologic manifestations, and fever [87]. Neuropathology shows hyaline thrombosis and occlusion of capillaries and arterioles without surrounding inflammatory reaction, which results in infarcts and petechial hemorrhages. Positive MRI findings may be seen in up to 82% of patients, with changes of posterior reversible encephalopathy syndrome occurring in about half of these patients. Additional MRI findings may include multifocal gray matter edema, infarction, and hemorrhage [88]. DW imaging can differentiate between these lesions (Fig. 11.26), which is important since some of the lesions seen on T2-weighted images may disappear following treatment with plasma exchange [89].

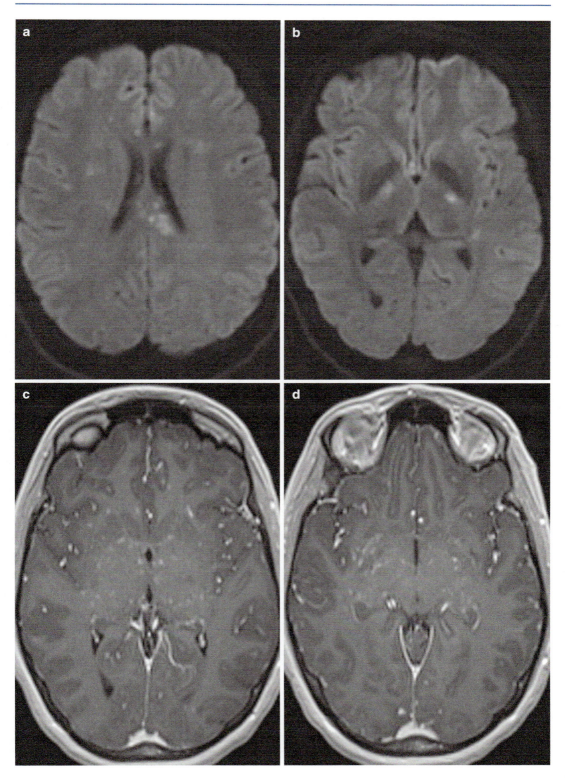

Fig. 11.23 Susac syndrome. Axial DWI images (**a**, **b**) reveal multiple acute infarcts involving the genu and splenium of corpus callosum, especially on the left side, as well as bilateral PVWM and PLIC. Axial post contrast images (**c**, **d**) reveal prominent bilateral perivascular enhancement and mild leptomeningeal enhancement

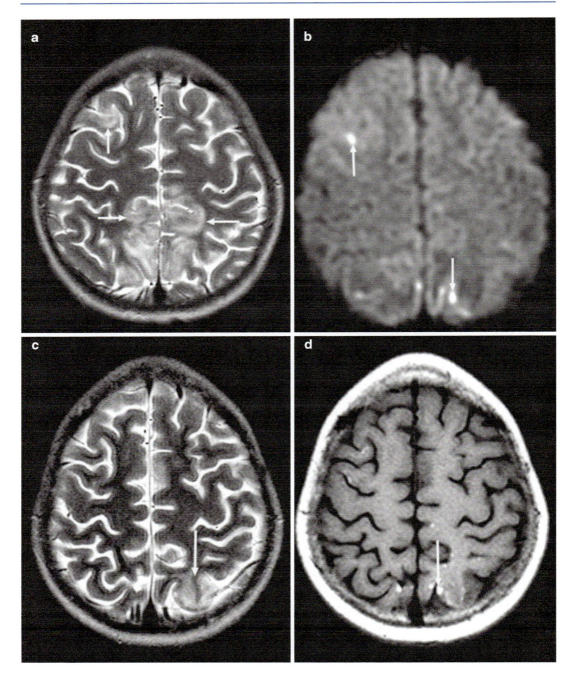

Fig. 11.24 Uremic encephalopathy in a 10-year-old girl with seizure. She improved after dialysis. (**a**) T2-weighted image shows hyperintense lesions in bilateral parietal and right frontal subcortical white matter and cortex (*arrows*). (**b**) DW image reveals punctate foci of high signal within T2 high signal area (*arrow*) in the right frontal lobe and an additional bright lesion in the left parietal lobe. (**c**) Follow-up T2-weighted image obtained 5 days later shows incomplete resolution of left parietal high signal area (*arrow*). (**d**) T1-weighted image reveals punctate foci of high signal corresponding to a high signal area on the initial DW image (*arrow*). (From [83])

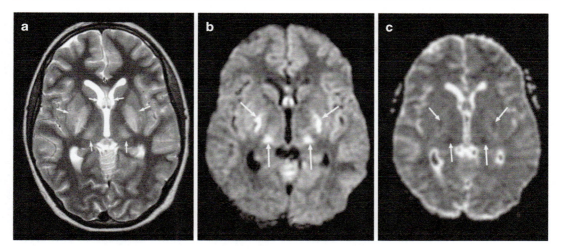

Fig. 11.25 Hemolytic uremic syndrome in a 12-year-old girl with bloody diarrhea. (**a**) T2-weighted image shows high signal intensity lesions in the bilateral basal ganglia, thalami, and fornices (*arrows*). (**b**) DW image shows these lesions as hyperintense (*arrows*). (**c**) ADC map shows these lesions as decreased ADC (*arrows*)

11.7.5.1 Cerebral Amyloid Angiopathy

Cerebral amyloid angiopathy is the most frequent cause of lobar ICH in the elderly and occurs secondary to deposition of beta-amyloid protein in the media and adventitia of small arteries and capillaries in the leptomeninges and cerebral cortex [90, 91]. Clinically, CAA is diagnosed using Boston criteria whose specificity varies between 88 and 92%. CAA is associated with Alzheimer disease (AD), and changes of CAA have been reported in nearly all AD patients, even though advanced CAA is only seen in about one-fourth of AD patients.

Even though hemorrhagic manifestations have traditionally been the focus of CAA, recent evidence from neuropathology as well as advanced and high-resolution imaging has expanded the spectrum of imaging findings in CAA to include micro-infarcts and white matter lesions (Fig. 11.27) [90–92]. In general, microhemorrhages are considered the hallmark of CAA and have been shown to most commonly involve the occipital lobe. In patients with multiple microhemorrhages, these tend to cluster in the same lobe. Other documented hemorrhagic manifestations include lobar hemorrhages and superficial siderosis. In general, the hemorrhagic manifestations are best seen on susceptibility weighted imaging and with higher strength magnets (Fig. 11.28) [91, 92].

With regard to the ischemic injury, most of these tend to be micro-infarcts and tend to be underrecognized on conventional thick scans on MRI studies performed at lower magnetic strength. However, the bright DW signal that may be seen with acute infarcts in the first 1–2 weeks can be appreciated. The reported frequency of micro-infarcts in pathologic studies varies between 37 and 100%, and these tend to localize to the cortical ribbon or the underlying subcortical white matter. These are seen in up to 15% of patients on the DWI images, which, based on mathematical modelling, translates to about eight new infarcts per year [91, 93]. Interestingly, the reported incidence in even higher with use of 7 T imaging and in ex vivo MRI studies of brain specimen. Not surprisingly, these do not correlate with known vascular risk factors but do seem to be associated with the burden of hemorrhagic lesions.

White matter hyperintensities are also considered part of the CAA spectrum and may show rapid increase over time in patients with advanced CAA. There is some evidence to suggest that these, at least partly, may reflect tiny infarcts

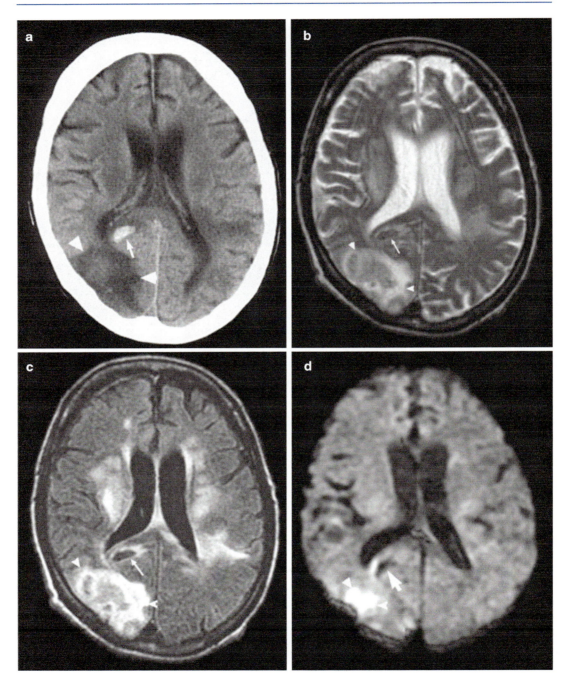

Fig. 11.26 Thrombotic thrombocytopenic purpura in a 53-year-old woman with altered mental status and seizures. (**a**) Computed tomography shows a hemorrhage in the right parieto-occipital area (*arrow*) and a wedged-shaped area of low density more peripherally in the right occipito-parietal area (*arrowheads*). (**b**) T2-weighted and (**c**) FLAIR images show corresponding hyperintense lesions in the deep white matter and right occipito-parietal area (*arrowheads*). Hemorrhage is seen as a hypointense lesion (*arrow*). (**d**) On DW image, deep white matter lesions are isointense, mainly representing vasogenic edema, while a cortical lesion in the right occipitoparietal area is hyperintense, representing acute infarction (*arrowheads*). Hemorrhage is hypointense with a hyperintense rim (*arrow*)

11 Vasculopathy and Vasculitis

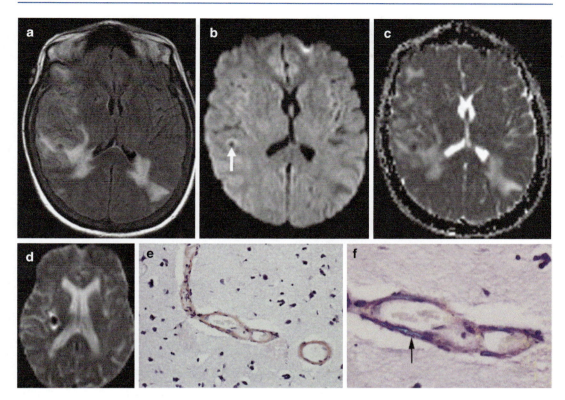

Fig. 11.27 Cerebral amyloid angiopathy with leukoencephalopathy in a 54-year-old woman (biopsy proven). (**a**) FLAIR image shows white matter hyperintensity in the right fronto-temporal and left temporo-occipital regions. A microhemorrhage is noted as a low signal spot in the right temporo-parietal white matter. (**b**, **c**) DW image shows the white matter lesions as isointense associated with increased ADC consistent with vasogenic edema (**d**). DW image also demonstrates the microbleed as a low signal spot (*arrow*). (**e**) Congo *red* stain shows β-amyloid deposits along the wall of the arteriole. (**f**) Congo *red* stain viewed with polarized light shows the classic yellow-green birefringence of the β-amyloid deposits (*arrow*)

which are beyond the resolution of imaging [90, 94]. Additional evidence supporting underlying vascular-related microscopic white matter injury in CAA comes from DTI-based studies which show that DTI abnormalities parallel the distribution of CAA pathology [90].

11.7.5.2 Amyloid Beta-Related Angiitis (ABRA)

ABRA refers to a rare form of angio-destructive, often granulomatous vasculitis triggered by immune response to Aβ protein. These cases are invariably associated with underlying CAA, with some authors proposing that ABRA likely represents a specific form of angiitis resulting from vascular deposition of Aβ in susceptible patients [13, 20]. The causative role of Aβ is also supported by the similar neuro-pathological findings in Aβ-immunization-related meningoencephalitis as well as Aβ-associated parenchymal inflammation.

Brain MRI is often positive (~98%), with bilateral white matter T2 hyperintense lesions being the most common. Associated cortical micro-hemorrhages (87%) and patchy enhancement (60%) may be seen (Fig. 11.29). About one-fourth of the patients may present with mass-like lesions which may show minimal or no enhancement [13]. White matter lesions often improve post therapy. Overall, presence of leptomeningeal enhancement and absence of lobar hemorrhages would favor ABRA over CAA [95]. In addition, patients with ABRA are often younger (mean age 67 years) when compared to those with non-inflammatory CAA (77 years).

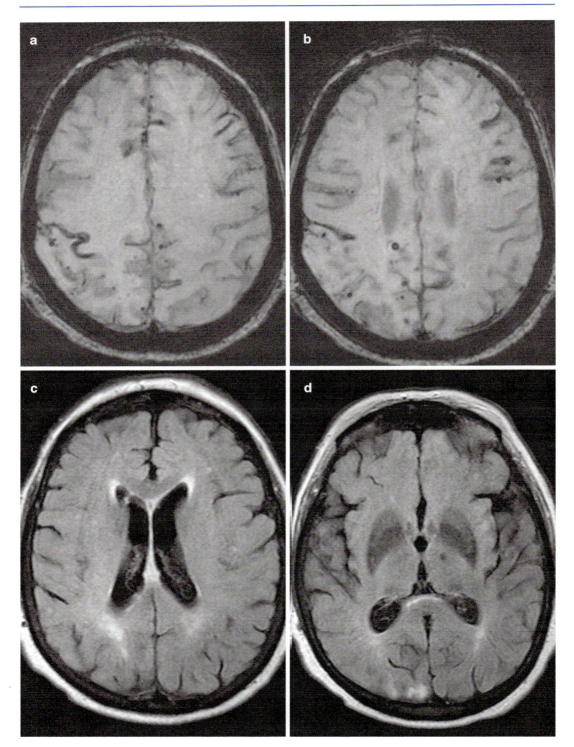

Fig. 11.28 Axial SWI images (**a**, **b**) show scattered microhemorrhages predominantly involving bilateral parietal lobes and left frontal lobe, as well as superficial siderosis along the right central sulcus and left frontal and parietal regions. Axial FLAIR images (**c**, **d**) reveal PVWM changes (**c**) and changes of old infarct in right occipital region (**d**)

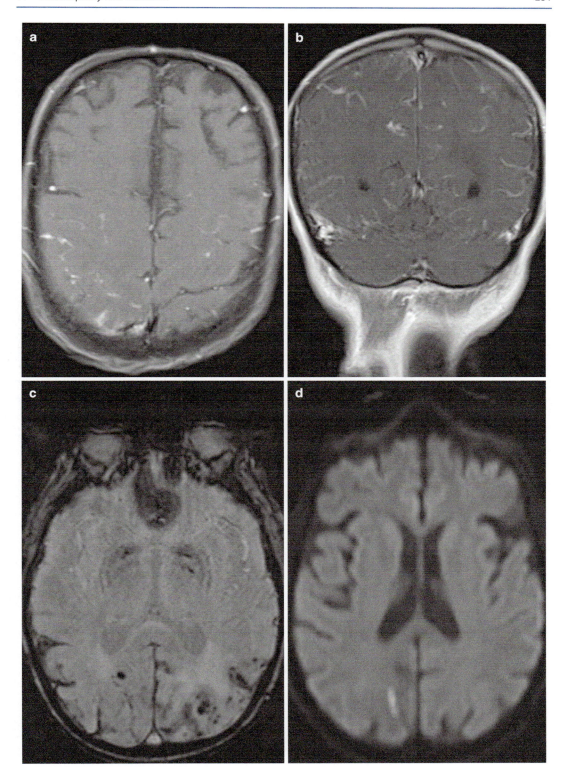

Fig. 11.29 Post contrast axial (**a**) and coronal (**b**) images in a patient with biopsy-proven ABRA demonstrate prominent leptomeningeal enhancement over bilateral cerebral convexities posteriorly. Axial SWI image (**c**) shows changes of superficial siderosis and scattered microhemorrhages in bilateral occipital lobes. Axial DWI image (**d**) at a slightly higher level shows an acute infarct in right parietal region

11.7.6 Hypereosinophilic Syndrome

Hypereosinophilia (HE) is characterized by an eosinophil count of more than 1500/μL on more than two occasions which are at least 4 weeks apart. Alternately, existence of tissue HE (defined as percentage of eosinophils in bone marrow >20%, pathological confirmation of extensive eosinophilic tissue infiltration or marked tissue deposition of eosinophilic granule proteins) also constitutes HE. A hypereosinophilic syndrome (HES) exists when there is peripheral blood HE along with evidence of organ damage/dysfunction attributable to tissue HE in the absence of alternate explanations [96]. On imaging, patients may have cerebrovascular manifestations, meningoencephalitis, demyelination, or leukoencephalopathy (Fig. 11.30). Cerebrovascular manifestations are most commonly seen (64%) and often present as multi-focal involvement/infarctions of bilateral internal border zone (45%). Additionally, patients may show non-borderzone infarctions, hemorrhage, and sinus thrombosis. The underlying etiology of infarctions remains unclear since the cardiac workup frequently does not show endomyocardial disease, and brain eosinophilic infiltration on pathological studies is rare in patients with infarctions [97]. However, parenchymal eosinophilic infiltration has been reported in some cases with meningoencephalitis [98]. CNS vasculitis in association with HES has also been reported. Interestingly, however, the authors noted prominent lymphocytic infiltration without eosinophils [99].

11.7.7 Radiation-Induced Vasculopathy

Larger cerebral vessels may develop stenotic and/or occlusive vasculopathy secondary to radiation. These usually occur over year or even decades after radiation therapy and are a well-recognized delayed complication (Fig. 11.31). MR imaging may show wall thickening and enhancement of the involved vessels [39, 100].

11.7.8 Miscellaneous Vasculopathies

Changes of vasculopathy may also be seen with various drugs (sulphonamides thiouracil, amphetamines, etc.), HIV vasculopathy, and neurofibromatosis type I, to name a few. HIV vasculopathy can involve both large- and medium-sized arteries, as well as veins, and may present with fusiform aneurysms, stroke secondary to embolic disease or with venous thrombosis [39]. Patients with NF-I most often have Moya-Moya syndrome (discussed above). Occasionally, these patients may present with vascular ectasias or stenosis (Fig. 11.32). Overall, vasculopathy has been reported in up to 18% of NF-I patients who undergo cerebral imaging [101].

11.8 Conclusion

Diffusion-weighted imaging is useful in patients with CNS vasculitis and vasculopathy to detect acute infarctions and to differentiate diseases that show cytotoxic edema from those with vasogenic edema. Overall, lesions demonstrating cytotoxic edema are usually irreversible and those with vasogenic edema are often reversible. Thus, DW imaging is an important tool to establish a prognosis and to determine the best treatment.

11.9 Treatment of CNS Vasculitis and Vasculopathy

Sadhana Murali and Mollie McDermott

11.9.1 Primary Angiitis of the Central Nervous System

Primary angiitis of the central nervous system (PACNS) can rapidly progress to neurological deterioration and death. Given this aggressive course, prompt diagnosis is important so that immediate treatment can be initiated. There are no randomized controlled trial (RCT) data to

11 Vasculopathy and Vasculitis

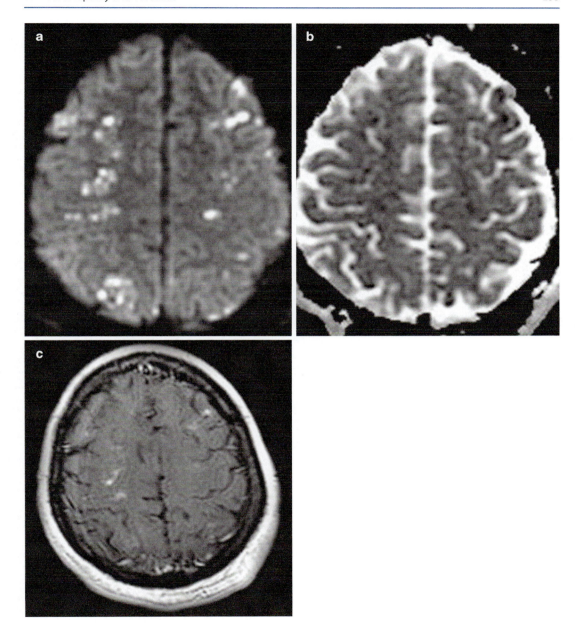

Fig. 11.30 Hypereosinophilic syndrome without evident cardiac abnormality. (**a**, **b**) DW image shows multiple hyperintense foci associated with the decreased ADC in bilateral watershed areas. (**c**) Postcontrast T1-weighted image shows multiple enhancing foci consistent with acute- to subacute-phase infarcts

guide treatment of PACNS. Given the rarity of the disease and the complexity surrounding diagnosis, high-level RCT data is unlikely to be forthcoming.

However, some observational data exist. One retrospective cohort study evaluated 163 patients who were diagnosed with PACNS between 1983 and 2011 at the Mayo Clinic, both in the inpatient and outpatient settings, based on either a positive brain biopsy or a conventional angiogram highly suggestive of vasculitis. This study found that patients had an improvement in their modified

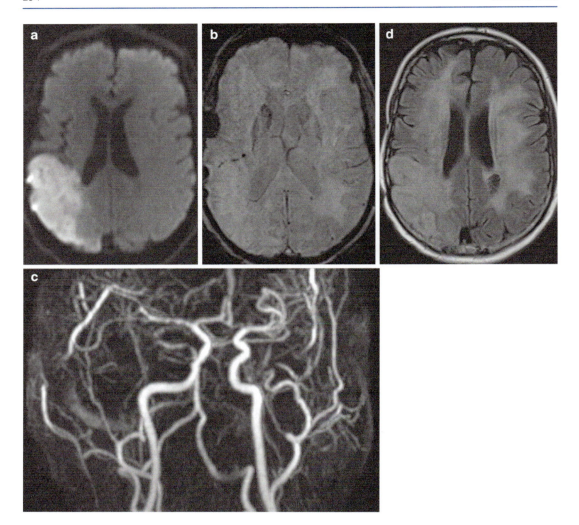

Fig. 11.31 Axial DWI image (**a**) reveals a large right MCA distribution infarct. Axial SWI image (**b**) shows linear focus of susceptibility over right temporal region which likely reflects an intravascular distal MCA thrombus. MIP image of the contrast enhanced MRA (**c**) reveals multiple areas of vascular stenosis involving the right M1 MCA and right PCA. Axial FLAIR image (**d**) reveals extensive areas of T2 prolongation involving bilateral PVWM, likely related to prior therapy. Chronic left posterior PVWM infarct is also noted. Patient had a prior history of metastatic lung cancer and had received whole brain radiation therapy

Rankin scale score after treatment with either prednisone alone or prednisone with cyclophosphamide [102]. In general practice, intravenous (IV) corticosteroids are started immediately after diagnosis followed by prednisone at a dose of 1 milligram (mg) per kilogram (kg) [103]. While no trials have evaluated steroid-sparing immunosuppressive agents, there are case reports of patients experiencing resolution of headache and focal neurological symptoms for up to 1–2 years after treatment with cyclophosphamide in conjunction to prednisone [103, 104]. Treatment with either cyclophosphamide and prednisone or prednisone alone generally continues until complete remission of symptoms has been achieved.

11 Vasculopathy and Vasculitis

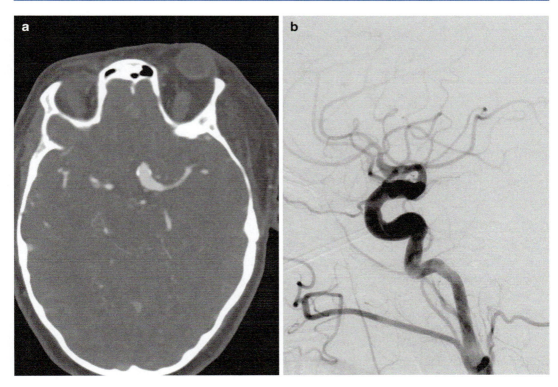

Fig. 11.32 Axial CTA image (in a patient with NF-I) at the level of circle of Willis (**a**) reveals ectatic left supraclionoid ICA. DSA of the left ICA injection (**b**) reconfirms the vascular ectasia that also extends into the proximal ACA

11.9.2 Giant Cell (Temporal) Arteritis

Urgent empiric treatment with steroids even prior to temporal artery biopsy is important when a diagnosis of giant cell arteritis (GCA) is suspected to prevent worsened vision loss. The British Society of Rheumatology (BSR) guidelines for the management of GCA recommend that 40–60 mg of prednisolone should be started in cases of uncomplicated GCA (no jaw claudication or visual disturbance). In cases of evolving vision loss or amaurosis fugax, the guidelines recommend that IV methylprednisolone should be initiated for 3 days followed by transition to oral steroids (prednisone or dexamethasone). In patients with established vision loss, 60 mg of prednisolone should be started to prevent contralateral eye involvement. Treatment should be continued for at least 3–4 weeks based on clinical response and inflammatory marker trend [105].

11.9.3 Takayasu Arteritis (Aortitis Syndrome)

In Takayasu arteritis (TA), aggressive control of vessel inflammation is pursued to prevent systemic complications such as ischemic and hemorrhagic stroke. Initial treatment generally consists of high-dose steroids based on observational data from case series [106]. As in PACNS, no RCT-level data exist to guide treatment. One observational study of 48 patients with TA found that patients with ischemic events used antiplatelet agents such as aspirin less frequently than patients without ischemic events [107]. Steroid-sparing agents such as cyclophosphamide, methotrexate, azathioprine, and mycophenolate are often used when steroids alone are insufficient. Surgical options include carotid artery bypass grafts, stent placement, and angioplasty [108]; however, evidence regarding the risks and benefits of surgery is based only on observational data and case reports at this time [109]. Guidelines generally recommend that surgical interventions should not be performed during the active phase of the disease.

11.9.4 Polyarteritis Nodosa and Churg-Strauss Disease

Treatment of polyarteritis nodosa (PAN) consists of steroids alone or in combination with cyclophosphamide for at least 12 months. In cases of PAN associated with hepatitis, antivirals are often added [42]. Pulse-dose cyclophosphamide is often used rather than oral cyclophosphamide, given increased toxicities associated with oral cyclophosphamide regimens, including neutropenia, hemorrhagic cystitis, and alopecia [110].

In Churg-Strauss Disease (CSD), pulse-dose steroids are the initial treatment of choice [111]. Steroids are continued for 1–3 days followed by transition to daily prednisone until clinical remission has been achieved. While data on steroid-sparing agents in CSD is limited, cyclophosphamide may be considered in progressive disease. One RCT found that adding plasmapheresis to a regimen of steroids and cyclophosphamide did not change outcomes in patients with PAN or CSD [112].

11.9.5 Henoch-Schonlein Purpura

Treatment for patients with Henoch-Schonlein purpura (HSP) is often symptomatic and targeted toward relief of pain and fever. One systematic review of relevant RCTs was inconclusive regarding the benefit of steroids, cyclophosphamide, and other immunosuppressants on non-neurological symptoms associated with HSP [112]. One case report describes a 46-year-old patient with HSP who developed sudden-onset right-sided weakness and showed clinical improvement in hemiparesis after 1 month of treatment with pulse cyclophospha-

mide and methylprednisolone [113]. Another case report describes a 12-year-old boy who developed symptoms consistent with HSP and subsequently developed cerebral vasculitis and seizures. His clinical symptoms resolved soon after initiation of treatment with oral steroids [114]. While there are case reports that describe improvement in neurologic symptoms in patients with stroke and HSP who receive treatment with steroids and cyclophosphamide, the data are overall inconclusive.

11.9.6 Microscopic Polyangiitis

Similarly, while there are case reports of treatment of microscopic polyangiitis (MPA)-related cerebral vasculitis, no controlled trial results are available. One case report describes a 12-year-old girl diagnosed with MPA and found to have multiple intraparenchymal hematomas thought to be sequelae of small-vessel cerebral vasculitis. She was treated with IV steroids, pulse cyclophosphamide, and maintenance azathioprine and eventually had both clinical remission as well as improvement of her myeloperoxidase antineutrophil cytoplasmic antibody levels [115].

11.9.7 Cryoglobulinemia

Evidence regarding the treatment of the CNS manifestations of cryoglobulinemia is limited to case reports as well. One case report describes a 61-year-old woman with hepatitis C and mixed cryoglobulinemia who was diagnosed with cerebral vasculitis based on imaging studies. She was treated with methylprednisolone and cyclophosphamide and had improvement in both her clinical symptoms and laboratory studies [116]. For non-neurological symptoms related to cryoglobulinemia, one RCT compared rituximab to steroids, azathioprine, cyclophosphamide, or plasmapheresis and found that rituximab was as effective as and even superior to other treatments in terms of clinical improvement [117].

11.9.8 Hypersensitivity (Leukocytoclastic) Vasculitis

A few case reports describe the treatment of hypersensitivity vasculitis with steroids. One case report describes a 70-year-old male who presented with rapidly progressive dementia over 2 weeks and was diagnosed with leukocytoclastic vasculitis by brain biopsy. He was treated with a course of oral prednisolone and had no further decline in cognition over a 6-month period after treatment [118]. Overall, the prognosis for hypersensitivity vasculitis has been reported to be good in terms of non-neurological symptoms, even without treatment. A retrospective study of 95 patients with non-neurologic manifestations of hypersensitivity vasculitis found that 54 patients did not require treatment, 26 patients were treated with non-steroidal anti-inflammatory drugs (NSAIDs), and 14 patients were treated with corticosteroids. All but two patients had complete recovery [119]. As with many rare diseases, data regarding the prognosis of patients with CNS involvement are limited.

11.9.9 Behcet's Disease

11.9.9.1 General Management

Neuro-Behcet's disease is further divided into parenchymal involvement and non-parenchymal involvement, the latter of which includes cerebral venous sinus thrombosis (CVST) and arterial stenosis. A patient's CSF profile may correlate with the clinical course of neuro-Behcet's disease. A retrospective analysis evaluated 200 patients with a diagnosis of Behcet's disease who developed neurological symptoms with either parenchymal or non-parenchymal involvement based on imaging elevated CSF protein level, and CSF pleocytosis were associated with a worse prognosis over a 3-year period [120].

11.9.9.2 Corticosteroids

One case series of eight patients noted a significant pleocytosis in patients with neuro-Behcet's compared to control patients without disease. An improvement in the pleocytosis was observed after treatment with oral corticosteroids; this improvement in CSF pleocyotsis is also correlated with clinical improvement [121].

For CSVT associated with neuro-Behcet, there are case series and case reports that describe clinical and radiographic improvement after treatment with anticoagulation and steroids [122, 123]. In one case series of 25 patients, 19 received both therapeutic heparin and oral prednisone, three patients received steroids alone, and three patients received heparin alone. Two of the patients did not receive treatment initially due to delayed diagnosis and experienced relapse of symptoms, while none of the patients who received treatment demonstrated relapse [122]. Per the 2018 update of the European League Against Rheumatism (EULAR) guidelines for the management of neuro-Behcet's disease, it is recommended that the first episode of cerebral venous thrombosis should be treated with high-dose glucocorticoids followed by tapering. Anticoagulation may be added for a short duration [124].

In terms of the treatment for arterial involvement, specific treatment is not well studied. It has been suggested that this entity may respond to corticosteroids and an immunosuppressant such as azathioprine [125]. Data regarding surgical management of neuro-Behcet's are limited.

11.9.10 Scleroderma

While the treatment for non-neurological manifestations of scleroderma is better studied, the treatment for the CNS manifestations is less well understood. For the non-neurological symptoms, EULAR guidelines recommend that calcium channel blockers such as nifedipine as well as steroid-sparing immunosuppression should be considered [126]. One case report describes a 45-year-old woman with a diagnosis of CREST syndrome who presented with several days of headaches and was found to have a subarachnoid hemorrhage. Conventional angiography was performed and was notable for numerous areas of stenosis concerning for secondary CNS vasculitis. She was initially treated with IV methylprednisolone but was transitioned to cyclophosphamide due to side effects with steroids. The patient did have clinical improvement while on cyclophosphamide, but she had recurrence of symptoms when the cyclophosphamide was held secondary to side effects, suggestive of an overall benefit while on cyclophosphamide [127].

11.9.11 Rheumatoid Arthritis

CNS vasculitis is a rare entity in rheumatoid arthritis (RA) that is thought to be related to systemic inflammation. Given the rarity of the condition, only case reports exist regarding potential management. One case report describes a 52-year-old woman with a 20-year history of seropositive RA who developed new-onset headache, right-sided visual field defects, and ataxia. Imaging was notable for multifocal infarcts, and cerebral vasculitis was eventually diagnosed in the setting of beading and stenoses found on conventional angiography. She was started on pulse-dose IV cyclophosphamide which was transitioned to azathioprine as well as IV methylprednisolone which was transitioned to oral prednisolone. She did not have any further neurological events after being started on immunosuppression though her presenting deficits continued to persist without improvement [128]. Two case reports note a clinical improvement in RA-associated cerebral vasculitis with glucocorticoids and cyclophosphamide [129]. One case report notes a clinical improvement with high-dose glucocorticoids and another case report notes improvement with the combination of high-dose glucocorticoids [130, 131]. Several case reports note improvement with methotrexate therapy [56, 132].

11.9.12 Infectious Vasculitides

In general, bacterial and fungal vasculitides should be treated with the appropriate antimicro-bial agent [133]. The role of steroids in conjunction with antimicrobial treatment is not well studied.

11.9.12.1 Viral-Related Vasculitides

Cytomegalovirus (CMV) and human immunodeficiency virus (HIV) cause the only virus-related vasculitides with specific treatments available. Evidence for HIV vasculopathy is mainly based on case reports; however, it is recommended by the Infectious Diseases Society of America (IDSA) that HAART treatment should be initiated if all other potential causes of vasculitis such as coinfection have been ruled out [133]. One case report describes a patient with brain biopsy-proven HIV vasculopathy who was treated with HAART after infectious causes had been ruled out and showed clinical improvement of neurological symptoms over a 9-week period [134]. Another case report describes a patient with HIV and left MCA territory infarcts found to have multiple areas of intra- and extracranial stenosis that were noted to radiographically improve after a course of treatment with steroids [135].

In VZV-related vasculopathy, patients should be treated with IV acyclovir for 14 days [133]. The role of steroids and other immunosuppressant medications is uncertain. One case series assessed the treatment and outcomes of 30 patients with VZV vasculopathy. Fifteen patients were treated with IV acyclovir for 10–28 days without steroids. Nine of the patients improved immediately, one patient clinically stabilized, two patients died, and three patients worsened until steroids were initiated and then showed clinical improvement. 12 patients were treated with both IV acyclovir and prednisone or prednisolone, of which 8 had a clinical improvement, 1 remained stable, and 3 worsened [136]. Recommended treatment for CMV-related cerebral vasculitis consists of ganciclovir and foscarnet [133].

11.9.12.2 Bacterial-Related Vasculitides

In tuberculous cerebral vasculitis, patients are generally treated with a 2-month course of a four-drug regimen (rifampicin, isoniazid, pyrazinamide, and ethambutol) [133] though the evidence for the efficacy of this treatment is derived from case series [137]. The role of corticosteroids is not clear based on these case series as some patients receiving corticosteroids in conjunction with four-drug treatment improved whereas others did not [137].

Neuroborreliosis is rarely associated with cerebral vasculitis. The recommended treatment consists of IV ceftriaxone for 4 weeks. Oral doxycycline may be a reasonable alternative [133]. Case reports describe both clinical and CSF profile improvement in neuroborreliosis with vasculitis after treatment with IV ceftriaxone [138]. A retrospective study of 11 patients with this diagnosis found that a 2- to 3-week course of IV ceftriaxone led to a complete recovery in 3 of the 11 patients and an incomplete recovery in one of the patients. The remaining patients had recurrent basilar artery thrombosis, systemic thrombosis, sinus thrombosis, or meningoencephalitis [139]. Another retrospective study of 115 patients diagnosed with neuroborreliosis-related CNS symptoms, including vasculitis, evaluated the efficacy of doxycycline. All patients had a clinical improvement after treatment on doxycycline and a decrease in CSF mononuclear cell counts was observed [140].

Suggested treatment for neurosyphilis-related cerebral vasculitis consists of a 2-week course of IV penicillin or alternatively a 2-week course of IV ceftriaxone for patients with an allergy to penicillin [133]. One case report describes clinical improvement on a combination of penicillin and corticosteroids [141]. However, there are also case reports of clinical improvement on penicillin treatment alone without concurrent corticosteroid treatment, so the role of corticosteroids in disease recovery is not known [142, 143].

11.9.12.3 Fungal-Related Vasculitides

Fungal infections such as candidiasis, histoplasmosis, cryptococcosis, and aspergillosis causing vasculitis should be treated with the appropriate anti-fungal agent. Aspergillosis is treated with a course of amphotericin B followed by a voriconazole or itraconazole. Cryptococcosis and candidiasis are treated with amphotericin B and flucytosine. Histoplasmosis is treated with amphotericin B and itraconazole [133]. These regimens are not specifically well-studied in cerebral vasculitis, so recommendations are extrapolated from general treatment guidelines and case reports.

Rare case reports describe patients with candidiasis infection and brain biopsy-proven vasculitis; however, the effect of treatment on the patients' recovery is not clear in these reports [144, 145]. Several case reports describe clinical improvement of cerebral vasculitis related to histoplasmosis after initial treatment with amphotericin later transitioned to voriconazole and then itraconazole [146]. For cerebral vasculitis related to aspergillus, one case report describes a patient who was started on amphotericin B after a delayed diagnosis of aspergillosis vasculitis was confirmed. The patient continued to have progression of neurological symptoms despite being transitioned to IV caspofungin and eventually died [147]. Similarly, there are case reports of patients with a delayed diagnosis of cryptococcus infection-related cerebral vasculitis who were started on amphotericin B and flucytosine, but despite treatment continued to have clinical worsening and died [148, 149]. However, other case reports describe clinical improvement on amphotericin B and flucytosine [150]. Given the limited number of such reports and the general acuity of such patients, it is not clear if cases of clinical deterioration are secondary to treatment failure versus the underlying illness itself.

11.9.13 Drug-Induced Vasculitis/ Vasculopathy, Including Illicit Drugs

Both chemotherapy agents and illicit drugs can lead to ischemic and hemorrhagic infarcts through a variety of mechanisms. Cocaine, methamphetamine, and heroin have been associated with stroke. Treatment includes abstention from illicit drug use and counseling. In chemotherapy-associated vasculopathy, the offending chemotherapeutic agent must often be stopped and replaced with an alternative agent.

11.10 Vasculopathy

11.10.1 Systemic Lupus Erythematosus

There are several mechanisms by which systemic lupus erythematosus (SLE) can lead to ischemic strokes, including vasculitis/vasculopathy, Libman-Sacks endocarditis, or a hypercoagulable state in the setting of antiphospholipid antibody syndrome. Given that SLE-related vasculitis is relatively uncommon, the EULAR guidelines recommend that a typical workup for stroke risk factors be pursued and managed with the appropriate secondary prevention. In cases where antiphospholipid antibody syndrome is diagnosed, antiplatelet versus anticoagulation therapy should be considered. However, if SLE-related cerebrovascular disease is thought to be due to vasculitis or vasculopathy from an underlying inflammatory state, glucocorticoids or other immunosuppressants should be initiated [151]. Many studies of SLE patients with neurologic manifestations group stroke with other entities such as seizures, headaches, cognitive symptoms, and polyneuropathy, which obscures the effect of treatment on stroke specifically [152–154].

11.10.2 Moyamoya Disease

11.10.2.1 Antiplatelets

Currently, there is no treatment for the underlying pathology that leads to Moyamoya disease. Initial management is focused on secondary prevention and can include antiplatelet therapy and typical stroke risk factor modification, though the effect of either on Moyamoya disease specifically is not well studied. One non-randomized prospective study evaluated the effects of antiplatelet therapy on stroke recurrence rate and found no difference in ischemic stroke recurrence in patients who received antiplatelet therapy versus those who did not. A significant decrease in the rate of cerebral hemorrhage was observed in patients not treated with antiplatelets [155].

11.10.2.2 Calcium Channel Blockers

There are case reports of patients demonstrating clinical improvement with calcium channel blockers such as nimodipine [156], verapamil [157], and nifedipine [158]. Acute management may consist of aggressive hydration and treatment of hypotension [159], administration of supplemental oxygen [160], and measures to avoid hypo and hypercapnia [159]; however, support for these treatments is derived primarily from observational data.

11.10.2.3 Revascularization Surgery

In patients with progressive disease, surgical intervention may be considered. Surgical interventions consist of both direct and indirect revascularization. Direct revascularization involves the creation of a superficial temporal artery bypass to the middle cerebral artery (MCA) or the middle meningeal artery. Indirect revascularization consists of placing a scalp artery directly over the surface of the brain to promote regional collateralization. However, the data to support surgery is limited. One prospective study of patients who underwent surgery versus patients who did not found that patients who underwent revascularization had a significant decrease in recurrence of ischemic strokes, but no difference in hemorrhage stroke recurrence [155]. One retrospective study that evaluated 29 children with Moyamoya disease specifically found that clinical symptoms resolved in 74% of patients and markedly decreased in 14% of patients who underwent indirect revascularization surgery [161]. Patients who had good collateral formation were more likely to improve than patients who had insufficient collateral formation [161]. Another retrospective study of 60 adult patients who underwent combined (indirect and direct revascularization) found that clinical status improved for 6 months after surgery and revascularization improved on imaging repeated several years after surgery [162].

11.10.3 Sickle Cell Disease

11.10.3.1 Transcranial Doppler Screening

For primary prevention of stroke related to sickle cell disease (SCD), guidelines strongly recommend that children be screened annually with transcranial dopplers starting at 2 years of age [163]. One cohort study followed 315 children with SCD and no prior history of stroke. In these children, the highest MCA/ICA velocity (Vmax) was an independent predictor of future risk of stroke, especially velocities >200 cm/s [164].

11.10.3.2 Exchange Transfusions

Stroke related to SCD is often acutely managed with serial exchange transfusions. The frequency of transfusions is dependent on the complete blood cell count and quantitative measurement of fetal hemoglobin. One observational study found that children with SCD and stroke who received transfusions for a target Hgb S level of <30% had a significant decrease in the risk of stroke recurrence compared to those who did not receive any transfusion [165, 166]. The American Heart Association/American Stroke Association recommends that patients with sickle cell disease and a prior history of ischemic stroke or TIA undergo chronic blood transfusions to reduce hemoglobin S levels to <30% of the total hemoglobin level (Class I, Level of Evidence B) [167].

11.10.3.3 Hydroxyurea

Daily hydroxyurea is often recommended in addition to or in place of exchange transfusions, depending on disease severity [163]. A case series of five patients between the ages of 3 and 16 years with recent stroke or TIA who were started on hydroxyurea at a dose of 30–40 mg/kg day found no recurrent stroke after 42–112 months of follow-up [168].

11.10.4 Neurosarcoidosis

11.10.4.1 General

The management outlined below is primarily for neurosarcoidosis without vasculitis given that neurosarcoidosis-related vasculitis is a rare entity in an already rare disorder. There are several case reports that describe neurosarcoidosis-related vasculopathies with various attempted treatments [169, 170]. One case report describes a patient with a moymoya-like vasculopathy in the setting of neurosarcoidosis who was successfully treated with methylprednisolone and ventriculoperitoneal shunting for hydrocephalus [171]. However, as it is difficult to generalize treatment for neurosarcoidosis-related vasculopathy based on these case reports, the rest of the section below will describe the treatment for neurosarcoidosis in general.

11.10.4.2 Immunosuppression

Corticosteroids are considered to be first-line treatment for active neurosarcoidosis. Prednisone is usually dosed at 0.5–1 mg/kg day for 2 weeks or longer depending on clinical status. In cases of severe neurological symptoms, IV methylprednisolone should be considered for the first 1–3 days of treatment [172]. In patients who are refractory to corticosteroids, other steroid-sparing agents such as infliximab, methotrexate, azathioprine, cyclosporine, leflunomide, and cyclophosphamide can be considered.

One retrospective study included 206 patients with neurosarcoidosis treated with a variety of immunosuppressants. Patients in this study had been diagnosed with neurosarcoidosis based on neurological symptoms in the presence of systemic sarcoid involvement or had brain biopsy-proven neurosarcoidosis. Patients who were treated with corticosteroid doses <10 mg/day often had relapse of symptoms. Methotrexate was used in three of the patients, but only one patient had a good clinical response. Other patients were treated with corticosteroids, azathioprine, or cyclosporine with variable clinical responses. This study did not find one particular treatment to be specifically correlated with clinical improvement [173]. There are several case reports of patients with refractory neurosarcoidosis having a good clinical response to infliximab [174, 175]. There is one case report of refractory neurosarcoidosis successfully treated with rituximab [176]. One case series describes the use of chloroquine or hydroxycholoroquine as monotherapy or in conjunction to corticosteroids with variable results [177].

11.10.4.3 Radiation Therapy

There are only case reports of radiation therapy being used for patients with neurosarcoidosis who are refractory to steroids and other immunosuppressant agents. In the retrospective study described above, three patients were treated with radiation therapy. Only one patient had a clinical response to treatment and had received a higher dose and longer duration of radiation treatment [173]. There are also several case reports of neurosarcoidosis refractory to steroids and immunosuppressants subsequently treated with radiation therapy with clinical remission [178, 179].

11.10.4.4 Surgical Intervention

While neurosarcoid-related cerebral vasculitis is associated with ischemic lesions, neurosarcoidosis itself can be associated with inflammatory mass lesions. In these clinical situations, resection could be considered if mass lesions persist despite medical management as stated above. Ventricular drains or shunts can be considered in the setting of acute hydrocephalus related to neurosarcoidosis [180]. Finally, there is one case report of neurosarcoidosis-related large vessel vasculitis of the M1 segment of the MCA being treated with balloon angioplasty. The patient in this report had immediate improvement of his left MCA syndrome and at 5-month follow-up had a marked clinical improvement [181]. However, given that these interventions have not been well studied with controlled trials, there is insufficient data to confidently recommend such interventions to patients.

11.10.5 Posterior Reversible Encephalopathy Syndrome/ Hypertensive Encephalopathy

11.10.5.1 General Management

Given that there are many different causes for posterior reversible encephalopathy syndrome (PRES), the management should focus on treating the underlying etiology or removing potential offending triggers or medications. Often, the clinical and radiographic findings of PRES are fully reversed within weeks after blood pressure control has been achieved and offending agents have been removed.

11.10.5.2 Blood Pressure Management

Blood pressure goals are not well established; however, in general, with cases of hypertensive emergency, it is recommended that mean arterial pressures not be acutely dropped by more than 25% per hour to avoid cerebral ischemia and other end-organ damage [182].

11.10.6 Reversible Cerebral Vasoconstriction Syndrome (RCVS)

11.10.6.1 General Management

There are theories that RCVS may be along a spectrum of disorders that also includes PRES and preeclampsia/eclampsia with similar pathophysiology. Similar to PRES, there are many potential triggers including medications, pregnancy [183, 184], chemotherapy, illicit drugs [185], and malignancy. Potential medication triggers include ergots [186], triptans [187], selective serotonin reuptake inhibitors (SSRIs) [188], serotonin norepinephrine reuptake inhibitors (SNRIs), chemotherapy agents such as tacrolimus [189] and cyclophosphamide [190], indomethacin [191], and various cough suppressants [192]. General management includes a thorough evaluation for potential triggers and removing potential offending agents and medications. There are case reports of patients improving after removal of offending agents without any other additional treatment [188].

11.10.6.2 Immunosuppressants

There are no guidelines for the treatment of RCVS, and the role of immunosuppressants is not well understood. One single-center, retrospective study of 162 patients with RCVS evaluated potential factors predicting clinical and radiologic prognosis and found that glucocorticoid use was independently associated with clinical worsening defined as an mRS 4–5 or death [193].

11.10.6.3 Calcium Channel Blockers

The usage of calcium channel blockers in patients with RCVS is not well studied. One retrospective study of nine patients with RCVS, PACNS, and moyamoya treated with intra-arterial nimodipine found that only the patients with RCVS had radiologic improvement of vasoconstriction, while the patients with PACNS or moyamoya did not have improvement [194]. One case report describes a patient diagnosed with RCVS who was treated with an IV nimodipine infusion and later transitioned to oral nifedipine who had both radiographic and clinical improvement of symptoms within several weeks of treatment being initiated [195]. However, several prospective trials found that treatment with nimodipine did not lead to early improvement of cerebral vasoconstriction [196, 197].

11.10.7 Preeclampsia/Eclampsia

11.10.7.1 General Management and Monitoring

The American College of Obstetricians and Gynecologists task force recommends serial assessments of maternal and fetal symptoms, serial measurements of blood pressure twice weekly, and assessments of platelets and liver enzymes weekly in patients with symptoms of preeclampsia or eclampsia [198]. In patients with severe preeclampsia, maternal stabilization and delivery are recommended if the patient is at ≥34 weeks of gestation. In patients with preeclampsia without severe features, delivery is recommended when the patient is ≥37 weeks of gestation [198, 199].

11.10.7.2 Blood Pressure Management

The ACOG task force recommends that in patients with blood pressures above 160/110, antihypertensives can be considered [198]. One retrospective study of 28 patients with preeclampsia and stroke found an association between systolic blood pressures between 155 and 160 and stroke, but did not find an association between the diastolic pressure and stroke [200].

11.10.7.3 Antiplatelets

Low-dose aspirin (60–80 mg) for primary prevention of preeclampsia was evaluated in a meta-analysis of 30,822 patients that found that patients receiving aspirin had a lower risk of developing preeclampsia compared to patients who did not receive aspirin [201]. The American College of Obstetricians and Gynecologists task force recommends that women who have a history of prior pregnancies complicated by preeclampsia should be started on daily low-dose aspirin starting in the late first trimester [198]. The US Preventive Services Task Force recommends that pregnant women who are at high risk for preeclampsia should be prescribed aspirin 81 mg daily after week 12 of gestation [202]. The effect of aspirin on reducing the risk of stroke associated with preeclampsia is not known.

11.10.7.4 Magnesium

Magnesium is recommended in the acute treatment of preeclampsia to treat seizures and to lower the risk of eclampsia [203]. However, the effect of magnesium on the occurrence of stroke in patients with preeclampsia is not well understood.

11.10.8 Hemolytic Uremic Syndrome

Currently, there is no specific treatment for stroke associated with hemolytic uremic syndrome (HUS), and management is focused on treating the underlying infection and correcting the resulting acute kidney injury with hydration or dialysis, depending on severity of the renal injury. Evidence for management of stroke related to HUS is based primarily on case reports. One case report describes a 2-year-old girl with left hemispheric infarcts in the setting of HUS. She was started on peritoneal dialysis and was also transfused with packed red blood cells and frozen plasma. She developed seizures during her hospital admission and was treated with phenobarbital with no further seizure activity. In follow-up a year later, her renal function had normalized and she did not have any recurrence of stroke [204]. Similarly, other case reports describe resolution of cerebrovascular disease after improvement of renal function [205, 206].

11.10.9 Cerebral Amyloid Angiopathy

11.10.9.1 Anticoagulation and Antiplatelets

In general, it is recommended that anticoagulation and antiplatelets be avoided in cerebral amyloid angiopathy (CAA) unless there is a clear indication and the risks/benefits have been discussed with the patient. However, there is no clear method of stratifying the risks and benefits to determine which patients are at higher risk for bleeding while on anticoagulation or antiplatelets. One single-center prospective cohort study of 104 patients with probable CAA and primary lobar ICH found that while aspirin was not associated with lobar ICH recurrence in univariate analysis, aspirin was associated with lobar ICU recurrence in the multivariate analyses that adjusted for baseline clinical predictors [207]. Another study found that the odds ratio of CAA associated with warfarin-related ICH was 3.8 (95% CI 1.0–14.6) [208] compared to patients on warfarin without a history of ICH.

11.10.9.2 Blood Pressure Control

In general, careful blood pressure management is recommended for patients with CAA, though there are no specific guidelines regarding target blood pressure parameters. A secondary analysis was performed in the PROGRESS trial which evaluated the effects of lower blood pressure on ICH with perindopril in patients with CAA. This randomized, placebo-controlled trial found that perindopril reduced the risk of CAA-related ICH by 77% [209]. This suggests an overall positive effect of blood pressure control on hemorrhage risk, though more studies are needed to clarify the appropriate blood pressure parameters.

11.10.9.3 Immunosuppression

The use of steroids or other immunosuppressants in CAA is described in case reports and case series with equivocal clinical benefit reported. Some case reports describe clinical and radiographic improvement with a course of steroids such as dexamethasone or prednisone [210–217], while other case reports describe no improvement with corticosteroid treatment [218, 219]. Case reports of patients with CAA being treated with a combination of corticosteroids and cyclophosphamide describe clinical and radiological improvement [20, 211, 215, 220–223]. One case report also found clinical and radiographic improvement with cyclophosphamide treatment alone [221]. However, in many of these case reports, patients also had brain biopsies positive for vasculitis, suggesting an alternative or additional diagnosis of PACNS, GCA, or CAA-related inflammation.

11.10.10 Susac Syndrome

11.10.10.1 Immunosuppressants

There are no randomized control trials or guidelines for the treatment of Susac syndrome given the rarity of the disease. Several case reports describe clinical improvement without any treatment [224, 225]. One case series found that early treatment with corticosteroids was associated with good prognosis and clinical improvement [225]. However, other case reports have found no improvement on high-dose prednisone [226, 227]. There are case reports of clinical improvement on cyclophosphamide [226, 228, 229] as well as one case report that showed no response to cyclophosphamide treatment [226]. There are also case reports of clinical improvement after treatment with intravenous immunoglobulin (IVIG) [230], mycophenolate mofetil [231], and cyclosporine [232]. However, given reports of clinical improvement without any treatment, further studies with a control group are needed.

11.10.10.2 Anticoagulation and Antiplatelets

While there are no guidelines on the use of antiplatelets and anticoagulation with Susac syndrome, it is generally recommended that patients should be evaluated for typical stroke risk factors and be started on aspirin when appropriate [233]. In a case series of nine patients, eight patients were treated with antiplatelets and corticosteroids, and all nine of the patients were treated with therapeutic anticoagulation as well. All patients had neurological improvement with no recurrent vascular events. One patient who was on aspirin and not anticoagulation initially did have relapse of neurological symptoms and was then started on anticoagulation without any further relapse. Two patients had new retinal artery occlusions after anticoagulation was discontinued, prompting reinitiation. However, as there was overlap between various treatments in this case series, it is difficult to determine the true effect of individual treatments on clinical improvement [234].

11.10.11 Hypereosinophilic Syndrome

In hypereosinophilic syndrome (HES), the goal of treatment is to reduce the absolute eosinophil count and improve clinical symptoms and progression. There are different myeloid variants of HES, and treatment varies depending on a given patient's causative mutation.

11.10.11.1 Imatinib

Imatinib is a platelet-derived growth factor that is the first-line treatment in patients who have the FIP1L1-PDGFRA mutation variant of HES. Several studies have found complete hematological response to imatinib, though the benefit in terms of decreased stroke recurrence is not known [235, 236].

11.10.11.2 Corticosteroids

For patients who are FIP1L1-PDGFRA mutation-negative, prednisone is considered to be first-line treatment. There are a few case series that describe partial or complete remission of symptoms and marked reduction in the absolute eosinophil count [235, 237]. One case report describes a 43-year-old male with primary eosinophilia who developed bilateral multifocal cerebral strokes. He was initially started on aspirin 100 mg daily and had some improvement of his neurological deficits over weeks. However, he returned with new neurological symptoms and was found to have recurrent cerebral ischemia. He was then started on IV hydrocortisone and transitioned to oral prednisone 60 mg for 2 weeks and no recurrences of stroke or eosinophilia over a 2-year follow-up period [238].

11.10.11.3 Steroid-Sparing Agents

For imatinib and corticosteroid-refractory patients, hydroxyurea or interferon alfa could be considered. One case series describes several patients with stroke in the setting of HES with mixed responses to various treatments. One patient was treated with hydroxyurea and warfarin with an initial improvement in eosinophil count, but eventually developed acute lymphoblastic leukemia and passed away. Another patient in the same case series was treated long term with low-dose corticosteroids and hydroxyurea and had remission of his clinical symptoms [239]. Given the lack of controlled trial data, it is difficult to ascertain the effect of any of these treatments on clinical response and stroke recurrence.

References

1. Berlit P (1994) The spectrum of vasculopathies in the differential diagnosis of vasculitis. Semin Neurol 14(4):370–379
2. Lie JT (1997) Classification and histopathologic spectrum of central nervous system vasculitis. Neurol Clin 15(4):805–819
3. Ebisu T et al (1993) Discrimination between different types of White-matter Edema with diffusion-weighted Mr-imaging. JMRI 3(6):863–868
4. Aisen AM, Gabrielsen TO, McCune WJ (1985) MR imaging of systemic lupus erythematosus involving the brain. AJR Am J Roentgenol 144(5):1027–1031
5. Moritani T et al (2001) Diffusion-weighted echo-planar MR imaging of CNS involvement in systemic lupus erythematosus. Acad Radiol 8(8):741–753

6. Kocer N et al (1999) CNS involvement in neuro-Behcet syndrome: an MR study. AJNR Am J Neuroradiol 20(6):1015–1024
7. Woolfenden AR et al (1998) Encephalopathy complicating Henoch-Schonlein purpura: reversible MRI changes. Pediatr Neurol 19(1):74–77
8. Hinchey J et al (1996) A reversible posterior leukoencephalopathy syndrome. N Engl J Med 334(8):494–500
9. John S, Hajj-Ali RA (2014) CNS vasculitis. Semin Neurol 34(4):405–412
10. Mandell DM et al (2017) Intracranial Vessel Wall MRI: principles and expert consensus recommendations of the American Society of Neuroradiology. AJNR Am J Neuroradiol 38(2):218–229
11. White ML et al (2007) Analysis of central nervous system vasculitis with diffusion-weighted imaging and apparent diffusion coefficient mapping of the normal-appearing brain. AJNR Am J Neuroradiol 28(5):933–937
12. Bathla G et al (2018) Cerebrovascular manifestations in neurosarcoidosis: how common are they and does perivascular enhancement matter? Clin Radiol 73(10):907 e15–907 e23
13. Danve A, Grafe M, Deodhar A (2014) Amyloid beta-related angiitis--a case report and comprehensive review of literature of 94 cases. Semin Arthritis Rheum 44(1):86–92
14. Birnbaum J, Hellmann DB (2009) Primary angiitis of the central nervous system. Arch Neurol 66(6):704–709
15. Pagnoux C, Hajj-Ali RA (2016) Pharmacological approaches to CNS vasculitis: where are we at now? Expert Rev Clin Pharmacol 9(1):109–116
16. Salvarani C, Pipitone N, Hunder GG (2016) Management of primary and secondary central nervous system vasculitis. Curr Opin Rheumatol 28(1):21–28
17. Jennette JC et al (2012) Revised international Chapel Hill consensus conference nomenclature of Vasculitides. Arthritis Rheum, 2013 65(1):1–11
18. Lie JT (1992) Primary (granulomatous) angiitis of the central nervous system: a clinicopathologic analysis of 15 new cases and a review of the literature. Hum Pathol 23(2):164–171
19. Schwab P et al (2003) Cerebral amyloid angiopathy associated with primary angiitis of the central nervous system: report of 2 cases and review of the literature. Arthritis Rheum 49(3):421–427
20. Scolding NJ et al (2005) Abeta-related angiitis: primary angiitis of the central nervous system associated with cerebral amyloid angiopathy. Brain 128(Pt 3):500–515
21. Salvarani C, Brown RD Jr, Hunder GG (2012) Adult primary central nervous system vasculitis. Lancet 380(9843):767–777
22. Harris KG et al (1994) Diagnosing intracranial vasculitis: the roles of MR and angiography. AJNR Am J Neuroradiol 15(2):317–330
23. Campi A et al (2001) Primary angiitis of the central nervous system: serial MRI of brain and spinal cord. Neuroradiology 43(8):599–607
24. Ay H et al (2002) Primary angiitis of the central nervous system and silent cortical hemorrhages. AJNR Am J Neuroradiol 23(9):1561–1563
25. Moritani T et al (2004) CNS vasculitis and vasculopathy: efficacy and usefulness of diffusion-weighted echoplanar MR imaging. Clin Imaging 28(4):261–270
26. Moore PM (1989) Diagnosis and management of isolated angiitis of the central nervous system. Neurology 39(2 Pt 1):167–173
27. MacLaren K et al (2005) Primary angiitis of the central nervous system: emerging variants. QJM 98(9):643–654
28. Rinagel M et al (2018) Diagnostic performance of temporal artery ultrasound for the diagnosis of giant cell arteritis: a systematic review and meta-analysis of the literature. Autoimmun Rev
29. Hunder GG et al (1990) The American College of Rheumatology 1990 criteria for the classification of giant cell arteritis. Arthritis Rheum 33(8):1122–1128
30. Siemonsen S et al (2015) 3T MRI reveals extra- and intracranial involvement in giant cell arteritis. AJNR Am J Neuroradiol 36(1):91–97
31. McKinney AM et al (2007) Posterior reversible encephalopathy syndrome: incidence of atypical regions of involvement and imaging findings. AJR Am J Roentgenol 189(4):904–912
32. Brack A et al (1999) Disease pattern in cranial and large-vessel giant cell arteritis. Arthritis Rheum 42(2):311–317
33. Cho HJ, Bloomberg J, Nichols J (2017) Giant cell arteritis. Dis Mon 63(3):88–91
34. Klink T et al (2014) Giant cell arteritis: diagnostic accuracy of MR imaging of superficial cranial arteries in initial diagnosis-results from a multicenter trial. Radiology 273(3):844–852
35. Ironi G et al (2018) Diffusion-weighted magnetic resonance imaging detects Vessel Wall inflammation in patients with Giant cell arteritis. JACC Cardiovasc Imaging
36. Yamada I et al (1998) Takayasu arteritis: evaluation of the thoracic aorta with CT angiography. Radiology 209(1):103–109
37. Abdel Razek AA et al (2014) Imaging spectrum of CNS vasculitis. Radiographics 34(4):873–894
38. Bond KM et al (2017) Intracranial and Extracranial neurovascular manifestations of Takayasu arteritis. AJNR Am J Neuroradiol 38(4):766–772
39. Garg A (2011) Vascular brain pathologies. Neuroimaging Clin N Am 21(4):897–926, ix
40. Provenzale JM, Allen NB (1996) Neuroradiologic findings in polyarteritis nodosa. AJNR Am J Neuroradiol 17(6):1119–1126
41. Sehgal M et al (1995) Neurologic manifestations of Churg-Strauss syndrome. Mayo Clin Proc 70(4):337–341

42. Berlit P (2010) Diagnosis and treatment of cerebral vasculitis. Ther Adv Neurol Disord 3(1):29–42
43. Liou HH et al (1997) Churg-Strauss syndrome presented as multiple intracerebral hemorrhage. Lupus 6(3):279–282
44. Murphy JM et al (1999) Wegener granulomatosis: MR imaging findings in brain and meninges. Radiology 213(3):794–799
45. Mehdipoor G et al (2018) Imaging manifestations of Behcet's disease: key considerations and major features. Eur J Radiol 98:214–225
46. Hiwatashi A et al (2003) Diffusion-weighted MR imaging of neuro-Behcet's disease: a case report. Neuroradiology 45(7):468–471
47. Castillo M (1994) Magnetic resonance imaging of meningitis and its complications. Top Magn Reson Imaging 6(1):53–58
48. DeLone DR et al (1999) Disseminated aspergillosis involving the brain: distribution and imaging characteristics. AJNR Am J Neuroradiol 20(9):1597–1604
49. Lexa FJ (1995) Drug-induced disorders of the central nervous system. Semin Roentgenol 30(1):7–17
50. Gradon JD, Wityk R (1995) Diagnosis of probable cocaine-induced cerebral vasculitis by magnetic resonance angiography. South Med J 88(12):1264–1266
51. Krendel DA et al (1990) Biopsy-proven cerebral vasculitis associated with cocaine abuse. Neurology 40(7):1092–1094
52. Mandell DM et al (2012) Vessel wall MRI to differentiate between reversible cerebral vasoconstriction syndrome and central nervous system vasculitis: preliminary results. Stroke 43(3):860–862
53. Kaichi Y et al (2014) Brain MR findings in patients with systemic lupus erythematosus with and without antiphospholipid antibody syndrome. AJNR Am J Neuroradiol 35(1):100–105
54. Morgen K, McFarland HF, Pillemer SR (2004) Central nervous system disease in primary Sjogrens syndrome: the role of magnetic resonance imaging. Semin Arthritis Rheum 34(3):623–630
55. Unnikrishnan G et al (2018) Cerebral large-vessel Vasculitis in Sjogren's syndrome: utility of high-resolution magnetic resonance Vessel Wall imaging. J Clin Neurol 14(4):588–590
56. Akrout R et al (2012) Cerebral rheumatoid vasculitis: a case report. J Med Case Rep 6:302
57. Bathla G et al (2018) Cerebrovascular manifestations of Neurosarcoidosis: an Underrecognized aspect of the imaging Spectrum. AJNR Am J Neuroradiol 39(7):1194–1200
58. Bathla G et al (2019) Neuroimaging findings in intracranial Sarcoid phlebitis: a case report. J Stroke Cerebrovasc Dis 28(2):369–370
59. Jennette JC, Falk RJ, Milling DM (1994) Pathogenesis of vasculitis. Semin Neurol 14(4):291–299
60. Vajkoczy P (2009) Moyamoya disease: collateralization is everything. Cerebrovasc Dis 28(3):258
61. Hallemeier CL et al (2006) Clinical features and outcome in north American adults with moyamoya phenomenon. Stroke 37(6):1490–1496
62. Qin Y et al (2015) High incidence of asymptomatic cerebral microbleeds in patients with hemorrhagic onset-type moyamoya disease: a phase-sensitive MRI study and meta-analysis. Acta Radiol 56(3):329–338
63. Yamada I et al (1999) Moyamoya disease: evaluation with diffusion-weighted and perfusion echo-planar MR imaging. Radiology 212(2):340–347
64. Moritani T et al (2004) Sickle cell cerebrovascular disease: usual and unusual findings on MR imaging and MR angiography. Clin Imaging 28(3):173–186
65. Thust SC, Burke C, Siddiqui A (2014) Neuroimaging findings in sickle cell disease. Br J Radiol 87(1040):20130699
66. Moran CJ, Siegel MJ, DeBaun MR (1998) Sickle cell disease: imaging of cerebrovascular complications. Radiology 206(2):311–321
67. Guilliams KP et al (2017) Large-vessel vasculopathy in children with sickle cell disease: a magnetic resonance imaging study of infarct topography and focal atrophy. Pediatr Neurol 69:49–57
68. Casey SO et al (2000) Posterior reversible encephalopathy syndrome: utility of fluid-attenuated inversion recovery MR imaging in the detection of cortical and subcortical lesions. AJNR Am J Neuroradiol 21(7):1199–1206
69. Bathla G, Hegde AN (2013) MRI and CT appearances in metabolic encephalopathies due to systemic diseases in adults. Clin Radiol 68(6):545–554
70. Bathla G, Policeni B (2018) Posterior reversible encephalopathy syndrome. In: Noujaim DL et al (eds) Neuroradiology: Spectrum and Evolution of Disease. Elsevier, Philadelphia, PA, pp 20–32
71. Bartynski WS, Zeigler Z, Spearman MP, Lin L, Shadduck RK, Lister J (2001) Etiology of cortical and white matter lesions in cyclosporin-a and FK-506 neurotoxicity. AJNR Am J Neuroradiol 22:1901–1914
72. Ducros A (2012) Reversible cerebral vasoconstriction syndrome. Lancet Neurol 11(10):906–917
73. Miller TR et al (2015) Reversible cerebral vasoconstriction syndrome, part 2: diagnostic work-up, imaging evaluation, and differential diagnosis. AJNR Am J Neuroradiol 36(9):1580–1588
74. Arrigan MT, Heran MKS, Shewchuk JR (2018) Reversible cerebral vasoconstriction syndrome: an important and common cause of thunderclap and recurrent headaches. Clin Radiol 73(5):417–427
75. Tikka S et al (2014) CADASIL and CARASIL. Brain Pathol 24(5):525–544
76. Zhu S, Nahas SJ (2016) CADASIL: imaging characteristics and clinical correlation. Curr Pain Headache Rep 20(10):57
77. Di Donato I et al (2017) Cerebral autosomal dominant Arteriopathy with subcortical infarcts and Leukoencephalopathy (CADASIL) as a model of small vessel disease: update on clinical, diagnostic, and management aspects. BMC Med 15(1):41
78. Kang HG, Kim JS (2015) Intracranial arterial disease in CADASIL patients. J Neurol Sci 359(1–2):347–350

79. Garcia-Carrasco M, Mendoza-Pinto C, Cervera R (2014) Diagnosis and classification of Susac syndrome. Autoimmun Rev 13(4–5):347–350

80. Kleffner I et al (2016) Diagnostic criteria for Susac syndrome. J Neurol Neurosurg Psychiatry 87(12):1287–1295

81. Engisch R et al (2016) Susac's syndrome: Leptomeningeal enhancement on 3D FLAIR MRI. Mult Scler 22(7):972–974

82. Marrodan M et al (2018) Clinical and imaging features distinguishing Susac syndrome from primary angiitis of the central nervous system. J Neurol Sci 395:29–34

83. Okada J et al (1991) Reversible MRI and CT findings in uremic encephalopathy. Neuroradiology 33(6):524–526

84. Kim DM, Lee IH, Song CJ (2016) Uremic encephalopathy: MR imaging findings and clinical correlation. AJNR Am J Neuroradiol 37(9):1604–1609

85. Schmidt S et al (2001) Brain involvement in haemolytic-uraemic syndrome: MRI features of coagulative necrosis. Neuroradiology 43(7):581–585

86. Wengenroth M et al (2013) Central nervous system involvement in adults with epidemic hemolytic uremic syndrome. AJNR Am J Neuroradiol 34(5):1016–21, S1

87. Bakshi R et al (1999) Thrombotic thrombocytopenic purpura: brain CT and MRI findings in 12 patients. Neurology 52(6):1285–1288

88. Burrus TM et al (2010) Renal failure and posterior reversible encephalopathy syndrome in patients with thrombotic thrombocytopenic purpura. Arch Neurol 67(7):831–834

89. D'Aprile P et al (1994) Thrombotic thrombocytopenic purpura: MR demonstration of reversible brain abnormalities. AJNR Am J Neuroradiol 15(1):19–20

90. Reijmer YD, van Veluw SJ, Greenberg SM (2016) Ischemic brain injury in cerebral amyloid angiopathy. J Cereb Blood Flow Metab 36(1):40–54

91. Viswanathan A, Greenberg SM (2011) Cerebral amyloid angiopathy in the elderly. Ann Neurol 70(6):871–880

92. van Veluw SJ et al (2016) Microbleed and microinfarct detection in amyloid angiopathy: a high-resolution MRI-histopathology study. Brain 139(Pt 12):3151–3162

93. Kimberly WT et al (2009) Silent ischemic infarcts are associated with hemorrhage burden in cerebral amyloid angiopathy. Neurology 72(14):1230–1235

94. Conklin J et al (2014) Are acute infarcts the cause of leukoaraiosis? Brain mapping for 16 consecutive weeks. Ann Neurol 76(6):899–904

95. Salvarani C et al (2016) Imaging findings of cerebral amyloid Angiopathy, Abeta-related Angiitis (ABRA), and cerebral amyloid Angiopathy-related inflammation: a single-institution 25-year experience. Medicine (Baltimore) 95(20):e3613

96. Valent P et al (2012) Contemporary consensus proposal on criteria and classification of eosinophilic disorders and related syndromes. J Allergy Clin Immunol 130(3):607–612 e9

97. Lee D, Ahn TB (2014) Central nervous system involvement of hypereosinophilic syndrome: a report of 10 cases and a literature review. J Neurol Sci 347(1–2):281–287

98. Kanamori M et al (2009) A case of idiopathic hypereosinophilic syndrome with leptomeningeal dissemination and intraventricular mass lesion: an autopsy report. Clin Neuropathol 28(3):197–202

99. Rice CM et al (2015) Idiopathic hypereosinophilic syndrome: a new cause of vasculitis of the central nervous system. J Neurol 262(5):1354–1359

100. Aoki S et al (2002) Radiation-induced arteritis: thickened wall with prominent enhancement on cranial MR images report of five cases and comparison with 18 cases of Moyamoya disease. Radiology 223(3):683–688

101. Kaas B et al (2013) Spectrum and prevalence of vasculopathy in pediatric neurofibromatosis type 1. J Child Neurol 28(5):561–569

102. Salvarani C et al (2015) Adult primary central nervous system vasculitis treatment and course: analysis of one hundred sixty-three patients. Arthritis Rheumatol 67:1637–1645

103. Salvarani C, Brown RD Jr, Hunder GG (2012) Adult primary central nervous system vasculitis: an update. Curr Opin Rheumatol 24:46–52

104. Cupps TR, Moore PM, Fauci AS (1983) Isolated angiitis of the central nervous system. Prospective diagnostic and therapeutic experience. Am J Med 74:97–105

105. Dasgupta B et al (2010) BSR and BHPR guidelines for the management of giant cell arteritis. Rheumatology (Oxford) 49:1594–1597

106. Fraga A, Mintz G, Valle L, Flores-Izquierdo G (1972) Takayasu's arteritis: frequency of systemic manifestations (study of 22 patients) and favorable response to maintenance steroid therapy with adrenocorticosteroids (12 patients). Arthritis Rheum 15:617–624

107. de Souza AW et al (2010) Antiplatelet therapy for the prevention of arterial ischemic events in takayasu arteritis. Circ J 74:1236–1241

108. Bali HK, Jain S, Jain A, Sharma BK (1998) Stent supported angioplasty in Takayasu arteritis. Int J Cardiol 66(Suppl 1):S213–S217; discussion S219–220

109. Kerr GS et al (1994) Takayasu arteritis. Ann Intern Med 120:919–929

110. Gayraud M et al (1997) Treatment of good-prognosis polyarteritis nodosa and Churg-Strauss syndrome: comparison of steroids and oral or pulse cyclophosphamide in 25 patients. French cooperative study Group for Vasculitides. Br J Rheumatol 36:1290–1297

111. Guillevin L et al (1995) Corticosteroids plus pulse cyclophosphamide and plasma exchanges versus corticosteroids plus pulse cyclophosphamide alone in the treatment of polyarteritis nodosa and Churg-Strauss syndrome patients with factors predicting poor prognosis. A prospective, randomized trial in sixty-two patients. Arthritis Rheum 38:1638–1645

112. Chartapisak W, Opastiraku S, Willis NS, Craig JC, Hodson EM (2009) Prevention and treatment of renal disease in Henoch-Schonlein purpura: a systematic review. Arch Dis Child 94:132–137

113. Ghosh K, Chatterjee A, Sau JT, Dey S (2012) Stroke and skin rash: a rare case of Henoch-Schonlein purpura. Ann Indian Acad Neurol 15:307–309

114. Bakkaloglu SA et al (2000) Cerebral vasculitis in Henoch-Schonlein purpura. Nephrol Dial Transplant 15:246–248

115. Iglesias E, Eleftheriou D, Mankad K, Prabhakar P, Brogan PA (2014) Microscopic polyangiitis presenting with hemorrhagic stroke. J Child Neurol 29:NP1–NP4

116. Arena MG, Ferlazzo E, Bonanno D, Quattrocchi P, Ferlazzo B (2003) Cerebral vasculitis in a patient with HCV-related type II mixed cryoglobulinemia. J Investig Allergol Clin Immunol 13:135–136

117. De Vita S et al (2012) A randomized controlled trial of rituximab for the treatment of severe cryoglobulinemic vasculitis. Arthritis Rheum 64:843–853

118. Pires C, Foreid H, Barroso C, Ferro JM (2011) Rapidly progressive dementia due to leukocytoclastic vasculitis of the central nervous system. BMJ Case Rep 2011. https://doi.org/10.1136/bcr.08.2011.4619

119. Martinez-Taboada VM, Blanco R, Garcia-Fuentes M, Rodriguez-Valverde V (1997) Clinical features and outcome of 95 patients with hypersensitivity vasculitis. Am J Med 102:186–191

120. Akman-Demir G, Serdaroglu P, Taşçi B (1999) Clinical patterns of neurological involvement in Behçet's disease: evaluation of 200 patients. The Neuro-Behçet study group. Brain 122(Pt 11):2171–2182

121. Nakamura S, Takase S, Itahara K (1980) Cytological examination of cerebrospinal fluid in eight patients with neuro-Behçet's disease. Tohoku J Exp Med 132:421–430

122. Wechsler B et al (1992) Cerebral venous thrombosis in Behcet's disease: clinical study and long-term follow-up of 25 cases. Neurology 42:614–618

123. Bank I, Weart C (1984) Dural sinus thrombosis in Behcet's disease. Arthritis Rheum 27:816–818

124. Hatemi G et al (2018) 2018 update of the EULAR recommendations for the management of Behcet's syndrome. Ann Rheum Dis 77:808–818

125. Borhani Haghighi A (2009) Treatment of neuro-Behcet's disease: an update. Expert Rev Neurother 9:565–574

126. Kowal-Bielecka O et al (2009) EULAR recommendations for the treatment of systemic sclerosis: a report from the EULAR scleroderma trials and research group (EUSTAR). Ann Rheum Dis 68:620–628

127. Pathak R, Gabor AJ (1991) Scleroderma and central nervous system vasculitis. Stroke 22:410–413

128. Spath NB, Amft N, Farquhar D (2014) Cerebral vasculitis in rheumatoid arthritis. QJM 107:1027–1029

129. Rodriguez Uranga JJ, Chinchon Espino D, Serrano Pozo A, Hernandez FG (2006) Pseodotumoral central nervous system vasculitis in rheumatoid arthritis. Med Clin (Barc) 127:438–439

130. Mrabet D, Meddeb N, Ajlani H, Sahli H, Sellami S (2007) Cerebral vasculitis in a patient with rheumatoid arthritis. Joint Bone Spine 74:201–204

131. Caballol Pons N et al (2010) Isolated cerebral vasculitis associated with rheumatoid arthritis. Joint Bone Spine 77:361–363

132. Ohno T, Matsuda I, Furukawa H, Kanoh T (1994) Recovery from rheumatoid cerebral vasculitis by low-dose methotrexate. Intern Med 33:615–620

133. Carod Artal FJ (2016) Clinical management of infectious cerebral vasculitides. Expert Rev Neurother 16:205–221

134. Cutfield NJ, Steele H, Wilhelm T, Weatherall MW (2009) Successful treatment of HIV associated cerebral vasculopathy with HAART. J Neurol Neurosurg Psychiatry 80:936–937

135. Bermel C, Spuntrup E, Fink G, Nowak DA (2009) Stroke in an adult with HIV infection due to carotid artery stenosis successfully treated with steroids: HIV-associated arteritis? J Neurol 256:1563–1565

136. Nagel MA et al (2008) The varicella zoster virus vasculopathies: clinical, CSF, imaging, and virologic features. Neurology 70:853–860

137. Javaud N et al (2011) Tuberculous cerebral vasculitis: retrospective study of 10 cases. Eur J Intern Med 22:e99–104

138. Topakian R, Stieglbauer K, Nussbaumer K, Aichner FT (2008) Cerebral vasculitis and stroke in Lyme neuroborreliosis. Two case reports and review of current knowledge. Cerebrovasc Dis 26:455–461

139. Back T et al (2013) Neuroborreliosis-associated cerebral vasculitis: long-term outcome and health-related quality of life. J Neurol 260:1569–1575

140. Bremell D, Dotevall L (2014) Oral doxycycline for Lyme neuroborreliosis with symptoms of encephalitis, myelitis, vasculitis or intracranial hypertension. Eur J Neurol 21:1162–1167

141. Mageau A et al (2018) Treatment of syphilis-associated cerebral Vasculitis: reappearance of an old question. Am J Med 131:1516–1519

142. Abkur TM, Ahmed GS, Alfaki NO, O'Connor M (2015) Neurosyphilis presenting with a stroke-like syndrome. BMJ Case Rep 2015. https://doi.org/10.1136/bcr-2014-206988

143. Kakumani PL, Hajj-Ali RA (2009) A forgotten cause of central nervous system vasculitis. J Rheumatol 36:655

144. Grouhi M, Dalal I, Nisbet-Brown E, Roifman CM (1998) Cerebral vasculitis associated with chronic mucocutaneous candidiasis. J Pediatr 133:571–574

145. Pichon N et al (2008) Fatal-stroke syndrome revealing fungal cerebral vasculitis due to Arthrographis kalrae in an immunocompetent patient. J Clin Microbiol 46:3152–3155

146. Nguyen FN, Kar JK, Zakaria A, Schiess MC (2013) Isolated central nervous system histoplasmosis presenting with ischemic pontine stroke and meningitis in an immune-competent patient. JAMA Neurol 70:638–641

147. Martins HS, da Silva TR, Scalabrini-Neto A, Velasco IT (2010) Cerebral vasculitis caused by Aspergillus simulating ischemic stroke in an immunocompetent patient. J Emerg Med 38:597–600

148. Rosario M, Song SX, McCullough LD (2012) An unusual case of stroke. Neurologist 18:229–232

149. Satish S, Rajesh R, Shashikala S, Kurian G, Unni VN (2010) Cryptococcal sepsis in small vessel vasculitis. Indian J Nephrol 20:159–161

150. Zimelewicz Oberman D, Patrucco L, Cuello Oderiz C (2018) Central nervous system Vasculitis for Cryptococcosis in an Immunocompetent patient. Diseases 6(3):75

151. Bertsias GK et al (2010) EULAR recommendations for the management of systemic lupus erythematosus with neuropsychiatric manifestations: report of a task force of the EULAR standing committee for clinical affairs. Ann Rheum Dis 69:2074–2082

152. Stojanovich L, Stojanovich R, Kostich V, Dzjolich E (2003) Neuropsychiatric lupus favourable response to low dose i.v. cyclophosphamide and prednisolone (pilot study). Lupus 12:3–7

153. Barile-Fabris L et al (2005) Controlled clinical trial of IV cyclophosphamide versus IV methylprednisolone in severe neurological manifestations in systemic lupus erythematosus. Ann Rheum Dis 64:620–625

154. Neuwelt CM (2003) The role of plasmapheresis in the treatment of severe central nervous system neuropsychiatric systemic lupus erythematosus. Ther Apher Dial 7:173–182

155. Yamada S et al (2016) Effects of surgery and antiplatelet therapy in ten-year follow-up from the registry study of research committee on Moyamoya disease in Japan. J Stroke Cerebrovasc Dis 25:340–349

156. Spittler JF, Smektala K (1990) Pharmacotherapy in moyamoya disease. Hokkaido Igaky Zasshi 65:235–240

157. McLean MJ, Gebarski SS, van der Spek AF, Goldstein GW (1985) Response of moyamoya disease to verapamil. Lancet 1:163–164

158. Sarenur T et al (1994) Twins with moyamoya disease. Acta Paediatr Jpn 36:705–708

159. Iwama T, Hashimoto N, Yonekawa Y (1996) The relevance of hemodynamic factors to perioperative ischemic complications in childhood moyamoya disease. Neurosurgery 38:1120–1125; discussion 1125–1126

160. Fujiwara J, Nakahara S, Enomoto T, Nakata Y, Takita H (1996) The effectiveness of O2 administration for transient ischemic attacks in moyamoya disease in children. Childs Nerv Syst 12:69–75

161. Matsushima T et al (1989) Surgical treatment for paediatric patients with moyamoya disease by indirect revascularization procedures (EDAS, EMS, EMAS). Acta Neurochir 98:135–140

162. Cho WS et al (2014) Long-term outcomes after combined revascularization surgery in adult moyamoya disease. Stroke 45:3025–3031

163. Yawn BP et al (2014) Management of sickle cell disease: summary of the 2014 evidence-based report by expert panel members. JAMA 312:1033–1048

164. Adams RJ et al (1997) Long-term stroke risk in children with sickle cell disease screened with transcranial Doppler. Ann Neurol 42:699–704

165. Pegelow CH et al (1995) Risk of recurrent stroke in patients with sickle cell disease treated with erythrocyte transfusions. J Pediatr 126:896–899

166. Ware RE et al (2004) Prevention of secondary stroke and resolution of transfusional iron overload in children with sickle cell anemia using hydroxyurea and phlebotomy. J Pediatr 145:346–352

167. Kernan WN et al (2014) Guidelines for the prevention of stroke in patients with stroke and transient ischemic attack: a guideline for healthcare professionals from the American Heart Association/American Stroke Association. Stroke 45:2160–2236

168. Sumoza A, de Bisotti R, Sumoza D, Fairbanks V (2002) Hydroxyurea (HU) for prevention of recurrent stroke in sickle cell anemia (SCA). Am J Hematol 71:161–165

169. Agca R et al (2017) EULAR recommendations for cardiovascular disease risk management in patients with rheumatoid arthritis and other forms of inflammatory joint disorders: 2015/2016 update. Ann Rheum Dis 76:17–28

170. Pawate S, Moses H, Sriram S (2009) Presentations and outcomes of neurosarcoidosis: a study of 54 cases. QJM 102:449–460

171. Ko JK, Lee SW, Choi CH (2009) Moyamoyalike vasculopathy in neurosarcoidosis. J Korean Neurosurg Soc 45:50–52

172. Hoitsma E, Drent M, Sharma OP (2010) A pragmatic approach to diagnosing and treating neurosarcoidosis in the 21st century. Curr Opin Pulm Med 16:472–479

173. Agbogu BN, Stern BJ, Sewell C, Yang G (1995) Therapeutic considerations in patients with refractory neurosarcoidosis. Arch Neurol 52:875–879

174. Morcos Z (2003) Refractory neurosarcoidosis responding to infliximab. Neurology 60:1220–1221; author reply 1220–1221

175. Pettersen JA, Zochodne DW, Bell RB, Martin L, Hill MD (2002) Refractory neurosarcoidosis responding to infliximab. Neurology 59:1660–1661
176. Bomprezzi R, Pati S, Chansakul C, Vollmer T (2010) A case of neurosarcoidosis successfully treated with rituximab. Neurology 75:568–570
177. Sharma OP (1997) Neurosarcoidosis: a personal perspective based on the study of 37 patients. Chest 112:220–228
178. Motta M et al (2008) Remission of refractory neurosarcoidosis treated with brain radiotherapy: a case report and a literature review. Neurologist 14:120–124
179. Sundaresan P, Jayamohan J (2008) Stereotactic radiotherapy for the treatment of neurosarcoidosis involving the pituitary gland and hypothalamus. J Med Imaging Radiat Oncol 52:622–626
180. Westhout FD, Linskey ME (2008) Obstructive hydrocephalus and progressive psychosis: rare presentations of neurosarcoidosis. Surg Neurol 69:288–292; discussion 292
181. Brisman JL, Hinduja A, McKinney JS, Gerhardstein B (2006) Successful emergent angioplasty of neurosarcoid vasculitis presenting with strokes. Surg Neurol 66:402–404
182. Vaughan CJ, Delanty N (2000) Hypertensive emergencies. Lancet 356:411–417
183. Raroque HG Jr, Tesfa G, Purdy P (1993) Postpartum cerebral angiopathy. Is there a role for sympathomimetic drugs? Stroke 24:2108–2110
184. Skeik N, Porten BR, Kadkhodayan Y, McDonald W, Lahham F (2015) Postpartum reversible cerebral vasoconstriction syndrome: review and analysis of the current data. Vasc Med 20:256–265
185. Surpur SS, Govindarajan R (2017) Extracranial four-vessel dissection with reversible cerebral vasoconstriction syndrome in a habitual cocaine user presenting with thunderclap headache. J Vasc Interv Neurol 9:54
186. Henry PY, Larre P, Aupy M, Lafforgue JL, Orgogozo JM (1984) Reversible cerebral arteriopathy associated with the administration of ergot derivatives. Cephalalgia 4:171–178
187. Kato Y et al (2016) Triptan-induced reversible cerebral vasoconstriction syndrome: two case reports with a literature review. Intern Med 55:3525–3528
188. Westover MB, Cohen AB (2013) Reversible vasoconstriction syndrome with bilateral basal ganglia hemorrhages. J Neuroimaging 23:122–125
189. Kodama S et al (2017) Tacrolimus-induced reversible cerebral vasoconstriction syndrome with delayed multi-segmental vasoconstriction. J Stroke Cerebrovasc Dis 26:e75–e77
190. Sayegh J et al (2010) Reversible cerebral vasoconstriction syndrome in a female patient with systemic lupus erythematosus. Rheumatology (Oxford) 49:1993–1994
191. Calic Z, Choong H, Schlaphoff G, Cappelen-Smith C (2014) Reversible cerebral vasoconstriction syndrome following indomethacin. Cephalalgia 34:1181–1186
192. Tark BE, Messe SR, Balucani C, Levine SR (2014) Intracerebral hemorrhage associated with oral phenylephrine use: a case report and review of the literature. J Stroke Cerebrovasc Dis 23:2296–2300
193. Singhal AB, Topcuoglu MA (2017) Glucocorticoid-associated worsening in reversible cerebral vasoconstriction syndrome. Neurology 88:228–236
194. Linn J et al (2011) Intra-arterial application of nimodipine in reversible cerebral vasoconstriction syndrome: a diagnostic tool in select cases? Cephalalgia 31:1074–1081
195. Nowak DA et al (2003) Reversible segmental cerebral vasoconstriction (call-Fleming syndrome): are calcium channel inhibitors a potential treatment option? Cephalalgia 23:218–222
196. Chen SP et al (2008) Transcranial color doppler study for reversible cerebral vasoconstriction syndromes. Ann Neurol 63:751–757
197. Ducros A et al (2007) The clinical and radiological spectrum of reversible cerebral vasoconstriction syndrome. A prospective series of 67 patients. Brain 130:3091–3101
198. O. American College of, Gynecologists, P. Task Force on Hypertension in, Hypertension in pregnancy (2013) Report of the American College of Obstetricians and Gynecologists' task Force on hypertension in pregnancy. Obstet Gynecol 122:1122–1131
199. Koopmans CM et al (2009) Induction of labour versus expectant monitoring for gestational hypertension or mild pre-eclampsia after 36 weeks' gestation (HYPITAT): a multicentre, open-label randomised controlled trial. Lancet 374:979–988
200. Martin JN Jr et al (2005) Stroke and severe pre-eclampsia and eclampsia: a paradigm shift focusing on systolic blood pressure. Obstet Gynecol 105:246–254
201. Askie LM, Duley L, Henderson-Smart DJ, Stewart LA, P. C. Group (2007) Antiplatelet agents for prevention of pre-eclampsia: a meta-analysis of individual patient data. Lancet 369:1791–1798
202. LeFevre ML, Force USPST (2014) Low-dose aspirin use for the prevention of morbidity and mortality from preeclampsia: U.S. preventive services task Force recommendation statement. Ann Intern Med 161:819–826
203. Duley L, Gulmezoglu AM, Henderson-Smart DJ, Chou D (2010) Magnesium sulphate and other anticonvulsants for women with pre-eclampsia. Cochrane Database Syst Rev:CD000025
204. Steinberg A, Ish-Horowitcz M, el-Peleg O, Mor J, Branski D (1986) Stroke in a patient with hemolytic-uremic syndrome with a good outcome. Brain and Development 8:70–72
205. DiMario FJ Jr, Bronte-Stewart H, Sherbotie J, Turner ME (1987) Lacunar infarction of the basal ganglia as a complication of hemolytic-uremic syndrome.

206. Rasoulpour M, Leichtner A, San Jorge M, Hyams J (1985) Cerebral vascular accident during the recovery phase of hemolytic uremic syndrome. Int J Pediatr Nephrol 6:287–288

207. Biffi A et al (2010) Aspirin and recurrent intracerebral hemorrhage in cerebral amyloid angiopathy. Neurology 75:693–698

208. Rosand J, Hylek EM, O'Donnell HC, Greenberg SM (2000) Warfarin-associated hemorrhage and cerebral amyloid angiopathy: a genetic and pathologic study. Neurology 55:947–951

209. Arima H et al (2010) Effects of perindopril-based lowering of blood pressure on intracerebral hemorrhage related to amyloid angiopathy: the PROGRESS trial. Stroke 41:394–396

210. Ginsberg L, Geddes J, Valentine A (1988) Amyloid angiopathy and granulomatous angiitis of the central nervous system: a case responding to corticosteroid treatment. J Neurol 235:438–440

211. Mandybur TI, Balko G (1992) Cerebral amyloid angiopathy with granulomatous angiitis ameliorated by steroid-cytoxan treatment. Clin Neuropharmacol 15:241–247

212. Ortiz O, Reed L (1996) Cerebral amyloid angiopathy presenting as a nonhemorrhagic, infiltrating mass. Neuroradiology 38:449–452

213. Streichenberger N et al (1999) Giant cell angiitis of the central nervous system with amyloid angiopathy. A case report and review of the literature. Clin Exp Pathol 47:311–317

214. Hoshi K et al (2000) Cessation of cerebral hemorrhage recurrence associated with corticosteroid treatment in a patient with cerebral amyloid angiopathy. Amyloid 7:284–288

215. Schwab P, Lidov HG, Schwartz RB, Anderson RJ (2003) Cerebral amyloid angiopathy associated with primary angiitis of the central nervous system: report of 2 cases and review of the literature. Arthritis Rheum 49:421–427

216. Oh U et al (2004) Reversible leukoencephalopathy associated with cerebral amyloid angiopathy. Neurology 62:494–497

217. Machida K et al (2008) Cortical petechial hemorrhage, subarachnoid hemorrhage and corticosteroid-responsive leukoencephalopathy in a patient with cerebral amyloid angiopathy. Amyloid 15:60–64

218. Silbert PL et al (1995) Cortical petechial hemorrhage, leukoencephalopathy, and subacute dementia associated with seizures due to cerebral amyloid angiopathy. Mayo Clin Proc 70:477–480

219. Osumi AK, Tien RD, Felsberg GJ, Rosenbloom M (1995) Cerebral amyloid angiopathy presenting as a brain mass. AJNR Am J Neuroradiol 16:911–915

220. Fountain NB, Eberhard DA (1996) Primary angiitis of the central nervous system associated with cerebral amyloid angiopathy: report of two cases and review of the literature. Neurology 46:190–197

221. Fountain NB, Lopes MB (1999) Control of primary angiitis of the CNS associated with cerebral amyloid angiopathy by cyclophosphamide alone. Neurology 52:660–662

222. Masson C, Henin D, Colombani JM, Dehen H (1998) A case of cerebral giant-cell angiitis associated with cerebral amyloid angiopathy. Favorable evolution with corticosteroid therapy. Rev Neurol (Paris) 154:695–698

223. Kinnecom C et al (2007) Course of cerebral amyloid angiopathy-related inflammation. Neurology 68:1411–1416

224. Gordon DL, Hayreh SS, Adams HP Jr (1991) Microangiopathy of the brain, retina, and ear: improvement without immunosuppressive therapy. Stroke 22:933–937

225. Turner BW, Digre KB, Shelton C (1998) Susac syndrome. Otolaryngol Head Neck Surg 118:866–867

226. Monteiro ML et al (1985) A microangiopathic syndrome of encephalopathy, hearing loss, and retinal arteriolar occlusions. Neurology 35:1113–1121

227. Bogousslavsky J et al (1989) Encephalopathy, deafness and blindness in young women: a distinct retinocochleocerebral arteriolopathy? J Neurol Neurosurg Psychiatry 52:43–46

228. O'Halloran HS, Pearson PA, Lee WB, Susac JO, Berger JR (1998) Microangiopathy of the brain, retina, and cochlea (Susac syndrome). A report of five cases and a review of the literature. Ophthalmology 105:1038–1044

229. Petty GW, Matteson EL, Younge BR, McDonald TJ, Wood CP (2001) Recurrence of Susac syndrome (retinocochleocerebral vasculopathy) after remission of 18 years. Mayo Clin Proc 76:958–960

230. Fox RJ et al (2006) Treatment of Susac syndrome with gamma globulin and corticosteroids. J Neurol Sci 251:17–22

231. Hahn JS, Lannin WC, Sarwal MM (2004) Microangiopathy of brain, retina, and inner ear (Susac's syndrome) in an adolescent female presenting as acute disseminated encephalomyelitis. Pediatrics 114:276–281

232. Gruhn N, Pedersen LK, Nielsen NV (2005) Susac's syndrome: the first case report in a Nordic country, with an 8-year follow-up. Acta Ophthalmol Scand 83:757–758

233. Rennebohm RM, Egan RA, Susac JO (2008) Treatment of Susac's syndrome. Curr Treat Options Neurol 10:67–74

234. Aubart-Cohen F et al (2007) Long-term outcome in Susac syndrome. Medicine (Baltimore) 86:93–102

235. Ogbogu PU et al (2009) Hypereosinophilic syndrome: a multicenter, retrospective analysis of clinical characteristics and response to therapy. J Allergy Clin Immunol 124:1319–1325 e1313

236. Baccarani M et al (2007) The efficacy of imatinib mesylate in patients with FIP1L1-PDGFRalpha-positive hypereosinophilic syndrome. Results of a multicenter prospective study. Haematologica 92:1173–1179

237. Khoury P, Abiodun AO, Holland-Thomas N, Fay MP, Klion AD (2018) Hypereosinophilic syndrome subtype predicts responsiveness to glucocorticoids. J Allergy Clin Immunol Pract 6:190–195

238. Chang WL, Lin HJ, Cheng HH (2008) Hypereosinophilic syndrome with recurrent strokes: a case report. Acta Neurol Taiwanica 17:184–188

239. Aida L et al (2013) Embolism and impaired wash-out: a possible explanation of border zone strokes in hypereosinophilic syndrome. J Neurol Sci 325:162–164

Epilepsy

12

Aristides A. Capizzano, and Toshio Moritani

Hiroto Kawasaki

12.1 Definition

Epilepsy is a chronic brain disorder, which has a wide spectrum of underlying causes. It is characterized by recurrent seizures due to excessive neuronal discharges and is associated with a variety of clinical and laboratory manifestations [1]. Epileptic seizures are defined as the clinical manifestation of abnormal excessive neuronal activity.

12.2 Classification

Since the prior edition of this book, the International League Against Epilepsy (ILEA) proposed a new classification of seizure types (Table 12.1) [1]. As in the previous nomenclature, seizure classification first takes into account

---

A. A. Capizzano (✉)
Division of Neuroradiology, Department of Radiology, University of Michigan,
Ann Arbor, MI, USA
e-mail: capizzan@med.umich.edu

T. Moritani
Division of Neuroradiology, Department of Radiology, Clinical Neuroradiology Research, University of Michigan, Ann Arbor, MI, USA
e-mail: tmoritan@med.umich.edu

H. Kawasaki
University of Iowa Hospitals & Clinics,
Iowa City, IA, USA
e-mail: hiroto-kawasaki@uiowa.edu

if the initial manifestations of the seizure are either focal or generalized. For focal seizures, the degree of awareness during the seizure is included in the seizure type; thus retained awareness during a focal seizure corresponds to the prior term "simple partial seizure." Contrariwise, focal impaired awareness seizure corresponds to the prior term "complex partial seizure." Focal aware or impaired awareness seizures may be further characterized by motor or non-motor onset symptoms, reflecting the first prominent sign or symptom in the seizure, for example, focal impaired awareness myoclonic seizure. Generalized seizures are divided into motor and non-motor (absence) seizures. Further subdivisions are similar to those of the 1981 classification, with the addition of myoclonic–atonic seizures.

After diagnosis of the seizure type, the next step is diagnosis of epilepsy type. The ILEA classification of the epilepsies was therefore also recently updated [2]. It includes focal epilepsy, generalized epilepsy, combined generalized and focal epilepsy, and also an unknown epilepsy group. The third level is that of epilepsy syndrome, which refers to a cluster of features incorporating seizure types, EEG and imaging features that tend to occur together (i.e., childhood absence epilepsy). The new classification incorporates etiology along each stage, emphasizing the need to consider etiology at each step of diagnosis as it often carries significant treatment implications. Etiology is broken into six

---

© Springer Nature Switzerland AG 2021
T. Moritani, A. A. Capizzano (eds.), *Diffusion-Weighted MR Imaging of the Brain, Head and Neck, and Spine*, https://doi.org/10.1007/978-3-030-62120-9_12

Table 12.1 Classification of seizures types (from [1])

Focal onset		Generalized onset	Unknown onset
Preserved awareness	Impaired awareness		
Motor Onset		*Motor*	*Motor*
Automatisms		Tonic–clonic	Tonic–clonic
Atonic		Clonic	Epileptic spasms
Clonic		Tonic	
Epileptic spasms		Myoclonic	
Hyperkinetic		Myoclonic–tonic–clonic	
Myoclonic		Myoclonic–atonic	
Tonic		Atonic	
		Epileptic spasms	
Nonmotor Onset		*Nonmotor (absence)*	*Nonmotor*
Autonomic		Typical	Behavior arrest
Behavior arrest		Atypical	
Cognitive		Myoclonic	
Emotional		Eyelid myoclonia	
Sensory			
Focal to bilateral tonic–clonic			*Unclassified*

Table 12.2 Classification of epilepsies (modified from [2])

Co-morbidities	*Seizure types*				Etiology
	Focal	Generalized	Unknown		Structural
	Epilepsy types				Genetic
	Focal	Generalized	Generalized and focal	Unknown	Infectious
					Metabolic
	Epilepsy syndromes				Immune
					Unknown

subgroups: structural, genetic, infectious, metabolic, immune, and unknown (Table 12.2).

The international classification of epileptic seizures is useful to describe the patient's symptoms, but this is often only the first step in the diagnostic process (Table 12.1) [2]. If the clinical characteristics are associated with a recognizable group of features, such as age of onset, genetic background, and course, they may constitute an epileptic syndrome. The international classification of epilepsies and epileptic syndromes classifies epilepsy as localized or generalized, and idiopathic, cryptogenic, or symptomatic (Table 12.2) [2].

Idiopathic epilepsies are the most common and occur in otherwise normal children who have underlying genetic etiology with age-related, specific seizures and classic EEG patterns. Most of these are related to genetically determined defects in ion-channel function: channelopathies (which may affect calcium, sodium, or potassium channels or Ach receptor, GABA receptors).

Symptomatic epilepsies are those in which seizures are related to abnormalities that are clearly defined by imaging, metabolic, or genetic testing.

12.3 Mechanisms and Pathophysiology of Seizures

The fundamental mechanisms of epilepsy are studied at the basic level of the molecular environment of the cell. This involves subcellular systems such as membrane channels, receptors, different cell populations, and their interactions. Several neurotransmitter systems are important for epilepsy. Glutamate is the main excitatory synaptic transmitter in the cerebral cortex and hippocampus. Glutamate has many types and subtypes of receptors (GluRs), belonging to two main families: ionotropic and metabotropic glutamate receptors. Ionotropic glutamate receptors (iGluRs) are ion channel receptors activated by glutamate. There are three main types of iGluRs: AMPA, NMDA, and kainate receptors, and each of these iGluR types has several subtypes. Second, the metabotropic glutamate receptors (mGluRs) are G-protein-coupled receptors [3].

NMDA receptors are the principal receptors in the CNS that control synaptic plasticity and memory and are heavily represented in the hippocampus, particularly at the CA1 sector [4]. NMDA activation results in voltage-dependent Na and Ca entry into the cell, and exit of K ions out of the cell. Excessive activation of the NMDA receptor leads to abnormally high level of Ca that enter the cells and activates a number of enzymes, including phospholipases, endonucleases, and also proteases such as calpain. These enzymes go on to damage several cell structures and result in cell death [3]. NMDA receptor concentration is higher in regions that are susceptible to excitotoxic damage such as the hippocampus (Fig. 12.1) [5, 6]. Astrocytes play a key role in regulation of extracellular glutamate, with 80–90% of extracellular glutamate uptake in brain being through astrocytic glutamate transporters [7]. In some models of epileptogenesis, it has been possible to block bursts of discharges by NMDA channel antagonists [8].

Gamma-aminobutyric acid (GABA) is the main inhibitory transmitter in the cerebral cortex. Loss of GABAergic inhibition can generate epileptiform activity, which is believed to be important in chronic epilepsy [9]. Interestingly, excitatory action of GABA may also occur in adult mammals in pathological states from activation of GABA A receptors and is the rule at the early stages of ontogeny. As in pathological states, the excitatory action of GABA early in ontogeny is explained by a higher reversal potential for chloride ions in immature neurons [10].

The onset of epileptiform activity presupposes that an epileptic focus exists where the seizure originates. The epileptic focus almost always exists in the cortex usually near structural brain abnormalities such as dysplasia or tumor, but it could be located far from the lesion, in the contralateral side, or in the absence of an identifiable lesion. The epileptic focus may exist in a discrete group of neurons, such as the CA1 pyramidal cells in the cornu ammonis, or over a larger cortical region [6]. The seizure activity is associated with abnormal electric discharges in populations of synchronously hyperactive neurons. The spread of the seizure is associated with accumulation of extracellular substances, such as potassium ions or excitotoxic amines, and electrical gating mechanisms among neurons.

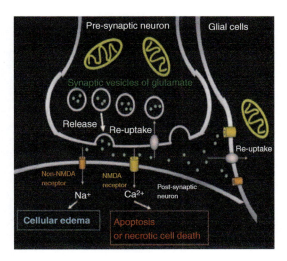

Fig. 12.1 Excitotoxic mechanisms in the neuron and astrocyte. In the neuron, glutamate is released from the presynaptic terminal into the synaptic cleft. The glutamate binding to NMDA receptors allows entry of Ca^{2+} into the postsynaptic neuron, which when excessive can result in necrotic cell death or apoptosis. The glutamate binding to non-NMDA receptors allows entry of Na^+ into the postsynaptic neuron, resulting in cytotoxic edema of the neuron. Reuptake of extracellular glutamate takes place at the pre-synaptic terminals and in adjacent astrocytes. Similar mechanisms also cause cytotoxic edema in the astrocyte

12.4 Anatomy of the Limbic Lobe on MRI

The limbic lobe generates synchronized physiological electric rhythms in the normal brain, notably in the theta rhythm, and the faster beta and gamma oscillations and sharp-wave ripples [4]. In the epileptic brain, synchronization becomes pathological thus generating seizures and several kinds of interictal electric activity [11]. Following the nomenclature of Vogt and

Vogt from 1919, the six-layered isocortex forms the bulk of the cortical mantle while the allocortex, confined to the medio-basal aspect of the hemisphere, is thinner and consists of three cell layers [12]. The limbic lobe can be defined on developmental terms as including all the non-isocortical regions of the cerebral mantle [13]. It thus encompasses the olfactory and hippocampal allocortex, the transitional cortex of the parahippocampal and cingulate gyri, and insular, orbitofrontal, and temporo-polar cortices as well as the cortical-like laterobasal and cortical amygdala [13]. These regions can be divided into a central limbic core and a surrounding belt. The central core consists of the allocortex of the hippocampus and prepiriform-periamygdaloid region and of subcortical amygdaloid and septal gray matter. The transitional (mesocortical) limbic belt includes the cingulate and parahippocampal gyri, which form a continuous semicircular convolution around the corpus callosum; the gyrus fornicatus [4].

Originally described by Chrisfried Jakob [15], the so-called circuit of Papez [16] connects the hippocampus via the fornices to the mamillary bodies of the caudal hypothalamus (Fig. 12.2). The loop continues via the mamillothalamic tract to the anterior nuclei of the thalamus; via the thalamocingulate fasciculus to the cingulate gyrus, via the cingulate fasciculus to the parahippocampal gyrus and the piriform area of the temporal lobe; and from there via the perforant tract of Cajal back to the hippocampus (Ammon's horn).

The hippocampus proper or cornu ammonis (Ammon's horn) is classically divided into tangential sectors CA1, CA2, CA3, and CA4 after Lorente de No [4] (Fig. 12.3). Recent high-resolution DWIs with 1 mm isotropic voxels averaged over 128 diffusion directions showed excellent anatomic detail of the hippocampal architecture including its subregions and reported increased MD and low FA of the stratum lacunosum moleculare in the deep cornu ammonis [17] (Fig. 12.4).

The radiologic evaluation of the pathologic limbic lobe is facilitated by the ability of MRI to distinguish the signal of allocortical (hippocampus and amygdala) and mesocortical (parahippocampus and cingulate gyri) limbic regions, which exhibit higher FLAIR and DWI signal compared with the isocortex [18–20] (Fig. 12.5). The increased DWI signal of the paralimbic cortices

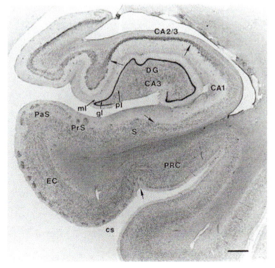

Fig. 12.3 Coronal section from a normal right rostral hippocampus stained with thionin. Arrows at borders between regions. *CA1* and *CA2/3* refer to the CA fields of the hippocampus. *DG* dentate gyrus, *ml* molecular layer of the dentate gyrus, *gl* granule cell layer, *pl* polymorphic layer, *S* subiculum, *PrS* presubiculum, *PaS* parasubiculum, *EC* entorhinal cortex, *cs* collateral sulcus, *PRC* perirhinal cortex. Scale bar, 1 mm. Nancy L. Rempel-Clower et al. J. Neurosci. 1996;16:5233–5255

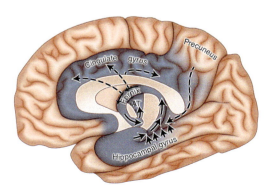

Fig. 12.2 The circuit of Papez in Paul Mac Lean's concept of the limbic system [14]. *M* mammillary body, *AT* anterior thalamic nuclei

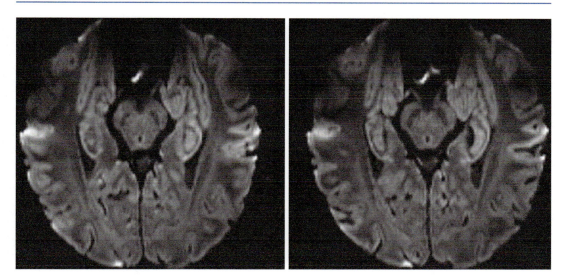

Fig. 12.4 Mean diffusion-weighted images with 1 mm isotropic spatial resolution acquired in 6 min for a healthy 30-year-old male. From Treit et al., Neuroimage 2018 [17]

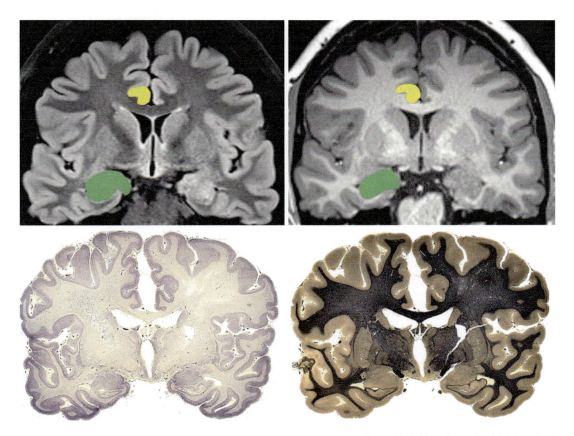

Fig. 12.5 Coronal, sagittal, and axial MRI (FLAIR, T1, and TRACE diffusion) outlining the amygdalo-hippocampal region (green) and cingulate gyrus (yellow) and corresponding cell (left) and myelin (right) stained slices, modified from the Yakovlev collection (http://neurosciencelibrary.org/index.html)

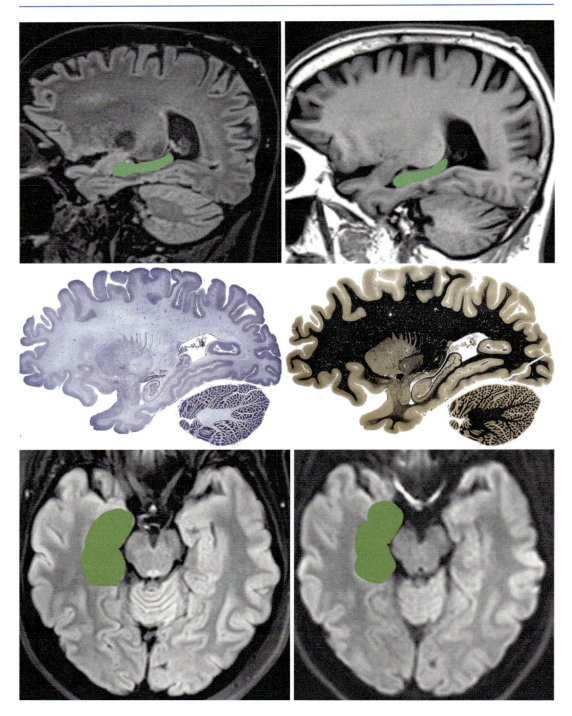

Fig. 12.5 (continued)

12 Epilepsy

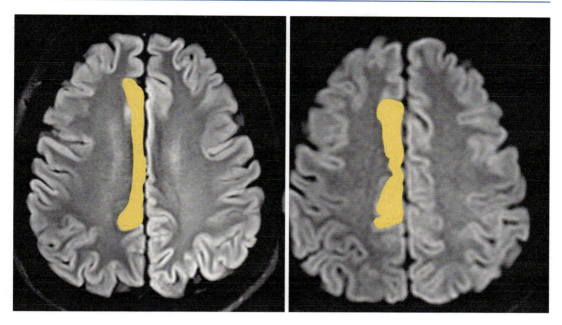

Fig. 12.5 (continued)

of the cingulate and insula is associated with ADC values similar to those of the cortex of the middle frontal gyrus and is thought to result from prolonged T2 relaxation [20].

12.5 Hippocampal Malrotation (HIMAL)

HIMAL refer to an atypical appearance of the hippocampus with abnormal medial location along the choroid fissure, round hippocampal shape on the coronal plane and verticalization of the collateral sulcus (Fig. 12.6). HIMAL results from incomplete infolding of mesial temporal structures, and its appearance is similar to the fetal hippocampus at gestation age 14–20 weeks. HIMAL is present in up to 24% of normal controls [21], therefore represents a common anatomic variant rather than a pathologic finding.

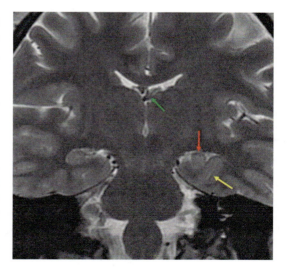

Fig. 12.6 Left HIMAL. Note round shape of the left hippocampus (red arrow), vertical orientation of the collateral sulcus (yellow arrow) and lower position of the left fornix (green arrow). Modified from Dr. Derek Smith, Radiopaedia.org, rID: 56216

12.6 MR Imaging of Epilepsy Substrates

The characterization and localization of the epileptogenic lesion are the first objectives of imaging in epilepsy. This is particularly relevant in surgical candidates. The identification of functionally relevant cortical areas and white matter tracts is also typically performed as part of the preoperative assessment of refractory epilepsy patients.

Cortical dysplasia is the most frequent histopathologic epilepsy substrate in children under 18 years of age that undergo epilepsy surgery, followed by tumors, atrophic lesions, and hippocampal sclerosis [22]. In adults, hippocampal sclerosis is the most common pathologic substrate, followed by tumors and cortical dysplasia.

12.6.1 Hippocampal Sclerosis (HS)

Temporal lobe epilepsy (TLE) is the most common form of drug-resistant epilepsy and most frequently presents on neuropathology examination and neuroimaging with ipsilateral HS. HS, also known as mesial temporal sclerosis (MTS), is the histopathological hallmark of TLE and the most common underlying etiology of refractory epilepsy in adults. It is characterized by neuronal loss and astrocytic gliosis in the hippocampal formation. Since early pathological descriptions [23], it has been recognized that the cornu ammonis (CA) subfields, with the exception of CA2, and the dentate gyrus (DG) present marked neuronal depletion in HS. The imaging correlates of HS are atrophy, prolonged T2 relaxation and blurring of the hippocampal architecture. Hippocampal atrophy on imaging correlates with pathological grades of hippocampal cell loss [24], while high T2 signal relates to glial cell count, particularly in the dentate gyrus [25] (Fig. 12.7).

When imaging findings coincide with electrophysiologic localization, patients with medically refractory epilepsy have an approximately 70% chance of becoming seizure free after resection of the seizure focus [26]. On the other hand, approximately 30% of drug-resistant TLE patients have normal brain MRIs, and have poorer surgical outcomes compared to TLE with HS [27], while a positive brain MRI carries favorable prognosis of postoperative seizure control. Furthermore, MRI-negative TLE patients frequently require invasive electrophysiologic evaluations, which carry significant morbidity, to localize the seizure focus preoperatively.

HS patients have higher ADC values in the ipsilateral vs. contralateral mesial temporal lobe as well as compared to controls [28], suggesting structural disorganization with expansion of the extracellular space. This, in turn, may be secondary to neuronal loss, reduction of dendritic branching, and astrocytic gliosis associated with epileptogenesis [28–30]. Mean diffusivity (MD) is the most significant MRI predictor of neuronal density other than hippocampal volume, being negatively correlated with neuronal density in HS [31]. TLE patients had significantly altered tissue diffusion characteristics of the ipsilateral temporal lobe inferior-longitudinal, uncinate, and superior longitudinal fasciculi and cingulum relative to controls. Furthermore, diffusion alterations of ipsilateral temporal lobe tracts were significantly related to age at onset of epilepsy, duration of epilepsy, and epilepsy burden [32]. Patients with intractable temporal lobe epilepsy and unilateral hippocampal sclerosis have bilateral reduction of the cingulum association fibers projecting from the cingulate gyrus to the parahippocampal gyrus as measured with DTI [33].

Apart from white matter abnormalities within the affected temporal lobe and limbic lobe, DTI studies in TLE with HS have also shown changes involving the extra-temporal and contralateral white matter [29]. HS patients displayed decreased fractional anisotropy (FA) and increased MD and radial diffusivity (RD) in the anterior, mid-posterior, and posterior segments of the corpus callosum, with more significant changes in patients with history of febrile seizures [34]. Combining FA values in the corpus callosum, cingulate bundle and fornix, correct lateralization of the seizure focus was obtained in all of 31 TLE patients [35].

12 Epilepsy

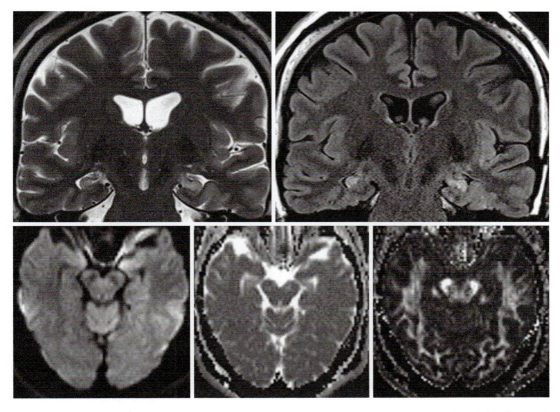

Fig. 12.7 Bilateral MTS. Characteristic imaging on coronal T2 and FLAIR images (top) and axial DWI, ADC map and FA map (bottom). FLAIR shows best the hippocampal hyperintensity

12.6.2 Amygdala Enlargement (AE)

AE as defined on brain MRI ipsilateral to the seizure focus has recently been found in a putatively different subtype of non-lesional mesial temporal lobe epilepsy (mTLE) [36–42]. Originally, AE was recognized in "imaging negative" mTLE using amygdala volumetry [41]. Radiologically, the abnormal side displays subtle expansion of the uncus of the temporal lobe with T2 hyperintensity with ill-defined borders that blend with the adjacent normal brain (Fig. 12.8). However, no significant differences in ADC were seen between the amygdalae of AE patients and controls [43]. Pathologic findings in AE include dysplasia with hypertrophic, clustered neurons, and/or astrocytic gliosis [38]. Both pathologic and imaging findings suggest wider involvement of the anterior hippocampus, amygdala, temporal pole, and adjacent temporal isocortex, key components of the limbic network involved in mTLE [44].

12.6.3 Malformations of Cortical Development (MCD)

The ILAE classification of malformations of cortical development is based primarily on histopathology, not imaging [45]. It recognizes three types: FCD type I refers to isolated lesions, with either radial (FCD Ia) or tangential (FCD Ib) architectural dyslamination of the neocortex. FCD type II is an isolated lesion characterized by cortical dyslamination and dysmorphic neurons without (type IIa) or with balloon cells (type IIb). Under type III are listed instances of combined (dual) pathology where dysplastic lesions appear in association with HS, tumors, vascular lesions, or epileptogenic lesions acquired in early life.

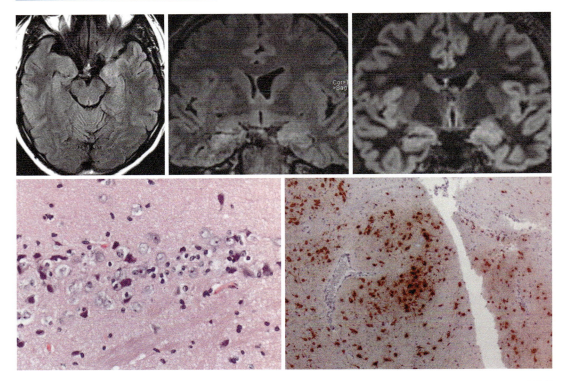

Fig. 12.8 AE. 26-year-old man with left temporal lobe epilepsy. FLAIR and double inversion recovery (DIR) images (top) showing subtle expansion and hyperintensity of the left uncus. Clustered, dystrophic neurons on H&E (bottom left) and Neu-N (bottom right) stains

Type IIb dysplasias are more commonly positive on MRI than other dysplasia types, presenting with white-gray matter junction blurring [46] and the transmantle sign best demonstrated on FLAIR images [47] (Fig. 12.9).

Patients with MCD have significant reductions of FA, with increase in MD and perpendicular diffusivity in all segments of the corpus callosum as compared to controls. This finding suggests that patients with epilepsy secondary to MCD present widespread white matter changes that extend beyond the macroscopic MRI-visible lesions [48].

12.6.4 Brain Tumors Associated with Epilepsy

The term LEATs ("long-term epilepsy-associated tumors") encompasses those CNS tumors that manifest mainly by early-onset epilepsy. The majority of LEATs are represented by gangliogliomas (GG) and dysembryoplastic neuroepithelial tumors (DNT), followed by rarer entities. While rare among all CNS neoplasms, LEATs are frequent as cause of pharmacoresistant focal seizures [49]. DNTs (Fig. 12.10) are pediatric and young adult benign brain tumors which display very high ADC values (mean ADC value of 1.62 mm^2/s), significantly higher than other epileptogenic lesions such as focal cortical dysplasia or GG [50]. The minimum ADC value of GG, on the other hand, was significantly higher than that of low- or high-grade astrocytomas (mean ADC of GG of 1.45 mm^2/s) [51].

Limbic and paralimbic tumors were recognized by Yaşargil [52], who proposed a classification thereof into *mediobasal temporal* involving the amygdala, hippocampus, or parahippocampus gyrus (Figs. 12.11 and 12.12), *insular-temporo-opercular*,

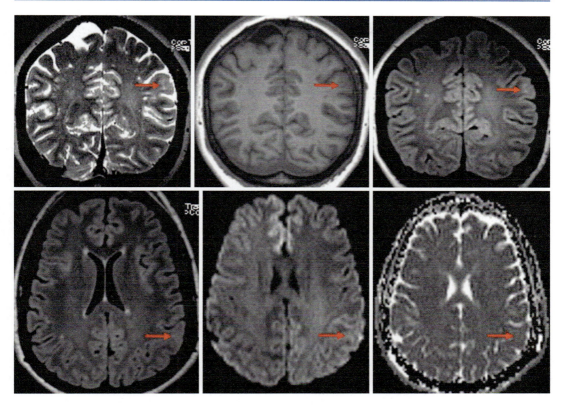

Fig. 12.9 Type IIb cortical dysplasia. 44-year-old female with epilepsy for 30 years. Left parietal focal blurring of the gray/white matter interphase on coronal T2 (top left), T1 (top center) and FLAIR (top right) and axial FLAIR (bottom left) images. DWI (bottom center) and ADC map (bottom right) with facilitated diffusion

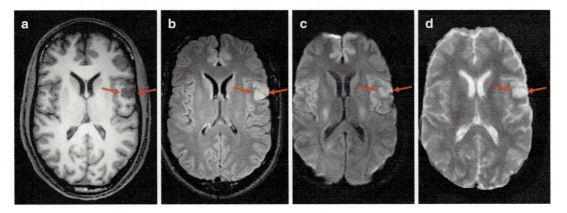

Fig. 12.10 DNT in a 24-year old man with seizures. Left frontal cortical-based lesion (arrows) hypointense on T1 (**a**) and hyperintense on FLAIR (**b**). Trace DWI (**c**) and ADC map (**d**) reveal facilitated diffusion with ADC measured at 1.16 mm^2/s

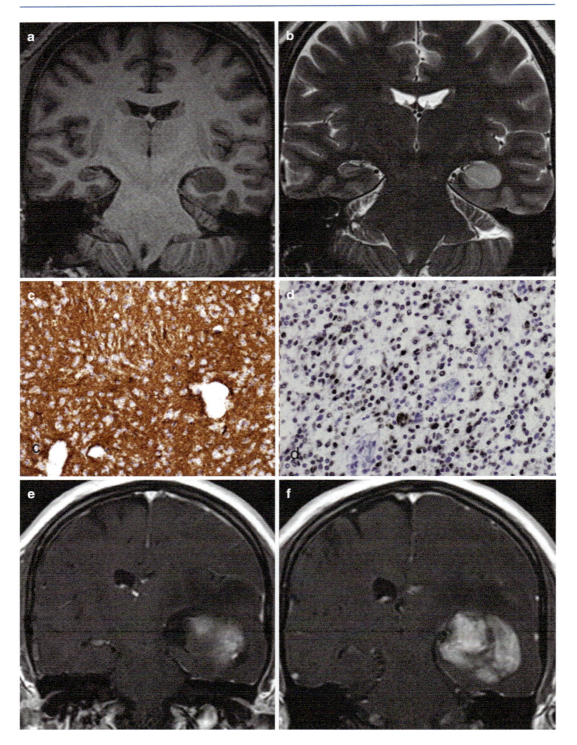

Fig. 12.11 Left hippocampal tumor in a 36-year-old man with seizures (**a**, **b**). Intensely positive synaptophysin stain (**c**), and positive NeuN stain (**d**) in this atypical extraventricular neurocytoma. Postcontrast T1-weighted images (**e**, **f**) 25 months later with marked tumor growth

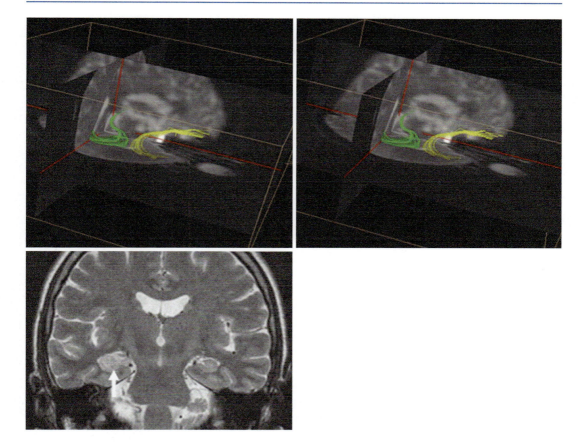

Fig. 12.12 Glioma in the hippocampus in a 66-year-old woman. *Bottom:* Coronal T2-weighted image show a focal hyperintense mass lesion in the right hippocampus (*arrow*). *Top:* DT imaging tractography images (stereo view) demonstrate the relationship between the tumor and uncinate fasciculus (*yellow*) and optic radiation (*green*). The uncinate fasciculus and optic radiation appear to be kissing at the temporal stem. (Courtesy of Toshiaki Taoka, MD, PhD)

fronto-orbital anterior insular-temporopolar, and *cingulate* tumors. The majority of patients with limbic and paralimbic tumors have epilepsy and have a more than 80% chance of becoming seizure-free after tumor resection [52]. Furthermore, limbic tumor has stereotyped patterns of tumor growth following white matter bundles [53].

Diffusion tensor tractography DTI is also used for presurgical planning of refractory TLE cases treated with anterior temporal lobectomy (ATL). DTI demonstrates the relationship between the target lesion and relevant fiber tracts such as the corticospinal tract, uncinate fasciculus, and optic radiation (Fig. 12.12), which is useful in preoperative planning. In particular, the Meyer's loop is the anterior bundle of the optic radiation which sweeps back on itself lateral to the temporal horn. Visual field defects after ATL cause denser medial than lateral deficits, and when the lateral sector is spared it leads to an incomplete superior quadrantanopia. DTI of the Meyer's loop before ATL may reduce the risk for postoperative visual field defect [54]. DTI can predict the risk of postoperative field cut when the anterior limit of the Meyer's loop is 35 mm or less from the temporal pole [55].

12.7 MR Imaging of Seizure Activity

On routine MRI, signal alterations related to postictal status can be misdiagnosed as infarctions, tumors, inflammatory, or demyelinating diseases. This may occur because routine MR sequences will not distinguish vasogenic edema from cytotoxic edema. Such misdiagnoses may result in unnecessary invasive treatments. DWI is helpful in evaluating postictal encephalopathy, as it will detect cytotoxic edema and can differentiate between cytotoxic and vasogenic edema in ictal and postictal lesions of the brain. Variable MR findings have been reported in the brain in the ictal or postictal stage [56, 57]. These findings include transient increase in T2 signal and swelling of the cerebral cortex, subcortical white matter and medial temporal lobe (including hippocampus), thalamus (anterior, medial dorsal thalamic nuclei, pulvinar), fornix, claustrum, and cerebellar hemispheres (Figs. 12.13, 12.14, and 12.15). The medial pulvinar of the thalamus has rich and reciprocal connections with the temporal lobe cortex [58] and is involved in the maintenance and propagation of epileptic seizures (corticothalamic coupling or thalamocortical synchrony through epileptogenic networks), hence the frequent association of postictal DWI hyperintensity in this location particularly after status epilepticus [59, 60]. Despite the ability of DWI to show postictal cytotoxic edema, the localization value of this findings in TLE has been limited in clinical practice [61]. Postictal cortical or subcortical lesions can be uni- or bilateral, and they are predominantly found in the fronto-parietal regions. Whether peri-ictal lesions are reversible or irreversible on MRI seems to depend on the duration and/or severity of the seizures.

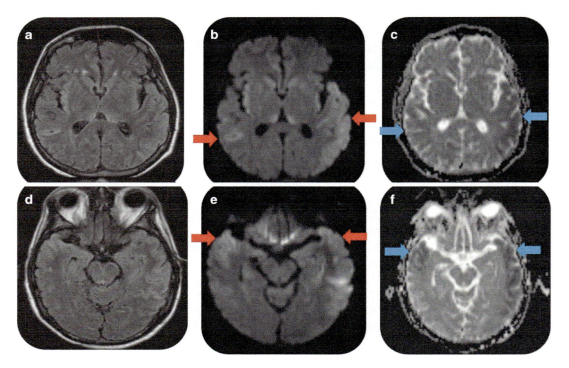

Fig. 12.13 Postictal changes after tonic–clonic seizure in patient with Cryptococcus meningitis. Axial FLAIR (**a**, **d**), DWI (**b**, **e**) and ADC map (**c**, **f**). High DWI signal in lateral temporal cortex and posterior thalami (**b**, **e**) with matching low ADC values (**c**, **f**), *arrows*

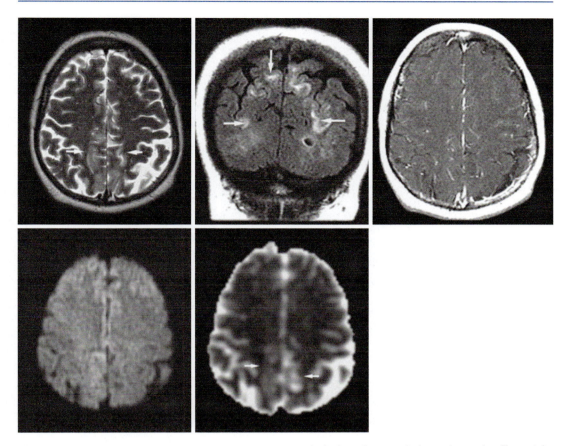

Fig. 12.14 Postictal encephalopathy lesion following partial seizure in a 64-year-old woman with generalized seizure secondary to hyperglycemia. *Top left:* T2-weighted image 24 h after seizures shows hyperintense lesions in bilateral medial fronto-parietal cortex (*arrows*). *Top center:* Coronal FLAIR image also shows cortical and subcortical hyperintense lesions (*arrows*). *Top right:* Gadolinium-enhanced T1-weighted image shows no abnormal enhancement. *Bottom left:* DW image shows these lesions as isointense with increased ADC *Bottom right:* (*arrows*), representing vasogenic edema

12.7.1 Ictal Stage to Peri-ictal Stage

During a seizure, there is an increase in metabolism with higher oxygen and glucose consumption in the seizure focus. This hypermetabolic state results in consumptive hypoxia, hypercarbia, and lactic acidosis, which impair vascular autoregulation in the affected areas of the cortex, leading to vasogenic edema and disruption of the blood–brain barrier [57]. If the seizures are not too prolonged, the peri-ictal brain lesions will only show transient T2 hyperintensity, mainly representing vasogenic edema. However, if the seizures are severe or prolonged, cytotoxic edema can develop, which usually results in cortical and/or subcortical white matter hyperintensity on DW imaging associated with decreased ADC [62]. This is often seen in patients with generalized tonic–clonic seizure or status epilepticus (Figs. 12.16 and 12.17). Whether these lesions show enhancement or not depends on the degree of blood–brain barrier disruption. Vasogenic edema in peri-ictal brain lesions has variable signal intensity on DW imaging, which is associated with an increase in ADC.

Fig. 12.15 Postictal lesion involving the pulvinar of the thalamus with intraparenchymal hemorrhage in a 65-year-old man. *Top left:* T2-weighted image shows a subacute phase hemorrhage in the left temporoparietal cortex. Mild hyperintensity is noted in the ipsilateral pulvinar of the thalamus *(arrow)*. *Top right:* DW image shows the left pulvinar lesion as hyperintense associated with decreased ADC *(bottom left)* and slightly decreased FA *(bottom right)*. The hemorrhage is very high on the DW image with decreased ADC and partially increased FA (**d**). (Courtesy of Edip Gurol, MD)

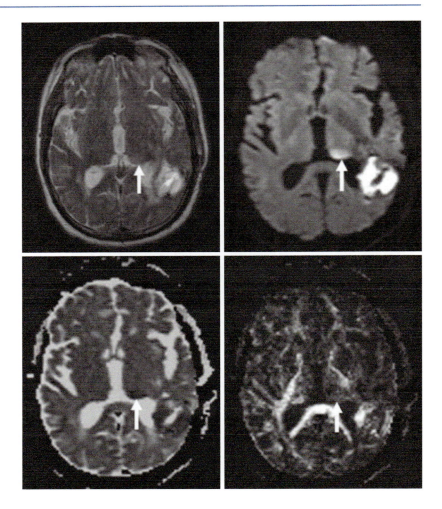

12.8 Status Epilepticus (SE)

Status epilepticus is defined as continuous seizure activity that lasts longer than 30 min, or two or more sequential seizures that together last longer than 30 min and without full recovery of consciousness between the seizure attacks [63]. Convulsive status epilepticus is an emergency and therefore should be treated aggressively, as the mortality associated with status epilepticus is about 8% in children and 30% in adults [63, 64]. Furthermore, febrile status epilepticus is a known cause of HS in children [65]. In status epilepticus, neuronal injury is thought to result primarily from an excitotoxic mechanism mediated by neuronal seizure activity. This is supported by the effect of kainic acid (an excitotoxic analog of glutamate), as shown in animal studies [66, 67]. Seizure activity increases the release of glutamate from the pre-synaptic terminal. The released glutamate crosses the synaptic cleft to bind to NMDA receptors of the postsynaptic neurons, resulting in cytotoxic edema.

12.8.1 Cytotoxic Edema in Status Epilepticus

Cytotoxic edema following status epilepticus can be at least partially reversible [57], as compared to cerebral ischemia, where these changes are usually irreversible. In cerebral ischemia, a significant compromise of blood supply leads to irreversible

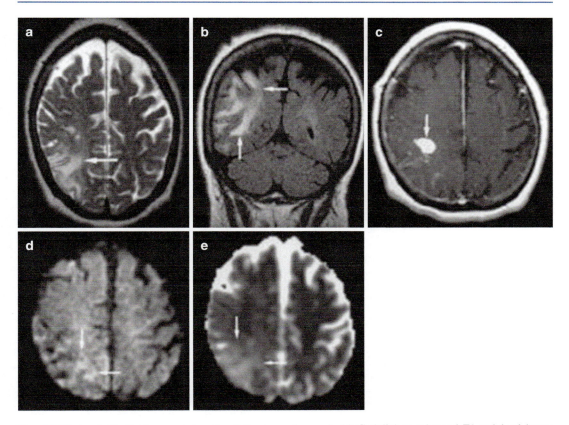

Fig. 12.16 (**a–e**) Postictal encephalopathy following partial seizures with or without secondary generalization in a 75-year-old woman. (**a**) T2-weighted image at 4 days after seizures shows hyperintense lesions in the right fronto-parietal region (*arrow*). (**b**) Coronal FLAIR image shows cortical and subcortical hyperintense lesions (*arrows*). (**c**) Gadolinium-enhanced T1-weighted image shows a densely enhancing nodule (*arrow*) and leptomeningeal enhancement (**d**) DW image shows these lesions as isointense to slightly hyperintense (*arrows*), with increased ADC (*arrows*) (**e**). Brain biopsy was performed and proved the lesions to be acute ischemic changes

failure of energy metabolism. In sustained seizures, there is increased cerebral metabolism with matched increase in cerebral blood flow. This will maintain the energy state of the neuron provided there is sufficient oxygen supply.

The regions of the human brain that are most vulnerable to excitotoxicity include the hippocampus (specifically the CA1 and CA3 fields, and the hilus), amygdala, pyriform cortex, thalamus, cerebellum, and cerebral cortex. NMDA receptors are predominantly located in the CA1 of the hippocampus [4] and layers 3 and 4 in the cerebral cortex [68, 69]. The Purkinje cell loss of the cerebellum, seen in severe epilepsy, may be explained by an increased demand for inhibition, resulting in GABA depletion and subsequent influx of calcium into neurons [70]. Unilateral cerebellar hemispheric involvement is occasionally seen in status epilepticus.

Transient and reversible MR signal changes have been reported in patients following status epilepticus [57, 59, 62, 71] (Figs. 12.18, 12.19, and 12.20). On the other hand, other lesions have been proven irreversible, resulting in selective neuronal necrosis, gliosis, and delayed neuronal death with subsequent atrophy and development of mesial temporal sclerosis [72–74] (Fig. 12.21).

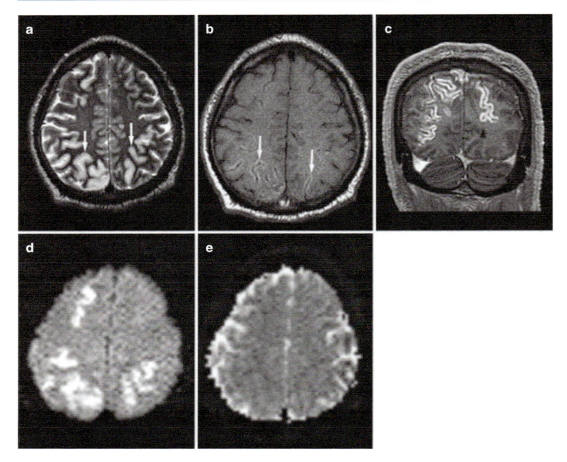

Fig. 12.17 Postictal encephalopathy following generalized tonic–clonic seizure in a 42-year-old man with alcohol withdrawal. (**a**) T2-weighted image shows hyperintense lesions (*arrows*) in bilateral fronto-parietal cortex. (**b**) T1-weighted image 8 days after the seizure shows gyriform high signal intensity in these lesions, representing cortical laminar necrosis (*arrows*). (**c**) Coronal gadolinium-enhanced T1-weighted image shows gyriform enhancement of these lesions. (**d**) DW image shows corresponding regions of hyperintensity. (**e**) ADC map shows almost normal ADC values of these lesions, suggesting a subacute phase of ischemia

Diffusion-weighted imaging and ADC maps are more sensitive than conventional MR imaging to show both gray and white matter involvement, and discriminate between cytotoxic and vasogenic edema following status epilepticus [57, 59, 60, 62, 65, 71, 75]. In experimental status epilepticus models, ADC decrease was first seen at about 3 h and lasted until 48 h after the onset of seizures, after which time it normalized or even increased [76, 77]. The definite time course of DW imaging changes in humans is unknown, but the signal abnormalities on DW imaging and ADC are seen in cytotoxic edema following status epilepticus, which are sometimes reversible, as mentioned above [57]. Over 25% of SE patients had peri-ictal DWI restriction and had a consistent EEG pattern characterized by periodic lateralized epileptiform discharges and intermittent seizure patterns [71]. Furthermore, patients with peri-ictal diffusion restriction had more often impairment of consciousness compared to those without it.

12 Epilepsy

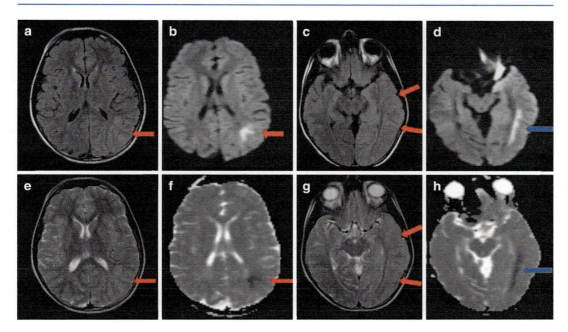

Fig. 12.18 12-year-old post SE 1 week before. Left temporo-occipital gyral thickening on FLAIR (**a, c, e, g**, arrows) and high DWI signal in the subcortical white matter (**b, d**, arrows) with corresponding low ADC (**f, h**) consistent with intramyelinic cytotoxic edema

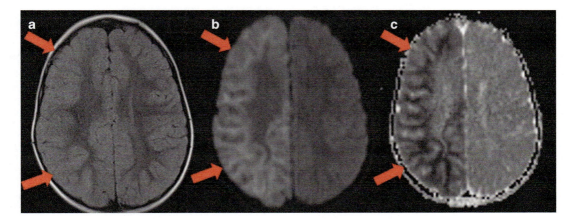

Fig. 12.19 3-year-old female with SE with right hemispheric subcortical white matter restricted diffusion (arrows). Axial FLAIR (**a**), DWI (**b**) and ADC map (**c**)

12.9 Acute Encephalopathy with Biphasic Seizures and Late Reduced Diffusion (AESD)

AESD is a recently described encephalopathy subtype, which is characterized by biphasic seizures and disturbances of consciousness in the acute stage, followed by restricted diffusion in the subcortical white matter in the subacute stage, finally resulting in cerebral atrophy and development of post-encephalopathy epilepsy [78] (Fig. 12.22). AESD is a leading cause of convulsive encephalopathy among children in Japan. Although the exact pathogenesis of AESD is uncertain, the etiology of AESD has been attributed to viral and bac-

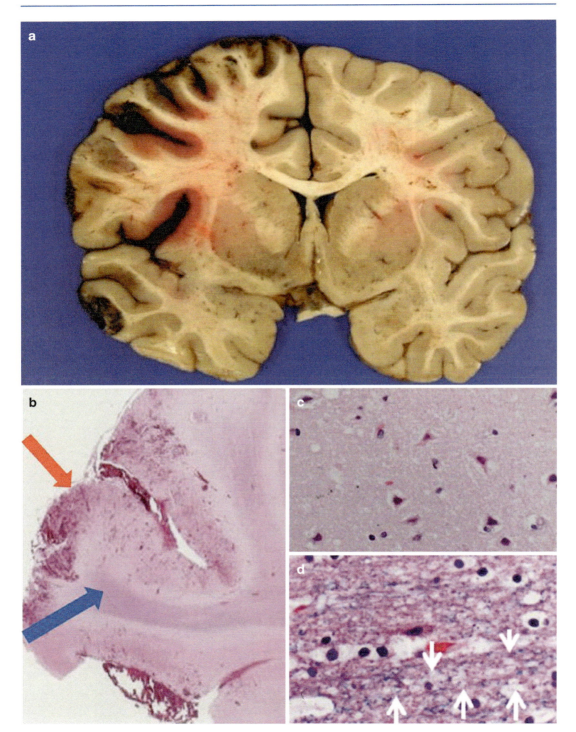

Fig. 12.20 The patient died from brain herniation. Macroscopic coronal brain cut view shows right frontal cortical and subcortical hemorrhage and edema (**a**, **b**). Microscopic assessment of H&E stain of the involved cortex (**c**) shows necrotic neurons. Subcortical white matter (**d**) with spongiform changes and intramyelinic edema (arrows)

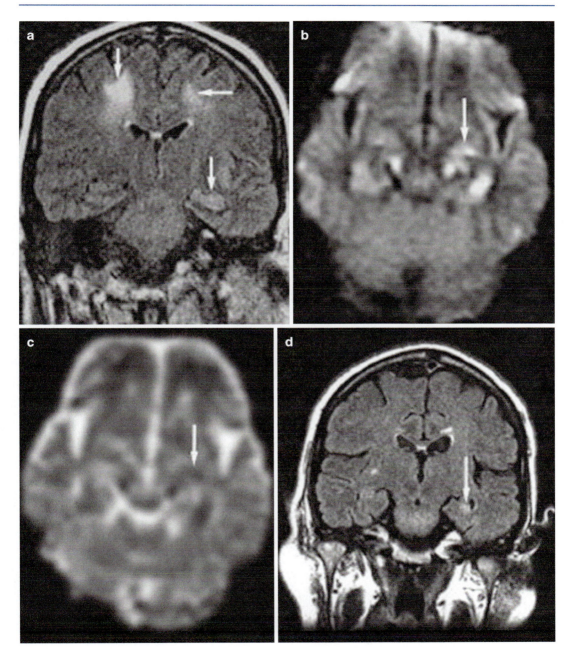

Fig. 12.21 Hippocampal lesion following status epilepticus in a 55-year-old man with prolonged seizures associated with tacrolimus toxicity. (**a**) FLAIR image at 2 days after seizure shows high signal areas in the bilateral frontal deep white matter and the left hippocampus (*arrows*). (**b**) DW image (*y axis*) shows high signal in the left hippocampus (*arrow*). (**c**) ADC (*y axis*) shows low signal intensity (*arrow*) consistent with cytotoxic edema. (**d**) Seven-month follow-up coronal FLAIR image shows the resolution of white matter changes and residual high signal intensity with atrophy in the left hippocampus (*arrow*)

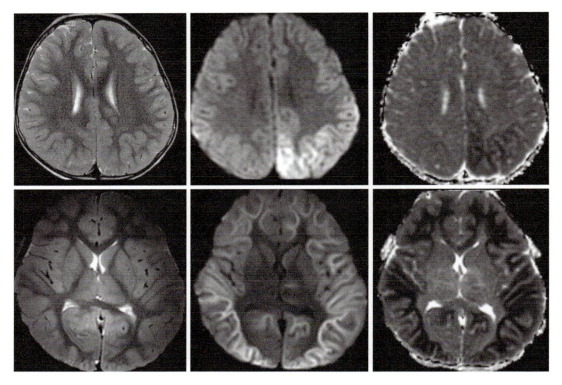

Fig. 12.22 4 y/o male with status epilepticus and MRI changes on presentation (top) and 17 days later (bottom) with delayed, subcortical white matter restricted diffusion consistent with AESD. Axial T2 (left), DWI (center) and ADC map (right)

terial infections [79]. Excitotoxic neuronal damage is thought to play a significant role in the pathogenesis of AESD, and elevation of glutamate signal on MRS was seen during the subacute phase of the condition [80]. CSF tau levels increase from day 3 of the disease between the initial and the secondary seizures and may hence represent a sensitive biomarker of axonal damage in AESD [81]. The main differential diagnosis of AESD is complex febrile seizure in the early phase [82].

12.10 Hemiconvulsion-Hemiplegia Epilepsy Syndrome and Rasmussen Encephalitis

Hemiconvulsion-hemiplegia epilepsy (HHE) syndrome is one of the recognized sequela of convulsive status epilepticus in infancy and early childhood. Main features are as follows: (1) Prevalent before 4 years of age; (2) prolonged seizures with unilateral predominance; and (3) sequelae of hemi-convulsion and hemiparesis [83, 84]. It is thought to represent a rare complication of febrile childhood seizures [85]. MR imaging shows signal abnormalities in the entire hemisphere. DW imaging shows diffuse cytotoxic edema confined to one hemisphere (Fig. 12.23).

Rasmussen encephalitis, characterized by seizures, progressive hemiplegia, and psychomotor deterioration is a chronic progressive inflammation of childhood of unknown etiology. The cardinal symptoms are progressive neurological deficits and intractable seizures, often in the form of epilepsia partialis continua and recurring status epilepticus [86]. Glutamate receptor 3 (GluR3) autoimmunity, associated with persistent viral infection has been proposed as a cause [87]. Diagnosis is confirmed by pathology, showing laminar spongiform degeneration, perivascular

12 Epilepsy

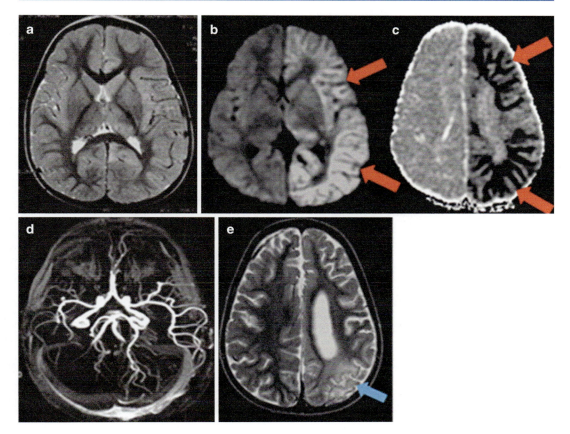

Fig. 12.23 Hemiplegic hemiconvulsion epilepsy syndrome in a 2-year-old girl with partial status epilepticus involving the right face and hand. (**a**) T2-weighted image 24 h after seizure shows diffuse cortical hyperintense lesions in the entire left cerebral hemisphere, including the basal ganglia, and thalamus (anterior and medial area, pulvinar). (**b**) DW image shows diffuse left-sided cortical and subcortical hyperintense lesions with decreased ADC (*arrows*) (**c**), representing cytotoxic edema. (**d**) MR angiography reveals dilatation of the left middle cerebral and posterior cerebral artery branches representing hyperperfusion. (**e**) Diffuse atrophy with ventricular dilatation and hyperintense lesions in the left hemisphere seen on 5-month follow-up T2-weighted image

T-cell lymphocyte cuffing, neuronal loss, gliosis, and microglial nodules. MR imaging shows T2 prolongation and progressive atrophy in the affected regions of the brain often involving the holohemisphere predominating in the perisylvian region with T2 hyperintensity including the basal ganglia (Fig. 12.24) [88, 89]. DW imaging usually shows increased ADC values [90] in the hemispheric lesion, but may show partially restricted diffusion areas [91, 92]. Adolescent and adult-onset RE cases have more recently been described, with better outcome and favorable response to immunomodulatory treatment [93].

12.11 Limbic Encephalitis

Paraneoplastic limbic encephalitis affecting the temporal lobe and limbic structures was first described by the British neuropathologist Corsellis in 1968 after identifying chronic inflammatory changes in the mesial temporal lobes of lung cancer patients with progressive memory loss [94]. Limbic encephalitis is an increasingly recognized cause of acute or subacute onset of confusion, temporal lobe seizures, short-term memory loss, and psychiatric symptoms [95]. Limbic encephalitis is now known to be a rela-

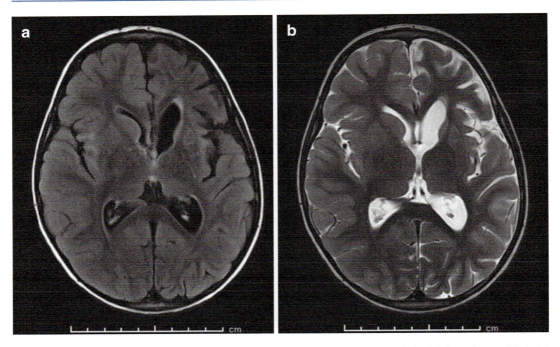

Fig. 12.24 Rasmussen encephalitis in a 5-year-old with refractory seizures and right-sided weakness. (**a**) Axial FLAIR, (**b**) Axial T2

tively frequent autoimmune encephalitis [96]. It is associated with various antibodies including paraneoplastic antibodies (Hu, Yo, Ri, Mal, Ma2, Cv2/CRMP5, Tr, amphiphysin) and non-paraneoplastic antibodies such as voltage-gated potassium channel (VGKC), N-methyl D-aspartate receptor (NMDAr) among others [97].

Antibody-mediated encephalitides can also be classified according to the location of their neuronal antigens with group I antibodies targeting intracellular antigens and group II antibodies targeting antigens on the cell surface [98]. Among group I, anti-Hu encephalitis is the most common paraneoplastic autoimmune encephalitis, has poor prognosis, and is associated with small-cell lung cancer in most cases [99]. Anti-Ma (Ma1/Ma2/Ma3) encephalitis has a better prognosis than anti-Hu and is strongly associated with testicular tumors in young men. Other group I entity is anti-glutamic acid decarboxylase (GAD) encephalitis, which is not typically associated with malignancy but is associated with other non-neoplastic autoimmune conditions such as type 1 diabetes. In group II, NMDAr encephalitis is one of the most common and best characterized autoimmune encephalitis classically seen in young women. Reported symptoms include psychiatric or cognitive impairment, speech dysfunction, seizures, dyskinesia, decreased consciousness, and autonomic dysfunction [100]. While no tumors are seen in males, ovarian teratomas were present in 56% of women older than 18 and 9% in girls of 14-year-old or younger [101]. Furthermore, it is increasingly recognized that a few weeks after HSV encephalitis, an immune reaction may trigger NMDAr encephalitis [102].

Also in group II, voltage-gated potassium channel (VGKC) encephalitis is one of the most common autoimmune encephalitis, which can demonstrate classic features of limbic encephalitis but is primarily defined by the early and prominent development of medically intractable epilepsy. More recently, two different entities were recognized within the VGKC group: anti-leucine-rich glioma-inactivated 1 (LGI1) and contactin-associated protein-like 2 (Caspr2) encephalitis. In anti-LGI1 encephalitis, faciobrachial dystonic seizures are highly specific, while patients also may have dyscognitive/autonomic or generalized seizures [103]. Caspr2

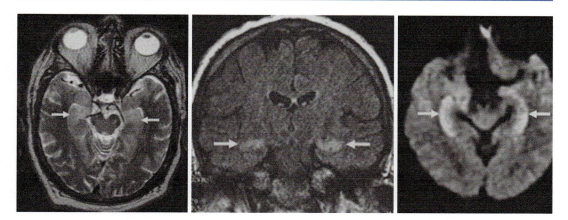

Fig. 12.25 Limbic encephalitis (non-paraneoplastic) in a 45-year-old woman. Axial T2-weighted (*left*) and coronal FLAIR (*center*) show hyperintense lesions in the bilateral hippocampi (*arrow*). DW image (*right*) shows these lesions as hyperintense (*arrows*) associated with slightly increased ADC (not shown)

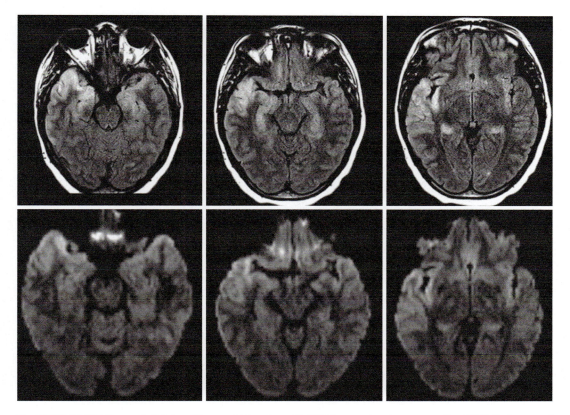

Fig. 12.26 NMDAR encephalitis in a 27-year-old female with poor outcome despite treatment with steroids and IVIG with delta brush on EEG. Presented with seizures, consciousness impairment, and left arm weakness. Axial FLAIR (top row) and corresponding DWI (bottom row) displaying right predominant temporo-insular and hippocampal hyperintesities

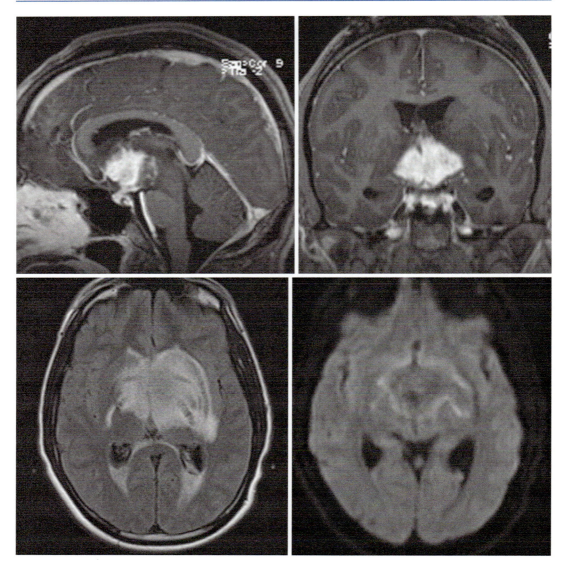

Fig. 12.27 Anti Ma2 encephalitis in 31-year-old man with mediastinal germinoma. Found unconscious with prior sleep abnormalities and hyponatremia. Biopsy showed classic demyelination changes in the diencephalon with foamy macrophages. Post-contrast T1 images (top row) and FLAIR (lower left) and TRACE DWI (lower right) showing involvement centered at the diencephalon. Note peripheral rim of high DWI signal

encephalitis is seen in more than 80% in males with cognitive dysfunction and/or seizures. Tumors are found in 10% of LGI1 and 20–30% of Caspr2 encephalitis [103].

On MRI, limbic encephalitis presents with T2 hyperintensity, best recognized on FLAIR, and enlargement of mesial temporal structures (Figs. 12.25 and 12.26). Anti-Ma2 encephalitis frequently involves the diencephalon (Fig. 12.27). VGKC encephalitis is followed by development of mesial temporal sclerosis in about half of the cases [104]. Among the latter, the majority had shown before contrast enhancement and/or restricted diffusion in the hippocampus. Imaging changes are otherwise frequently reversible. Apart from limbic T2 hyperintensity, mild contrast enhancement was reported in NMDAr and LGl1 encephalitides

[105]. Quantitative T2 prolongation of the amygdala and hippocampus was verified in probable and possible limbic encephalitis compared to controls and performed better than visual ratings [106]. Among NMDAr patients, MRI abnormalities have been reported only in 23–50% of the patients [105]. Using DTI, there is evidence of brain structural changes beyond the limbic lobe in immune-mediated encephalitis. In LGl1 encephalitis, DTI during follow-up showed widespread changes in the cerebral and cerebellar white matter, most prominent in the anterior corona radiata, capsula interna, and corpus callosum as well as global brain atrophy [107]. Furthermore, widespread changes of fractional anisotropy were seen in GAD-associated limbic encephalitis, whereas no changes were found in VGKC-complex-associated limbic encephalitis [108].

Neuropathologic features are dominant T-cell infiltration, neuronal loss, activated microglia, neuronophagia, and reactive astrocytosis. MR imaging contributes to the diagnosis by showing T2 and FLAIR high signal and swelling in the medial temporal lobe which is more often bilateral than unilateral. Contrast enhancement is rare. Significant atrophy is visible approximately 1 year after symptom onset with extralimbic involvement occasionally seen [105].

12.12 Focal Reversible Lesion of the Splenium of the Corpus Callosum

An stereotyped, ovoid, reversible DWI hyperintense lesion in the central portion of the splenium of the corpus callosum has been associated with different neurologic conditions, originally considered a peri-ictal phenomenon [109] (Figs. 12.28, 12.29, and 12.30). The cause of this focal lesion, however, is not known. It has been speculated to represent transient focal edema, related to the transhemispheric propagation of generalized seizure activity [109, 110]. Interhemispheric propagation of the seizure activity involves the splenial callosal fibers. The splenium contains fibers originating in the temporal lobe, which are likely to be involved in a secondarily generalized seizure. Furthermore, the lesion may be related to toxic effects of antiepileptic drugs such as phenytoin, carbamazepine, and vigabatrin [111]. Abrupt withdrawal and dose reduction of antiepileptic drugs may contribute to the transient edema, mediated by the influence of these drugs on fluid balance systems, namely arginine–vasopressin [112]. However, reversible splenial lesions are apparent in a wide spectrum of diseases and conditions, including infectious encephalitis/meningitis, encephalopathy, alcoholism and malnutrition, hypoglycemia, osmotic myelinolysis, trauma, medications (5-FU, metro-

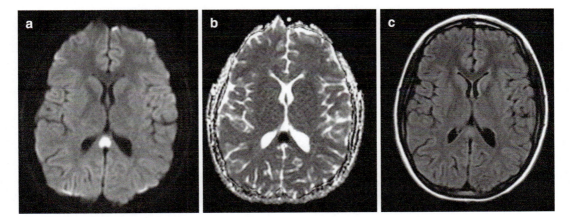

Fig. 12.28 12-year-old girl with 1-day history of intermittent blurry vision and dizziness. Patient was PCR positive for influenza virus. TRACE DWI (**a**), ADC map (**b**), and FLAIR (**c**)

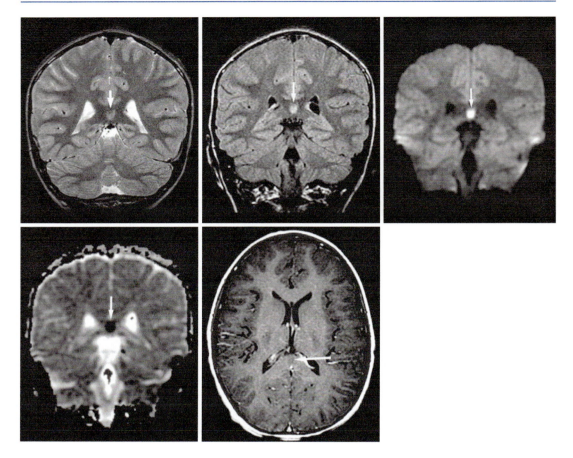

Fig. 12.29 Focal lesion in the splenium of the corpus callosum in epilepsy in a 9-year-old patient presenting with intractable partial seizures since the age of 4 years. Coronal T2-weighted (*top left*) and FLAIR (*top center*) images 3 days after seizure show a small round hyperintense lesion in the central portion of the splenium of the corpus callosum *(arrow)*. Coronal DW image (*top right*) shows this lesion *(arrow)* as hyperintense associated with decreased ADC (*bottom left*). Gadolinium-enhanced T1-weighted image reveals mild hypointense lesion with no abnormal enhancement (*bottom right, arrow*)

nidazole, IVIG), systemic lupus erythematosus, and leptomeningeal malignancy [110, 113–117]. The cause of the reversible splenial lesions should be related to more integrated mechanisms such as CNS cytokinopathy and excitotoxic mechanisms [110, 118–120]. The reason for the anatomic predilection for the splenium of the corpus callosum is unclear. It has been hypothesized to result from the high concentration of cytokine, glutamate, and drug receptors in the splenium [110], or be related to its relative lack of adrenergic tone, making it susceptible to hypoxic vasodilation and autoregulation failure [121].

Conventional MR imaging shows a non-hemorrhagic, hyperintense lesion on T2-weighted and FLAIR images, which is slightly hypointense on T1-weighted images. DW imaging shows an hyperintense lesion in the splenium of the corpus callosum, with decreased ADC. Three morphologic patterns of splenial lesion have been reported: small round or oval lesion in the center of the splenium, lesion centered in the splenium but extending laterally into the adjacent white matter, or a lesion centered in the splenium but extending into the anterior portion of the corpus callosum [110]. There is no enhancement after

12 Epilepsy

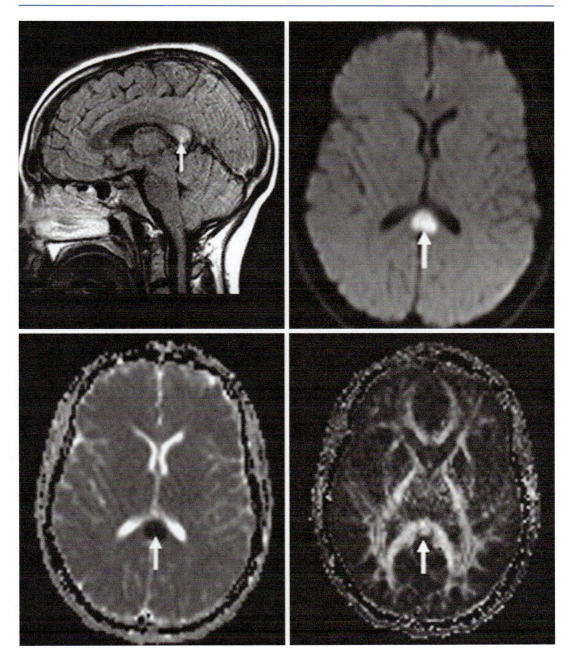

Fig. 12.30 Focal lesion in the splenium of the corpus callosum with intractable epilepsy in a 25-year-old patient. Sagittal FLAIR image *(top left)* shows hyperintense lesion in the splenium of the corpus callosum *(arrow)*. DW image *(top right)* shows an oval-shaped splenium lesion as hyperintense associated with decreased ADC *(bottom left)* and preserved normal FA values *(bottom right, arrow)*

administration of intravenous gadolinium. Fractional anisotropy (FA) map shows preserved FA values in the lesion. These findings indicate that the lesion represents cytotoxic edema in myelinated tracts (intramyelinic edema) in the corpus callosum. The lesion typically (although not always) resolves on follow-up imaging within 1 month without sequela [110, 120].

12.13 Conclusion

Routine MR imaging is widely used to evaluate various primary brain diseases that cause seizures as well as to evaluate patients with epilepsy. Seizures can be present with stroke, anoxic injury, trauma, tumor, infections, demyelination, congenital anomaly, and other causes. The typical MR finding in post-ictal patients is an area of T2 hyperintensity with restricted diffusion, often located in the cerebral cortex and hippocampus but also thalamus, subcortical white matter, and/or cerebellum. DW imaging can provide additional information concerning the brain edema and tell whether it is primarily cytotoxic or vasogenic. This is important since cytotoxic edema following seizures indicates a more serious injury and, although often reversible, may result in brain atrophy and necrosis.

12.14 Treatment of Epilepsy

Hiroto Kawasaki

12.14.1 Treatment

Epilepsy renders various disadvantages in daily life, for example, increased risks of injury, restriction in obtaining driver's license, and limitation in types of jobs patients can have. Sudden unexpected death in epilepsy (SUDEP) is another tremendous risk that occurs in about 1–2 per 100 epilepsy person-year [123]. These disadvantages warrant treatment of epilepsy, which includes seizure medications (anti-epileptic drugs (AEDs)), diet, and surgery. The first line of treatment is AEDs. Once epilepsy is diagnosed, treatment with single AED (monotherapy) is started [124]. Selection of AED is individualized according to various factors, such as type of seizures, comorbidities, age, and gender. AEDs have a variety of medical and

Table 12.3 [122]

Focal epilepsy	Focal and generalized epilepsy	Generalized epilepsy
Oxcarbazepine	Lamotrigine	Ethosuximide (absence seizures)
Carbamazepine	Levetiracetam	
Phenytoin	Valproate	
Eslicarbazepine	Topiramate	
Lacosamide	Zonisamide	
Gabapentin	Perampanel	
	Clobazam	
	Clonazepam	

psychiatric side effects. AEDs should be effective and well-tolerated. Table 12.3 summarizes commonly used AEDs and indications for focal, generalized, and both types of epilepsies. If the first AED does not work or is not well tolerated, then the first AED is replaced by the next AED or in some case a second AED may be added. Usually administering new AED give approximately 20% chance of suppression of seizures. Overall seizures can be controlled in 60–70% of epilepsy patients. However, if patients fail to respond to two AEDs, chance for their seizure symptoms being controlled with another AEDs is diminished progressively as the number of failed AEDs increases [122].

If patients have a prolonged seizure or are not conscious enough to take oral intake, AEDs may be administered through intravenous (benzodiazepines, levetiracetam, vimpat), intranasal (benzodiazepine), or rectal (benzodiazepine, levetiracetam, phenobarbital) routes. In case of status epilepticus general anesthetics such as propofol or barbiturate may be administered continuously through i.v. drip. In such situation, airway protection and respiration support are necessary because respiration is often suppressed by anti-seizure medications and also by the seizure.

12.14.2 Diet

Dietary therapy with low carbohydrate and high fat food, which is called ketogenic diet, has been used for many years [125–129]. Nearly half of patients experience at least 50% reduction of frequency of seizures. Ketogenic diet is usually pre-

12.14.3 Immunotherapy

Autoimmune mechanisms against components of the brain is considered to be involved in generation of seizures in many epilepsy patients [130]. Inflammation due to autoimmune reaction often causes encephalitis in the limbic system (limbic encephalitis), most typically in the medial temporal lobe, and also causes more diffuse cerebral encephalitis. Seizures are one of major symptoms of autoimmune encephalitis along with other symptoms such as memory impairment, behavioral changes, ataxia, and hemiparesis.

Paraneoplastic limbic encephalitis is associated with malignant tumors outside of the central nervous system [131]. Sometimes patients exhibit symptoms of encephalitis before the primary malignant disease is found. It is often seen in small cell lung cancer and also in a variety of other cancers such as thymoma, breast cancer, testicular cancer, or lymphoma. Treatment of underlying malignant disease may improve neurologic symptoms.

Many different antibodies causing autoimmune encephalitis were discovered, and the number of antibodies is increasing [130]. Some of them target ion components of ion channels, such as voltage-gated potassium channel, voltage-gated calcium channel, receptors, such as NMDA receptor and GABA-A receptor. Many of the encephalitis show limbic predilection and are often preceded by non-specific febrile illness. Antibodies can be found in the CSF. Firstline treatment is administration of steroids and IVIG; however, more aggressive treatment with immunosuppressant may be necessary [132]. Systemic autoimmune diseases can have cerebral involvement that cause seizures. Systemic lupus erythematosus, the antiphospholipid syndrome, and type 1 diabetes mellitus are most often associated with epilepsy.

12.14.4 Surgery

If non-surgical treatment is not effective, some patients may be treated with surgery [133]. There are several different types of surgical procedures. General principle of surgery is either, to remove seizure onset zone, to destroy/ablate seizure onset zone, or to disconnect seizure onset zones from rest of the brain.

Before surgical indication is determined, these patients undergo extensive presurgical epilepsy work up which includes detailed history of epilepsy, past, and current history of other diseases, genetic background or family history, social and academic background, observation of epilepsy symptoms, a brief EEG recording while patients are not having seizures and a long-term video EEG recording which ideally captures EEG during seizure (ictal EEG), magnetoencehalography (MEG) [134], brain MRI [135], brain metabolism study (PET or SPECT), neuropsychology evaluation, evaluation of language dominance, and memory reserve with Wada test [136] or functional MRI.

If results of these presurgical evaluations are all concordant to localize a single seizure onset zone, patients may be good candidates for the epilepsy surgery to surgically remove the seizure focus. The medial temporal epilepsy and epilepsy associated with a well-delineated lesion are examples of good indication [137]. If results of presurgical evaluations are not clearly conclusive, long-term video EEG monitoring with intracranial electrodes is conducted. Electrodes are surgically implanted over the surface of the brain with subdural strip and grid electrodes, or deep brain structures are covered with depth electrodes. Different types of electrodes are used separately or in combination. Subdural electrodes are placed with open craniotomy procedure. Depth electrodes can be placed with either open craniotomy or percutaneously [138, 139]. If video EEG recording can identify resectable seizure focus, the patient is eligible for the seizure focus removal surgery.

Removal of seizure onset zone is performed for focal epilepsy when the seizure onset zone is located in the surgically removable area, which means surgical resection of the seizure onset zone will not cause debilitating neurological deficit. Removal of a large area of brain tissue is performed in more severe epilepsy. Removal surgery is also performed when patients have well-delineated lesions such as brain tumor, cortical dysplasia, or vascular malformation, concurrently removing lesion and seizure onset zone [140].

Ablation is the surgical technique to destroy the seizure onset zone using thermocoagulation or radiation. Thermocoagulation ablates the brain tissue by heating. Heat is generated by either laser [141] or radiofrequency electric current. Laser is delivered through a thin fiberoptic probe, and radiofrequency electric current is delivered through an electrode, both of which are inserted toward the deep seizure onset zone using stereotactic navigation. They are minimally invasive approaches that would cause only a limited injury to the area around the seizure onset zone and track of the fiberoptic probe or the electrode. Radiation is delivered using focused radiation technology [142, 143]. Ablation is performed when a seizure onset zone is deep seated in the brain. In such case, open surgical access to the seizure onset zone may cause destruction of surrounding brain which would result in neurological deficit. MTLE, hypothalamic hamartoma, periventricular heterotopia, and subependymal tuber in tuberous sclerosis are representative cases that are indicated for ablation surgery.

Disconnection is performed when a relatively large area of the brain is involved in generation and propagation of seizures. Hemispherectomy is the most extreme form of removal surgery with which the entire cortex of one hemisphere is removed or disconnected [144]. This approach is used for seizures when one hemisphere is diffusely involved. Epileptic seizures associated with Rasmussen's encephalitis, Sturge-Weber syndrome, large hemispheric stroke, or trauma are indications for hemispherectomy. Corpus callosotomy is the surgery to cut the corpus callosum at the midline either the anterior two-thirds or in its entirety [145]. This surgery is performed when one hemisphere has diffuse or multiple sei-

zure onsets and the seizures propagate to the other hemisphere. Seizure onset zones may exist in both hemispheres independently. It is used often for epilepsy with drop attacks [146].

12.14.4.1 Medial Temporal Lobe Epilepsy

By far the best surgical indication is medial temporal lobe epilepsy (MTLE) with unilateral hippocampal sclerosis [147, 148]. In such cases, all presurgical work up data concordantly suggest that seizure onset zone locates in the unilateral medial temporal lobe. A typical patient has medial temporal lobe epilepsy symptoms, such as déjà vu, olfactory hallucination of bad smell, lip smacking, and automatisms, neuropsychological impairment of same side of temporal lobe function, such as impaired verbal memory and naming scores for language dominant side of MTLE, impaired visual memory and impaired visuospatial processing for non-dominant side, hippocampal atrophy with FLAIR high intensity on MRI, decreased metabolism of medial temporal lobe on PET, and epileptic discharges in unilateral temporal area on interictal EEG and ictal EEG. There are several surgical approaches to treat this condition. Common to all approaches is removal or destruction of the medial temporal structures that include amygdala, hippocampus, and parahippocampal gyrus. Anterior temporal lobectomy involves resection of temporal cortex and removal of the medial temporal structures. With this approach, 70–80% of patients are expected to become seizure-free at 1 year after the surgery. Selective amygdalohippocampectomy is the surgical approach to reduce surgical injury to the temporal cortex aiming for more preservation of temporal cortical function than traditional anterior temporal lobectomy [149]. Surgical efficacy of controlling seizure has been reported comparable to that of anterior temporal lobectomy, and postoperative cognition appeared to be slightly better [150, 151]. In recent years, laser interstitial thermal therapy (LiTT) is increasingly utilized [152]. This is the less invasive surgical approach to destroy medial temporal structures using heat generated by a laser which is delivered through a small diameter fiber optic applicator introduced in the brain through a tiny twist drill hole. Temperature monitoring with MRI makes it possible to precisely control the extent of ablation. Efficacy for seizure control appears slightly lower than that of the conventional surgical approach. Finally, stereotactic radiosurgery (SRS) is as effective as ATL in selected mesial temporal lobe epilepsy cases [142].

12.14.5 Electrical Stimulation

There are three different types of electrical stimulation therapy for epilepsy.

- *Vagus nerve stimulation (VNS)*: VNS is indicated for patients with AED treatment-resistant epilepsy who are either not candidates for epilepsy surgery or who have failed surgery [153]. Representative cases include multifocal epilepsy, bilateral onset focal epilepsy, generalized epilepsy with diffuse epileptogenic abnormalities, recurrent or continued seizures after seizure focus resection surgery. Approximately half of patients who are treated with VNS shows effectiveness which defined by reduction of seizure frequency 50% or more compared to presurgical frequency. It is unlikely to become completely free of seizures.
- *Responsive Neurostimulation (RNS)*: RNS controls seizures by electrically stimulating brain tissue close to seizure onset zone [154]. It detects seizure activity then delivers electrical pulses to suppress it, thus it is called "responsive." It can stimulate up to two seizure foci [155]. Neocortical epilepsy with seizure onset in the eloquent cortex such as Broca's area or motor cortex, MTLE of language-dominant side with preserved verbal memory, and MTLE with bilateral onset are considered to be good indications. Seizure onset zone has to be localized before the placement of the device, therefore, usually it requires intracranial seizure monitoring or patients with clear MRI lesion whose location is concordant to scalp EEG seizure localization.

- *Deep Brain Stimulation (DBS)*: Electrical stimulation of the bilateral anterior thalamic nuclei is used for treatment of medically refractory focal-onset epilepsy [156]. It appears DBS works better for MTLE and limbic epilepsy than focal epilepsy with onset in other regions [157].

References

1. Fisher RS et al (2017) Operational classification of seizure types by the international league against epilepsy: position paper of the ILAE commission for classification and terminology. Epilepsia 58(4):522–530
2. Scheffer IE et al (2017) ILAE classification of the epilepsies: position paper of the ILAE commission for classification and terminology. Epilepsia 58(4):512–521
3. Levite M (2014) Glutamate receptor antibodies in neurological diseases: anti-AMPA-GluR3 antibodies, anti-NMDA-NR1 antibodies, anti-NMDA-NR2A/B antibodies, anti-mGluR1 antibodies or anti-mGluR5 antibodies are present in subpopulations of patients with either: epilepsy, encephalitis, cerebellar ataxia, systemic lupus erythematosus (SLE) and neuropsychiatric SLE, Sjogren's syndrome, schizophrenia, mania or stroke. These autoimmune anti-glutamate receptor antibodies can bind neurons in few brain regions, activate glutamate receptors, decrease glutamate receptor's expression, impair glutamate-induced signaling and function, activate blood brain barrier endothelial cells, kill neurons, damage the brain, induce behavioral/psychiatric/cognitive abnormalities and ataxia in animal models, and can be removed or silenced in some patients by immunotherapy. J Neural Transm (Vienna) 121(8):1029–1075
4. Gloor P (1997) The temporal lobe and limbic system, in the temporal lobe and limbic system. Oxford University Press, New York
5. Vyklicky V et al (2014) Structure, function, and pharmacology of NMDA receptor channels. Physiol Res 63(Suppl 1):S191–S203
6. Babb TL et al (1984) Distribution of pyramidal cell density and hyperexcitability in the epileptic human hippocampal formation. Epilepsia 25(6):721–728
7. Coulter DA, Eid T (2012) Astrocytic regulation of glutamate homeostasis in epilepsy. Glia 60(8):1215–1226
8. Herron CE, Williamson R, Collingridge GL (1985) A selective N-methyl-D-aspartate antagonist depresses epileptiform activity in rat hippocampal slices. Neurosci Lett 61(3):255–260
9. Wasterlain CG et al (1993) Pathophysiological mechanisms of brain damage from status epilepticus. Epilepsia 34(Suppl 1):S37–S53

10. Ben-Ari Y (2002) Excitatory actions of gaba during development: the nature of the nurture. Nat Rev Neurosci 3(9):728–739
11. Jefferys JGR et al (2012) Limbic network synchronization and temporal lobe epilepsy. In: Noebels JL, Avoli M, Rogawski MA, Delgado-Escueta AV, Olsen RW (eds) Jasper's basic mechanisms of the epilepsies, 4th edn. National Center for Biotechnology Information (US), Bethesda, MD
12. Vogt Cc, Vogt O (1919) Allgemeine Ergebnisse unserer Hirnforschung, Journal für Psychologie und Neurologie.Bd. 25. Ergänzungsheft I. J.A. Barth, Leipzig. 190 p
13. Heimer L, Van Hoesen GW (2006) The limbic lobe and its output channels: implications for emotional functions and adaptive behavior. Neurosci Biobehav Rev 30(2):126–147
14. MacLean PD (1990) The triune brain in evolution: role in paleocerebral functions. Plenum Press, New York. xxiv, 672 p
15. Triarhou LC (2008) Centenary of Christfried Jakob's discovery of the visceral brain: an unheeded precedence in affective neuroscience. Neurosci Biobehav Rev 32(5):984–1000
16. Papez JW (1995) A proposed mechanism of emotion. 1937. J Neuropsychiatry Clin Neurosci 7(1):103–112
17. Treit S et al (2018) High resolution in-vivo diffusion imaging of the human hippocampus. NeuroImage 182:479–487
18. Bendersky M et al (2003) Magnetic resonance imaging identifies cytoarchitectonic subtypes of the normal human cerebral cortex. J Neurol Sci 211(1–2):75–80
19. Hirai T et al (2000) Limbic lobe of the human brain: evaluation with turbo fluid-attenuated inversion-recovery MR imaging. Radiology 215(2):470–475
20. Asao C et al (2008) Human cerebral cortices: signal variation on diffusion-weighted MR imaging. Neuroradiology 50(3):205–211
21. Tsai MH et al (2016) Hippocampal malrotation is an anatomic variant and has no clinical significance in MRI-negative temporal lobe epilepsy. Epilepsia 57(10):1719–1728
22. Lerner JT et al (2009) Assessment and surgical outcomes for mild type I and severe type II cortical dysplasia: a critical review and the UCLA experience. Epilepsia 50(6):1310–1335
23. Margerison JH, Corsellis JA (1966) Epilepsy and the temporal lobes. A clinical, electroencephalographic and neuropathological study of the brain in epilepsy, with particular reference to the temporal lobes. Brain 89(3):499–530
24. Cascino GD et al (1991) Magnetic resonance imaging-based volume studies in temporal lobe epilepsy: pathological correlations. Ann Neurol 30(1):31–36
25. Briellmann RS et al (2002) Hippocampal pathology in refractory temporal lobe epilepsy: T2-weighted signal change reflects dentate gliosis. Neurology 58(2):265–271

26. Hu WH et al (2013) Selective amygdalohippocampectomy versus anterior temporal lobectomy in the management of mesial temporal lobe epilepsy: a meta-analysis of comparative studies. J Neurosurg 119(5):1089–97
27. Immonen A (2010) Long-term epilepsy surgery outcomes in patients with MRI-negative temporal lobe epilepsy. Epilepsia 51(11):2260–9.
28. Yoo SY et al (2002) Apparent diffusion coefficient value of the hippocampus in patients with hippocampal sclerosis and in healthy volunteers. AJNR Am J Neuroradiol 23(5):809–812
29. Yogarajah M, Duncan JS (2008) Diffusion-based magnetic resonance imaging and tractography in epilepsy. Epilepsia 49(2):189–200
30. Wehner T et al (2007) The value of interictal diffusion-weighted imaging in lateralizing temporal lobe epilepsy. Neurology 68(2):122–127
31. Goubran M et al (2016) In vivo MRI signatures of hippocampal subfield pathology in intractable epilepsy. Hum Brain Mapp 37(3):1103–1119
32. Kreilkamp BA et al (2017) Automated tractography in patients with temporal lobe epilepsy using TRActs Constrained by UnderLying Anatomy (TRACULA). Neuroimage Clin 14:67–76
33. Urbach H et al (2017) Bilateral cingulum fiber reductions in temporal lobe epilepsy with unilateral hippocampal sclerosis. Eur J Radiol 94:53–57
34. Lyra KP et al (2017) Corpus callosum diffusion abnormalities in refractory epilepsy associated with hippocampal sclerosis. Epilepsy Res 137:112–118
35. Nazem-Zadeh MR et al (2016) DTI-based response-driven modeling of mTLE laterality. Neuroimage Clin 11:694–706
36. Mitsueda-Ono T et al (2011) Amygdalar enlargement in patients with temporal lobe epilepsy. J Neurol Neurosurg Psychiatry 82(6):652–657
37. Beh SM, Cook MJ, D'Souza WJ (2016) Isolated amygdala enlargement in temporal lobe epilepsy: a systematic review. Epilepsy Behav 60:33–41
38. Minami N et al (2015) Surgery for amygdala enlargement with mesial temporal lobe epilepsy: pathological findings and seizure outcome. J Neurol Neurosurg Psychiatry. 86(8):887–94, https://doi.org/10.1136/jnnp-2014-308383
39. Lv RJ et al (2014) Temporal lobe epilepsy with amygdala enlargement: a subtype of temporal lobe epilepsy. BMC Neurol 14:194
40. Kim DW et al (2012) Clinical features and pathological characteristics of amygdala enlargement in mesial temporal lobe epilepsy. J Clin Neurosci 19(4):509–512
41. Bower SP et al (2003) Amygdala volumetry in "imaging-negative" temporal lobe epilepsy. J Neurol Neurosurg Psychiatry 74(9):1245–1249
42. Takaya S et al (2014) Temporal lobe epilepsy with amygdala enlargement: a morphologic and functional study. J Neuroimaging 24(1):54–62
43. Capizzano AA et al (2018) Amygdala enlargement in mesial temporal lobe epilepsy: an alternative imag-

ing presentation of limbic epilepsy. Neuroradiology 61:119–127

44. Abel TJ et al (2018) Role of the temporal pole in temporal lobe epilepsy seizure networks: an intracranial electrode investigation. J Neurosurg 129(1):165–173

45. Blumcke I et al (2011) The clinicopathologic spectrum of focal cortical dysplasias: a consensus classification proposed by an ad hoc Task Force of the ILAE Diagnostic Methods Commission. Epilepsia 52(1):158–174

46. Knerlich-Lukoschus F et al (2017) Clinical, imaging, and immunohistochemical characteristics of focal cortical dysplasia Type II extratemporal epilepsies in children: analyses of an institutional case series. J Neurosurg Pediatr 19(2):182–195

47. Wang DD et al (2013) Transmantle sign in focal cortical dysplasia: a unique radiological entity with excellent prognosis for seizure control. J Neurosurg 118(2):337–344

48. Andrade CS et al (2014) Diffusion abnormalities of the corpus callosum in patients with malformations of cortical development and epilepsy. Epilepsy Res 108(9):1533–1542

49. Kasper BS, Kasper EM (2017) New classification of epilepsy-related neoplasms: the clinical perspective. Epilepsy Behav 67:91–97

50. Fellah S et al (2012) Epileptogenic brain lesions in children: the added-value of combined diffusion imaging and proton MR spectroscopy to the presurgical differential diagnosis. Childs Nerv Syst 28(2):273–282

51. Kikuchi T et al (2009) Minimum apparent diffusion coefficient for the differential diagnosis of ganglioglioma. Neurol Res 31(10):1102–1107

52. Yasargil MG et al (1992) Tumours of the limbic and paralimbic systems. Acta Neurochir 118(1–2):40–52

53. Capizzano AA, Kirby P, Moritani T (2015) Limbic tumors of the temporal lobe: radiologic-pathologic correlation. Clin Neuroradiol 25(2):127–135

54. Lilja Y et al (2014) Visualizing Meyer's loop: A comparison of deterministic and probabilistic tractography. Epilepsy Res 108(3):481–490

55. James JS et al (2015) Diffusion tensor imaging tractography of Meyer's loop in planning resective surgery for drug-resistant temporal lobe epilepsy. Epilepsy Res 110:95–104

56. Silverstein AM, Alexander JA (1998) Acute postictal cerebral imaging. AJNR Am J Neuroradiol 19(8):1485–1488

57. Kim JA et al (2001) Transient MR signal changes in patients with generalized tonicoclonic seizure or status epilepticus: periictal diffusion-weighted imaging. AJNR Am J Neuroradiol 22(6):1149–1160

58. Rosenberg DS et al (2006) Involvement of medial pulvinar thalamic nucleus in human temporal lobe seizures. Epilepsia 47(1):98–107

59. Nakae Y et al (2016) Relationship between cortex and pulvinar abnormalities on diffusion-weighted imaging in status epilepticus. J Neurol 263(1):127–132

60. Ohe Y et al (2014) MRI abnormality of the pulvinar in patients with status epilepticus. J Neuroradiol 41(4):220–226

61. Diehl B et al (2001) Postictal diffusion-weighted imaging for the localization of focal epileptic areas in temporal lobe epilepsy. Epilepsia 42(1):21–28

62. Mendes A, Sampaio L (2016) Brain magnetic resonance in status epilepticus: a focused review. Seizure 38:63–67

63. Treatment of convulsive status epilepticus (1993) Recommendations of the Epilepsy Foundation of America's Working Group on Status Epilepticus. JAMA 270(7):854–859

64. Hauser WA (1990) Status epilepticus: epidemiologic considerations. Neurology 40(5 Suppl 2):9–13

65. Lewis DV et al (2014) Hippocampal sclerosis after febrile status epilepticus: the FEBSTAT study. Ann Neurol 75(2):178–185

66. Sperk G et al (1983) Kainic acid induced seizures: neurochemical and histopathological changes. Neuroscience 10(4):1301–1315

67. Siesjo BK, Wieloch T (1986) Epileptic brain damage: pathophysiology and neurochemical pathology. Adv Neurol 44:813–847

68. Ingvar M, Morgan PF, Auer RN (1988) The nature and timing of excitotoxic neuronal necrosis in the cerebral cortex, hippocampus and thalamus due to flurothyl-induced status epilepticus. Acta Neuropathol 75(4):362–369

69. DeGiorgio CM et al (1992) Hippocampal pyramidal cell loss in human status epilepticus. Epilepsia 33(1):23–27

70. Dam M, Gram L (1991) Comprehensive epileptology. Raven Press, New York. xx, 844 p

71. Rennebaum F et al (2016) Status epilepticus: clinical characteristics and EEG patterns associated with and without MRI diffusion restriction in 69 patients. Epilepsy Res 120:55–64

72. Tien RD, Felsberg GJ (1995) The hippocampus in status epilepticus: demonstration of signal intensity and morphologic changes with sequential fast spin-echo MR imaging. Radiology 194(1):249–256

73. Men S et al (2000) Selective neuronal necrosis associated with status epilepticus: MR findings. AJNR Am J Neuroradiol 21(10):1837–1840

74. Warren DE et al (2012) Long-term neuropsychological, neuroanatomical, and life outcome in hippocampal amnesia. Clin Neuropsychol 26(2):335–369

75. Cole AJ (2004) Status epilepticus and periictal imaging. Epilepsia 45(Suppl 4):72–77

76. Zhong J et al (1993) Changes in water diffusion and relaxation properties of rat cerebrum during status epilepticus. Magn Reson Med 30(2):241–246

77. Wall CJ, Kendall EJ, Obenaus A (2000) Rapid alterations in diffusion-weighted images with anatomic correlates in a rodent model of status epilepticus. AJNR Am J Neuroradiol 21(10):1841–1852

78. Ito Y et al (2015) Seizure characteristics of epilepsy in childhood after acute encephalopathy with biphasic seizures and late reduced diffusion. Epilepsia 56(8):1286–1293

79. Bekci T et al (2014) A missed diagnosis: acute encephalopathy with biphasic seizures and late reduced diffusion. Clin Neurol Neurosurg 127:161–162

80. Takanashi J et al (2009) Excitotoxicity in acute encephalopathy with biphasic seizures and late reduced diffusion. AJNR Am J Neuroradiol 30(1):132–135

81. Tanuma N et al (2010) The axonal damage marker tau protein in the cerebrospinal fluid is increased in patients with acute encephalopathy with biphasic seizures and late reduced diffusion. Brain and Development 32(6):435–439

82. Yokochi T et al (2016) Prediction of acute encephalopathy with biphasic seizures and late reduced diffusion in patients with febrile status epilepticus. Brain and Development 38(2):217–224

83. Salih MA et al (1997) Hemiconvulsion-hemiplegia-epilepsy syndrome. A clinical, electroencephalographic and neuroradiological study. Childs Nerv Syst 13(5):257–263

84. Freeman JL et al (2002) Hemiconvulsion-hemiplegia-epilepsy syndrome: characteristic early magnetic resonance imaging findings. J Child Neurol 17(1):10–16

85. Albakaye M et al (2018) Clinical aspects, neuroimaging, and electroencephalography of 35 cases of hemiconvulsion-hemiplegia syndrome. Epilepsy Behav 80:184–190

86. Granata T, Andermann F (2013) Rasmussen encephalitis. Handb Clin Neurol 111:511–519

87. Whitney KD, McNamara JO (2000) GluR3 autoantibodies destroy neural cells in a complement-dependent manner modulated by complement regulatory proteins. J Neurosci 20(19):7307–7316

88. Geller E et al (1998) Rasmussen encephalitis: complementary role of multitechnique neuroimaging. AJNR Am J Neuroradiol 19(3):445–449

89. Chiapparini L et al (2003) Diagnostic imaging in 13 cases of Rasmussen's encephalitis: can early MRI suggest the diagnosis? Neuroradiology 45(3):171–183

90. Pradeep K et al (2014) Evolution of MRI changes in Rasmussen's encephalitis. Acta Neurol Scand 130(4):253–259

91. Sener RN (2003) Diffusion MRI and spectroscopy in Rasmussen's encephalitis. Eur Radiol 13(9):2186–2191

92. Arias M et al (2006) Rasmussen encephalitis in the sixth decade: magnetic resonance image evolution and immunoglobulin response. Eur Neurol 56(4):236–239

93. Dupont S et al (2017) Late-onset Rasmussen Encephalitis: a literature appraisal. Autoimmun Rev 16(8):803–810

94. Corsellis JA, Goldberg GJ, Norton AR (1968) "Limbic encephalitis" and its association with carcinoma. Brain 91(3):481–496

95. Graus F, Saiz A (2008) Limbic encephalitis: an expanding concept. Neurology 70(7):500–501

96. Irani S, Lang B (2008) Autoantibody-mediated disorders of the central nervous system. Autoimmunity 41(1):55–65

97. Iizuka T et al (2008) Anti-NMDA receptor encephalitis in Japan: long-term outcome without tumor removal. Neurology 70(7):504–511

98. Kelley BP et al (2017) Autoimmune encephalitis: pathophysiology and imaging review of an overlooked diagnosis. AJNR Am J Neuroradiol 38(6):1070–1078

99. Senties-Madrid H, Vega-Boada F (2001) Paraneoplastic syndromes associated with anti-Hu antibodies. Isr Med Assoc J 3(2):94–103

100. Graus F et al (2016) A clinical approach to diagnosis of autoimmune encephalitis. Lancet Neurol 15(4):391–404

101. Florance NR et al (2009) Anti-N-methyl-D-aspartate receptor (NMDAR) encephalitis in children and adolescents. Ann Neurol 66(1):11–18

102. Galli J, Clardy SL, Piquet AL (2017) NMDAR encephalitis following herpes simplex virus encephalitis. Curr Infect Dis Rep 19(1):1

103. Bastiaansen AEM, van Sonderen A, Titulaer MJ (2017) Autoimmune encephalitis with anti-leucine-rich glioma-inactivated 1 or anti-contactin-associated protein-like 2 antibodies (formerly called voltage-gated potassium channel-complex antibodies). Curr Opin Neurol 30(3):302–309

104. Kotsenas AL et al (2014) MRI findings in autoimmune voltage-gated potassium channel complex encephalitis with seizures: one potential etiology for mesial temporal sclerosis. AJNR Am J Neuroradiol 35(1):84–89

105. Heine J et al (2015) Imaging of autoimmune encephalitis—Relevance for clinical practice and hippocampal function. Neuroscience 309:68–83

106. Schievelkamp AH et al (2018) Limbic encephalitis in patients with epilepsy-is quantitative MRI diagnostic? Clin Neuroradiol 29(4):623–630

107. Szots M et al (2017) Global brain atrophy and metabolic dysfunction in LGI1 encephalitis: a prospective multimodal MRI study. J Neurol Sci 376:159–165

108. Wagner J et al (2016) Distinct white matter integrity in glutamic acid decarboxylase and voltage-gated potassium channel-complex antibody-associated limbic encephalitis. Epilepsia 57(3):475–483

109. Cohen-Gadol AA et al (2002) Transient postictal magnetic resonance imaging abnormality of the corpus callosum in a patient with epilepsy. Case report and review of the literature. J Neurosurg 97(3):714–717

110. Starkey J et al (2017) Cytotoxic lesions of the corpus callosum that show restricted diffusion: mechanisms, causes, and manifestations. Radiographics 37(2):562–576

111. Kim SS et al (1999) Focal lesion in the splenium of the corpus callosum in epileptic patients: antiepileptic drug toxicity? AJNR Am J Neuroradiol 20(1):125–129

112. Polster T, Hoppe M, Ebner A (2001) Transient lesion in the splenium of the corpus callosum: three further cases in epileptic patients and a pathophysiological hypothesis. J Neurol Neurosurg Psychiatry 70(4):459–463

113. Appenzeller S et al (2006) Focal transient lesions of the corpus callosum in systemic lupus erythematosus. Clin Rheumatol 25(4):568–571

114. Doherty MJ et al (2005) Clinical implications of splenium magnetic resonance imaging signal changes. Arch Neurol 62(3):433–437

115. Kim JH et al (2007) Reversible splenial abnormality in hypoglycemic encephalopathy. Neuroradiology 49(3):217–222

116. Takanashi J et al (2006) Widening spectrum of a reversible splenial lesion with transiently reduced diffusion. AJNR Am J Neuroradiol 27(4):836–838

117. Maeda M et al (2006) Reversible splenial lesion with restricted diffusion in a wide spectrum of diseases and conditions. J Neuroradiol 33(4):229–236

118. Moritani T et al (2005) Diffusion-weighted imaging of acute excitotoxic brain injury. AJNR Am J Neuroradiol 26(2):216–228

119. Bulakbasi N et al (2006) Transient splenial lesion of the corpus callosum in clinically mild influenza-associated encephalitis/encephalopathy. AJNR Am J Neuroradiol 27(9):1983–1986

120. Tada H et al (2004) Clinically mild encephalitis/encephalopathy with a reversible splenial lesion. Neurology 63(10):1854–1858

121. Garcia-Monco JC et al (2011) Reversible splenial lesion syndrome (RESLES): what's in a name? J Neuroimaging 21(2):e1–e14

122. Johnson EL (2019) Seizures and epilepsy. Med Clin North Am 103(2):309–324

123. Harden C et al (2017) Practice guideline summary: sudden unexpected death in epilepsy incidence rates and risk factors: Report of the Guideline Development, Dissemination, and Implementation Subcommittee of the American Academy of Neurology and the American Epilepsy Society. Neurology 88(17):1674–1680

124. Glauser T et al (2013) Updated ILAE evidence review of antiepileptic drug efficacy and effectiveness as initial monotherapy for epileptic seizures and syndromes. Epilepsia 54(3):551–563

125. Schwartz RH et al (1989) Ketogenic diets in the treatment of epilepsy: short-term clinical effects. Dev Med Child Neurol 31(2):145–151

126. Hassan AM et al (1999) Ketogenic diet in the treatment of refractory epilepsy in childhood. Pediatr Neurol 21(2):548–552

127. Sirven J et al (1999) The ketogenic diet for intractable epilepsy in adults: preliminary results. Epilepsia 40(12):1721–1726

128. D'Andrea Meira I et al (2019) Ketogenic diet and epilepsy: what we know so far. Front Neurosci 13:5

129. deCampo DM, Kossoff EH (2019) Ketogenic dietary therapies for epilepsy and beyond. Curr Opin Clin Nutr Metab Care 22(4):264–268

130. Dubey D et al (2017) Neurological autoantibody prevalence in epilepsy of unknown etiology. JAMA Neurol 74(4):397–402

131. Lucchinetti CF, Kimmel DW, Lennon VA (1998) Paraneoplastic and oncologic profiles of patients seropositive for type 1 antineuronal nuclear autoantibodies. Neurology 50(3):652–657

132. Gaspard N (2016) Autoimmune epilepsy. Continuum (Minneap Minn) 22(1 Epilepsy):227–245

133. Penfield W, Baldwin M (1952) Temporal lobe seizures and the technic of subtotal temporal lobectomy. Ann Surg 136(4):625–634

134. Tovar-Spinoza ZS et al (2008) The role of magnetoencephalography in epilepsy surgery. Neurosurg Focus 25(3):E16

135. Barkovich AJ, Rowley HA, Andermann F (1995) MR in partial epilepsy: value of high-resolution volumetric techniques. AJNR Am J Neuroradiol 16(2):339–343

136. Wada J, Rasmussen T (2007) Intracarotid injection of sodium amytal for the lateralization of cerebral speech dominance. 1960. J Neurosurg 106(6):1117–1133

137. Jobst BC, Cascino GD (2015) Resective epilepsy surgery for drug-resistant focal epilepsy: a review. JAMA 313(3):285–293

138. Bancaud J et al (1970) Functional stereotaxic exploration (SEEG) of epilepsy. Electroencephalogr Clin Neurophysiol 28(1):85–86

139. Nagahama Y et al (2018) Intracranial EEG for seizure focus localization: evolving techniques, outcomes, complications, and utility of combining surface and depth electrodes. J Neurosurg 130:1–13

140. Engel J Jr (1996) Surgery for seizures. N Engl J Med 334(10):647–652

141. Curry DJ et al (2012) MR-guided stereotactic laser ablation of epileptogenic foci in children. Epilepsy Behav 24(4):408–414

142. Regis J et al (2004) Gamma knife surgery in mesial temporal lobe epilepsy: a prospective multicenter study. Epilepsia 45(5):504–515

143. Barbaro NM et al (2009) A multicenter, prospective pilot study of gamma knife radiosurgery for mesial temporal lobe epilepsy: seizure response, adverse events, and verbal memory. Ann Neurol 65(2):167–175

144. Baumgartner JE et al (2017) Technical descriptions of four hemispherectomy approaches: from the pediatric epilepsy surgery meeting at Gothenburg 2014. Epilepsia 58(Suppl 1):46–55

145. Wilson DH, Reeves A, Gazzaniga M (1978) Division of the corpus callosum for uncontrollable epilepsy. Neurology 28(7):649–653

146. Graham D et al (2018) Seizure outcome after corpus callosotomy in a large paediatric series. Dev Med Child Neurol 60(2):199–206

147. Wiebe S et al (2001) A randomized, controlled trial of surgery for temporal-lobe epilepsy. N Engl J Med 345(5):311–318

148. Engel J Jr et al (2012) Early surgical therapy for drug-resistant temporal lobe epilepsy: a randomized trial. JAMA 307(9):922–930

149. Wieser HG, Yasargil MG (1982) Selective amygdalohippocampectomy as a surgical treatment of mesiobasal limbic epilepsy. Surg Neurol 17(6):445–457

150. Paglioli E et al (2006) Seizure and memory outcome following temporal lobe surgery: selective compared with nonselective approaches for hippocampal sclerosis. J Neurosurg 104(1):70–78

151. Wendling AS et al (2013) Selective amygdalohippocampectomy versus standard temporal lobectomy in patients with mesial temporal lobe epilepsy and unilateral hippocampal sclerosis. Epilepsy Res 104(1–2):94–104

152. Willie JT et al (2014) Real-time magnetic resonance-guided stereotactic laser amygdalohippocampotomy for mesial temporal lobe epilepsy. Neurosurgery 74(6):569–584; discussion 584-5

153. Uthman BM et al (2004) Effectiveness of vagus nerve stimulation in epilepsy patients: a 12-year observation. Neurology 63(6):1124–1126

154. Fountas KN, Smith JR (2007) A novel closed-loop stimulation system in the control of focal, medically refractory epilepsy. Acta Neurochir Suppl 97(Pt 2):357–362

155. Heck CN et al (2014) Two-year seizure reduction in adults with medically intractable partial onset epilepsy treated with responsive neurostimulation: final results of the RNS System Pivotal trial. Epilepsia 55(3):432–441

156. Herrman H et al (2019) Anterior thalamic deep brain stimulation in refractory epilepsy: a randomized, double-blinded study. Acta Neurol Scand 139(3):294–304

157. Li MCH, Cook MJ (2018) Deep brain stimulation for drug-resistant epilepsy. Epilepsia 59(2):273–290

Demyelinating Diseases

13

Aristides A. Capizzano, and Toshio Moritani

Andrew Romeo

13.1 Demyelinating Diseases

Demyelination refers to loss of myelin with relative preservation of axons. This results from diseases that damage myelin sheaths and/or the oligodendrocytes. Demyelinating diseases can be classified into two types: primary and secondary. Primary demyelination is defined as the abnormality or dysfunction of oligodendrocytes. Secondary demyelination is defined as myelin changes secondary to neuronal or axonal degeneration associated with ischemia, infection, or metabolic/toxic diseases. The term demyelinating disease usually refers to the primary type of demyelination, which pathologically represents inflammatory demyelination. Idiopathic inflammatory-demyelinating diseases comprise the spectrum of demyelinating diseases based on purely clinical considerations, including monophasic, multiphasic, and progressive disorders from a localized form to multifocal or diffuse variants [1, 2].

13.1.1 Multiple Sclerosis (MS)

Multiple sclerosis (MS) is the most common demyelinating disease characterized by relapses and remissions of neurological disturbances. It is classified according to the clinical course into the following types: (1) relapsing remitting (80%), (2) primary progressive (10%), (3) secondary progressive (10%) [2]. MS plaques are usually well-demarcated round-to-oval and frequently show finger-like extensions in the periphery that follow the pathway of a small- or medium-sized vein (Dawson's finger) [3], which was observed by Dr. Dawson (neuropathologist) in 1916.

MR imaging has become critical for the diagnosis of MS, which is integrated with clinical and paraclinical diagnostic methods in the McDonald's diagnostic criteria [4]. The cornerstone of imaging diagnosis of MS is to demonstrate *dissemination in space* (development of lesions in distinct anatomical locations within the CNS, indicating a multifocal process) and *dissemination in time* (development or appearance of new CNS lesions over time) with exclusion of other etiologies [4]. White matter lesions are assessed in the following locations: cortical-juxtacortical, periventricular, infratentorial, and spinal cord [4]. Spinal cord lesions in MS are discussed in Chap. 24.

A. A. Capizzano (✉)
Division of Neuroradiology, Department
of Radiology, University of Michigan,
Ann Arbor, MI, USA
e-mail: capizzan@med.umich.edu

T. Moritani
Division of Neuroradiology, Department of
Radiology, Clinical Neuroradiology Research,
University of Michigan, Ann Arbor, MI, USA
e-mail: tmoritan@med.umich.edu

A. Romeo
University of Michigan, Ann Arbor, MI, USA
e-mail: aromeo@umich.edu

© Springer Nature Switzerland AG 2021
T. Moritani, A. A. Capizzano (eds.), *Diffusion-Weighted MR Imaging of the Brain, Head and Neck, and Spine*, https://doi.org/10.1007/978-3-030-62120-9_13

Axial T2-weighted and fluid-attenuated inversion-recovery (FLAIR) images show well-demarcated round-to-oval lesions along white matter tracts. These MR sequences are sensitive for depicting focal lesions, but lack histopathologic specificity. Other histologic lesions such as inflammation, edema, reactive gliosis, axonal loss, and secondary demyelination may have a similar imaging appearance [5]. On sagittal FLAIR images, subcallosal striations and ependymal "dot-dash" signs have been reported as relatively specific early findings of MS (Fig. 13.1) [6, 7]. Enhancement in the MS plaque on post-contrast T1-weighted images is related to the activity of the plaque, which histologically represents inflammation with breakdown of the blood–brain barrier. Hypointense T1 lesions in MS are usually caused by extracellular matrix destruction and loss of axons [8]. The T1 hypointense MS lesion usually has a low magnetization transfer ratio (MTR), and correlates better with clinical disability than proton density/T2 hyperintense lesions [9].

The presence of a central vein within the white matter lesion, identified as a hypointensity relative to the surrounding lesion on T2*-weighted images and known as the central vein sign, is thought to be a specific biomarker of inflamma-

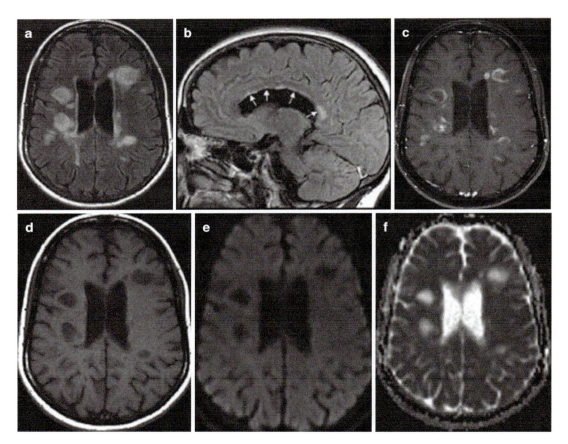

Fig. 13.1 (**a–g**) Multiple sclerosis (secondary progressive type) in a 33-year-old woman with lower extremity weakness. (**a**) Axial FLAIR image shows multiple well-demarcated and oval-shaped hyperintense lesions in the deep white matter. (**b**) Sagittal FLAIR demonstrates the dots and dash pattern of the lesions along the callosomarginal interface (*arrows*). (**c, d**) T1-weighted image shows the lesions as hypointense (**c**) with peripheral or open-ring enhancement representing active plaques (*arrows*) (**d**). (**e, f**) DW image (**e**) shows multiple hypointense lesions associated with increased ADCs. The peripheral enhancing area appears with less increased ADC values (**f**). (**g**) Fractional anisotropy (FA) map reveals decreased FA values in the plaques

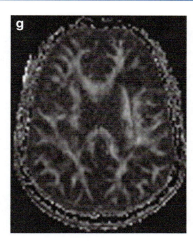

Fig. 13.1 (continued)

tory demyelination and, thus, of MS lesions [10]. The central vein sign is most prevalent in periventricular lesions and its prevalence decreases with proximity to the cortex. Another specific imaging marker of demyelination that may help in the differential diagnosis in difficult cases is the presence of high DWI signal at the edge of the lesion, manifesting as an ADC dark arc or ring at the lesion edge. Such peripheral diffusion restriction was found more commonly in ring-enhancing demyelinating lesions than in tumors or abscesses [11]. Interestingly, other non-inflammatory demyelinating conditions such as PML [12] and adrenoleukodystrophy [13] may present a similar DWI bright edge.

The correlation between contrast enhancement and restricted diffusion in demyelinating plaques has been investigated in the quest for an alternative biomarker of lesion activity. Lesions that visually restrict diffusion (hyperintense lesions in trace DWI images and hypointense in the ADC map) often enhance with gadolinium contrast, indicating high specificity. However, though most gadolinium-positive lesions quantitatively show decreased ADC values on quantitative analysis, it is difficult to visually appreciate diffusion restriction in these lesions. This results in low sensitivity to predict the presence of enhancement [15]. MS plaques can show hyper, iso, or hypointensity on DWI (with increased ADC) in contrast-enhancing active plaques (Figs. 13.1, 13.2, and 13.3) and chronic plaques alike. Therefore, the DWI/ADC combination is not a reliable surrogate marker for lesion activity as is contrast enhancement. Accordingly, in the 2017 McDonald's criteria, there is no mention of DWI changes as a marker of dissemination in time [4].

In cases of acute or subacute phase of MS, decreased ADC is observed in plaques (Figs. 13.2, 13.3, and 13.4) [16]. The decreased ADC value is presumably due to intramyelinic edema with inflammatory cell infiltration and accumulation of myelin breakdown products (cytotoxic plaque). The decreased ADC area can be located in the periphery of the plaque. Intramyelinic edema occurs in the myelin sheath itself and/or in the intramyelinic cleft. Some of the intramyelinic edema may be reversible. The enhancing portion of the MS plaques tends to have mildly increased ADC, representing prominent inflammation and blood–brain barrier breakdown with mild demyelination, while the non-enhancing portions tend to have increased ADC, representing scarring with mild inflammation and myelin loss [17, 18]. Moreover, MS plaques are reported to have decreased anisotropy [18, 19] (Fig. 13.1). The increased ADC and decreased fractional anisotropy (FA) in MS plaques are thought to relate to an increase in the extracellular space due to demyelination, perivascular inflammation with vasogenic edema, gliosis, and axonal loss. Furthermore, ADC values of MS plaques seem to be related to the severity of MS. The ADC values in secondary-progressive MS are higher than those in relapsing-remitting MS [20].

Several studies have depicted increased ADC or MD (mean diffusivity) values and decreased FA (fractional anisotropy) values in normal appearing white matter (NAWM) and also gray matter in MS patients [21–23]. Facilitated diffusion in NAWM may reflect demyelination or axonal loss, with consequent reduction of restricting

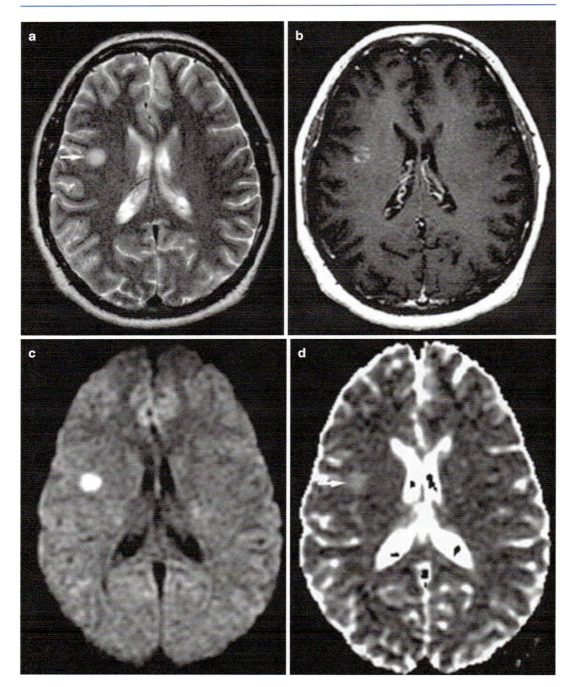

Fig. 13.2 (a–d) Multiple sclerosis (active plaque) in a 28-year-old man presenting with visual problems. (a) T2-weighted image shows a round hyperintense lesion in the right frontotemporal region (*arrow*). (b) Gadolinium T1-weighted image shows mild enhancement of this lesion, representing an active plaque. (c, d) DW image shows a hyperintense lesion associated with increased ADC (*arrow*), which represents T2 shine-through

13 Demyelinating Diseases

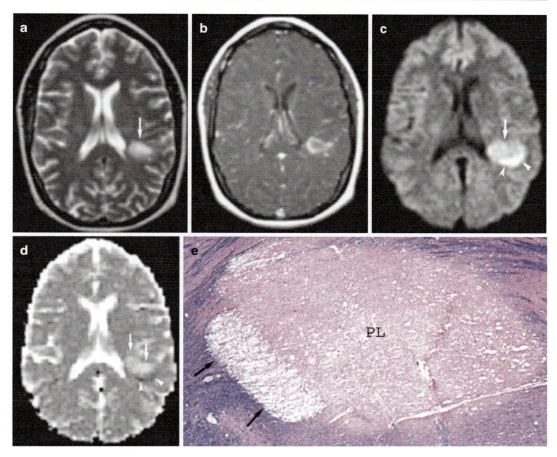

Fig. 13.3 (**a–e**) Multiple sclerosis (active plaque) in a 36-year-old woman presenting with subacute onset of progressive aphasia. (**a**) T2-weighted image shows an oval-shaped, hyperintense lesion in the left periventricular white matter (*arrow*). (**b**) Gadolinium T1-weighted image with magnetization transfer contrast shows rim enhancement of this lesion. (**c**) DW image shows combination of a moderately hyperintense (*arrow*) and a significantly hyperintense lesion (*arrowheads*). (**d**) The moderately hyperintense lesion on DW image with increased ADC may represent demyelination (*arrows*), and the very hyperintense lesion on DW image with decreased ADC may represent intramyelinic edema (*arrowheads*). (**e**) Histopathology of another case shows that intramyelinic edema (*arrows*) is located in the periphery of a plaque (*PL*) (Luxor fast blue PAS stain, original magnification ×40). (From [14])

structural barriers to water diffusion. Increased ADC and FA are also observed in cortical lesions in MS [24]. Therefore, diffusion metrics may provide more sensitive biomarkers of lesion load than T2-weighted images. Decreased MTR is also observed in NAWM in MS patients, indicating microscopic abnormalities beyond T2 hyperintense lesions [25].

13.1.2 Clinically Isolated Syndrome (CIS) and Radiologically Isolated Syndrome (RIS)

CIS is the first clinical episode of symptoms and signs suggestive of an inflammatory demyelinating disorder of the CNS. The episode should last for at least 24 h in the absence of fever, infection,

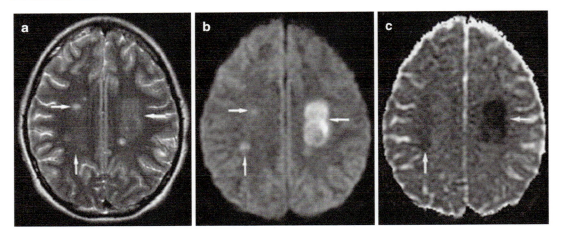

Fig. 13.4 (**a–c**) Multiple sclerosis (acute plaque) in a 13-year-old girl who presented with acute-onset right-sided weakness and dysarthria. (**a**) T2-weighted image shows multiple hyperintense lesions in the bilateral centrum semiovale (*arrows*). (**b**) DW image shows some lesions as hyperintense (*arrows*). (**c**) ADC is decreased representing acute cytotoxic plaques (*arrows*)

or encephalopathy [26]. Most commonly, CIS is isolated in time (monophasic) and space (monofocal) with clinical features of a lesion in the optic nerve (a common clinical presentation of CIS), spinal cord, brainstem or cerebellum, or the cerebral hemispheres. There is a wide range of reported clinical conversion rates from CIS to MS; for instance, for optic neuritis, follow-up studies have reported conversion to MS for 10–85% of patients [26]. 50–70% of adults with CIS have multiple asymptomatic white matter brain lesions, suggestive of previous asymptomatic demyelination. The long-term risk for clinically definite MS is 60–80% when other lesions are present vs. 20% when MRI is normal apart from the symptomatic lesion. Positive CSF oligoclonal bands further increase the risk of CIS developing to MS [27].

On the other hand, brain MRI features typical of demyelination fulfilling MRI criteria for MS are sometimes seen in asymptomatic individuals or patients with nonspecific symptoms, and have been termed radiologically isolated syndrome (RIS) [28]. Follow-up to 5 years have reported that 30% of RIS patients will develop a symptomatic demyelinating event. Involvement of the spinal cord, male gender, and age under 35 years are significant predictors for a future demyelinating event [29, 30]. Therefore, RIS stands at high risk for MS. RIS studies have reported whole brain and cortical atrophy in RIS patients. DTI studies have reported that RIS patients show altered microstructural white matter integrity compared to controls but only at the level of the T2 hyperintense focal lesions, suggesting a more limited pathology than in MS [29].

13.1.3 Baló's Concentric Sclerosis

Baló's concentric sclerosis is a rare demyelinating disease and a variant of multiple sclerosis [2, 31–33]. First described by Marburg in 1906, it became more widely known when, in 1928, the Hungarian neuropathologist Josef Baló published a report of a student with right hemiparesis and optic neuritis, who at autopsy had demyelinating lesions that he described as "encephalitis periaxialis concentrica" [34, 35]. It often has an acute monophasic course and is more common in individuals of Asian descent, suggesting a genetic predisposition. Baló-like lesions can occasionally be seen during an exacerbation of relapsing remitting MS with a non-fatal course [2].

MR imaging shows a multilayered appearance, mostly hyperintense on T2-weighted images, with alternating high and low signal concentric rings and variable degree of enhancement. DW images show hyperintensity with a reduced ADC in the acute phase of Baló's concentric sclerosis and Baló-like lesions (Fig. 13.5) [36–38] with a DWI hyperintense rim at the edge of the lesion [34]. Follow-up DW imaging shows increased ADC in the chronic lesion.

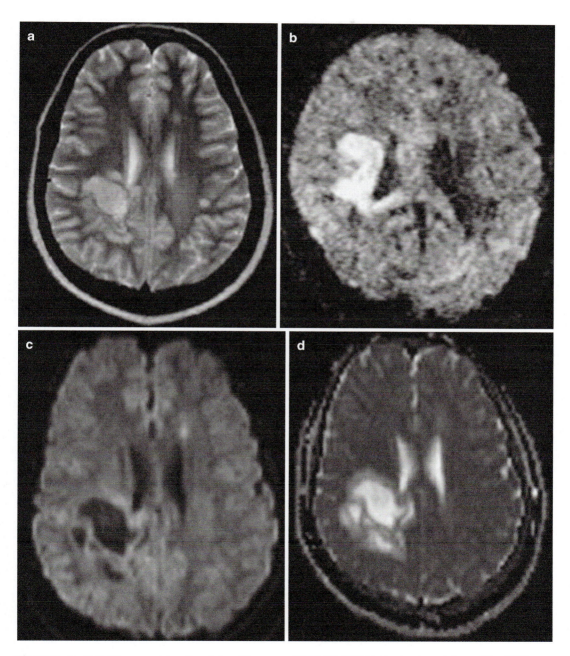

Fig. 13.5 (a–d) Baló's concentric sclerosis in a 17-year-old female patient who presented with stroke-like symptoms. (a) T2-weighted image shows a large hyperintense mass with a multilayered appearance in the right posterior periventricular and deep white matter. (b) DW image shows the lesions as very hyperintense. The ADC map was not obtained at this time. (c, d) A 2-month follow-up DW image shows the lesion as hypointense with increased ADC centrally and peripheral restricted diffusion

13.1.4 Myelinoclastic Diffuse Sclerosis (Schilder's Disease)

Myelinoclastic diffuse sclerosis, also known as inflammatory diffuse sclerosis and Schilder's disease, is a rare primary demyelination disorder and is now considered to be a variant of MS [2, 39, 40]. In 1912, Schilder described the case of a 14-year-old girl with mental deterioration who died after 19 weeks. An autopsy revealed large areas of sharply demarcated plaques of demyelination in both hemispheres. Schilder named this specific form "encephalitis periaxialis diffusa" [41, 42]. The characteristic pathological features are demyelination of the white matter, lymphocytic perivascular infiltrates, and microglial proliferation. Schider's disease can present together with Balo's-like findings in patients with MS, suggesting a pathologic continuum [43].

MR imaging shows large, mass-like T2 hyperintense lesions with irregular or smooth enhancing rims in the deep and subcortical white matter. The "open-ring" imaging sign is characteristic of tumefactive demyelination and is useful in differentiating it from a neoplasm or abscess [44]. The enhancement is shaped like an open-ring or a crescent circumscribed to the white matter, but the enhancement is not identified on the cortical side. DW imaging shows a thin, smooth, hyperintense rim with decreased ADC, and surrounding hypointense areas with increased ADC (Fig. 13.6).

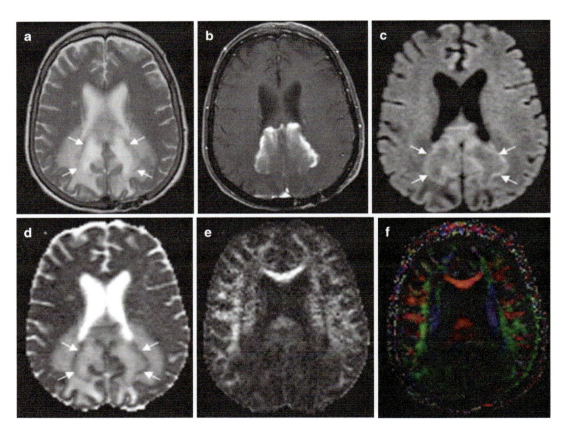

Fig. 13.6 (**a–f**) Myelinoclastic diffuse sclerosis in an 80-year-old woman with confusion. (**a**) T2-weighted image shows symmetric large hyperintense lesions with slightly low signal curvilinear areas (*arrows*) involving the posterior corpus callosum and occipital white matter bilaterally. (**b**) Post-contrast T1-weighted image shows symmetric irregular enhancement along the curvilinear T2 low signal areas. (**c, d**) DW image shows the curvilinear areas as isointense with iso ADC, corresponding to active demyelination (*arrows*). The surrounding areas are mildly hypointense on DW imaging with increased ADC, which probably represents vasogenic edema and demyelination. (**e, f**) FA and color maps show decreased anisotropy in both areas

13.1.5 MS Mimics

Given the lack of specificity of MRI findings in MS, several inflammatory and non-inflammatory neurologic conditions may present with white matter T2 hyperintensities (WMH) that may resemble MS and are thus considered MS imaging mimics [45]. Some of these entities will be discussed later in this chapter, such as NMOSD, ADEM, and PML. Toxic white matter diseases and osmotic demyelination are covered in Chap. 15. Vasculitis, sarcoidosis, and PRES are discussed in Chap. 11. Leukodystrophies are presented in Chap. 19.

In contradistinction to MS, WMH in subcortical ischemic vascular disease (SIVD) tend to spare the U-fibers, the corpus callosum, the temporal lobe white matter, and the spinal cord, all of which are commonly affected in MS. Furthermore, SIVD frequently involves the basal ganglia and central rather than the peripheral pons, and is associated with lacunar infarctions and microbleeds [46]. The characteristic distribution of age-related periventricular leukoaraiosis is in paraventricular bands parallel to the lateral ventricular walls and caps at the anterior frontal horns as opposed to the Dawson fingers seen in MS [47]. Migraine-associated white matter lesions are typically small and non-confluent in the deep white matter (sparing the U-fibers), and are more stable over time than MS lesions [45]. In the brainstem and cerebellum, several inflammatory conditions may present with WMH similar to MS including Behcet's disease, Lyme disease (neuroborreliosis), neurosarcoidosis, Whipple's disease, Listeria rhombencephalitis, Bickerstaff's brainstem encephalitis, and vasculitis due to SLE [48]. Susac's syndrome presents central "snowball" lesions within the thickness of the corpus callosum in association with the clinical triad of encephalopathy—with or without focal neurological signs-, branch retinal artery occlusions, and hearing loss [49] (Table 13.1).

13.1.6 Neuromyelitis Optica Spectrum Disorder (NMOSD)

Originally known as Devic's disease, NMOSD diagnosis was revolutionized with the discovery in 2004 of a pathogenic autoantibody targeting the astrocytic water channel protein aquaporin 4 [50]. New diagnostic criteria incorporate this biomarker in combination with core clinical and

Table 13.1 Mimics of MS

Inflammatory condition	Entity	MRI observations
YES	NMOSD	Optic neuritis, long segment myelitis, brain lesions next to third and fourth ventricles
	MOG-related demyelination	Anterior optic neuritis, myelitis with conus involvement
	ADEM	Monophasic demyelination
	Vasculitis (SLE, sarcoidosis, Behcet's, PACNS)	Variable from frequently normal in PACNS to different patterns of enhancing lesions in sarcoidosis
	Lyme disease	Meningeal and cranial nerve enhancement
	Susac syndrome	"Snowball" lesions of the corpus callosum
	CLIPPERS	Pontine perivascular enhancement
NO	SIVD, CADASIL	Deep white matter preference, association with lacunes and microhemorrhages
	Migraine-related	Small lesions, non-enhancing
	PML	Immunosuppression, lack of enhancement
	Leukodystrophies	Variable depending on specific disease
	Toxic	Variable, history of exposure (chemotherapy, illicit drugs, etc.) Corpus callosum involvement in Marchiafava Bignami.
	Neoplastic: Gliomatosis, lymphoma	Confluent lesions, enhancement, and mass effect

imaging features [51]. Aquaporin 4 (AQP4) IgG-associated NMOSD is regarded as an immune astrocytopathy. In patients with AQP4-IgG, a single clinical event referable to one of six neuroanatomically defined CNS regions (optic nerve, spinal cord, area postrema, brain stem, diencephalon, or cerebrum) is sufficient for diagnosis. A second autoantibody; myelin oligodendrocyte glycoprotein IgG (MOG) (seen in 25% of AQP4-IgG seronegative NMOSD), which targets myelin, leads to an NMOSD syndrome with clinical and radiologic features sometimes distinct from those of AQP4 IgG-associated NMOSD or MS.

On imaging, anti-AQP4 IgG seropositive NMOSD displays optic neuritis (ON) which is often severe and may involve the optic chiasm, and or acute myelitis which is longitudinally extensive (>3 vertebral segments) and preferentially involves the central gray matter. Area postrema lesions of the dorsal medulla associated with intractable hiccup, nausea, and vomiting are highly specific [52]. Diencephalic lesions, especially those in the hypothalamus, can develop in a number of anti-AQP4 IgG-seropositive patients and are commonly bilateral (Fig. 13.7). Cerebral lesions other than brainstem or diencephalic have also been reported in anti-AQP4 IgG NMOSD patients. WMH lesions are seen in half of anti-AQP4 IgG-seropositive patients.

The appearance of WMH is different from those in patients with MS, being typically extensive with irregular and indistinct borders (Fig. 13.8). Cerebral lesions in anti-AQP4 IgG-seropositive NMOSD usually appear in the deep and subcortical white matter, but are rare in the

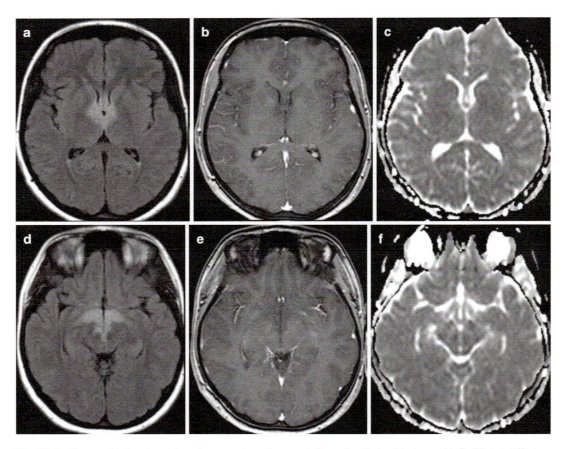

Fig. 13.7 19-year-old female with anti-aquaporin antibody + NMO. Axial FLAIR (**a**, **d**), post-contrast axial T1 (**b**, **e**) and ADC map (**c**, **f**) displaying non-enhancing diencephalic and optic tract lesions with facilitated diffusion. She responded favorably to rituximab

13 Demyelinating Diseases

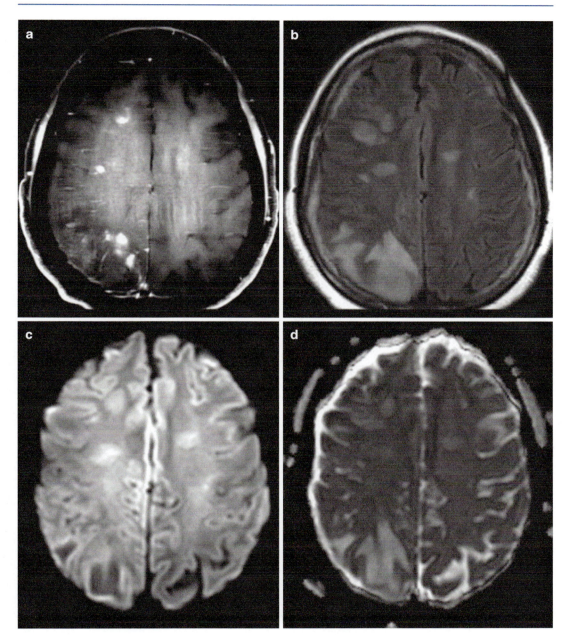

Fig. 13.8 NMO in a 56-year-old female with a history of lupus cerebritis and NMO with chronic bilateral leg weakness and neurogenic bladder who presents to the ED with a 1-day history of acute mental status change and left homonymous hemianopia. She was successfully treated with Rituximab. Post-contrast axial T1 (**a**) and FLAIR (**b**) displaying several enhancing white matter lesions, the largest in the right parietal lobe, with facilitated DWI. TRACE DWI (**c**) and ADC map (**d**)

cortical gray matter, in contradistinction to MS [53]. A comparative study of imaging of NMOSD vs. MS in a large retrospective sample reported that 17% of lesions were periventricular in NMOSD with 68% in the deep white matter, while MS had almost equal frequencies of lesions in these two locations (41% and 42%, respectively) [54]. In the spinal cord, NMOSD had more frequent lesions in the thoracic cord, which were longer than cervical cord lesions [54]. Therefore, the authors emphasized that spinal cord lesions may be short in NMOSD patients with spinal cord lesions only in the cervical region.

Multiple white matter areas had reduced FA in NMOSD patients vs. controls in the corona radiata, uncinate fasciculus, corpus callosum, optic radiation, internal and external capsules, and cerebral peduncles [55]. A significant decrease in DTI-derived FA values of NMOSD patients versus controls was also observed in the splenium of the corpus callosum and the left optic radiation [56], consistent with diffuse white matter involvement in NMOSD [57]. Thalamic gray matter atrophy and reduced FA was reported both in NMOSD and MS but with more severity in MS [58]. NMOSD-associated acute optic neuritis had statistically lower ADC values than MS-associated acute optic neuritis [59]. The decreased ADC value was correlated with optic nerve atrophy on 6-month follow-up. In the cervical spinal cord, FA in NMO patients was significantly reduced both in lesions and in normal appearing cord compared to controls and correlated with the Expanded Disability Status scale [60].

13.1.7 Anti-myelin Oligodendrocyte Glycoprotein Antibody (MOG)-Related Demyelination

MOG is a glycoprotein exclusively expressed on the surface of oligodendrocytes and myelin. MOG has long been a putative candidate autoantigen and autoantibody target in demyelination [61]. Anti-MOG antibodies are thought not to be associated with multiple sclerosis in adults. On the other hand, MOG antibody-associated demyelination has unique clinical, radiological, and therapeutic features. Anti-MOG disease encompasses almost 25% of patients with NMOSD negative for AQP4 IgG antibodies [62], and the most frequently observed clinical manifestation is optic neuritis. Optic nerve-MRI abnormalities consist in T2 hyperintensity and gadolinium enhancement that predominates in the anterior parts of the optic nerve sparing its posterior part and chiasm contrary to AQP4-IgG-positive NMOSD optic neuritis [63](Fig. 13.9). Anti-MOG also has a better treatment response than AQP4-IgG-positive NMOSD.

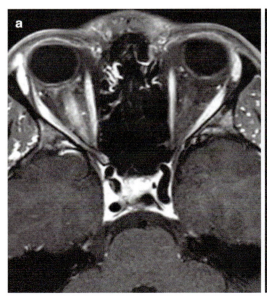

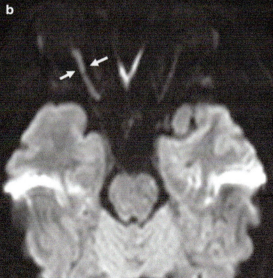

Fig. 13.9 Anti MOG-related demyelination in 20-year-old man with right optic neuritis and myelitis. Fat-saturated post-contrast axial MRI with right optic nerve enhancement (**a**) and TRACE DWI (**b**) displaying hyperintense signal in the right optic nerve (arrows). Sagittal (**c**) and axial (**d, e**) T2-weighted images of the cervicothoracic spine with long segment myelitis, which did not enhance. The patient improved after steroid and plasma exchange therapy

13 Demyelinating Diseases

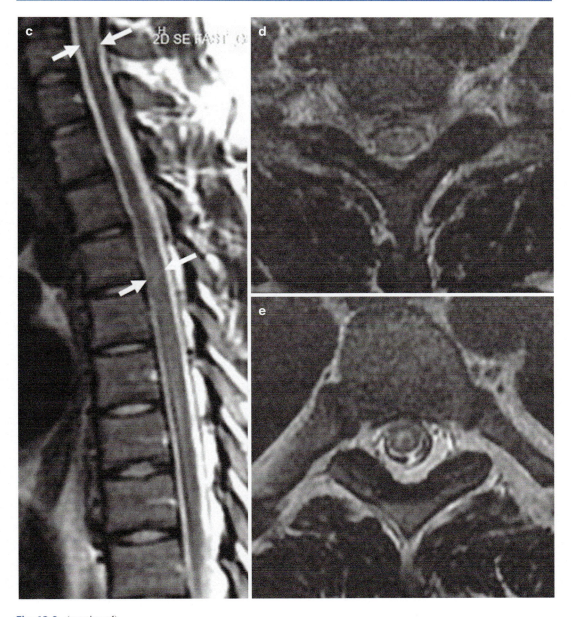

Fig. 13.9 (continued)

13.1.8 Tumefactive Demyelination (TD)

Patients present with symptoms and signs atypical for MS and have imaging findings suggestive of primary brain tumor or other space occupying lesions such as an abscess. The prevalence of TD is estimated to be approximately 1–2 per 1000 cases of MS [64]. Multiple lesions on MRI are present in 70% of cases, with the frontal and parietal lobes being the most common location followed by the corpus callosum [65]. Although most pathologically proven TD lesions have a closed ring appearance [66](Fig. 13.10), when present, an open ring of enhancement with the incomplete portion of the ring facing the gray matter side is an important diagnostic clue to TD as well as to other atypical demyelinating conditions [44]. Furthermore,

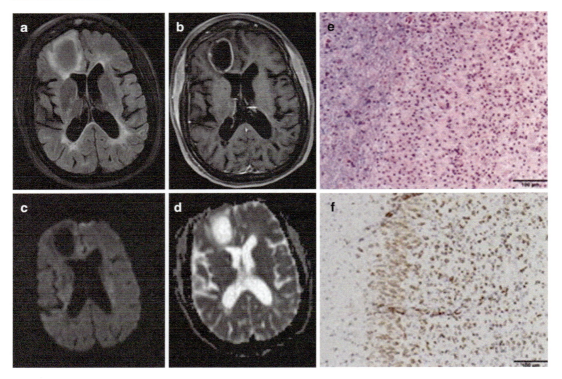

Fig. 13.10 50-year-old woman with history of secondary progressive MS diagnosed at age 20, presented with seizure without return to baseline mentation. (**a**) Axial FLAIR: large right frontal white matter lesion with hyperintense rim and isointense center. (**b**) Post-contrast T1: ring enhancement, (**c**) TRACE DWI and ADC map (**d**) with facilitated diffusion and rim of restricted diffusion. (**e**) Luxol fast blue/H&E stain shows sharp border between blue myelin and pink demyelination. (**f**) CD68 immunostaining shows macrophages in the area of demyelination

CT hypoattenuation of MR-enhancing regions was frequently observed in TD but rarely in patients with tumor. The CT attenuation of the MR enhancing regions was significantly lower for patients with TD than for those with tumor and improved the correct diagnosis of TD [67]. In a recent meta-analysis, the pooled sensitivity and specificity of MR imaging for differentiating TD lesions from primary brain tumor were 89% and 94%, respectively [68]. Open ring or incomplete rim enhancement showed a high specificity (98%–100%) in the distinction of TD from primary brain tumor.

When assessing diffusion metrics in TD, it is critical to distinguish the central non-enhancing vs. the peripheral, enhancing lesion components and the perilesional tissue. Tumefactive demyelinating lesions showed a central high ADC value with peripheral restricted diffusion, and low cerebral blood volume on PWI [68]. However, within the enhancing part of the lesion, the isotropic component of the diffusion tensor p was reduced in TD versus high-grade gliomas, which was attributed to differences in cellularity. The mean value of the anisotropic component of the diffusion tensor q was also decreased in TD compared with gliomas, which may reflect wider myelin loss in TD than in gliomas [69]. Interestingly, the ADC in the enhancing areas was lower in TD than in glioma, probably from the hypercellular inflammatory infiltrates [69]. On the other hand, minimum ADC values were significantly higher in TD than in lymphoma (Fig. 13.11) or high-grade gliomas [70, 71]. TD had also higher FA and lower MD values in the peripheral enhancing portions of the lesions compared with those of high-grade gliomas [72].

13 Demyelinating Diseases

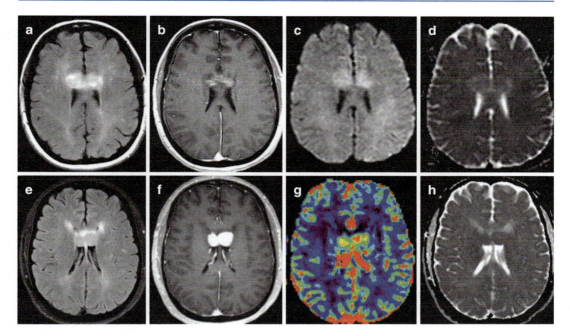

Fig. 13.11 54-year-old woman with new onset of Lhermitte phenomenon and body numbness below the neck. Imaging on presentation (upper row) shows anterior callosal lesion on FLAIR (**a**) with patchy enhancement (**b**), bright TRACE DWI (**c**) signal, and mild diffusion restriction on ADC map (**d**). Three months later, the lesion is more marginated on FLAIR (**e**) with intense enhancement (**f**), high blood volume (**g**), and restricted diffusion on ADC map (**h**). Pathology reported diffuse large B-cell lymphoma activated B cell type

13.1.9 Acute Disseminated Encephalomyelitis

Acute disseminated encephalomyelitis (ADEM) is an immune-mediated inflammatory disorder of the CNS, usually triggered by an inflammatory response to viral infections or vaccinations [73]. The neurologic picture of ADEM commonly reflects a multifocal but usually monophasic involvement, while MS is characterized by recurrent episodes with dissemination in time and space. The following findings were more commonly seen in ADEM compared with MS: prodromic infectious disease, polysymptomatic presentation, pyramidal signs, encephalopathy, bilateral optic neuritis, and seizures [74].

ADEM lesions tend to resolve, partially or completely, and new lesion formation rarely occurs (5–8%) [73]. Inflammatory demyelinating lesions are observed in the supratentorial and infratentorial white matter, brain stem, spinal cord, and also in the thalami and basal ganglia, especially in children. Involvement of the subcortical white matter is nearly a constant finding. Pathologic findings include perivenous demyelination, infiltration of lymphocytes and macrophages, hyperemia, edema, endothelial swelling, and hemorrhage.

MR imaging shows ill-defined T2 and FLAIR hyperintense lesions asymmetrically distributed in the white and gray matter. The incidence of gadolinium-enhancing lesions on T1-weighted sequences is quite variable, depending on the stage of inflammation. Magnetization transfer ratio and ADC values in NAWM of ADEM patients are similar to those of healthy control subjects [31]. DW imaging usually shows hyperintense lesions with increased ADC in the white matter due to expanded extracellular space with axonal loss, demyelination, and vasogenic edema [32] (Figs. 13.12 and 13.13). However, in the acute stage, ADEM lesions can show decreased ADC, presumably due to intramyelinic edema (Fig. 13.14) [33, 34]. Vasogenic edema, associ-

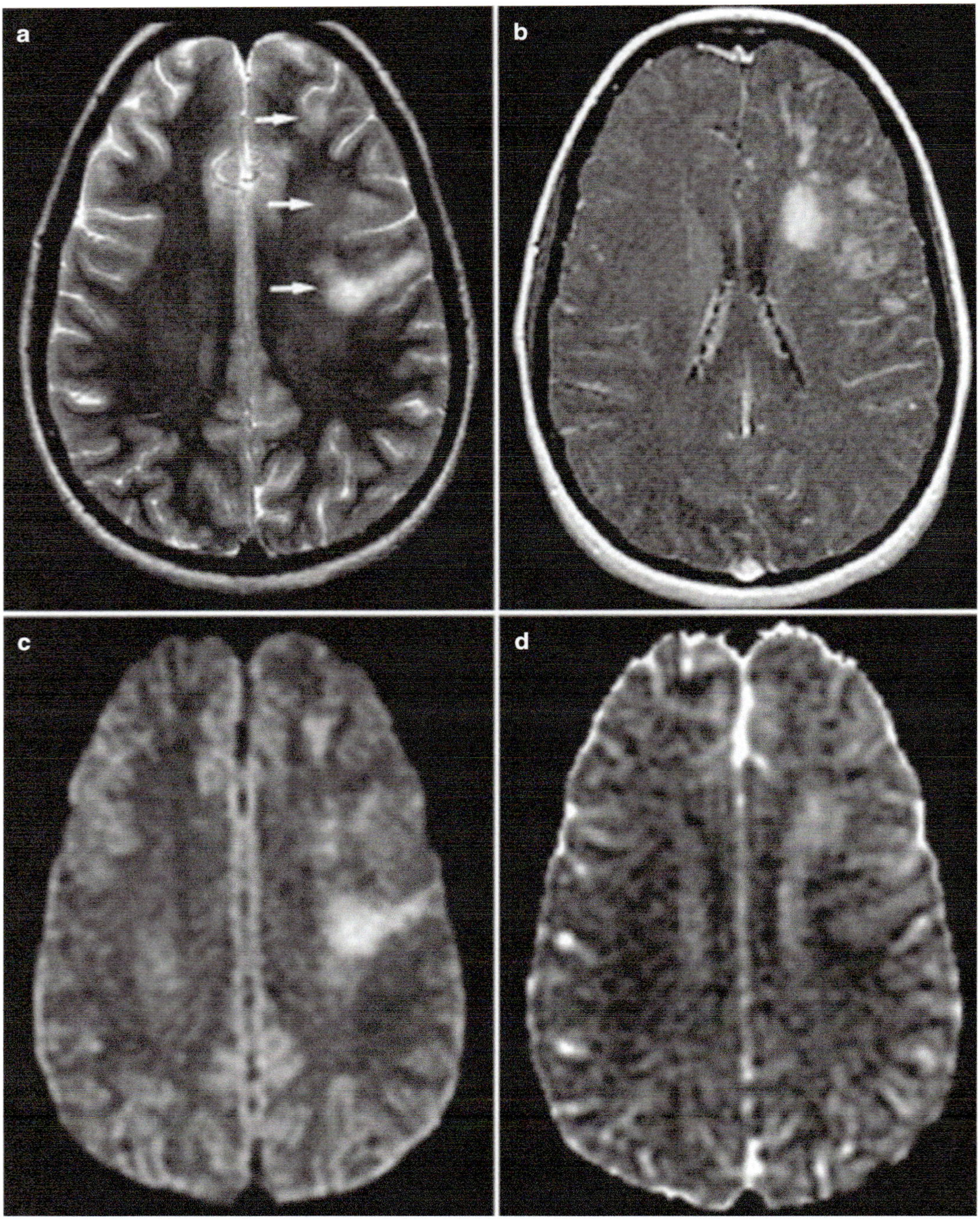

Fig. 13.12 (a–d) Acute disseminated encephalomyelitis in a 15-year-old male patient presenting with right hemiparesis. (a) T2-weighted image shows multiple ill-defined, hyperintense lesions in the left frontal lobe (*arrows*) (b) Gadolinium T1-weighted image with magnetization transfer contrast shows inhomogeneous enhancement of these lesions. (c) DW image shows left frontal lesions as hyperintense due to T2 shine-through. (d) ADC is increased

13 Demyelinating Diseases

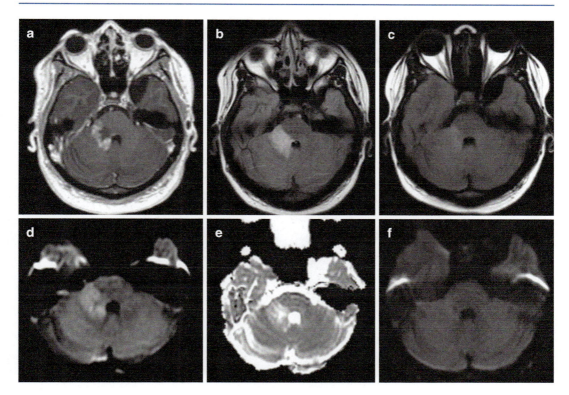

Fig. 13.13 ADEM in 19-year-old woman with numbness on the right side of her face, altered taste sensation, vertigo, sustained nystagmus, and ataxia. (**a**) Incomplete ring-enhancing lesion in right pons with high FLAIR (**b**), TRACE DWI (**c**), and ADC map (**d**) indicating vasogenic edema. Substantial clinical and imaging improvement followed under steroids treatment: (**e**) FLAIR and (**f**) TRACE DWI 4 months later

ated with high ADC values, was found in most evaluated ADEM patients [75]. Low FA and high RD occurred in MS pediatric patients compared with ADEM and controls, and hence DTI could distinguish between ADEM and MS at disease onset [76].

13.1.10 Acute Hemorrhagic Leukoencephalitis

Acute hemorrhagic leukoencephalitis (AHL; Hurst encephalitis) is an acute, rapidly progressive, and frequently fulminant inflammatory hemorrhagic demyelination, considered a hyperacute form of ADEM [1, 73]. It is unclear whether AHL is part of the spectrum of ADEM or a different clinical entity because of the paucity of AHL case reports [77]. It is usually triggered by upper respiratory tract infections. Most cases are fatal within 1 week from clinical onset. MR imaging shows large white matter lesions with extensive surrounding edema [78]. DW imaging shows restricted diffusion in the affected areas of the brain and hemorrhage, probably due to acute vasculitis with subsequent vessel occlusion (Fig. 13.15) [73, 79]. Pathologically, early features are hemorrhages, vessel fibrinoid necrosis, perivascular fibrin exudation, edema, and neutrophilic inflammation. Perivascular demyelination, microglial foci, and myelin-laden macrophages appear later. Pathological evidence of primary astrocyte damage with secondary demyelination has been reported in an AHL patient [80].

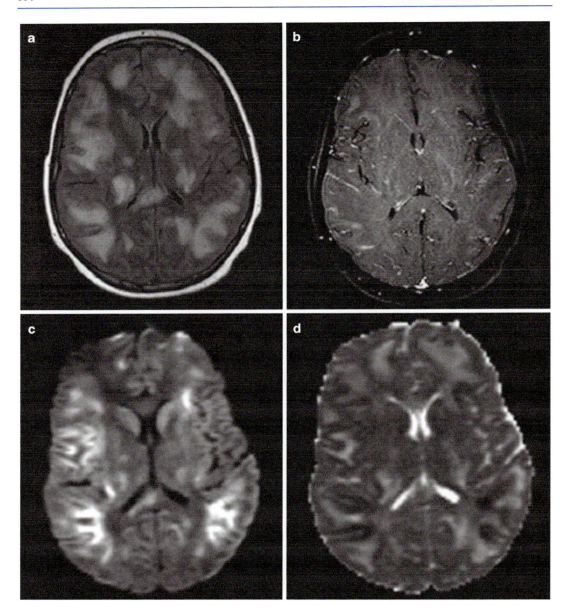

Fig. 13.14 (**a–d**) Acute disseminated encephalomyelitis in an 11-year-old boy with altered mental status. (**a**) FLAIR image shows multiple ill-defined, hyperintense lesions in the white matter, corpus callosum and basal ganglia, and thalami. (**b**) Post-contrast T1-weighted image shows mild enhancement in subcortical white matter lesions. (**c, d**) DW image shows multiple hyperintense lesions with increased ADC and partially decreased ADC in the peripheral area of the lesions, which probably represents a combination of vasogenic and cytotoxic edema with demyelination

13.2 Systemic Lupus Erythematosus (SLE)

SLE is discussed in Chap. 11 (Vasculopathy and Vasculitis); here emphasis is placed in its differential imaging diagnosis with demyelinating conditions. SLE is a chronic, immune-mediated, inflammatory disease affecting 0.1% of the general population [81]. Neuropsychiatric manifestations in SLE (NPSLE) have been more frequently recognized in recent years, occurring in up to 75% of patients during the disease course.

13 Demyelinating Diseases

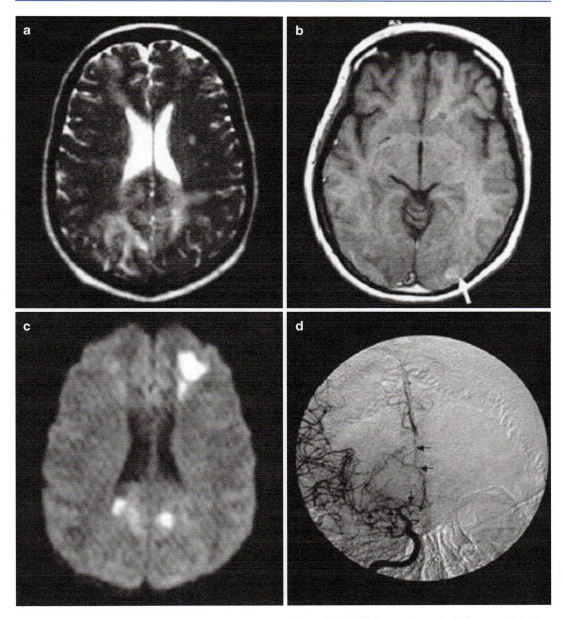

Fig. 13.15 (**a–d**) Acute hemorrhagic leukoencephalitis in a 48-year-old woman with altered mental status. (**a**) T2-weighted image shows multiple hyperintense lesions in the anterior and posterior white matter bilaterally. (**b**) T1-weighted image shows a hyperintense area in the left occipital lobe consistent with intracerebral hemorrhage (*arrows*). (**c**) DW image shows the lesions as mildly low or isointense signal intensity areas with multiple very hyperintense foci consistent with a combination of vasogenic and cytotoxic edema. (**d**) DSA shows multiple stenoses in the anterior and middle cerebral arteries (*arrows*). This patient died within 1 week

Brain atrophy and WMH are the main imaging presentations, and also stroke, hemorrhage, vasculitis, dural sinus thrombosis, myelitis, and aseptic meningitis have been reported [82]. The most common focal MRI abnormality in SLE are WMHs, which were observed in 57.1% of patients vs. 30.8% for gray matter T2 hyperintensities. Cerebral calcifications particularly in the basal ganglia and cerebellum have been reported [83]. Abnormal MRI findings were more commonly observed in SLE patients with antiphospholipid syndrome [84]. DW imaging shows either infarctions or vasogenic edema (Fig. 13.16) with or without microinfarcts [85]. Most imaging studies of SLE using DTI reported reduced FA and increased MD values in several white regions of both NPSLE and non-NPSLE patients compared to controls, indicating compromised white matter structural integrity [86–88]. Decreased FA values in NPSLE patients were reported mainly in the corpus callosum, frontal, and parietal white matter [86].

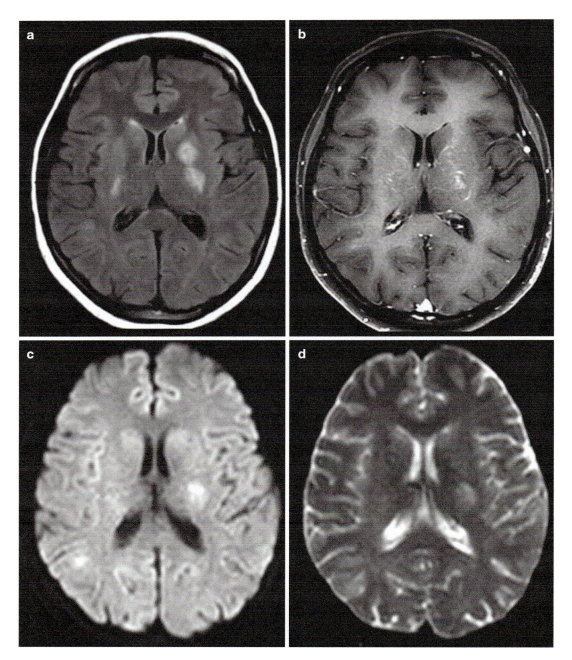

Fig. 13.16 31-year-old woman with SLE and meningoencephalitis. Axial FLAIR (**a**) shows hyperintense lesions of the left basal ganglia and right internal capsule with faint enhancement (**b**). TRACE DWI (**c**) and ADC MAP (**d**) with facilitated diffusion

13 Demyelinating Diseases

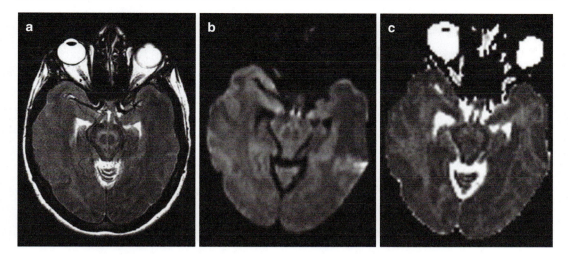

Fig. 13.17 (**a–c**) Hashimoto's encephalopathy in a 43-year-old woman with hypothyroidism. (**a**) T2-weighted image shows brain swelling and right temporal white matter hyperintensity. (**b, c**) DW imaging shows right temporal white matter hyperintensity with increased ADC consistent with vasogenic edema. Follow-up MR imaging (not shown) displayed improved swelling and edema (Courtesy of Dr. Limin Yang)

13.3 Steroid-Responsive Encephalopathy Associated with Autoimmune Thyroiditis (Hashimoto's Encephalopathy)

Steroid-responsive encephalopathy associated with autoimmune thyroiditis (SREAT), often termed Hashimoto's encephalopathy, is characterized by subacute relapsing-remitting neurologic and neuropsychiatric symptoms and increased titers of antithyroid antibodies (thyroperoxidase antibody) in the serum and CSF [89]. SREAT has a variety of clinical presentations including stroke-like symptoms, seizure, tremor, mental status changes, delirium, hallucination, and dementia. It is often misdiagnosed initially due to nonspecific symptoms. The pathogenesis is largely debated. Current hypotheses encompass autoimmunity (an immunological reaction to antineuronal antibodies against brain–thyroid antigens), autoimmune vasculitis, direct toxic effect by excessive thyrotropin-releasing hormone, global hypoperfusion, edema, and primary demyelination [89–96]. Since the disease responds to steroids, early diagnosis is important in conjunction with MR imaging, which can minimize the adverse outcome. Recently reported MR imaging findings include diffuse white matter lesions [97], involvement of the nucleus accumbens in the ventral striatum [98], hippocampal and medullary lesions, as well as cerebellar atrophy [99, 100]. DW imaging shows diffuse white matter lesions as isointense with increased ADC values (Fig. 13.17).

13.4 Chronic Lymphocytic Inflammation with Pontine Perivascular Enhancement Responsive to Steroids (CLIPPERS)

CLIPPERS is a recently defined inflammatory CNS disorder involving the brainstem and particularly the pons. The clinical symptoms are referable to the location of the brainstem pathology. On MRI there are punctate and curvilinear foci of intense gadolinium enhancement following a perivascular distribution in the pons (Fig. 13.18, [101]). Adjacent rhombencephalic structures such as the cerebellar peduncles, cerebellum, medulla, and the midbrain may also be involved. Enhancing lesions may additionally extend into the spinal cord and thalamus, basal ganglia, capsula interna, corpus callosum, and

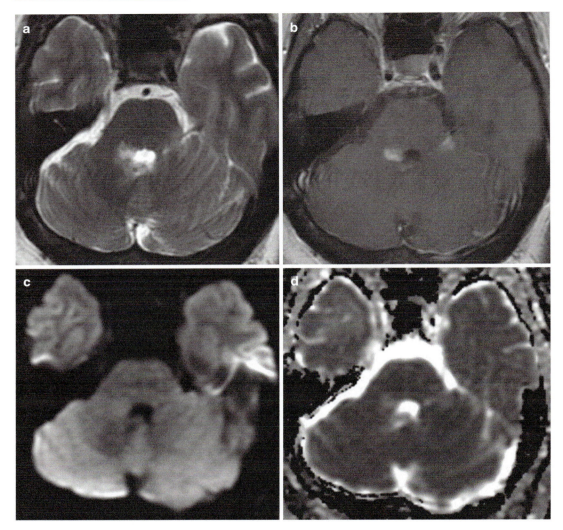

Fig. 13.18 CLIPPERS in a 52-year-old female with progressive bilateral body numbness, difficulty walking and hand clumsiness. Three serial lumbar punctures showed pleocytosis but negative cytology and oligoclonal bands. Responded favorably to steroid treatment. Axial T2 (**a**) and post-contrast T1 (**b**) with patchy enhancement and edema at the pons with facilitated diffusion on TRACE DWI (**c**) and ADC map (**d**)

the cerebral white matter. The visualization of the lesions is faint on T2-weighted and FLAIR sequences as compared to post-contrast T1-weighted images. Only 1 out of 22 CLIPPERS patients had minor DWI hyperintensity [102]. It has been reported that relapsing remitting MS patients may present imaging findings of CLIPPERS [103].

There is characteristic clinical and radiological responsiveness to glucocorticosteroid-based immunosuppression, as indicated in the name of the syndrome. Withdrawal of steroids commonly leads to disease exacerbation; hence long-term immunosuppressive therapy is frequently required. A specific serum or CSF biomarker for the disorder is currently not known. Brain neuropathology in CLIPPERS demonstrated strong CD3-positive T-lymphocyte, mild B-lymphocyte, and moderate macrophage perivascular infiltrates. There is also diffuse parenchymal lymphocytic infiltration in meninges, white and gray matter, associated with variable tissue destruction, astrogliosis, and secondary myelin loss [102]. No evidence of granulomas, infection, lymphoma, or vasculitis was seen on neuropathology [104]. There have been reports of lymphoma following diagnosis of CLIPPERS, but this is not the case for the majority of patients [102, 105, 106].

13.5 Miscellaneous Conditions

13.5.1 Erdheim Chester Disease (ECD)

ECD is rare form of non-Langerhans cells histiocytosis with multi-organ involvement. Individuals are more frequently affected in the fifth decade. ECD patients have mutations in the proto-oncogene BRAF [107]. Osseous involvement is the most frequent feature with bilateral symmetric osteosclerotic changes in long bone diaphyseal and metaphyseal regions, sparing epiphyses with increased bone scintigraphy uptake in almost all patients, even asymptomatic. Other classical features evocative of ECD include "coated" aorta and "hairy kidney" patterns from local histiocytic infiltration [108]. FDG-PET reveals increased glucose uptake in the long bones, mostly in the lower extremities (Fig. 13.19). Cerebellar ataxia and diabetes insipidus are the most common neurologic presentations. Neuroradiologic involvement can be seen in the dura, brainstem, cerebellum, spinal cord, hypothalamic-pituitary axis, and orbits [109]. WMHs in ECD are more frequently infratentorial (Fig. 13.19), also with frequent spinal cord involvement [110]. Skull base involvement with discrete solitary tumor lesions may resemble meningioma or schwannoma [111].

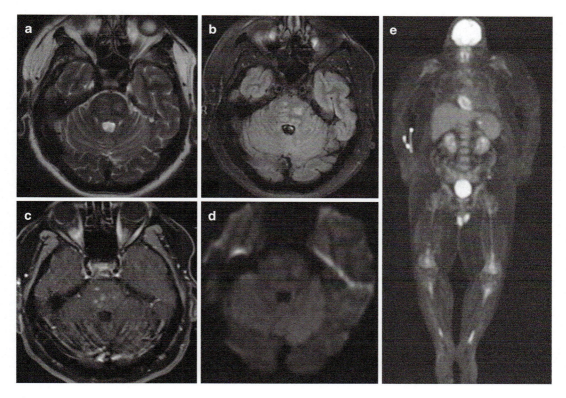

Fig. 13.19 Erdheim Chester disease in 48-year-old man with weakness, facial tingling and diplopia. Note similar enhancement pattern as CLIPPERS. (**a**) T2, (**b**) FLAIR, (**c**) T1 post-contrast, (**d**) DWI, (**e**) whole body FDG PET with increased uptake in the long bones

13.5.2 Hemophagocytic Lymphohistiocytosis (HLH)

HLH is a life-threatening disorder characterized by excessive activation of cytotoxic T lymphocytes, natural killer (NK) cells and macrophages resulting in a cytokine storm with injury of multiple organ systems. It affects both children and adults and may be either primary, driven by genetic mutations, or secondary to malignant, infectious, or autoimmune stimuli. Clinical and laboratory manifestations include fever, splenomegaly, neurologic dysfunction, coagulopathy, liver dysfunction, cytopenias, highly increased CSF protein, and hemophagocytosis [112]. Neurologic manifestations are reported in over 50% in pediatric [113] and 10% of adult [114] HLH patients with disturbance of consciousness, cranial nerve palsies, seizures, headache, limb paralysis, irritability, meningism, and memory loss [114]. Neuropathological findings consist of leptomeningeal inflammatory infiltrates, perivascular infiltration, and tissue infiltration with blood vessel destruction and necrosis [115]. On brain MRI, children with HLH, unlike patients with ADEM had symmetric periventricular WMHs without thalamic or brainstem involvement [116]. WMHs can be large or circumscribed areas of patchy T2 signal changes might correspond to demyelination, edema, and gliosis, with variable ring or nodular contrast enhancement [115] (Fig. 13.20).

13.6 Progressive Multifocal Leukoencephalopathy

Progressive multifocal leukoencephalopathy (PML) is a demyelinating disease of the central nervous system occurring in immunocompromised patients such as those with HIV infection or other conditions associated with impaired T-cell function [117]. Demyelination in PML results from the lytic infection of oligodendrocytes by JC papovavirus, spreading to adjacent oligodendrocytes. Diagnosis is established by the detection of JC virus DNA in the CSF.

MR imaging shows T2 and FLAIR hyperintense white matter lesions, often extending to subcortical U-fibers. The degree of contrast enhancement of the lesion depends on the patient's immunological status: it is absent in immunocompromised subjects and present in immune reconstitution inflammatory syndrome (IRIS). DW imaging usually shows mildly hyperintense lesions with increased ADC, which may have a central iso- or hypointense area. It occasionally shows hyperintensity with decreased ADC, especially at the margins of the lesion, reflecting different stages of the disease (Figs. 13.21, 13.22, and 13.23). These findings probably represent the sequential process of tissue injury with central areas of completed tissue injury with necrosis surrounded by a progressing rim of active tissue injury with cytotoxic edema [118]. High b value (3000 s/mm^2) DWI improves the contrast resolution between lesion rim, core, and normal-appearing white matter thus improving identification of the typical rim-and-core pattern of PML lesions. The peripheral hyperintensity rim on DW images with decreased ADC may represent JC virus-infected, swollen oligodendrocytes with viral intranuclear inclusions [117–119]. On DTI, an area of decreased FA is observed in PML, which represents abnormal microstructure of the myelin sheath. This change may be observed earlier than the increased ADC which represents secondary diffuse cell loss (Fig. 13.22) [118].

13.7 Conclusion

Magnetic resonance imaging with DWI and DTI including ADC and FA maps and fiber tractography are useful in characterizing demyelinating lesions of the brain. These imaging techniques can increase specificity and improve our understanding of the pathophysiology of these complex diseases.

13 Demyelinating Diseases

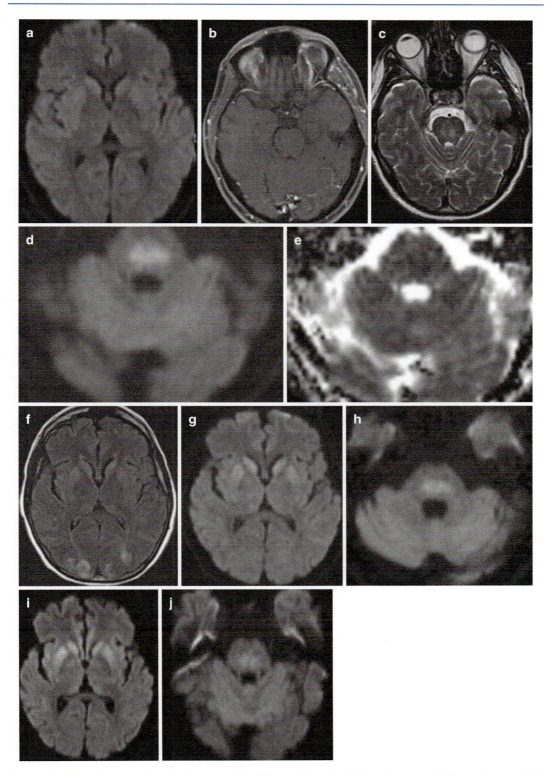

Fig. 13.20 Hemophagocytic lymphohistiocytosis in 37-year-old male viral meningoencephalitis causing systemic inflammatory response syndrome (SIRS). Imaging on day 14 of admission (**a–e**), on day 29 (**f–h**) and 43 (**i, j**)

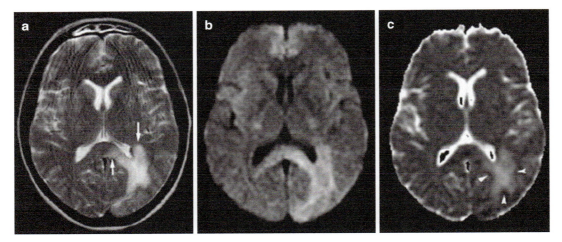

Fig. 13.21 (**a–c**) Progressive multifocal leukoencephalopathy in a 50-year-old woman presenting with right hemianopsia after chemotherapy for chronic lymphocytic leukemia. (**a**) T2-weighted image shows a hyperintense lesion in the left occipital white matter extending into the posterior corpus callosum (*arrows*). (**b**) DW image shows the lesion as hyperintense due to T2 shine-through. (**c**) ADC is increased. The peripheral area of the lesion seems to have relatively decreased ADC (*arrowheads*)

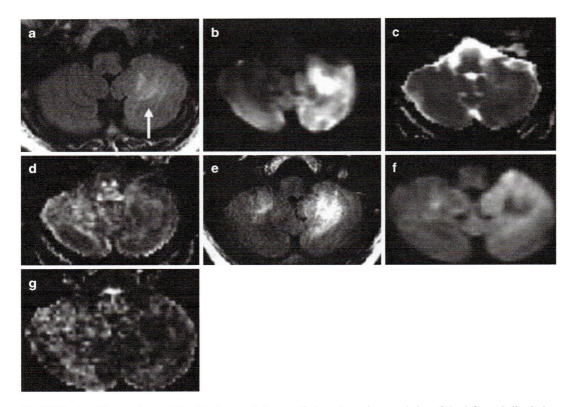

Fig. 13.22 (**a–g**) Progressive multifocal leukoencephalopathy (PML) in a 48-year-old man. (**a**) FLAIR image shows a hyperintense lesion in the left cerebellum (*arrow*). (**b, c**) DW imaging shows the lesion as hyperintense with iso or slightly increased ADC values, which suggests the early active phase of demyelination in PML. (**d**) FA is slightly decreased in this lesion. (**e**) Follow-up FLAIR image after 19 days shows increased size of the left cerebellar lesion extending to the right cerebellum. (**f**) DW image shows the left cerebellar lesion as mildly hyperintense with a central hypointensity, suggesting vasogenic edema, demyelination, and necrosis. (**g**) FA map showed a significantly enlarged area of decreased FA in the left cerebellum suggesting ongoing tissue damage. (Courtesy of Edip Gurol, MD)

13 Demyelinating Diseases

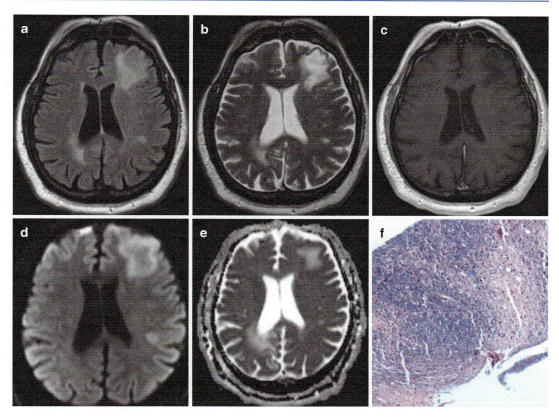

Fig. 13.23 PML in a 67-year-old man with history of diffuse large B-cell lymphoma on Rituximab presenting with new onset confusion. Axial T2 (**a**) and FLAIR (**b**): Ill-defined hyperintense left frontal lobe lesion sparing the cortex with no enhancement on post-GAD T1 images (**c**). TRACE DWI (**d**) and ADC map (**e**) display peripheral reduced diffusion and central facilitated diffusion. (**f**) Luxol fast blue stain showing patchy myelin loss

13.8 Treatment of Demyelinating Diseases Section

Andrew Romeo

13.8.1 Multiple Sclerosis Treatment

13.8.1.1 Acute Treatment of Multiple Sclerosis Relapses

Depending on the severity of symptoms, as well as patient and provider preference, MS relapses may be treated with high-dose pulses of corticosteroids to speed recovery [120]. Relapses which are disabling in some way (e.g., optic neuritis or paraparesis) are typically treated with corticosteroids. Pulse doses of corticosteroids may be administered for 3–5 days, either intravenous or oral, in bioequivalent doses (e.g., methylprednisolone 1000 mg IV daily or prednisone 1250 mg PO daily for 3–5 days) [121]. Therapeutic plasmapheresis (plasma exchange, PLEX) may be indicated for severe relapse if the response to corticosteroids is deemed inadequate [122].

13.8.1.2 Multiple Sclerosis Disease-Modifying Therapy

Relapsing Remitting Multiple Sclerosis Disease-Modifying Therapy

Relapse prevention is the basic goal of maintenance treatment in MS. Early treatment is believed to delay worsening of disability [148–151]. Some providers strive for "no evidence of disease activity" (NEDA), developed as a clinical trial outcome measure and defined as no clinical relapse, no sustained worsening on expanded disability status scale (EDSS), and no new lesions on MRI (no new T2 hyperintense lesions or new enhancing lesions) [150, 152]. Currently available disease-modifying therapies essentially fall into three categories: self-injection, oral, and infusion (Table 13.2). Most treatments have not been subjected to head-to-head randomized clinical trials. Two contrasting approaches to treatment selection have been proposed: escalation and induction [153]. Taking an escalation approach, a patient may start treatment with an injectable treatment, which has possibly lower efficacy but a more favorable safety profile. In the event of clinical relapse, or new lesions on surveillance imaging, therapy would be escalated to an oral therapy, and subsequently to an infusion therapy. Conversely, an induction approach would utilize an infusion therapy first-line, in hopes of yielding better long-term clinical outcomes (though this has yet to be definitively demonstrated) [151, 154]. In practice, treatment choices (initiation or switching) are not algorithmic, and should be made in partnership with the patient, guided by the patient's concerns and preferences regarding route of administration and potential/experienced adverse effects [149, 155].

Pertinent potential adverse effects of the available MS disease-modifying therapies are listed in Table 13.2; regular safety monitoring is essential, but specifics of safety monitoring remain provider- and practice-dependent. Peripartum treatment considerations merit dedicated discussion [156]. Even when disease-modifying therapy is well-managed, people with MS can suffer from a number of chronic or intermittent symptoms (e.g., neuropathic pain, depression, and neurogenic bladder impairment); treatment of these symptoms requires a nuanced approach, again in partnership with the patient [157].

Progressive Multiple Sclerosis Disease-Modifying Therapy

Ocrelizumab is currently the only approved therapy for primary progressive multiple sclerosis. In a randomized placebo-controlled trial, ocrelizumab was found to modestly slow dis-

ability progression (assessed via Expanded Disability Status Scale), with other positive imaging and clinical outcome measures [142]. It was suggested that gadolinium-enhancing lesions on baseline MRI may be a marker of ocrelizumab treatment response in PPMS, but the study was not adequately powered to demonstrate this [142].

Currently no available therapies are labeled for treatment of secondary progressive multiple sclerosis. Evidence for interferon beta in SPMS is mixed, but suggests that patients early in the transition to secondary progression and/or experiencing more inflammatory activity may benefit from therapy [158–160]. Siponimod is a selective sphingosine-1-phosphate receptor functional antagonist. In a randomized placebo-controlled trial, siponimod reduced confirmed disability progression at 3 and 6 months, and reduced brain volume loss [161].

13.8.1.3 Pediatric Multiple Sclerosis Treatment

The preceding discussion implicitly addressed treatment of multiple sclerosis relapses and disease-modifying therapy for adults. Data is more limited in the pediatric population. High-dose pulses of corticosteroids may be used to acutely treat relapses, with adjusted dosing (e.g., 20–30 mg/kg daily for 3–5 days) [162]. Injectable disease-modifying therapies (interferon beta and glatiramer acetate) have primarily been used to treat pediatric patients with relapsing multiple sclerosis (based on retrospective and uncontrolled prospective studies). Fingolimod was recently demonstrated to be superior to interferon beta-1a, reducing both annualized relapse rate and annualized rate of new or newly enlarged T2-hyperintense white matter lesions in pediatric MS patients [163]. More patients attained freedom from relapses with fingolimod, but there were more serious adverse events in the fingolimod group. Experience with other oral and infusion therapies is more limited in the pediatric population.

Table 13.2 Disease-modifying therapies for relapsing multiple sclerosis (approved in the United States)

Route of administration	Disease-modifying therapy	Efficacy	Mechanisms of action (Known or postulated)	Potential adverse effects
Self-injection	Interferon beta-1b subcutaneous, alternate day (Betaseron)	• Up to approximately 34% reduction in ARR compared to placebo at 2 years [123] • Up to 75% median reduction in new lesion formation compared to placebo [124]	Immunomodulation/Leukocyte Trafficking [125] • Decreases production of pro-inflammatory cytokines (e.g., IL-17 and osteopontin) • Increases production of anti-inflammatory cytokines (e.g., IL-10 and IL-4) • Inhibits leukocyte migration across blood–brain barrier	• Injection site reactions [125] • Flu-like symptoms • Transaminitis • Depression
	Interferon beta-1a intramuscular, once weekly (Avonex)	• Approximately 32% reduction in ARR compared to placebo [126]		
	Interferon beta-1a subcutaneous, three times weekly (Rebif)	• Up to 33% reduction in ARR compared to placebo [127]		
	Pegylated interferon every 2 weeks (Plegridy)	• Up to approximately 36% reduction in ARR compared to placebo [128] • Approximately 67% reduction in adjusted mean number of new or enlarged T2-hyperintense lesions [128]		
	Glatiramer acetate (Copaxone, Glatopa)	• 29% reduction in ARR compared to placebo at 24 months [129]	Immunomodulation [130] • Competes with other antigens to impede T-cell activation • Shifts T- and B-cell responses from pro-inflammatory to anti-inflammatory	• Injection site reactions [129, 131] • Self-limited systemic injection reaction with flushing, chest tightness, dyspnea, palpitations, and/or anxiety [129]

(continued)

Table 13.2 (continued)

Route of administration	Disease-modifying therapy	Efficacy	Mechanisms of action (Known or postulated)	Potential adverse effects
Oral	Fingolimod (Gilenya)	• 54% reduction in ARR compared to placebo at 24 months [132] • 50.5% had no new or enlarged T2-hyperintense lesions at 24 months (21.2% placebo) [132]	Leukocyte Trafficking [132] • Functional antagonist of sphingosine-1-phosphate receptor • Inhibits lymphocyte egress from lymph nodes	• Bradycardia (potentially atrioventricular conduction block) [132, 133] • Macular edema • VZV infection • Transaminitis • Dermatologic malignancy
	Dimethyl fumarate (Tecfidera)	• 44% reduction in ARR compared to placebo at 2 years [134] • 71% reduction in new or enlarged T2-hyperintense lesions compared to placebo at 2 years [134]	Immunosuppression/Antioxidant [135] • Induces lymphocyte apoptosis • Inhibits lymphocyte proliferation • Antioxidant effect via Nrf-2 pathway	• Flushing [134, 135] • Gastrointestinal (abdominal pain, diarrhea, nausea, vomiting) • Lymphopenia
	Teriflunomide (Aubagio)	• Approximately 31% reduction in ARR (with 7 mg or 14 mg daily dose) compared to placebo [136] • Approximately 36% reduction in ARR (with 14 mg daily dose) compared to placebo [137]	Immunosuppression [136] • Inhibits dihydroorotate dehydrogenase, an enzyme in de novo pyramidine synthesis pathway • Reduces T- and B-cell activation and proliferation • Inhibits lymphocyte response to autoantigens	• Alopecia [138] • Diarrhea, nausea • Transaminitis • Neutropenia and/or lymphopenia • Peripheral neuropathy

Infusion	Natalizumab (Tysabri)	• 68% reduction in ARR compared to placebo at 2 years [139] • 83% reduction in new or enlarged T2-hyperintense lesions compared to placebo at 2 years [139]	Leukocyte Trafficking [139] • Monoclonal antibody against $\alpha4$ subunit of $\alpha4\beta1$ and $\alpha4\beta7$ integrins on leukocytes, inhibiting interaction with VCAM-1 • Inhibits leukocyte migration across blood–brain barrier	Progressive multifocal leukoencephalopathy [140]
	Ocrelizumab (Ocrevus)	• 46% and 47% reduction in ARR compared to interferon beta-1a, at 96 weeks [141] • 94% and 95% reduction in mean number of gadolinium-enhancing lesions per T1-weighted MRI [141] • 77% and 83% reduction in mean number of new or enlarged hyperintense lesions per T2-weighted MRI [141]	Immunosuppression [141] • Monoclonal antibody against CD20 • Depletes B-cells	• Infusion-related reaction (throat irritation, pruritus, rash, flushing) [141] • Infection (upper respiratory tract, nasopharyngitis, or urinary tract) • Possible risk of malignancy [141, 142]
	Alemtuzumab (Lemtrada)	• Approximately 54% reduction in ARR compared to interferon-beta1a, when used as first-line or second-line therapy [143, 144] • Treatment efficacy may be sustained for multiple years following second course of treatment [145, 146]	Immunosuppression [143, 144, 147] • Monoclonal antibody against CD52 • Depletes B- and T-cells, and the repopulated immune phenotype is believed to be less inflammatory (with regard to MS disease activity)	• Infusion-related reaction (headache, nausea, rash, fever) [143, 144] • Infection (nasopharyngitis, upper respiratory tract, urinary tract, herpetic) [143, 144] • Secondary autoimmunity (thyroid disorders, ITP, and glomerulonephritis) [144–146] • Malignancy [146]

ARR annualized relapse rate, *CD* cluster of differentiation, *ITP* immune thrombocytopenic purpura, *VCAM-1* vascular-cell adhesion molecule 1, *VZV* varicella zoster virus

13.8.2 Acute Disseminated Encephalomyelitis (ADEM) Treatment

ADEM is traditionally considered a monophasic illness, and concepts of recurrent or multiphasic ADEM remain controversial [164]. Accordingly, this discussion will be limited to acute treatment of ADEM, for both pediatric and adult patients. No randomized trials of treatment of ADEM have been performed. The heterogeneity of clinical presentations subsumed under the label of ADEM may challenge generalizability of findings from available studies. High-dose corticosteroids are the first-line acute treatment for ADEM (e.g., methylprednisolone 1000 mg IV daily (for adults) or 20–30 mg/kg/day (for children) for 3–5 days). If there is failure of response to corticosteroids, of if corticosteroids are contraindicated, intravenous immunoglobulin may be administered (though in cases, IVIg has been administered concurrently with corticosteroids) [165–167]. Alternatively, PLEX may be indicated for treatment-refractory cases [167, 168].

13.8.3 Neuromyelitis Optica Spectrum Disorders (NMOSD) Treatment

13.8.3.1 Treatment of NMOSD Relapses

In contrast to multiple sclerosis relapses, NMOSD exacerbations always call for acute treatment, due to the potential for permanent disability [169]. High-dose corticosteroids (e.g., methylprednisolone 1000 mg IV for 3–5 days) are first line for treatment of NMOSD exacerbation. Recent data suggest that early initiation of PLEX may confer a more favorable recovery from NMOSD exacerbation [170–172].

13.8.3.2 NMOSD Maintenance Treatment

Rituximab, mycophenolate mofetil, azathioprine, and chronic corticosteroids have been conventionally utilized for prevention of NMOSD exacerbations [173]. Currently there are no published placebo-controlled randomized trials for NMOSD maintenance therapy. A recent randomized trial demonstrated superiority of rituximab over azathioprine for prevention of NMOSD exacerbations [174]. Maintenance treatment for 5 years following the first NMOSD exacerbation has been recommended [175].

13.8.4 Progressive Multifocal Leukoencephalopathy (PML) Treatment

PML is generally fatal or neurologically disabling, thus risk stratification and attempted prevention are crucial for multiple sclerosis patients on disease-modifying therapies which have been associated with PML (natalizumab, fingolimod, and dimethyl fumarate) [176]. Positive serum anti-JC virus antibody, treatment for more than 2 years (more than 24 infusions with standard dosing), and prior immunosuppressant use (e.g., azathioprine, mycophenolate mofetil, methotrexate, cyclophosphamide, and mitoxantrone) are key risk factors for PML in patients treated with natalizumab [177]. The level (index) of serum anti-JC virus antibody may further stratify the risk of PML [178]. Extending the natalizumab dosing interval (from every 4 weeks to every 6 weeks) may be a way to reduce PML risk, without reducing treatment efficacy [179, 180]. In practice, the risk of PML is sufficiently low in patients with negative serum anti-JC virus antibody, and natalizumab may be safely initiated. Testing for serum anti-JC virus antibody is repeated every 6 months, and in most cases a positive antibody result prompts strong consideration of switching MS therapies. For MS patients on dimethyl fumarate, absolute lymphocyte counts should be monitored regularly, and dimethyl fumarate should be discontinued if sustained lymphopenia develops [176].

Treatment of PML is largely supportive, while facilitating immune reconstitution or surveillance [181]. Highly-active antiretroviral therapy should be initiated for patients with AIDS that develop PML. Natalizumab must be discontinued if a treated patient develops PML. Plasma exchange

(PLEX) has been utilized to speed the elimination of natalizumab, but evidence is mounting against this practice as it may hasten or prolong PML-immune reconstitution inflammatory syndrome (PML-IRIS) [182, 183]. Corticosteroids are routinely used to treat PML-IRIS, though efficacy has not been definitively demonstrated [184, 185]. PML prognosis remains grim, no matter the pre-disposing condition [176].

References

1. Canellas AR, Gols AR, Izquierdo JR, Subirana MT, Gairin XM (2007) Idiopathic inflammatory-demyelinating diseases of the central nervous system. Neuroradiology 49(5):393–409
2. Poser CM, Brinar VV (2004) The nature of multiple sclerosis. Clin Neurol Neurosurg 106(3):159–171
3. Traboulsee AL, Li DK (2006) The role of MRI in the diagnosis of multiple sclerosis. Adv Neurol 98:125–146
4. Thompson AJ, Banwell BL, Barkhof F, Carroll WM, Coetzee T, Comi G et al (2018) Diagnosis of multiple sclerosis: 2017 revisions of the McDonald criteria. Lancet Neurol 17(2):162–173
5. Filippi M, Inglese M (2001) Overview of diffusion-weighted magnetic resonance studies in multiple sclerosis. J Neurol Sci 186(Suppl 1):S37–S43
6. Palmer S, Bradley WG, Chen DY, Patel S (1999) Subcallosal striations: early findings of multiple sclerosis on sagittal, thin-section, fast FLAIR MR images. Radiology 210(1):149–153
7. Lisanti CJ, Asbach P, Bradley WG Jr (2005) The ependymal "Dot-Dash" sign: an MR imaging finding of early multiple sclerosis. AJNR Am J Neuroradiol 26(8):2033–2036
8. van Walderveen MA, Lycklama ANGJ, Ader HJ, Jongen PJ, Polman CH, Castelijns JA et al (2001) Hypointense lesions on T1-weighted spin-echo magnetic resonance imaging: relation to clinical characteristics in subgroups of patients with multiple sclerosis. Arch Neurol 58(1):76–81
9. Loevner LA, Grossman RI, McGowan JC, Ramer KN, Cohen JA (1995) Characterization of multiple sclerosis plaques with T1-weighted MR and quantitative magnetization transfer. AJNR Am J Neuroradiol 16(7):1473–1479
10. Sati P, Oh J, Constable RT, Evangelou N, Guttmann CR, Henry RG et al (2016) The central vein sign and its clinical evaluation for the diagnosis of multiple sclerosis: a consensus statement from the North American Imaging in Multiple Sclerosis Cooperative. Nat Rev Neurol 12(12):714–722
11. Abou Zeid N, Pirko I, Erickson B, Weigand SD, Thomsen KM, Scheithauer B et al (2012) Diffusion-weighted imaging characteristics of biopsy-proven demyelinating brain lesions. Neurology 78(21):1655–1662
12. Finelli PF, Foxman EB (2014) The etiology of ring lesions on diffusion-weighted imaging. Neuroradiol J 27(3):280–287
13. Sener RN (2002) Atypical X-linked adrenoleukodystrophy: new MRI observations with FLAIR, magnetization transfer contrast, diffusion MRI, and proton spectroscopy. Magn Reson Imaging 20(2):215–219
14. Moritani T, Edema B (2009) In: Moritani TES, Westesson PL (eds) Diffusion-weighted MR imaging of the brain. Springer, Berlin, Heidelberg, pp 37–54
15. Abdoli M, Chakraborty S, MacLean HJ, Freedman MS (2016) The evaluation of MRI diffusion values of active demyelinating lesions in multiple sclerosis. Mult Scler Relat Disord 10:97–102
16. Rovira A, Pericot I, Alonso J, Rio J, Grive E, Montalban X (2002) Serial diffusion-weighted MR imaging and proton MR spectroscopy of acute large demyelinating brain lesions: case report. AJNR Am J Neuroradiol 23(6):989–994
17. Roychowdhury S, Maldjian JA, Grossman RI (2000) Multiple sclerosis: comparison of trace apparent diffusion coefficients with MR enhancement pattern of lesions. AJNR Am J Neuroradiol 21(5):869–874
18. Tievsky AL, Ptak T, Farkas J (1999) Investigation of apparent diffusion coefficient and diffusion tensor anisotrophy in acute and chronic multiple sclerosis lesions. AJNR Am J Neuroradiol 20(8):1491–1499
19. Horsfield MA, Larsson HB, Jones DK, Gass A (1998) Diffusion magnetic resonance imaging in multiple sclerosis. J Neurol Neurosurg Psychiatry 64(Suppl 1):S80–S84
20. Castriota Scanderbeg A, Tomaiuolo F, Sabatini U, Nocentini U, Grasso MG, Caltagirone C (2000) Demyelinating plaques in relapsing-remitting and secondary-progressive multiple sclerosis: assessment with diffusion MR imaging. AJNR Am J Neuroradiol 21(5):862–868
21. Zacharzewska-Gondek A, Pokryszko-Dragan A, Gondek TM, Koltowska A, Gruszka E, Budrewicz S et al (2019) Apparent diffusion coefficient measurements in normal appearing white matter may support the differential diagnosis between multiple sclerosis lesions and other white matter hyperintensities. J Neurol Sci 397:24–30
22. Ceccarelli A, Rocca MA, Falini A, Tortorella P, Pagani E, Rodegher M et al (2007) Normal-appearing white and grey matter damage in MS. J Neurol 254(4):513–518
23. Temel Ş, Keklİğkoğlu HD, Vural G, Deniz O, Ercan K (2013) Diffusion tensor magnetic resonance imaging in patients with multiple sclerosis and its relationship with disability. Neuroradiol J 26(1):3–17
24. Poonawalla AH, Hasan KM, Gupta RK, Ahn CW, Nelson F, Wolinsky JS et al (2008) Diffusion-tensor MR imaging of cortical lesions in multiple sclerosis: initial findings. Radiology 246(3):880–886

25. Loevner LA, Grossman RI, Cohen JA, Lexa FJ, Kessler D, Kolson DL (1995) Microscopic disease in normal-appearing white matter on conventional MR images in patients with multiple sclerosis: assessment with magnetization-transfer measurements. Radiology 196(2):511–515

26. Miller DH, Chard DT, Ciccarelli O (2012) Clinically isolated syndromes. Lancet Neurol. 11(2):157–169

27. Schwenkenbecher P, Sarikidi A, Bonig L, Wurster U, Bronzlik P, Suhs KW et al (2017) Clinically isolated syndrome according to McDonald 2010: intrathecal IgG synthesis still predictive for conversion to multiple sclerosis. Int J Mol Sci 18(10):2061

28. Okuda DT, Mowry EM, Beheshtian A, Waubant E, Baranzini SE, Goodin DS et al (2009) Incidental MRI anomalies suggestive of multiple sclerosis: the radiologically isolated syndrome. Neurology 72(9):800–805

29. Labiano-Fontcuberta A, Benito-Leon J (2016) Radiologically isolated syndrome: an update on a rare entity. Mult scler (Houndmills, Basingstoke, England) 22(12):1514–1521

30. Lebrun C, Kantarci OH, Siva A, Pelletier D, Okuda DT (2018) Anomalies characteristic of central nervous system demyelination: radiologically isolated syndrome. Neurol Clin 36(1):59–68

31. Caracciolo JT, Murtagh RD, Rojiani AM, Murtagh FR (2001) Pathognomonic MR imaging findings in Balo concentric sclerosis. AJNR Am J Neuroradiol 22(2):292–293

32. Capello E, Mancardi GL (2004) Marburg type and Balo's concentric sclerosis: rare and acute variants of multiple sclerosis. Neurol Sci 25(Suppl 4):S361–S363

33. Karaarslan E, Altintas A, Senol U, Yeni N, Dincer A, Bayindir C et al (2001) Balo's concentric sclerosis: clinical and radiologic features of five cases. AJNR Am J Neuroradiol 22(7):1362–1367

34. Hardy TA, Miller DH. Balo's concentric sclerosis. Lancet Neurol. 2014;13(7):740–746

35. BALO J (1928) Encephalitis periaxialis concentrica. Arch Neurol Psychiatr 19(2):242–264

36. Kavanagh EC, Heran MK, Fenton DM, Lapointe JS, Nugent RA, Graeb DA (2006) Diffusion-weighted imaging findings in Balo concentric sclerosis. Br J Radiol 79(943):e28–e31

37. Wiendl H, Weissert R, Herrlinger U, Krapf H, Kuker W (2005) Diffusion abnormality in Balo's concentric sclerosis: clues for the pathogenesis. Eur Neurol 53(1):42–44

38. Ball T, Malik O, Roncaroli F, Quest RA, Aviv RI (2007) Apparent diffusion coefficient changes and lesion evolution in Balo's type demyelination-correlation with histopathology. Clin Radiol 62(5):498–503

39. Miyamoto N, Kagohashi M, Nishioka K, Fujishima K, Kitada T, Tomita Y et al (2006) An autopsy case of Schilder's variant of multiple sclerosis (Schilder's disease). Eur Neurol 55(2):103–107

40. Obara S, Takeshima H, Awa R, Yonezawa H, Oyoshi T, Nagayama T et al (2003) Tumefactive myelinoclastic diffuse sclerosis—case report. Neurol Med Chir 43(11):563–566

41. Jahn M, Steinberg H (2018) First description of Schilder's disease: Paul Ferdinand Schilder and his struggle for the delimitation of a new entity. Nervenarzt 90(4):415–422

42. Schilder P (1912) Zur Kenntnis der sogenannten diffusen Sklerose. (Über Encephalitis periaxialis diffusa.). Zeitschrift für die gesamte Neurologie und Psychiatrie 10(1):1

43. Kurdi M, Ramsay D (2016) Balo's concentric lesions with concurrent features of Schilder's disease in relapsing multiple sclerosis: neuropathological findings. Autops Case Rep 6(4):21–26

44. Masdeu JC, Quinto C, Olivera C, Tenner M, Leslie D, Visintainer P (2000) Open-ring imaging sign: highly specific for atypical brain demyelination. Neurology 54(7):1427–1433

45. Geraldes R, Ciccarelli O, Barkhof F, De Stefano N, Enzinger C, Filippi M et al (2018) The current role of MRI in differentiating multiple sclerosis from its imaging mimics. Nat Rev Neurol 14(4):199–213

46. Aliaga ES, Barkhof F (2014) MRI mimics of multiple sclerosis. Handb Clin Neurol 122:291–316

47. Scheltens P, Erkinjunti T, Leys D, Wahlund LO, Inzitari D, del Ser T et al (1998) White matter changes on CT and MRI: an overview of visual rating scales. European task force on age-related white matter changes. Eur Neurol 39(2):80–89

48. Falini A, Kesavadas C, Pontesilli S, Rovaris M, Scotti G (2001) Differential diagnosis of posterior fossa multiple sclerosis lesions—neuroradiological aspects. Neurol Sci 22(Suppl 2):S79–S83

49. Kleffner I, Dorr J, Ringelstein M, Gross CC, Bockenfeld Y, Schwindt W et al (2016) Diagnostic criteria for Susac syndrome. J Neurol Neurosurg Psychiatry 87(12):1287–1295

50. Weinshenker BG, Wingerchuk DM (2017) Neuromyelitis spectrum disorders. Mayo Clin Proc 92(4):663–679

51. Wingerchuk DM, Banwell B, Bennett JL, Cabre P, Carroll W, Chitnis T et al (2015) International consensus diagnostic criteria for neuromyelitis optica spectrum disorders. Neurology 85(2):177–189

52. Akaishi T, Nakashima I, Sato DK, Takahashi T, Fujihara K (2017) Neuromyelitis optica spectrum disorders. Neuroimaging Clin N Am 27(2):251–265

53. Popescu BF, Parisi JE, Cabrera-Gomez JA, Newell K, Mandler RN, Pittock SJ et al (2010) Absence of cortical demyelination in neuromyelitis optica. Neurology 75(23):2103–2109

54. Tatekawa H, Sakamoto S, Hori M, Kaichi Y, Kunimatsu A, Akazawa K et al (2018) Imaging differences between neuromyelitis optica spectrum disorders and multiple sclerosis: a multi-institutional study in Japan. AJNR Am J Neuroradiol 39(7):1239–1247

55. Rueda Lopes FC, Doring T, Martins C, Cabral FC, Malfetano FR, Pereira VC et al (2012) The role of demyelination in neuromyelitis optica damage: diffusion-tensor MR imaging study. Radiology 263(1):235–242

56. Kimura MC, Doring TM, Rueda FC, Tukamoto G, Gasparetto EL (2014) In vivo assessment of white matter damage in neuromyelitis optica: a diffusion tensor and diffusion kurtosis MR imaging study. J Neurol Sci 345(1–2):172–175

57. Yu C, Lin F, Li K, Jiang T, Qin W, Sun H et al (2008) Pathogenesis of normal-appearing white matter damage in neuromyelitis optica: diffusion-tensor MR imaging. Radiology 246(1):222–228

58. Liu Y, Duan Y, Huang J, Ren Z, Ye J, Dong H et al (2015) Multimodal quantitative MR imaging of the thalamus in multiple sclerosis and neuromyelitis optica. Radiology 277(3):784–792

59. Wan H, He H, Zhang F, Sha Y, Tian G (2017) Diffusion-weighted imaging helps differentiate multiple sclerosis and neuromyelitis optica-related acute optic neuritis. J Magn Reson Imaging 45(6):1780–1785

60. Rivero RL, Oliveira EM, Bichuetti DB, Gabbai AA, Nogueira RG, Abdala N (2014) Diffusion tensor imaging of the cervical spinal cord of patients with Neuromyelitis Optica. Magn Reson Imaging 32(5):457–463

61. Ramanathan S, Dale RC, Brilot F (2016) Anti-MOG antibody: the history, clinical phenotype, and pathogenicity of a serum biomarker for demyelination. Autoimmun Rev 15(4):307–324

62. Jarius S, Ruprecht K, Kleiter I, Borisow N, Asgari N, Pitarokoili K et al (2016) MOG-IgG in NMO and related disorders: a multicenter study of 50 patients. Part 1: frequency, syndrome specificity, influence of disease activity, long-term course, association with AQP4-IgG, and origin. J Neuroinflammation 13(1):279

63. Biotti D, Bonneville F, Tournaire E, Ayrignac X, Dalliere CC, Mahieu L et al (2017) Optic neuritis in patients with anti-MOG antibodies spectrum disorder: MRI and clinical features from a large multicentric cohort in France. J Neurol 264(10):2173–2175

64. Hardy TA, Chataway J (2013) Tumefactive demyelination: an approach to diagnosis and management. J Neurol Neurosurg Psychiatry 84(9):1047–1053

65. Lucchinetti CF, Gavrilova RH, Metz I, Parisi JE, Scheithauer BW, Weigand S et al (2008) Clinical and radiographic spectrum of pathologically confirmed tumefactive multiple sclerosis. Brain J Neurol 131(Pt 7):1759–1775

66. Altintas A, Petek B, Isik N, Terzi M, Bolukbasi F, Tavsanli M et al (2012) Clinical and radiological characteristics of tumefactive demyelinating lesions: follow-up study. Mult Scler (Houndmills, Basingstoke, England) 18(10):1448–1453

67. Kim DS, Na DG, Kim KH, Kim JH, Kim E, Yun BL et al (2009) Distinguishing tumefactive demyelinating lesions from glioma or central nervous

system lymphoma: added value of unenhanced CT compared with conventional contrast-enhanced MR imaging. Radiology 251(2):467–475

68. Suh CH, Kim HS, Jung SC, Choi CG, Kim SJ (2018) MRI Findings in tumefactive demyelinating lesions: a systematic review and meta-analysis. AJNR Am J Neuroradiol 39(9):1643–1649

69. Hiremath SB, Muraleedharan A, Kumar S, Nagesh C, Kesavadas C, Abraham M et al (2017) Combining diffusion tensor metrics and DSC perfusion imaging: can it improve the diagnostic accuracy in differentiating tumefactive demyelination from high-grade glioma? AJNR Am J Neuroradiol 38(4):685–690

70. Mabray MC, Cohen BA, Villanueva-Meyer JE, Valles FE, Barajas RF, Rubenstein JL et al (2015) Performance of apparent diffusion coefficient values and conventional MRI features in differentiating tumefactive demyelinating lesions from primary brain neoplasms. Am J Roentgenol 205(5):1075–1085

71. Wen JB, Huang WY, Xu WX, Wu G, Geng DY, Yin B (2017) Differentiating primary central nervous system lymphomas from glioblastomas and inflammatory demyelinating pseudotumor using relative minimum apparent diffusion coefficients. J Comput Assist Tomogr 41(6):904–909

72. Toh CH, Wei KC, Ng SH, Wan YL, Castillo M, Lin CP (2012) Differentiation of tumefactive demyelinating lesions from high-grade gliomas with the use of diffusion tensor imaging. AJNR Am J Neuroradiol 33(5):846–851

73. Tenembaum S, Chitnis T, Ness J, Hahn JS (2007) Acute disseminated encephalomyelitis. Neurology 68(16 Suppl 2):S23–S36

74. Dale RC, de Sousa C, Chong WK, Cox TC, Harding B, Neville BG (2000) Acute disseminated encephalomyelitis, multiphasic disseminated encephalomyelitis and multiple sclerosis in children. Brain J Neurol 123(Pt 12):2407–2422

75. Zuccoli G, Panigrahy A, Sreedher G, Bailey A, EJt L, La Colla L et al (2014) Vasogenic edema characterizes pediatric acute disseminated encephalomyelitis. Neuroradiology 56(8):679–684

76. Aung WY, Massoumzadeh P, Najmi S, Salter A, Heaps J, Benzinger TLS et al (2018) Diffusion tensor imaging as a biomarker to differentiate acute disseminated encephalomyelitis from multiple sclerosis at first demyelination. Pediatr Neurol 78:70–74

77. Yae Y, Kawano G, Yokochi T, Imagi T, Akita Y, Ohbu K et al (2018) Fulminant acute disseminated encephalomyelitis in children. Brain Dev 41(4):373–377

78. Gibbs WN, Kreidie MA, Kim RC, Hasso AN (2005) Acute hemorrhagic leukoencephalitis: neuroimaging features and neuropathologic diagnosis. J Comput Assist Tomogr 29(5):689–693

79. Mader I, Wolff M, Niemann G, Kuker W (2004) Acute haemorrhagic encephalomyelitis (AHEM): MRI findings. Neuropediatrics 35(2):143–146

80. Robinson CA, Adiele RC, Tham M, Lucchinetti CF, Popescu BF (2014) Early and widespread injury of

astrocytes in the absence of demyelination in acute haemorrhagic leukoencephalitis. Acta Neuropathol Commun 2:52

81. Postal M, Lapa AT, Reis F, Rittner L, Appenzeller S (2017) Magnetic resonance imaging in neuropsychiatric systemic lupus erythematosus: current state of the art and novel approaches. Lupus 26(5):517–521

82. Graham JW, Jan W (2003) MRI and the brain in systemic lupus erythematosus. Lupus 12(12):891–896

83. Raymond AA, Zariah AA, Samad SA, Chin CN, Kong NC (1996) Brain calcification in patients with cerebral lupus. Lupus 5(2):123–128

84. Kaichi Y, Kakeda S, Moriya J, Ohnari N, Saito K, Tanaka Y et al (2014) Brain MR findings in patients with systemic lupus erythematosus with and without antiphospholipid antibody syndrome. AJNR Am J Neuroradiol 35(1):100–105

85. Moritani T, Shrier DA, Numaguchi Y, Takahashi C, Yano T, Nakai K et al (2001) Diffusion-weighted echo-planar MR imaging of CNS involvement in systemic lupus erythematosus. Acad Radiol 8(8):741–753

86. Costallat BL, Ferreira DM, Lapa AT, Rittner L, Costallat LTL, Appenzeller S (2018) Brain diffusion tensor MRI in systematic lupus erythematosus: a systematic review. Autoimmun Rev 17(1):36–43

87. Correa DG, Zimmermann N, Pereira DB, Doring TM, Netto TM, Ventura N et al (2016) Evaluation of white matter integrity in systemic lupus erythematosus by diffusion tensor magnetic resonance imaging: a study using tract-based spatial statistics. Neuroradiology 58(8):819–825

88. Schmidt-Wilcke T, Cagnoli P, Wang P, Schultz T, Lotz A, McCune WJ et al (2014) Diminished white matter integrity in patients with systemic lupus erythematosus. NeuroImage Clin 5:291–297

89. Castillo P, Woodruff B, Caselli R, Vernino S, Lucchinetti C, Swanson J et al (2006) Steroid-responsive encephalopathy associated with autoimmune thyroiditis. Arch Neurol 63(2):197–202

90. Mahad DJ, Staugaitis S, Ruggieri P, Parisi J, Kleinschmidt-Demasters BK, Lassmann H et al (2005) Steroid-responsive encephalopathy associated with autoimmune thyroiditis and primary CNS demyelination. J Neurol Sci 228(1):3–5

91. Takahashi S, Mitamura R, Itoh Y, Suzuki N, Okuno A (1994) Hashimoto encephalopathy: etiologic considerations. Pediatr Neurol 11(4):328–331

92. Oide T, Tokuda T, Yazaki M, Watarai M, Mitsuhashi S, Kaneko K et al (2004) Anti-neuronal autoantibody in Hashimoto's encephalopathy: neuropathological, immunohistochemical, and biochemical analysis of two patients. J Neurol Sci 217(1):7–12

93. Nolte KW, Unbehaun A, Sieker H, Kloss TM, Paulus W (2000) Hashimoto encephalopathy: a brainstem vasculitis? Neurology 54(3):769–770

94. Sanchez Contreras A, Rojas SA, Manosalva A, Mendez Patarroyo PA, Lorenzana P, Restrepo JF et al (2004) Hashimoto encephalopathy (autoimmune encephalitis). J Clin Rheumatol 10(6):339–343

95. Irani S, Lang B (2008) Autoantibody-mediated disorders of the central nervous system. Autoimmunity 41(1):55–65

96. Tamagno G, Federspil G, Murialdo G (2006) Clinical and diagnostic aspects of encephalopathy associated with autoimmune thyroid disease (or Hashimoto's encephalopathy). Intern Emerg Med 1(1):15–23

97. Creutzfeldt CJ, Haberl RL (2005) Hashimoto encephalopathy: a do-not-miss in the differential diagnosis of dementia. J Neurol 252(10):1285–1287

98. Mancardi MM, Fazzini F, Rossi A, Gaggero R (2005) Hashimoto's encephalopathy with selective involvement of the nucleus accumbens: a case report. Neuropediatrics 36(3):218–220

99. McCabe DJ, Burke T, Connolly S, Hutchinson M (2000) Amnesic syndrome with bilateral mesial temporal lobe involvement in Hashimoto's encephalopathy. Neurology 54(3):737–739

100. Song YM, Seo DW, Chang GY (2004) MR findings in Hashimoto encephalopathy. AJNR Am J Neuroradiol 25(5):807–808

101. Dudesek A, Rimmele F, Tesar S, Kolbaske S, Rommer PS, Benecke R et al (2014) CLIPPERS: chronic lymphocytic inflammation with pontine perivascular enhancement responsive to steroids. Review of an increasingly recognized entity within the spectrum of inflammatory central nervous system disorders. Clin Exp Immunol 175(3):385–396

102. Tobin WO, Guo Y, Krecke KN, Parisi JE, Lucchinetti CF, Pittock SJ et al (2017) Diagnostic criteria for chronic lymphocytic inflammation with pontine perivascular enhancement responsive to steroids (CLIPPERS). Brain J Neurol 140(9):2415–2425

103. Ferreira RM, Machado G, Souza AS, Lin K, Correa-Neto Y (2013) CLIPPERS-like MRI findings in a patient with multiple sclerosis. J Neurol Sci 327(1–2):61–62

104. Pittock SJ, Debruyne J, Krecke KN, Giannini C, van den Ameele J, De Herdt V et al (2010) Chronic lymphocytic inflammation with pontine perivascular enhancement responsive to steroids (CLIPPERS). Brain J Neurol 133(9):2626–2634

105. Taieb G, Uro-Coste E, Clanet M, Lassmann H, Benouaich-Amiel A, Laurent C et al (2014) A central nervous system B-cell lymphoma arising two years after initial diagnosis of CLIPPERS. J Neurol Sci 344(1–2):224–226

106. De Graaff HJ, Wattjes MP, Rozemuller-Kwakkel AJ, Petzold A, Killestein J (2013) Fatal B-cell lymphoma following chronic lymphocytic inflammation with pontine perivascular enhancement responsive to steroids. JAMA Neurol 70(7):915–918

107. Campochiaro C, Tomelleri A, Cavalli G, Berti A, Dagna L (2015) Erdheim-Chester disease. Eur J Intern Med 26(4):223–229

108. Moulis G, Sailler L, Bonneville F, Wagner T (2014) Imaging in Erdheim-Chester disease: classic features and new insights. Clin Exp Rheumatol 32(3):410–414

109. Parks NE, Goyal G, Go RS, Mandrekar J, Tobin WO (2018) Neuroradiologic manifestations of Erdheim-Chester disease. Neurol Clin Pract 8(1):15–20

110. Chiapparini L, Cavalli G, Langella T, Venerando A, De Luca G, Raspante S et al (2018) Adult leukoencephalopathies with prominent infratentorial involvement can be caused by Erdheim-Chester disease. J Neurol 265(2):273–284

111. Marinelli JP, Peters PA, Vaglio A, Van Gompel JJ, Lane JI, Carlson ML (2019) Skull base manifestations of erdheim-chester disease: a case series and systematic review. Neurosurgery 80(S 01):S1–S244

112. Al-Samkari H, Berliner N (2018) Hemophagocytic lymphohistiocytosis. Annu Rev Pathol 13:27–49

113. Jovanovic A, Kuzmanovic M, Kravljanac R, Micic D, Jovic M, Gazikalovic S et al (2014) Central nervous system involvement in hemophagocytic lymphohistiocytosis: a single-center experience. Pediatr Neurol 50(3):233–237

114. Cai G, Wang Y, Liu X, Han Y, Wang Z (2017) Central nervous system involvement in adults with haemophagocytic lymphohistiocytosis: a single-center study. Ann Hematol 96(8):1279–1285

115. Rego I, Severino M, Micalizzi C, Faraci M, Pende D, Dufour C et al (2012) Neuroradiologic findings and follow-up with magnetic resonance imaging of the genetic forms of haemophagocytic lymphohistiocytosis with CNS involvement. Pediatr Blood Cancer 58(5):810–814

116. Deiva K, Mahlaoui N, Beaudonnet F, de Saint Basile G, Caridade G, Moshous D et al (2012) CNS involvement at the onset of primary hemophagocytic lymphohistiocytosis. Neurology 78(15):1150–1156

117. Mader I, Herrlinger U, Klose U, Schmidt F, Kuker W (2003) Progressive multifocal leukoencephalopathy: analysis of lesion development with diffusion-weighted MRI. Neuroradiology 45(10):717–721

118. Huisman TA, Boltshauser E, Martin E, Nadal D (2005) Diffusion tensor imaging in progressive multifocal leukoencephalopathy: early predictor for demyelination? AJNR Am J Neuroradiol 26(8):2153–2156

119. Ohta K, Obara K, Sakauchi M, Obara K, Takane H, Yogo Y (2001) Lesion extension detected by diffusion-weighted magnetic resonance imaging in progressive multifocal leukoencephalopathy. J Neurol 248(9):809–811

120. Filippini G, Brusaferri F, Sibley WA, Citterio A, Ciucci G, Midgard R et al (2000) Corticosteroids or ACTH for acute exacerbations in multiple sclerosis. Cochrane Database Syst Rev 4:CD001331

121. Lattanzi S, Cagnetti C, Danni M, Provinciali L, Silvestrini M (2017) Oral and intravenous steroids for multiple sclerosis relapse: a systematic review and meta-analysis. J Neurol 264(8):1697–1704

122. Weinshenker BG, O'Brien PC, Petterson TM, Noseworthy JH, Lucchinetti CF, Dodick DW et al (1999) A randomized trial of plasma exchange in acute central nervous system inflammatory demyelinating disease. Ann Neurol 46(6):878–886

123. Interferon (1993) beta-1b is effective in relapsing-remitting multiple sclerosis. I. Clinical results of a multicenter, randomized, double-blind, placebo-controlled trial. The IFNB Multiple Sclerosis Study Group. Neurology 43(4):655–661

124. Paty DW, Li DK (1993) Interferon beta-1b is effective in relapsing-remitting multiple sclerosis. II. MRI analysis results of a multicenter, randomized, double-blind, placebo-controlled trial. UBC MS/MRI Study Group and the IFNB Multiple Sclerosis Study Group. Neurology 43(4):662–667

125. Kieseier BC (2011) The mechanism of action of interferon-beta in relapsing multiple sclerosis. CNS Drugs 25(6):491–502

126. Jacobs LD, Cookfair DL, Rudick RA, Herndon RM, Richert JR, Salazar AM et al (1996) Intramuscular interferon beta-1a for disease progression in relapsing multiple sclerosis. The Multiple Sclerosis Collaborative Research Group (MSCRG). Ann Neurol 39(3):285–294

127. Randomised double-blind placebo-controlled study of interferon beta-1a in relapsing/remitting multiple sclerosis (1998) PRISMS (Prevention of Relapses and Disability by Interferon beta-1a Subcutaneously in Multiple Sclerosis) Study Group. Lancet 352(9139):1498–1504

128. Calabresi PA, Kieseier BC, Arnold DL, Balcer LJ, Boyko A, Pelletier J et al (2014) Pegylated interferon beta-1a for relapsing-remitting multiple sclerosis (ADVANCE): a randomised, phase 3, double-blind study. Lancet Neurol 13(7):657–665

129. Johnson KP, Brooks BR, Cohen JA, Ford CC, Goldstein J, Lisak RP et al (1995) Copolymer 1 reduces relapse rate and improves disability in relapsing-remitting multiple sclerosis: results of a phase III multicenter, double-blind placebo-controlled trial. The Copolymer 1 Multiple Sclerosis Study Group. Neurology 45(7):1268–1276

130. Aharoni R (2013) The mechanism of action of glatiramer acetate in multiple sclerosis and beyond. Autoimmun Rev 12(5):543–553

131. Boster AL, Ford CC, Neudorfer O, Gilgun-Sherki Y (2015) Glatiramer acetate: long-term safety and efficacy in relapsing-remitting multiple sclerosis. Expert Rev Neurother 15(6):575–586

132. Kappos L, Radue EW, O'Connor P, Polman C, Hohlfeld R, Calabresi P et al (2010) A placebo-controlled trial of oral fingolimod in relapsing multiple sclerosis. N Engl J Med 362(5):387–401

133. Thomas K, Proschmann U, Ziemssen T (2017) Fingolimod hydrochloride for the treatment of relapsing remitting multiple sclerosis. Expert Opin Pharmacother 18(15):1649–1660

134. Fox RJ, Miller DH, Phillips JT, Hutchinson M, Havrdova E, Kita M et al (2012) Placebo-controlled phase 3 study of oral BG-12 or glatiramer in multiple sclerosis. N Engl J Med 367(12):1087–1097

135. Dubey D, Kieseier BC, Hartung HP, Hemmer B, Warnke C, Menge T et al (2015) Dimethyl fumarate in relapsing-remitting multiple sclerosis: rationale,

135. mechanisms of action, pharmacokinetics, efficacy and safety. Expert Rev Neurother 15(4):339–346

136. O'Connor P, Wolinsky JS, Confavreux C, Comi G, Kappos L, Olsson TP et al (2011) Randomized trial of oral teriflunomide for relapsing multiple sclerosis. N Engl J Med 365(14):1293–1303

137. Confavreux C, O'Connor P, Comi G, Freedman MS, Miller AE, Olsson TP et al (2014) Oral teriflunomide for patients with relapsing multiple sclerosis (TOWER): a randomised, double-blind, placebo-controlled, phase 3 trial. Lancet Neurol 13(3):247–256

138. Comi G, Freedman MS, Kappos L, Olsson TP, Miller AE, Wolinsky JS et al (2016) Pooled safety and tolerability data from four placebo-controlled teriflunomide studies and extensions. Mult Scler Relat Disord 5:97–104

139. Polman CH, O'Connor PW, Havrdova E, Hutchinson M, Kappos L, Miller DH et al (2006) A randomized, placebo-controlled trial of natalizumab for relapsing multiple sclerosis. N Engl J Med 354(9):899–910

140. Delbue S, Comar M, Ferrante P (2017) Natalizumab treatment of multiple sclerosis: new insights. Immunotherapy 9(2):157–171

141. Hauser SL, Bar-Or A, Comi G, Giovannoni G, Hartung HP, Hemmer B et al (2017) Ocrelizumab versus interferon beta-1a in relapsing multiple sclerosis. N Engl J Med 376(3):221–234

142. Montalban X, Hauser SL, Kappos L, Arnold DL, Bar-Or A, Comi G et al (2017) Ocrelizumab versus placebo in primary progressive multiple sclerosis. N Engl J Med 376(3):209–220

143. Cohen JA, Coles AJ, Arnold DL, Confavreux C, Fox EJ, Hartung HP et al (2012) Alemtuzumab versus interferon beta 1a as first-line treatment for patients with relapsing-remitting multiple sclerosis: a randomised controlled phase 3 trial. Lancet 380(9856):1819–1828

144. Coles AJ, Twyman CL, Arnold DL, Cohen JA, Confavreux C, Fox EJ et al (2012) Alemtuzumab for patients with relapsing multiple sclerosis after disease-modifying therapy: a randomised controlled phase 3 trial. Lancet 380(9856):1829–1839

145. Havrdova E, Arnold DL, Cohen JA, Hartung HP, Fox EJ, Giovannoni G et al (2017) Alemtuzumab CARE-MS I 5-year follow-up: durable efficacy in the absence of continuous MS therapy. Neurology 89(11):1107–1116

146. Coles AJ, Cohen JA, Fox EJ, Giovannoni G, Hartung HP, Havrdova E et al (2017) Alemtuzumab CARE-MS II 5-year follow-up: efficacy and safety findings. Neurology 89(11):1117–1126

147. Cox AL, Thompson SA, Jones JL, Robertson VH, Hale G, Waldmann H et al (2005) Lymphocyte homeostasis following therapeutic lymphocyte depletion in multiple sclerosis. Eur J Immunol 35(11):3332–3342

148. Goodin DS, Bates D (2009) Treatment of early multiple sclerosis: the value of treatment initiation after a first clinical episode. Mult Scler 15(10):1175–1182

149. Montalban X, Gold R, Thompson AJ, Otero-Romero S, Amato MP, Chandraratna D et al (2018) ECTRIMS/EAN Guideline on the pharmacological treatment of people with multiple sclerosis. Mult Scler 24(2):96–120

150. University of California SFMSET, Cree BA, Gourraud PA, Oksenberg JR, Bevan C, Crabtree-Hartman E et al (2016) Long-term evolution of multiple sclerosis disability in the treatment era. Ann Neurol 80(4):499–510

151. Brown JWL, Coles A, Horakova D, Havrdova E, Izquierdo G, Prat A et al (2019) Association of initial disease-modifying therapy with later conversion to secondary progressive multiple sclerosis. JAMA 321(2):175–187

152. Rotstein DL, Healy BC, Malik MT, Chitnis T, Weiner HL (2015) Evaluation of no evidence of disease activity in a 7-year longitudinal multiple sclerosis cohort. JAMA Neurol 72(2):152–158

153. Giovannoni G, Turner B, Gnanapavan S, Offiah C, Schmierer K, Marta M (2015) Is it time to target no evident disease activity (NEDA) in multiple sclerosis? Mult Scler Relat Disord 4(4):329–333

154. Merkel B, Butzkueven H, Traboulsee AL, Havrdova E, Kalincik T (2017) Timing of high-efficacy therapy in relapsing-remitting multiple sclerosis: a systematic review. Autoimmun Rev 16(6):658–665

155. Rae-Grant A, Day GS, Marrie RA, Rabinstein A, Cree BAC, Gronseth GS et al (2018) Practice guideline recommendations summary: disease-modifying therapies for adults with multiple sclerosis: Report of the Guideline Development, Dissemination, and Implementation Subcommittee of the American Academy of Neurology. Neurology 90(17): 777–788

156. Voskuhl R, Momtazee C (2017) Pregnancy: effect on multiple sclerosis, treatment considerations, and breastfeeding. Neurotherapeutics 14(4):974–984

157. Crabtree-Hartman E (2018) Advanced symptom management in multiple sclerosis. Neurol Clin 36(1):197–218

158. Placebo-controlled multicentre randomised trial of interferon beta-1b in treatment of secondary progressive multiple sclerosis (1998) European Study Group on interferon beta-1b in secondary progressive MS. Lancet 352(9139):1491–1497

159. Panitch H, Miller A, Paty D, Weinshenker B, North American Study Group on Interferon beta-1b in Secondary Progressive MS (2004) Interferon beta-1b in secondary progressive MS: results from a 3-year controlled study. Neurology 63(10):1788–1795

160. Kappos L, Weinshenker B, Pozzilli C, Thompson AJ, Dahlke F, Beckmann K et al (2004) Interferon beta-1b in secondary progressive MS: a combined analysis of the two trials. Neurology 63(10):1779–1787

161. Kappos L, Bar-Or A, Cree BAC, Fox RJ, Giovannoni G, Gold R et al (2018) Siponimod versus placebo in secondary progressive multiple sclerosis (EXPAND): a double-blind, randomised, phase 3 study. Lancet 391(10127):1263–1273

162. Brenton JN, Banwell BL (2016) Therapeutic approach to the management of pediatric demyelinating disease: multiple sclerosis and acute disseminated encephalomyelitis. Neurotherapeutics 13(1):84–95
163. Chitnis T, Arnold DL, Banwell B, Bruck W, Ghezzi A, Giovannoni G et al (2018) Trial of Fingolimod versus interferon beta-1a in pediatric multiple sclerosis. N Engl J Med 379(11):1017–1027
164. Koelman DL, Mateen FJ (2015) Acute disseminated encephalomyelitis: current controversies in diagnosis and outcome. J Neurol 262(9):2013–2024
165. Shahar E, Andraus J, Savitzki D, Pilar G, Zelnik N (2002) Outcome of severe encephalomyelitis in children: effect of high-dose methylprednisolone and immunoglobulins. J Child Neurol 17(11):810–814
166. Ravaglia S, Piccolo G, Ceroni M, Franciotta D, Pichiecchio A, Bastianello S et al (2007) Severe steroid-resistant post-infectious encephalomyelitis: general features and effects of IVIg. J Neurol 254(11):1518–1523
167. Koelman DL, Chahin S, Mar SS, Venkatesan A, Hoganson GM, Yeshokumar AK et al (2016) Acute disseminated encephalomyelitis in 228 patients: a retrospective, multicenter US study. Neurology 86(22):2085–2093
168. Khurana DS, Melvin JJ, Kothare SV, Valencia I, Hardison HH, Yum S et al (2005) Acute disseminated encephalomyelitis in children: discordant neurologic and neuroimaging abnormalities and response to plasmapheresis. Pediatrics 116(2):431–436
169. Wingerchuk DM, Hogancamp WF, O'Brien PC, Weinshenker BG (1999) The clinical course of neuromyelitis optica (Devic's syndrome). Neurology 53(5):1107–1114
170. Bonnan M, Valentino R, Debeugny S, Merle H, Ferge JL, Mehdaoui H et al (2018) Short delay to initiate plasma exchange is the strongest predictor of outcome in severe attacks of NMO spectrum disorders. J Neurol Neurosurg Psychiatry 89(4):346–351
171. Jiao Y, Cui L, Zhang W, Zhang Y, Wang W, Zhang L et al (2018) Plasma exchange for neuromyelitis optica spectrum disorders in Chinese patients and factors predictive of short-term outcome. Clin Ther 40(4):603–612
172. Kleiter I, Gahlen A, Borisow N, Fischer K, Wernecke KD, Hellwig K et al (2018) Apheresis therapies for NMOSD attacks: a retrospective study of 207 therapeutic interventions. Neurol Neuroimmunol Neuroinflamm 5(6):e504
173. Papadopoulos MC, Bennett JL, Verkman AS (2014) Treatment of neuromyelitis optica: state-of-the-art and emerging therapies. Nat Rev Neurol 10(9):493–506
174. Nikoo Z, Badihian S, Shaygannejad V, Asgari N, Ashtari F (2017) Comparison of the efficacy of azathioprine and rituximab in neuromyelitis optica spectrum disorder: a randomized clinical trial. J Neurol 264(9):2003–2009
175. Wingerchuk DM, Weinshenker BG (2008) Neuromyelitis optica. Curr Treat Options Neurol 10(1):55–66
176. Bartsch T, Rempe T, Leypoldt F, Riedel C, Jansen O, Berg D et al (2019) The spectrum of progressive multifocal leukoencephalopathy: a practical approach. Eur J Neurol 26(4):566–e41
177. Bloomgren G, Richman S, Hotermans C, Subramanyam M, Goelz S, Natarajan A et al (2012) Risk of natalizumab-associated progressive multifocal leukoencephalopathy. N Engl J Med 366(20):1870–1880
178. Plavina T, Subramanyam M, Bloomgren G, Richman S, Pace A, Lee S et al (2014) Anti-JC virus antibody levels in serum or plasma further define risk of natalizumab-associated progressive multifocal leukoencephalopathy. Ann Neurol 76(6):802–812
179. Zhovtis Ryerson L, Frohman TC, Foley J, Kister I, Weinstock-Guttman B, Tornatore C et al (2016) Extended interval dosing of natalizumab in multiple sclerosis. J Neurol Neurosurg Psychiatry 87(8):885–889
180. Yamout BI, Sahraian MA, Ayoubi NE, Tamim H, Nicolas J, Khoury SJ et al (2018) Efficacy and safety of natalizumab extended interval dosing. Mult Scler Relat Disord 24:113–116
181. Pavlovic D, Patera AC, Nyberg F, Gerber M, Liu M (2015) Progressive Multifocal Leukoencephalopathy C. Progressive multifocal leukoencephalopathy: current treatment options and future perspectives. Ther Adv Neurol Disord 8(6):255–273
182. Clifford DB, De Luca A, Simpson DM, Arendt G, Giovannoni G, Nath A (2010) Natalizumab-associated progressive multifocal leukoencephalopathy in patients with multiple sclerosis: lessons from 28 cases. Lancet Neurol 9(4):438–446
183. Scarpazza C, Prosperini L, De Rossi N, Moiola L, Sormani MP, Gerevini S et al (2017) To do or not to do? plasma exchange and timing of steroid administration in progressive multifocal leukoencephalopathy. Ann Neurol 82(5):697–705
184. Tan IL, McArthur JC, Clifford DB, Major EO, Nath A (2011) Immune reconstitution inflammatory syndrome in natalizumab-associated PML. Neurology 77(11):1061–1067
185. Fournier A, Martin-Blondel G, Lechapt-Zalcman E, Dina J, Kazemi A, Verdon R et al (2017) Immune reconstitution inflammatory syndrome unmasking or worsening AIDS-related progressive multifocal leukoencephalopathy: a literature review. Front Immunol 8:577

Degenerative Diseases of the CNS

14

Aristides A. Capizzano, and Toshio Moritani

Juana Nicoll Capizzano

14.1 Alzheimer's Disease (AD)

AD is the most prevalent dementia with its main risk factor being older age. By 2050, the number of people living with AD in the United States is projected to reach 13.8 million, resulting in nearly 1 million new cases per year [1]. Although the sporadic rather than the familial forms of the disease is by far the most prevalent, 20 genes with common variants contribute to the risk of AD [2]. In particular, the occurrence of ε4 genotype of the apolipoprotein E is the strongest genetic risk factor for AD [3]. The pathologic lesions of AD are neuritic plaques (NPs) around a core of beta amyloid (Aβ) and intracellular neurofibrillary tangles (NFTs) composed of aggregates of hyperphosphorylated microtubule-associated tau protein. The "amyloid hypothesis of AD" states that the imbalance between production and clearance of Aβ42 and related Aβ peptides is the determining, very early factor in AD [4]. NFTs lesions have a sequential pattern of deposition in the brain, appearing first in the entorhinal cortex, later in the hippocampal formation and finally in isocortical association areas, which has been used to stage the disease [5].

Clinically, AD patients have an insidious onset of cognitive decline heralded by episodic amnesia. Executive dysfunction, visuospatial difficulties, aphasia, apraxia, and agnosia develop subsequently and variably. Patients with cognitive impairment that do not meet diagnosis of dementia are labeled as mild cognitive impairment (MCI), whose prevalence is estimated between 15 and 20% for 60 years and older [6]. MCI patients progress to AD at a yearly rate of 10–15%, and predictors of this conversion include whether the patient is a carrier of the ε4 allele of the apolipoprotein E (APOE) gene, clinical severity, brain atrophy on imaging, positive CSF biomarkers, cerebral glucose metabolism, and Aβ deposition [7]. Revised criteria for the diagnosis of AD recommend biomarkers derived from structural MRI, CSF analysis, and PET to complement clinical criteria with objective evidence of the underlying neuropathology [8].

The Alzheimer's Disease Neuroimaging Initiative (ADNI) led to the development of clinical, imaging, genetic, and biochemical biomarkers for the early detection and longitudinal assessment of control subjects, MCI, and AD patients [9]. The radiologic hallmark of AD is atrophy of mesial temporal structures, i.e., the hippocampus and parahippocampal gyrus, which is present at the MCI stage and progresses along with the disease [10] (Fig. 14.1). At the mild

---

A. A. Capizzano (✉) · T. Moritani
Division of Neuroradiology, University of Michigan, Ann Arbor, MI, USA
e-mail: capizzan@med.umich.edu;
tmoritan@med.umich.edu

J. N. Capizzano
University of Michigan, Ann Arbor, MI, USA
e-mail: jcapizza@umich.edu

© Springer Nature Switzerland AG 2021
T. Moritani, A. A. Capizzano (eds.), *Diffusion-Weighted MR Imaging of the Brain, Head and Neck, and Spine*, https://doi.org/10.1007/978-3-030-62120-9_14

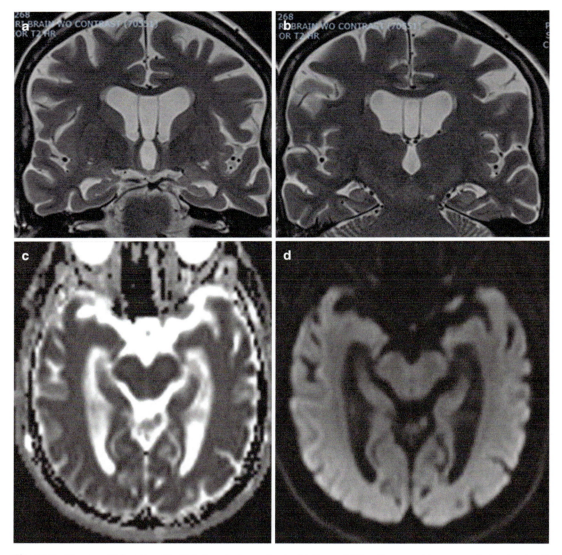

Fig. 14.1 66-year-old female with Alzheimer's dementia. (**a, b**) Coronal T2 with severe hippocampal atrophy. (**c, d**) Axial ADC map and trace DWI along the temporal horns

dementia stage of AD, hippocampal volume is reduced by 15–30% relative to controls, and in the amnestic variant of MCI hippocampal volume is reduced by 10–15% [10]. The topography of brain tissue loss correlates with cognitive deficits, both cross-sectionally and longitudinally, and recapitulates the Braak's pathology stages [5]. Apart from mesial temporal atrophy, whole-brain atrophy and ventricular enlargement predict underlying Aβ and tau pathology [11]. Furthermore, the annual rate of hippocampal volume loss distinguishes MCI patients that progress to dementia (accelerated atrophy) from those that remain stable (lower rate of atrophy) [12]. Apart from structural imaging, metabolic imaging biomarkers of AD are cortical hypometabolism and amyloid/tau accumulation on PET, the latter showing the earliest brain changes in AD [9].

The concept of AD being inevitable with advanced aging has been challenged since the neuropathology of dementia of the very old (over 95 years) shows stagnation in the incidence of AD while vascular dementia and hippocampal

14 Degenerative Diseases of the CNS

sclerosis of aging (HS aging), a TDP 43 proteinopathy, become increasingly prevalent [13]. The co-occurrence of AD and vascular brain injury (VBI) in the elderly is very common and contributes to cognitive dysfunction in an additive and independent fashion. White matter T2 signal hyperintensities (leukoaraiosis [14]), lacunar or large infarcts and hemorrhages are visible on MRI and currently constitute the most reliable biomarker for VBI [15].

14.1.1 DWI in AD

DWI is typically not part of the clinical diagnosis of AD but contributed significant value to the understanding of brain pathology in AD, particularly white matter involvement, by using DTI. Hippocampal atrophy, the MRI hallmark of AD, is related to subsequent disruption of the uncinate fasciculus and the cingulum bundle in amnestic MCI as determined by DTI tractography analysis. Fiber loss in these white matter tracts is also related to metabolic decrease in the posterior cingulate and medial orbitofrontal cortices [16]. This degeneration seems to be closely related with, and is possibly a consequence of, medial temporal atrophy. Hippocampal ADC is higher in MCI and AD patients [17, 18]. ADC values in the hippocampal formation are elevated before conventional MRI reflects early changes in the progression of AD. ADC of the temporal stem and posterior cingulate, occipital, and parietal white matter is higher in AD compared to controls. Widespread changes in DTI metrics have been reported in bilateral limbic and association white matter tracts at the MCI and mild AD stages of the disease [19]. Increased mean, axial, and radial diffusivity occur in normal-appearing white matter of AD patients, with less significant reduction in fractional anisotropy, and these changes were correlated with gray matter atrophy. In MCI, axial diffusivity was increased in the limbic network and the cortico-cortical pathways, whereas the mean diffusivity, fractional anisotropy, and radial diffusivity values were preserved [20]. Studies of the ADNI cohort have found both global and local changes of WM

tracts during AD progression with globally increased axial diffusivity and radial diffusivity in MCI patients, and further increase in these DTI measures, along with decreased global fractional anisotropy (FA) in demented subjects, consistent with widespread WM damage [21].

14.1.2 Atypical AD Variants

Clinical, radiological, and pathologically [22] atypical presentations of AD have been described, which tend to present in younger patients (under 65 years). These include the following:

- Posterior cortical atrophy (PCA) [23], presents with unusual visuoperceptual symptoms, such as diminished ability to interpret, locate, or reach for objects under visual guidance; visual agnosia and deficits in numeracy, literacy, and praxis. Episodic memory and insight are initially relatively preserved, but there is later progression to a more diffuse pattern of cognitive dysfunction. On imaging, there is predominantly posterior parietal cortical atrophy with relative preservation of the medial temporal lobe volume [24].
- Frontal variant AD, with prominent behavioral disturbances and apathy resembling FTLD and predominant frontal lobe atrophy [25].
- Language presentation with fluent or non-fluent aphasia and logopenic AD variant, with asymmetric left temporal lateral cortical atrophy [26].

14.1.3 Other Tauopathies

Hyperphosphorylated aggregates of the microtubule-associated protein tau are the main component of the intracellular inclusions seen in the neurodegenerative diseases known as tauopathies. These include AD, frontotemporal dementia with parkinsonism-17 (FTDP-17), Pick disease (PiD), progressive supranuclear palsy (PSP), and corticobasal degeneration (CBD) [27].

14.1.3.1 Corticobasal Degeneration (CBD)

CBD has varied clinical presentations. Typically presents with the corticobasal syndrome: asymmetric parkinsonism with a variable combination of ideomotor apraxia, rigidity, myoclonus, and dystonia, often associated with the presence of an alien limb phenomenon (involuntary motor activity of a limb with feeling of estrangement from that limb) [28]. On macroscopic exam and structural imaging, there is hemiatrophy or bilateral asymmetrical cortical atrophy, which predominates in the perirolandic or in the perisylvian areas (Fig. 14.2). The recent development of selective in vivo tau PET imaging ligands such as [(18)F]THK523 provides support for diagnosis of CBD and other tauopathies [29]. The characteristic microscopic hallmark of CBD is the swollen ballooned neuron and more specifically the astrocytic plaque, a non-amyloid cortical plaque composed of abnormal tau in the distal processes of astrocytes [30].

14.1.3.2 Progressive Supranuclear Palsy (PSP)

PSP presents most characteristically with a constellation of supranuclear gaze palsy (although seen only a minority of patients), progressive axial rigidity, pseudobulbar palsy, and dementia [31]. Tufted astrocytes filled with tau inclusions are the characteristic microscopic lesion [30]. On structural imaging and using simple measurements, the reduced area of the midbrain relative to the pons [32] or the enlarged third ventricle [33] allows distinction of PSP from controls and Parkinson's disease (PD) patients with high specificity (Fig. 14.3). The superior cerebellar peduncle (SCP) is also atrophic in PSP, which contrasts with the relative sparing of the middle cerebellar peduncle (MCP). These features were incorporated into the MR Parkinsonism index (MRPI), which takes into account both the midbrain-pons area ratio (P/M) and the ratio of the MCP to SCP width, thus: [(P/M)*(MCP/SCP)]. The MRPI is typically

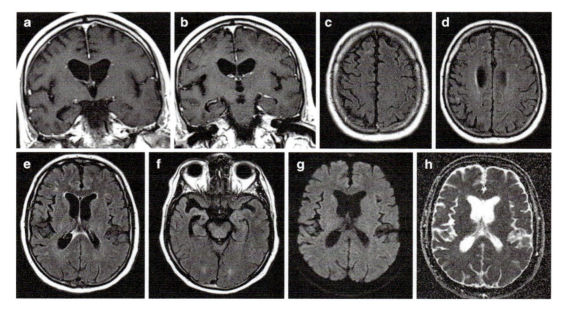

Fig. 14.2 CBD. 64-year-old patient with a history of dementia, left-sided weakness, numbness, dysarthria, mild dystonia, hyperreflexia, and apraxia worse on left side and involuntary alien limb movements. (**a, b**) Coronal T1, (**c-f**) Axial FLAIR, (**g**) trace DWI, and (**h**) ADC map. Asymmetric right cortical atrophy. **FDG PET of same CBD** patient (**i** axial, **j** coronal images) with right frontotemporal hypometabolism

14 Degenerative Diseases of the CNS

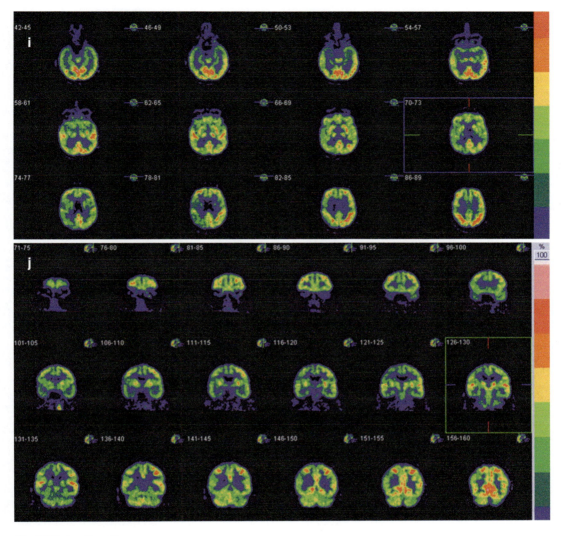

Fig. 14.2 (continued)

increased in PSP compared to controls, MSA-P and PD, and sensitivity and specificity values for the differential diagnosis of PSP from MSA-P, PD, and vascular parkinsonism have been reported between 80 and 100% [34]. Furthermore, a meta-analysis of studies with a total of 159 PSP patients showed significant white matter volume reductions compared to controls in the midbrain, pons, and the regions close to the basal ganglia [35].

14.2 Dementia with Lewy Body Disease (LBD)

LBD is the second most prevalent degenerative dementia after AD. The essential clinical feature of LBD is dementia, with prominent deficits in attention, executive function, and visuospatial skills. The revised LBD consensus criteria distinguish clearly between clinical features and diagnostic biomarkers, including neuroimaging

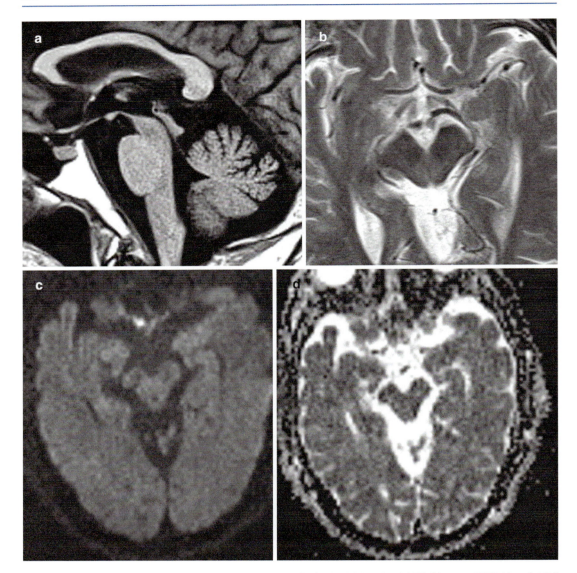

Fig. 14.3 PSP. 69-year-old. Male with PSP cardinal features including pseudobulbar palsy, rigidity, bradykinesia, masked facies, and ocular paresis with down and up gaze. Sagittal T1 (**a**) and axial T2 (**b**), trace DWI (**c**) and ADC map (**d**) with midbrain tegmental atrophy and subtle T2 hyperintensity

[36]. Core clinical features are fluctuating cognition, recurrent visual hallucinations, and parkinsonism, which distinguish LBD from AD. Main differential diagnostic considerations of LBD are Parkinson's disease with dementia (PDD) and AD. Diagnostic criteria indicate that dementia should occur before or concurrently with parkinsonism to diagnose LBD [37], while PDD is diagnosed when parkinsonism is present for 12 months or more before the onset of dementia [38]. Imaging provides indicative diagnostic biomarkers of LBD, such as reduced dopamine transporter uptake in the basal ganglia on SPECT or PET, preserved medial temporal lobe volume on structural imaging and low SPECT/PET brain uptake in the occipital cortex [36]. The characteristic pathologic lesion in LBD is the Lewy body (LB) cytoplasmic neuronal inclusion, which is immunoreactive to the presynaptic protein α-synuclein [39]. Therefore,

LBD is counted among the α-synucleinopathies together with PD and multiple system atrophy (MSA). Cortical LBs progression starts in the amygdala, then spreads to the limbic cortex and finally to the neocortex [40]. Apart from LBs, other histopathological features of LBD are Lewy-related neurites, AD-type pathology (plaques and tangles), spongiform changes, and synapse loss [41].

14.2.1 Imaging

Atrophic changes are less conspicuous and differently distributed in LBD compared to AD. Volume loss in LBD involves the dorsal midbrain, hypothalamus, and substantia innominata with sparing of the hippocampus and temporo-parietal cortex [42]. In comparison with PDD, in LBD there is more frontotemporal gray matter atrophy that correlated with neuropsychological impairment [43]. Occipital hypoperfusion and hypometabolism in LBD have been reported using SPECT and FDG-PET, respectively [44] (Fig. 14.4). Dopaminergic dysfunction assessed with SPECT or PET has become a suggestive feature of the diagnosis of LBD under the consensus criteria. LBD and PDD patients display severely reduced dopaminergic uptake in the caudate and putamen compared to controls and AD patients [45].

14.2.2 DTI

LBD is characterized by increased ADC values in the precuneus [46]. Using tract-based spatial statistics (TBSS), a voxelwise approach to DTI data in the style of VBM, LBD displayed lower FA of parieto-occipital white matter compared to controls with significantly fewer changes in frontal regions. AD subjects on the other hand had more diffuse reductions in FA on both sides of the central sulcus. Mean diffusivity (MD) changes were widespread in both conditions. The DTI changes in LBD correlated with episodic memory, letter fluency, and parkinsonian signs [47]. DLB is characterized by a loss of parieto-occipital white matter integrity (lower FA) with associated cortical glucose hypometabolism [48].

14.3 Parkinson's Disease (PD)

Parkinsonism is defined as bradykinesia, in combination with either rest tremor, rigidity, or both and is the prerequisite for clinical diagnosis of PD. Non-motor manifestations of PD such as anosmia, sleep disturbance, orthostatic hypotension, and cognitive impairment are also included in the diagnostic criteria. Movement Disorder Society PD criteria [49] use motor parkinsonism as the core feature of the diagnosis, defined as bradykinesia plus rest tremor or rigidity. After determination of parkinsonism, diagnosis of PD uses three categories of diagnostic features: absolute exclusion criteria (which rule out PD), red flags (which must be counterbalanced by additional supportive criteria to allow diagnosis of PD), and supportive criteria (positive features that increase confidence of the PD diagnosis). Normal functional imaging of the presynaptic dopaminergic system is one of the absolute exclusion criteria, whose presence rules out PD. 75–95% of patients diagnosed with PD by clinical experts have their diagnosis confirmed on autopsy [49]. Sporadic PD involves multiple neuronal systems and results from changes developing in a few susceptible types of nerve cells. Essential for neuropathological diagnosis are α-synuclein-immunopositive Lewy neurites and Lewy bodies. The pathological process starts in the dorsal motor nucleus of the glossopharyngeal and vagal nerves and anterior olfactory nucleus. Thereafter, the disease process propagates along the brain stem with an ascending course leading to the midbrain [50]. Degeneration of nigrostriatal neurons is responsible for the classical motor manifestations of PD. The underlying pathophysiology includes α-synuclein deposition in Lewy bodies, found in residual neurons in affected areas such as the substantia nigra pars compacta (SNpc), and in dystrophic neurons in striatal or cortical regions (Lewy neurites).

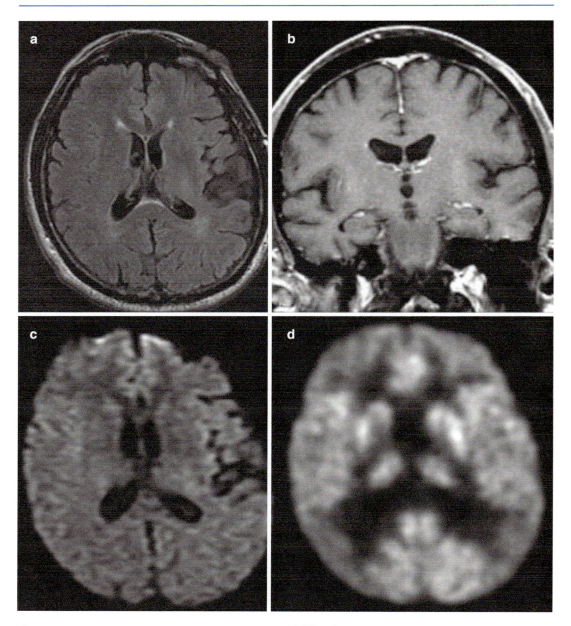

Fig. 14.4 75-year-old male with probable Lewy body disease. Axial FLAIR (**a**) and coronal T1 (**b**) show lack of obvious cortical atrophy or vascular brain damage. Trace DWI (**c**) is unremarkable. Axial FDG PET (**d**) with bilateral temporo-occipital hypometabolism

14.3.1 Imaging

Historically, MRI has contributed little to the assessment of PD, except to rule out vascular lesions. Different metabolic imaging approaches may be used to assess the altered function of the nigrostriatal dopaminergic nerve terminals. The most widely used approach is a marker for the dopamine transporter (DAT) (Fig. 14.5). Several positron or photon-emitting molecules are available with PET or SPECT, respectively. Striatal DAT binding correlates with loss of nigrostriatal dopamine terminals, but only correlates with nigral neuron density when neuron loss does not

14 Degenerative Diseases of the CNS

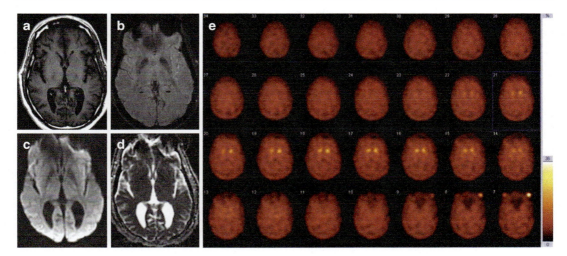

Fig. 14.5 59-year-old man with Parkinson's disease. Axial T1 (**a**) and SWI (**b**) at the level of the basal ganglia. Trace DWI (**c**) and ADC map (**d**) are grossly unremarkable. [I-123] FPCIT DAT imaging (**e**) with right greater than left decreased uptake in the bilateral putamen

exceed 50%. Therefore, striatal DAT may not reflect disease progression beyond the mild-to-moderate stage [51].

Advanced MRI approaches have disclosed potential markers that are useful in research and clinical diagnosis of PD. The loss of the normal nigrosome-1 hyperintensity against the dark SN on iron-sensitive SWI constitutes the basis of the "swallow tail" sign in PD [52]. Using SWI MRI, healthy controls consistently display a hyperintense, ovoid area within the dorsolateral border of the otherwise hypointense SNpc. Across studies, the signal loss in this region had a high sensitivity (79–100%) and specificity (84.6–100%) to separate PD from HC [53]. T1-weighted images are sensitive to the paramagnetic properties of neuromelanin, a pigment contained in the SNpc that appears as an area of high signal intensity on T1-weighted images. The neuromelanin pigmented neurons of the SNpc are particularly vulnerable to neurodegeneration in PD where the neuronal loss is earliest in the ventral–lateral tier of the SN, resulting in a rostro-caudal gradient of reduction of nigrostriatal projections. T1-weighted FSE imaging has consistently demonstrated significant reduction in the neuromelanin-associated T1 hyperintensity of the SN in PD compared to healthy controls [54].

14.3.2 DWI in PD

In a meta-analysis [55] of 39 studies on DTI in PD vs. controls, five anatomic regions demonstrated significant differences between PD patients and healthy controls in FA and MD. Four of these regions showed a decrease of FA and an increase of MD: the SN, the corpus callosum, the cingulate, and the temporal cortices. On the other hand, the corticospinal tract showed an opposite change: increased FA and decreased MD.

14.4 Multiple System Atrophy (MSA)

MSA is a sporadic, adult-onset neurodegenerative disease that presents with a combination of parkinsonism, cerebellar ataxia, and autonomic failure. Based on the dominant clinical presentation, it is subdivided into MSA-P, the parkinsonian phenotype that is the most common, MSA-C, the cerebellar type, and MSA-A or autonomic failure. Olivo-ponto-cerebellar atrophy and striatonigral degeneration are found at postmortem examination [56]. Neurodegenerative changes also involve the central autonomic nuclei, including the hypothalamus, noradrenergic, and serotoninergic brain-stem nuclei, the dorsal nucleus of the vagus, nucleus ambiguus, and intermediolateral columns of the spinal cord. Proteinaceous oligodendroglial cytoplasmic inclusions (Papp–Lantos bodies) are the histologic hallmark of MSA. The constituent of these inclusions is misfolded α-synuclein; therefore, MSA is counted among the α-synucleinopathies together with PD and LBD, although in the former two diseases α-synuclein deposits are primarily intraneuronal.

On conventional MRI, MSA-P exhibits putaminal atrophy, T2* hypointensity, and "slit-like" marginal FLAIR hyperintensities (Fig. 14.6), whereas MSA-C shows atrophy of

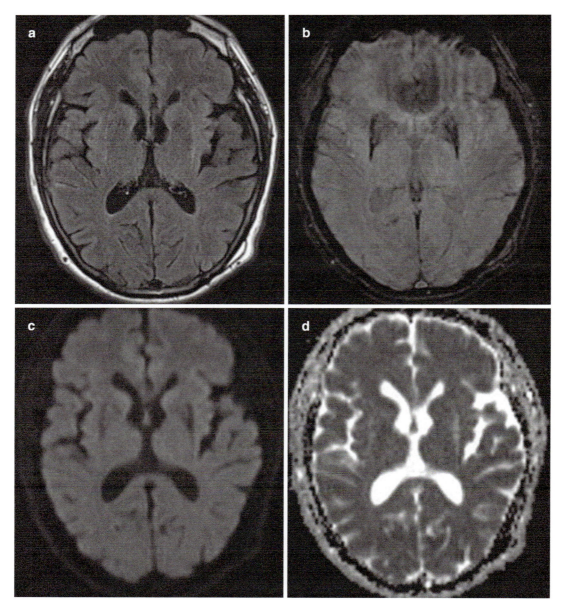

Fig. 14.6 63-year-old man with **MSA-P**. Diagnosed with parkinsonian syndrome 4 years before without benefit from carbidopa/levodopa. Axial FLAIR (**a**) and SWI (**b**) with lateral putaminal hyper and hypointensity, respectively. Trace DWI (**c**) and ADC map (**d**)

14 Degenerative Diseases of the CNS

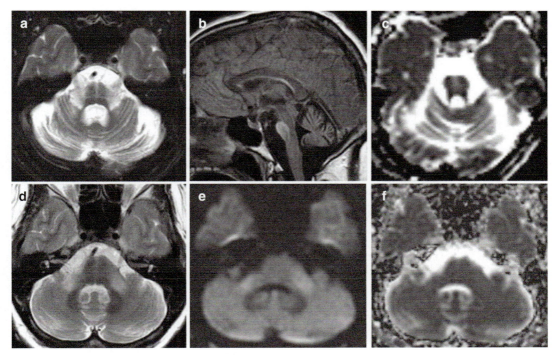

Fig. 14.7 53-year-old woman with a 5-year history of gradually progressive cerebellar ataxia, dysarthria, and balance difficulties. Axial T2 with hot cross bun sign (**a**), sagittal FLAIR with pontine atrophy and hyperintensity (**b**), and ADC map (**c**). Imaging 3 years 9 months earlier with T2 hyperintensity of middle cerebellar peduncles (**d**) with high signal on trace DWI (**e**) ADC map (**f**)

the lower brainstem, pons, middle cerebellar peduncles, vermis, with pontine cruciform T2-weighted hyperintensity (hot cross bun sign) (Fig. 14.7) [52]. SWI signal values of the putamen and pulvinar show more iron deposition in MSA-P, differentiating MSA-P from PD [57]. As already mentioned for PD, the loss of the dorsolateral normal nigral SWI hyperintensity was seen unilaterally in all patients with MSA or PSP, in 83 of 90 patients with PD, but only in 1 of 42 controls; therefore, it has been proposed as an imaging biomarker for neurodegenerative parkinsonism [58].

14.4.1 DWI in MSA

A recent meta-analysis of putaminal diffusivity on high-field DWI showed discrimination of PD from MSA-P, which has higher ADC values, with sensitivity of 90 and 93% specificity [59]. DTI reveals lower FA and higher MD in the middle cerebellar peduncles of MSA patients, while diffusivity is increased at the decussation of the superior cerebellar peduncles in PSP [60].

14.5 Frontotemporal Lobar Degeneration

14.5.1 Introduction

Frontotemporal lobar degeneration (FTLD) includes heterogeneous neurodegenerative disorders clinically characterized by progressive behavioral changes, language disturbances and focal brain atrophy. The average age at clinical onset is 50–60 years, i.e., younger than for sporadic AD. FTLD encompasses three main clinical syndromes: behavioral variant frontotemporal dementia (bvFTD), semantic dementia (SD), and progressive non-fluent aphasia (PNFA) [61].

Primary progressive aphasia includes three clinical subtypes (non-fluent, semantic, and logopenic variants). Furthermore, there is a strong association between FTLD and amyotrophic lateral sclerosis (ALS): half of ALS patients have cognitive impairment of the frontal type, while 50% of FTLD patients have clinical features of ALS [62].

FTLD is pathologically heterogeneous, but an early common feature is gross circumscribed atrophy of the frontal or anterior temporal lobes. The pattern of atrophy shown by clinical imaging correlates with the specific clinical syndrome. Prefrontal atrophy leads to bvFTD, anterior temporal atrophy correlates with SD and left perisylvian atrophy with PNFA. From the molecular standpoint, three subtypes of FTLD are recognized [63]: (1) tau-positive pathology (Pick's disease); (2) tau-negative with ubiquitin-positive inclusions of transactive response DNA-binding protein of 43 kDa (TDP-43) (the most common type of FTLD diseases); and (3) tau-negative, ubiquitin-negative pathology.

14.5.1.1 Imaging

There is characteristic atrophy on clinical CT and MRI studies which correlates with the clinical syndrome [64]. In bvFTD there is an anteroposterior gradient of atrophy involving the frontal and temporal lobes with sparing of the parietal and occipital lobes, often asymmetrical (Fig. 14.8). A meta-analysis of VBM studies in bvFTD demonstrated significant gray matter loss in prefrontal regions compared to controls, with the most significant changes in the medial frontal lobes with volume reductions also in the insula and striatum [65]. However, hippocampal and amygdalar atrophy that are characteristic of AD are also seen with bvFTD [66].

SD shows consistent left anterior temporal lobe atrophy, also involving inferior and mesial temporal lobe regions, with an anteroposterior gradient (more atrophy seen anteriorly) which distinguishes SD from AD [67] (Fig. 14.9). PNFA leads to cortical thinning and atrophy of the left inferior frontal lobe including Broca's area, superior temporal lobe, and insula. The patterns of cortical thinning

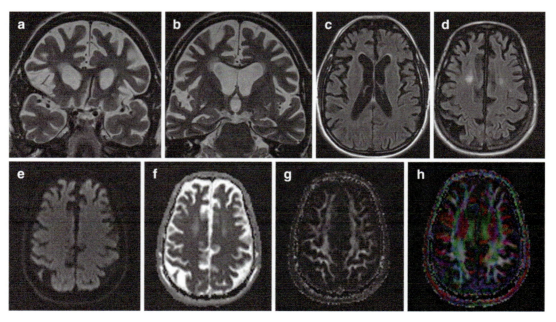

Fig. 14.8 53-year-old man who, in less than 1 year, progressed from cognitively normal to first behavioral changes followed by broad cognitive deficits including prominently reduced fluency. (**a**, **b**) Coronal T2 and (**c**, **d**) axial FLAIR show bilateral frontotemporal cortical atrophy with wide sylvian fissures. (**e**) trace DWI, (**f**) ADC map, (**g**) FA map, (**h**) DTI color map

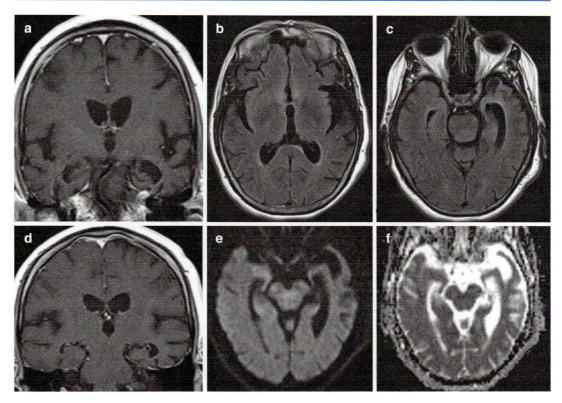

Fig. 14.9 61-year-old woman with frontotemporal dementia, behavioral variant with significant semantic deficits that developed later in the course of the disease. (**a**, **d**) Coronal T1, (**b**, **c**) axial FLAIR, (**e**): trace DWI and (**f**) ADC map show left perisylvian and prominent left hippocampal atrophy

differ between PNFA and SD, with more frontal and parietal atrophy in PNFA vs. bilateral temporal cortical atrophy in SD [68]. Nuclear medicine clinical imaging studies in FTLD demonstrate abnormal brain perfusion and glucose metabolism using SPECT and PET, respectively. A pattern of bilaterally reduced frontal CBF in the absence of parietal hypoperfusion is characteristic in pathologically confirmed FTLD [64].

14.5.1.2 DTI

The diffusivity of gray matter is increased in regions affected in FTLD, suggesting disruption of the cytoarchitecture of remaining tissue. Furthermore, damage was identified in white matter tracts that interconnect affected regions [69]. DTI studies in bvFTD showed bilateral involvement of white matter tracts connecting the frontal lobes such as the anterior cingulum, superior longitudinal fasciculus, and genu of the corpus callosum [70]. PPA patients displayed more focal white matter involvement compared to bvFTD, with differential involvement in the non-fluent, semantic, and logopenic variants of PPA. White matter disorganization in FTLD likely results from axonal degeneration secondary to neuronal body death, as supported by the correlation between white matter changes and cortical atrophy.

14.6 Vascular Dementia

Although not considered among neurodegenerative diseases, vascular dementia is the second cause of dementia after Alzheimer's disease, causing around 15% of cases [71]. Pathological studies showed that subcortical ischemic vascular disease (SIVD), rather than large cortical infarcts, accounts for most cases of vascular dementia

[72]. SIVD results from small-vessel disease, with arteriolar occlusion and lacunar infarctions or widespread incomplete infarction of white matter due to critical stenosis of medullary arterioles and hypoperfusion. Binswanger disease represents the most severe form of SIVD with sparing only of the subcortical U fibers (Fig. 14.10).

The imaging appearance of the progressively confluent white matter T2 hyperintensities with facilitated DWI is best described as leukoaraiosis, i.e., white matter rarefaction [73]. With progressive aging, mixed dementia that results from a combination of neurodegenerative and vascular lesions becomes more prevalent than pure forms [74]. Cerebral amyloid angiopathy is highly prevalent in these pathologically mixed dementia cases, while lacunar infarctions are characteristic of SIVD [74]. Although rare among cases of vascular dementia, cerebral autosomal dominant arteriopathy with subcortical infarcts and leukoencephalopathy (CADASIL) has a defined genetic cause from a frameshift mutation in the notch gene on chromosome 19 [75].

14.7 Fragile X Syndrome (FXS)

FXS is the most common cause of inherited intellectual disability and the leading form of the monogenic cause of autism. FXS is caused by a triplet expansion that inhibits expression of the mental retardation type 1 (FMR1) gene; its gene product, FMRP, regulates mRNA metabolism in the brain. Expansion in this triplet sequence gives rise to FXS, which is the prototype of unstable triplet expansion disorders [76]. Fragile X FMR1 gene premutation (with number of CGG repeats ranging from 55 to 200) is the first single-gene cause of primary ovarian failure and one of the most common causes of ataxia (fragile X-associated tremor/ataxia syndrome [FXTAS]) [77].

Neuroimaging features include T2 hyperintense lesions in the middle cerebellar peduncles as the main imaging criterion and cerebellar white matter hyperintensities, cerebellar and callosal atrophy with ventricular enlargement and white matter T2 hyperintensities [78]. Hyperintensity of the splenium of the corpus callosum is also frequently observed and can suggest the diagnosis even in the absence of hyperintensities of the brachium pontis [79] (Fig. 14.11).

14.8 Creutzfeldt-Jakob Disease (CJD)

CJD is one of the prion diseases characterized by rapidly progressive degenerative dementia, myoclonus, and ataxia. However, the initial clinical presentation is sometimes nonspecific and variable such as visual disturbance (Heidenhain variant), deafness, and hemiparesis [80]. The cause of neurodegeneration is thought to be an accumulation of an abnormal form of human prion protein (infectious proteinaceous scrapie particles, PrP^{Sc}). There are four forms of CJD: sporadic, iatrogenic, familial, and variant [81]. Iatrogenic cases include contaminated neurosurgical instruments, administration of human growth hormone, cadaver-derived gonadotrophin, and dura matter (Fig. 14.12) and corneal grafts [81]. Histological features include spongiform degeneration of the gray matter, characterized by clustered, 5–25 micrometer large prion protein-containing vacuoles in the neuronal and glial elements, and neuronal loss, presumably due to apoptosis and gemistocytic astrocytosis [82] (Fig. 14.13). Electron microscopy shows these vacuoles as focal swelling of neuritic processes, both axonal and dendritic swelling (cellular edema), which may cause decreased ADC [83].

DWI is the most sensitive MRI technique for diagnosing CJD, and is included in the clinical diagnostic criteria [84–87] (Fig. 14.12). Specifically, DWI or FLAIR hyperintensity in the basal ganglia (both caudate nucleus and putamen) or in at least two cortical regions (either the temporal, parietal, or occipital cerebral cortices) is one of the supportive tests for CJD diagnosis, together with detection of 14-3-3 protein in CSF

14 Degenerative Diseases of the CNS

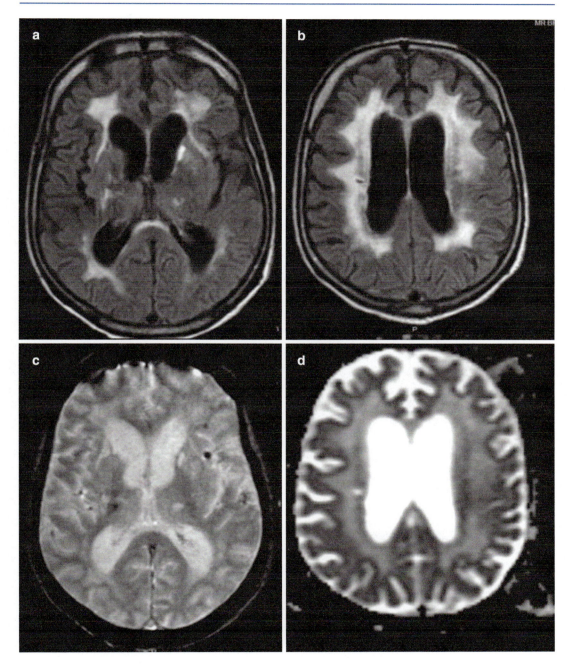

Fig. 14.10 Severe SIVD consistent with Binswanger disease. FLAIR (**a**, **b**), GRE (**c**), and ADC map (**d**) in 71-year-old male with essential hypertension and systemic vasculopathy

and presence of periodic sharp wave complexes on EEG [88] (Figs. 14.12, 14.13, and 14.14). A newer in vitro protein assay system for the detection of prion protein in CSF is real-time quaking-induced conversion assay (RT-QuIC), which has sensitivity of 80–95% and specificity of 99% for CJD diagnosis when applied in symptomatic patients in clinical setting [89].

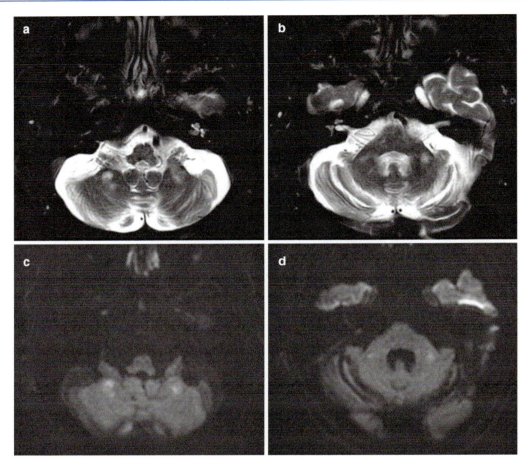

Fig. 14.11 FXS in 71-year-old man with tremor, balance issues, and cognitive impairment with maternal inheritance pattern and FXS premutation status (with 93 CGG repeats at the FMR1 gene). (**a**, **b**) Axial T2, (**c**, **d**) axial trace DWI displaying characteristic involvement of the middle cerebellar peduncles

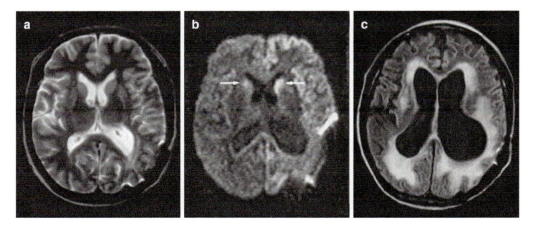

Fig. 14.12 Creutzfeldt–Jakob disease in a 57-year-old woman with progressive dementia 10 years after surgery using cadaver dura matter. (**a**) T2-weighted image shows postoperative change in the left temporo-occipital region with mild ventricular dilatation. (**b**) DW image reveals bilateral hyperintensity in the caudate nuclei (*arrows*) and mild increased signal diffusely in the left hemisphere. (**c**) A 4-month follow-up FLAIR image shows extensive white matter hyperintensity and diffuse atrophy

14 Degenerative Diseases of the CNS

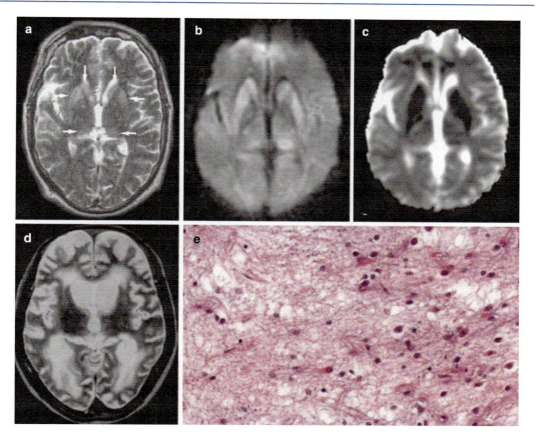

Fig. 14.13 Creutzfeldt–Jakob disease in a 51-year-old man with progressive dementia. (**a**) T2-weighted image demonstrates mild hyperintensity bilaterally in the caudate nuclei, putamina, and pulvinar of the thalami (*arrows*). (**b**) DW image clearly demonstrates these lesions as hyperintense. (**c**) ADC is decreased. (**d**) A 6-month follow-up T2-weighted image shows prominent diffuse atrophy and white matter hyperintensity. (**e**) Pathological specimen of another case shows spongiform degeneration and reactive astrocytosis. (Courtesy of Ukisu R, MD, Showa University, School of Medicine, Japan)

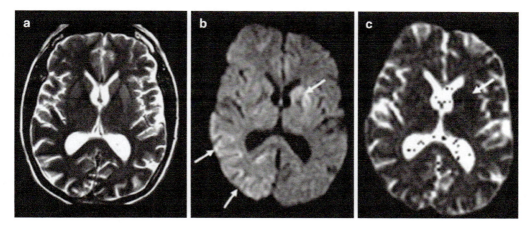

Fig. 14.14 Creutzfeldt–Jakob disease in a 58-year-old woman with altered mental status and visual symptoms (Heidenhain variant). (**a**) T2-weighted image shows questionable hyperintensities in the basal ganglia bilaterally. (**b**) DW image demonstrates hyperintensities only in the left basal ganglia (*arrows*). Hyperintense lesions are also noted in the right temporo-occipital cortices, which does not correspond to a single vascular territory (*arrows*). (**c**) ADC is partially decreased in these lesions (*arrows*)

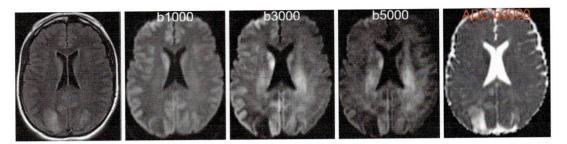

Fig. 14.15 Diffusion restriction in the right caudate and bilateral cerebral hemispheres at three different b values in a CJD case with concurrent PRES

MRI is very important for diagnosis in the context of the clinical criteria because 10% of cases are RT-QuIC negative [89]. T2-weighted and FLAIR images show subtle hyperintense lesions in the cerebral cortex and bilateral basal ganglia in patients with CJD, usually seen 2–5 months after the onset of symptoms. The lesions often involve the bilateral thalami (pulvinar sign) and periaqueductal areas in patients with variant CJD [90], but this finding is also seen in sporadic CJD [91] (Fig. 14.13) Cerebral white matter T2 hyperintensity is considered to be primary degeneration, and first occurs in the periventricular area 4–5 months after the onset and rapidly extends to the deep and subcortical white matter during the following several months [92].

The cortical involvement is usually asymmetric, which does not correspond to arterial territories. Bilateral basal ganglia or thalamic involvement is usually symmetric, but can be asymmetric (Figs. 14.12, 14.13, and 14.14). The lesions are hyperintense on DW images and often associated with decreased ADC [83, 87, 93]. High b values of 2000 s/mm^2 or 3000 s/mm^2 [94] have been found to be more sensitive to detect spongiform pathology in variant and sporadic CJD (Fig. 14.15). Caution should be exercised, though, when comparing DWI studies acquired at different b values because higher b factors change the absolute value of the measured ADC, which is important for lesion detection [95]. In the late stages, abnormal hyperintense signals disappear with prominent brain atrophy, histologically representing neuronal loss and marked fibrillary gliosis [93].

14.9 Neuronal Intranuclear Inclusion Disease (NIID)

Neuronal intranuclear inclusion disease (NIID) is a recently described, rare neurodegenerative disease pathologically characterized by eosinophilic hyaline intranuclear inclusions in the central, peripheral, and autonomic nervous system and visceral organs [96, 97]. NIID has been considered a heterogeneous disease because of the highly variable clinical manifestations, with sporadic and familial forms. Adult-onset NIID develops with progressive dementia, but may also have stroke-like episodes and seizures. Muscle weakness and sensory disturbance have also been observed, particularly in early-onset cases.

On MRI, there is high signal intensity in the corticomedullary junction on diffusion-weighted images in both sporadic and familial NIID cases, which is a strong clue to the diagnosis (Fig. 14.16). Spongiotic white matter changes on pathology co-localize with subcortical DWI high signals [98]. Other findings are cerebellar atrophy and high FLAIR signal in the paramedian cerebellar hemispheres [99]. Biphasic perfusion changes with initially reduced blood flow followed by hyperperfusion have been reported [96]. Skin biopsy is diagnostic with demonstration of eosinophilic, ubiquitin-immunoreactive, and p62-immunoreactive intranuclear inclusions.

14   Degenerative Diseases of the CNS

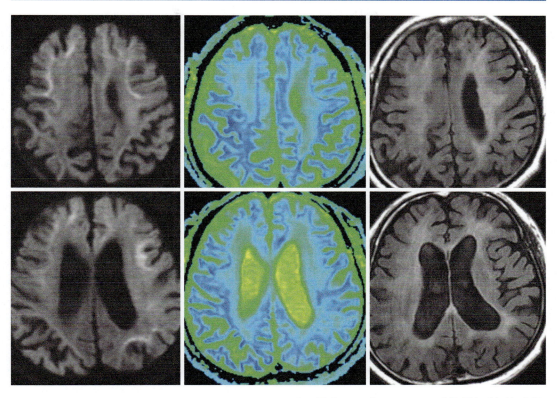

Fig. 14.16 NIID. 60-year-old male with aphasia and incomplete right hemiparesis 2 years before onset of dementia. Subcortical white matter restricted diffusion on color ADC map. Case courtesy of Dr. Takashi Abe MD, PhD, Department of Radiology, Faculty of Medicine, Tokushima University, Japan

14.10 Hereditary Diffuse Leukoencephalopathy with Axonal Spheroids (HDLS)

HDLS is a rare, autosomal dominant disease clinically characterized by adult onset of progressive dementia and behavioral changes, apraxia, apathy, impaired balance, parkinsonism, spasticity, and epilepsy [100]. The underlying genetic defect has been linked to mutations in the colony stimulating factor 1 receptor (CSF1R) gene, primarily expressed in microglia [101]. On imaging, patients display frontal T2 hyperintensity in the periventricular, deep, and subcortical white matter, small white matter calcifications, thinning of the corpus callosum and T2 hyperintensity of the corticospinal tracts with central atrophy, but no significant gray matter abnormality [102]. MRS revealed decreased NAA and glutamate concentrations in the affected white matter, which probably reflected neuronal loss [103]. Differential diagnoses include multiple sclerosis [104], cerebral autosomal dominant arteriopathy with subcortical infarcts and leukoencephalopathy (CADASIL) and other leukoencephalopathies such as late-onset metachromatic leukodystrophy (MLD), X-linked adrenoleukodystrophy (x-ALD), and Krabbe disease [105]. Microscopically, the white matter abnormalities are characterized by loss of myelin and axons and the presence of numerous round to sausage-shaped axonal swellings: the neuroaxonal spheroids [106]. On DWI weighted imaging, small, persistent, and increasing foci of diffusion restriction are seen within the white matter lesions, presumably reflecting intramyelinic edema in regions of neurodegeneration (Fig. 14.17) [107]. Thus, persistent foci of restricted diffusion constitute a characteristic imaging feature of HDLS [100, 102, 105], not seen in other leukoencephalopathies.

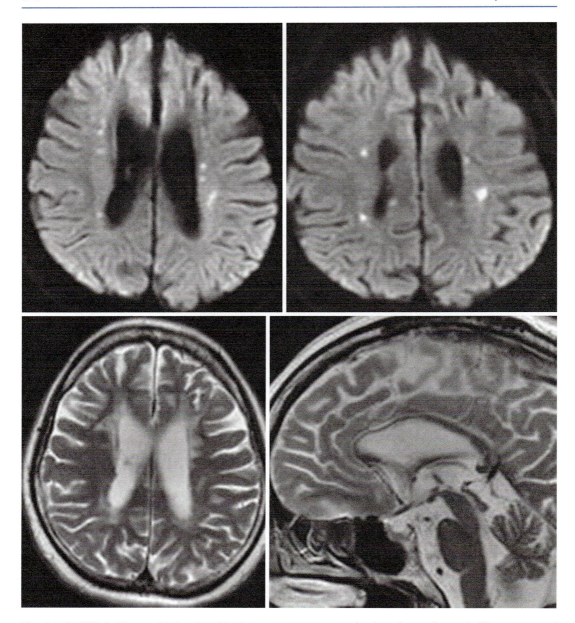

Fig. 14.17 HDLS 55-year-old female with dementia: Foci of longstanding restricted diffusion in the deep white matter (top) and T2 hyperintensity with volume loss of the centrum semiovale and genu (bottom). (Case courtesy of Dr.Takashi Abe MD, PhD, Department of Radiology, Faculty of Medicine, Tokushima University, Japan)

14.11 Amyotrophic Lateral Sclerosis (ALS)

Amyotrophic lateral sclerosis (ALS) is a neurodegenerative, heterogeneous syndrome that is currently conceptualized as a continuum between frontotemporal dementia and motor neuron disease and is strongly associated with expansion mutations in the *C9orf72* gene [108]. ALS affects both upper and lower motor neurons and their projections. It often afflicts middle-aged patients and is characterized by progressive muscle weakness, limb and truncal atrophy associated with bulbar signs and symptoms. The disease progression is relentless, and half of the patients die within 3 years. Degeneration of upper motor neurons usually starts in the primary motor cortex, and secondary degeneration of motor fibers and gliosis occurs along the corticospinal tract with TDP-43 pathology.

MR images of ALS are characterized by high T2 signal along the large myelinated pyramidal tract fibers in the posterior limb of the internal capsule and cerebral peduncles. On DW imaging there are typically increased ADC values and decreased fractional anisotropy in the corticospinal tracts [109]. DTI is useful in analyzing the extent and severity of axonal degeneration quantitatively in ALS (Fig. 14.18) [110–113]. Compared to controls, ALS patients showed a significant decrease of FA and fiber length and density in the corticospinal tracts (CSTs) and in the corpus callosum (CC) [114] and in other white matter regions including the brainstem [115]. Clinical functional scales correlate with corticospinal DTI measures along the clinical spectrum of *C9orf72* mutation carriers [113]. Reduced FA in the pyramidal tracts in ALS was associated with poor prognosis and FA reduction follows disease progression [116]. DTI can also be used for segmentation of white matter tracts, particularly the CST and corticobulbar tract (CBT) (Fig. 14.19), which may enable differentiation of clinical subtypes of ALS. For instance, FA values along the corticobulbar tract of bulbar-onset type are significantly lower than that of limb-onset type (Fig. 14.19) [110].

14.12 Huntington Disease (HD)

HD is an autosomal dominant disorder characterized by motor, cognitive, and behavioral disturbances. Age of diagnosis varies inversely with the expanded number of polyglutamine (cytosine-adenine-guanine or CAG) repeats in the huntingtin gene. Anatomically, HD primarily affects striatal neurons, with bilateral caudate atrophy being the most consistent imaging finding. Motor onset usually occurs in midlife, with a duration of 15–20 years after diagnosis. Striatal volume loss is present years before clinical diagnosis; however, white matter degradation is also prevalent and has been investigated as putative biomarker of the neurodegeneration. Increases in mean dif-

fusivity (MD) and radial diffusivity (RD) in HD relative to controls were seen in inferior and lateral prefrontal cortex regions, which were seen at the prodromal stage of HD and tracked with baseline disease progression [117]. DTI metrics in selected tracts connecting the primary motor, primary somato-sensory, and premotor areas of the cortex with the subcortical caudate and putamen also suggested white matter degeneration, which were present up to a decade before predicted HD diagnosis [118]. Over a 2-year follow-up period, volumetric MRI was more sensitive to striatal degeneration in early symptomatic HD than DWI [119].

14.13 Secondary Neuronal Degeneration (Wallerian, Transneuronal, and Retrograde Degeneration)

There are three major types of secondary neuronal degenerations: (1) Wallerian degeneration (antegrade), (2) transneuronal/trans-synaptic degeneration (antegrade or retrograde), and (3) retrograde degeneration (Fig. 14.20) [120]. Wallerian degeneration is an antegrade degeneration of the axons and myelin sheath resulting from injury of the proximal portion of the axons or cell bodies. It is most commonly recognized in the corticospinal tract secondary to middle cerebral artery infarction. Wallerian degeneration can also be seen in corticobulbar and corticopontine tracts, the corpus callosum, and middle cerebral peduncles [121]. Energy depletion in layer 5 neurons may lead to failure of ion channel activity in the axolemma [122]. This results in axonal swelling followed by disintegration of the intra-axonal organelles. This in turn is followed by collapse of the myelin sheath and ensuing gliosis. DW imaging shows the acute phase of Wallerian degeneration as hyperintense signal associated with decreased ADC, presumably representing axonal and reactive astrocytic swelling [123, 124] (Fig. 14.21). DW high signals can be observed after more than 24 h following the associated territorial infarction [125]. In DTI, FA is reduced in the corticospinal tract, and may correlate with

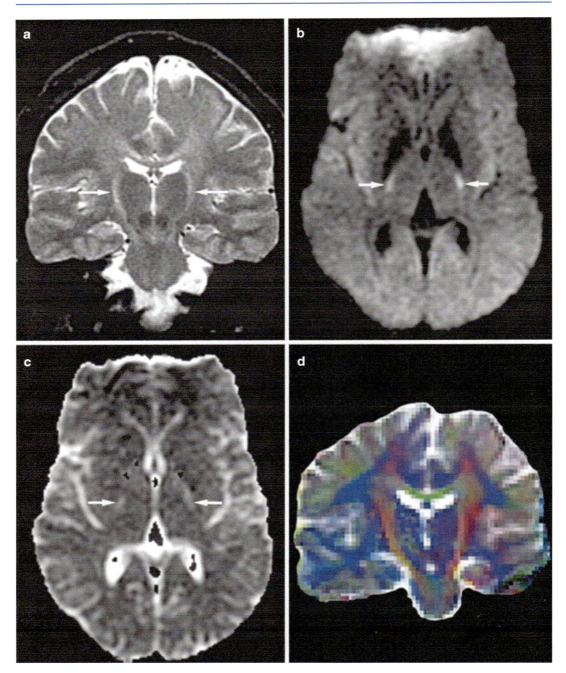

Fig. 14.18 Amyotrophic lateral sclerosis in a 27-year-old man with progressive weakness and dysphagia. (**a**) Coronal spin-echo T2-weighted image shows bilateral symmetrical hyperintensity along the corticospinal tract (*arrows*), extending into the white matter of the motor area. (**b**) DW image shows mild hyperintensity in bilateral corticospinal tracts. (**c**) ADC is increased (*arrows*). Hyperintensity and distortion in the frontal region are due to susceptibility artifact from air in the frontal sinuses. (**d**) Coronal diffusion tensor image with color mapping reveals decreased anisotropy along bilateral corticospinal tracts

14 Degenerative Diseases of the CNS

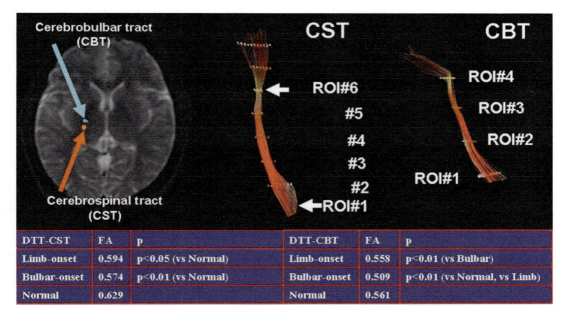

Fig. 14.19 Tract-specific analysis of the corticospinal and corticobulbar tracts in amyotrophic lateral sclerosis. (Courtesy of Aoki S. MD, The University of Tokyo, Japan)

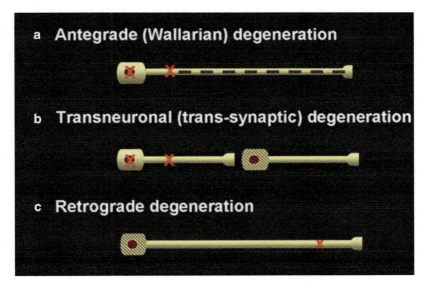

Fig. 14.20 Three major types of secondary degenerations. (**a**) Wallerian degeneration; an antegrade degeneration of the axons and myelin sheath resulting from injury of the proximal portion of the axons or cell bodies. (**b**) Transneuronal/trans-synaptic degeneration (antegrade type); a degeneration of the distal neuron via the synapse resulting from injury of the proximal portion of the axons or cell bodies. (**c**) Retrograde degeneration; a degeneration of the proximal neuron resulting from injury of the distal portion of the axons

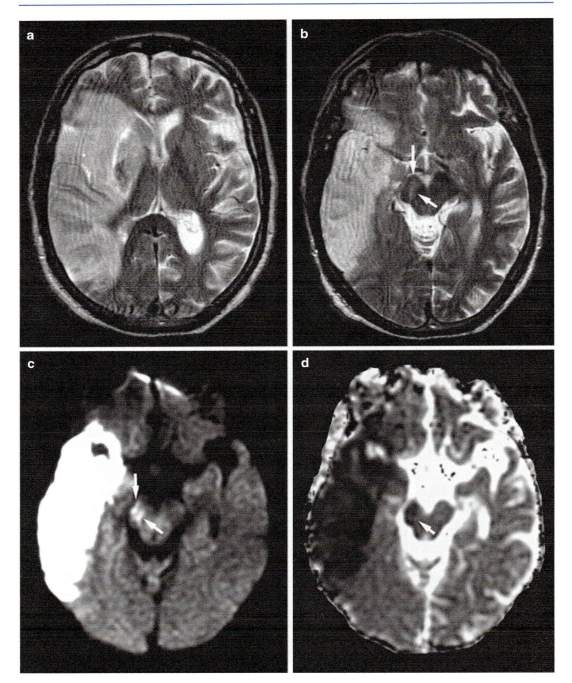

Fig. 14.21 Wallerian and transneuronal degeneration (acute phase) in a 76-year-old man with a large infarct in the right middle cerebral artery (MCA) territory (6 days after onset). (**a**) T2-weighted image shows a right MCA infarct as hyperintense, including the left putamen. (**b**) T2-weighted image at the level of the midbrain reveals a slightly hyperintense lesion in the right cerebral peduncle including the substantia nigra (*arrows*), as well as a right MCA infarct in the temporal area. (**c**) DW image shows hyperintensity in the T2 hyperintense foci seen in (**b**) (*arrows*). (**d**) ADC is decreased involving both the right cerebral peduncle and the right substantia nigra (*arrow*)

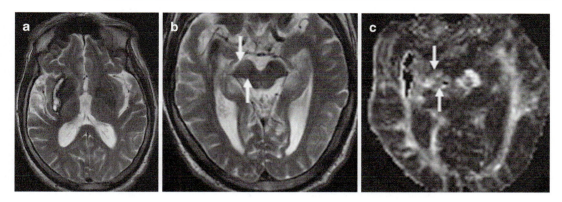

Fig. 14.22 Wallerian and transneuronal degeneration in a 78-year-old woman with right chronic putaminal hemorrhage. (**a**) T2-weighted image shows a right old putaminal hemorrhage as hypointense. (**b**) T2-weighted image at the level of the midbrain reveals mild hyperintense lesion in the right cerebral peduncle, including the substantia nigra (*arrows*). (**c**) FA map shows decreased anisotropy in the right cerebral peduncle (*arrows*)

impairment of motor function [126, 127] (Fig. 14.19). DT imaging is more sensitive than DW imaging in detecting chronic Wallerian degeneration [128].

Transneuronal (trans-synaptic) degeneration in the substantia nigra can occur secondary to striatal stroke [129]. This occurs along fiber connections originating in the caudate and putamen projecting over the substantia nigra (striatonigral pathway) [130]. Loss of inhibitory GABAergic output from the ischemic lesion can induce a postsynaptic long-term potentiation or a continuous excitatory state in the substantia nigra, resulting in neuronal swelling and cell death [131]. DW imaging shows hyperintensity associated with decreased ADC in the substantia nigra (Figs. 14.21 and 14.22) [132]. The decreased ADC of these lesions is thought to represent cellular edema of astrocytes or neurons in the substantia nigra. Diffusion abnormalities in the striatum or thalamus secondary to external capsular hemorrhage have also been reported, which are presumably related to antegrade transneuronal degeneration of the striatum (cortico-striatal fibers) and retrograde transneuronal degeneration of the thalamus (thalamostriate fibers) (Fig. 14.22) [133].

A distinct type of transneuronal degeneration relevant in neuroimaging is hypertrophic olivary degeneration (HOD). HOD ensues after damage to the dentato-rubro-olivary pathway, also known as the Guillain-Mollaret triangle. It results in palatal or oculopalatal myoclonus and cerebellar dysfunction [134]. HOD is a unique type of degeneration in that the degenerating olivary nuclei become transiently hypertrophic rather than atrophic and T2 hyperintense (Fig. 14.23). Interestingly, over 40% of HOD patients may not present an MRI-detectable lesion in the Guillain-Mollaret triangle [135].

Retrograde thalamic degeneration is usually seen in anterior and dorsomedial nuclei secondary to ipsilateral large infarction or hemorrhage. It is thought to be a retrograde degeneration through the thalamo-cortical pathways [136, 137]. DW imaging shows hyperintensity in the thalamic nuclei (Fig. 14.24).

14.14 Treatment Section: Treatment of Dementia

Juana Nicoll Capizzano

Introduction: New advances in the understanding of the pathophysiology of dementia illnesses have changed the management of patients with these disorders. The mainstay of management is still symptomatic; however, since there are no disease-modifying treatments currently available for any of the neurodegenerative dementias. However, it has been estimated that approximately 35% of AD

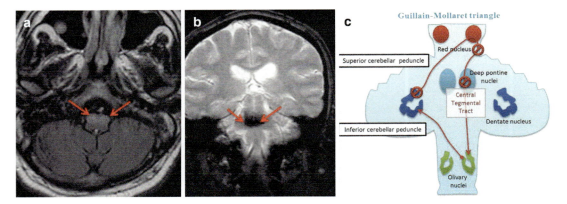

Fig. 14.23 (a) Hypertrophic olivary degeneration in patient with pontine hematoma (b). (c) Guillain-Mollaret triangle: Injury to the dentate nucleus, superior cerebellar peduncle, or central tegmental tract will result in transneuronal hypertrophic olivary degeneration

risk is modifiable with early life education and mid and late life control of vascular risk factors having a significant protective effect against late-life dementia [138]. The future promises disease-specific and, hopefully, disease-modifying treatments. Currently, the first step in dementia management is an accurate diagnosis of the type of dementia.

14.14.1 Alzheimer's Disease (AD)

It is the most prevalent neurodegenerative disease of aging, and it affects over 26 million people worldwide with this number continuously increasing [1, 139, 140]. The USA Food and Drug Administration (FDA) has approved five drugs for treatment of AD (Table 14.1). Three of these drugs are cholinesterase inhibitors, one is an N-Methyl-D-aspartate (NMDA) antagonist, and one is a combination of these two mechanisms. Additionally, addressing the treatment of behavioral and sleep problems is an important aspect of the care of patients with dementia.

Cholinesterase Inhibitors (ACHEIs): Patients with AD have reduced cerebral content of choline acetyl-transferase, which leads to a decrease in acetylcholine synthesis and impaired cortical cholinergic function. Cholinesterase inhibitors increase cholinergic transmission by inhibiting cholinesterase at the synaptic cleft. Evidence suggests that ACHEIs moderately improve cognitive and global function status of mild to moderate AD and DLB patients [141]. However, the efficacy wanes with long-term treatment due to side effects such as weight loss, diarrhea, and syncope [141]. On the other hand, ACHEIs may worsen behavioral symptoms in frontotemporal lobar degeneration (FTLD) [142].

N-methyl-D-aspartate (NMDA) receptor antagonists: Memantine blocks over-excited NMDA glutamate receptors, thereby inhibiting excitotoxicity [143]. Memantine alone or in combination with ACHEIs (Namzaric) has been approved for treatment of moderate to severe AD patients [144]. It has not been shown to be of benefit in mild AD. There is some evidence that it may be effective in vascular dementia and LBD/PDD [138].

Nonpharmacologic Therapy and Supportive Care: Non-pharmacologic interventions like diet, exercise, cognitive training, sleep hygiene, and vitamin supplementation have protective effects against cognitive decline and have been studied in AD prevention trials. The most promising dietary intervention has been the Mediterranean diet rich in fruits and vegetables, combined with olive oil and fish. The Three-City (3C) study suggested that participants who adhered to the Mediterranean diet had a slower rate of decline on the mini-mental status examination (MMSE) but not the other cognitive tests [145]. Furthermore, it has

14 Degenerative Diseases of the CNS

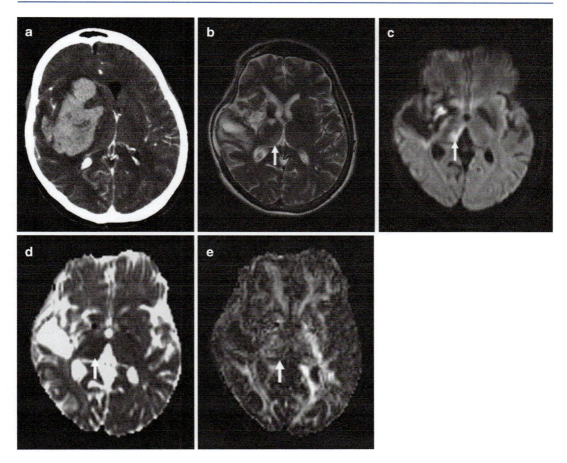

Fig. 14.24 Retrograde degeneration in the dorsomedial thalamus in a 56-year-old woman with right large putaminal hemorrhage. (**a**) Postcontrast CT shows a large hematoma in the right putamen extending into the frontotemporal region with edema and a mass effect. (**b**) The 2-month follow-up T2-weighted image shows a high signal intensity in the dorsomedial thalamus (*arrow*). Right craniectomy and extensive encephalomalacia are also noted. (**c, d**) DW image shows a hyperintense lesion with decreased ADC in the right dorsomedial thalamus (*arrow*). (**e**) FA map shows decreased anisotropy in the right internal capsule and dorsomedial thalamus (*arrow*). (Courtesy of Lee HK, MD, The University of Iowa Hospitals and Clinics, USA)

Table 14.1 Current US Food and Drug Administration-Approved Drugs for treating AD

Drug name	Trade name	Mechanism of action	Indication	Approval year
Donepezil	Aricept	Cholinesterase Inhibitor	Mild, moderate, and severe AD	1996
Rivastigmine	Exelon	Cholinesterase Inhibitor	Mild to moderate AD	2006
Galantamine	Razadyne	Cholinesterase Inhibitor	Mild to moderate AD	2001
Memantine	Namenda	NMDA antagonist	Moderate to severe AD	2003
Memantine plus Donepezil	Namzaric	NMDA antagonist and cholinesterase inhibitor	Moderate to severe AD	2014

also been shown that the Mediterranean Dietary Approach to Systolic Hypertension (DASH) intervention for neurodegenerative delay (MIND) diet may reduce the risk of Alzheimer's by up to 50%, and the protective effects persist until later time even when diet recommendations were not followed rigorously [146, 147].

Several studies have demonstrated that formal exercise programs may improve physical functioning and at least slow the progression of functional decline in patients with AD; however, current evidence is insufficient to provide detailed recommendations regarding specific physical exercise linked to AD prevention, e.g., type, frequency, intensity, and duration of exercise [148]. Overall, it is indicated that physical activities combined with social and cognitive stimulation or diet modification may be more beneficial at reducing risk of AD [148].

In the past decade more attention has been brought to the use of supplements such as vitamin E, Gingko biloba, and omega-3 fatty acids for AD prevention. Based on recent systematic reviews, there is no evidence suggesting any beneficial effects of vitamin E on preventing MCI conversion into AD or improving cognitive function of MCI or AD patients [149]. However, results from a single study of combined vitamin E and memantine therapy in AD suggest that vitamin E may delay functional decline in these patients by 19% per year versus placebo [150, 151].

Cognitive interventions hold promise for the mitigation of cognitive symptoms in dementias. Strategies include cognitive stimulation and neurorehabilitation. However, the evidence for their efficacy is lacking. Finally, it is paramount that caregivers be taught about what to expect from the course of the disease, the underlying causes of behavior changes, and be trained on how to problem solve situations with regard to dementia [138].

14.14.2 Vascular Dementia (VaD)

Vascular cognitive impairment (VCI) is defined as cognitive impairment associated with clinical stroke or subclinical vascular brain injury and ranges from mild cognitive impairment (MCI) to its most severe form, vascular dementia (VaD)

[152]. VCI is the second most common type of dementia after AD. VCI has received significant attention recently as a potentially preventable and treatable cause of cognitive impairment [153, 154].

Acetylcholinesterase inhibitors are believed to improve cognition in patients with AD by increasing the availability of acetylcholine in the synaptic cleft. There is also evidence that these medications increase cerebral blood flow [152, 155, 156]. Therefore, these drugs are considered as a potential treatment option in patients with VCI. However, in clinical trials, dose–response effects to acetylcholinesterase inhibitors in VCI have not been consistent. Moreover, no definitive benefit is seen in patients with VaD in global functioning when treated, thus, no acetylcholinesterase inhibitors has received FDA approval for use in VaD.

Herbal Medicines: There is a long history of herbal medicine used to boost memory and cognitive functions and to manage behavioral and psychological symptoms associated with neurodegenerative or vascular dementia. Some of the most commonly used and studied herbs include Ginkgo biloba, Huperzia serrata, Curcuma longa, Panax notoginseng, and Bacopa nonnieri. Gingko Biloba is one of the most studied medicinal herbs. Ginkgo leaf extract is widely used for aging-related memory disorders in many European and Asian countries. The principal constituents of ginkgo include flavonol glycosides and terpenoids [157]. Preclinical studies suggest that ginkgo decreases oxygen radical discharge and proinflammatory functions of macrophages (antioxidant and anti-inflammatory), reduces corticosteroid production (antianxiety), and increases glucose uptake and utilization and adenosine triphosphate (ATP) production [158].

In animal studies, the effects of ginkgo leaf extracts on neuroprotection and cognitive dysfunction have been demonstrated in various cerebral ischemia models in rats, mice, and gerbils [159, 160]. In healthy young adults, ginkgo treatment has been shown to improve speed of processing, working memory, executive function, and cognition [161]. The evidence to support the use of gingko for dementia remains controversial. Although clinical studies failed to show a significant difference between ginkgo and placebo in dementia groups [162], there are

14 Degenerative Diseases of the CNS

potentially beneficial effects for dementia when it is administered at doses greater than 200 mg/day for at least 5 months [163]. Given the lower quality of the evidence, further rigorously designed, multicenter-based, large-scale RCTs are warranted.

14.14.3 Dementia with Lewy Bodies (DLB)

DLB is characterized by dementia, cognitive fluctuations, visual hallucinations, parkinsonism, and rapid eye movement (REM) sleep behavior disorder [36]. It was first described as separate disease entity by Kosaka and colleagues [164]. DLB has a marked clinicopathologic overlap with Parkinson's disease dementia (PDD) posing challenges to distinguish between DLB and PDD in clinical practice.

14.14.3.1 Symptomatic Treatment Options for DLB

- **Dementia, visual hallucinations, and other neuropsychiatric disturbances**: Cognitive impairment is usually the initial symptom of DLB, and cognition can exhibit a more rapid decline as compared with AD. Cholinesterase inhibitors (AChEIs) rivastigmine and donepezil are the first-line treatment recommended for cognitive disturbances in DLB [165]. However, despite the cholinergic hypothesis, cholinesterase inhibitor drugs have demonstrated limited effectiveness in clinical practice.
- **Neuropsychiatric symptoms**: These are associated with the higher distress that DLB caregivers experience, and they include visual hallucinations, delusions, depression, apathy, anxiety, psychomotor excitement, and agitation. Neuropsychiatric symptoms are attributed to dysfunctional, decreased serotonergic, and cholinergic neurotransmission [166]. None of the AChEIs has been found to be better than other because there are no head-to-head trials comparing their efficacy in DLB. Japanese authors described in several

reports the complete disappearance of visual hallucinations after treatment with donepezil, suggesting a dose-dependent effect and recommending donepezil as the first-choice drug for the treatment of DLB-related psychotic symptoms [167].
- The use of antipsychotics for the acute management of substantial behavioral disturbances, delusions, or visual hallucinations comes with significant mortality risks in patients with dementia, and they should be avoided whenever possible, given the increased risk of a serious neuroleptic sensitivity reaction [168]. Low-dose quetiapine may be relatively safer that other antipsychotics and is widely used. In alignment with general advice on depression in dementia, selective serotonin reuptake inhibitors, serotonin-norepinephrine reuptake inhibitors, and mirtazapine are options in DLB with treatment guided by individual patient tolerability and response.
- **Motor symptoms**: Parkinsonism is often less responsive to dopaminergic treatments in DLB than in Parkinson's disease, and their use may be associated with an increased risk of psychosis. Levodopa is generally well-tolerated in modest doses by DLB patients, without producing neuropsychiatric side effects [168]. Patients at risk of falling may benefit from safety assessment as well as bone mineral density screening, and assessment of vitamin D status to manage risk of fractures. Sleep disorders can be managed with melatonin as a possible safe option. Clonazepam carries a risk of worsening cognition and gait impairment and should be avoided [169].

14.14.4 Parkinson's Disease (PD)

Is the second most common neurodegenerative disorder after AD affecting more than 6 million people worldwide [170]. Management remains complicated over the course of the disease and should be individualized based on the patient's quality of life at each stage of the disease. Dopaminergic medica-

Table 14.2 Current US Food and Drug Administration-Approved Drugs for treating PD

Agent	Mechanism of action	Side effects	Typical dose	Level of evidence
Levodopa (with carbidopa or benserazide)[a] (Sinemet, Levocarb, Prolopa)	Metabolizes to dopamine	Nausea, vomiting, constipation, psychosis, hallucinations, hypotension, and dyskinesias.	300–1200 mg (higher if tolerated)/day (Divided tid,qid,q3h,q2h)	A
Dopamine agonists (Ropinirole, Pramipezole and Rotigotine patch)	Directly stimulate dopamine receptors	As above, plus leg edema, reward-seeking behavior, daytime sleepiness, and sudden-onset sleep. Skin reactions with the rotigotine patch	Ropinirole: 3–24 mg/day (TID) Pramipexole: 1.5–4.5 mg/day (TID) Rotigotine: 4–8 mg/24 h (patch)	A
Catechol-O-methyltransferase (COMT) inhibitors (Entacapone)	Blocks peripheral COMT activity	Related to increased levodopa delivery: diarrhea, urine discoloration.	200 mg pill, up to 8 times/day (given with each dose of levodopa)	A
Monoamine Oxidase (MAO) Inhibitors (Selegiline, Rasagiline)	Blocks MAO-B to reduce metabolism of dopamine (central and peripheral)	Nausea, hypotension, confusion, hallucinations.	Rasagline: 0.5–1 mg/day (od) Selegiline: 5–10 mg/day (BID) early in the day.	A
Amantadine	Blocks NMDA and acetylcholine receptors.	Confusion, hallucinations, leg edema, rash (livedo reticularis)	100 mg od to 100 mg (TID)	C
Anticholinergics (e.g., trihexyphenidyl)	Blocks acetylcholine receptors	Dry eyes and mouth urinary retention, confusion, worsening of glaucoma	Trihexiphenadyl: 1–6 mg/day (TID)	U

Levels of evidence are derived from the American Academy of Neurology recommendations: A = established effective, B = probably effective, C = possibly effective, U = date inadequate or conflicting
[a]Levodopa should be taken 1 h prior to, or 2 h after, meals containing protein, to improve absorption. Sinemet CR (controlled release 100/25 and 200/50 mg) cannot be used to reduce frequency of immediate-release levodopa administration

tions are the mainstay of symptomatic therapy for motor symptoms. The mechanism of action, starting and target doses and adverse effects are summarized in Table 14.2 [171].

Anticholinergics, such as trihexyphenidyl, may be used in patients with early-onset Parkinson disease and severe tremor, but not as a first choice owing to limited efficacy and propensity of neuropsychiatric adverse effects. Recent data show that injections of botulinum toxin may effectively treat the tremor from of Parkinson disease [172].

Drugs that should be avoided in PD: Drugs that block dopamine receptors can result in parkinsonism or substantially worsen motor symptoms in patient with PD and may lead to neuroleptic malignant syndrome. These include neuroleptics such as haloperidol, thioridazine, chlorpromazine, promethazine, fluphenazine, ris-

peridone, and olanzapine. Antiemetics such as prochlorperazine and metoclopramide, tetrabenazine and antihypertensives, such as methyldopa [173]. Meperidine should be avoided in those receiving monoamine oxidase B inhibitors [173].

Deep Brain Stimulation: Approved in 2002 as an adjunctive therapy for reducing motor fluctuation in advanced PD. The globus pallidus interna and the subthalamic nucleus are accepted targets for this procedure.

Good candidates are those patients with adequate response to dopaminergic therapy, presence of on–off fluctuations, age <70 years, and dyskinesia impairing quality of life and medication-resistant tremor. Poor candidates are those with severe dementia, severe autonomic dysfunction, poor dopaminergic response, atypical parkinsonism, unstable psychiatric disease or absence of a dedicated caregiver.

Patients should be considered for deep brain stimulation only if adequate trials of multiple medications for PD have been unsuccessful [174]. Although duration of therapy is not clearly established, patients who undergo deep brain stimulation may have sustained benefit for at least 10 years [174].

Levodopa-carbidopa intestinal gel: For patients who are not candidates for or decline deep brain stimulation, levodopa-carbidopa intestinal gel may be considered. This gel is pumped into the jejunum via a percutaneous tube insertion, recently approved for the treatment of motor fluctuations in PD [175]. Administration of the gel has been shown to result in faster absorptions, comparable bioavailability and reduced intra-subject variability in levodopa concentrations compared with oral levodopa-carbidopa [176].

References

1. (2016) 2016 Alzheimer's disease facts and figures. Alzheimers Dement 12(4):459–509
2. Naj AC, Schellenberg GD (2017) Genomic variants, genes, and pathways of Alzheimer's disease: an overview. Am J Med Genet B Neuropsychiatr Genet 174(1):5–26
3. Pericak-Vance MA, Bebout JL, Gaskell PC, Yamaoka LH, Hung WY, Alberts MJ et al (1991) Linkage studies in familial Alzheimer disease: evidence for chromosome 19 linkage. Am J Hum Genet 48(6):1034–1050
4. Selkoe DJ, Hardy J (2016) The amyloid hypothesis of Alzheimer's disease at 25 years. EMBO Mol Med 8(6):595–608
5. Braak H, Braak E (1995) Staging of Alzheimer's disease-related neurofibrillary changes. Neurobiol Aging 16(3):271–278; discussion 8–84
6. Petersen RC (2016) Mild cognitive impairment. Continuum (Minneapolis, Minn) 22(2 Dementia):404–418
7. Petersen RC, Roberts RO, Knopman DS, Boeve BF, Geda YE, Ivnik RJ et al (2009) Mild cognitive impairment: ten years later. Arch Neurol 66(12):1447–1455
8. McKhann GM, Knopman DS, Chertkow H, Hyman BT, Jack CR Jr, Kawas CH et al (2011) The diagnosis of dementia due to Alzheimer's disease: recommendations from the National Institute on Aging-Alzheimer's Association workgroups on diagnostic guidelines for Alzheimer's disease. Alzheimers Dement 7(3):263–269
9. Weiner MW, Veitch DP, Aisen PS, Beckett LA, Cairns NJ, Cedarbaum J et al (2015) 2014 update of the Alzheimer's disease neuroimaging initiative: a review of papers published since its inception. Alzheimers Dement 11(6):e1–120
10. Frisoni GB, Fox NC, Jack CR Jr, Scheltens P, Thompson PM (2010) The clinical use of structural MRI in Alzheimer disease. Nat Rev Neurol 6(2):67–77
11. Dallaire-Theroux C, Callahan BL, Potvin O, Saikali S, Duchesne S (2017) Radiological-pathological correlation in Alzheimer's disease: systematic review of Antemortem magnetic resonance imaging findings. JAD 57(2):575–601
12. Risacher SL, Shen L, West JD, Kim S, McDonald BC, Beckett LA et al (2010) Longitudinal MRI atrophy biomarkers: relationship to conversion in the ADNI cohort. Neurobiol Aging 31(8):1401–1418
13. Nelson PT, Head E, Schmitt FA, Davis PR, Neltner JH, Jicha GA et al (2011) Alzheimer's disease is not "brain aging": neuropathological, genetic, and epidemiological human studies. Acta Neuropathol 121(5):571–587
14. Hachinski VC, Potter P, Merskey H (1987) Leukoaraiosis. Arch Neurol 44(1):21–23
15. Chui HC, Ramirez-Gomez L (2015) Clinical and imaging features of mixed Alzheimer and vascular pathologies. Alzheimers Res Ther 7(1):21
16. Villain N, Fouquet M, Baron JC, Mezenge F, Landeau B, de La Sayette V et al (2010) Sequential relationships between grey matter and white matter atrophy and brain metabolic abnormalities in early Alzheimer's disease. Brain J Neurol 133(11):3301–3314
17. Kantarci K, Jack CR Jr, Xu YC, Campeau NG, O'Brien PC, Smith GE et al (2001) Mild cognitive impairment and Alzheimer disease: regional diffusivity of water. Radiology 219(1):101–107
18. Schwartz RB (2001) Apparent diffusion coefficient mapping in patients with Alzheimer disease or mild cognitive impairment and in normally aging control subjects: present and future. Radiology 219(1):8–9
19. Remy F, Vayssiere N, Saint-Aubert L, Barbeau E, Pariente J (2015) White matter disruption at the prodromal stage of Alzheimer's disease: relationships with hippocampal atrophy and episodic memory performance. NeuroImage Clinical 7:482–492
20. Agosta F, Pievani M, Sala S, Geroldi C, Galluzzi S, Frisoni GB et al (2011) White matter damage in Alzheimer disease and its relationship to gray matter atrophy. Radiology 258(3):853–863
21. Weiner MW, Veitch DP, Aisen PS, Beckett LA, Cairns NJ, Green RC et al (2017) Recent publications from the Alzheimer's disease neuroimaging initiative: reviewing progress toward improved AD clinical trials. Alzheimers Dement 13(4):e1–e85

22. Kawakatsu S, Kobayashi R, Hayashi H (2017) Typical and atypical appearance of early-onset Alzheimer's disease: a clinical, neuroimaging and neuropathological study. Neuropathology 37(2):150–173

23. Crutch SJ, Schott JM, Rabinovici GD, Murray M, Snowden JS, van der Flier WM et al (2017) Consensus classification of posterior cortical atrophy. Alzheimers Dement 13(8):870–884

24. Moller C, van der Flier WM, Versteeg A, Benedictus MR, Wattjes MP, Koedam EL et al (2014) Quantitative regional validation of the visual rating scale for posterior cortical atrophy. Eur Radiol 24(2):397–404

25. Blennerhassett R, Lillo P, Halliday GM, Hodges JR, Kril JJ (2014) Distribution of pathology in frontal variant Alzheimer's disease. JAD. 39(1):63–70

26. Rogalski E, Sridhar J, Rader B, Martersteck A, Chen K, Cobia D et al (2016) Aphasic variant of Alzheimer disease: clinical, anatomic, and genetic features. Neurology 87(13):1337–1343

27. Gao YL, Wang N, Sun FR, Cao XP, Zhang W, Yu JT (2018) Tau in neurodegenerative disease. Annals of translational medicine 6(10):175

28. Grijalvo-Perez AM, Litvan I (2014) Corticobasal degeneration. Semin Neurol 34(2):160–173

29. Dani M, Brooks DJ, Edison P (2016) Tau imaging in neurodegenerative diseases. Eur J Nucl Med Mol Imaging 43(6):1139–1150

30. Yoshida M (2014) Astrocytic inclusions in progressive supranuclear palsy and corticobasal degeneration. Neuropathology 34(6):555–570

31. Agarwal S, Gilbert R (2018) Progressive Supranuclear palsy. StatPearls Publishing LLC, Treasure Island, FL

32. Oba H, Yagishita A, Terada H, Barkovich AJ, Kutomi K, Yamauchi T et al (2005) New and reliable MRI diagnosis for progressive supranuclear palsy. Neurology 64(12):2050–2055

33. Quattrone A, Morelli M, Nigro S, Quattrone A, Vescio B, Arabia G et al (2018) A new MR imaging index for differentiation of progressive supranuclear palsy-parkinsonism from Parkinson's disease. Parkinsonism Relat Disord 54:3–8

34. Whitwell JL, Hoglinger GU, Antonini A, Bordelon Y, Boxer AL, Colosimo C et al (2017) Radiological biomarkers for diagnosis in PSP: where are we and where do we need to be? Mov Disord 32(7):955–971

35. Yang J, Shao N, Li J, Shang H (2014) Voxelwise meta-analysis of white matter abnormalities in progressive supranuclear palsy. Neurol Sci 35(1):7–14

36. McKeith IG, Boeve BF, Dickson DW, Halliday G, Taylor JP, Weintraub D et al (2017) Diagnosis and management of dementia with Lewy bodies: fourth consensus report of the DLB consortium. Neurology 89(1):88–100

37. McKeith IG, Dickson DW, Lowe J, Emre M, O'Brien JT, Feldman H et al (2005) Diagnosis and manage-ment of dementia with Lewy bodies: third report of the DLB consortium. Neurology 65(12):1863–1872

38. Emre M, Aarsland D, Brown R, Burn DJ, Duyckaerts C, Mizuno Y et al (2007) Clinical diagnostic criteria for dementia associated with Parkinson's disease. Mov Disord 22(12):1689–1707; quiz 837

39. Jellinger KA (2009) Formation and development of Lewy pathology: a critical update. J Neurol 256(Suppl 3):270–279

40. Marui W, Iseki E, Nakai T, Miura S, Kato M, Ueda K et al (2002) Progression and staging of Lewy pathology in brains from patients with dementia with Lewy bodies. J Neurol Sci 195(2):153–159

41. McKeith IG, Galasko D, Kosaka K, Perry EK, Dickson DW, Hansen LA et al (1996) Consensus guidelines for the clinical and pathologic diagnosis of dementia with Lewy bodies (DLB): report of the consortium on DLB international workshop. Neurology 47(5):1113–1124

42. Whitwell JL, Weigand SD, Shiung MM, Boeve BF, Ferman TJ, Smith GE et al (2007) Focal atrophy in dementia with Lewy bodies on MRI: a distinct pattern from Alzheimer's disease. Brain : a journal of neurology 130(Pt 3):708–719

43. Sanchez-Castaneda C, Rene R, Ramirez-Ruiz B, Campdelacreu J, Gascon J, Falcon C et al (2009) Correlations between gray matter reductions and cognitive deficits in dementia with Lewy bodies and Parkinson's disease with dementia. Mov Disord 24(12):1740–1746

44. Taylor JP, O'Brien J (2012) Neuroimaging of dementia with Lewy bodies. Neuroimaging Clin N Am 22(1):67–81. viii

45. McKeith I, O'Brien J, Walker Z, Tatsch K, Booij J, Darcourt J et al (2007) Sensitivity and specificity of dopamine transporter imaging with 123I-FP-CIT SPECT in dementia with Lewy bodies: a phase III, multicentre study. The Lancet Neurology. 6(4):305–313

46. O'Donovan J, Watson R, Colloby SJ, Blamire AM, O'Brien JT (2014) Assessment of regional MR diffusion changes in dementia with Lewy bodies and Alzheimer's disease. Int Psychogeriatr 26(4):627–635

47. Watson R, Blamire AM, Colloby SJ, Wood JS, Barber R, He J et al (2012) Characterizing dementia with Lewy bodies by means of diffusion tensor imaging. Neurology 79(9):906–914

48. Nedelska Z, Schwarz CG, Boeve BF, Lowe VJ, Reid RI, Przybelski SA et al (2015) White matter integrity in dementia with Lewy bodies: a voxel-based analysis of diffusion tensor imaging. Neurobiol Aging 36(6):2010–2017

49. Postuma RB, Berg D, Stern M, Poewe W, Olanow CW, Oertel W et al (2015) MDS clinical diagnostic criteria for Parkinson's disease. Mov Disord 30(12):1591–1601

50. Braak H, Del Tredici K, Rub U, de Vos RA, Jansen Steur EN, Braak E (2003) Staging of brain pathology

related to sporadic Parkinson's disease. Neurobiol Aging 24(2):197–211

51. Strafella AP, Bohnen NI, Perlmutter JS, Eidelberg D, Pavese N, Van Eimeren T et al (2017) Molecular imaging to track Parkinson's disease and atypical parkinsonisms: new imaging frontiers. Mov Disord 32(2):181–192

52. Brooks DJ, Tambasco N (2016) Imaging synucleinopathies. Mov Disord 31(6):814–829

53. Lehericy S, Vaillancourt DE, Seppi K, Monchi O, Rektorova I, Antonini A et al (2017) The role of high-field magnetic resonance imaging in parkinsonian disorders: pushing the boundaries forward. Mov Disord 32(4):510–525

54. Martin-Bastida A, Pietracupa S, Piccini P (2017) Neuromelanin in parkinsonian disorders: an update. Int J Neurosci 127(12):1116–1123

55. Atkinson-Clement C, Pinto S, Eusebio A, Coulon O (2017) Diffusion tensor imaging in Parkinson's disease: review and meta-analysis. NeuroImage Clinical. 16:98–110

56. Fanciulli A, Wenning GK (2015) Multiple-system atrophy. N Engl J Med 372(3):249–263

57. Wang Y, Butros SR, Shuai X, Dai Y, Chen C, Liu M et al (2012) Different iron-deposition patterns of multiple system atrophy with predominant parkinsonism and idiopathic Parkinson diseases demonstrated by phase-corrected susceptibility-weighted imaging. AJNR Am J Neuroradiol 33(2):266–273

58. Reiter E, Mueller C, Pinter B, Krismer F, Scherfler C, Esterhammer R et al (2015) Dorsolateral nigral hyperintensity on 3.0T susceptibility-weighted imaging in neurodegenerative parkinsonism. Mov Disord 30(8):1068–1076

59. Bajaj S, Krismer F, Palma JA, Wenning GK, Kaufmann H, Poewe W et al (2017) Diffusion-weighted MRI distinguishes Parkinson disease from the parkinsonian variant of multiple system atrophy: a systematic review and meta-analysis. PLoS One 12(12):e0189897

60. Blain CR, Barker GJ, Jarosz JM, Coyle NA, Landau S, Brown RG et al (2006) Measuring brain stem and cerebellar damage in parkinsonian syndromes using diffusion tensor MRI. Neurology 67(12):2199–2205

61. Neary D, Snowden JS, Gustafson L, Passant U, Stuss D, Black S et al (1998) Frontotemporal lobar degeneration: a consensus on clinical diagnostic criteria. Neurology 51(6):1546–1554

62. Lomen-Hoerth C, Anderson T, Miller B (2002) The overlap of amyotrophic lateral sclerosis and frontotemporal dementia. Neurology 59(7):1077–1079

63. Cairns NJ, Bigio EH, Mackenzie IR, Neumann M, Lee VM, Hatanpaa KJ et al (2007) Neuropathologic diagnostic and nosologic criteria for frontotemporal lobar degeneration: consensus of the consortium for Frontotemporal lobar degeneration. Acta Neuropathol 114(1):5–22

64. Lu PH, Mendez MF, Lee GJ, Leow AD, Lee HW, Shapira J et al (2013) Patterns of brain atrophy in

clinical variants of frontotemporal lobar degeneration. Dement Geriatr Cogn Disord 35(1–2):34–50

65. Pan PL, Song W, Yang J, Huang R, Chen K, Gong QY et al (2012) Gray matter atrophy in behavioral variant frontotemporal dementia: a meta-analysis of voxel-based morphometry studies. Dement Geriatr Cogn Disord 33(2–3):141–148

66. Munoz-Ruiz MA, Hartikainen P, Koikkalainen J, Wolz R, Julkunen V, Niskanen E et al (2012) Structural MRI in frontotemporal dementia: comparisons between hippocampal volumetry, tensor-based morphometry and voxel-based morphometry. PLoS One 7(12):e52531

67. Chan D, Fox NC, Scahill RI, Crum WR, Whitwell JL, Leschziner G et al (2001) Patterns of temporal lobe atrophy in semantic dementia and Alzheimer's disease. Ann Neurol 49(4):433–442

68. Rohrer JD, Warren JD, Modat M, Ridgway GR, Douiri A, Rossor MN et al (2009) Patterns of cortical thinning in the language variants of frontotemporal lobar degeneration. Neurology 72(18):1562–1569

69. Whitwell JL, Avula R, Senjem ML, Kantarci K, Weigand SD, Samikoglu A et al (2010) Gray and white matter water diffusion in the syndromic variants of frontotemporal dementia. Neurology 74(16):1279–1287

70. Agosta F, Scola E, Canu E, Marcone A, Magnani G, Sarro L et al (2012) White matter damage in frontotemporal lobar degeneration spectrum. Cerebral cortex (New York, NY : 1991) 22(12):2705–2714

71. O'Brien JT, Thomas A (2015) Vascular dementia. Lancet (London, England) 386(10004):1698–1706

72. Roman GC, Erkinjuntti T, Wallin A, Pantoni L, Chui HC (2002) Subcortical ischaemic vascular dementia. The Lancet Neurology 1(7):426–436

73. Streifler JY, Eliasziw M, Benavente OR, Alamowitch S, Fox AJ, Hachinski V et al (2003) Development and progression of leukoaraiosis in patients with brain ischemia and carotid artery disease. Stroke 34(8):1913–1916

74. De Reuck J, Maurage CA, Deramecourt V, Pasquier F, Cordonnier C, Leys D et al (2018) Aging and cerebrovascular lesions in pure and in mixed neurodegenerative and vascular dementia brains: a neuropathological study. Folia Neuropathol 56(2): 81–87

75. Herve D, Chabriat H (2010) CADASIL. J Geriatr Psychiatry Neurol 23(4):269–276

76. Bagni C, Tassone F, Neri G, Hagerman R (2012) Fragile X syndrome: causes, diagnosis, mechanisms, and therapeutics. J Clin Invest 122(12):4314–4322

77. Mila M, Alvarez-Mora MI, Madrigal I, Rodriguez-Revenga L (2018) Fragile X syndrome: an overview and update of the FMR1 gene. Clin Genet 93(2):197–205

78. Brunberg JA, Jacquemont S, Hagerman RJ, Berry-Kravis EM, Grigsby J, Leehey MA et al (2002) Fragile X premutation carriers: characteristic MR imaging findings of adult male patients with pro-

gressive cerebellar and cognitive dysfunction. AJNR Am J Neuroradiol 23(10):1757–1766

79. Renaud M, Perriard J, Coudray S, Sevin-Allouet M, Marcel C, Meissner WG et al (2015) Relevance of corpus callosum splenium versus middle cerebellar peduncle hyperintensity for FXTAS diagnosis in clinical practice. J Neurol 262(2):435–442

80. Tsuji Y, Kanamori H, Murakami G, Yokode M, Mezaki T, Doh-ura K et al (2004) Heidenhain variant of Creutzfeldt-Jakob disease: diffusion-weighted MRI and PET characteristics. J Neuroimaging 14(1):63–66

81. Johnson RT, Gibbs CJ Jr (1998) Creutzfeldt-Jakob disease and related transmissible spongiform encephalopathies. N Engl J Med 339(27):1994–2004

82. Brown P, Preece M, Brandel JP, Sato T, McShane L, Zerr I et al (2000) Iatrogenic Creutzfeldt-Jakob disease at the millennium. Neurology 55(8):1075–1081

83. Murata T, Shiga Y, Higano S, Takahashi S, Mugikura S (2002) Conspicuity and evolution of lesions in Creutzfeldt-Jakob disease at diffusion-weighted imaging. AJNR 23(7):1164–1172

84. Matsusue E, Kinoshita T, Sugihara S, Fujii S, Ogawa T, Ohama E (2004) White matter lesions in panencephalopathic type of Creutzfeldt-Jakob disease: MR imaging and pathologic correlations. AJNR 25(6):910–918

85. Shiga Y, Miyazawa K, Sato S, Fukushima R, Shibuya S, Sato Y et al (2004) Diffusion-weighted MRI abnormalities as an early diagnostic marker for Creutzfeldt-Jakob disease. Neurology 63(3):443–449

86. Young GS, Geschwind MD, Fischbein NJ, Martindale JL, Henry RG, Liu S et al (2005) Diffusion-weighted and fluid-attenuated inversion recovery imaging in Creutzfeldt-Jakob disease: high sensitivity and specificity for diagnosis. AJNR 26(6):1551–1562

87. Kallenberg K, Schulz-Schaeffer WJ, Jastrow U, Poser S, Meissner B, Tschampa HJ et al (2006) Creutzfeldt-Jakob disease: comparative analysis of MR imaging sequences. AJNR 27(7):1459–1462

88. Zerr I, Kallenberg K, Summers DM, Romero C, Taratuto A, Heinemann U et al (2009) Updated clinical diagnostic criteria for sporadic Creutzfeldt-Jakob disease. Brain J Neurol 132(Pt 10):2659–2668

89. Hermann P, Laux M, Glatzel M, Matschke J, Knipper T, Goebel S et al (2018) Validation and utilization of amended diagnostic criteria in Creutzfeldt-Jakob disease surveillance. Neurology 91(4):e331–e3e8

90. Zeidler M, Sellar RJ, Collie DA, Knight R, Stewart G, Macleod MA et al (2000) The pulvinar sign on magnetic resonance imaging in variant Creutzfeldt-Jakob disease. Lancet (London, England) 355(9213):1412–1418

91. Molloy S, O'Laoide R, Brett F, Farrell M (2000) The "Pulvinar" sign in variant Creutzfeldt-Jakob disease. AJR 175(2):555–556

92. Haik S, Brandel JP, Oppenheim C, Sazdovitch V, Dormont D, Hauw JJ et al (2002) Sporadic CJD clinically mimicking variant CJD with bilateral increased signal in the pulvinar. Neurology 58(1):148–149

93. Mittal S, Farmer P, Kalina P, Kingsley PB, Halperin J (2002) Correlation of diffusion-weighted magnetic resonance imaging with neuropathology in Creutzfeldt-Jakob disease. Arch Neurol 59(1):128–134

94. Hyare H, Thornton J, Stevens J, Mead S, Rudge P, Collinge J et al (2010) High-b-value diffusion MR imaging and basal nuclei apparent diffusion coefficient measurements in variant and sporadic Creutzfeldt-Jakob disease. AJNR 31(3):521–526

95. Lee H, Hoffman C, Kingsley PB, Degnan A, Cohen O, Prohovnik I (2010) Enhanced detection of diffusion reductions in Creutzfeldt-Jakob disease at a higher B factor. AJNR 31(1):49–54

96. Fujita K, Osaki Y, Miyamoto R, Shimatani Y, Abe T, Sumikura H et al (2017) Neurologic attack and dynamic perfusion abnormality in neuronal intranuclear inclusion disease. Neurology Clinical practice 7(6):e39–e42

97. Sone J, Mori K, Inagaki T, Katsumata R, Takagi S, Yokoi S et al (2016) Clinicopathological features of adult-onset neuronal intranuclear inclusion disease. Brain J Neurol 139(Pt 12):3170–3186

98. Yokoi S, Yasui K, Hasegawa Y, Niwa K, Noguchi Y, Tsuzuki T et al (2016) Pathological background of subcortical hyperintensities on diffusion-weighted images in a case of neuronal intranuclear inclusion disease. Clin Neuropathol 35(6):375–380

99. Sugiyama A, Sato N, Kimura Y, Maekawa T, Enokizono M, Saito Y et al (2017) MR imaging features of the cerebellum in adult-onset neuronal Intranuclear inclusion disease: 8 cases. AJNR 38(11):2100–2104

100. Kleinfeld K, Mobley B, Hedera P, Wegner A, Sriram S, Pawate S (2013) Adult-onset leukoencephalopathy with neuroaxonal spheroids and pigmented glia: report of five cases and a new mutation. J Neurol 260(2):558–571

101. Sundal C, Van Gerpen JA, Nicholson AM, Wider C, Shuster EA, Aasly J et al (2012) MRI characteristics and scoring in HDLS due to CSF1R gene mutations. Neurology 79(6):566–574

102. Konno T, Kasanuki K, Ikeuchi T, Dickson DW, Wszolek ZK (2018) CSF1R-related leukoencephalopathy: a major player in primary microgliopathies. Neurology 91(24):1092–1104

103. Abe T, Kawarai T, Fujita K, Sako W, Terasawa Y, Matsuda T et al (2017) MR spectroscopy in patients with hereditary diffuse Leukoencephalopathy with spheroids and asymptomatic carriers of Colony-stimulating factor 1 receptor mutation. Magn Reson Med Sci 16(4):297–303

104. Inui T, Kawarai T, Fujita K, Kawamura K, Mitsui T, Orlacchio A et al (2013) A new CSF1R mutation presenting with an extensive white matter lesion

mimicking primary progressive multiple sclerosis. J Neurol Sci 334(1–2):192–195

105. Bender B, Klose U, Lindig T, Biskup S, Nagele T, Schols L et al (2014) Imaging features in conventional MRI, spectroscopy and diffusion weighted images of hereditary diffuse leukoencephalopathy with axonal spheroids (HDLS). J Neurol 261(12):2351–2359

106. van der Knaap MS, Naidu S, Kleinschmidt-Demasters BK, Kamphorst W, Weinstein HC (2000) Autosomal dominant diffuse leukoencephalopathy with neuroaxonal spheroids. Neurology 54(2):463–468

107. Terasawa Y, Osaki Y, Kawarai T, Sugimoto T, Orlacchio A, Abe T et al (2013) Increasing and persistent DWI changes in a patient with hereditary diffuse leukoencephalopathy with spheroids. J Neurol Sci 335(1–2):213–215

108. Burrell JR, Halliday GM, Kril JJ, Ittner LM, Gotz J, Kiernan MC et al (2016) The frontotemporal dementia-motor neuron disease continuum. Lancet (London, England) 388(10047):919–931

109. Ellis CM, Simmons A, Jones DK, Bland J, Dawson JM, Horsfield MA et al (1999) Diffusion tensor MRI assesses corticospinal tract damage in ALS. Neurology 53(5):1051–1058

110. Aoki S, Iwata NK, Masutani Y, Yoshida M, Abe O, Ugawa Y et al (2005) Quantitative evaluation of the pyramidal tract segmented by diffusion tensor tractography: feasibility study in patients with amyotrophic lateral sclerosis. Radiat Med 23(3):195–199

111. Iwata NK, Aoki S, Okabe S, Arai N, Terao Y, Kwak S et al (2008) Evaluation of corticospinal tracts in ALS with diffusion tensor MRI and brainstem stimulation. Neurology 70(7):528–532

112. Abe O, Yamada H, Masutani Y, Aoki S, Kunimatsu A, Yamasue H et al (2004) Amyotrophic lateral sclerosis: diffusion tensor tractography and voxel-based analysis. NMR Biomed 17(6):411–416

113. Floeter MK, Danielian LE, Braun LE, Wu T (2018) Longitudinal diffusion imaging across the C9orf72 clinical spectrum. J Neurol Neurosurg Psychiatry 89(1):53–60

114. Trojsi F, Caiazzo G, Di Nardo F, Fratello M, Santangelo G, Siciliano M et al (2017) High angular resolution diffusion imaging abnormalities in the early stages of amyotrophic lateral sclerosis. J Neurol Sci 380:215–222

115. Muller HP, Turner MR, Grosskreutz J, Abrahams S, Bede P, Govind V et al (2016) A large-scale multicentre cerebral diffusion tensor imaging study in amyotrophic lateral sclerosis. J Neurol Neurosurg Psychiatry 87(6):570–579

116. Fukui Y, Hishikawa N, Sato K, Nakano Y, Morihara R, Shang J et al (2018) Detecting spinal pyramidal tract of amyotrophic lateral sclerosis patients with diffusion tensor tractography. Neurosci Res 133:58–63

117. Matsui JT, Vaidya JG, Johnson HJ, Magnotta VA, Long JD, Mills JA et al (2014) Diffusion

weighted imaging of prefrontal cortex in prodromal Huntington's disease. Hum Brain Mapp 35(4):1562–1573

118. Shaffer JJ, Ghayoor A, Long JD, Kim RE, Lourens S, O'Donnell LJ et al (2017) Longitudinal diffusion changes in prodromal and early HD: evidence of white-matter tract deterioration. Hum Brain Mapp 38(3):1460–1477

119. Vandenberghe W, Demaerel P, Dom R, Maes F (2009) Diffusion-weighted versus volumetric imaging of the striatum in early symptomatic Huntington disease. J Neurol 256(1):109–114

120. Yamada K, Patel U, Shrier DA, Tanaka H, Chang JK, Numaguchi Y (1998) MR imaging of CNS tractopathy: wallerian and transneuronal degeneration. AJR 171(3):813–818

121. Gupta RK, Saksena S, Hasan KM, Agarwal A, Haris M, Pandey CM et al (2006) Focal Wallerian degeneration of the corpus callosum in large middle cerebral artery stroke: serial diffusion tensor imaging. JMRI 24(3):549–555

122. Mazumdar A, Mukherjee P, Miller JH, Malde H, McKinstry RC (2003) Diffusion-weighted imaging of acute corticospinal tract injury preceding Wallerian degeneration in the maturing human brain. AJNR 24(6):1057–1066

123. Castillo M, Mukherji SK (1999) Early abnormalities related to postinfarction Wallerian degeneration: evaluation with MR diffusion-weighted imaging. J Comput Assist Tomogr 23(6):1004–1007

124. Kang DW, Chu K, Yoon BW, Song IC, Chang KH, Roh JK (2000) Diffusion-weighted imaging in Wallerian degeneration. J Neurol Sci 178(2):167–169

125. Pierpaoli C, Barnett A, Pajevic S, Chen R, Penix LR, Virta A et al (2001) Water diffusion changes in Wallerian degeneration and their dependence on white matter architecture. NeuroImage 13(6 Pt 1):1174–1185

126. Thomalla G, Glauche V, Weiller C, Rother J (2005) Time course of wallerian degeneration after ischaemic stroke revealed by diffusion tensor imaging. J Neurol Neurosurg Psychiatry 76(2):266–268

127. Thomalla G, Glauche V, Koch MA, Beaulieu C, Weiller C, Rother J (2004) Diffusion tensor imaging detects early Wallerian degeneration of the pyramidal tract after ischemic stroke. NeuroImage 22(4):1767–1774

128. Werring DJ, Toosy AT, Clark CA, Parker GJ, Barker GJ, Miller DH et al (2000) Diffusion tensor imaging can detect and quantify corticospinal tract degeneration after stroke. J Neurol Neurosurg Psychiatry 69(2):269–272

129. Ogawa T, Okudera T, Inugami A, Noguchi K, Kado H, Yoshida Y et al (1997) Degeneration of the ipsilateral substantia nigra after striatal infarction: evaluation with MR imaging. Radiology 204(3):847–851

130. Abe O, Nakane M, Aoki S, Hayashi N, Masumoto T, Kunimatsu A et al (2003) MR imaging of post-ischemic neuronal death in the substantia nigra and

thalamus following middle cerebral artery occlusion in rats. NMR Biomed 16(3):152–159

131. Kinoshita T, Moritani T, Shrier DA, Wang HZ, Hiwatashi A, Numaguchi Y et al (2002) Secondary degeneration of the substantia nigra and corticospinal tract after hemorrhagic middle cerebral artery infarction: diffusion-weighted MR findings. Magn Reson Med Sci 1(3):175–178

132. Nakane M, Tamura A, Miyasaka N, Nagaoka T, Kuroiwa T (2001) Astrocytic swelling in the ipsilateral substantia nigra after occlusion of the middle cerebral artery in rats. AJNR Am J Neuroradiol 22(4):660–663

133. Moon WJ, Na DG, Kim SS, Ryoo JW, Chung EC (2005) Diffusion abnormality of deep gray matter in external capsular hemorrhage. AJNR 26(2):229–235

134. Tilikete C, Desestret V (2017) Hypertrophic Olivary degeneration and palatal or Oculopalatal tremor. Front Neurol 8:302

135. Gu CN, Carr CM, Kaufmann TJ, Kotsenas AL, Hunt CH, Wood CP (2015) MRI findings in Nonlesional hypertrophic Olivary degeneration. J Neuroimaging 25(5):813–817

136. Nakane M, Tamura A, Sasaki Y, Teraoka A (2002) MRI of secondary changes in the thalamus following a cerebral infarct. Neuroradiology 44(11):915–920

137. Ogawa T, Yoshida Y, Okudera T, Noguchi K, Kado H, Uemura K (1997) Secondary thalamic degeneration after cerebral infarction in the middle cerebral artery distribution: evaluation with MR imaging. Radiology 204(1):255–262

138. Tisher A, Salardini A (2019) A comprehensive update on treatment of dementia. Semin Neurol 39(2):167–178

139. Minino AM, Murphy SL, Xu J, Kochanek KD (2011) Deaths: final data for 2008. Natl Vital Stat Rep 59(10):1–126

140. (2013) 2013 Alzheimer's disease facts and figures. Alzheimers Dement 9(2):208–245

141. Buckley JS, Salpeter SR (2015) A risk-benefit assessment of dementia medications: systematic review of the evidence. Drugs Aging 32(6):453–467

142. O'Brien JT, Burns A (2011) Clinical practice with anti-dementia drugs: a revised (second) consensus statement from the British Association for Psychopharmacology. Journal of psychopharmacology (Oxford, England) 25(8):997–1019

143. Johnson JW, Kotermanski SE (2006) Mechanism of action of memantine. Curr Opin Pharmacol 6(1):61–67

144. Patel L, Grossberg GT (2011) Combination therapy for Alzheimer's disease. Drugs Aging 28(7):539–546

145. Feart C, Samieri C, Rondeau V, Amieva H, Portet F, Dartigues JF et al (2009) Adherence to a Mediterranean diet, cognitive decline, and risk of dementia. JAMA 302(6):638–648

146. Morris MC, Tangney CC, Wang Y, Sacks FM, Bennett DA, Aggarwal NT (2015) MIND diet asso-

ciated with reduced incidence of Alzheimer's disease. Alzheimers Dement 11(9):1007–1014

147. Morris MC, Tangney CC, Wang Y, Sacks FM, Barnes LL, Bennett DA et al (2015) MIND diet slows cognitive decline with aging. Alzheimers Dement 11(9):1015–1022

148. Stephen R, Hongisto K, Solomon A, Lonnroos E (2017) Physical activity and Alzheimer's disease: a systematic review. J Gerontol A Biol Sci Med Sci 72(6):733–739

149. Farina N, Llewellyn D, Isaac M, Tabet N (2017) Vitamin E for Alzheimer's dementia and mild cognitive impairment. Cochrane Database Syst Rev 4:Cd002854

150. Dysken MW, Sano M, Asthana S, Vertrees JE, Pallaki M, Llorente M et al (2014) Effect of vitamin E and memantine on functional decline in Alzheimer disease: the TEAM-AD VA cooperative randomized trial. JAMA 311(1):33–44

151. Dysken MW, Guarino PD, Vertrees JE, Asthana S, Sano M, Llorente M et al (2014) Vitamin E and memantine in Alzheimer's disease: clinical trial methods and baseline data. Alzheimers Dement 10(1):36–44

152. Gorelick PB, Scuteri A, Black SE, Decarli C, Greenberg SM, Iadecola C et al (2011) Vascular contributions to cognitive impairment and dementia: a statement for healthcare professionals from the american heart association/american stroke association. Stroke 42(9):2672–2713

153. Gorelick PB (2015) World stroke day proclamation 2015: call to preserve cognitive vitality. Stroke 46(11):3037–3038

154. Hachinski V (2015) Stroke and potentially preventable dementias proclamation: updated world stroke day proclamation. Stroke 46(11):3039–3040

155. Grantham C, Geerts H (2002) The rationale behind cholinergic drug treatment for dementia related to cerebrovascular disease. J Neurol Sci 203–204:131–136

156. Gottfries CG, Blennow K, Karlsson I, Wallin A (1994) The neurochemistry of vascular dementia. Dementia (Basel, Switzerland) 5(3–4):163–167

157. Smith JV, Luo Y (2004) Studies on molecular mechanisms of Ginkgo biloba extract. Appl Microbiol Biotechnol 64(4):465–472

158. Chan PC, Xia Q, Fu PP (2007) Ginkgo biloba leave extract: biological, medicinal, and toxicological effects. J Environ Sci Health C Environ Carcinog Ecotoxicol Rev 25(3):211–244

159. Saleem S, Zhuang H, Biswal S, Christen Y, Dore S (2008) Ginkgo biloba extract neuroprotective action is dependent on heme oxygenase 1 in ischemic reperfusion brain injury. Stroke 39(12):3389–3396

160. Koh PO (2010) Gingko biloba extract (EGb 761) prevents cerebral ischemia-induced p70S6 kinase and S6 phosphorylation. Am J Chin Med 38(4):727–734

161. Scholey AB, Kennedy DO (2002) Acute, dose-dependent cognitive effects of Ginkgo biloba, Panax

ginseng and their combination in healthy young volunteers: differential interactions with cognitive demand. Hum Psychopharmacol 17(1):35–44

162. DeKosky ST, Williamson JD, Fitzpatrick AL, Kronmal RA, Ives DG, Saxton JA et al (2008) Ginkgo biloba for prevention of dementia: a randomized controlled trial. JAMA 300(19):2253–2262

163. Yuan Q, Wang CW, Shi J, Lin ZX (2017) Effects of Ginkgo biloba on dementia: an overview of systematic reviews. J Ethnopharmacol 195:1–9

164. Kosaka K, Yoshimura M, Ikeda K, Budka H (1984) Diffuse type of Lewy body disease: progressive dementia with abundant cortical Lewy bodies and senile changes of varying degree--a new disease? Clin Neuropathol 3(5):185–192

165. Stinton C, McKeith I, Taylor JP, Lafortune L, Mioshi E, Mak E et al (2015) Pharmacological Management of Lewy Body Dementia: a systematic review and meta-analysis. Am J Psychiatry 172(8):731–742

166. Ballard C, Aarsland D, Francis P, Corbett A (2013) Neuropsychiatric symptoms in patients with dementias associated with cortical Lewy bodies: pathophysiology, clinical features, and pharmacological management. Drugs Aging 30(8):603–611

167. Ukai K, Fujishiro H, Iritani S, Ozaki N (2015) Long-term efficacy of donepezil for relapse of visual hallucinations in patients with dementia with Lewy bodies. Psychogeriatrics 15(2):133–137

168. McKeith I, Fairbairn A, Perry R, Thompson P, Perry E (1992) Neuroleptic sensitivity in patients with senile dementia of Lewy body type. BMJ (Clinical research ed) 305(6855):673–678

169. Aurora RN, Zak RS, Maganti RK, Auerbach SH, Casey KR, Chowdhuri S et al (2010) Best practice guide for the treatment of REM sleep behavior disorder (RBD). JCSM 6(1):85–95

170. (2017) Global, regional, and national incidence, prevalence, and years lived with disability for 328 diseases and injuries for 195 countries, 1990–2016: a systematic analysis for the global burden of disease study 2016. Lancet (London, England) 390(10100):1211–1259

171. Rizek P, Kumar N, Jog MS (2016) An update on the diagnosis and treatment of Parkinson disease. CMAJ 188(16):1157–1165

172. Rahimi F, Samotus O, Lee J, Jog M (2015) Effective Management of Upper Limb Parkinsonian Tremor by IncobotulinumtoxinA injections using sensor-based biomechanical patterns. Tremor and Other Hyperkinetic Movements (New York, NY) 5:348

173. Nicholson G, Pereira AC, Hall GM (2002) Parkinson's disease and anaesthesia. Br J Anaesth 89(6):904–916

174. Okun MS (2012) Deep-brain stimulation for Parkinson's disease. N Engl J Med 367(16):1529–1538

175. Pickut BA, van der Linden C, Dethy S, Van De Maele H, de Beyl DZ (2014) Intestinal levodopa infusion: the Belgian experience. Neurol Sci 35(6):861–866

176. Othman AA, Dutta S (2014) Population pharmacokinetics of levodopa in subjects with advanced Parkinson's disease: levodopa-carbidopa intestinal gel infusion vs. oral tablets. Br J Clin Pharmacol 78(1):94–105

Toxic and Metabolic Diseases

15

Aristides A. Capizzano, and Toshio Moritani
Yang Mao-Draayer, Brian Chang, and Deema Fattal

15.1 Toxic Disease

15.1.1 Chemotherapy-Induced Leukoencephalopathy

Intrathecal or intravenous methotrexate, with or without radiation therapy, can cause diffuse white matter changes [1]. There are two types of methotrexate-related leukoencephalopathy: (1) disseminated necrotizing leukoencephalopathy (DNL) and (2) mild leukoencephalopathy [2]. DNL indicates a rapidly deteriorating clinical course, with irreversible extensive white matter damage. Mild leukoencephalopathy is usually transient. MR imaging findings are different in these two types. In DNL, MR imaging shows

multifocal T2 and FLAIR hyperintensities in the white matter with small irregular low-signal foci and contrast enhancement. DW imaging shows slightly increased ADC in the center of the lesion and increased ADC in the perilesional vasogenic edema [3] (Fig. 15.1). In mild leukoencephalopathy MR imaging shows diffuse T2 hyperintensity in the white matter. DW imaging shows the diffuse white matter as hyperintense with decreased apparent diffusion coefficient (ADC), even before conventional MR imaging can detect the lesions (Fig. 15.2). Pathologically the white matter lesion represents intramyelinic edema.

High-dose chemotherapy including carmustine (BCNU), cyclophosphamide, cisplatin, 5-fluorouracil (5-FU), and carmofur (a derivative of 5-FU) can also cause diffuse white matter disease. The lesions are hyperintense on T2-weighted images as well as on DW images, and ADC is decreased [4–6] (Fig. 15.3). Chemotherapeutic agents such as 5-FU and carmofur can have direct toxic effects on myelin, which causes intramyelinic edema [7]. Chemotherapy-associated leukoencephalopathy can be fatal and early diagnosis and discontinuation of the offending drug is therefore necessary. Leukoencephalopathy was found in 30% of long-term ALL survivors treated with methotrexate and persisted in 80% [8]. Furthermore, mean diffusivity in the genu of the corpus callosum, corona radiata, and the superior fronto-occipital fasciculi was associated with global neurocognitive impairment [8, 9].

A. A. Capizzano (✉) · T. Moritani
Division of Neuroradiology, University of Michigan, Ann Arbor, MI, USA
e-mail: capizzan@med.umich.edu;
tmoritan@med.umich.edu

Y. Mao-Draayer
University of Michigan, Ann Arbor, MI, USA
e-mail: maodraay@umich.edu

B. Chang
University of Michigan Medical School, Ann Arbor, MI, USA
e-mail: bkchang@med.umich.edu

D. Fattal
University of Iowa Hospitals & Clinics, Iowa City, IA, USA
e-mail: deema-fattal@uiowa.edu

© Springer Nature Switzerland AG 2021
T. Moritani, A. A. Capizzano (eds.), *Diffusion-Weighted MR Imaging of the Brain, Head and Neck, and Spine*, https://doi.org/10.1007/978-3-030-62120-9_15

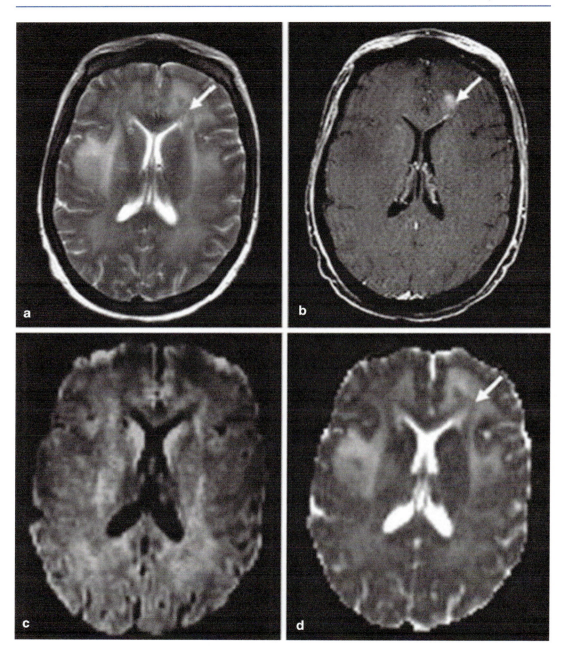

Fig. 15.1 Disseminated necrotizing leukoencephalopathy in a 43-year-old woman with leptomeningeal metastasis from breast carcinoma treated with methotrexate and radiation. (**a**) T2-weighted image shows multifocal hyperintensities in the deep white matter with small irregular low-signal foci in the left frontal area (*arrow*). (**b**) Postcontrast T1-weighted image reveals enhancement in the foci (*arrow*) in the left frontal white matter consistent with necrosis. (**c, d**) DWI image shows mild hyperintensity in the white matter lesions associated with diffuse increased ADC and mild increased ADCs in the left frontal foci, consistent with diffuse vasogenic edema and necrotic foci (*arrow*). (Courtesy of Policeni B, MD, University of Iowa Hospitals and Clinics, USA)

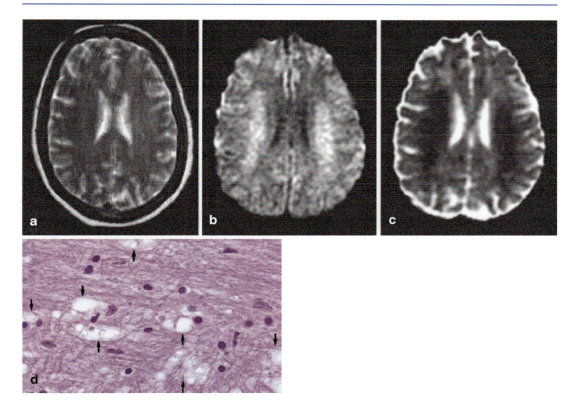

Fig. 15.2 Methotrexate leukoencephalopathy (high dose) in a 50-year-old woman. (**a**) T2-weighted image does not demonstrate an appreciable abnormality in the white matter. (**b**) DWI image shows symmetric hyperintensity in the bilateral corona radiata extending into the central semiovale. (**c**) ADC map shows white matter lesions as decreased ADC, which represents intramyelinic edema. (**d**) Pathology shows spongiform change representing intramyelinic edema (*arrows*) diffusely in white matter. Astrocytes are relatively spared (hematoxylin–eosin stain, original magnification ×200)

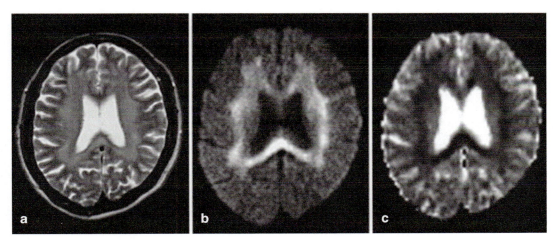

Fig. 15.3 Carmofur leukoencephalopathy in a 58-year-old woman. (**a**) T2-weighted image shows symmetric hyperintensity in the periventricular white matter including the corpus callosum. (**b**, **c**) DW image shows these lesions as hyperintense with decreased ADC, presumably related to intramyelinic edema

15.1.2 Carbon Monoxide Intoxication

The affinity of hemoglobin for carbon monoxide (CO) is approximately 250 times that of oxygen. The carboxyhemoglobin reduces the oxygen-carrying capacity of blood, causing tissue hypoxia. CO also inhibits the mitochondrial electron transport enzyme system and activates polymorphonuclear leukocytes, which causes brain lipid peroxydation and myelin breakdown. The globus pallidus is the most common site of involvement. The putamen, caudate nucleus, thalamus, hippocampus, and substantia nigra are also occasionally involved [10]. The globus pallidus and the pars reticulata of the substantia nigra contain the highest iron concentration in the brain. CO directly binds heme-iron in these areas, which is the cause of the histotoxicity and selective vulnerability of the pallidoreticularis [11]. DW imaging shows hyperintensity with decreased ADC in these lesions in the acute phase (Fig. 15.4). Cerebral white matter involvement is common and usually presents as delayed anoxic encephalopathy. It is usually seen in the late subacute phase after recovery from the acute stage of CO poisoning (with a lucid interval of usually 2–3 weeks). DW imaging shows diffuse hyperintensity with decreased ADC in the periventricular white matter and centrum semiovale [12, 13].

15.1.3 Cocaine, Phencyclidine Hydrochloride, Amphetamines, and Related Catecholaminergics

Cocaine, phencyclidine hydrochloride, amphetamines, and related catecholaminergics can cause hemorrhage or infarction due to vasculitis, vasculopathy, or acute hypertensive effects [1]. DW imaging can be useful for the detection of these lesions (see also Chap. 11).

15.1.4 Opiods (Morphine, Methadone, Oxycodone, Heroin)

Opioid overdose has been reported as a cause of delayed hypoxic leukoencephalopathy, cerebellar white matter edema (particularly with heroin and methadone) [14, 15] and symmetric pallidal and hippocampal-restricted DWI [14, 16–21]. Narcotic-induced leukoencephalopathy is not only secondary to hypoxia but to direct toxicity to the myelin-rich white matter by lipophilic drugs [22]. This toxic leukoencephalopathy may be reversible [23]. The inhalation of black-market heroin vapors (pyrolysate), practice known as "chasing the dragon," as well as intravenous consumption of heroin can lead to toxic leukoencephalopathy [24]. The leukoencephalopathy is pathologically characterized by spongiform degeneration of the white matter as a result of fluid accumulation within the myelin sheaths (intramyelinic edema). Electron microscopy shows vacuoles between the myelin lamellae by splitting of the intraperiod lines [25]. On brain MRI, it displays symmetric white matter T2 hyperintensities in the cerebrum, cerebellum, and brainstem [26] with facilitated diffusion [27] also involving the cerebral peduncles, corticospinal tracts, lemniscus medialis, and solitary tracts [28–30]. The accumulation of restricted fluid between the layers of myelin lamellae may cause hyperintensity on DW imaging with decreased ADC [31] (Figs. 15.5 and 15.6). Because the myelin itself and the blood–brain barrier are intact in cases of less severe heroin-induced leukoencephalopathy, the changes in the DW signal may be reversible on follow-up MR imaging [21].

15.1.5 Metronidazole Induced Encephalopathy

Metronidazole is an antimicrobial agent used in the treatment of protozoal and anaerobic bacterial infections and is often used in hepatic encephalopathy. Metronidazole toxicity can cause both peripheral neuropathy and central nervous system dysfunction with ataxic gait, dysarthria, seizures, and encephalopathy, which may result from both short-term and chronic use of this drug and is collectively referred to as "metronidazole induced encephalopathy." Neuroimaging is essential for the diagnosis of this uncommon entity. Typical anatomical sites of involvement include the cerebellum, midbrain, brainstem, and corpus callosum. Symmetric T2 hyperintensity of the dentate nuclei is the most suggestive feature (Fig. 15.7) [32, 33]. Diffusion restriction at the abovementioned sites has been mentioned, but ADC values

15 Toxic and Metabolic Diseases

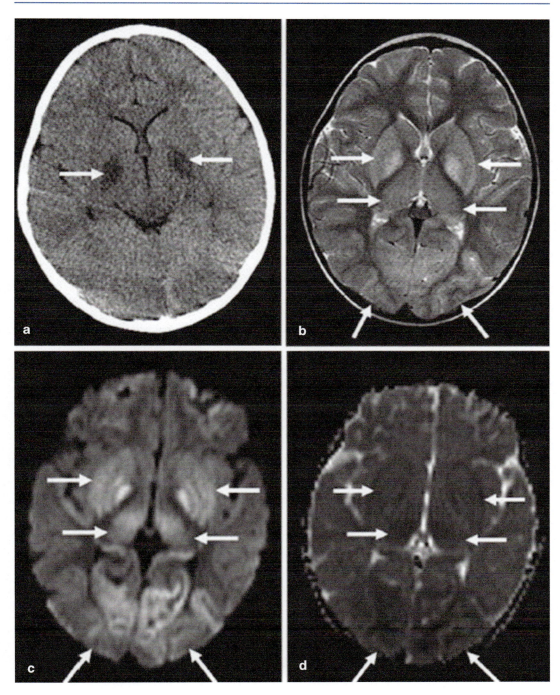

Fig. 15.4 Carbon monoxide poisoning in a 4-year-old boy. (**a**) CT shows symmetric low-density areas in the globi pallidi. (**b**) T2-weighted imaging shows symmetric extensive hyperintense lesions in the basal ganglia, thalami, hippocampi, and posterior cerebral cortices. (**c**, **d**) DW image shows these areas as hyperintense with decreased ADC

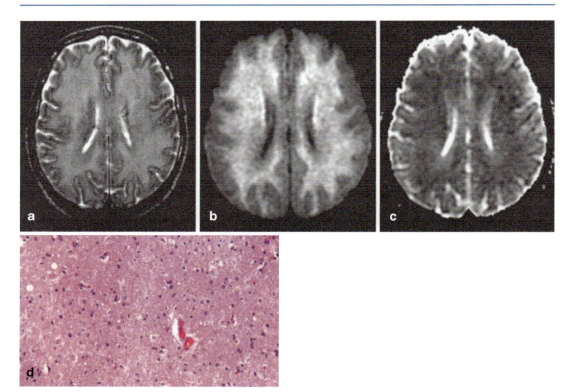

Fig. 15.5 Heroin-induced leukoencephalopathy in a 55-year-old man. (**a**) T2-weighted image shows diffuse hyperintensity in the white matter including U fibers. (**b**, **c**) DWI image shows these lesions as diffusely hyperintense with mildly decreased ADC. (**d**) Pathology shows intramyelinic edema and reactive astrogliosis, consistent with the subacute phase of heroin-induced leukoencephalopathy (hematoxylin–eosin stain, original magnification ×200)

have been variable. DWI showed increased ADC value consistent with vasogenic edema in lesions of the midbrain, pons, medulla, and cerebellar dentate nuclei, which involve mainly gray matter, but decreased ADC values indicating cytotoxic edema in lesions of the corpus callosum [34]. Improvement in clinical symptoms and imaging findings after discontinuation of metronidazole is noticed in the majority of cases; however, reversibility is not universal [33, 35].

15.1.6 Marchiafava–Bignami Disease

Marchiafava–Bignami disease is a rare complication of chronic alcoholism characterized by demyelination of the corpus callosum [36]. The genu of the corpus callosum is more frequently involved, but the degeneration can extend throughout the entire corpus callosum. Occasionally, optic chiasm and the visual tracts, putamen, anterior commissure, cerebellar peduncles, cortical gray matter, and U fibers may be involved. Clinical signs include seizures, impairment of consciousness, and signs of interhemispheric disconnection, but they are nonspecific.

The corpus callosum appears hypodense on CT and hyperintense on T2-weighted and FLAIR MR images, which is essential to confirm the diagnosis. These lesions can be partially reversible with treatment [37]. DW imaging shows lesions in the early phase as hyperintense with decreased ADC [38] representing cytotoxic edema, mainly in the myelin sheaths (intramyelinic edema). In the subacute phase, the lesions are hyperintense on DW imaging with increased ADC representing demyelination or necrosis (Fig. 15.8). DTI demonstrates reduced FA in the corpus callosum, and fiber-tracking demonstrates disruption of axonal

15 Toxic and Metabolic Diseases

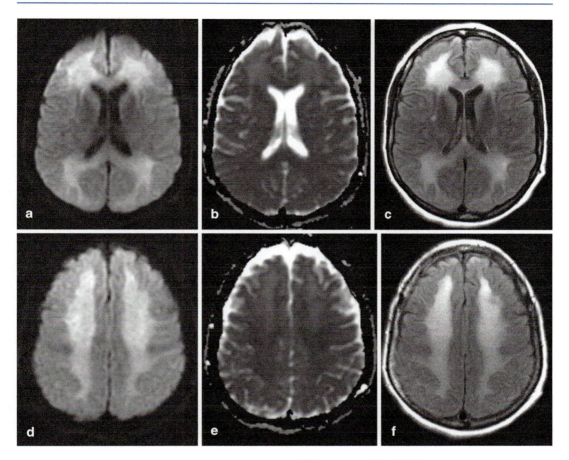

Fig. 15.6 49-year-old female with acute encephalopathy and positive urine screening for methadone. She had clinical recovery with no imaging follow-up (**a**, **d**: DWI, **b**, **e**: ADC map, **c**, **e**: FLAIR). Note simultaneous occurrence of facilitated diffusion anteriorly and restricted diffusion posteriorly in the ADC map

fiber bundles, most marked within the body of the corpus callosum [39]. The prognosis of Marchiafava–Bignami disease may be good even in cases with severe diffusion restriction of the entire corpus callosum if treatment with parenteral thiamine is initiated early, leading to imaging and clinical reversibility [40, 41].

15.2 Metabolic Diseases

15.2.1 Hypoxic–Ischemic Encephalopathy

Hypoxic-ischemic encephalopathy (HIE) is the result of decreased global perfusion or oxygenation. The distribution of HIE varies according to the duration, degree, and abruptness of the hypoxic and/or ischemic insults, basal blood flow, and metabolic activity in the areas of ischemia, temperature, and serum glucose levels [42, 43]. Hypoxia basically causes cardiac decompensation within minutes, resulting in global hypoperfusion and ischemic brain injury. However, pure anoxic encephalopathy may exist in some patients who are found early after the insult or who have suffered less severe anoxia [44]. In pure anoxia, cerebral blood flow is preserved allowing effective supply of nutrients and removal of toxic products such as lactic acid. Neurons tolerate pure anoxia for a longer duration than ischemia. Coma and other clinical findings can result from synaptic dysfunction.

DW imaging often depicts acute or subacute ischemic lesions when conventional MR imaging

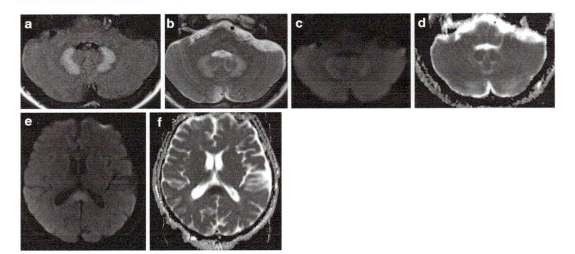

Fig. 15.7 69-year-old male with history of perforated appendix with phlegmon as well as pneumonia who has been on more than 2 months of metronidazole and moxifloxacin. He presented with 2–3 weeks of paresthesias in the bilateral feet, fall within the previous week with contusion to the head, dysarthria, and dysmetria for the past 3 days. FLAIR (**a**), T2-weighted (**b**), DWI (**c**), and ADC map (**d**) showing symmetric hyperintense lesions of the dentate nuclei. Additionally, there was a splenial lesion with restricted diffusion (**e–f**). (Courtesy Dr. Atsuhiko Handa, MD, University of Iowa Hospitals & Clinics)

and CT scans show only subtle abnormalities [45]. Layers 3 and 5 of the cerebral cortex, the CA1 field of the hippocampus, Purkinje neurons of the cerebellar cortex, and the watershed zones are most sensitive to ischemia [46]. Cortical laminar necrosis is observed as hyperintensity on T2-weighted, FLAIR images (variably seen as early as 1 day after injury) and on T1-weighted images from the subacute to chronic phase of HIE. DW imaging often depicts acute or subacute ischemic lesions when other MR sequences, and CT scans are still normal or show only subtle abnormalities [45]. DW hyperintensity throughout the cerebral cortex suggests devastating diffuse hypoxic-ischemic necrosis, whereas a pattern of basal ganglia or thalamic hyperintensity suggests primary hypoxic injury or mild HIE (Figs. 15.9 and 15.10). The prognosis of HIE depends on the extension of the cytotoxic edema, which is usually irreversible. DW imaging is helpful in establishing both the diagnosis and prognosis, and also in the management of HIE [47, 48]. High-b-value (3000 s/mm^2) DW imaging with long TE improves accuracy in the early detection of the HIE lesions [49].

15.2.2 Delayed Postanoxic Encephalopathy

Delayed postanoxic encephalopathy is a condition in which patients appear to make a complete clinical recovery after an episode of anoxia or hypoxia and then develop progressive neuropsychiatric symptoms and/or neurological deficits [50]. The incidence has been reported to range from 1 to 28 per 1000 suffering from hypoxic or anoxic events. It is most commonly associated with CO poisoning [51], but has also been reported after hypoxic events related to childbirth, surgery and anesthesia, drug overdose, exposure to toxins, anaphylaxis, seizures, cyanosis, and strangulation [52, 53]. The prognosis is variable from a full recovery to permanent neurologic sequelae, personality changes, and death. The pathogenesis is presumably related to programmed cell death/apoptosis of the oligodendrocytes triggered by hypoxia.

DW imaging shows diffuse hyperintensity with decreased ADC in the periventricular white matter and centrum semiovale, pathologically

15 Toxic and Metabolic Diseases

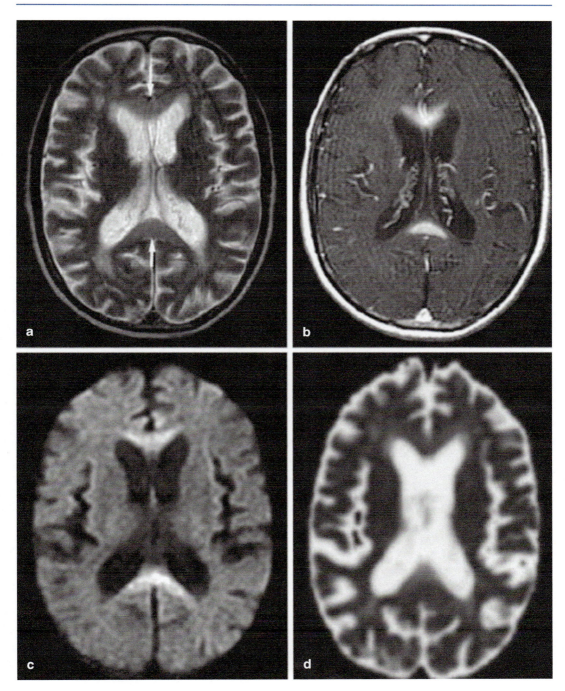

Fig. 15.8 Marchiafava–Bignami disease in a 58-year-old man. (**a**) T2-weighted image shows hyperintensity in the anterior and posterior corpus callosum (*arrows*) and in the periventricular white matter. (**b**) Gadolinium-enhanced T1-weighted image with magnetization transfer contrast reveals enhancing lesions in the anterior and posterior corpus callosum. (**c**, **d**) DW image shows hyperintense lesions with increased ADC in the corpus callosum, representing demyelination and necrosis in the subacute phase

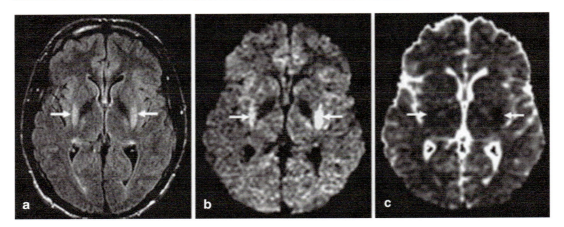

Fig. 15.9 Hypoxic-ischemic encephalopathy in an 18-year-old male patient after hanging himself. (**a**) FLAIR image shows hyperintensity in the posterior part of the putamina bilaterally. (**b, c**) DW image shows these lesions as hyperintense with the decreased ADC

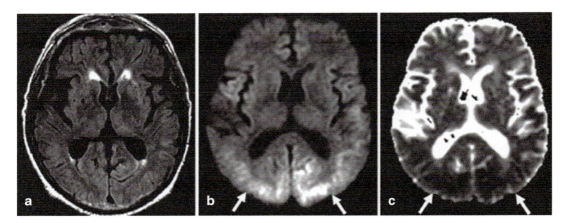

Fig. 15.10 Hypoxic-ischemic encephalopathy in an 83-year-old man with a cardiac arrest. (**a**) No obvious abnormality seen on FLAIR. (**b, c**) DW image shows extensive diffuse hyperintense lesions in the temporo-occipital cortices bilaterally (*arrows*) with decreased ADC values

consistent with cytotoxic edema in the myelin sheath (intramyelinic edema) (Fig. 15.11).

15.2.3 Brain Death

Brain death is defined as the irreversible cessation of all brain function [54]. Brain death criteria that most countries have commonly accepted are [55]: deep unresponsive coma; absence of brain stem function and reflexes; positive apnea test despite pCO_2 greater than 60 mmHg. The irreversibility of such criteria must be confirmed. Brain electrical activity (EEG, brain stem evoked potentials) may be inaccurate in comatose patients with drug-induced hypothermia or intoxication. The absence of cerebral blood flow is accepted as a confirmatory sign of brain death.

Conventional angiography was considered the gold standard until the 1990s, but it is an invasive method and may damage transplantable organs. MR imaging and MR angiography have been

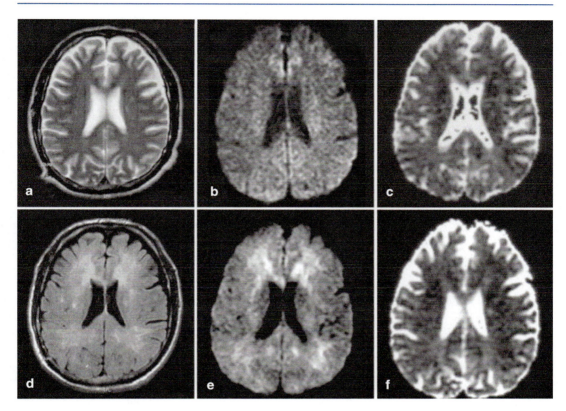

Fig. 15.11 Delayed postanoxic encephalopathy in a 53-year-old man with progressive mental status changes for 3–4 days. There was a history of narcotic overdose 2 weeks earlier. (a) T2-weighted image shows no abnormal signal intensity in the brain. (b, c) DW image shows very subtle hyperintensity with mild decreased ADC in the corona radiata. (d) Follow-up MR imaging was performed 14 days after the onset. FLAIR image shows high signal intensity in the deep white matter bilaterally. (e) DW images revealed diffuse hyperintensity with decreased ADC (f). The patient continued to deteriorate and died about 20 days later, 46 days after the overdose. Autopsy was performed. (g–i) Pathology shows myelin discoloration in the periventricular white matter and caudate nucleus. Pathology shows neuronal axonal spheroids (*arrows*) in the gray matter (h) and varying degrees of myelin loss with spongiform changes in the white matter, reflecting intramyelinic edema in the deep white matter (i)

reported as reliable methods in demonstrating absence of cerebral blood flow and determining brain death [54, 56, 57]. MR findings in brain death include (1) central and tonsillar herniation, (2) absent intracranial vascular flow voids, (3) poor gray matter/white matter differentiation, (4) no intracranial contrast enhancement, (5) carotid artery gadolinium enhancement (intravascular enhancement sign), and (6) prominent nasal and scalp enhancement (MR hot nose sign) [56]. MR angiogram shows no intracranial flow above the supra-clinoid carotid arteries due to the increased intracranial pressure. DW imaging shows diffuse hyperintense areas in the gray and white matter including the brain stem (Figs. 15.12 and 15.13). A massive drop in ADC values in the hemispheres has been reported (<50% of normal values) [58]. The ADC value of the white matter is significantly lower than that of the gray matter [59]. Diffusion restriction usually extends to the brain stem and, variably, the cerebellum [60]. Severe ADC reduction in gray and white matter probably reflects global irreversible cytotoxic edema.

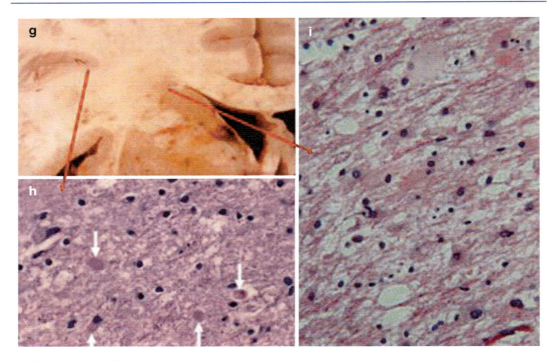

Fig. 15.11 (continued)

15.2.4 Hypoglycemia and Hyperglycemia

Glucose is the main energy substrate of the brain. Hypoglycemia is caused by overuse of insulin, oral hypoglycemic agents, insulinoma, sepsis, renal or hepatic failure, or Addison disease. Neurologic signs of hypoglycemia are nonspecific including weakness, confusion, seizures, and coma. Sequelae of hypoglycemic coma are rare, but they include profound memory loss, persistent vegetative state, and death in 2–4% of cases. MR imaging of hypoglycemia shows lesions that involve the cerebral cortex, particularly the temporal lobe, hippocampus, and basal ganglia [61]. The most severely affected patients manifest basal ganglia involvement. DW imaging shows hyperintense lesions with decreased ADC similar to hypoxic–ischemic encephalopathy (Fig. 15.14) [61, 62]. Reversible lesions on DW imaging have also been reported, which often involve the bilateral internal capsules, corona radiata, and corpus callosum [63, 64]. This pattern may be the result of a different pathophysiologic process from glucose starvation such as a release of excitatory amino acids into the extracellular space [65].

Hyperglycemia can disrupt the blood–brain barrier and produce decreased cerebral blood flow, intracellular acidosis, accumulation of extracellular glutamate, and decreased activity of GABAergic neurons. Hemichorea-hemiballismus associated with hyperglycemia is characterized by hyperintensities in the striatum on T1-weighted images and CT studies. The process is either unilateral or bilateral. The T1 high signal is probably related to manganese (Mn) accumulation accompanied by induction of Mn superoxide dismutase (MN-SOD) and glutamine synthetase (GS) with rich protein contents in the reactive swollen astrocytes (gemistocytes) [66–68]. Increased viscosity was also proposed as a potential basis for the high T1 signal, which could also explain restricted diffusion [67]. DW imaging has been

15 Toxic and Metabolic Diseases

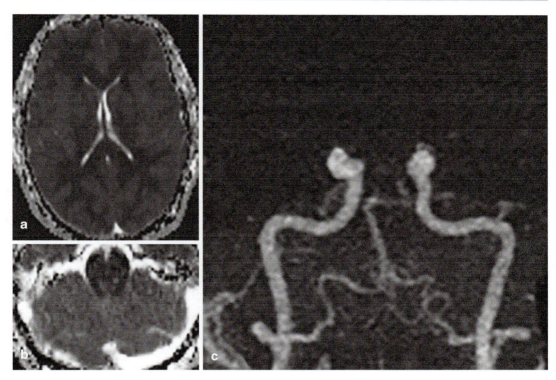

Fig. 15.12 32-year-old man with brain death. (**a**) ADC map reveals marked decreased ADC in the white matter (0.21 × 10⁻³ mm²/s) and decreased ADC in the cortex (0.51 × 10⁻³ mm²/s). Note diffuse obliteration of cortical sulci. (**b**) Decreased ADC is observed in the pons (0.30 × 10⁻⁵ mm²/s) but not in the cerebellum. (**c**) Dynamic contrast MR angiography shows loss of vascular flow in the supraclinoid internal carotid arteries but reveals opacification of intracranial vertebral and basilar arteries

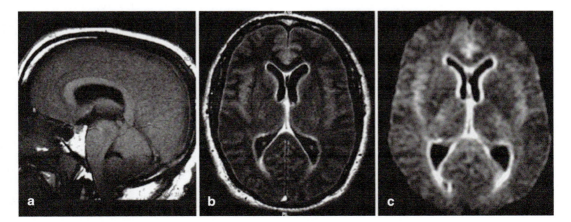

Fig. 15.13 Brain death in a 48-year-old man. (**a**) Sagittal T1-weighted image shows central and tonsillar herniation. (**b**) FLAIR image shows diffuse hyperintensity in the cortex, deep gray matter, and periventricular white matter. (**c**) DW image shows extensive diffuse hyperintensity in the brain, especially the periventricular white matter. (**d**) The ADC values of the brain are diffusely decreased in the cortex (0.51 × 10⁻³ mm²/s) and white matter (0.25 × 10⁻³ mm²/s). (**e**) MR angiography shows non-visualization of intracranial vessels above the supraclinoid carotid arteries

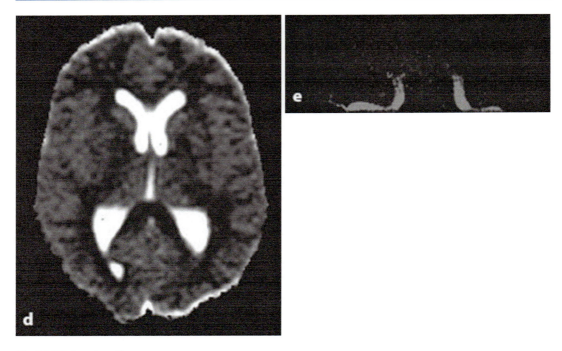

Fig. 15.13 (continued)

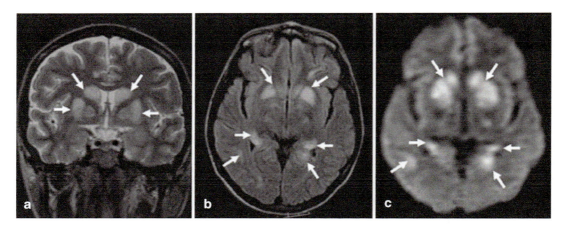

Fig. 15.14 Hypoglycemic encephalopathy in a 53-year-old man. (**a, b**) Coronal T2-weighted and axial FLAIR images show symmetric hyperintense lesions in the basal ganglia, hippocampi, and temporo-occipital lobes (*arrows*). (**c**) DW image shows these areas as hyperintensity lesions (*arrows*)

reported to detect early ischemic damage as areas of heterogeneous signal intensity with decreased ADC (Fig. 15.15) [67–69]. On the other hand, diabetic ketoacidosis with prolonged hyperglycemia may cause subtle FLAIR and diffusion abnormalities in the cortex (Fig. 15.16) associated with elevations in glucose, myoinositol, taurine, and ketones in MR spectroscopy [70].

15 Toxic and Metabolic Diseases

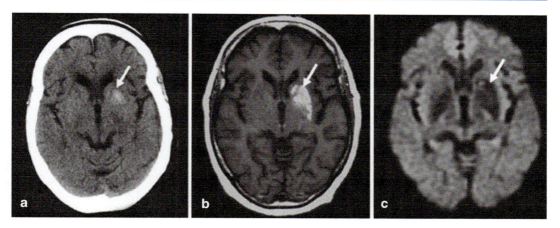

Fig. 15.15 Hemichorea-hemiballismus associated with hyperglycemia in a 69-year-old woman with type 2 diabetes. (**a**) CT shows high-density areas in the left caudate head and anterior part of the putamen (*arrow*). (**b**) T1-weighted image shows hyperintensity in the left entire striatum (*arrows*). (**c**) DW image shows these lesions as low-signal intensity with an isointense area in the left caudate head (*arrows*)

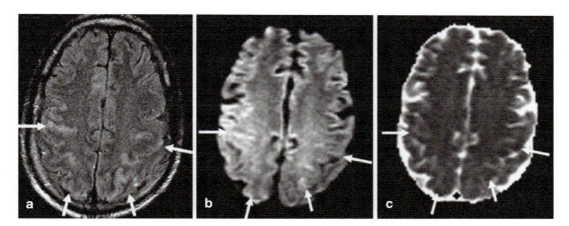

Fig. 15.16 Diabetic ketoacidosis with type 1 diabetes in a 28-year-old man (blood sugar 1500 mg/dl). (**a**) FLAIR image shows symmetric hyperintense lesions in the parietal cortices bilaterally. (**b**, **c**) DW image shows these areas as hyperintense with mildly decreased ADC

15.2.5 Osmotic Demyelination (OD)

OD encompasses previously reported central pontine myelinolysis (CPM) and extrapontine myelinolysis (EPM), which represent destruction of myelin sheaths in characteristic locations within the brain stem and cerebrum. The most common location is the central part of the basis pontis, followed by a combined type with central and extrapontine areas of myelinolysis. Isolated EPM is the least common presentation [71]. A symmetric trident-shaped hyperintensity in the central pons is the characteristic finding on T2-weighted and FLAIR MR images. The ventrolateral pons and the corticospinal tracts typically are spared [72]. The basal ganglia, thalamus, geniculate bodies, internal and external capsules, corpus callosum, cerebellum, cerebellar peduncles, and gray–white matter junction are possible sites of EPM [73–76]. The cortico-subcortical junction, especially at the crown of the cortical gyri, is vulnerable to osmotic demyelination syndrome [77, 78]. The synonyms include osmotic myelinolysis and osmotic demyelination syndrome. Symptoms include acute confusional state, pseudobulbar affect, stupor, coma, and occasionally locked-in syndrome, intermingled with prominent motor manifestations of flaccid evolving to spastic quadriparesis, dysarthria, and dysphagia [79–81].

Pathological findings show destruction of myelin sheaths, though the nerve cells and axons are relatively spared. The underlying etiology and pathogenesis are unknown, but the hypotheses include osmotic endothelial injury, microglia-derived cytokines, excessive brain dehydration, and metabolic compromise [82]. Organic osmolytes, including glutamate, glutamine, myoinositol, and taurine, have been implicated in the pathogenesis of myelinolysis [83]. The most common osmotic insult is a rapid correction of compensated subacute hyponatremia. However, CPM and EPM can also occur in normo- or hypernatremic states in patients with chronic alcoholism, post-liver transplantation, malnutrition, burns, hyperemesis gravidarum, and AIDS [84–86].

MR imaging has a fundamental role in the diagnosis and discloses hyperintense lesions on T2-weighted images, with or without enhancement on gadolinium-enhanced T1-weighted images. DW imaging is useful in detecting the lesions in the early phase as hyperintense with decreased ADC, which represents cytotoxic edema (Figs. 15.17, 15.18, and 15.19) [87]. Cytotoxic edema in CPM and EPM occur not only in myelin sheaths but also in neurons, axons, and astrocytes [88]. The clinical outcome of CPM and EPM is highly variable, and both fatal and clinically reversible cases may be associated with this kind of cytotoxic edema.

15.2.6 Wernicke's Encephalopathy

Thiamine (vitamin B1) deficiency can cause Wernicke encephalopathy, characterized by confusion, ataxia, and abnormal eye movements, but the classical clinical triad is not always present. It is frequently associated with chronic alcohol abuse. Nonalcoholic Wernicke encephalopathy includes many other conditions such as tumors and bypass surgery of the gastrointestinal tract, gastroplasty, pancreatitis, anorexia nervosa, voluntary food starvation, hyperemesis gravidarum, chronic uremia, dialysis, HIV infection, and thyrotoxicosis [89–91]. Without thiamine, the Krebs and pentose phosphate cycles cannot metabolize glucose. Thiamine is also essential in maintaining osmotic gradients across cell membranes. Cellular homeostasis will soon fail resulting in release of glutamate into the extracellular space leading to NMDA receptor mediated excitotoxicity. Pathologic features are edema, swelling of capillary endothelial cells and astrocytes, hemorrhage, necrosis, and decreased myelination. The lesions are commonly seen in the mamillary bodies (57–75%), medial thalamic and hypothalamic nuclei, periaqueductal

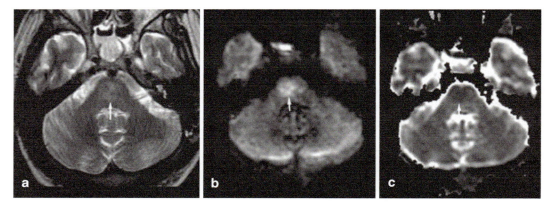

Fig. 15.17 Central pontine myelinolysis in a 33-year-old man. (**a**) T2-weighted image shows a hyperintense lesion in the center of the pons (*arrow*). (**b**, **c**) DW image shows this lesion as hyperintense with decreased ADC

15 Toxic and Metabolic Diseases

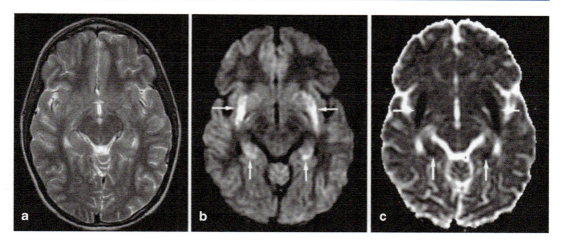

Fig. 15.18 Extrapontine myelinolysis in an 11-year-old boy. (**a**) T2-weighted image shows no appreciable abnormality in the external capsules and hippocampi. (**b**, **c**) DW image demonstrates bilateral symmetrical hyperintense lesions with decreased ADC in the external capsules and hippocampi (*arrows*), representing cytotoxic edema

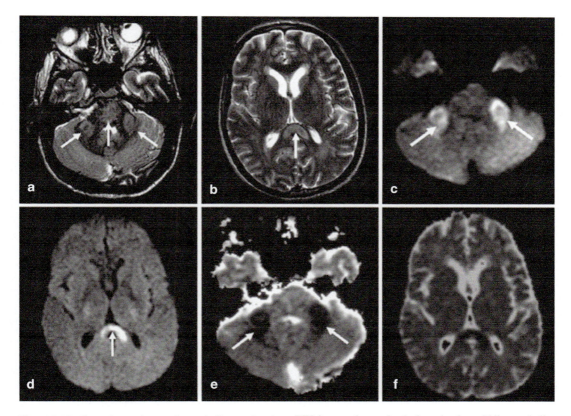

Fig. 15.19 Central pontine and cerebellar peduncle myelinolysis in a 54-year-old man with slurred speech and confusion. (**a**, **b**) T2-weighted image shows hyperintense lesions in the center of the pons, middle cerebellar peduncles (**a**), and corpus callosum. (**b**) (*arrows*). (**c–f**) DW image shows the lesions in the middle cerebellar peduncles and corpus callosum as hyperintense with decreased ADC (*arrows*), and the pontine lesion as isointense with increased ADC

gray matter, tectal plate, walls of the third and floor of the fourth ventricle, and less commonly in the caudate nuclei, frontal, and parietal cortex, pons, dorsal medulla, red nuclei, corpus callosum, cerebellum, and dentate nuclei [91–95].

MR imaging shows symmetrical hyperintense lesions of these areas on FLAIR and T2-weighted images [96]. They may or may not show enhancement on T1weighted images following contrast agent injection, depending on local disruption of the blood–brain barrier [91, 97]. Mammillary body involvement and enhancement are often seen in Wernicke encephalopathy with alcohol abuse but are less frequent in nonalcoholic Wernicke encephalopathy [89–91]. With intravenous thiamine treatment, these lesions may resolve. DW imaging shows these lesions as hyperintense with decreased or increased ADC. Lesions with decreased ADC are thought to represent cytotoxic edema of neurons or astrocytes, while lesions with increased ADC may represent vasogenic edema (Figs. 15.20 and 15.21) [95, 98–100]. Both types of lesion can be reversible [98]. The important differential diagnosis of symmetric lesions in the medial thalami includes ischemia due to occlusion of the artery of Percheron and deep cerebral vein thrombosis.

15.2.7 Hyperammonemic Encephalopathy

Hyperammonemia is the end result of several metabolic derangements such as hepatic encephalopathy, deficiencies of urea cycle enzymes, Reye's syndrome, and other toxic encephalopathies [102]. FLAIR and DWI display abnormalities in the thalami, posterior limb of the internal capsule, periventricular white matter, dorsal brainstem, or diffuse cortical involvement. Restricted diffusion involving the insular and cingulate cortices and thalamus bilaterally is characteristic (Fig. 15.22) [103]. FLAIR and DWI changes correlate with plasma ammonia level, which is a strong predictor of outcome [104]. The combination of facilitated and restricted diffusion suggests the presence of both intracellular and extracellular components of cerebral edema in patients with acute-on-chronic liver failure [105]. The time course of ADC changes is reminiscent of HIE, with pseudonormalization at 8 days [101]. In well-compensated cirrhosis patients free of overt hepatic encephalopathy, ADC values were significantly increased in the genu and body of the corpus callosum suggesting increase in extracellular fluid [106].

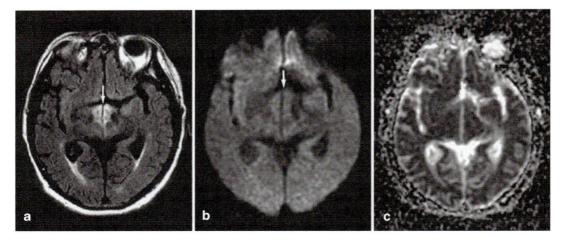

Fig. 15.20 Wernicke encephalopathy with alcohol abuse in a 75-year-old man. (a) FLAIR shows a symmetrical hyperintense lesion in the hypothalamus (*arrow*). (b, c) DW image shows isointense lesions with increased ADC in the hypothalamus, which may represent vasogenic edema (*arrow*)

15 Toxic and Metabolic Diseases

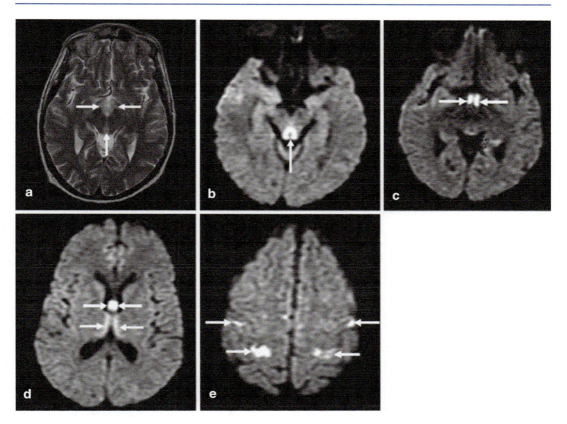

Fig. 15.21 Wernicke encephalopathy with thyrotoxicosis in a 36-year-old man. (**a**) T2-weighted image shows symmetric hyperintense lesions in the mammillary bodies, hypothalamus, and periaqueductal region (*arrows*). (**b–e**) DW imaging shows hyperintense lesions in the hypothalamus, midbrain tectum, periaqueductal region, medial thalami, fornices, and pre- and postcentral gyri (*arrows*), associated with partially decreased ADC (not shown)

15.2.8 Wilson's Disease (WD)

The incidence of WD is approximately 1:30,000. The underlying mechanism of WD is a defect in ATP7B, a copper transporting ATPase that is mainly expressed in hepatocytes. This leads to accumulation of copper, which eventually overwhelms safe storage capacity and cellular injury occurs. Most WD patients present with liver disease during their first and second decades of life with neurologic or psychiatric symptoms in the second and third decades or later on [107]. Neurologic disease most often presents with tremor and progresses with gait imbalance, dysarthria, drooling, and parkinsonism. Psychiatric disease may range from mild mood disturbance to frank psychosis.

On T2-weighted images, neurological WD patients show high signal changes in the putamen, followed by involvement of the caudate, midbrain, thalamus, and cerebral cortex (Fig. 15.23) [108, 109]. The appearance of axial T2-weighted images at the midbrain has been linked to a "giant panda" face sign [110]. On DWI images, restricted diffusion in the putamen can be detected before the occurrence of neurologic manifestations in WD. In contrast, an increase in diffusion is detected after the occurrence of symptoms within the putamen, pallidum, internal capsule, and subcortical white matter, which parallel the signal changes seen on FLAIR [111].

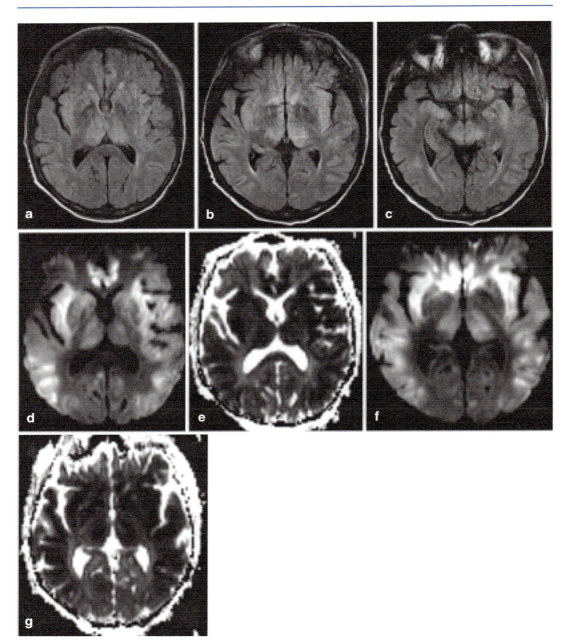

Fig. 15.22 Hyperammonemic encephalopathy in a 55-year-old man with cirrhosis, subsequently fatal, with initial plasma ammonia level (PAL) of 410 µM/L. (**a–c**) Axial FLAIR symmetric hyperintensities in thalami, upper midbrain, insula and external capsule and temporal cortex. DWI trace images (**d** and **f**) and ADC map (**e** and **g**) display extensive restricted DWI in those areas. The graph shows temporal evolution of ADC changes with pseudonormalization at 8 days [101]

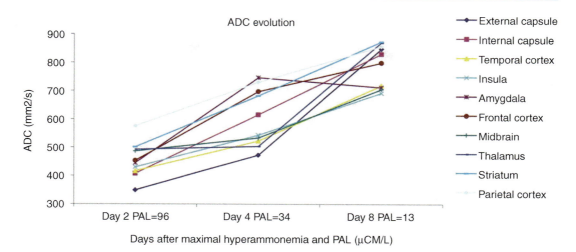

Fig. 15.22 (continued)

15.2.9 Mitochondrial Encephalopathies

Mitochondrial encephalopathies are a heterogeneous group of disorders affecting primarily the central nervous system and skeletal muscles that result from mutations in the mitochondrial DNA that are inherited through the maternal line. Two main hypotheses attempt to explain the cerebral lesions: (a) mitochondrial dysfunction, which results in anaerobic metabolism and neuronal death from acidosis and (b) metabolic damage of the endothelium, which leads to small-vessel occlusion and secondary neuronal death [112].

Mitochondrial encephalomyopathy, lactic acidosis, and stroke-like episodes (MELAS) is one of the most frequent mitochondrial disorders. MELAS syndrome is a multi-organ disease with stroke-like episodes, dementia, epilepsy, lactic acidemia, myopathy, recurrent headaches with vomiting, hearing impairment, diabetes, and short stature [112]. 80% of MELAS cases are associated with the m.3243A > G mutation in the MT-TL1 gene encoding the mitochondrial tRNA$^{Leu(UUR)}$ (Fig. 15.24). On the other hand, Leigh syndrome displays a wide variety of presentations, from severe neurologic symptoms to subtle abnormalities. Most frequently, the central nervous system is affected with psychomotor retardation, seizures, nystagmus, ophthalmoparesis, optic atrophy, ataxia, dystonia, or respiratory failure. Some patients also present with peripheral nervous system involvement, including polyneuropathy or myopathy, or non-neurologic abnormalities, e.g., diabetes, short stature, cardiomyopathy, anemia, renal failure, vomiting, or diarrhea (Leigh-like syndrome) [113]. Onset is in early childhood, but in a small number of cases, adults are affected (Fig. 15.25).

T2-weighted images occasionally show increased signal intensity in the cortex and subcortical white matter, with features reminiscent of stroke but not respecting vascular territories. Cerebellar atrophy may be a hint to a preexisting abnormality (Figs. 15.24 and 15.25). Proton MR spectroscopy is useful in the diagnosis by detecting elevated lactate peak. DW imaging often shows the stroke-like lesions in MELAS as hyperintense with restricted diffusion initially and later facilitated diffusion [114]. They have increased or normal ADC, which presumably represents vasogenic edema, however, decreased ADC in these lesions representing cytotoxic edema can be observed [114] (Fig. 15.25).

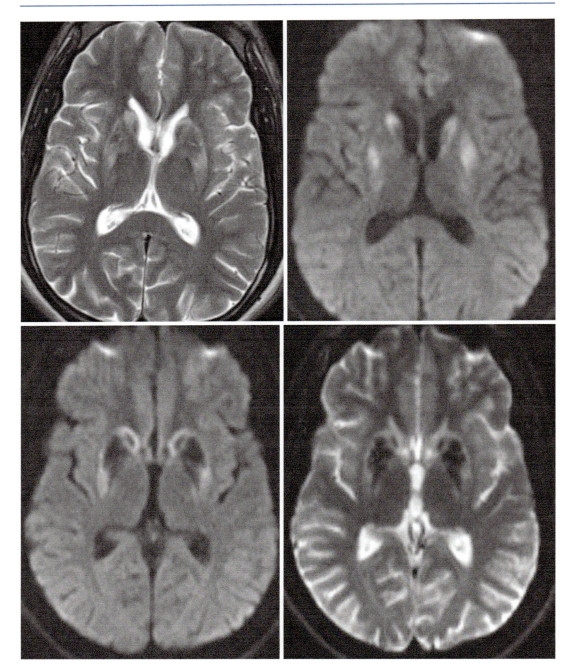

Fig. 15.23 Wilson disease 19 year/o male with slurred speech, change in behavior, depression, and low ceruloplasmin. Symmetric T2 and DWI hyperintensities with facilitated diffusion in the striatum

15.2.10 SMART Syndrome

SMART syndrome (stroke-like migraine attacks after radiation therapy) is a rare condition that involves complex migraines with focal neurologic findings in patients following cranial irradiation for central nervous system malignancies. It may be diagnosed up to 35 years (on average 20 years) after high-dose radiation (>5000 centi Gray) treatment for intracranial neoplasms. It

15 Toxic and Metabolic Diseases

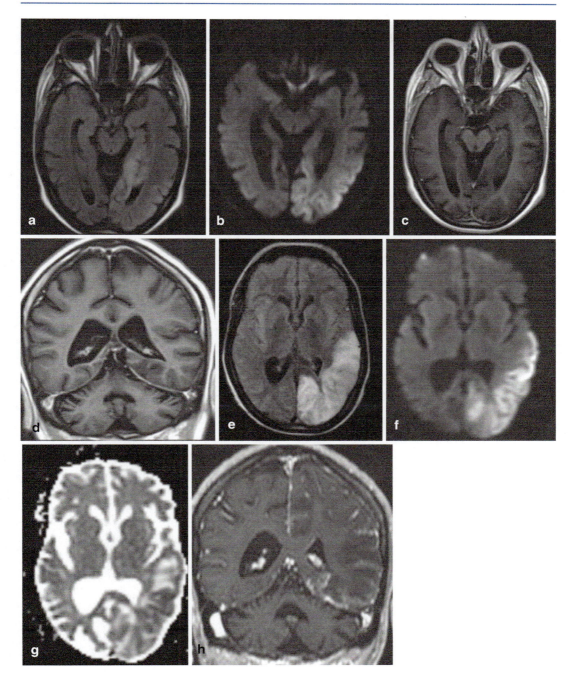

Fig. 15.24 MELAS 42-year-old female with headache, blurry vision, and altered mental status. Hereditary deafness in maternal line. m.3243A > G pathogenic variant in the MT-TL1 gene. (**a–d**) At presentation, (**e–h**) follow-up with worsening cortical-based restricted DWI (**f–g**), and cortical enhancement (**h**)

involves complicated migraine symptoms consisting of transient neurologic deficits such as hemiparesis, aphasia, and sensory disturbances [115]. On imaging, it may resemble subacute infarction or MELAS on post-contrast images (Fig. 15.26): unilateral gyriform enhancement on MR imaging that develops within 2–7 days and resolves in 2–5 weeks. On the other hand,

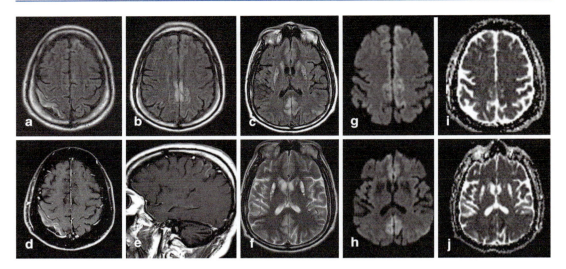

Fig. 15.25 **Adult Leigh syndrome**. 42-year-old man with a pathogenic mutation in MTATP6. Had recurrent stroke-like episodes, imaging evidence of necrotizing encephalopathy, decompensation at the time of infectious illness, chronic migraine, sensorineural hearing loss, and psychotic symptoms. Also had lifelong progressive muscle weakness, ataxia, cerebral and cerebellar atrophy, and visual problems. Symmetric gray matter symmetric involvement with high FLAIR signal in cortex and basal ganglia (**a–c**), with cortical enhancement (**d–e**) and restricted DWI (**g–j**). Note basal ganglia (**c–f**) and cerebellar (**e**) atrophy

DWI abnormalities primarily demonstrated T2 shine through without convincing evidence of restricted diffusion as opposed to mitochondrial diseases. Although considered reversible, up to 45% of SMART cases had incomplete neurologic recovery with imaging or clinical sequelae such as dysphasia, cognitive impairment, or hemiparesis [116].

15.3 Treatment of Toxic and Metabolic Diseases

Yang Mao-Draayer and Brian Chang

15.3.1 Chemotherapy-Induced Leukoencephalopathy

The most commonly implicated agent associated with leukoencephalopathy is methotrexate, and there is no standardized treatment for methotrexate-induced leukoencephalopathy [117]. Some case reports have suggested benefit with aminophylline and a retrospective series of patients with subacute encephalopathy found improvement with dextromethorphan [118, 119]. However, whether methotrexate in general should even be stopped should be assessed with relation to many mitigating factors, including determination of why the affected patient was more at risk for toxicity, whether leukoencephalopathy was symptomatic or not, how extensive the leukoencephalopathy was, and how much the patient would benefit from continuing methotrexate [120]. Other methotrexate-induced neurotoxicities—specifically transverse myelopathy and disseminated necrotizing leukoencephalopathy—require immediate discontinuation of methotrexate [121, 122]. A case report of the former has documented improvement with high doses of metabolites of the methyl-transfer pathway including S-adenosylmethionine, folinate, cyanocobalamin, and methionine [123]. The latter has been associated with poor outcomes, with supportive treatment as the only therapeutic management [2].

While less common, other chemotherapies associated with leukoencephalopathy include bortzemoib, gemcitabine, sunitinib, cisplatin, and oxiplatin [124–131]. Treatment for these

15 Toxic and Metabolic Diseases

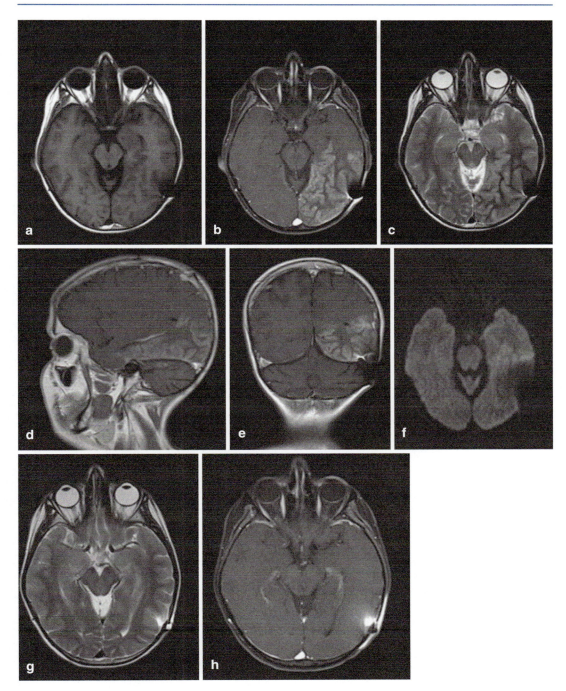

Fig. 15.26 SMART syndrome. 30-year-old male with VP shunt presents with progressive left-sided headache, language difficulties, right arm numbness, and weight loss. History of medulloblastoma status-post excision, chemotherapy and radiation 24 years before. **Right**: Imaging on presentation with pre contrast T1 (**a**) and gyriform cortical enhancement in the left temporo-occipital region (**b, d, e**) and no definite restricted DWI (**f**). **Left**: Imaging resolution on follow-up (**g h**)

neurotoxicities as detailed in case reports generally involve removal of the offending agent, supportive care including anti-seizure medications, and control of comorbidities, especially hypertension.

15.3.2 Heroin-Induced Spongiform Leukoencephalopathy

There is no proven treatment for heroin-induced spongiform leukoencephalopathy. However, some manuscripts have reported varying levels of improvement with antioxidants including coenzyme Q10 on its own or in combination with vitamin E and vitamin C [132, 133].

15.3.3 Cocaine, Phencyclidine Hydrochloride, Amphetamines, and Related Catecholaminergics

Management for these toxicities begins first and foremost with establishment of airway, breathing, and circulation. Should intubation be required, succinylcholine should be avoided, as it is a strong acetylcholine receptor agonist that produces sustained depolarization and has a well-established risk of rhabdomyolysis as compared to non-depolarizing neuromuscular blocking drugs [134].

Following resuscitation, treatment relies largely on attenuating CNS release of catecholamines and treating the sequelae of sympathetic activation. Intermediate to long-acting benzodiazepines including lorazepam and diazepam are first-line agents for acute cocaine, phencyclidine hydrochloride, and amphetamine toxicity, lowering blood pressure, attenuating hyperthermia, and decreasing agitation [135–137]. For hypertension resistant to benzodiazepines, short-acting vasodilators including nitroglycerin and nitroprusside are employed, while residual tachycardia may be treated with calcium channel blockers. If myocardial infarction is suspected or diagnosed, appropriate therapeutic steps should be taken.

15.3.4 Hypoxic–Ischemic Encephalopathy

Management of hypoxic-ischemic encephalopathy (HIE) varies by age. In adults, supportive and preventive care is the standard [138–140]. Seizures may be treated with appropriate anti-seizure medications, and myoclonic seizures specifically may be treated with valproate or clonazepam [141]. Patients may also present with post-hypoxic myoclonus, which case reports have been responsive to phenytoin, phenobarbitone, or benzodiazepines [142]. Limited evidence exists for the treatment of subclinical seizures [143].

In neonates, the only protective strategy that has shown consistently benefit has been therapeutic hypothermia, started within the first 6 h after delivery [144]. Mechanistically, it is thought to reduce free radicals and glutamate levels, decrease oxygen demand, and decrease apoptosis [145]. This should be supplemented with supportive care, including volume support, management of seizures with phenobarbital, lorazepam, fosphenytoin, or levetiracetam, and respiratory therapy for infants with persistent pulmonary hypertension to maintain oxygenation.

15.3.5 Hypoglycemia and Hyperglycemia

Treatment is specific to etiology of the glucose imbalance (Table 15.1).

First, we consider hypoglycemia in patients with type 1 or type 2 diabetes. By far, the most commonly implicated etiology is medication. Preventive strategies around this include setting glycemic targets, establishing consistent medication regimens, recognizing signs and symptoms of hypoglycemia early, and ingesting bedtime snacks to prevent nocturnal hypoglycemia. If hypoglycemia does arise, treatment may vary from ingesting fast-acting carbohydrates and retesting blood glucose if the patient is asymptomatic or mildly symptomatic to administering glucagon or IV dextrose if the patient is severely symptomatic [146, 147].

15 Toxic and Metabolic Diseases

Table 15.1 Etiologies of hypo- and hyperglycemia by diabetes status

	Without diabetes	With diabetes
Hypoglycemia	Medications Alcohol Cortisol deficiency Insulinoma/excess insulin Critical illness/sepsis	Medications
Hyperglycemia	Stress-induced Acute myocardial infarction	Type 1 diabetes Type 2 diabetes Hyperosmotic hyperglycemia state (HHS)/diabetic ketoacidosis (DKA)

Next, we address patients with diabetes who present with hyperglycemia. In patients with type I diabetes, physicians should adjust their insulin regimen and address their dietary habits. In patients with type II diabetes, management begins with lifestyle changes including diet, exercise, and weight loss. Should this be unsuccessful, the first-line treatment is metformin, with a glycemic treatment goal of HgbA1c goal of <7.0 in younger adults without complications or 8–8.5 depending on advanced age, comorbidities, and life expectancy [148, 149]. If within 3 months, the glycemic treatment goal is not achieved with metformin along with lifestyle intervention, a second agent may be prescribed. Following that, triple agent therapy and bariatric surgery are third-tier options, though recurrences of diabetes in the latter are not uncommon and microvascular and macrovascular complications are comparable to those of medical therapy [150, 151]. Medications should be prescribed as tolerated with additional comorbidities (such as obesity) in mind. In patients in diabetic ketoacidosis (DKA) or hyperosmotic hyperglycemic state (HHS), the overriding principles are to correct fluid and electrolyte abnormalities, administer insulin, and monitor laboratory parameters closely until the anion gap closes [152]. The use of sodium bicarbonate has been widely debated, as side effects include peripheral hypoxemia, paradoxical CNS acidosis, and cerebral edema in children and young adults [153–155]. However, a general consensus has been formed around its use strictly in adults when arterial pH is less than 7.0 or when potentially life-threatening hyperkalemia (>6.4 mEq/l) is present [156–158].

If hypoglycemia occurs in patients without diabetes, treatment should be targeted at the underlying etiology of the low blood sugar. Again, medications are a widely implicated cause. A number of common medications have a known side effect of hypoglycemia, such as pentamidine, quinine, and indomethacin [159]. Other medications less commonly but still associated with hypoglycemia include lithium and IGF-1 [160]. Physicians should adjust medication regimens as appropriate, titrating therapeutic effects to each patient. Chronic alcoholism is also associated with hypoglycemia, and should be treated with dietary counseling and support around alcohol cessation [161]. Cortisol deficiency secondary to Addison's disease may be treated with cortisone therapy, and sepsis should be managed with appropriate resuscitation and treatment of the offending organism. While a relatively uncommon cause of hypoglycemia, insulinomas may be treated with resection of primary tumor, ethanol ablation, or medical management with diazoxide, octreotide/lanreotide if refractory to diazoxide, or verapamil [162–164].

Finally, hyperglycemia in patients without diabetes and with appropriately drawn labs could be attributable to stress-induced hyperglycemia (SIH), an enhanced metabolic state induced after trauma [165]. Attempts at tight glycemic control in both ICU and non-ICU patients do not improve outcomes, and the ideal glucose parameters under this condition are unclear as spontaneous improvement in fasting blood glucoses is inconsistently found in some patients with SIH [166]. However, a general target range between 100 and 180 mg/dl has been suggested by experts [167].

15.3.6 Carbon Monoxide Intoxication

If exposed to excessive quantities of carbon monoxide (CO), patients should be immediately removed from the source of the CO and administered 100%, high-flow oxygen via a nonrebreather mask. In most cases, such treatment will be successful in resolving symptoms. However, patients with persistent symptoms or EKG or lab findings suggestive of severe poisoning should be hospitalized. Additionally, if patients become comatose or unable to protect their airway, they should be intubated immediately [168].

The benefit of hyperbaric oxygen is unclear. Randomized control trials have shown mixed effects of hyperbaric treatment, and one meta-analysis conducted in 2011 demonstrated no statistically significant difference between treatment and control [169, 170]. However, studies have been heterogeneous, with variable outcome measures. In general, hyperbaric treatment is recommended if any of the following are present: loss of consciousness, new neurologic impairments, end-organ ischemia, or pregnancy [171].

15.3.7 Delayed Postanoxic Encephalopathy

Following emergence of delayed postanoxic encephalopathy, treatment is supportive with active rehabilitation [172]. If Parkinsonian symptoms arise, case reports have described successful use of carbidopa and haloperidol [50, 173, 174]. Outcomes are generally positive.

15.3.8 Osmotic Demyelination

Prevention is crucial toward avoiding these demyelination syndromes, with slow (less than 6–8 mEq/l correction every 24-h period) correction in patients with hyponatremia lasting more than 2 days or with hyponatremia of unknown duration. Should an osmotic demyelinating syndrome arise, treatment is largely supportive, with careful monitoring of serum sodium concentration every 2–3 h initially.

While less commonly employed, case reports have demonstrated benefit from lowering sodium levels [175–177]. As such, desmopressin has been administered for its antidiuretic effects along with fluid replacement with dextrose if excessive urinary-free water loss is present [178, 179]. Additionally, one case report detailed symptomatic improvement in two of three patients following plasmapheresis. However, imaging remained unchanged, and spontaneous self-resolution of neurologic impairment has been previously observed [180].

15.3.9 Wernicke Encephalopathy

Immediate parenteral administration of thiamine is required after diagnosis, with a transition to oral vitamin B1 as tolerated [181]. Even after treatment, patients with thiamine insensitivity may necessitate higher than normal levels of thiamine [182]. If patients are hypoglycemic as well, case reports and series have suggested that glucose administration prior to thiamine might be a risk factor for development of Wernicke encephalopathy [183]. Regardless, correction of hypoglycemia should be either concurrent with or immediately preceded by administration of thiamine. Following appropriate management, patients should be counseled on dietary requirements of B vitamins and alcohol cessation if abuse or overuse is present.

15.3.10 Marchiafava–Bignami Disease

Similar to Wernicke encephalopathy, Marchiafava-Bignami disease is associated with chronic alcoholism, so treatment aimed at correcting underlying nutritional and vitamin imbalances is often

15.4 Brain Death Management

Deema Fatal

15.4.1 History of Brain Death Concept

employed. Parenteral thiamine has been associated with better outcomes, especially during the acute phase of the illness compared to chronic disease. Additionally, a case report has documented benefit with steroids. However, the disease has poor prognosis overall, therapeutic failure is often seen even after supplementation of B1, and a case series by Hillbom et al. showed no statistically significant improvement in 150 patients with steroid treatment [41, 184, 185]. A subset of surviving patients develops subsequent dementia, though partial or complete spontaneous recovery has been reported in some of these cases [184].

15.3.11 Steroid-Responsive Encephalopathy Associated with Autoimmune Thyroiditis (Hashimoto's Encephalopathy)

A vast majority of patients respond well to high-dose steroids with duration and tapering titrated to improvement in symptoms [186]. Other therapeutics including IV immunoglobulins, plasmapheresis, and immunomodulators such as methotrexate, azathioprine, and mycophenolate have been used with variable success in patients who have been steroid-intolerant [187–190].

Disclosures/Conflict of Interest
BC is currently being funded through the NIH TL1 grant. YMD has received consulting and/or speaker fees from Biogen, Bayer Pharmaceutical, Novartis, Celgene, Teva, Genentech, Sanofi-Genzyme, and EMD Serono. YMD has also received research support from NIH NINDS R01-NS080821, NIAID Autoimmune Center of Excellence UM1-AI110557, PCORI, Sanofi-Genzyme, Novartis, and Chugai.

Funding
This research did not receive any specific grant from funding agencies in the public, commercial, or not-for-profit sectors.

Brain death criteria is a new concept that was developed in the twentieth century as a result of improvements in intensive care of comatose patients, including unresponsive patients. The concept of brain death was first noted in the medical literature in 1959 by Mollaret and Goulon, which they called irreversible coma (coma dépassé) [191]. During the 1950s, advances in positive pressure ventilators led to patients, who would have died otherwise, to remain alive but without being responsive. As a result of such situations, neurologists had ongoing debates about these patients throughout the 1960s, and such debates were ongoing across the globe too, in Great Britain, Switzerland, South Africa, and Australia [192]. In 1967, anesthesiologist Henry Beecher led a committee to review the "ethical problems created by the hopelessly unconscious patient" [192]. This culminated in 1968 in the Harvard report on brain death [193]. This report was the first to put forth specific criteria for brain death [192]. The purpose of the report was to "define irreversible coma as a new criterion for death" and to discuss the ethical issue of procuring organs from such patients for transplantation; and both these issues were mentioned in the final report: "(1) the burden is great on patients who suffer permanent loss of intellect, on their families, on the hospitals, and on those in need of hospital beds already occupied by these comatose patients; (2) obsolete criteria for the definition of death can lead to controversy in obtaining organs for transplantation" [193]. The Harvard report's brain death criteria were the following: a person can be declared dead if there is (1) unreceptivity and unresponsivity even to the most intensely painful stimuli; (2) No movements (observed for 1 h) or breathing (upon turning off the ventilator for 3 min); (3) No reflexes (pupil, calorics, dolls eyes, corneal, and pharyngeal reflexes, and no swallow, yawning, or vocalization); and no stretch reflexes; (4) Flat EEG recorded for at least 10 min [193]; all this should be repeated 24 h later. Moreover, hypothermia <90 °F and depressants such as barbiturates should be excluded [193].The Harvard criteria were not legally binding [192]. Yet over the ensuing decade, the concept of brain death spread and during the 1970s some states started to develop brain death criteria, making it possible to be alive in one state and dead in another [192].

To overcome the confusion related to brain death across the states, there was a need for regulation at the federal level. In 1981, The President's Commission report for the "Study of Ethical Problems in Medicine and Biomedical and Behavioral Research" led to a proposal for a legal definition for brain death, which, in turn, resulted in the Uniform Determination of Death Act (UDDA) [194]. UDDA states that "An individual who has sustained either (1) irreversible cessation of circulatory and respiratory functions, or (2) irreversible cessation of all functions of the entire brain, including the brain stem, is dead. A determination of death must be made with accepted medical standards" [195]. Over time, all 50 states adopted one version or another of UDDA.

Though brain death was now defined in all states, confusion related to the exact criteria of brain death remained. The UDDA did not define "accepted medical standards." So in 1995, the American Academy of Neurology (AAN) published practice parameter to delineate the medical standards for the determination of brain death [196] and updated them in 2010 [197].

15.4.2 Diagnostic Criteria for Brain Death

To define brain death, three specified parameters need to be followed which are (1) Coma: irreversible cessation of all functions of the entire brain, including the brain stem due to a known condition that can cause brain death; (2) absence of brainstem reflexes; and (3) apnea. In other words, brain death is declared when "brainstem reflexes, motor responses, and respiratory drive are absent in a normothermic, non-drugged comatose patient with a known irreversible massive brain lesion and no contributing metabolic derangements" [198]. Typically, cardiac death occurs within few days of brain death [199], but not uniformly—the case of Jahi McMath [192]. It is important to note that once the AAN criteria for brain death determination were followed completely, no one has been reported to recover [197].

15.4.3 Neuropathology

In the past, the neuropathology of brain-dead patients showed total brain necrosis, so-called respirator brain [200]. But, with the advent of transplantation protocols, brain fixation is occurring in a timely fashion. In 2008, Wijdicks and Pfeifer reviewed neuropathology of 41 brains from brain dead patients where the autopsy was done within 36 h of brain death [200]. The findings were the following: (1) there are no pathognomonic feature; and (2) severe pathology was not uniform; in fact, mild changes were seen in as much as one-third of cerebral hemispheres and half of the brainstems [200].

15.4.4 Brain Death Causes

Known causes of brain death are intracranial hemorrhage, subarachnoid hemorrhage, large strokes with edema and herniation, hypoxic-ischemic injury, severe trauma, and fulminant hepatic necrosis with cerebral edema and increased intracranial pressure [201]. In fact, 90% of brain death causes are brain trauma, intracranial hemorrhage, subarachnoid hemorrhage, stroke, and anoxia [202].

15.4.5 Brain Death Mimickers

Severe clinical conditions can present in coma and could potentially be confused with brain

Table 15.2 Brain death examination

Unresponsive to verbal/pain stimuli
Temperature > 36 °C
Systolic blood pressure BP ≥ 100
Pupils fixed mid position
No corneal reflex
No gag, cough reflexes
No oculocephalic or oculovestibular reflexes
No grimace to facial pain
No response to pain to all limbs

death: fulminant Guillain-Barré syndrome, organophosphate intoxication, high cervical spinal cord injury, lidocaine toxicity, baclofen overdose, and delayed vecuronium clearance [197]. Yet review of these cases showed that none had a complete brain death examination using the AAN practice parameters [197].

15.4.6 Determination of Brain Death

To determine brain death, using AAN 2010 guidelines [197], the following criteria are needed:

1. Known irreversible cause
2. No confounding factors (such as no paralytic agents, sedatives, hypnotics, drugs, alcohol, or severe electrolytes, acid base, or endocrine disturbances)
3. Complete brain death examination—see Table 15.2.
4. Apnea test

The lack of need for a second exam was shown in a study by Lustbader et al. [203]. They studied 1229 brain dead adult bodies and 82 pediatrics. None regained brainstem function upon repeat examination. The time between the two exams was 19 h. Consent for organ donation decreased from 57 to 45% as the brain death declaration interval increased. Twelve percent sustained cardiac arrest between the first and second examination.

It is important to note that the apnea test cannot be completed in about 10% [204]. This is where the role of radiological tests may become relevant.

15.4.7 Future Directions

The biggest consequence of brain death criteria has been the ability to procure organs and save lives. But the definition of brain death has remained challenging. First, many versions of brain death criteria exist across the USA and the globe [198, 205]. In one study, 80 countries were surveyed and major discrepancies were found, such as PCO2 target was recommended in only 59% of the protocols [198]. Second, the concept of brain death has been difficult to conceptualize. Is the brain essential for the function of the whole organism, so that a dead brain means a dead organism [206]? This argument did not hold water over time since brain dead patients, with support of artificial feeding and ventilation, can remain stable for years, and can even give birth, negating the claim that the brain is essential for the functioning of the whole body [207]. In 2008, president's council on bioethics addressed this issue in its white paper "controversies in the determination of death" [208]. Although brain dead patients can remain stable and maintain "integrated functioning," they are still dead because "they have ceased to perform the fundamental vital work of a living organism" [192]. However, this concept too is on shaky grounds: the lack of ability to perform a vital function as criteria for death is confusing since a patient who has pneumonia and needs a ventilator cannot perform a vital function yet s/he is not dead. As 3-D printing of organs and tissues and xenotransplantation science continues to evolve, it is possible that the need for organ donation will become obsolete, making brain death definition less important in the future [192]. Until then, brain death concept remains, 50 years later, "well settled, yet still unresolved" [192].

References

1. Lexa FJ (1995) Drug-induced disorders of the central nervous system. Semin Roentgenol 30(1):7–17
2. Oka M, Terae S, Kobayashi R, Sawamura Y, Kudoh K, Tha KK et al (2003) MRI in methotrexate-related leukoencephalopathy: disseminated necrotising leukoencephalopathy in comparison with mild leukoencephalopathy. Neuroradiology 45(7):493–497

3. Raghavendra S, Nair MD, Chemmanam T, Krishnamoorthy T, Radhakrishnan VV, Kuruvilla A (2007) Disseminated necrotizing leukoencephalopathy following low-dose oral methotrexate. Eur J Neurol 14(3):309–314
4. Tha KK, Terae S, Sugiura M, Nishioka T, Oka M, Kudoh K et al (2002) Diffusion-weighted magnetic resonance imaging in early stage of 5-fluorouracil-induced leukoencephalopathy. Acta Neurol Scand 106(6):379–386
5. Fujikawa A, Tsuchiya K, Katase S, Kurosaki Y, Hachiya J (2001) Diffusion-weighted MR imaging of Carmofur-induced leukoencephalopathy. Eur Radiol 11(12):2602–2606
6. Brown MS, Stemmer SM, Simon JH, Stears JC, Jones RB, Cagnoni PJ et al (1998) White matter disease induced by high-dose chemotherapy: longitudinal study with MR imaging and proton spectroscopy. AJNR 19(2):217–221
7. Matsumoto S, Nishizawa S, Murakami M, Noma S, Sano A, Kuroda Y (1995) Carmofur-induced leukoencephalopathy: MRI. Neuroradiology 37(8):649–652
8. Sabin ND, Cheung YT, Reddick WE, Bhojwani D, Liu W, Glass JO et al (2018) The impact of persistent Leukoencephalopathy on brain White matter microstructure in long-term survivors of acute lymphoblastic Leukemia treated with chemotherapy only. AJNR 39(10):1919–1925
9. Edelmann MN, Krull KR, Liu W, Glass JO, Ji Q, Ogg RJ et al (2014) Diffusion tensor imaging and neurocognition in survivors of childhood acute lymphoblastic leukaemia. Brain J Neurol 137(Pt 11):2973–2983
10. Lo CP, Chen SY, Lee KW, Chen WL, Chen CY, Hsueh CJ et al (2007) Brain injury after acute carbon monoxide poisoning: early and late complications. AJR 189(4):W205–W211
11. Kinoshita T, Sugihara S, Matsusue E, Fujii S, Ametani M, Ogawa T (2005) Pallidoreticular damage in acute carbon monoxide poisoning: diffusion-weighted MR imaging findings. AJNR 26(7):1845–1848
12. Kim JH, Chang KH, Song IC, Kim KH, Kwon BJ, Kim HC et al (2003) Delayed encephalopathy of acute carbon monoxide intoxication: diffusivity of cerebral white matter lesions. AJNR 24(8):1592–1597
13. Murata T, Kimura H, Kado H, Omori M, Onizuka J, Takahashi T et al (2001) Neuronal damage in the interval form of CO poisoning determined by serial diffusion weighted magnetic resonance imaging plus 1H-magnetic resonance spectroscopy. J Neurol Neurosurg Psychiatry 71(2):250–253
14. Rando J, Szari S, Kumar G, Lingadevaru H (2016) Methadone overdose causing acute cerebellitis and multi-organ damage. Am J Emerg Med 34(2):343.e1–343.e3
15. Kass-Hout T, Kass-Hout O, Darkhabani MZ, Mokin M, Mehta B, Radovic V (2011) "Chasing the

dragon"—heroin-associated spongiform leukoencephalopathy. J Med Toxicol 7(3):240–242
16. Ramirez-Zamora A, Ramani H, Pastena G (2015) Neurological picture. Bilateral pallidal and medial temporal lobe ischaemic lesions after opioid overdose. J Neurol Neurosurg Psychiatry 86(12):1383–1384
17. Morales Odia Y, Jinka M, Ziai WC (2010) Severe leukoencephalopathy following acute oxycodone intoxication. Neurocrit Care 13(1):93–97
18. Huisa BN, Gasparovic C, Taheri S, Prestopnik JL, Rosenberg GA (2013) Imaging of subacute blood-brain barrier disruption after methadone overdose. J Neuroimaging 23(3):441–444
19. Carroll I, Heritier Barras AC, Dirren E, Burkhard PR, Horvath J (2012) Delayed leukoencephalopathy after alprazolam and methadone overdose: a case report and review of the literature. Clin Neurol Neurosurg 114(6):816–819
20. Bileviciute-Ljungar I, Haglund V, Carlsson J, von Heijne A (2014) Clinical and radiological findings in methadone-induced delayed leukoencephalopathy. J Rehabil Med 46(8):828–830
21. Barnett MH, Miller LA, Reddel SW, Davies L (2001) Reversible delayed leukoencephalopathy following intravenous heroin overdose. J Clin Neurosci 8(2):165–167
22. Reisner A, Hayes LL, Holland CM, Wrubel DM, Kebriaei MA, Geller RJ et al (2015) Opioid overdose in a child: case report and discussion with emphasis on neurosurgical implications. J Neurosurg Pediatr 16(6):752–757
23. Cerase A, Leonini S, Bellini M, Chianese G, Venturi C (2011) Methadone-induced toxic leukoencephalopathy: diagnosis and follow-up by magnetic resonance imaging including diffusion-weighted imaging and apparent diffusion coefficient maps. J Neuroimaging 21(3):283–286
24. Maschke M, Fehlings T, Kastrup O, Wilhelm HW, Leonhardt G (1999) Toxic leukoencephalopathy after intravenous consumption of heroin and cocaine with unexpected clinical recovery. J Neurol 246(9):850–851
25. Wolters EC, van Wijngaarden GK, Stam FC, Rengelink H, Lousberg RJ, Schipper ME et al (1982) Leucoencephalopathy after inhaling "heroin" pyrolysate. Lancet (London, England) 2(8310):1233–1237
26. Halloran O, Ifthikharuddin S, Samkoff L (2005) Leukoencephalopathy from "chasing the dragon". Neurology 64(10):1755
27. Offiah C, Hall E (2008) Heroin-induced leukoencephalopathy: characterization using MRI, diffusion-weighted imaging, and MR spectroscopy. Clin Radiol 63(2):146–152
28. Tan TP, Algra PR, Valk J, Wolters EC (1994) Toxic leukoencephalopathy after inhalation of poisoned heroin: MR findings. AJNR 15(1):175–178
29. Hagel J, Andrews G, Vertinsky T, Heran MK, Keogh C (2005) "Chasing the dragon"--imaging of heroin

30. Keogh CF, Andrews GT, Spacey SD, Forkheim KE, Graeb DA (2003) Neuroimaging features of heroin inhalation leukoencephalopathy. Can Assoc Radiol J 56(4):199–203

30. Keogh CF, Andrews GT, Spacey SD, Forkheim KE, Graeb DA (2003) Neuroimaging features of heroin inhalation toxicity: "chasing the dragon". AJR 180(3):847–850

31. Chen CY, Lee KW, Lee CC, Chin SC, Chung HW, Zimmerman RA (2000) Heroin-induced spongiform leukoencephalopathy: value of diffusion MR imaging. J Comput Assist Tomogr 24(5):735–737

32. Roy U, Panwar A, Pandit A, Das SK, Joshi B (2016) Clinical and Neuroradiological Spectrum of metronidazole induced encephalopathy: our experience and the review of literature. JCDR 10(6):Oe01–Oe09

33. Patel L, Batchala P, Almardawi R, Morales R, Raghavan P (2019) Acute metronidazole-induced neurotoxicity: an update on MRI findings. Clin Radiol 75(3):202–208

34. Kim E, Na DG, Kim EY, Kim JH, Son KR, Chang KH (2007) MR imaging of metronidazole-induced encephalopathy: lesion distribution and diffusion-weighted imaging findings. AJNR 28(9):1652–1658

35. Goolsby TA, Jakeman B, Gaynes RP (2018) Clinical relevance of metronidazole and peripheral neuropathy: a systematic review of the literature. Int J Antimicrob Agents 51(3):319–325

36. Gambini A, Falini A, Moiola L, Comi G, Scotti G (2003) Marchiafava-Bignami disease: longitudinal MR imaging and MR spectroscopy study. AJNR 24(2):249–253

37. Gass A, Birtsch G, Olster M, Schwartz A, Hennerici MG (1998) Marchiafava-Bignami disease: reversibility of neuroimaging abnormality. J Comput Assist Tomogr 22(3):503–504

38. Inagaki T, Saito K (2000) A case of Marchiafava-Bignami disease demonstrated by MR diffusion-weighted image. No to shinkei = Brain Nerve 52(7):633–637

39. Sair HI, Mohamed FB, Patel S, Kanamalla US, Hershey B, Hakma Z et al (2006) Diffusion tensor imaging and fiber-tracking in Marchiafava-Bignami disease. J Neuroimaging 16(3):281–285

40. Wenz H, Eisele P, Artemis D, Forster A, Brockmann MA (2014) Acute Marchiafava-Bignami disease with extensive diffusion restriction and early recovery: case report and review of the literature. J Neuroimaging 24(4):421–424

41. Hillbom M, Saloheimo P, Fujioka S, Wszolek ZK, Juvela S, Leone MA (2014) Diagnosis and management of Marchiafava-Bignami disease: a review of CT/MRI confirmed cases. J Neurol Neurosurg Psychiatry 85(2):168–173

42. Siesjo BK, Katsura K, Mellergard P, Ekholm A, Lundgren J, Smith ML (1993) Acidosis-related brain damage. Prog Brain Res 96:23–48

43. Busto R, Dietrich WD, Globus MY, Ginsberg MD (1989) The importance of brain temperature in cerebral ischemic injury. Stroke 20(8):1113–1114

44. Singhal AB, Topcuoglu MA, Koroshetz WJ (2002) Diffusion MRI in three types of anoxic encephalopathy. J Neurol Sci 196(1–2):37–40

45. McKinney AM, Teksam M, Felice R, Casey SO, Cranford R, Truwit CL et al (2004) Diffusion-weighted imaging in the setting of diffuse cortical laminar necrosis and hypoxic-ischemic encephalopathy. AJNR 25(10):1659–1665

46. Sieber FE, Palmon SC, Traystman RJ, Martin LJ (1995) Global incomplete cerebral ischemia produces predominantly cortical neuronal injury. Stroke 26(11):2091–2095; discussion 6

47. Els T, Kassubek J, Kubalek R, Klisch J (2004) Diffusion-weighted MRI during early global cerebral hypoxia: a predictor for clinical outcome? Acta Neurol Scand 110(6):361–367

48. Wijdicks EF, Campeau NG, Miller GM (2001) MR imaging in comatose survivors of cardiac resuscitation. AJNR 22(8):1561–1565

49. Tha KK, Terae S, Yamamoto T, Kudo K, Takahashi C, Oka M et al (2005) Early detection of global cerebral anoxia: improved accuracy by high-b-value diffusion-weighted imaging with long echo time. AJNR 26(6):1487–1497

50. Custodio CM, Basford JR (2004) Delayed postanoxic encephalopathy: a case report and literature review. Arch Phys Med Rehabil 85(3):502–505

51. Kwon OY, Chung SP, Ha YR, Yoo IS, Kim SW (2004) Delayed postanoxic encephalopathy after carbon monoxide poisoning. EMJ 21(2):250–251

52. Shprecher D, Mehta L (2010) The syndrome of delayed post-hypoxic leukoencephalopathy. NeuroRehabilitation 26(1):65–72

53. Katyal N, Narula N, George P, Nattanamai P, Newey CR, Beary JM (2018) Delayed post-hypoxic Leukoencephalopathy: a case series and review of the literature. Cureus 10(4):e2481

54. Karantanas AH, Hadjigeorgiou GM, Paterakis K, Sfiras D, Komnos A (2002) Contribution of MRI and MR angiography in early diagnosis of brain death. Eur Radiol 12(11):2710–2716

55. Wijdicks EF, Varelas PN, Gronseth GS, Greer DM (2010) Evidence-based guideline update: determining brain death in adults: report of the quality standards Subcommittee of the American Academy of neurology. Neurology 74(23):1911–1918

56. Orrison WW Jr, Champlin AM, Kesterson OL, Hartshorne MF, King JN (1994) MR 'hot nose sign' and 'intravascular enhancement sign' in brain death. AJNR 15(5):913–916

57. Ishii K, Onuma T, Kinoshita T, Shiina G, Kameyama M, Shimosegawa Y (1996) Brain death: MR and MR angiography. AJNR 17(4):731–735

58. Lovblad KO, Bassetti C (2000) Diffusion-weighted magnetic resonance imaging in brain death. Stroke 31(2):539–542

59. Nakahara M, Ericson K, Bellander BM (2001) Diffusion-weighted MR and apparent diffusion coefficient in the evaluation of severe brain injury.

Acta radiologica (Stockholm, Sweden: 1987) 42(4):365–369

60. Selcuk H, Albayram S, Tureci E, Hasiloglu ZI, Kizilkilic O, Cagil E et al (2012) Diffusion-weighted imaging findings in brain death. Neuroradiology 54(6):547–554

61. Finelli PF (2001) Diffusion-weighted MR in hypoglycemic coma. Neurology 57(5):933

62. Lo L, Tan AC, Umapathi T, Lim CC (2006) Diffusion-weighted MR imaging in early diagnosis and prognosis of hypoglycemia. AJNR 27(6):1222–1224

63. Albayram S, Ozer H, Gokdemir S, Gulsen F, Kiziltan G, Kocer N et al (2006) Reversible reduction of apparent diffusion coefficient values in bilateral internal capsules in transient hypoglycemia-induced hemiparesis. AJNR 27(8):1760–1762

64. Aoki T, Sato T, Hasegawa K, Ishizaki R, Saiki M (2004) Reversible hyperintensity lesion on diffusion-weighted MRI in hypoglycemic coma. Neurology 63(2):392–393

65. Auer RN (2004) Hypoglycemic brain damage. Metab Brain Dis 19(3–4):169–175

66. Fujioka M, Taoka T, Matsuo Y, Mishima K, Ogoshi K, Kondo Y et al (2003) Magnetic resonance imaging shows delayed ischemic striatal neurodegeneration. Ann Neurol 54(6):732–747

67. Chu K, Kang DW, Kim DE, Park SH, Roh JK (2002) Diffusion-weighted and gradient echo magnetic resonance findings of hemichorea-hemiballismus associated with diabetic hyperglycemia: a hyperviscosity syndrome? Arch Neurol 59(3):448–452

68. Shan DE (2005) An explanation for putaminal CT, MR, and diffusion abnormalities secondary to nonketotic hyperglycemia. AJNR 26(1):194; author reply-5

69. Wintermark M, Fischbein NJ, Mukherjee P, Yuh EL, Dillon WP (2004) Unilateral putaminal CT, MR, and diffusion abnormalities secondary to nonketotic hyperglycemia in the setting of acute neurologic symptoms mimicking stroke. AJNR 25(6):975–976

70. Cameron FJ, Kean MJ, Wellard RM, Werther GA, Neil JJ, Inder TE (2005) Insights into the acute cerebral metabolic changes associated with childhood diabetes. Diabet Med 22(5):648–653

71. Gocht A, Colmant HJ (1987) Central pontine and extrapontine myelinolysis: a report of 58 cases. Clin Neuropathol 6(6):262–270

72. Howard SA, Barletta JA, Klufas RA, Saad A, De Girolami U (2009) Best cases from the AFIP: osmotic demyelination syndrome. Radiographics 29(3):933–938

73. Mangat KS, Sherlala K (2002) Cerebellar peduncle myelinolysis: case report. Neuroradiology 44(9):768–769

74. Kim J, Song T, Park S, Choi IS (2007) Cerebellar peduncular myelinolysis in a patient receiving hemodialysis. J Neurol Sci 253(1–2):66–68

75. Hagiwara K, Okada Y, Shida N, Yamashita Y (2008) Extensive central and extrapontine myelinolysis in a case of chronic alcoholism without

hyponatremia: a case report with analysis of serial MR findings. Internal medicine (Tokyo, Japan) 47(5):431–435

76. Huq S, Wong M, Chan H, Crimmins D (2007) Osmotic demyelination syndromes: central and extrapontine myelinolysis. J Clin Neurosci 14(7):684–688

77. Hagiwara A, Yamazaki M, Onoda N (2017) Crown abnormality in osmotic demyelination syndrome. J Neuroradiol 44(5):344–345

78. Tatewaki Y, Kato K, Tanabe Y, Takahashi S (2012) MRI findings of corticosubcortical lesions in osmotic myelinolysis: report of two cases. Br J Radiol 85(1012):e87–e90

79. Kleinschmidt-Demasters BK, Rojiani AM, Filley CM (2006) Central and extrapontine myelinolysis: then...And now. J Neuropathol Exp Neurol 65(1):1–11

80. Ho VB, Fitz CR, Yoder CC, Geyer CA (1993) Resolving MR features in osmotic myelinolysis (central pontine and extrapontine myelinolysis). AJNR 14(1):163–167

81. Sterns RH, Riggs JE, Schochet SS Jr (1986) Osmotic demyelination syndrome following correction of hyponatremia. N Engl J Med 314(24):1535–1542

82. Norenberg MD (1983) A hypothesis of osmotic endothelial injury. A pathogenetic mechanism in central pontine myelinolysis. Arch Neurol 40(2):66–69

83. Lien YH (1995) Role of organic osmolytes in myelinolysis. A topographic study in rats after rapid correction of hyponatremia. J Clin Invest 95(4):1579–1586

84. Miller RF, Harrison MJ, Hall-Craggs MA, Scaravilli F (1998) Central pontine myelinolysis in AIDS. Acta Neuropathol 96(5):537–540

85. Rodriguez J, Benito-Leon J, Molina JA, Ramos A, Bermejo F (1998) Central pontine myelinolysis associated with cyclosporin in liver transplantation. Neurologia (Barcelona, Spain) 13(9):437–440

86. Mascalchi M, Cincotta M, Piazzini M (1993) Case report: MRI demonstration of pontine and thalamic myelinolysis in a normonatremic alcoholic. Clin Radiol 47(2):137–138

87. Cramer SC, Stegbauer KC, Schneider A, Mukai J, Maravilla KR (2001) Decreased diffusion in central pontine myelinolysis. AJNR 22(8):1476–1479

88. Anderson AW, Zhong J, Petroff OA, Szafer A, Ransom BR, Prichard JW et al (1996) Effects of osmotically driven cell volume changes on diffusion-weighted imaging of the rat optic nerve. Magn Reson Med 35(2):162–167

89. Zhong C, Jin L, Fei G (2005) MR imaging of nonalcoholic Wernicke encephalopathy: a follow-up study. AJNR 26(9):2301–2305

90. Fei GQ, Zhong C, Jin L, Wang J, Zhang Y, Zheng X et al (2008) Clinical characteristics and MR imaging features of nonalcoholic Wernicke encephalopathy. AJNR 29(1):164–169

91. Zuccoli G, Gallucci M, Capellades J, Regnicolo L, Tumiati B, Giadas TC et al (2007) Wernicke enceph-

alopathy: MR findings at clinical presentation in twenty-six alcoholic and nonalcoholic patients. AJNR 28(7):1328–1331

92. Morcos Z (2003) Diffusion abnormalities and Wernicke encephalopathy. Neurology 60(4):727–728; author reply -8

93. Loh Y, Watson WD, Verma A, Krapiva P (2005) Restricted diffusion of the splenium in acute Wernicke's encephalopathy. J Neuroimaging 15(4):373–375

94. Bae SJ, Lee HK, Lee JH, Choi CG, Suh DC (2001) Wernicke's encephalopathy: atypical manifestation at MR imaging. AJNR 22(8):1480–1482

95. Doherty MJ, Watson NF, Uchino K, Hallam DK, Cramer SC (2002) Diffusion abnormalities in patients with Wernicke encephalopathy. Neurology 58(4):655–657

96. Manzo G, De Gennaro A, Cozzolino A, Serino A, Fenza G, Manto A (2014) MR imaging findings in alcoholic and nonalcoholic acute Wernicke's encephalopathy: a review. Biomed Res Int 2014:503596

97. Sparacia G, Anastasi A, Speciale C, Agnello F, Banco A (2017) Magnetic resonance imaging in the assessment of brain involvement in alcoholic and nonalcoholic Wernicke's encephalopathy. World J Radiol 9(2):72–78

98. Bergui M, Bradac GB, Zhong JJ, Barbero PA, Durelli L (2001) Diffusion-weighted MR in reversible wernicke encephalopathy. Neuroradiology 43(11):969–972

99. White ML, Zhang Y, Andrew LG, Hadley WL (2005) MR imaging with diffusion-weighted imaging in acute and chronic Wernicke encephalopathy. AJNR 26(9):2306–2310

100. Oka M, Terae S, Kobayashi R, Kudoh K, Chu BC, Kaneko K et al (2001) Diffusion-weighted MR findings in a reversible case of acute Wernicke encephalopathy. Acta Neurol Scand 104(3):178–181

101. Capizzano AA, Sanchez A, Moritani T, Yager J (2012) Hyperammonemic encephalopathy: time course of MRI diffusion changes. Neurology 78(8):600–601

102. Sureka J, Jakkani RK, Panwar S (2012) MRI findings in acute hyperammonemic encephalopathy resulting from decompensated chronic liver disease. Acta Neurol Belg 112(2):221–223

103. Rosario M, McMahon K, Finelli PF (2013) Diffusion-weighted imaging in acute hyper-ammonemic encephalopathy. Neurohospitalist 3(3):125–130

104. McKinney AM, Lohman BD, Sarikaya B, Uhlmann E, Spanbauer J, Singewald T et al (2010) Acute hepatic encephalopathy: diffusion-weighted and fluid-attenuated inversion recovery findings, and correlation with plasma ammonia level and clinical outcome. AJNR 31(8):1471–1479

105. Zhang LJ, Zhong J, Lu GM (2013) Multimodality MR imaging findings of low-grade brain edema in hepatic encephalopathy. AJNR 34(4):707–715

106. Grover VP, Crossey MM, Fitzpatrick JA, Saxby BK, Shaw R, Waldman AD et al (2016) Quantitative magnetic resonance imaging in patients with cirrhosis: a cross-sectional study. Metab Brain Dis 31(6):1315–1325

107. Schilsky ML (2017) Wilson disease: diagnosis, treatment, and follow-up. Clin Liver Dis 21(4):755–767

108. Hermann W (2014) Morphological and functional imaging in neurological and non-neurological Wilson's patients. Ann N Y Acad Sci 1315:24–29

109. Zhong W, Huang Z, Tang X (2019) A study of brain MRI characteristics and clinical features in 76 cases of Wilson's disease. J Clin Neurosci 59:167–174

110. Sinha S, Taly AB, Ravishankar S, Prashanth LK, Venugopal KS, Arunodaya GR et al (2006) Wilson's disease: cranial MRI observations and clinical correlation. Neuroradiology 48(9):613–621

111. Favrole P, Chabriat H, Guichard JP, Woimant F (2006) Clinical correlates of cerebral water diffusion in Wilson disease. Neurology 66(3):384–389

112. El-Hattab AW, Adesina AM, Jones J, Scaglia F (2015) MELAS syndrome: clinical manifestations, pathogenesis, and treatment options. Mol Genet Metab 116(1–2):4–12

113. Finsterer J (2008) Leigh and Leigh-like syndrome in children and adults. Pediatr Neurol 39(4):223–235

114. Tzoulis C, Bindoff LA (2009) Serial diffusion imaging in a case of mitochondrial encephalomyopathy, lactic acidosis, and stroke-like episodes. Stroke 40(2):e15–e17

115. Armstrong AE, Gillan E, DiMario FJ Jr (2014) SMART syndrome (stroke-like migraine attacks after radiation therapy) in adult and pediatric patients. J Child Neurol 29(3):336–341

116. Black DF, Morris JM, Lindell EP, Krecke KN, Worrell GA, Bartleson JD et al (2013) Stroke-like migraine attacks after radiation therapy (SMART) syndrome is not always completely reversible: a case series. AJNR 34(12):2298–2303

117. Boogerd W, vd Sande JJ, Moffie D (1988) Acute fever and delayed leukoencephalopathy following low dose intraventricular methotrexate. J Neurol Neurosurg Psychiatry 51(10):1277–1283

118. Bernini JC, Fort DW, Griener JC, Kane BJ, Chappell WB, Kamen BA (1995) Aminophylline for methotrexate-induced neurotoxicity. Lancet 345(8949):544–547

119. Afshar M, Birnbaum D, Golden C (2014) Review of dextromethorphan administration in 18 patients with subacute methotrexate central nervous system toxicity. Pediatr Neurol 50(6):625–629

120. Salkade PR, Lim TA (2012) Methotrexate-induced acute toxic leukoencephalopathy. J Cancer Res Ther 8(2):292–296

121. Kim JY, Kim ST, Nam DH, Lee JI, Park K, Kong DS (2011) Leukoencephalopathy and disseminated necrotizing leukoencephalopathy following intrathecal methotrexate chemotherapy and radiation therapy for central nerve system lymphoma or leukemia. J Korean Neurosurg Soc 50(4):304–310

122. Levin G, Chill HH, Rottenstreich A (2017) Transverse myelitis following methotrexate treatment of ectopic pregnancy: a case report. Eur J Contracept Reprod Health Care 22(6):476–478

123. Ackermann R, Semmler A, Maurer GD, Hattingen E, Fornoff F, Steinbach JP et al (2010) Methotrexate-induced myelopathy responsive to substitution of multiple folate metabolites. J Neuro-Oncol 97(3):425–427

124. Ho CH, Lo CP, Tu MC (2014) Bortezomib-induced posterior reversible encephalopathy syndrome: clinical and imaging features. Intern Med 53(16):1853–1857

125. Larsen FO, Hansen SW (2004) Severe neurotoxicity caused by gemcitabine treatment. Acta Oncol 43(6):590–591

126. Cioffi P, Laudadio L, Nuzzo A, Belfiglio M, Petrelli F, Grappasonni I (2012) Gemcitabine-induced posterior reversible encephalopathy syndrome: a case report. J Oncol Pharm Pract 18(2):299–302

127. Han CH, Findlay MP (2010) Chemotherapy-induced reversible posterior leucoencephalopathy syndrome. Intern Med J 40(2):153–159

128. Martin G, Bellido L, Cruz JJ (2007) Reversible posterior leukoencephalopathy syndrome induced by sunitinib. J Clin Oncol 25(23):3559

129. Padhy BM, Shanmugam SP, Gupta YK, Goyal A (2011) Reversible posterior leucoencephalopathy syndrome in an elderly male on sunitinib therapy. Br J Clin Pharmacol 71(5):777–779

130. Palma JA, Gomez-Ibanez A, Martin B, Urrestarazu E, Gil-Bazo I, Pastor MA (2011) Nonconvulsive status epilepticus related to posterior reversible leukoencephalopathy syndrome induced by cetuximab. Neurologist 17(5):273–275

131. Terwiel E, Hanrahan R, Lueck C, D'Rozario J (2010) Reversible posterior encephalopathy syndrome associated with bortezomib. Intern Med J 40(1):69–71

132. Hedley-Whyte ET (2000) Leukoencephalopathy and raised brain lactate from heroin vapor inhalation. Neurology 54(10):2027–2028

133. Kriegstein AR, Shungu DC, Millar WS, Armitage BA, Brust JC, Chillrud S et al (1999) Leukoencephalopathy and raised brain lactate from heroin vapor inhalation ("chasing the dragon"). Neurology 53(8):1765–1773

134. Barrons RW, Nguyen LT (2018) Succinylcholine-induced Rhabdomyolysis in adults: case report and review of the literature. J Pharm Pract. https://doi.org/10.1177/0897190018795983

135. Richards JR, Garber D, Laurin EG, Albertson TE, Derlet RW, Amsterdam EA et al (2016) Treatment of cocaine cardiovascular toxicity: a systematic review. Clin Toxicol (Phila) 54(5):345–364

136. Bey T, Patel A (2007) Phencyclidine intoxication and adverse effects: a clinical and pharmacological review of an illicit drug. Cal J Emerg Med 8(1):9–14

137. Wodarz N, Krampe-Scheidler A, Christ M, Fleischmann H, Looser W, Schoett K et al (2017) Evidence-based guidelines for the pharmacological Management of Acute Methamphetamine-Related Disorders and Toxicity. Pharmacopsychiatry 50(3):87–95

138. Chalela JA, Kasner SE (2018) Acute toxic-metabolic encephalopathy in adults. December 28. https://www.uptodate.com/contents/acute-toxic-metabolic-encephalopathy-in-adults

139. Weinhouse GL, Young B (2018) Hypoxic-ischemic brain injury in adults: evaluation and prognosis. December 28. https://www.uptodate.com/contents/hypoxic-ischemic-brain-injury-in-adults-evaluation-and-prognosis

140. Khot S, Tirschwell DL (2006) Long-term neurological complications after hypoxic-ischemic encephalopathy. Semin Neurol 26(4):422–431

141. Patel R, Jha S (2004) Intravenous valproate in post-anoxic myoclonic status epilepticus: a report of ten patients. Neurol India 52(3):394–396

142. Gupta HV, Caviness JN (2016) Post-hypoxic myoclonus: current concepts, neurophysiology, and treatment. Tremor Other Hyperkinet Mov (N Y) 6:409

143. van Rooij LG, Toet MC, van Huffelen AC, Groenendaal F, Laan W, Zecic A et al (2010) Effect of treatment of subclinical neonatal seizures detected with aEEG: randomized, controlled trial. Pediatrics 125(2):e358–e366

144. Tagin MA, Woolcott CG, Vincer MJ, Whyte RK, Stinson DA (2012) Hypothermia for neonatal hypoxic ischemic encephalopathy: an updated systematic review and meta-analysis. Arch Pediatr Adolesc Med 166(6):558–566

145. Roka A, Azzopardi D (2010) Therapeutic hypothermia for neonatal hypoxic ischaemic encephalopathy. Early Hum Dev 86(6):361–367

146. Oyer DS (2013) The science of hypoglycemia in patients with diabetes. Curr Diabetes Rev 9(3):195–208

147. Rickels MR, Ruedy KJ, Foster NC, Piche CA, Dulude H, Sherr JL et al (2016) Intranasal glucagon for treatment of insulin-induced Hypoglycemia in adults with type 1 Diabetes: a randomized crossover noninferiority study. Diabetes Care 39(2):264–270

148. Davies MJ, D'Alessio DA, Fradkin J, Kernan WN, Mathieu C, Mingrone G et al (2018) Management of Hyperglycemia in type 2 Diabetes, 2018. A consensus report by the American Diabetes Association (ADA) and the European Association for the Study of Diabetes (EASD). Diabetes Care 41(12):2669–2701

149. Halter JB, Musi N, McFarland Horne F, Crandall JP, Goldberg A, Harkless L et al (2014) Diabetes and cardiovascular disease in older adults: current status and future directions. Diabetes 63(8):2578–2589

150. Brito JP, Montori VM, Davis AM (2017) Metabolic surgery in the treatment algorithm for type 2 Diabetes: a joint statement by international Diabetes organizations. JAMA 317(6):635–636

151. American Diabetes A (2018) 7. Obesity Management for the Treatment of type 2 Diabetes: standards of medical Care in Diabetes-2018. Diabetes Care 41(Suppl 1):S65–S72

152. Fayfman M, Pasquel FJ, Umpierrez GE (2017) Management of Hyperglycemic Crises: diabetic ketoacidosis and Hyperglycemic hyperosmolar state. Med Clin North Am 101(3):587–606

153. Lever E, Jaspan JB (1983) Sodium bicarbonate therapy in severe diabetic ketoacidosis. Am J Med 75(2):263–268

154. Bureau MA, Begin R, Berthiaume Y, Shapcott D, Khoury K, Gagnon N (1980) Cerebral hypoxia from bicarbonate infusion in diabetic acidosis. J Pediatr 96(6):968–973

155. Kannan CR (1999) Bicarbonate therapy in the management of severe diabetic ketoacidosis. Crit Care Med 27(12):2833–2834

156. Kraut JA, Madias NE (2012) Treatment of acute metabolic acidosis: a pathophysiologic approach. Nat Rev Nephrol 8(10):589–601

157. Fraley DS, Adler S (1977) Correction of hyperkalemia by bicarbonate despite constant blood pH. Kidney Int 12(5):354–360

158. Hale PJ, Crase J, Nattrass M (1984) Metabolic effects of bicarbonate in the treatment of diabetic ketoacidosis. Br Med J (Clin Res Ed) 289(6451):1035–1038

159. Murad MH, Coto-Yglesias F, Wang AT, Sheidaee N, Mullan RJ, Elamin MB et al (2009) Clinical review: drug-induced hypoglycemia: a systematic review. J Clin Endocrinol Metab 94(3):741–745

160. Desimone ME, Weinstock RS (2000) Non-diabetic Hypoglycemia. In: De Groot LJ, Chrousos G, Dungan K, Feingold KR, Grossman A, Hershman JM et al (eds) . Endotext, South Dartmouth, MA

161. Tetzschner R, Norgaard K, Ranjan A (2018) Effects of alcohol on plasma glucose and prevention of alcohol-induced hypoglycemia in type 1 diabetes-a systematic review with GRADE. Diabetes Metab Res Rev 34(3):e2965

162. Gill GV, Rauf O, MacFarlane IA (1997) Diazoxide treatment for insulinoma: a national UK survey. Postgrad Med J 73(864):640–641

163. Caliri M, Verdiani V, Mannucci E, Briganti V, Landoni L, Esposito A et al (2018) A case of malignant insulinoma responsive to somatostatin analogs treatment. BMC Endocr Disord 18(1):98

164. Hirshberg B, Cochran C, Skarulis MC, Libutti SK, Alexander HR, Wood BJ et al (2005) Malignant insulinoma: spectrum of unusual clinical features. Cancer 104(2):264–272

165. Marik PE, Bellomo R (2013) Stress hyperglycemia: an essential survival response! Crit Care Med 41(6):e93–e94

166. Kwon S, Thompson R, Dellinger P, Yanez D, Farrohki E, Flum D (2013) Importance of perioperative glycemic control in general surgery: a report from the surgical care and outcomes assessment program. Ann Surg 257(1):8–14

167. Evans CH, Lee J, Ruhlman MK (2015) Optimal glucose management in the perioperative period. Surg Clin North Am 95(2):337–354

168. Hampson NB, Piantadosi CA, Thom SR, Weaver LK (2012) Practice recommendations in the diagnosis, management, and prevention of carbon monoxide poisoning. Am J Respir Crit Care Med 186(11):1095–1101

169. Rose JJ, Wang L, Xu Q, McTiernan CF, Shiva S, Tejero J et al (2017) Carbon monoxide poisoning: pathogenesis, management, and future directions of therapy. Am J Respir Crit Care Med 195(5):596–606

170. Buckley NA, Juurlink DN, Isbister G, Bennett MH, Lavonas EJ (2011) Hyperbaric oxygen for carbon monoxide poisoning. Cochrane Database Syst Rev 4:CD002041

171. Buboltz JB, Robins M (2018) Hyperbaric, carbon monoxide toxicity. StatPearls, Treasure Island (FL

172. Shah MK, Al-Adawi S, Dorvlo AS, Burke DT (2004) Functional outcomes following anoxic brain injury: a comparison with traumatic brain injury. Brain Inj 18(2):111–117

173. Weinberger LM, Schmidley JW, Schafer IA, Raghavan S (1994) Delayed postanoxic demyelination and arylsulfatase-a pseudodeficiency. Neurology 44(1):152–154

174. Wang WC, Yang HC, Chen YJ (2015) Acute multiple focal neuropathies and delayed postanoxic encephalopathy after alcohol intoxication. Neuropsychiatr Dis Treat 11:1781–1784

175. Sterns RH (2018) Treatment of severe Hyponatremia. Clin J Am Soc Nephrol 13(4):641–649

176. Soupart A, Ngassa M, Decaux G (1999) Therapeutic relowering of the serum sodium in a patient after excessive correction of hyponatremia. Clin Nephrol 51(6):383–386

177. Oya S, Tsutsumi K, Ueki K, Kirino T (2001) Reinduction of hyponatremia to treat central pontine myelinolysis. Neurology 57(10):1931–1932

178. Perianayagam A, Sterns RH, Silver SM, Grieff M, Mayo R, Hix J et al (2008) DDAVP is effective in preventing and reversing inadvertent overcorrection of hyponatremia. Clin J Am Soc Nephrol 3(2):331–336

179. MacMillan TE, Cavalcanti RB (2018) Outcomes in severe Hyponatremia treated with and without Desmopressin. Am J Med 131(3):317 e1–317e10

180. Bibl D, Lampl C, Gabriel C, Jungling G, Brock H, Kostler G (1999) Treatment of central pontine myelinolysis with therapeutic plasmapheresis. Lancet 353(9159):1155

181. Cook CC, Hallwood PM, Thomson AD (1998) B vitamin deficiency and neuropsychiatric syndromes in alcohol misuse. Alcohol Alcohol 33(4):317–336

182. Manzardo AM, Penick EC (2006) A theoretical argument for inherited thiamine insensitivity as one possible biological cause of familial alcoholism. Alcohol Clin Exp Res 30(9):1545–1550

183. Schabelman E, Kuo D (2012) Glucose before thiamine for Wernicke encephalopathy: a literature review. J Emerg Med 42(4):488–494

184. Carrilho PE, Santos MB, Piasecki L, Jorge AC (2013) Marchiafava-Bignami disease: a rare entity with a poor outcome. Rev Bras Ter Intensiva 25(1):68–72

185. Haas L, Tjan D, Van Die J, Vos A, van Zanten A (2006) Coma in an alcoholic: Marchiafava-Bignami disease. N Z Med J 119(1244):U2280

186. Castillo P, Woodruff B, Caselli R, Vernino S, Lucchinetti C, Swanson J et al (2006) Steroid-responsive encephalopathy associated with autoimmune thyroiditis. Arch Neurol 63(2):197–202

187. Marshall GA, Doyle JJ (2006) Long-term treatment of Hashimoto's encephalopathy. J Neuropsychiatry Clin Neurosci 18(1):14–20

188. Olmez I, Moses H, Sriram S, Kirshner H, Lagrange AH, Pawate S (2013) Diagnostic and therapeutic aspects of Hashimoto's encephalopathy. J Neurol Sci 331(1–2):67–71

189. Drulovic J, Andrejevic S, Bonaci-Nikolic B, Mijailovic V (2011) Hashimoto's encephalopathy: a long-lasting remission induced by intravenous immunoglobulins. Vojnosanit Pregl 68(5):452–454

190. Boers PM, Colebatch JG (2001) Hashimoto's encephalopathy responding to plasmapheresis. J Neurol Neurosurg Psychiatry 70(1):132

191. Mollaret GM (1959) The depassed coma (preliminary memoir). Rev Neurol (Paris) 101:3–15

192. Truog RD, Pope TM, Jones DS (2018) The 50-Year Legacy of the Harvard Report on Brain Death. JAMA 320(4):335–336

193. Ad Hoc Committee of the Harvard Medical School to Examine the Definition of Brain Death (1968) A definition of irreversible coma. JAMA 205(6):337–340

194. Guidelines for the determination of death: Report of the medical consultants on the diagnosis of death to the President's commission for the study of ethical problems in medicine and biochemical and behavioral research (1981). JAMA 246:2184–2186

195. Uniform Law Commission (2008) Uniform Determination of Death Act, 12A uniform laws annotated 777. June 1. http://www.uniformlaws.org/Act.aspx?title=Determination%20of%20Death%20Act

196. Practice parameters for determining brain death in adults (summary statement) (1995) The Quality Standards Subcommittee of the American Academy of Neurology. Neurology May 45(5):1012–1014

197. Wijdicks EF, Varelas PN, Gronseth GS, Greer DM, American Academy of Neurology (2010) Evidence-based guideline update: determining brain death in adults: report of the quality standards Subcommittee of the American Academy of neurology. Neurology 74(23):1911–1918

198. Wijdicks EF (2002) Brain death worldwide: accepted fact but no global consensus in diagnostic criteria. Neurology 58(1):20–25

199. Black PM (1978) Brain death (first of two parts). N Engl J Med 299(7):338–344

200. Wijdicks EF, Pfeifer EA (2008) Neuropathology of brain death in the modern transplant era. Neurology 70(15):1234–1237

201. Wijdicks EF (1995) Determining brain death in adults. Neurology 45(5):1003–1011

202. Fugate JE, Rabinstein AA, Wijdicks EF (2011) Blood pressure patterns after brain death. Neurology 77(4):399–401

203. Lustbader D, O'Hara D, Wijdicks EF, MacLean L, Tajik W, Ying A, Berg E, Goldstein M (2011) Second brain death examination may negatively affect organ donation. Neurology 76(2):119–124

204. Wijdicks EF, Rabinstein AA, Manno EM, Atkinson JD (2008) Pronouncing brain death: Contemporary practice and safety of the apnea test. Neurology 71(16):1240–1244

205. Greer DM, Wang HH, Robinson JD, Varelas PN, Henderson GV, Wijdicks EF (2016) Variability of brain death policies in the United States. JAMA Neurol 73(2):213–218

206. Bernat JL, Culver CM, Gert B (1981) On the definition and criterion of death. Ann Intern Med 94(3):389–394

207. Shewmon DA (1998) Chronic "brain death": meta-analysis and conceptual consequences. Neurology 51(6):1538–1545

208. The President's Council on Bioethics (2008) Controversies in the determination of death: a white paper by the President's Council on Bioethics. June 1. https://bioethicsarchive.georgetown.edu/pcbe/reports/death/

Infectious Diseases

16

Toshio Moritani, Yoshiaki Ota, and Patricia A. Kirby

Eiyu Matsumoto

16.1 Overview of Brain Infections

Infections of the brain are caused by bacteria, virus, fungi, or parasites. Bacterial infections are often related to septic emboli and extracranial infections spreading intracranially and intra-axially. This can result in cerebritis and brain abscesses. Viral infections are more diffuse and cause encephalitis and vasculitis. Toxoplasmosis, which is the most common parasitic infection of the brain, causes encephalitis and abscesses, while disseminated aspergillosis causes vasculitis-mediated infarctions resulting in extensive cerebritis and/or abscess formation.

The pathophysiology and the imaging findings vary greatly depending on the organism causing the infection. Diffusion-weighted (DW) imaging is useful for the diagnosis of infectious conditions of the brain by means of differentiat-ing vasogenic edema from cytotoxic edema [1]. DW imaging can also separate abscesses from cystic and necrotic tumors [2–6].

16.2 Bacterial Infection

16.2.1 Brain Abscess and Cerebritis

Bacterial brain abscesses are potentially fatal, but can often be medically and surgically treated if detected early. Symptoms are often nonspecific and vague, and imaging is therefore necessary for detection and characterization.

A brain abscess begins as a focal area of microvascular injury, usually at the gray–white matter junction or deeper in the white matter. Pathologically the initial stage of a brain abscess is a focal area of cerebritis or presuppurative encephalitis. This is characterized by early necrosis of the cerebral parenchyma, vascular congestion, petechial hemorrhage, neutrophil infiltration, and vasogenic edema [7–9]. DW imaging shows a variety of signal characteristics in the area of the cerebritis with mildly increased or decreased ADC, presumably depending on the degree of inflammatory cell infiltration and types of edema (cytotoxic or vasogenic).

Late cerebritis is characterized by a necrotic and purulent center. This evolves into frank abscess formation, which is characterized by central pus, inflammatory granulation tissue, and a fibrous capsule. The pus usually consists of both

T. Moritani (✉)
Division of Neuroradiology, University of Michigan, Ann Arbor, MI, USA
e-mail: tmoritan@med.umich.edu

Y. Ota
Department of Radiology, University of Michigan, Ann Arbor, MI, USA
e-mail: yoshiako@umich.edu

P. A. Kirby · E. Matsumoto
University of Iowa Hospitals & Clinics, Iowa City, IA, USA
e-mail: patricia-kirby@uiowa.edu;
eiyu-matsumoto@uiowa.edu

© Springer Nature Switzerland AG 2021
T. Moritani, A. A. Capizzano (eds.), *Diffusion-Weighted MR Imaging of the Brain, Head and Neck, and Spine*, https://doi.org/10.1007/978-3-030-62120-9_16

dead and viable neutrophils, necrosis, and bacteria. Even in the chronic phase of an abscess, neutrophils and necrosis can still be found (Fig. 16.1).

The early phase of the brain abscess has a homogeneous, bright signal on DW imaging associated with decreased apparent diffusion coefficient (ADC) (Figs. 16.2 and 16.3). The late phase of an abscess can still show hyperintensity on DW images, but ADC values are partially increased (Fig. 16.1) [10]. A possible explanation for the high signal on DW imaging is restriction of water mobility due to the high viscosity of coagulative necrosis and the prominence of polynucleated neutrophils in the pus. DW imaging is superior to conventional MR imaging in evaluating the success or failure of abscess therapy [11].

A brain abscess cavity shows regions of increased fractional anisotropy (FA) values with restricted mean diffusivity (Fig. 16.3) [12]. Geometrical analysis shows that a planar shape of the diffusion tensor is more frequently observed in the abscess than that in the normal

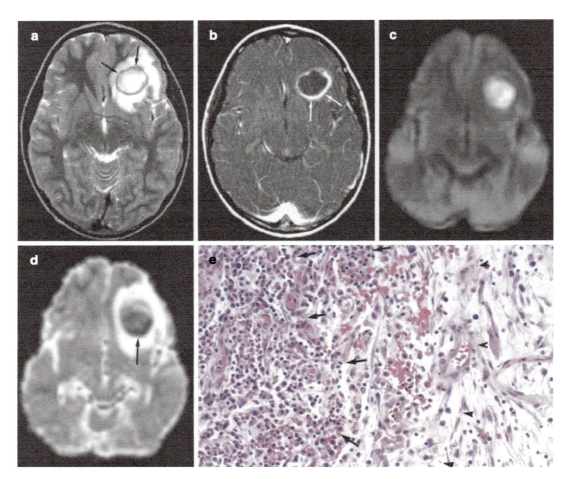

Fig. 16.1 Streptococcal brain abscess in a 7-year-old boy presenting with a week-long severe headache. (**a**) T2-weighted image shows a central hyperintense mass lesion with low-signal rim (*black arrows*) and peripheral edema in the left frontal lobe. (**b**) Gadolinium-enhanced T1-weighted image with magnetization transfer contrast shows this mass with ring enhancement. (**c**) DW image shows a central cystic component as hyperintense. (**d**) ADC map shows a fluid–fluid level and partially decreased ADC of this component, which is sometimes observed in the late phase of the abscess. (**e**) Pathology shows numerous neutrophils (*arrows*) in the center of the abscess with surrounding granulation tissue and organizing fibrous capsule, and in the pus and granulomatous fibrous capsules (*arrowheads*) in a chronic abscess

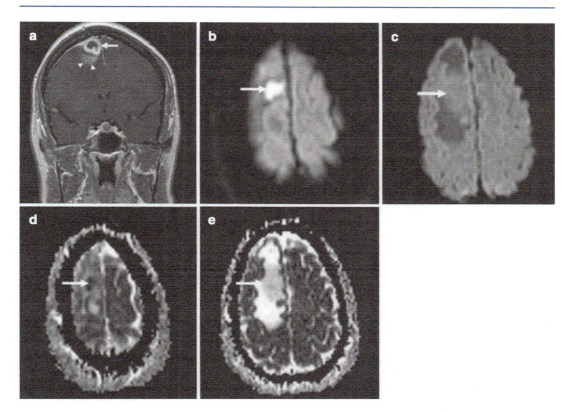

Fig. 16.2 Streptococcal brain abscess in a 48-year-old woman presenting with headache. (**a**) Gadolinium-enhanced coronal T1-weighted image shows a ring-enhancing mass (*arrow*) and enhancement (*arrowheads*) in the surrounding edema, consistent with abscess and cerebritis. There is an incidental finding of a Rathke's cleft cyst in the pituitary gland. (**b, c**) DW image shows an abscess as hyperintense (*arrow*) (**b**) and cerebritis as isointense (*arrow*) (**c**). (**d, e**) ADC map shows the abscess as decreased ADC (*arrow*) (**d**) and the cerebritis as mildly increased ADC (*arrow*) which is lower than the surrounding edema (**e**)

white matter tract in which the diffusion tensor is predominantly of a linear shape. This phenomenon presumably reflects adherent inflammatory cells, tangled up with each other, inside the abscess cavity [13].

16.2.2 Septic Emboli

The main risk factors for brain abscesses are bacterial endocarditis and chronic suppurative intrathoracic infections [14]. If septic emboli of sufficient size are lodged in an intracerebral arterial vessel, infarction can occur. Infarctions are bright on DW imaging, with decreased ADC (Fig. 16.4). Septic infarctions usually occur in the distal cortical branch territories, while small septic emboli are characteristically found in the cortical-white matter junction. It can take a few weeks and up to several months for septic emboli to develop into an abscess. Serial DW imaging is therefore often useful in patients at risk for septic encephalopathy. By means of repeated DW imaging, it is possible to identify the initial infarction and the subsequent cerebritis/abscess evolution [15]. This allows for early treatment.

16.2.3 Brain Abscess Caused by Unusual Bacteria

The classical finding in a brain abscess is a cystic lesion with marked enhancement following contrast medium injection. On DW imaging,

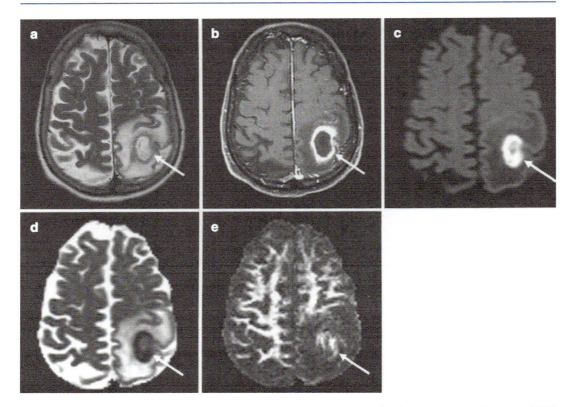

Fig. 16.3 Brain abscess with mixed anaerobe bacteria in an 86-year-old woman presenting with right upper and lower extremity weakness and seizures. (**a**) T2-weighted image shows a central hyperintense mass with low-signal rim and peripheral edema in the left frontoparietal region (*arrow*). (**b**) Gadolinium-enhanced T1-weighted image shows this mass with ring enhancement (*arrow*), (**c**) DW image shows a central cystic component as hyperintense. (**d**) ADC map shows decreased ADC of this component (*arrow*). (**e**) FA map shows increased FA values in the abscess (*arrow*)

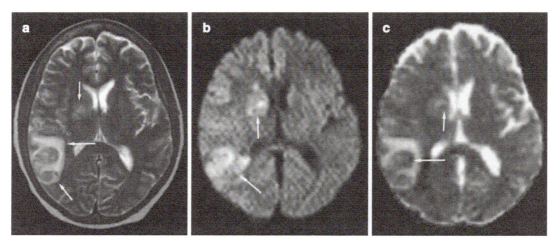

Fig. 16.4 Septic emboli from staphylococcus endocarditis in a 44-year-old woman presenting with left hemiparesis of 3 days' duration. (**a**) T2-weighted image shows hyperintense lesions in the right basal ganglia and posteriorly in the middle cerebral artery territory (*arrows*). (**b**) DW image shows these lesions as hyperintense (*arrows*). (**c**) ADC map shows these lesions as decreased ADC, mainly representing infarcts (*arrows*)

the cystic area shows a high signal and ADC is reduced. However, the characteristics of brain abscess appear to be related to the type of organism and the immunity of the host. Thus, in an immunodeficient patient with sepsis, multiple micro-abscesses are often observed. Multiple micro-abscesses may involve basal ganglia bilaterally and mimic small infarcts (Fig. 16.5) [16].

Listeria monocytogenes is a facultative intracellular non-spore-forming gram-positive bacillus. Listeria infection, usually seen in immunocompromised hosts, is often associated with extensive parenchymal involvement, especially in the brain stem and basal ganglia [17]. The ability to cross the meninges and blood–brain barrier is thought to be the result of endothelial cell or macrophage phagocytosis of the organisms, which use the host-cell contractile system to migrate to and grow within the brain. A central small abscess may be seen as high signal on DW imaging with decreased ADC with the surrounding vasogenic edema (Fig. 16.6).

Nocardia asteroides is an aerobic acid-fast branching gram-positive bacterium. Nocardia infection is under-reported and often goes unrecognized. Nocardia brain abscesses have mortality rates three times higher than usual bacterial brain abscesses. It may be curable with long-term trimethoprim–sulfamethoxazole. Immunodeficiency makes the prognosis poorer than in immunocompetent patients [18, 19]. DW imaging shows some lesions as low ADC and others as iso ADC (Fig. 16.7).

Tuberculous abscess has been reported to be seen as hyperintensity with low ADC, probably due to the presence of intact inflammatory cells in the pus [20, 21]. The diffusion abnormality of the caseous necrosis may be variable depending on the degree of liquefaction [22].

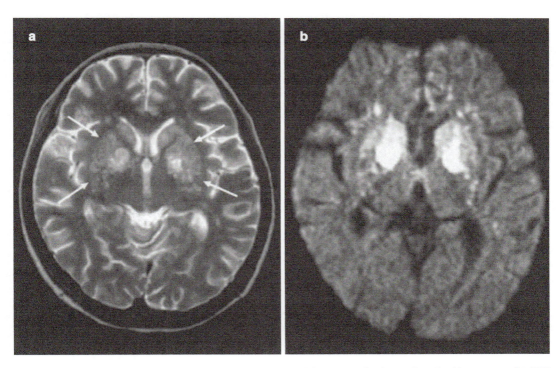

Fig. 16.5 Brain abscesses due to gram-negative rod bacteria in a 28-year-old woman with Crohn's disease and long-term steroid use presenting with headache. Blood culture showed gram-negative rods. (**a**) T2-weighted image shows multiple small hyperintense lesions in bilateral basal ganglia (*arrows*) and white matter. (**b**) DW image shows these lesions as very hyperintense with decreased ADC (not shown). This finding mimics multiple small infarcts, but it represents multiple small abscesses

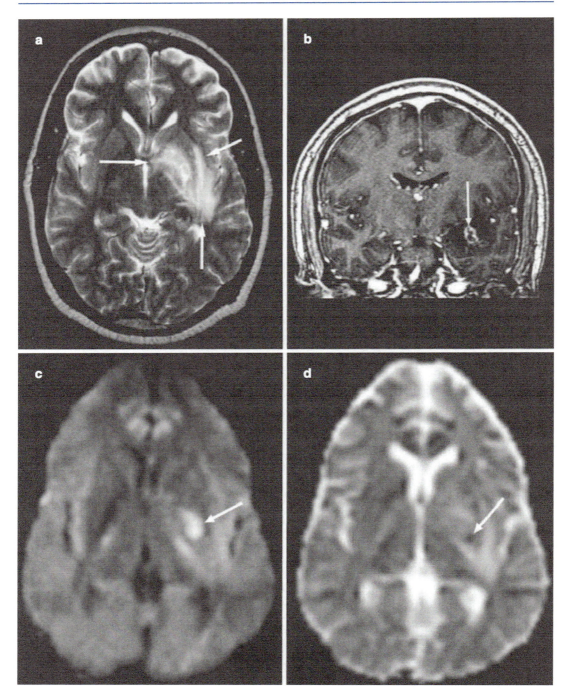

Fig. 16.6 Listeria meningoencephalitis after bone marrow transplantation for chronic myeloblasts leukemia in a 31-year-old man presenting with a 2-day history of severe headache. (**a**) T2-weighted image shows hyperintense lesions in the left basal ganglia, internal capsule, and white matter in the temporal lobe, representing encephalitis (*arrows*). (**b**) Coronal gadolinium-enhanced T1-weighted image shows an irregular ring-enhancing lesion (*arrow*). (**c**) DW image shows a central cystic component as hyperintense with decreased ADC (**d**) (*arrow*), representing an abscess

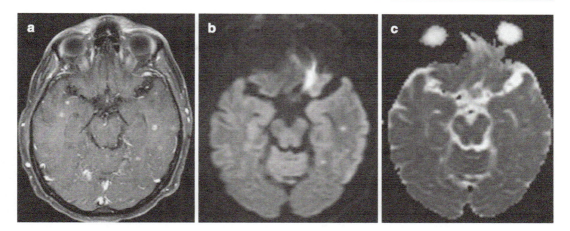

Fig. 16.7 Nocardia abscess in a 50-year-old man with alcohol abuse. (**a**) Gadolinium-enhanced T1-weighted image shows multiple small ring-enhancing lesions in the bilateral temporo-occipital lobes. (**b**, **c**) DW image shows these lesions as hyperintense with decreased ADC (**c**), representing small abscesses

16.2.3.1 Differential Diagnosis

DW imaging can discriminate brain abscesses from cystic or necrotic tumors, which is often difficult with conventional MR imaging (Fig. 16.8) [2–6]. Cystic and necrotic components of the tumor are usually dark on DW images associated with increased ADC. However, there are exceptions; central necrosis of a primary tumor or metastasis can occasionally show the same characteristics with hyperintensity on DW imaging with iso or low ADC values (Fig. 16.9) [23–25]. Sterile and coagulative necrosis, hemorrhage, and viscous mucinous components are possible causes for this finding. The sensitivity and specificity in differentiating cystic/necrotic neoplasms from bacterial abscesses are reported as 85% and 95%, respectively, at the threshold of 1.39 ADC ratio (dividing the ADC values of the nonenhancing portion of the mass by those of contralateral normal-appearing white matter) [23].

Pure coagulative necrosis typically develops after radiofrequency thalamotomy [26]. The lesion often shows hyperintensity on DW imaging, with decreased ADC (Fig. 16.10). Although imaging characteristics are very similar to those of an abscess, the history of the patient and the symptomatology can usually help to differentiate postsurgical lesions from abscesses.

16.2.4 Bacterial Abscess in the Extra-Axial Space

Infections can enter the extra-axial spaces by a variety of mechanisms, including direct spread from an adjacent focus, retrograde septic thrombophlebitis, hematogenous seeding, and sequela of purulent leptomeningitis [27]. Abscesses can occur in epidural (Fig. 16.11), subdural (Fig. 16.12), subarachnoid (Fig. 16.13), or intraventricular spaces (Fig. 16.14) [28, 29]. Wherever they occur, DW imaging shows pus in the abscess as hyperintense, with relatively low ADC values. An exception to the rule can be found in some cases of extra-axial pus collections where the ADC value varies from low to high. Regions of increased ADC presumably represent dilution of the pus with the cerebrospinal fluid or exudate.

16.2.4.1 Differential Diagnosis

Hematomas and epidermoids occasionally have imaging characteristics similar to those of an extra-axial abscess on DW imaging. The hematomas often show hyperintensity with decreased ADC, probably because of the hypercellularity or hyperviscosity (Fig. 16.15) [30, 31]. Epidermoids also show an extra-axial hyperintense lesion on DW imaging (Fig. 16.16) caused by high viscos-

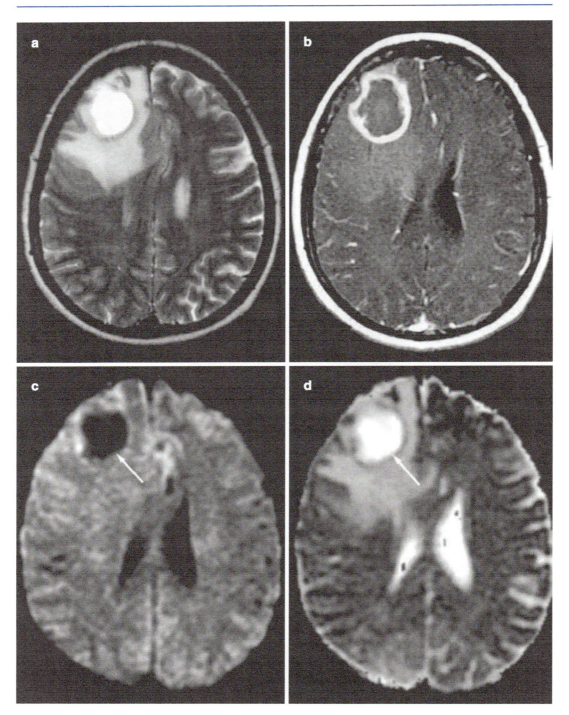

Fig. 16.8 Glioblastoma in a 69-year-old woman. (**a**) T2-weighted image shows a central hyperintense mass lesion with low-signal rim and peripheral edema in the right frontal lobe. (**b**) Gadolinium-enhanced T1-weighted image with magnetization transfer contrast shows this mass with irregular ring enhancement. (**c**) DW image shows a central cystic component as hypointense (*arrow*). (**d**) ADC map shows increased ADC of this cystic component (*arrow*)

16 Infectious Diseases

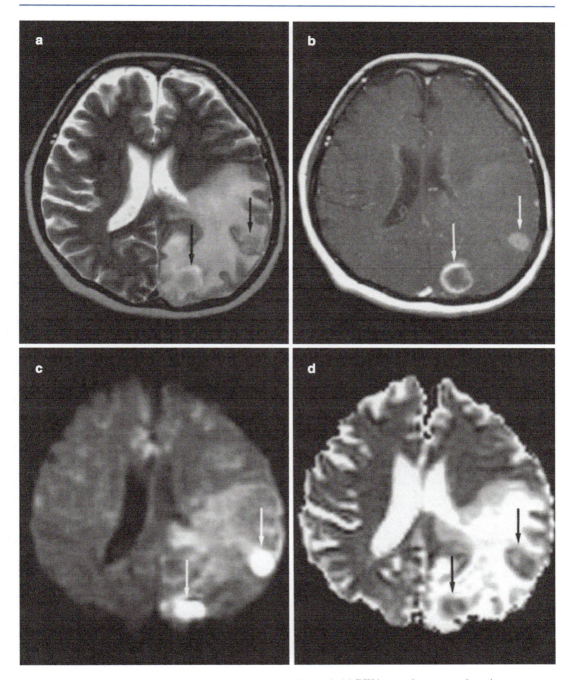

Fig. 16.9 Brain metastasis from adenocarcinoma of the lung in a 44-year-old man. (**a**) T2-weighted image shows multiple mass lesions and peripheral edema in the left parieto-occipital lobe. (**b**) Gadolinium-enhanced T1-weighted image with magnetization transfer contrast shows these lesions with irregular ring enhancement (*arrows*). (**c**) DW image shows central cystic components as hyperintense (*arrows*). (**d**) ADC map shows relative low ADC values of cystic components, presumably representing coagulative necrosis or mucinous substance (*arrows*)

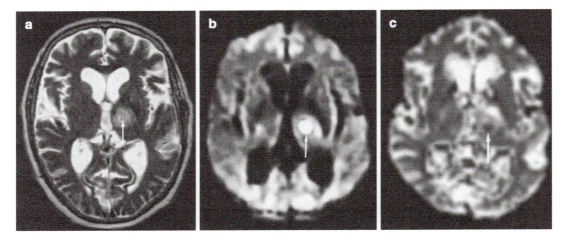

Fig. 16.10 Coagulative necrosis 4 weeks after radiofrequency thalamotomy for essential tremor in a 70-year-old man. (**a**) T2-weighted image shows a hyperintense lesion with mild peripheral edema in the left thalamus (*arrow*). (**b**) DW image shows a central cystic component as hyperintense. (**c**) ADC map shows this component as decreased ADC, probably representing coagulative necrosis. This lesion was decreased in size on follow-up MR imaging without antibiotic treatment

ity keratohyalin-containing materials, which are arranged in layers, as in an onion bulb. ADC maps usually show slightly increased ADC as compared with normal brain parenchyma [32].

16.2.5 Bacterial Vasculitis

Cerebral infarctions secondary to meningitis are well documented in the pediatric age group. Thus, *Streptococcus* B meningitis in neonates can result in infarction, a condition that is rare in adults. The blood–brain/blood–cerebrospinal fluid (CSF) barrier and the mechanical integrity of meninges are immature in young infants, which may explain the preponderance for these changes to occur in babies and young infants [33]. Both arteries and veins can be involved by infection via the perivascular space. Pial arteriolar occlusion causes infarction of the subpial cortex (Fig. 16.17). Although vasculitic changes occur early, they only become prominent resulting in an infarction by the second to third week after onset of the meningeal infection. DW imaging is useful in early detection of the infarction, which is bright on DW imaging, with low ADC.

16.2.6 Whipple Disease

Whipple disease (WD) is a rare bacterial infection and caused by tropheryma whippelii. It predominantly occurs to middle-aged Caucasian male, but precise epidemiology is still unknown [34, 35]. Whipple disease is a systematic disorder, and gastrointestinal, cardia, and CNS systems are mainly involved. WD patients may experience CNS symptoms such as hypersomnia, ophthalmoplegia, myoclonus, ataxia, or upper motor neuron sign without gastrointestinal symptoms such as abdominal pain, malabsorption with diarrhea, and weight loss. Pathophysiology is poorly understood, but the histologic specimens of brain of WD patients revealed that PAS-positive rods and sickle-shaped inclusions in macrophages in central necrosis area and hemorrhage. The prognosis of patients with CNS involvement of WD is poor and approximately 25% of patient died within 4 years, and the cur-

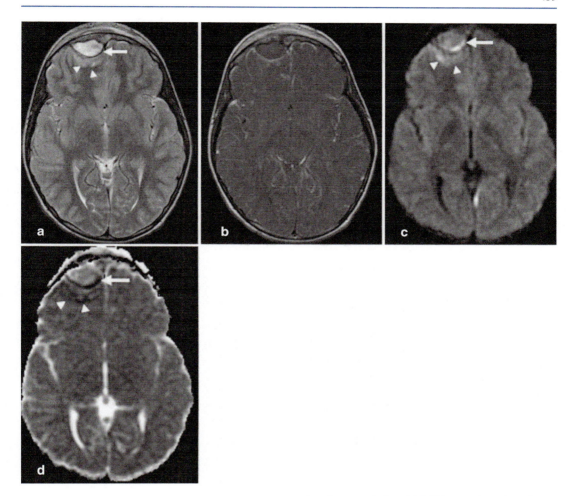

Fig. 16.11 Epidural empyema in a 21-year-old man. (**a**) T2-weighted image shows an epidural hyperintense mass in the right frontal region (*arrows*) and an area of mild hyperintensity noted in the underlying frontal cortex (*arrowheads*). (**b**) Gadolinium-enhanced T1-weighted image with magnetization transfer contrast shows a rim-enhancing mass lesion. (**c**) DW image shows hyperintensity in the epidural empyema (*arrows*) and underlying cerebritis (*arrowhead*). (**d**) ADC map shows the empyema as slightly increased ADC with layer of decreased ADC (*arrow*), and the underlying cerebritis shown as the decreased ADC (*arrowheads*)

rent treatment recommendation for CNS involvement is ceftriaxone, 2 g, intravenously every 12 h for 2 weeks followed by oral trimethoprim-sulfamethoxazole for 1–2 years.

Common findings of MR images are diffuse bilateral hyperintensity on T2WI and FLAIR sequences within midbrain, middle cerebellar peduncle, fronto-temporo-parietal cortex and mesial temporal lobe, hypothalamus, and the corticospinal tracts. Diffusion-weighted image may show restriction (Fig. 16.18).

16.3 Parasitic Infection

16.3.1 Toxoplasmosis

Toxoplasma abscesses consist of ischemic necrosis of the brain tissue associated with sclerosing endoarteritis and a variety of inflammatory reactions. Toxoplasma abscesses are more commonly seen in immunocompromised patients, such as patients with acquired immunodeficiency syndrome (AIDS). In fact, toxoplasma abscesses in

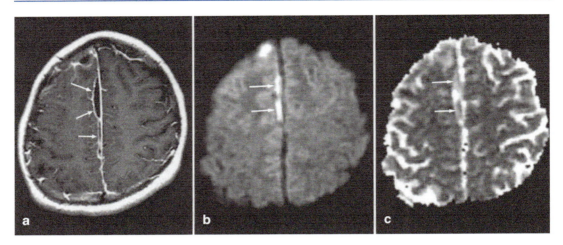

Fig. 16.12 Subdural empyema in a 16-year-old male patient. (**a**) Gadolinium-enhanced T1-weighted image with magnetization transfer contrast shows rim-enhancing lesions along the falx (*arrows*). Mild meningeal enhancement is also seen. (**b**) DW image shows these lesions as hyperintense, representing subdural abscesses (*arrows*). (**c**) ADC map shows these lesions as relatively decreased ADC (*arrows*) compared with CSF. (Courtesy of Morikawa M MD, Nagasaki University, School of Medicine, Japan)

Fig. 16.13 Purulent leptomeningitis in a 77-year-old man. Pneumococcus was proven by CSF examination. (**a**) Coronal fluid-attenuated inversion-recovery image shows hyperintense lesions in subarachnoid space in the right fronto-parietal region (*arrow*). (**b**) Gadolinium-enhanced T1-weighted image with magnetization transfer contrast shows irregular enhancement of these lesions (*arrows*). (**c**) DW image shows these lesions as hyperintense, representing purulent leptomeningitis (*arrows*). (**d**) ADC map shows these lesions as decreased ADC (*arrows*)

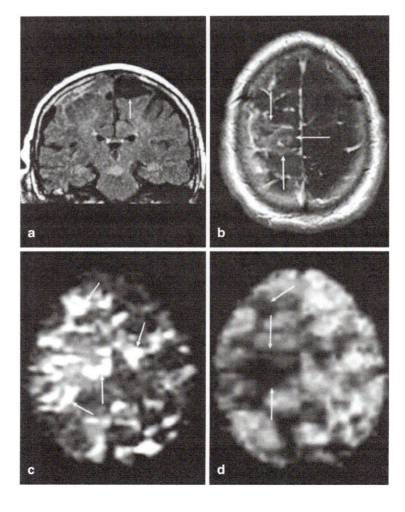

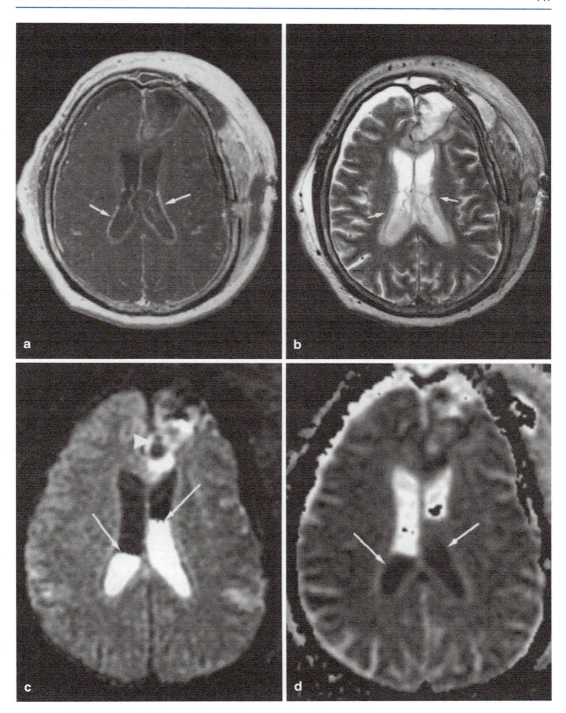

Fig. 16.14 Purulent ventriculitis after surgery in a 60-year-old man. (**a**) Gadolinium-enhanced T1-weighted image with magnetization transfer contrast shows linear enhancement along the ventricle (*arrows*). There are postsurgical changes in the left frontal lobe and extracranially on the left. (**b**) T2-weighted image shows a fluid–fluid level in bilateral lateral ventricles (*arrows*) and postoperative changes in the left frontal lobe (*arrowhead*). (**c**) DW image shows the fluid (*arrows*) as hyperintense, representing purulent ventriculitis, and postoperative changes in the left frontal lobe (*arrowhead*). (**d**) ADC map shows these lesions as decreased ADC

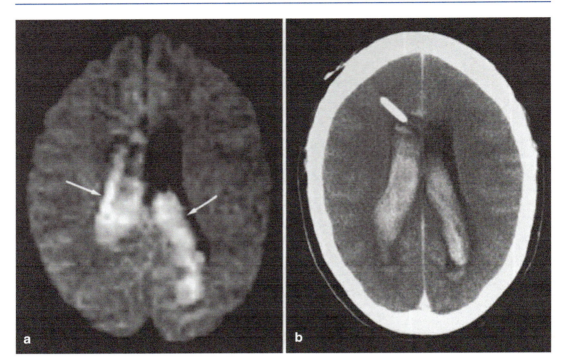

Fig. 16.15 Intraventricular hemorrhage due to arteriovenous malformation in a 29-year-old man. (**a**) DW image shows hyperintense lesions (*arrows*) with decreased ADC (not shown), similar to the finding seen in purulent intraventriculitis. (**b**) Computed tomography shows the high density of intraventricular hemorrhage

AIDS patients were once so common that they were morphologically grouped into three subtypes: (1) poorly circumscribed areas of necrosis (necrotizing abscess), (2) a central area of coagulative necrosis surrounded by macrophages and organism (organizing abscess), and (3) well-demarcated cystic spaces (chronic abscess) [36]. Central necrosis in toxoplasma abscesses does not contain as many inflammatory cells as regular bacterial abscesses.

DW imaging of a toxoplasma abscess has been reported to show no water restriction in the core of the rim-enhancing area, which is helpful in differentiating them from bacterial abscesses and possibly lymphomas (Figs. 16.19 and 16.21) [37, 38]. However, there are exceptions; DW imaging may show a variety of signal characteristics (Fig. 16.20) [38, 39]. Abscesses with different characteristics are occasionally seen in the same patient. This probably reflects the different pathologic/morphologic subtypes such as coagulative or liquefactive necrosis (Fig. 16.20).

16.3.1.1 Differential Diagnosis

The main differential diagnosis is lymphoma. In AIDS patients, central nervous system lymphoma is often associated with central necrosis. This is occasionally liquefactive, presumably related to hypoxia or apoptosis of tumor cells. The enhancing portion of the lesion usually shows hyperintensity on DW imaging, with relatively low ADC due to hypercellularity of lymphomas (Fig. 16.21). A central necrosis typically shows hypointensity on DW imaging with increased ADC [39]. However, a non-enhancing central core may show relatively lower ADC values than those in toxoplasmosis, reflecting the hypercellularity of lymphoma, especially in AIDS patients [37].

16.3.2 Neurocysticercosis

Cysticercosis is the most common parasitic infection of the central nervous system, and it is caused

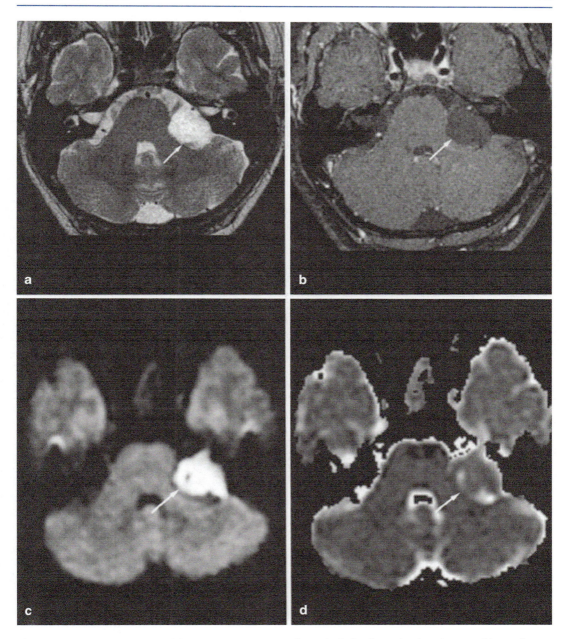

Fig. 16.16 Epidermoid in a 29-year-old man. (**a**) T2-weighted image shows a hyperintense mass (*arrow*) in the left cerebello-pontine angle. (**b**) Gadolinium-enhanced T1 weighted image with magnetization transfer contrast shows the lesion (*arrow*) as hypointense with no enhancement. (**c**) DW image shows this lesion (*arrow*) as hyperintense. (**d**) ADC map shows almost similar ADC value to the cerebellar parenchyma

by *Taenia solium*. Pathologically, there are four forms: (1) parenchymal cysticerci (Fig. 16.22), (2) leptomeningitis, (3) intraventricular cysticerci (Fig. 16.23), and (4) racemose cysts. DW imaging shows cystic lesions in neurocysticercosis as low-signal intensity with high ADC values, which is useful in differentiating them from bacterial or tuberculous abscess [21]. The scolex may be detectable as a hyperintense nodule on DW imaging (Figs. 16.22 and 16.23) [40].

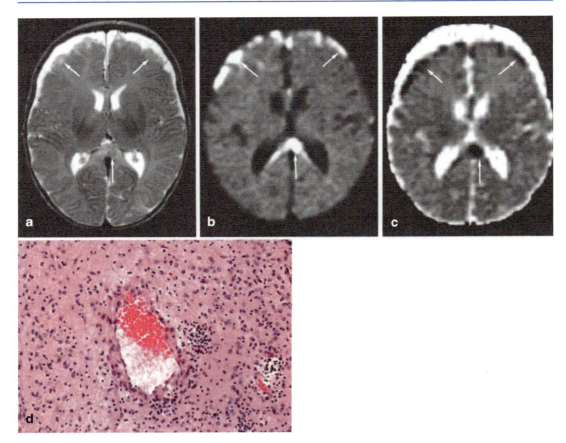

Fig. 16.17 Group B *Streptococcus* meningitis in a 5-week-old boy. (**a**) T2-weighted image shows bifrontal subdural effusion and hyperintense lesions in bilateral frontal superficial cortices and posterior corpus callosum (*arrows*). (**b**) DW image shows these cortical and corpus callosal lesions (*arrows*) as hyperintense. (**c**) ADC map shows the cortical lesions (*arrows*) as decreased ADC, representing acute infarcts and cerebritis of the subpial cortex. (**d**) Infection spreads via the perivascular space into the veins and arteries causing vasculitis, infarction, and cerebritis. Neutrophil infiltrations are noted in the venous and arterial walls

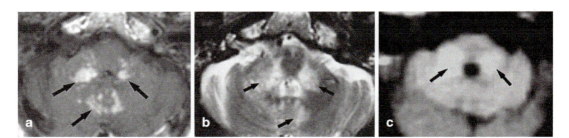

Fig. 16.18 Whipple disease in a 72-year-old male presented with a 6-month history of progressive dysphagia, anorexia, hypersomnia, 60-lb weight loss, and ophthalmoplegia. (**a, b**) T2-weighed image and FLAIR shows diffuse hyperintense lesions within bilateral middle cerebellar peduncles and vermis. (**c**) DW image shows restriction within bilateral middle cerebellar peduncles (from Ref. [35])

16 Infectious Diseases   445

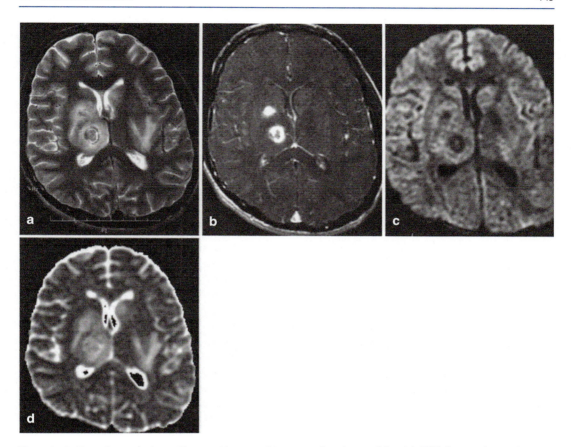

Fig. 16.19 Toxoplasmosis in a 43-year-old man with AIDS. (**a**) T2-weighted image shows mass lesions with vasogenic edema in the bilateral basal ganglia. (**b**) Gadolinium-enhanced T1-weighted image with magnetization transfer contrast shows a ring-enhancing mass and an enhancing nodule. (**c**) DW image shows the non-enhancing central cystic area as isointense, and the enhancing rim and nodule as hypointense with peripheral isointense vasogenic edema. (**d**) ADC map shows increased ADC of these areas

16.3.3 Cerebral Malaria

Malaria has infected humans for over 50,000 years. There are 300–500 million cases per year and 2 million people die of the disease (90% in Africa). It is transmitted by Anopheles mosquitoes. Cerebral malaria (2% of cases) is responsible for most malaria deaths, and Plasmodium falciparum (tropical malaria) is the most common parasite. The diagnosis of malaria is based on a blood smear which shows ring-stage trophozoites. If malaria load in the blood smear is more than 10%, about 50% of the patients die. Moreover, 15–25% of patients with cerebral malaria die despite treatment. Two main mechanisms have been suggested in cerebral malaria: (1) Infected RBCs adhered to the endothelium cause blockage of the capillaries, and (2) cerebral toxicity by cytokines [41].

CT is normal in 30–50% of cases. MR imaging demonstrates diffuse cytotoxic or vasogenic cerebral edema (70%) or infarcts in the white matter, especially involving the corpus callosum, basal ganglia, thalami, brain stem, and cerebellum [42]. DW imaging shows these areas as hyperintense with reduced ADC (Fig. 16.24) [43]. Diffuse petechial hemorrhages in the cortex and subcortical white matter are well visualized on gradient T2*-weighted images (Fig. 16.24).

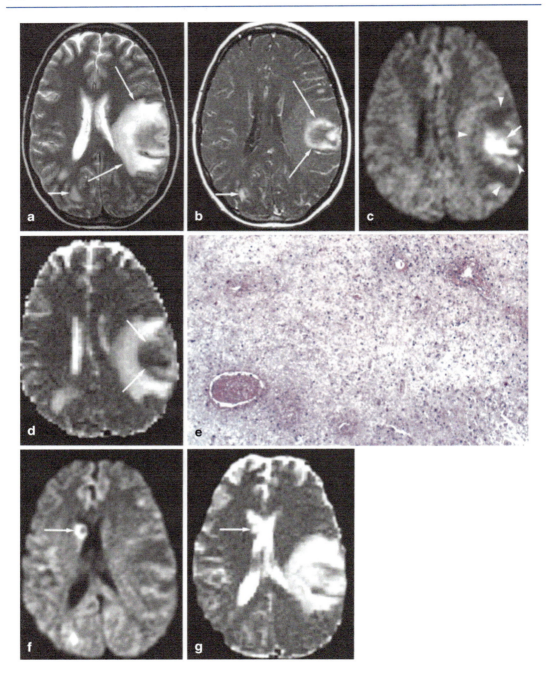

Fig. 16.20 Toxoplasmosis in an 18-year-old female patient with acute myeloblastic leukemia. (**a**) T2-weighted image shows a mass lesion with vasogenic edema in the leftfronto-temporal region (*long arrows*). Hyperintense lesions are also seen in the right occipital area (*short arrow*). (**b**) Gadolinium-enhanced T1-weighted image with magnetization transfer contrast shows a ring-enhancing mass (*long arrows*) and an enhancing nodule (*short arrow*). (**c**) DW image shows the non-enhancing cystic central area as hyperintense (*arrow*), and the enhancing rim and peripheral vasogenic edema as hypointense (*arrowheads*). (**d**) ADC map shows decreased ADC of this cystic component (*arrows*). (**e**) Biopsy specimen shows coagulative necrosis of this cystic component (hematoxylin-eosin stain). (**f, g**) DW image shows a small cystic lesion (*arrow*) as hypointense with increased ADC (**g**) in the right caudate nucleus (*arrow*), which may indicate the different phase of toxoplasma abscess. Leftfronto-temporal mass and multiple hyperintense nodules are also seen

16 Infectious Diseases

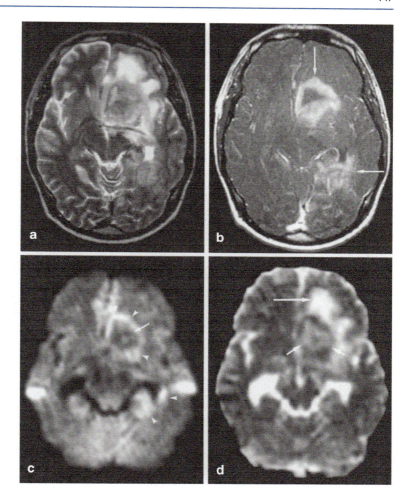

Fig. 16.21 AIDS-related lymphoma in a 23-year-old man. (**a**) T2-weighted image shows a necrotic mass in the left frontal lobe extending into the temporo-occipital lobe. (**b**) Gadolinium-enhanced T1-weighted image magnetization transfer contrast shows these lesions (*arrows*) with irregular ring enhancement. (**c**) DW image shows enhancing solid components as hyperintensity (*arrowheads*), and a necrotic component as hypointensity (*arrow*). (**d**) ADC map shows central necrosis as increased ADC (*arrow*) and the solid components (*arrowheads*) as relatively low ADC compared to the central necrosis

16.4 Fungal Infection

16.4.1 Aspergillosis

Aspergillosis is the most common intracranial fungal infection, commonly seen in immunocompromised patients. In disseminated aspergillosis, *Aspergillus* infiltrates and destroys the internal elastic lamina of cerebral arteries and causes vasculitis [44]. This leads initially to acute infarction or hemorrhage. Most of the process extends into the surrounding tissue as cerebritis and may evolve into an abscess. Infection of already infarcted brain tissue is often aggressive with rapid progression. MR imaging shows round lesions often involving the basal ganglia and gray–white matter junction with absence or minimal peripheral enhancement. Ring or parenchymal enhancement of the lesion can be seen in less severely immunocompromised patients. DW imaging is useful for early detection of this vasculopathy-mediated septic infarction and abscess (Fig. 16.25) [20, 41, 42, 45, 46]. The mortality rate is estimated between 85 and 100%. New antifungal therapies (triazole) have made effective treatment possible.

16.4.2 Mucormycosis

Rhinocerebral mucormycosis often occurs in diabetic patients, especially with diabetic ketoacidosis, which is an excellent medium for this fungus in an environment of elevated glucose and acidic pH [47]. DW imaging shows the lesion as restricted water diffusion typically located in the inferior frontal lobe (Fig. 16.26) [48].

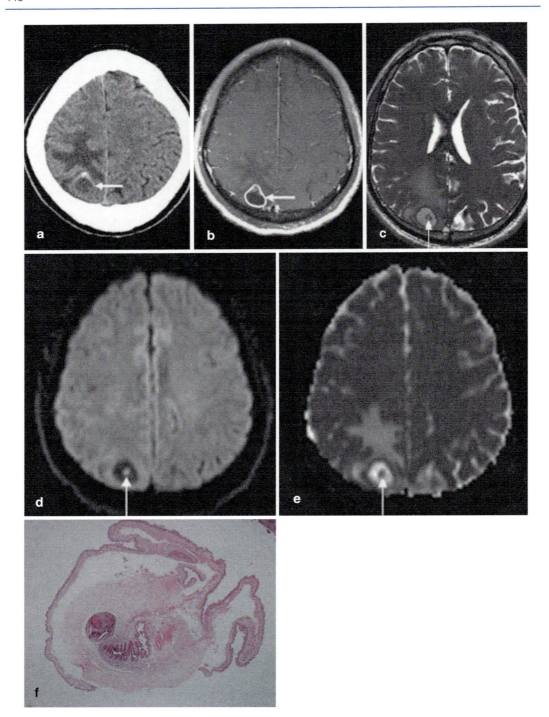

Fig. 16.22 Neurocysticercosis (parenchymal cysticerci) in an 18-year-old man. (**a**) CT shows a calcified cystic mass with the surrounding edema in the right parietal area (*arrow*). (**b**) Gadolinium-enhanced T1-weighted image shows ring enhancement (*arrow*). (**c**) CISS image shows a low-signal spot in the center of the cyst representing a scolex (*arrow*). (**d**) DW image shows a cystic component as low signal with a small hyperintensity in the center of the cyst (*arrow*). (**e**) ADC map shows the cyst as increased ADC and the scolex as a low ADC spot (*arrow*). (**f**) Pathology specimen in another case demonstrates a scolex in the cyst

16 Infectious Diseases

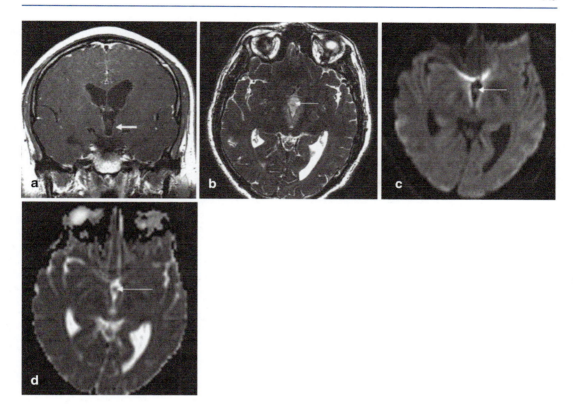

Fig. 16.23 Neurocysticercosis (intraventricular cysticerci) in a 29-year-old man. (**a**) Coronal gadolinium-enhanced T1-weighted image shows a cystic lesion in the third ventricle with ependymal enhancement (*arrow*). (**b**) CISS image shows a low-signal spot (*arrow*) in the center of the cyst and the surrounding edema. (**c**) DW image shows a cystic component as low signals with a small hyperintensity in the center of the cyst (*arrow*). (**d**) ADC map shows the cyst as increased ADC with a central low ADC spot (*arrow*). Pathology showed a degenerating Cysticercus

16.4.3 Cryptococosis

Cryptococcus infection shows enhancing or non-enhancing lesions involving the basal ganglia and posterior fossa (Fig. 16.27). The cystic lesions are usually isosignal to CSF on T2-weighted and DW images (Fig. 16.28) [49]. While meningitis is also more common overall, in the basal ganglia, localized pockets of organisms up to several millimeters in size may develop with a pathognomonic appearance of gelatinous pseudocyst formation, known as a cryptococcoma (Fig. 16.29). Gelatinous pseudocysts are T1 hypointense and T2 hyperintense lesion with T2 hypointense ring. The outer T2 hypointense ring may represent methemoglobin blood products in the capsule wall or activated macrophages producing free radicals and paramagnetic susceptibility artifact. The pseudocyst center often lacks enhancement owing to its avascular nature and may or may not cause reduced diffusion. A large pseudocyst may convert into a frank abscess with enhancement and reduced diffusion [50].

16.4.4 Candidiasis

Neurocandidiasis usually results from systemic candida infection in immunosuppressed patients or related to intravascular catheter infections [50–52]. Neurocandidiasis most frequently appears as ring-enhancing or non-enhancing microabscess, measuring <3 mm, often found in the gray–white junction, basal

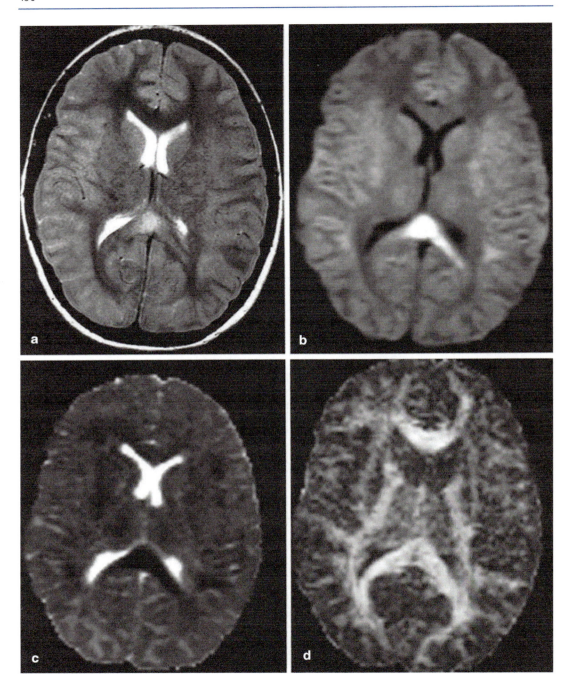

Fig. 16.24 Cerebral malaria in a 19-year-old female patient with headache, fever, and jaundice. (**a**) T2-weighted image shows diffuse hyperintensity and swelling in the brain, especially of the gray matter and the splenium of the corpus callosum. (**b**) DW image shows hyperintense lesions in the white matter, thalami, basal ganglia, and the splenium of the corpus callosum. (**c**) ADC map shows these areas as decreased ADC consistent with cytotoxic edema. (**d**) Fractional anisotropy is preserved in these areas. (**e**) Gradient T2*-weighted image shows petechial hemorrhage in the cortico-white matter junction postmortem (Courtesy of Kim J MD, The University of Iowa Hospitals and Clinics, USA). (**f**) Blood smear shows ring-stage trophozoites. (**g**) Pathological specimen shows diffuse brain edema and petechial hemorrhage in the cortico-white matter junction (*arrows*). (**h**) Luxol Fast *Blue* stain shows ring hemorrhage at the cortico-white matter junction and Durck's granulomas in the white matter. (**i**) Malarial trophoziotes and hematoidin pigment are noted in the red blood cell in the capillary (*arrows*)

16 Infectious Diseases

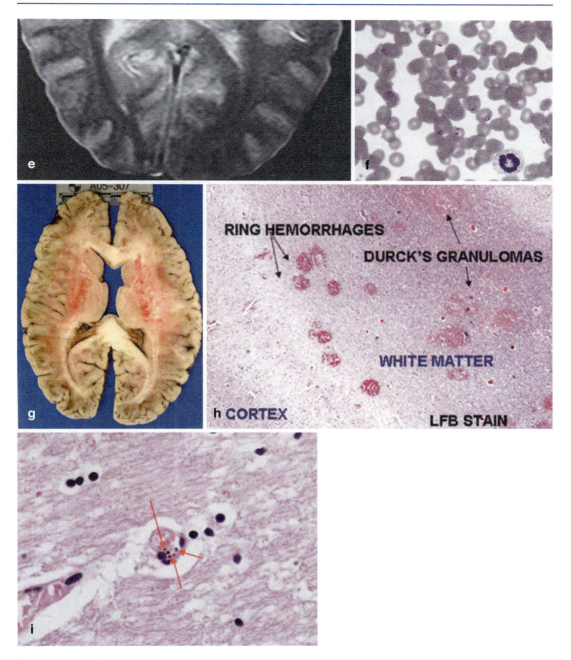

Fig. 16.24 (continued)

ganglia, and cerebellum (Fig. 16.30). Neonatal candidemia occurs in 4–15% of extremely low birth weight infants. DW imaging can play an important role in the diagnosis of cerebral candida abscess in premature infants (see Chap. 19, Fig. 19.22).

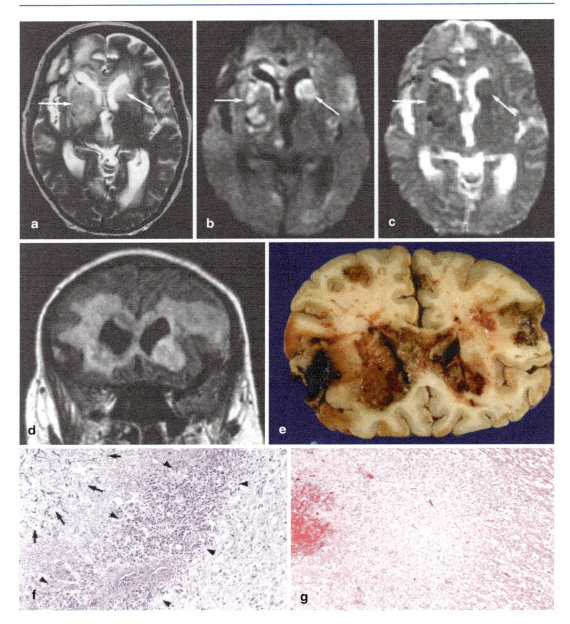

Fig. 16.25 Disseminated aspergillosis in a 55-year-old woman with fever and mental status change. She had hepatitis C and underwent liver transplantation. (**a**) T2-weighted image shows multiple hyperintense round lesions (*arrows*) in bilateral basal ganglia, right thalamus, and cerebral white matter and cortex. Subdural hematoma is also seen in the right frontal region. (**b**) DW image shows these lesions as very high signal intensity (*arrows*), representing infarction, hemorrhage, and abscess, (**c**) ADC maps show decreased ADC in these lesions (*arrows*). (**d**) Coronal FLAIR image shows extensive hyperintense lesions in the frontal lobes. (**e**) Brain specimen with the same slice of the FLAIR image demonstrates extensive hemorrhagic necrotic lesions. (**f**) Pathological specimen of the right thalamus shows *Aspergillus* hyphae (*arrows*) and infiltration of neutrophils and macrophages (*arrowheads*) in an abscess (hematoxylin-eosin stain). (**g**) Pathological specimen of left frontal area shows necrosis due to vasculitis-mediated acute septic infarction and hemorrhage (hematoxylin-eosin stain)

16 Infectious Diseases

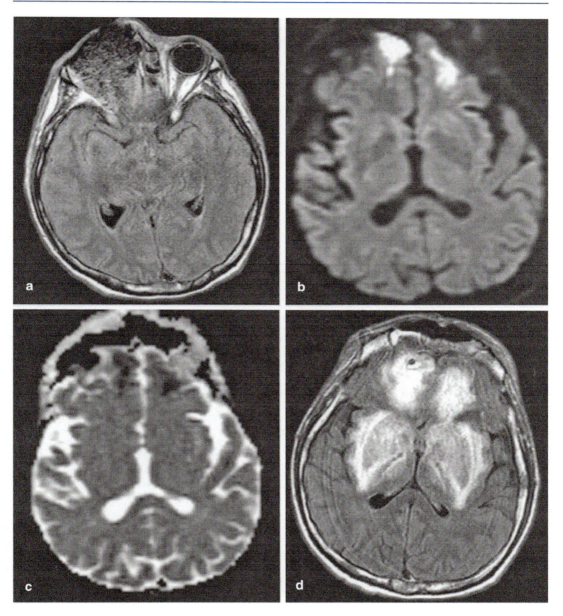

Fig. 16.26 Rhinocerebral mucormycosis in a 48-year-old man with diabetes mellitus type 1 and ketoacidosis. (**a**) FLAIR image shows postoperative changes of invasive fungal infection in the right orbit and paranasal sinus. (**b**) DW image shows hyperintense lesions in the bilateral frontal bases. (**c**) Decreased ADCs of these lesions are noted, consistent with cerebritis. (**d**) On a 1-week follow-up MR image, the lesions extend into the frontal lobes and basal ganglia shown as hyperintense lesions on the FLAIR image

16.4.5 Histoplasmosis

Histoplasmosis may show ring-enhancing lesions on the brain MR images. DW imaging may show various signals depending on the presence of inflammatory cells and the type of necrosis, i.e., coagulative or liquefactive (Fig. 16.31) [53].

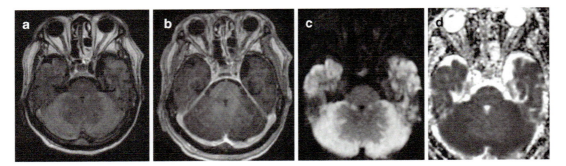

Fig. 16.27 Cryptococcus meningoencephalitis in a 93-year-old man presented with fever and altered level of consciousness. (**a**) FLAIR image shows hyperintense lesions in the bilateral cerebellar hemispheres and temporal lobes. (**b**) Axial postcontrast T1-image shows mild leptomeningeal enhancement along the cerebellar folia. (**c**) DWI shows diffusion restriction in the lesions with decreased ADC (**d**). (Courtesy of Dr. Ryo Kurokawa, The University of Tokyo)

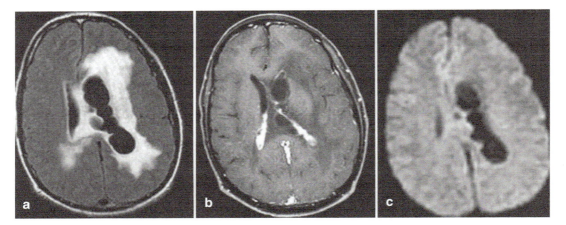

Fig. 16.28 Cryptococcus ependymitis and choroid plexitis in a 40-year-old man with AIDS. (**a**) FLAIR image shows multiloculated cystic lesions in the lateral ventricles with extensive periventricular and deep white matter edema. (**b**) Gadolinium-enhanced T1-weighted image shows thin-wall-enhancing intraventricular cystic lesions and ependymal enhancement. (**c**) DW image shows the cystic lesions as hypointense with increased ADC (not shown)

16.4.6 Blastomycosis

Blastomycosis is caused by the dimorphic fungus *Blastomyces dermatitidis*. It exists as a mold in the environment and a yeast at body temperatures. Infections are usually sporadic. The only recognized risk factor is living in endemic areas of the midwestern USA, classically near the states surrounding the Ohio or Mississippi river. Presentation is nonspecific with headache, AMS, fever, vision changes, and seizures. The lungs are affected most often following introduction of spores by inhalation. However, the organism can infect the skin, genitourinary system, and CNS, and isolated CNS infection can be seen in patients with diabetes or immunosuppression. The few available case reports suggest that leptomeningeal enhancement and enhancing mass lesions are common. Reduced diffusion may be central (Fig. 16.32) [50].

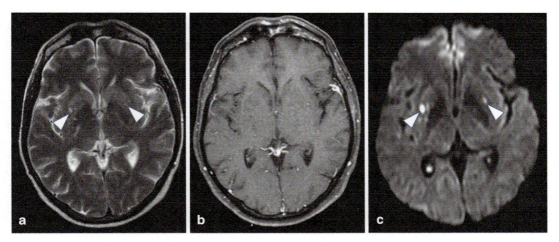

Fig. 16.29 Gelatinous pseudocyst formation (cryptococcoma) in a 40-year-old HIV-positive man with a CD4 count of 22 and viral load of 1.3 million. (**a**) Axial T1-weighted image shows hyperintense punctate lesions within the ganglia (arrowheads). (**b**) Axial postcontrast T1-weighted image shows no enhancement, typical of cryptococcal infection with severe immune suppression. (**c**) DWI shows reduced diffusion within the basal ganglia (arrowheads) (from Ref. [50])

16.4.7 Coccidioidomycosis

Coccidioides immitis is a fungus found in the soil and endemic to the southwestern USA and northern Mexico. It produces spores and is dimorphic. Because the *C. immitis* is geographically limited to the southwest USA, the strongest risk factor is living in an endemic area. Pulmonary infection is common, while CNS involvement is distinctly uncommon, and only a few cases of CNS infection are reported in the literature. Patients usually present with headaches, lethargy, and fevers. CNS involvement is usually secondary to hematogenous dissemination from the lungs. The meninge is the most common site of infection, but parenchymal infection is also seen (Fig. 16.33). Approximately 4–5% of symptomatic patients may develop disseminated disease with high morbidity and mortality, with dissemination more common in immunocompromised patients. Contrast enhancement of the basal cisterns is typical in coccidioidomycosis meningitis. DWI with peripheral lesion restriction has been reported. [50]

16.5 Viral Infection

16.5.1 Herpes Simplex Encephalitis (HSE) Infection

HSE is the most common cause of sporadic fatal encephalitis, accounting for 10–20% of encephalitic viral infections. Pathologically, herpes encephalitis has both cytotoxic and vasogenic edema associated with massive tissue necrosis and petechial or even confluent hemorrhage, typically in the limbic system and the insular cortex. In adults, the medial temporal lobes, inferior frontal lobes, and insula, encompassing limbic and paralimbic areas, are commonly involved. Predominantly cortical involvement may extend into the white matter. In infants and young children, the lesions tend to extend into frontoparietal lobes. In neonatal HSE, cerebral cortex and white matter are involved in a more global fashion [54, 55]. Restricted diffusion of herpes encephalitides is attributed to direct cytotoxicity that results in neuronal swelling. DW imaging is more sensitive than conventional MR imaging in detecting early changes of herpes encephalitis

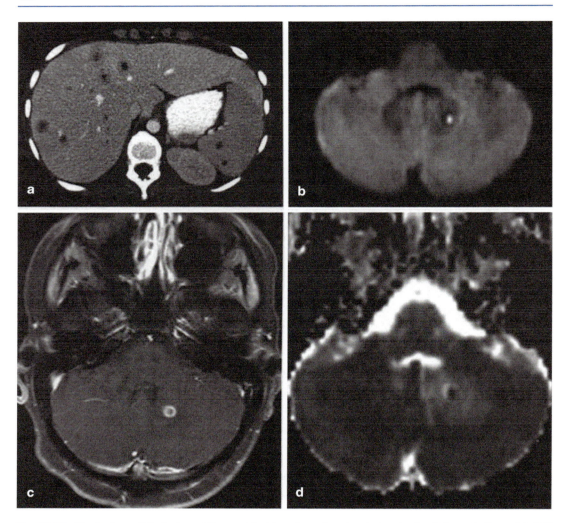

Fig. 16.30 Cerebral candidiasis in a 17-year-old girl with pre-B-cell acute lymphoblastic leukemia and fungal sepsis. (**a**) Contrast-enhanced abdominal CT shows multiple abscesses in the liver and spleen. (**b**) Gadolinium-enhanced T1-weighted image shows a small ring-enhancing lesion in the left cerebellum. (**c**) DW image shows very small hyperintensity representing a small abscess. (**d**) ADC map shows decreased ADC in the abscess

(Figs. 16.34, 16.35, and 16.36) [56–60]. This is important for early diagnosis, as treatment with acyclovir reduces mortality at 18 months from 70 to 30%. Herpes encephalitis often affects the temporal lobes, which occasionally can make the detection of lesions in the middle cranial fossa difficult on DW imaging because of susceptibility artifacts.

16.5.2 Varicella Zoster Virus (VZV) Infection

VZV is a ubiquitous human DNA virus. Primary infection occurs via respiratory aerosols or contact with vesicles from an infected individual and results in the disseminated rash of chickenpox [54, 55]. A parainfectious, immune-mediated

16 Infectious Diseases

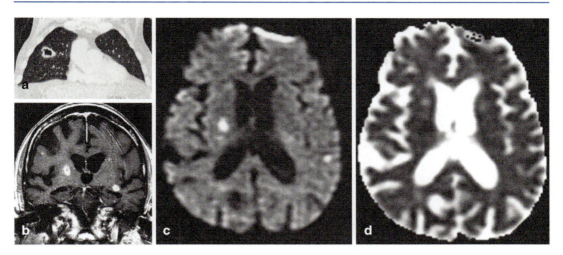

Fig. 16.31 Histoplasmosis in an 81-year-old man with diabetic mellitus and alcoholism. (**a**) Contrast-enhanced chest CT with coronal reconstruction shows a cavitary lesion in the right lung. (**b**) Coronal gadolinium-enhanced T1-weighted image shows multiple ring-enhancing lesions in the brain. (**c, d**) DW image shows the lesions as hyperintense with the decreased ADC

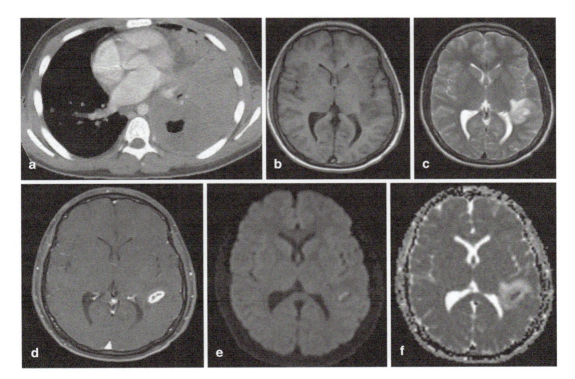

Fig. 16.32 Blastomycosis in a 17-year-old male with cough, left chest pain, low grade fever, and weight loss after 4-wheel trip with family in Wisconsin. (**a**) Chest CT shows left lobar consolidation with air bronchogram and pleural effusion. (**b, c**) T1-weighted image shows hypointensity and T2-weighted image shows hyperintensity within the left temporal lobe. The lesion exerts minimal mass effect on the posterior horn of the left lateral ventricle. (**d**) Axial T1 postcontrast image shows thick ring enhancement. (**e, f**) Axial DWI and ADC show mild central reduced diffusion (from Ref. [50])

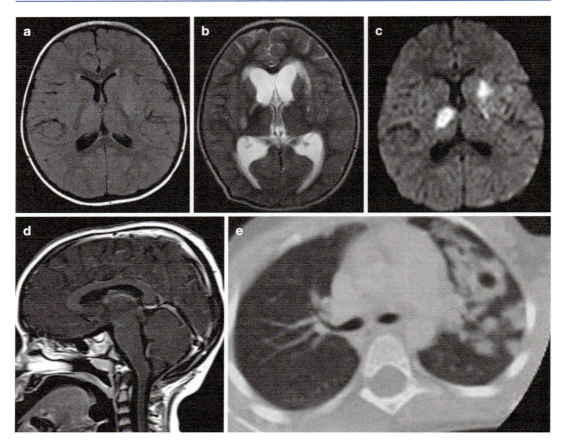

Fig. 16.33 Coccidioidomycosis in a 4-year-old girl with a history of recurrent rashes who had a sudden onset of acute neurologic deficits following 3 days of nausea, vomiting, and dehydration with persistent headaches and "fuzzy" vision. (**a**) FLAIR shows mild hyperintensity in the right thalamus and left basal ganglia. (**b**) DWI shows reduce diffusion in the same areas suggestive of acute infarction. (**c**) Sagittal gadolinium-enhanced T1-weighted image shows no enhancement of the basal cistern. (**d**) Follow-up T2-weighted image reveals multuple old infarcts and hydrocephalus. (**e**) Chest CT shows multiple ill-defined nodules, cavitation and segmental consolidation in the left lung (from Ref. [50])

syndrome with cerebellar ataxia is the most common CNS manifestation of chickenpox (0.1%). Acute varicella encephalitis is rare (0.05%). VZV becomes latent in the cranial nerve ganglia, spinal dorsal root ganglia, and autonomic ganglia. VZV reactivation commonly manifests as herpes zoster (shingles). Herpes zoster meningoencephalitis, myelitis, or polyradiculopathy usually occurs in elderly and immunocompromised patients. The diagnostic value of anti-VZV immunoglobulin G in CSF (93% sensitivity) is greater than that of VZV DNA by PCR in CSF (30% sensitivity). Negative results for both tests tend to exclude VZV infection. Pathologic findings in varicella zoster encephalitis include perivascular lymphocytic cuffing and focal demyelination within trinuclear inclusion bodies in endothelial cells, neurons, and glial cells. Granulomatous angiitis can be seen.

MR imaging of herpes zoster meningoencephalitis shows multifocal cortical and white matter lesions with leptomeningeal enhancement. Contrast enhancement is patchy and mild in varicella-zoster encephalitis. VZV vasculopathy results from productive viral infection of arteries. VZV can affect both large and small arteries,

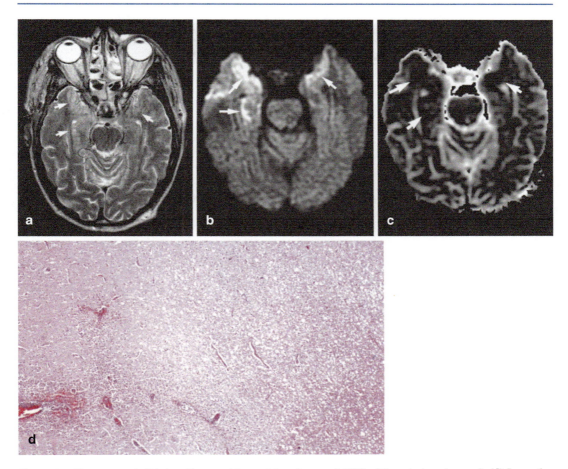

Fig. 16.34 Herpes encephalitis in a 48-year-old man. (**a**) T2-weighted image shows hyperintense lesions in bilateral temporal lobes (*arrows*). (**b**) DW image shows these lesions as hyperintense. (**c**) ADC map shows partially decreased ADC of these lesions (*arrows*). (**d**) In another patient with herpes encephalitis, pathological specimen shows cytotoxic edema, necrosis, and hemorrhage

which results in aneurysm formation, arterial ectasia, dissection, subarachnoid hemorrhage, infarction, and hemorrhage (Fig. 16.37). Thirty-seven percent of VZV vasculopathy cases do not have the characteristic varicella or zoster rash. VZV vasculopathy occurs more frequently late in the course of AIDS, especially when there is significant CD41 depletion. MR imaging with DWI is useful to detect ischemic stroke, which often involves gray matter–white matter junctions. MR or CT angiogram is useful to detect vascular abnormalities [54, 55]. MRI findings of encephalitis are seen in cerebral cortex, basal ganglia, deep white matter, and periventricular white lesion with hyperintensities on T2W/FLAIR sequences, usually seen in severely immune compromised host. Restriction is usually seen on DWI (Fig. 16.38).

16.5.3 Epstein-Barr Virus (EBV) Infection

EBV is a ubiquitous virus and epidemiologically important because it asymptomatically infects more than 90% of the world's population [54, 55]. Acute infectious mononucleosis is the commonest manifestation of EBV, and is usually a self-limiting condition. Chronic active EBV infection is rare but often fatal. CNS complica-

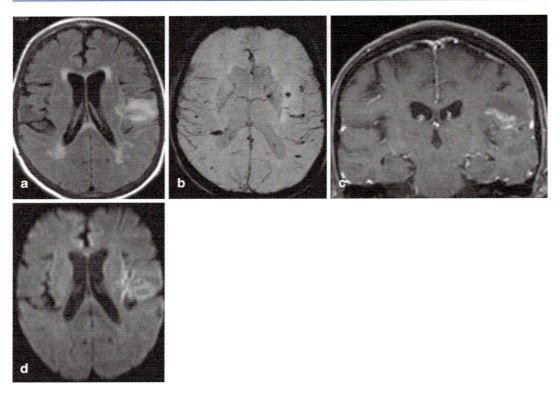

Fig. 16.35 Herpes simplex encephalitis in a 63-year-old female. (**a**) FLAIR image shows hyperintensity in the left insula area. (**b**) Gradient echo (GRE) reveals hemorrhage predominantly in the lesion. (**c**) T1 post-gadolinium image reveals leptomeningeal and gyral enhancement in the lesion. (**d**) DWI shows hyperintensity in the cortical lesions extending into the white. The lesion starts from insula area with spare of medial temporal lobe. Gyral enhancement pattern with diffusion restriction and microhemorrhage are suggestive of herpes encephalitis

tions of EBV infection range from 0.4 to 7.3% and include meningitis, encephalitis, myelitis, cerebellitis, ADEM, reversible encephalitis, Guillain-Barré syndrome, and neuropsychiatric disturbances. EBV meningoencephalitis is usually mild with personality changes, depressed level of consciousness, and abnormal movements, and fatal cases secondary to brain encephalitis have been reported (Fig. 16.39). Acyclovir and corticosteroids have been recommended for treatment of EBV encephalitis, but the effectiveness is uncertain. The diagnosis of EBV infection is made with a positive PCR for EBV DNA in CSF and specific EBV immunoglobulin (Ig) M antibodies against viral capsid antigen in serum.

Virus-associated hemophagocytic syndrome (VAHS), also called hemophagocytic lymphohistiocytosis (HLH), is a multisystem disorder characterized with aggressive proliferation of macrophages and histiocytes showing hemophagocytosis with an upregulation of the inflammatory cytokines, including macrophage colony-stimulating factor, by T-helper cells. HLH can be primary (familial, autosomal recessive) or secondary. EBV is the most common cause of VAHS (secondary HLH). VAHS often follows a brief of viral illness. VAHS affects the CNS in 10–73% of patients with variable neurologic symptoms including irritability, seizures, hemiparesis, and coma. The CSF is normal in approximately 50%. [54, 55] Pathology shows initial leptomeningeal and intraparenchymal perivascular lymphocytic infiltration with astrogliosis affecting mainly white matter, followed by areas of necrosis and focal demyelination. MR imaging findings are parenchymal volume loss with focal necrosis and/or white matter abnormalities (Fig. 16.40). Leptomeningeal and perivascular

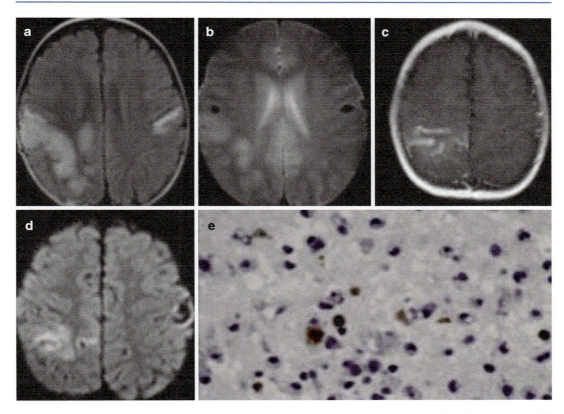

Fig. 16.36 Herpes simplex encephalitis in a 2-year-old girl with seizures. (**a**) FLAIR image shows bilateral frontoparietal cortical lesions. (**b**) Gradient echo (GRE) reveals hemorrhage in the lesions. (**c**) T1 post-gadolinium image reveals leptomeningeal and gyral enhancement. (**d**) DWI shows hyperintensity in the cortical lesions extending into the white. (**e**) HSV stain was positive (original magnification ×1000) (from Ref. [54])

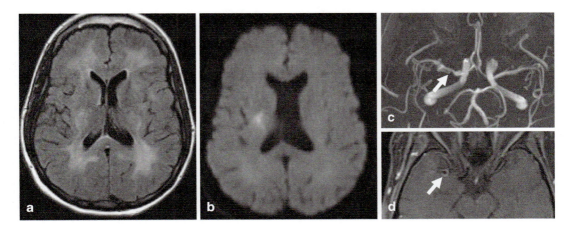

Fig. 16.37 Varicella-zoster vasculitis in a 26-year-old man with a stroke and a history of HIV infection. (**a**) FLAIR image shows diffuse white matter hyperintensity consistent with HIV encephalopathy. (**b**) DWI shows hyperintensity in the posterior internal capsule. (**c**) MR angiography reveals an ectatic M1 portion of the right middle cerebral artery. (**d**) T1 post-gadolinium image shows enhancement of the wall of ectatic right middle cerebral artery consistent with arteritis (from Ref. [54])

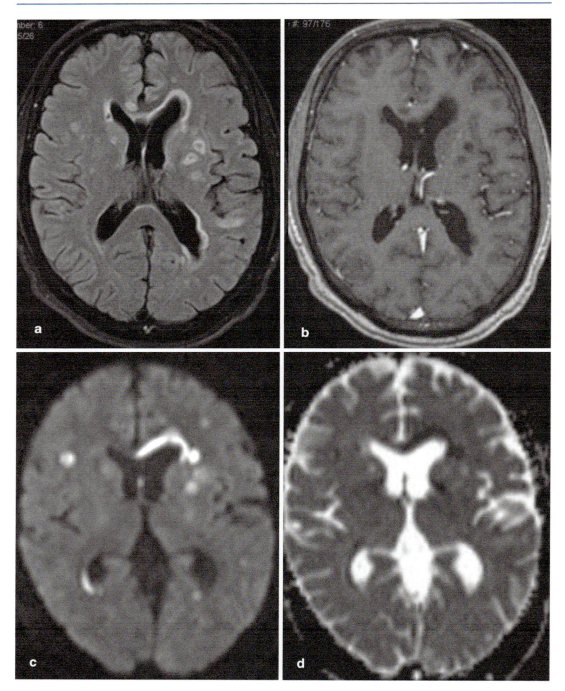

Fig. 16.38 VZV encephalitis in a 44-year-old HIV-positive male with altered mental status with a CD4 count of 19. (**a**) FLAIR image shows hyperintensity in bilateral deep white matter, periventricular white lesion, and left putamen. (**b**) Postcontrast T1-weighted image shows no enhancement of meninges, gray matter, and white matter with hypointensity in genu of corpus callosum and left putamen. (**c**, **d**) DWI and ADC show restriction in bilateral deep white matter, periventricular white lesion, and left putamen

16 Infectious Diseases 463

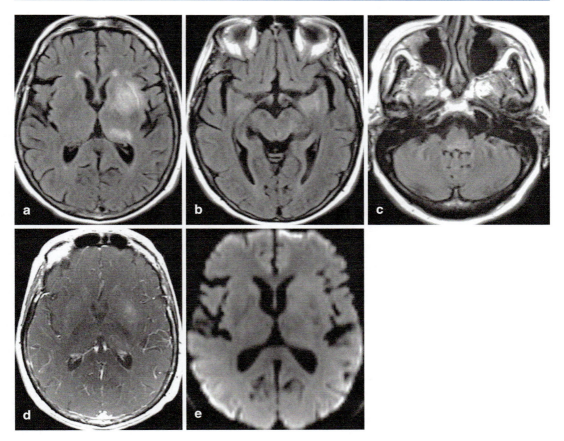

Fig. 16.39 EBV meningoencephalitis in a 76-year-old female with worsening vertigo, double vision, speech difficulties, gait difficulties. CSF: EBV PCR was 19,000 IU/ml (**a**, **b**, **c**) FLAIR image shows hyperintensity in the left putamen and globus pallitus. Consistent with HIV encephalopathy. (**d**) Postcontrast T1-weighted image shows meningeal enhancement. (**e**) DWI shows no hyperintensity (from Ref. [54])

enhancement is frequently seen. Multiple enhancing lesions have also been described. Treatment consists of immunosuppression chemotherapy, including corticosteroids and cyclosporine A, combined with etoposide and, ultimately, bone marrow transplantation. VAHS/HLH may have a relapsing and remitting course, or it may rapidly progress to multiorgan failure and death. Between 30 and 40% of patients with VAHS have poor clinical outcomes.

EBV was the first human tumor virus to be discovered and identified in Burkitt lymphoma (in 1964). When EBV infects B cells in vitro, lymphoblastoid cell lines eventually emerge that are capable of indefinite growth. EBV is associated with several lymphomas and lymphoproliferative disorders that include B-cell, T-cell, and NK-cell neoplasias. These include posttransplant lymphoproliferative disease (PTLD) (Fig. 16.41), lymphomatoid granulomatosis (LYG) (Fig. 16.42), and AIDS-related CNS lymphoma (Fig. 16.43). EBER in situ hybridization is positive and diagnostically useful for EBV-associated lymphoma and lymphoproliferative disorder [54, 55].

16.5.4 Human Herpesvirus-6 (HHV6) Infection

HHV6 is a ubiquitous neurotropic virus latent in most adults, also known to be the cause of exanthem subitum or roseola infantum [61, 62]. HHV-6-associated encephalitis/encephalopathy has

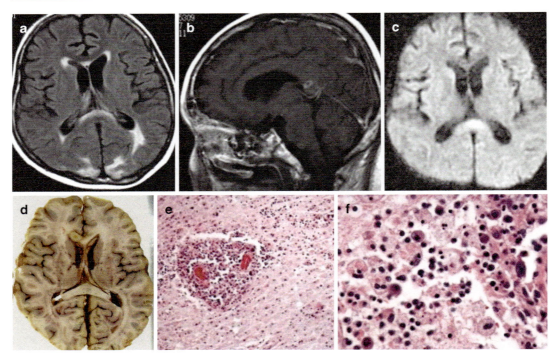

Fig. 16.40 EBV-associated hemophagocytic syndrome in a 13-year-old boy with mental status change, hepatosplenomegaly, and hypercytokinemia. (**a, c**) FLAIR image and DWI show a splenial lesion as hyperintense. FLAIR hyperintense lesions in bilateral occipital lobes represent posterior reversible encephalopathy syndrome caused by the treatment of cyclosporine A. (**b**) Sagittal postcontrast T1-weighted image reveals enhancement in the splenial lesion. The patient died with multiorgan failure. (**d**) Brain at autopsy reveals infiltration of hemophagocytic histiocytes and atypical lymphocytes with edema in the splenial lesion (hematoxylin-eosin, original magnification (**e**) ×400, (**f**) ×1000). (Courtesy of Dr. Nobuo Kobayashi, MD, St. Luke's International Hospital, Tokyo, Japan.) (from Ref. [54])

been increasingly recognized as a serious complication in immunocompromised patients. MR imaging often shows mesial temporal lobe abnormalities. Abnormal high signal intensity with ADC reduction is observed to be consistent with cytotoxic edema (Fig. 16.44). In transplantation, acyclovir is routinely administered but not effective against HHV-6 because of the lack of virus-specific thymidine kinase. Ganciclovir and foscarnet can be effective in therapy.

16.5.5 Brain Stem Encephalitis

Brain stem encephalitis, mesenrhombencephalitis, is a rare life-threatening inflammatory disorder involving the brain stem and cerebellum. It was initially described by Bickerstaff and Cloake in 1951 [63]. The etiology is frequently undetermined but thought to be an immune-mediated process. It often follows viral infection (herpes simplex virus, influenza A, enterovirus 71, adenovirus). In some cases, bacteria (Listeria, Mycoplasma, Legionella) and parasites or paraneoplastic syndromes have been implicated. MR imaging shows a T2- and FLAIR-hyperintense lesion in the brain stem, and enhancement in the lesion can be seen post-contrast on T1-weighted images [64]. DW imaging shows hyperintensity in the lesion with decreased or increased ADC, depending on whether there is cytotoxic or vasogenic edema (Fig. 16.45) [65].

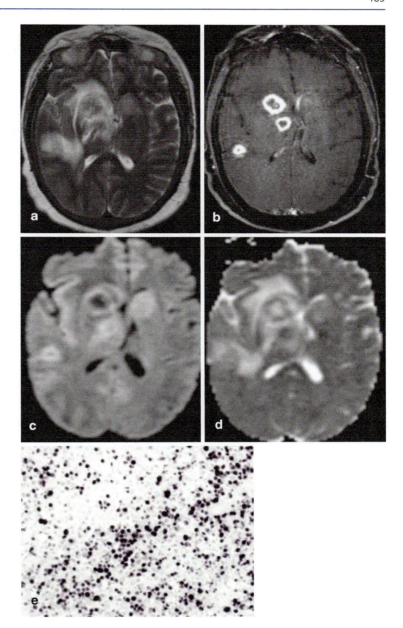

Fig. 16.41 Posttransplant lymphoproliferative disease in a 54-year-old man after renal transplantation. (**a**) T2-weighted image shows multiple mildly hyperintense masses with vasogenic edema in the white matter. (**b**) Postcontrast T1-weighted image shows ring or heterogeneous enhancement. (**c**) DWI shows hyperintensity in the ring-enhancing solid portion and hypointensity in the central necrosis. (**d**) ADC map shows partially decreased ADC of the solid portion of the mass. (**e**) Brain biopsy reveals a hypercellular atypical lymphoid infiltrate with mitosis and nuclear pleomorphism. In situ hybridization analysis of EBER was positive([e] original magnification ×400) (from Ref. [54])

16.5.6 West Nile Encephalitis

West Nile virus (WNV) is a single-stranded RNA flavivirus, and part of the Japanese encephalitis serocomplex. It is transmitted by Culex species mosquitoes. WNV can infect birds, humans, horses, dogs, cats, bats, chipmunks, skunks, squirrels, and rabbits.

Four other transmissions have been reported: (1) transfusion, (2) transplanted organ, (3) transplacental, and (4) breast feeding. The incubation period is around 3–14 days. One in 150 patients with WNV develops meningoencephalitis. The clinical symptoms include fever, headache, altered mental status, tremor, and flaccid paralysis and poliomyelitis associated

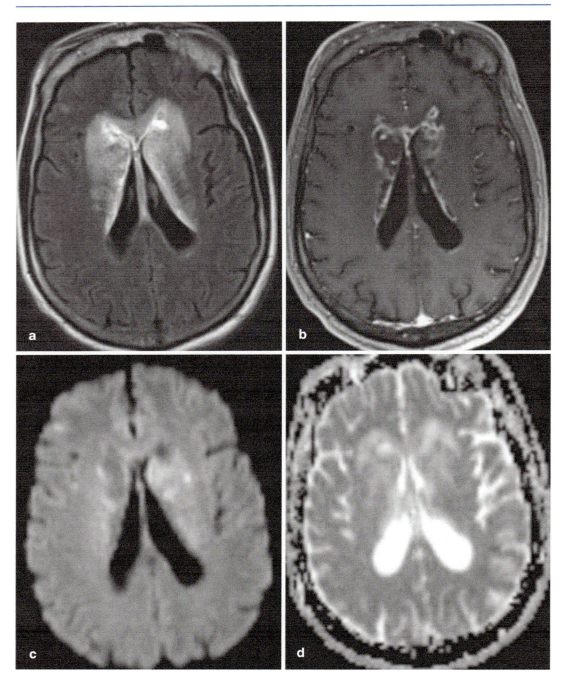

Fig. 16.42 Lymphomatoid granulomatosis in a 56-year-old man with mental status changes. (**a**) FLAIR image shows symmetric periventricular hyperintensity. (**b**) post-contrast T1-weighted image reveals heterogeneous enhancement in the lesions. (**c**) DWI shows mixed hyperintensity, and (**d**) hypointensity associated with heterogeneous ADC values representing cellular infiltration and necrosis. In situ hybridization (EBER) was positive for EBV (not shown) (from Ref. [54])

16 Infectious Diseases

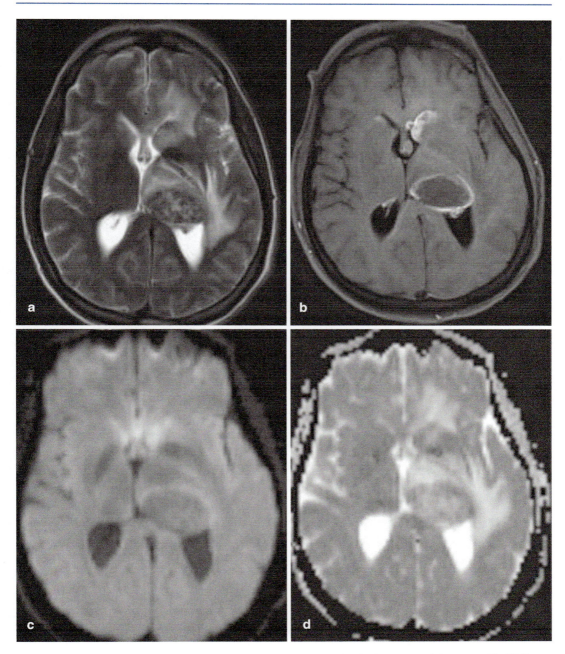

Fig. 16.43 AIDS-related lymphoma in a 42-year-old man. (**a**) T2-weighted image shows mildly hyperintense or hypointense masses in the left periventricular region with vasogenic edema in the white matter. (**b**) Postcontrast T1-weighted image shows ring or heterogeneous enhancement. (**c**) DWI reveals hyperintensity in the ring and hypointensity in the center of the mass. (**d**) ADC map shows partially decreased ADC of the solid portion of the mass. Brain biopsy reveals lymphoma with necrosis. In situ hybridization (EBER) was positive for EBV (not shown) (from Ref. [54])

Fig. 16.44 Human herpesvirus-6 encephalitis in a 28-year-old woman with acute lymphoblastic leukemia after allogeneic stem cell transplant. (**a**) FLAIR image shows a hyperintense lesion in the left temporal lobe. (**b**) Gadolinium-enhanced T1-weighted image shows mild enhancement in the lesion. (**c**) DW image shows the lesion as hyperintense. (**d**) ADC map shows decreased ADC of the lesion

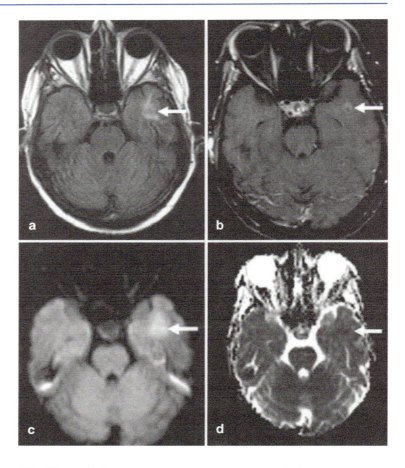

with spinal cord involvement. The diagnosis is based on detection of an WNV IgM antibody in the CSF. MR imaging shows mild hyperintense lesions on T2 and FLAIR studies in the basal ganglia, thalami, mesial temporal lobe, white matter, cerebellum, brain stem, especially the substantia nigra and medulla, and the spinal cord with or without enhancement (Fig. 16.46). Leptomeningeal enhancement and FLAIR hyperintensity in the CSF can also be seen. However, 30% of cases have normal MR images. DW imaging shows these parenchymal lesions as hyperintense with reduced ADC [66–70]. Pathology demonstrates lymphocytic neutropholis, perivascular lymphocytic cuffing, microglial nodules, spongiotic changes, and necrosis (Fig. 16.46). Treatment is conservative with IV fluid and respiratory support. Interferon-α2b or ribavirin may be used.

16.5.7 Human Immunodeficiency Virus Infection

The pathological hallmark of human immunodeficiency virus (HIV) encephalopathy is multinucleated giant cells in the white matter [71]. MR imaging typically shows diffuse periventricular white matter lesions, but brain stem and basal ganglia can also be involved. DW imaging usually shows mild hyperintensity with increased ADC which is secondary to a T2 shine-through effect (Fig. 16.47).

Cerebral infarction in HIV patients is common and has been seen on MR imaging in up to 18% of the patients [72]. The infarctions are caused by opportunistic infections, drug use, and primary HIV vasculitis. AIDS-related bilateral basal ganglia lesions are reported to be numerous microinfarcts on postmortem neuropathological

16 Infectious Diseases

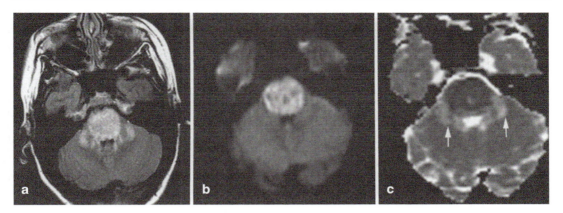

Fig. 16.45 Brain stem encephalitis in a 29-year-old woman diagnosed with a viral syndrome. (**a**) FLAIR image shows hyperintense lesions diffusely in the pons and bilateral middle cerebellar peduncles. (**b, c**) DW image shows the diffuse pontine lesion as hyperintense with decreased ADC which represents cytotoxic edema, and the bilateral middle cerebellar peduncles as isointense with increased ADC representing vasogenic edema (*arrows*)

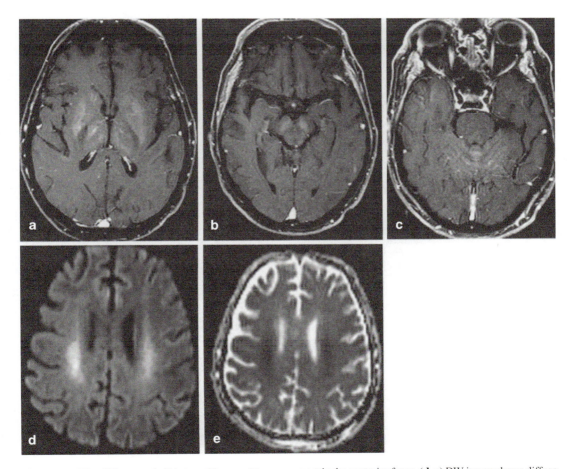

Fig. 16.46 West Nile encephalitis in a 56-year-old man with fever and tremors with a history of renal transplant. (**a–c**) Gadolinium-enhanced T1-weighted image shows symmetric mild enhancement in the basal ganglia, thalami, and substantia nigra, and leptomeningeal enhancement in the posterior fossa. (**d, e**) DW image shows diffuse symmetric hyperintense lesions with decreased ADC only in the deep white matter. (**f, g**) Pathological specimens of the brain biopsy show perivascular lymphocytic cuffing (**f**) and microglial nodules (**g**)

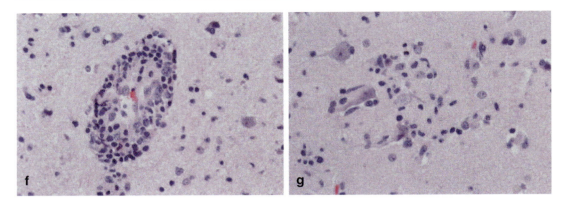

Fig. 16.46 (continued)

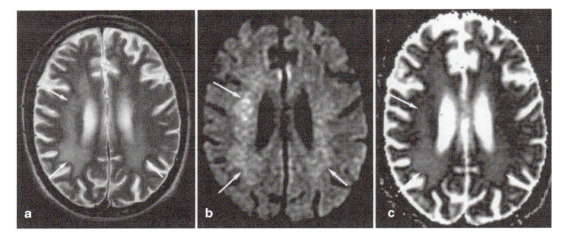

Fig. 16.47 HIV encephalopathy in a 60-year-old man. (a) T2-weighted image shows periventricular hyperintense lesions (*arrows*). (b) DW image shows these lesions as mild hyperintensity (*arrows*). (c) ADC map shows these lesions as increased ADC. Mild hyperintensity on DW imaging is due to T2 shine-through effect (*arrows*)

examination [73]. DW imaging can show numerous hyperintense lesions in bilateral basal ganglia, presumably representing microinfarcts (Fig. 16.48).

16.5.8 Progressive Multifocal Leukoencephalopathy (PML)

PML is a noninflammatory demyelinating disease first described in 1958, associated with oligodendrocytes infected with John Cunningham virus (JCV). JCV is a ubiquitous human pathogen [50, 74, 75]. Primary asymptomatic infection with JCV is presumed to occur during childhood. The reservoir of the virus is thought to be established in the kidneys and B lymphocytes. Reactivation and dissemination may occur under impaired T-cell function. How and when JCV reaches the CNS remains unknown. The symptoms of PML are often psychiatric/behavioral changes or progressive neurologic deficits. HIV accounts for approximately 80% of PML cases. Other causes of immunodeficiency are organ/stem cell transplant, hematologic malignancy, autoimmune disease or multiple sclerosis treated with immune modulators including monoclonal antibodies (natalizumab, efalizumab, rituximab), and primary immunodeficiency syndrome. The pathology of PML typically shows demyelination without evidence of inflammation, swollen oligodendrocytes with densely basophilic nuclear inclusion bodies, and astrocytes with enlarged hyperchromatic nuclei (bizarre astrocytes) resembling neoplastic cells. In advanced cases, lesions may have cavitary necrosis. PML is, rarely, associated with a marked inflammatory reaction characterized by perivascular mononuclear infiltrates. There are different settings of this type of PML: in patients with HIV with HAART (PML-IRIS), patients with HIV without HAART, or patients without HIV. Three other subtypes of JCV-associated disease have been recently recognized: (1) JCV infecting only cerebellar granule cell neurons (JCVGCN), (2) JCV meningoencephalitis, and (3) JCV preferentially infecting cortical pyramidal neurons and astrocytes (JCV encephalopathy [JCE]). In the HAART era for the treatment of HIV infection, imaging has become more important in the diagnosis of PML. MR imaging is the most sensitive imaging tool for PML. Supratentorial white matter lesions are typically asymmetric, multifocal, bilateral, sometimes with confluent lobar involvement, but can be unilateral or there may be a single lesion. The lesions characteristically extend into the subcortical U fibers (Figs. 16.49, 16.50, and 16.51). PML can involve deep gray matter such as the thalamus and basal ganglia. Posterior fossa lesions are common and typically affect the middle cerebellar peduncles, adjacent pons, and cerebellar hemisphere (Figs. 16.51 and 16.52), and can extend into the midbrain and medulla. Spinal cord involvement is extremely rare. Initial MRI and newer margins in spreading lesions on follow-up MRI show a diffuse pale hyperintensity and/or numerous discrete hyperintense dots on T2-weighted images, so-called Milky Way appearance [75]. The degree of enhancement depends on the patient's immunologic status. The peripheral hyperintensity rim on DWI with reduced ADC may represent JCV-infected, swollen oligodendrocytes in the active margin of the lesions. JCVGCN presents with isolated cerebellar atrophy. JCE is initially restricted to hemispheric gray matter with extension to the subcortical white matter. Differential diagnosis includes other opportunistic infection, encephalitis/encephalopathy, lymphoma, or other demyelinating disease. There is no specific treatment of JCV infection. HAART is the best treatment in patients with HIV. HAART increased the 1-year survival rate by 10–50%. In HIV-negative patients, reduction of the cause of immunosuppression is indicated as much as is clinically allowable [50, 75].

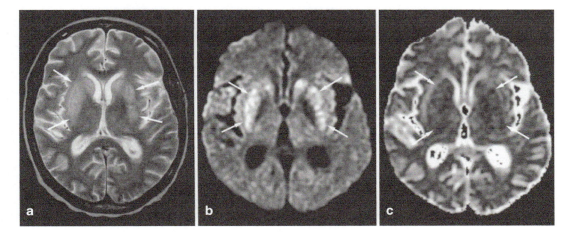

Fig. 16.48 AIDS-related bilateral basal ganglia lesions in a 38-year-old woman with multiple small infarcts. (**a**) T2-weighted image shows hyperintense lesions in bilateral caudate nuclei and putamina (*arrows*). (**b**) DW image demonstrates these lesions as numerous hyperintense spots, probably representing microinfarcts associated with HIV infection and/or drug abuse (*arrows*). (**c**) ADC map shows these lesions as partially decreased ADC (*arrows*)

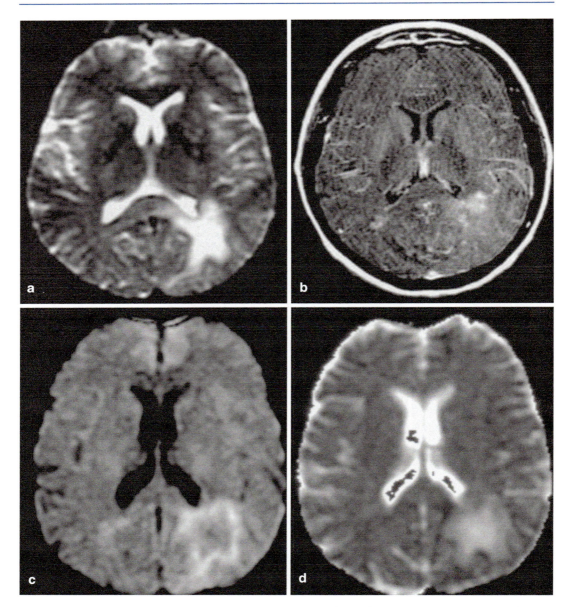

Fig. 16.49 Progressive multifocal leukoencephalopathy (PML) in a 50-year-old woman with right hemianopsia after chemotherapy and bone marrow transplant for chronic lymphocytic leukemia. (**a**) T2 hyperintense lesions are seen in the posterior part of the corpus callosum and left parieto-occipital white matter extending into the U fibers. (**b**) Postcontrast T1-weighted image reveals multiple patchy enhancement in the white matter lesion. (**c, d**) DWI reveals a peripheral rim of hyperintensity associated with slightly decreased ADC (from Ref. [50])

16.5.9 Coronavirus Disease 2019 (COVID-19)

Severe acute respiratory syndrome coronavirus 2 (SARS-CoV-2) emerged in December 2019, causing human COVID-19, which has now spread into a worldwide pandemic. A variety of brain imaging findings of COVID-19 has been reported including (1) ischemic infarct with micro- or macrothrombus, (2) intraparenchymal hemorrhage, (3) involvement of the mesial temporal lobe likely related seizures, (4) non-confluent multifocal WM lesions on FLAIR and DWI with variable enhancement

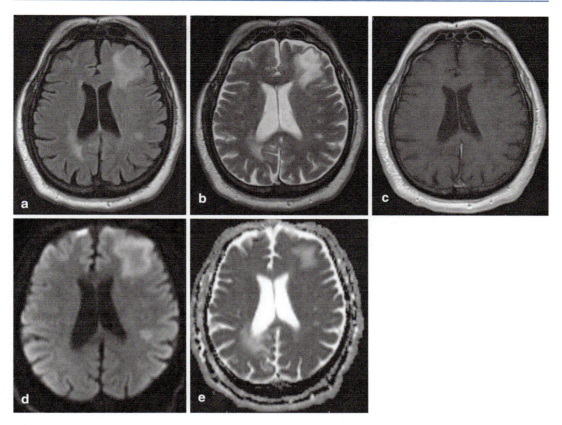

Fig. 16.50 PML in a 67-year-old male with a history of diffuse large B-cell lymphoma on Rituximab presenting with new onset confusion. (**a, b**) FLAIR and T2-weighted image show hyperintense ill-defined lesions in left frontal lobe involving the cortex. (**c**) T1-weighed image shows hypointensity in the lesion. (**d, e**) The lesions demonstrate peripheral reduced diffusion and central facilitated diffusion

and hemorrhagic lesions, possibly related to cytokine storm-induced vasculitis/vasculopathy (Fig. 16.53), (5) extensive (juxtacallosal/callosal) or isolated WM microhemorrhages (Fig. 16.54), (6) diffuse leukoencephalopathy which may be related to delayed post-anoxic leukoencephalopathy, (7) olfactory bulbs and gyrus rectus involvement, (8) cortical involvement possibly related to autoimmune encephalopathy, and (9) acute hemorrhagic necrotizing encephalopathy [76–83]. Posterior reversible encephalopathy, mild encephalitis, meningitis/encephalopathy with a reversible splenial lesion (MERS)/cytotoxic lesions of the corpus callosum, cerebral sinus vein thrombosis, Guillian-Barre syndrome (GBS) has also been reported. Positive SARS-CoV-2 RNA in the CSF is rare (Fig. 16.54).

16.6 Treatment of Infectious Diseases

Eiyu Matsumoto

16.6.1 Brain Abscess and Other Intracranial Suppurative Diseases (Subdural Empyema, Epidural Abscess, Ventriculitis)

16.6.1.1 Bacterial Brain Abscess

Prior to developing a fulminant brain abscess, microorganisms need to reach the brain. There are several pathways for that. The most common pathogenic mechanism is spread from a contiguous focus of infection most often in the middle

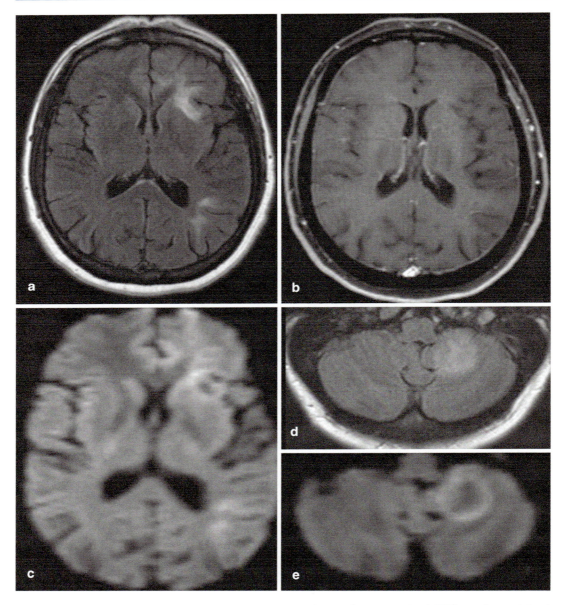

Fig. 16.51 PML in a 43-year-old HIV-positive woman with ataxia. (**a**, **d**) FLAIR image shows hyperintense lesions in left deep white matter extending to U fibers and the left cerebellum. (**b**) Postcontrast T1-weighted image reveals no enhancement. (**c**, **e**) DWI reveals a peripheral rim of hyperintensity in left cerebellar hemisphere (from Ref. [50])

ear, mastoid cells, or paranasal sinuses. Dental infections can also spread in this manner. An otogenic brain abscess most commonly locates in the temporal lobe and cerebellum [84]. On the other hand, an odontogenic abscess tends to occur in the frontal lobe. Another mechanism for brain abscess formation is hematogenous dissemination of organisms from other organs. Common sources of infection include pyogenic lung abscess, empyema, endocarditis, and intraabdominal infections. Trauma/surgery is a third pathogenic mechanism [85]. These

16 Infectious Diseases

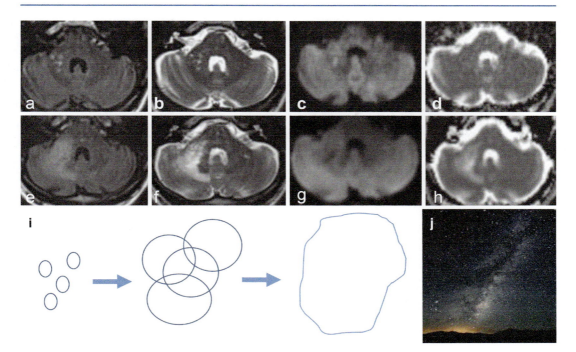

Fig. 16.52 PML in a 56-year-old man with multiple sclerosis on Natalizumab. (**a, b**) T2/FLAIR shows hyperintense small dots in the right cerebellar penduncle. (**c, d**) DWI and ADC map shows no restriction in the lesions. (**e–h**) Three months later, the lesions in the right cerebellar peduncle become confluent and involve the right cerebellar hemisphere. Facilitated diffusion is demonstrated in the lesion. (**i**) Numerous early demyelinating foci of PML become confluent large demyelinated lesions. Initial MRI and newer margins in spreading lesions on the follow-up MRI show diffuse pale hyperintensity and/or discrete T2 hyperintense dots called "Milky Way appearance" (**j**). (Courtesy of Dr Mio Sakai)

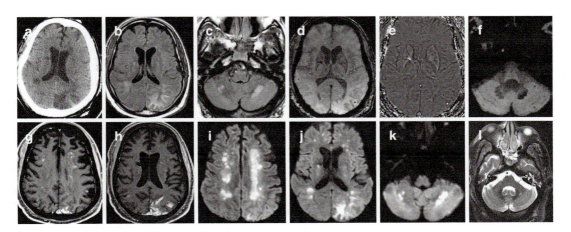

Fig. 16.53 COVID-19 with non-confluent multifocal white matter lesions with variable enhancement and microhemorrhage in a 57-year-old male, presented with altered mental status in the setting of ARDS requiring invasive ventilation. History of end-stage renal disease, coronary artery disease, and hypertension. (**a**) CT shows multiple low-density areas in the white matter and left parieto-occipital region. FLAIR (**b, c**) and DWI (**i–k**) show non-confluent multifocal WM lesions with variable enhancement on postcontrast T1-weighted image (**g, h**) and microhemorrhages (**d–f**). (**l**) Prominent pan-paranasal sinusitis

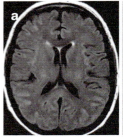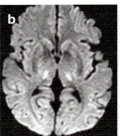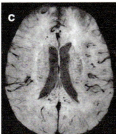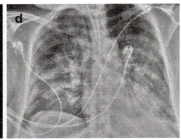

Fig. 16.54 COVID-19 with extensive white matter (juxtacallosal and callosal) microhemorrhages in a 59-year-old female, presented with altered mental status in the setting of ARDS requiring invasive ventilation. History of hypertension and asthma. (**a**) FLAIR shows mild hyperintensity in the thalami and splenium of the corpus callosum. (**b**) DWI show diffusion restriction in the thalamic lesions. (**c**) Susceptibility-weighted image demonstrates extensive juxtacallosal and callosal microhemorrhages. (**d**) Chest radiograph shows bilateral interstitial shadows consistent with COVID-19 pneumonia

distinctions (contiguous vs. hematogenous vs. trauma/surgery) are clinically very important to determine the management strategy. For example, if septic emboli to the brain are suspected, a superior radiologist can advise a clinician to evaluate for further infections besides CNS involvement (e.g., echocardiogram). This also means that antimicrobial coverage of *Staphylococcus aureus* (e.g., vancomycin) is mandatory since it is one of the most predominant etiologic agents.

The clinical course of brain abscess ranges from indolent to fulminant. Symptomatology is generally nonspecific. If imaging is suggestive of brain abscess, the first step is both HIV testing and blood cultures. The purpose of HIV testing is to narrow the differential diagnosis of pathogens (e.g., *Toxoplasma gondii* in HIV-positive population). Once HIV is ruled out, the patient should be considered for surgery if single or multiple ring-enhancing lesions are found. Lumbar puncture and CSF examination are contraindicated since the decompression of the CSF pressure below the tentrium can result in brainstem herniation, although inadvertently performed lumbar puncture may occur.

All lesions >2.5 cm in diameter should be excised or stereotactically aspirated. Specimens should be sent to microbiology for analysis. This should include gram stain, routine aerobic and anaerobic cultures, cultures for mycobacteria and fungi and pathology laboratories. When abscess material has been obtained for microbiologic and histopathologic studies, empirical antimicrobial therapy should be initiated on the basis of the patient's predisposing conditions and the presumed pathogenesis of abscess formation [85]. For patients with a brain abscess derived from an odontogenic, otogenic, or sinus causes, typical initial regimen is metronidazole plus either penicillin G or ceftriaxone. The intention of this regimen is to cover most common organisms in those disease sources such as streptococci, *Haemophilus influenzae*, *Moraxella catalaris*, and anaerobes.

For a brain abscess from suspected hematogenous spread, vancomycin needs to be started since *S. aureus* is the most common pathogen. For a brain abscess in a postoperative neurosurgical or otolaryngological patient, coverage of both *S. aureus* and nosocomial gram-negative organisms such as *Pseudomonas aeruginosa* is recommended. Therefore, vancomycin plus high-dose cefepime or anti-pseudomonal carbapenem such as meropenem would be often the empirical choice of therapy. Most of pyogenic brain abscess can be treated with 6–8 weeks of high-dose intravenous antimicrobial agents with an anticipated cure rate of more than 90% [85]. A higher mortality rate is reported in the brain abscess with hematogenous mechanism. Repeat imaging for follow-up purpose is commonly performed. MRI may show persistent abnormalities despite sterilization of abscess which could lead to unnecessary long antibiotic duration [86]. Contrast enhancement in MRI at the site of abscess may persist for several months [87]. CT scan may be more useful for therapeutic monitoring purpose.

16.6.1.2 Fungal Brain Abscess

The incidence of fungal brain abscess has increased in the modern era as a result of increased immunocompromised hosts. Risk factors for fungal brain abscess include administration of immunosuppressive agents, broad-spectrum antimicrobial therapy, prolonged neutropenia, and organ transplant. Common causative organisms include *Candida* spp., *Aspergillus* spp., *Mucor* spp., and *Scedosporium* spp. [85].

Fungal brain abscesses are primarily diagnosed by brain biopsy. The optimal therapy for fungal brain abscesses usually requires a combined medical and surgical intervention. Surgical options mean either excision or drainage. Despite the advancement in diagnosis and therapy, the prognosis of fungal brain abscess remains generally poor. Table 16.1 summarizes each organism and the typical therapeutic choice.

16.6.1.3 Subdural Empyema and Epidural Abscess

Subdural empyema refers to a collection of pus in the space between the dura and arachnoid. In contrast, epidural abscess refers to a localized collection of pus between the dura mater and the overlying skull or vertebral column. Although the anatomical locations of these diseases are different, the bacterial etiology and pathogenesis of both conditions are similar. The most common pathogenesis is direct extension of infection from a contiguous focus (e.g., otogenic infection) or from inadvertent inoculation of microorganism during trauma or neurosurgical procedure. Therefore, most common pathogens are streptococci, gram-negative bacilli, and anaerobes.

Table 16.1 Antimicrobial treatment of fungal infection

Organism	Antimicrobial choice
Candida spp.	Amphotericin B and 5-flucytosine
Aspergillus spp.	Voriconazole
Mucor spp.	Amphotericin B
Scedosporium spp.	Voriconazole

Clinically, those patient presents with headache, fever, meningeal irritation, seizure, and focal neurological deficit. CSF analysis is contraindicated with a concern of possible brain herniation. The diagnosis heavily relies on radiological studies such as CT and MRI. The general principle for the treatment is initiation of early empiric antimicrobial administration and surgical drainage. One therapeutic example for a suspected otogenic subdural empyema is the combination of ceftriaxone plus metronidazole to cover streptococci, *H. influenzae*, *M. catalaris*, and anaerobes. For a postsurgical case, methicillin-resistant *S. aureus* and pseudomonal species must be at least initially covered. Therefore, vancomycin plus meropenem would be an example of standard regimen. Antibiotic should be ultimately tailored based on microbiological information. The antibiotic duration is typically 3–6 weeks in cases without concomitant osteomyelitis. With osteomyelitis, 6–8 weeks would be the standard [88]. The presence (or absence) of osteomyelitis is determined by both radiological and intraoperative findings.

16.6.1.4 Pyogenic Ventriculitis

Pyogenic ventriculitis is bacterial infection of the ventricles in the brain. Common causes of ventriculitis include trauma with CFS leak, ventricular drains or shunts, and ruptured brain abscess. Clinical presentation varies depending on the virulence of pathogen. For example, ventriculitis from gram-negative bacilli derived from contaminated postoperative extraventricular device can cause dramatic decline in one's mental status. On the other hand, CNS shunt device infection from *Cutibacterium acnes* (formerly called as *Propionibacterium acnes*) often causes chronic headache without mounting systemic fever or mental status changes. CSF culture and chemistry panel are the corner stones for diagnosis. Of note, positive CSF culture does not necessarily mean the presence of infection. Given the high frequency of the infection from skin commensurate (e.g., coagulase-negative staphylococci and *C. acnes*) associated with retained man-made material (e.g., extraventricular device and shunt tube) in this disease entity, distinguishing contamination of organism from true infection should be carefully made. Although it is not always clear cut, infection is favored if gram stain is positive, CSF glucose level is low (<25 mg/dl), CSF protein level is high (>50 mg/dl), or a finding of neutrophilic pleocytosis (>10 cells/microl). For the evaluation of ambiguous cases, obtaining an infectious disease expert consultation is recommended. In the fulminant cases of postoperative ventriculitis, systemic antibiotic with better CNS penetration can be life-saving. Intraventricular antibiotic should be considered in severe cases. Antibiotic duration is typically for 1–3 weeks depending on the causative organism. If a new shunt system is needed after the treatment, CSF should be analyzed again while off antibiotic ensuring absence of infection. Practical clinical guidelines from Infectious Diseases Society of America (IDSA) are available online for a reference purpose [89].

16.6.2 Meningitis

Acute meningitis is clinically defined as a syndrome characterized by the onset of meningeal symptoms over the course of hours to up to several days. Symptoms include headache, fever, and meningismus, often later complicated by mental status change. Routine blood work is often unhelpful. At least two sets of blood cultures should be obtained from all patients prior to the initiation of antimicrobial therapy. More than 50 percent of patient with bacterial meningitis have positive blood cultures. Antibiotic administration for suspected bacterial meningitis should be initiated as soon as possible. CSF examination should be routinely performed for evaluation unless contraindicated [90].

Table 16.2 shows typical CSF findings in patients with selected infectious causes of men-

ingitis. Although most acute meningitis cases follow the pattern, some cases can be very difficult to establish or reject the diagnosis of acute bacterial meningitis. Of note, multiplex or panel-based PCR tests have emerged that test for multiple viral and bacterial pathogens simultaneously in a single CSF sample. These tests are highly sensitive and specific, although both false-positive and false-negative results can occur. Multiplex tests do not detect all the causes of CNS infection or perform susceptibility testing for the causative organism. Therefore, conventional culture method will continue to be used.

Chronic meningitis is defined as at least 4 weeks of symptoms with signs of inflammation in the CSF. This condition typically takes an indolent onset. Although the depending on the report, the three most common causes are sarcoidosis, cryptococcosis, and tuberculosis. Other less common etiologies include syphilis, Lyme disease, coccidioidomycosis, histoplasmosis, blastomycosis, sporotrichosis, acanthamebiasis, lymphoma, and Vogt-Koyanagi-Harada syndrome. No empiric treatment is typically needed unless there is high suspicion for severe tuberculous meningitis. Management is depending on the etiology.

16.6.2.1 Acute Bacterial Meningitis

There have been remarkable changes in regard to the etiology of acute bacterial meningitis over the last several decades. In the United States, following the initiation of routine infant immunization with the conjugate *Haemophilus influenzae* type b vaccine in 1990 and the 7-valent *Streptococcus pneumoniae* conjugate vaccine in 2000, the incidence of meningitis under 5 years old has dramatically decreased. Another big change is emergence of penicillin- or cephalosporin-resistant strain in *S. pneumoniae*.

Table 16.2 CSF study of meningitis

Cause of meningitis	White blood cell count (cells/mm^3)	Primary cell type	Glucose (mg/dl)	Protein (mg/dl)
Viral	50–1000	Mononuclear	>45	<200
Bacterial	100–5000	Neutrophilic	<40	100–500
Tuberculous	50–300	Mononuclear	<45	50–300
Cryptococcal	20–500	Mononuclear	<40	>45

16 Infectious Diseases

The causative organism is depending on age and immune status (Table 16.3). Empiric antibiotic regimen should be selected accordingly. *S. pneumoniae*, *H. influenzae*, *Neisseria meningitidis* are the three most common pathogens in many age groups. Therefore, ceftriaxone would be the first line. For the coverage of penicillin-resistant *S. pneumoniae*, vancomycin should be added. *Listeria monocytogenes* is a unique pathogen seen in very young, pregnant, and older (age ≥ 50) patients. For the coverage, a clinician needs to add ampicillin to the regimen since listeria is intrinsically resistant to cephalosporins. There is a consensus on the use of corticosteroids (dexamethasone 0.15 mg/kg every 6 h for 2–4 days) in *S. pneumoniae* meningitis in all ages. Corticosteroids should be stopped if the acute meningitis is caused by other organisms. Clinicians are often afraid of the possibility of brain herniation upon lumbar puncture.

Table 16.3 Antimicrobial treatment of bacterial infection

Predisposing factor	Common bacterial pathogen	Typical antimicrobial therapy
Age		
<1 month	*Streptococcus agalactiae*	Ampicillin plus aminoglycoside
	Escherichia coli	Ampicillin plus a third-generation cephalosporin
	Listeria monocytogenes	
1–23 months	*Streptococcus pneumoniae*	Vancomycin plus a third-generation cephalosporin
	Neisseria meningitidis	
	S. agalactiae	
2–50 years	*S. pneumoniae*	Vancomycin plus a third-generation cephalosporin
	N. meningitidis	
≥50 years	*S. pneumoniae*	Vancomycin plus ampicillin plus a third-generation cephalosporin
	N. meningitidis	
	L. monocytogenes	
	Aerobic gram-negative bacilli	

However, the incidence of herniation is very low. Obtaining CT before performing lumbar puncture should be limited to the patients with suspected bacterial meningitis if a patient is either immunocompromised, has CNS diseases, papilledema, or focal neurologic deficit. Empiric antibiotic should not be delayed pending lumbar puncture if bacterial meningitis is suspected. Typical duration of antimicrobial therapy for bacterial meningitis is as follows. 7 days: *Neisseria meningitidis*, 7 days: *Haemophilus influenzae*, 10–14 days: *Streptococcus pneumoniae*, 14–21 days: *Streptococcus agalactiae*, 21 days: aerobic gram-negative bacilli, 21 days ≥ *Listeria monocytogenes*. In the patients with bacterial meningitis who have responded appropriately to antimicrobial therapy, repeated CSF analysis to document CSF sterilization and improvement of CSF parameters is not routinely indicated. However, repeated CSF analysis should be performed for any patient who has not responded clinically after 48 h of appropriate antimicrobial therapy [90].

16.6.3 Management of Encephalitis and Viral Infections

Encephalitis is defined as an inflammatory process of the brain parenchyma associated with clinical or laboratory evidence of neurologic dysfunction. It can be caused by infectious processes, predominantly viruses, or noninfectious causes such as autoimmune, paraneoplastic, or collagen vascular diseases. Herpes simplex virus (HSV) is the most common agent for sporadic encephalitis. Other viral causes of acute encephalitis include the other herpesviruses (e.g., varicella-zoster virus, cytomegalovirus, and human herpesvirus 6), arboviruses (e.g., West Nile, eastern equine, St. Louis, La Crosse, and Japanese encephalitis viruses), HIV, rabies virus, and the enteroviruses. Nonviral causes of encephalitis include *L. monocytogenes*, *Rickettsia* spp., *Ehrlichia* spp., *Bartonella* spp., *Mycoplasma pneumoniae*, and *Toxoplasma gondii*. Several free-living amebae (e.g., *Naegleria fowleri*, *Acanthoamoeba* spp., and *Balamuthia mandril-*

laris) have also been reported to cause encephalitis. Despite a modern advance in medicine with a multitude of expensive diagnostic tests, one-third to two-thirds of encephalitis cases remain of unknown etiology even with very extensive comprehensive investigational protocols [91]. Therefore, many infectious disease experts tend to focus on treatable diseases, likely diseases, and diseases that cannot be missed. Clinical guidelines are available [92].

16.6.3.1 Herpes Simplex Virus (HSV)

HSV is the most common cause of sporadic encephalitis in the United States. HSV-1 accounts for more than 90% of all cases of HSV encephalitis with the remainder caused by HSV-2. Identification of HSV encephalitis is clinically important since it is one of the few causes of viral encephalitis that is treatable by antimicrobial medications. Polymerase chain reaction (PCR) of HSV DNA in the CSF is the procedure of choice for the diagnosis of HSV encephalitis. CSF HSV PCR has a sensitivity of 98% and a specificity of 94% compared with gold standard of brain biopsy [93]. Although these numbers seem high, they are not perfect since misdiagnosis can result in a dreadful outcome. HSV PCR tends to be falsely negative especially when the specimen was obtained <3 days from the symptom onset. MRI and electroencephalogram (EEG) are important adjunctive for diagnosis in those cases. Typical HSV encephalitis predominantly involves the temporal lobe. One study showed that MRI revealed abnormalities of the temporal lobes in 89% of cases confirmed by CSF HSV PCR. EEG pattern seen in HSV encephalitis is often nonspecific, but focal EEG abnormalities have been reported in 81% of biopsy-proven HSV encephalitis cases, and temporal lobe abnormalities occur in 75% of PCR-proven cases [94]. Therefore, if MRI or EEG findings are typical for HSV encephalitis with negative initial CSF HSV PCR, clinicians should consider testing for second CSF HSV PCR to be sure for the absence of HSV encephalitis. For this reason, MRI read from a radiologist can be extremely important. Once confirmed, HSV encephalitis is typically treated by 2–3 weeks of intravenous acyclovir.

16.6.3.2 Varicella-Zoster Virus (VZV)

Varicella-zoster virus (VZV) causes two clinically distinct diseases. The primary infection to a susceptible individual primarily occurs in pediatric population, known as chicken pox. Like all other herpesviruses, VZV demonstrates latency following primary infection with subsequent reactivation manifested as shingles.

CNS complications with varicella occurs approximately 1–3 per 10, 000 cases. The CNS manifestations most frequently associated with chickenpox are cerebellar ataxia and encephalitis. Children can develop acute cerebellar ataxia from several days before to 2 weeks after the onset of rash. Symptoms are vomiting, headache, lethargy, fever, seizures, and ataxia. In uncomplicated cases, the diagnosis can be made clinically without further investigation. It is a self-limited disease which typically resolves in 1–3 weeks from the onset. Mortality is essentially zero [95].

Neurologic complications of herpes zoster can occur during the acute eruption or weeks to months after the episode of rash. These include encephalitis, herpes zoster ophthalmicus with delayed contralateral hemiparesis, transverse myelitis, cranial and peripheral nerve palsies, acute retinal necrosis, and postherpetic neuralgia. VZV is one of the most common causes of encephalitis. Typical VZV encephalitis includes increased opening pressure, increased protein, and lymphocytic pleocytosis. PCR is the most sensitive diagnostic tool for zoster encephalitis. Caution should be made in interpreting the spinal fluid findings because pleocytosis is also present in up to 50 percent of uncomplicated herpes zoster. There is no controlled trial in the management of neurologic complications of herpes zoster. Based on the anecdotal experience and in vitro data, use of intravenous acyclovir is a common practice [96].

16.6.3.3 Human Herpesvirus Types 6 (HHV-6)

Human herpesviruses 6 is one of members of the beta herpes virus subfamily. It is ubiquitous. In pediatric population it can cause exanthema subium (or roseola infantum). In immunocompromised hosts such as hematopoietic stem cell transplant (HSCT), recipients are at risk for reactivation of the virus causing diseases. One of the best documented manifestations of HHV-6 in immunosuppressed patients is limbic encephalitis. The disease is especially common in transplant recipients receiving cord blood, up to 8.5 percent. Most common symptoms are short-term memory loss and insomnia. Diagnosis of HHV-6 as the cause of symptoms in immunocompromised patients is often a challenge because HHV-6 frequently reactivates in a large proportion of these patients regardless of presence or absence of HHV-6 encephalitis. Typical finding of MRI findings can be suggestive of the diagnosis. CSF shows elevated protein in two-thirds of cases with a mild lymphocytic pleocytosis. A high or a rising level of viral DNA or RNA in the blood is more likely suggestive of HHV-6 disease, but not always. Detection of HHV-6 in the CSF is strongly suggestive of CNS disease, but again is not definite. The use of PCR for the diagnosis of HHV-6 is further complicated by the fact that HHV-6 is integrated into chromosomal DNA in 0.7–1.5 percent of persons. HHV-6 is sensitive to ganciclovir, foscarnet, and cidofovir in vitro. There are no controlled studies available. Based on anecdotal reports, a 7-day course of single or dual agents is utilized [97].

16.6.3.4 Progressive Multifocal Leukoencephalopathy (PML)

JC virus or John Cunningham virus is a type of human polyomavirus. It is ubiquitous in most human populations throughout the world, and up to 86 percent of the general adult population is seropositive. JC virus does not cause disease in immunocompetent individuals, but it can cause multifocal demyelination of the white matter of the CNS known as progressive multifocal leukoencephalopathy (PML) as the reactivation process in immunosuppressed individuals. In a recent study, 82 percent of patients with PML had AIDS, 8.4 percent had hematologic malignant diseases, 2.8 percent had solid-organ transplant recipients, 0.95 percent had chronic inflammatory diseases, and 6 percent had no defined risk factor for PML [98]. Of note, natalizumab, an immunomodulatory drug for multiple sclerosis or Crohn's disease, is associated with PML [99]. Initial symptoms of PML can vary greatly depending on the location of white matter affected; however, coordination difficulties, gait disturbance, cognitive dysfunction, visual problems, and limb paresis are common. In general, these symptoms are irreversible. Diagnosis of PML is essentially made by MRI findings. Although CSF chemistry profile for PML is non-specific, JCV PCR assay is known to be helpful with a sensitivity of 72–92 percent and a specificity of 92–100 percent. There is no established treatment exists for PML [100]. Boosting the immune system is the single established treatment. In HIV-positive patient cohort, initiation of optimization of anti-retroviral treatment was associated with an increased survival rate at 1 year from 10 percent to 50 percent. Adjunctive corticosteroids are commonly used when brain swelling and mass effect are present. More recently, successful use of monoclonal antibody therapy has been reported [101].

16.6.4 HIV

Neurologic manifestations are common in human immunodeficiency virus (HIV) infection. Before the era of combined antiretroviral therapy (cART), neurologic disease was seen in 10 percent at initial presentation and in 30–50 percent during the course [102]. It seems like the incidence of neurological complication has decreased with wide use of cART [103].

Acute aseptic meningitis may be the initial presentation for acute HIV infection. Patients typically presents with headache, stiff neck, and fever. It is a self-limited disease that subsides spontaneously. A high index of suspicion and sexual history are the key for making the diagnosis.

16.6.4.1 Opportunistic Infections (Cryptococcal Meningitis)

Numerous opportunistic infections can invade CNS in HIV patients. Cryptococcal meningitis, syphilitic meningitis, CNS toxoplasmosis may be the most common presentations. Here below, cryptococcal meningitis will be described. Please refer to the next subchapter "4.2 Management of Brain Mass Lesions in a HIV Positive Patient" for the management of CNS toxoplasmosis.

Cryptococcal meningitis is the most common opportunistic meningitis in AIDS. This illness typically occurs in individuals with CD4+ T-lymphocyte counts of <200 cells/microl. The presentation consists of subacute headache, fever, confusion, blindness, and altered mental status. The characteristics of CSF profile include markedly elevated opening pressure, mononuclear pleocytosis, elevated protein, and decreased glucose concentration. The detection of *Cryptococcus neoformans* antigen titers by enzyme immunoassay in the CSF provides a rapid diagnosis. Brain imaging is usually negative. Treatment should be initiated with amphotericin B with 5-flucotosine until the patient is clearly responding and for no <2 weeks. Lipid formulations of amphotericin are commonly used to decrease renal toxicity. After amphotericin use, consolidation therapy with higher dose of fluconazole, followed by maintenance dose of fluconazole for a total of 12 months of duration is recommended. Secondary prevention by fluconazole is recommended until recovery of CD4 count rises above the certain level. Besides antibiotic therapy, there are two issues in the management of cryptococcal meningitis. The first one is management of intracranial pressure. Intracranial pressure greater than 200 mm H_2O is a well-known complication occurring almost in all patients. It should be recognized and treated aggressively by repeat lumbar punctures, temporary external lumbar drainage, or intraventricular shunts since elevated pressure is negatively correlated with prognosis. The second challenge is the timing of initiation of cART. Neurologic deterioration after commencing ART occurs in 26 percent of patients as the result of immune reconstitution inflammatory syndrome (IRIS). Although corticosteroids can alleviate the phenomenon, some patient may die during the phase [104].

16.6.4.2 Management of Brain Mass Lesions in a HIV-Positive Patient (CNS Toxoplasmosis and CNS Lymphoma)

Neurologic manifestations are frequent in HIV-1 infection. Among those, CNS mass lesions may be one of the most common clinical entities. Depending on the CD4+ T-lymphocyte count, the most common two etiologies of mass lesions are toxoplasmosis and lymphoma. Distinction of these two entities is important given the different management strategies. Typical toxoplasma encephalitis occurs in a patient with CD4+ T-lymphocyte counts <200 cells/microl. If MRI findings are typical (multiple lesions, corticomedullary junction, white matter, basal ganglia) and/or serum *Toxoplasma gondii*, IgG is positive and/or CSF *Toxoplasma gondii* DNA PCR is positive, a targeted treatment for toxoplasmosis with antimicrobial agent for 2 weeks followed by repeat MRI is recommended. If the follow-up MRI does not show any improvement or the initial MRI findings are atypical for toxoplasmosis, immediate brain biopsy is recommended. For the treatment of toxoplasma encephalitis, 6 weeks of combination antimicrobial therapy is utilized, followed by secondary maintenance therapy which should be continued for 3 months beyond the patient's achievement of CD4+ T-cell counts higher than 200 cells/microl. If the diagnosis is made in a timely fashion with smooth treatment course, toxoplasma encephalitis has a relatively high therapeutic success rate and death is usually caused by other complications of AIDS [105].

16.6.4.3 HIV-Associated Neurocognitive Disorder (HAND)

HIV-associated neurocognitive disorder (HAND), so-called AIDS dementia complex can occur as the first manifestation of the HIV disease in 3–10 percent of cases. The clinical characteristics of this disorder can be subdivided into three main categories: cognitive, behavioral, and motor. The onset of the illness is insidious. Numerous groups have detected early neurologic dysfunction in HIV-1-infected asymptomatic patients. Diagnosis is made by combination of

16 Infectious Diseases

HIV testing result, MRI, and clinical manifestation. There is no role of brain biopsy. Although the use of cART with a profile of high CSF penetration of the drug is a common practice in the case of HAND, cognitive dysfunction persists regardless of presence of cART or the selection. There is no proven treatment for the condition to date [106].

References

1. Ebisu T, Naruse S, Horikawa Y et al (1993) Discrimination between different types of white matter edema with diffusion-weighted MR imaging. J Magn Reson Imaging 3:863–868
2. Ebisu T, Tanaka C, Umeda M et al (1996) Discrimination of brain abscess from necrotic or cystic tumors by diffusion-weighted echo planar imaging. Magn Reson Imaging 14:1113–1116
3. Kim YJ, Chang KH, Song IC et al (1998) Brain abscess and necrotic or cystic brain tumor: discrimination with signal intensity on diffusion-weighted MR imaging. AJR Am J Roentgenol 171:1487–1490
4. Desprechins B, Stadnik T, Koerts G et al (1999) Use of diffusion-weighted MR imaging in differential diagnosis between intracerebral necrotic tumors and cerebral abscesses. AJNR Am J Neuroradiol 20:1252–1257
5. Noguchi K, Watanabe N, Nagayoshi T et al (1999) Role of diffusion-weighted echo-planar MRI in distinguishing between brain Tadayoshi abscess and tumour: a preliminary report. Neuroradiology 41:171–174
6. Castillo M (1999) Imaging brain abscesses with diffusion-weighted and other sequences. AJNR Am J Neuroradiol 20:1193–1194
7. F G PN (1997) Bacterial infections. In: DI G, PL L (eds) Greenfield's neuropathology, 6th edn, pp 114–129
8. Falcone S, Post MJ (2000) Encephalitis, cerebritis, and brain abscess: pathophysiology and imaging findings. Neuroimaging Clin N Am 10:333–353
9. Hatta S, Mochizuki H, Kuru Y et al (1994) Serial neuroradiological studies in focal cerebritis. Neuroradiology 36:285–288
10. Ketelslegers E, Duprez T, Ghariani S et al (2000) Time dependence of serial diffusion-weighted imaging features in a case of pyogenic brain abscess. J Comput Assist Tomogr 24:478–481
11. Cartes-Zumelzu FW, Stavrou I, Castillo M et al (2004) Diffusion-weighted imaging in the assessment of brain abscesses therapy. AJNR Am J Neuroradiol 25:1310–1317
12. Gupta RK, Hasan KM, Mishra AM et al (2005) High fractional anisotropy in brain abscesses versus other cystic intracranial lesions. AJNR Am J Neuroradiol 26:1107–1114
13. Kumar M, Gupta RK, Nath K et al (2008) Can we differentiate true white matter fibers from pseudo-fibers inside a brain abscess cavity using geometrical diffusion tensor imaging metrics? NMR Biomed 21:581–588
14. Bakshi R, Wright PD, Kinkel PR et al (1999) Cranial magnetic resonance imaging findings in bacterial endocarditis: the neuroimaging spectrum of septic brain embolization demonstrated in twelve patients. J Neuroimaging 9:78–84
15. Hollinger P, Zurcher R, Schroth G et al (2000) Diffusion magnetic resonance imaging findings in cerebritis and brain abscesses in a patient with septic encephalopathy. J Neurol 247:232–234
16. Nagase T, Wada S, Nakamura R et al (1995) Magnetic resonance imaging of multiple brain abscesses of the bilateral basal ganglia. Intern Med 34:554–558
17. Southwick FS, Purich DL (1996) Intracellular pathogenesis of listeriosis. N Engl J Med 334:770–776
18. Fleetwood IG, Embil JM, Ross IB (2000) Nocardia asteroides cerebral abscess in immunocompetent hosts: report of three cases and review of surgical recommendations. Surg Neurol 53:605–610
19. Shin JH, Lee HK (2003) Nocardial brain abscess in a renal transplant recipient. Clin Imaging 27:321–324
20. Luthra G, Parihar A, Nath K et al (2007) Comparative evaluation of fungal, tubercular, and pyogenic brain abscesses with conventional and diffusion MR imaging and proton MR spectroscopy. AJNR Am J Neuroradiol 28:1332–1338
21. Gupta RK, Prakash M, Mishra AM et al (2005) Role of diffusion weighted imaging in differentiation of intracranial tuberculoma and tuberculous abscess from cysticercus granulomas-a report of more than 100 lesions. Eur J Radiol 55:384–392
22. Sadeghi N, Rorive S, Lefranc F (2003) Intracranial tuberculoma: is diffusion-weighted imaging useful in the diagnosis? Eur Radiol 13:2049–2050
23. Holtas S, Geijer B, Stromblad LG et al (2000) A ring-enhancing metastasis with central high signal on diffusion-weighted imaging and low apparent diffusion coefficients. Neuroradiology 42:824–827
24. Hartmann M, Jansen O, Heiland S et al (2001) Restricted diffusion within ring enhancement is not pathognomonic for brain abscess. AJNR Am J Neuroradiol 22:1738–1742
25. Tung GA, Evangelista P, Rogg JM et al (2001) Diffusion-weighted MR imaging of rim-enhancing brain masses: is markedly decreased water diffusion specific for brain abscess? AJR Am J Roentgenol 177:709–712
26. Friedman DP, Goldman HW, Flanders AE (1997) MR imaging of stereotaxic pallidotomy and thalamotomy. AJR Am J Roentgenol 169:894–896
27. Ackerman LL, Traynelis VC (1999) Dural space infection: cranial subdural empyema and cranial epidural abscess. In: Osenbach RK, Zeidman SM

(eds) Infections in neurological surgery. Lippincott-Raven, Philadelphia, pp 85–99

28. Ramsay DW, Aslam M, Cherryman GR (2000) Diffusion-weighted imaging of cerebral abscess and subdural empyema. AJNR Am J Neuroradiol 21:1172

29. Rana S, Albayram S, Lin DD et al (2002) Diffusion-weighted imaging and apparent diffusion coefficient maps in a case of intracerebral abscess with ventricular extension. AJNR Am J Neuroradiol 23:109–112

30. Ebisu T, Tanaka C, Umeda M et al (1997) Hemorrhagic and nonhemorrhagic stroke: diagnosis with diffusion-weighted and T2-weighted echo-planar MR imaging. Radiology 203:823–828

31. Atlas SW, DuBois P, Singer MB et al (2000) Diffusion measurements in intracranial hematomas: implications for MR imaging of acute stroke. AJNR Am J Neuroradiol 21:1190–1194

32. Tsuruda JS, Chew WM, Moseley ME et al (1990) Diffusion-weighted MR imaging of the brain: value of differentiating between extraaxial cysts and epidermoid tumors. AJNR Am J Neuroradiol 11:925–931; discussion 932–924

33. Moodley M, Bullock MR (1985) Severe neurological sequelae of childhood bacterial meningitis. S Afr Med J 68:566–570

34. Black DF, Aksamit AJ, Morris JM (2010) MR imaging of central nervous system Whipple disease: a 15-year review. AJNR Am J Neuroradiol 31:1493–1497

35. Jared W, Nelson MLW, Zhang Y, Moritani T (2005) Proton magnetic resonance spectroscopy and diffusion-weighted imaging of central nervous system Whipple disease. J Comput Assist Tomogr 29:320–32234

36. Navia BA, Petito CK, Gold JW et al (1986) Cerebral toxoplasmosis complicating the acquired immune deficiency syndrome: clinical and neuropathological findings in 27 patients. Ann Neurol 19:224–238

37. Camacho DL, Smith JK, Castillo M (2003) Differentiation of toxoplasmosis and lymphoma in AIDS patients by using apparent diffusion coefficients. AJNR Am J Neuroradiol 24:633–637

38. Chong-Han CH, Cortez SC, Tung GA (2003) Diffusion-weighted MRI of cerebral toxoplasma abscess. AJR Am J Roentgenol 181:1711–1714

39. Schroeder PC, Post MJ, Oschatz E et al (2006) Analysis of the utility of diffusion-weighted MRI and apparent diffusion coefficient values in distinguishing central nervous system toxoplasmosis from lymphoma. Neuroradiology 48:715–720

40. do Amaral LL, Ferreira RM, da Rocha AJ et al (2005) Neurocysticercosis: evaluation with advanced magnetic resonance techniques and atypical forms. Top Magn Reson Imaging 16:127–144

41. Cordoliani YS, Sarrazin JL, Felten D et al (1998) MR of cerebral malaria. AJNR Am J Neuroradiol 19:871–874

42. Patankar TF, Karnad DR, Shetty PG et al (2002) Adult cerebral malaria: prognostic importance of imaging findings and correlation with postmortem findings. Radiology 224:811–816

43. Sakai O, Barest GD (2005) Diffusion-weighted imaging of cerebral malaria. J Neuroimaging 15:278–280

44. DeLone DR, Goldstein RA, Petermann G et al (1999) Disseminated aspergillosis involving the brain: distribution and imaging characteristics. AJNR Am J Neuroradiol 20:1597–1604

45. Charlot M, Pialat JB, Obadia N et al (2007) Diffusion-weighted imaging in brain aspergillosis. Eur J Neurol 14:912–916

46. Gaviani P, Schwartz RB, Hedley-Whyte ET et al (2005) Diffusion-weighted imaging of fungal cerebral infection. AJNR Am J Neuroradiol 26:1115–1121

47. Simmons JH, Zeitler PS, Fenton LZ et al (2005) Rhinocerebral mucormycosis complicated by internal carotid artery thrombosis in a pediatric patient with type 1 diabetes mellitus: a case report and review of the literature. Pediatr Diabetes 6:234–238

48. Tung GA, Rogg JM (2003) Diffusion-weighted imaging of cerebritis. AJNR Am J Neuroradiol 24:1110–1113

49. Ho TL, Lee HJ, Lee KW et al (2005) Diffusion-weighted and conventional magnetic resonance imaging in cerebral cryptococcoma. Acta Radiol 46:411–414

50. Starkey J, Moritani T, Kirby P (2014) MRI of CNS fungal infections: review of aspergillosis to histoplasmosis and everything in between. Clin Neuroradiol 24:217–230

51. Mao J, Li J, Chen D, Zhang J et al (2012) MRI-DWI improves the early diagnosis of brain abscess induced by Candida Albicans in preterm infants. Transl Pediatr 2:76–84

52. Lin DJ, Sacks A, Shen J et al (2013) Neurocandidiasis: a case report and consideration of the causes of restricted diffusion. Radiology Case 7(5):1–5

53. Smith JS, Quinones-Hinojosa A, Phillips JJ et al (2006) Limitations of diffusion-weighted imaging in distinguishing between a brain tumor and a central nervous system histoplasmoma. J Neuro-Oncol 79:217–218

54. Moritani T, Capizzano A, Kirby P et al (2014) Viral infections and white matter lesions. Radiol Clin N Am 52:355–382

55. Jayaraman K, Rangasami R, Chandrasekharan A (2018) Magnetic resonance imaging findings in viral encephalitis: a pictorial essay. J Neurosci Rural Pract 9:556–560

56. Sener RN (2001) Herpes simplex encephalitis: diffusion MR imaging findings. Comput Med Imaging Graph 25:391–397

57. Tsuchiya K, Katase S, Yoshino A et al (1999) Diffusion-weighted MR imaging of encephalitis. AJR Am J Roentgenol 173:1097–1099

58. Obeid M, Franklin J, Shrestha S et al (2007) Diffusion-weighted imaging findings on MRI as the sole radiographic findings in a child with

proven herpes simplex encephalitis. Pediatr Radiol 37:1159–1162

59. Kuker W, Nagele T, Schmidt F et al (2004) Diffusion-weighted MRI in herpes simplex encephalitis: a report of three cases. Neuroradiology 46:122–125

60. Heiner L, Demaerel P (2003) Diffusion-weighted MR imaging findings in a patient with herpes simplex encephalitis. Eur J Radiol 45:195–198

61. Noguchi T, Mihara F, Yoshiura T et al (2006) MR imaging of human herpesvirus-6 encephalopathy after hematopoietic stem cell transplantation in adults. AJNR Am J Neuroradiol 27:2191–2195

62. Gorniak RJ, Young GS, Wiese DE et al (2006) MR imaging of human herpesvirus-6-associated encephalitis in 4 patients with anterograde amnesia after allogeneic hematopoietic stem-cell transplantation. AJNR Am J Neuroradiol 27:887–891

63. Wasenko JJ, Park BJ, Jubelt B et al (2002) Magnetic resonance imaging of mesenrhombencephalitis. Clin Imaging 26:237–242

64. Soo MS, Tien RD, Gray L et al (1993) Mesenrhombencephalitis: MR findings in nine patients. AJR Am J Roentgenol 160:1089–1093

65. Weidauer S, Ziemann U, Thomalske C et al (2003) Vasogenic edema in Bickerstaff's brainstem encephalitis: a serial MRI study. Neurology 61:836–838

66. Ali M, Safriel Y, Sohi J et al (2005) West Nile virus infection: MR imaging findings in the nervous system. AJNR Am J Neuroradiol 26:289–297

67. Petropoulou KA, Gordon SM, Prayson RA et al (2005) West Nile virus meningoencephalitis: MR imaging findings. AJNR Am J Neuroradiol 26:1986–1995

68. Kraushaar G, Patel R, Stoneham GW (2005) West Nile virus: a case report with flaccid paralysis and cervical spinal cord: MR imaging findings. AJNR Am J Neuroradiol 26:26–29

69. Zak IT, Altinok D, Merline JR et al (2005) West Nile virus infection. AJR Am J Roentgenol 184:957–961

70. Rosas H, Wippold FJ 2nd. (2003) West Nile virus: case report with MR imaging findings. AJNR Am J Neuroradiol 24:1376–1378

71. Flowers CH, Mafee MF, Crowell R et al (1990) Encephalopathy in AIDS patients: evaluation with MR imaging. AJNR Am J Neuroradiol 11:1235–1245

72. Connor MD, Lammie GA, Bell JE et al (2000) Cerebral infarction in adult AIDS patients: observations from the Edinburgh HIV autopsy cohort. Stroke 31:2117–2126

73. Meltzer CC, Wells SW, Becher MW et al (1998) AIDS-related MR hyperintensity of the basal ganglia. AJNR Am J Neuroradiol 19:83–89

74. Bag AK, Curé JK, Chapman PR et al (2010) JC virus infection of the brain. AJNR Am J Neuroradiol 31(9):1564–1576

75. Sakai M, Inoue Y, Aoki S et al (2009) Follow-up magnetic resonance imaging findings in patients with progressive multifocal leukoencephalopathy: evaluation of long-term survivors under highly active antiretroviral therapy. Jpn J Radiol 27:69–77

76. Kremer S, Lersy F, de Sèze J et al (2020) Brain MRI findings in severe COVID-19: a retrospective observational study [published online ahead of print, 2020 Jun 16]. Radiology:202222. https://doi.org/10.1148/radiol.2020202222

77. Radmanesh A, Derman A, Lui YW et al (2020) COVID-19-associated diffuse Leukoencephalopathy and Microhemorrhages [published online ahead of print, 2020 may 21]. Radiology:202040. https://doi.org/10.1148/radiol.2020202040

78. Kandemirli SG, Dogan L, Sarikaya ZT et al (2020) Brain MRI findings in patients in the intensive care unit with COVID-19 infection [published online ahead of print, 2020 may 8]. Radiology:201697. https://doi.org/10.1148/radiol.2020201697

79. Paterson RW, Brown RL, Benjamin L et al (2020) The emerging spectrum of COVID-19 neurology: clinical, radiological and laboratory findings [published online ahead of print, 2020 Jul 8]. Brain:awaa240. https://doi.org/10.1093/brain/awaa240

80. Dogan L, Kaya D, Sarikaya T et al (2020) Plasmapheresis treatment in COVID-19-related autoimmune meningoencephalitis: case series. Brain Behav Immun 87:155–158. https://doi.org/10.1016/j.bbi.2020.05.022

81. Poyiadji N, Shahin G, Noujaim D, Stone M, Patel S, Griffith B (2020) COVID-19-associated acute Hemorrhagic necrotizing encephalopathy: CT and MRI features [published online ahead of print, 2020 Mar 31]. Radiology:201187. https://doi.org/10.1148/radiol.2020201187

82. Abdel-Mannan O, Eyre M, Löbel U et al (2020) Neurologic and radiographic findings associated with COVID-19 infection in children [published online ahead of print, 2020 Jul 1]. JAMA Neurol:e202687. https://doi.org/10.1001/jamaneurol.2020.2687

83. Chougar L, Shor N, Weiss N et al (2020) Retrospective observational study of brain magnetic resonance imaging findings in patients with acute SARS-CoV-2 infection and neurological manifestations [published online ahead of print, 2020 Jul 17]. Radiology:202422. https://doi.org/10.1148/radiol.2020202422

84. Sennaroglu L, Sozeri B (2000) Otogenic brain abscess: review of 41 cases. Otolaryngol Head Neck Surg 123(6):751–755

85. Brouwer M, Tunkel A, Mckhann G, Beek D (2014) Brain abscess. N Engl J Med 371:447–456

86. Helweg-Larsen J, Astradsson A, Richhall H, Erdal J, Laursen A, Brennum J (2012) Pyogenic brain abscess, a 15 year survey. BMC Infect Dis 12:332

87. Cavuşoglu H, Kaya RA, Türkmenoglu ON, Colak I, Aydin Y (2008) Brain abscess: analysis of results in a series of 51 patients with a combined surgical and medical approach during an 11-year period. Neurosurg Focus 24(6):E9

88. Bockova J, Rigamonti D (2000) Intracranial Empyema. Pediatr Infect Dis J 19(8):735–737

89. Tunkel AR, Hasbun R, Bhimraj A, Byers K, Kaplan SL, Scheld WM et al (2017) Infectious Diseases

Society of America's clinical practice guidelines for healthcare-associated Ventriculitis and meningitis*. Clin Infect Dis 64(6):e34–e65

90. Tunkel AR, Hartman BJ, Kaplan SL, Kaufman BA, Roos KL, Scheld WM et al (2004) Practice guidelines for the management of bacterial meningitis. Clin Infect Dis 39(9):1267–1284

91. Glaser C, Gilliam S, Schnurr D, Forghani B, Honarmand S, Khetsuriani N, Fischer M, Cossen C, Anderson L (2003) In search of encephalitis Etiologies: diagnostic challenges in the California encephalitis project, 1998–2000. Clin Infect Dis 36:731–742

92. Tunkel A, Glaser C, Bloch K, Sejvar J, Marra C, Roos K, Hartman B, Kaplan S, Scheld W, Whitley R (2008) The Management of Encephalitis: clinical practice guidelines by the Infectious Diseases Society of America. Clin Infect Dis 47:303–327

93. Lakeman F, Whitley R (1995) Diagnosis of herpes simplex encephalitis: application of polymerase chain reaction to cerebrospinal fluid from brain-biopsied patients and correlation with disease. J Infect Dis 171:857–863

94. Domingues R, Tsanaclis A, Pannuti C, Mayo M, Lakeman F (1997) Evaluation of the range of clinical presentations of herpes simplex encephalitis by using polymerase chain reaction assay of cerebrospinal fluid samples. Clin Infect Dis 25:86–91

95. Bozzola E, Bozzola M, Tozzi AE, Calcaterra V, Longo D, Krzystofiak A et al (2014) Acute cerebellitis in varicella: a ten year case series and systematic review of the literature. Ital J Pediatr 40:57

96. Steiner I, Benninger F (2018) Manifestations of herpes virus infections in the nervous system. Neurol Clin 36(4):725–738

97. Pellett Madan R, Hand J Human herpesvirus 6, 7, and 8 in solid organ transplantation: guidelines from the American Society of Transplantation infectious diseases Community of Practice. Clin Transpl. https://doi.org/10.1111/ctr.13518

98. Gheuens S, Wüthrich C, Koralnik IJ (2013) Progressive multifocal leukoencephalopathy: why gray and white matter. Annu Rev Pathol 8:189–215

99. Van Assche G, Van Ranst M, Sciot R, Dubois B, Vermeire S, Noman M et al (2005) Progressive multifocal leukoencephalopathy after natalizumab therapy for Crohn's disease. N Engl J Med 353(4):362–368

100. Cinque P, Scarpellini P, Vago L, Linde A, Lazzarin A (1997) Diagnosis of central nervous system complications in HIV-infected patients: cerebrospinal fluid analysis by the polymerase chain reaction. AIDS 11(1):1–17

101. Rauer S, Marks R, Urbach H, Warnatz K, Nath A, Holland S et al (2019) Treatment of progressive multifocal Leukoencephalopathy with Pembrolizumab. N Engl J Med 380(17):1676–1677

102. Snider WD, Simpson DM, Nielsen S, Gold JW, Metroka CE, Posner JB (1983) Neurological complications of acquired immune deficiency syndrome: analysis of 50 patients. Ann Neurol 14(4):403–418

103. d'Arminio Monforte A, Cinque P, Mocroft A, Goebel FD, Antunes F, Katlama C et al (2004) Changing incidence of central nervous system diseases in the EuroSIDA cohort. Ann Neurol 55(3):320–328

104. Saag MS, Graybill RJ, Larsen RA, Pappas PG, Perfect JR, Powderly WG et al (2000) Practice guidelines for the management of cryptococcal disease. Infectious Diseases Society of America. Clin Infect Dis 30(4):710–718

105. (2019) Guidelines for the prevention and treatment of opportunistic infections in HIV-infected adults and adolescents. In: AIDSinfo. https://aidsinfo.nih.gov/guidelines/html/4/adult-and-adolescent-opportunistic-infection/0. Accessed 25 Jan 2019

106. Kaplan JE, Benson C, Holmes KK, Brooks JT, Pau A, Masur H (2009) Guidelines for prevention and treatment of opportunistic infections in HIV-infected adults and adolescents: recommendations from CDC, the National Institutes of Health, and the HIV medicine Association of the Infectious Diseases Society of America. MMWR Recomm Rep 58(RR-4):1–207; quiz CE1–4

Trauma

17

Vikas Jain, and Toshio Moritani

Hiroto Kawasaki

17.1 Introduction

Traumatic brain injuries (TBI) are a common cause of significant morbidity and mortality worldwide. They are the most common cause of death and permanent disability in the early decades of life. Approximately 1.7 million people are affected by TBI in the USA every year, out of which 275,000 patients are admitted. TBI leads to approximately 52,000 deaths annually in the USA [1, 2]. The victims vary widely with regard to their etiology, clinical presentation, pathophysiology, and optimal treatment strategies.

Traumatic brain injuries may be focal or diffuse or a combination of both. Focal brain injuries are usually due to direct impact and result in contusions and extra axial hematomas. Diffuse brain injuries are usually caused by acceleration/deceleration injuries and are typically seen following high velocity vehicular accidents or shaken baby syndrome. The clinical sequelae can include concussions and/or diffuse axonal injury. Traumatic axonal injury (TAI) results from shear injuries that reflect sudden acceleration and deceleration as well as rotational strain which result in hemorrhagic and nonhemorrhagic foci at gray-white matter junctions, in the corpus callosum and in the dorsolateral aspect of the brainstem. The term diffuse axonal injury (DAI) is defined by three or more lesions in two or more lobes and corpus callosum [2].

Many of the survivors may suffer significant long-term consequences. DAI is a major pathologic substrate of unconsciousness, persistent vegetative state, neurological deficits, and cognitive decline.

Diagnostic neuroimaging plays a pivotal role in the management of these injuries. Non-contrast CT scan of the head is the initial modality of choice by consensus and provides extremely valuable information for triage and trauma patient management. Head CT is excellent for showing traumatic lesions which require immediate surgical intervention such as decompressive craniotomy or craniectomy, hematoma evacuation, and ventriculostomy catheter placement. However, CT is very insensitive in the detection of TAI/DAI and grossly underestimates nonhemorrhagic contusions especially in the acute setting. MRI, particularly diffusion-weighted image (DWI), fluid attenuated inversion recovery (FLAIR),

V. Jain (✉)
Department of Radiology, MetroHealth Medical Center, Case Western Reserve University, Cleveland, OH, USA

T. Moritani
Department of Radiology, Division of Neuroradiology, Clinical Neuroradiology Research, University of Michigan, Ann Arbor, MI, USA
e-mail: tmoritan@med.umich.edu

H. Kawasaki
University of Iowa Hospitals & Clinics, Iowa City, IA, USA
e-mail: hiroto-kawasaki@uiowa.edu

© Springer Nature Switzerland AG 2021
T. Moritani, A. A. Capizzano (eds.), *Diffusion-Weighted MR Imaging of the Brain, Head and Neck, and Spine*, https://doi.org/10.1007/978-3-030-62120-9_17

T2*-weighted gradient-echo (GRE), and susceptibility-weighted image (SWI) sequences, is much more sensitive than CT scan for the detection of such TAI/DAI. MR is however performed in relatively few selected patients, generally where there is mismatch between the CT findings and neurological symptoms or clinical examination [3–5].

17.2 Diffuse Axonal Injury

Strich and colleagues first described DAI in 1956 and it was later characterized by Adams and coworkers, who linked the histopathological features of post-traumatic damage in the axons to rotational acceleration-deceleration forces to the head that result in stretch injuries [6, 7].

DAI refers to the shear injury at the tissue interfaces with different density and is classically located at gray white matter junctions such as the centrum semiovale, corpus callosum, internal capsules, fornix, posterolateral aspect of the upper brainstem, and cerebellar peduncles. DAI may be confined to the white matter of the frontal and temporal lobes in mild head trauma (Fig. 17.1). Lesions in the posterior half of the corpus callosum indicate more severe injury. With even more severe injuries, DAI lesions may be seen in the anterior corpus callosum and dorsolateral aspect of the upper brainstem (Figs. 17.2 and 17.3). DAI lesions may also be seen, but less commonly, in other areas of the brain such as the parietal and occipital lobes, internal and external capsules, basal ganglia, thalami, fornix, and septum pellucidum (Fig. 17.4). Intraventricular hemorrhage may be seen in some patients due to disruption of the subependymal plexus of capillaries and veins lining the ventricular surface of the corpus callosum, septum pellucidum, and fornix [4, 8, 9].

DAI lesions are usually multiple, diffuse, small (5–15 mm), and mainly T2-hyperintense foci which are generally limited to white matter and are rarely seen on standard CT scans. 10–30% of the DAI lesions are hemorrhagic [4, 8] (Fig. 17.3).

DAI is a common finding in patients suffering from severe TBI and is a more important predictor of poor neurological outcome and long-term outcome with respect to cognition and behavior impairment than focal TBI [10]. The consequences are often devastating, and the presence of DAI is a major adverse prognostic factor in the majority of affected patients. These patients also usually develop global atrophy after few months.

Clinically, DAI typically manifests as impaired consciousness and coma shortly after trauma due to acute injury to the axons. While the axons are injured on initial impact due to shearing injury, major damage to the axons continues to propagate after the traumatic event because of delayed activation of complex biochemical processes in the cells [11].

Pathologically, injury related to DAI is always much more extensive microscopically than at gross examination or as seen on imaging. Microscopically, shearing injuries initially produce multiple, characteristic axonal bulbs, or retraction balls, as well as numerous foci of perivascular hemorrhage [1, 12, 13].

17.3 Grading of DAI and Location

There are three grades of DAI in the Adams classification which was first proposed by J.H. Adams and associates in 1989; these grades are based on the anatomic distribution of the injury and have been shown to have a direct relationship to the severity of injury and adverse outcomes [6].

Grade I is presence of lesions at gray white matter junctions, which are most commonly seen in the parasagittal regions of the frontal lobes and periventricular temporal lobes. Parietal and occipital lobes, cerebellum, and internal capsules are less commonly involved. DAI may be confined to the white matter of the frontal and temporal lobes in mild head trauma [9] (Fig. 17.5).

Grade II includes involvement of the corpus callosum in addition to grade I lesions and is seen in approximately 20% of patients. The posterior body and splenium of the corpus callosum are most commonly affected with progression anteriorly as the severity increases (Fig. 17.6).

Grade III is defined by lesions in the dorsolateral brainstem (Fig. 17.7).

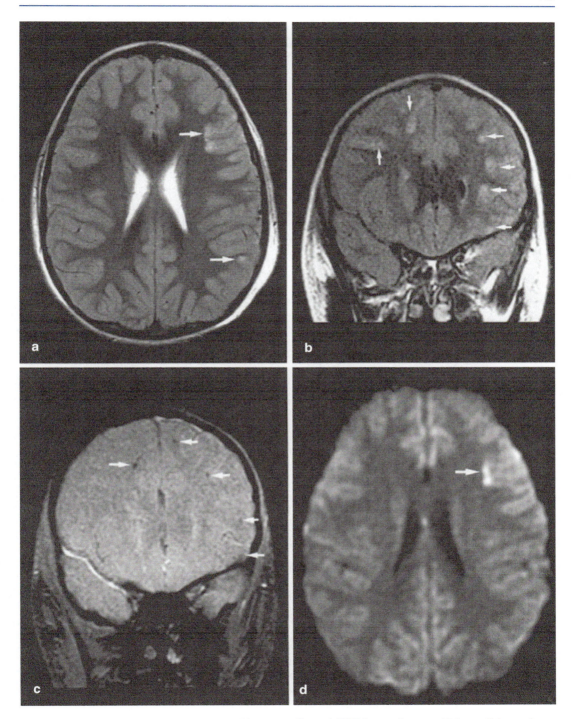

Fig. 17.1 (a–d) Diffuse axonal injury in gray-white matter junction in a 7-year-old boy after a motor vehicle accident. (a, b) T2-weighted and coronal FLAIR images show multiple hyperintense lesions in the gray-white matter junction of bilateral frontoparietal lobes (*arrows*). (c) Coronal GRE image shows multiple small hemorrhages as low signal in these lesions (*arrows*). (d) DW image demonstrates diffuse axonal injury as high signal intensity (*arrow*) with decreased ADC (not shown), representing cytotoxic edema

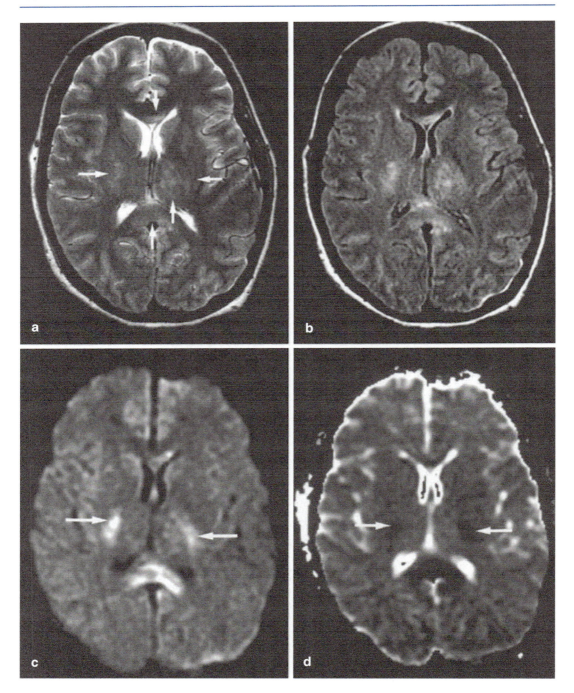

Fig. 17.2 (**a**–**d**) Diffuse axonal injury in the corpus callosum, internal capsule, and thalamus in a 29-year-old woman after a motor vehicle accident. (**a**, **b**) T2-weighted and FLAIR images show multiple hyperintense lesions in the anterior and posterior corpus callosum, internal capsules, and left thalamus (*arrows*). (**c**, **d**) DW image demonstrates these lesions as high signal intensity with decreased ADC (*arrows*)

17 Trauma

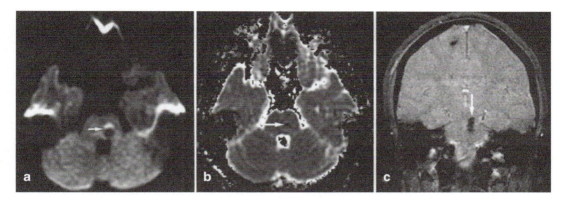

Fig. 17.3 (**a–c**) Diffuse axonal injury in the brain stem in a 28-year-old man after a motor vehicle accident. (**a**) DW image shows a hypointense lesion with a hyperintense rim in the dorsolateral aspect of the midbrain, representing a hemorrhagic lesion of diffuse axonal injury (*arrow*). (**b**) ADC map shows decreased ADC of this lesion (*arrow*). This might be due to a paramagnetic susceptibility artifact. (**c**) Coronal GRE image clearly shows hemorrhagic lesions as hypointense in the brain stem (*arrow*) and in the right frontoparietal region

Intraventricular hemorrhage can accompany these findings. They have the same mechanical origin and are due to disruption of the subependymal plexus of capillaries and veins that lie along the ventricular surface of the corpus callosum, fornix, and septum pellucidum [8, 9, 14, 15] (Figs. 17.8 and 17.14).

Hamdeh et al. conducted a study on 30 patients with severe DAI (Glasgow Motor Scale of <6) examined with MRI within one-week post injury and concluded after multivariate analysis that there was an independent indicator of poor outcome for patients with lesions in the substantia nigra and tegmentum on SWI. They found that lesions seen in these areas have a worse outcome than patients with lesions in other parts of the brainstem [10].

Once it was thought that edema following traumatic brain injury was vasogenic, but recent experimental studies using diffusion-weighted imaging (DWI) have shown that edema after head trauma consists of both vasogenic and cytotoxic edema [3, 16–19]. Since DW imaging is also very sensitive in detecting small lesions of cytotoxic edema and can differentiate cytotoxic from vasogenic edema, it has become especially useful in the evaluation and staging of patients with DAI.

17.4 Computed Tomography (CT) and Magnetic Resonance (MR) Imaging

Few DAI lesions are visible on head CT. Only large lesions or those that are grossly hemorrhagic are seen. MR imaging has been proven to be more sensitive for detection as well as for characterization of DAI lesions. Conventional MR imaging shows multiple, small, deeply situated elliptical lesions that spare the overlying cortex. MRI is also more sensitive to detect subtle and early ischemic changes and contusions on the surface of the brain (Figs. 17.7 and 17.9). FLAIR images are more sensitive than T2-weighted images to detect small hyperintense lesions adjacent to the cerebrospinal fluid, such as in the fornix and septum pellucidum [4, 14, 20, 21]. DWI has been found to be equally or more sensitive than FLAIR in multiple studies.

Nonhemorrhagic lesions (NHL) are more numerous than hemorrhagic lesions. While DWI can also detect some hemorrhagic lesions, GRE and SWI are more sensitive for detecting hemorrhagic lesions. Small hemorrhagic lesions are seen in 10–30% of all DAI lesions and are best detected on GRE images because of their susceptibility effects. SWI uses the magnetic sus-

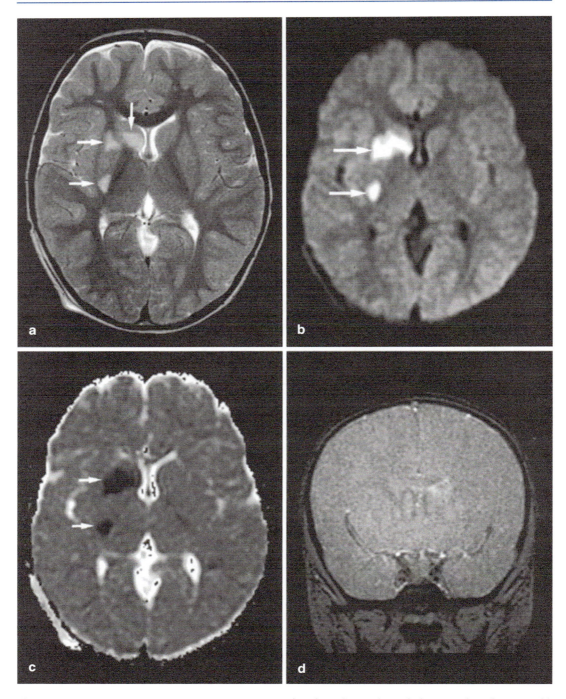

Fig. 17.4 (**a–d**) Diffuse axonal injury in the basal ganglia in a 3-year-old boy after a motor vehicle accident. (**a**) T2-weighted image shows hyperintense lesions in the right lentiform and caudate nucleus (*arrows*). (**b, c**) DW imaging shows these lesions as hyperintense with decreased ADC (*arrows*). (**d**) Coronal GRE image clearly shows no hemorrhagic foci in these lesions

17 Trauma

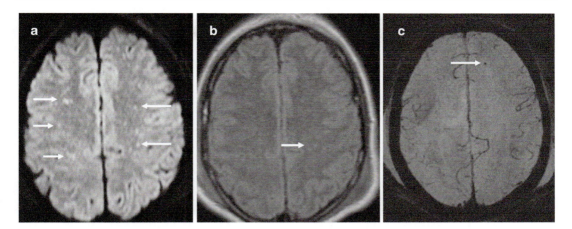

Fig. 17.5 (**a–c**) DAI grade 1 in a 34-year-old male after MVA. CT head was negative (not shown). (**a**) DWI shows multiple tiny foci of RD (decreased ADC not shown) in bilateral cerebral hemispheres. (**b**) FLAIR shows fewer lesions which are very subtle. (**c**) SWI shows only one lesion in the left frontal lobe which was also seen on the DWI. Adam's grade I DAI as lesions are seen only in the cerebral hemispheres, without involvement of the corpus callosum or brainstem

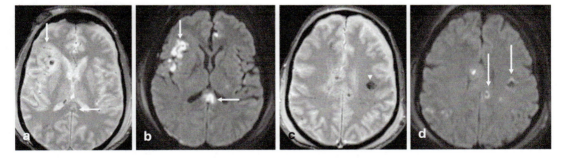

Fig. 17.6 (**a–d**) DAI grade 2. 25-year-old female after high-speed MVA. Multiple nonhemorrhagic and hemorrhagic (arrowhead in **c**) lesions seen on DWI (**b**, **d**) and GRE (**a**, **c**) sequences. The nonhemorrhagic DAI lesions in the splenium of the corpus callosum (**b**) and near the right sylvian fissure (**b**) are better seen on DWI. DWI is more sensitive for nonhemorrhagic lesions. DWI can also detect hemorrhagic DAI lesions but is less sensitive than GRE. Hemorrhagic DAI lesions appear as central areas of hypointensity surrounded by peripheral halo of hyperintensity on DWI images (long arrows in **d**)

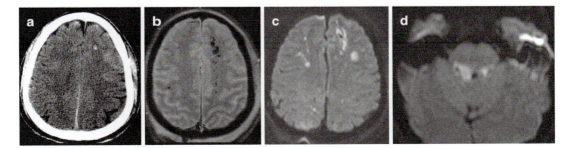

Fig. 17.7 (**a–d**) DAI grade III. 25-year-old male with altered metal status after high-speed MCC. A mixture of hemorrhagic and nonhemorrhagic DAI in bilateral frontal lobes. CT (**a**) shows only one hemorrhagic lesion. Many nonhemorrhagic lesions seen on DWI (**c**) are not seen on GRE (**b**). Multiple DAI lesions seen in the cerebral hemispheres and in the posterior aspect of the brainstem on both sides (**c** and **d**). DAI lesions in the brainstem (**d**) indicates Adam's Grade III DAI and are associated with a poorer prognosis

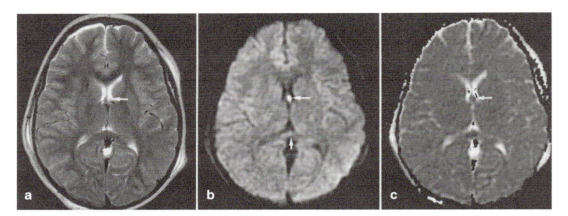

Fig. 17.8 (a–c) Diffuse axonal injury in the fornix of an 11-year-old girl after a motor vehicle accident. (a) On T2-weighted image, it is difficult to detect a small hyperintense lesion in the fornix (*arrow*). (b, c) DW image shows the lesion in the fornix and posterior corpus callosum as hyperintense with decreased ADC (*arrows*)

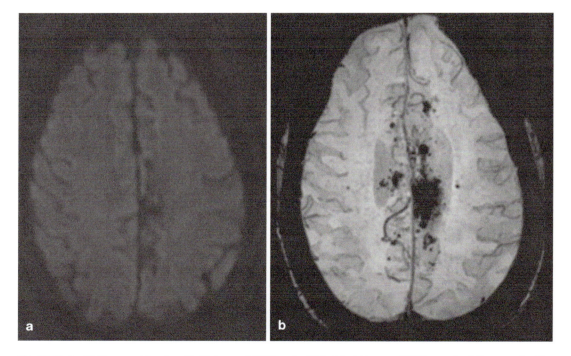

Fig. 17.9 (a–d) 32-year-old male with high-speed MVA presenting with altered mental status. Acute to subacute SDH can appear hyperintense on DWI (a) and hypointense on ADC maps (b). The T1 image (c) shows curvilinear hyperintensity and CT scan (d) shows curvilinear hyperdensity because of SDH over the left convexity. The underlying brain parenchyma adjacent to the SDH also shows RD (arrows in **a** and **b**) suggestive of ischemic injury secondary to SDH and trauma

ceptibility differences between various tissues, which gives phase differences between the regions which contain paramagnetic deoxygenated blood products and normal surrounding tissues. SWI is 3–6 times more sensitive than GRE in detecting the size, number, volume, and distribution of hemorrhagic foci of DAI. However, even these MR imaging sequences are thought

17 Trauma

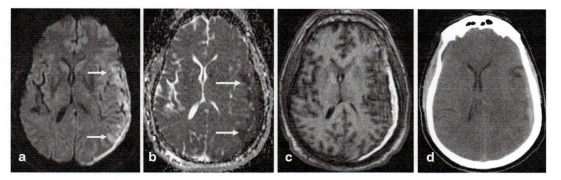

Fig. 17.10 (**a–b**) MRI of a 55-year-old male after MVA shows multiple hemorrhagic foci in bilateral cerebral hemispheres seen on SWI (**b**) which were not as conspicuous on DWI (**a**). SWI or GRE are more sensitive for detecting hemorrhagic lesions

to underestimate the true extent of DAI [20–23] (Fig. 17.10).

Traumatic midline SAH in the perimesencephalic cistern and interhemispheric fissure on the initial CT scan after trauma has been found to strongly implicate shearing injury and severe DAI in a study conducted by Meta-Mbemba et al. They reported sensitivity of 60.8% and specificity of 81.7% for severe DAI in a study on 270 patients with history of head trauma [24].

17.5 Diffusion-Weighted Imaging (DWI)

DWI measures a unique physiological parameter characterized by random microscopic motion of water molecules in the tissues which can define types of edema in various conditions. DWI can detect lesions with both increased/ facilitated diffusion and restricted diffusion (RD). Lesions with increased/ facilitated diffusion are bright on both DWI and ADC maps and have increased extracellular water where water molecules are more mobile. This finding reflects vasogenic edema which is usually reversible. These lesions appear hyperintense on DWI due to T2 shine through. The diffusion maps are generated with combined input from diffusion-weighted and T2-weighted properties and therefore lesions with long T2 relaxation time will also be bright on DWI. This effect is removed on ADC maps, which represent the apparent diffusion coefficient [25–28].

The lesions with cytotoxic edema show restricted diffusion and are bright on DWI and dark on ADC maps; this is the classic pattern of acute infarcts. This phenomenon results from the shift of freely mobile water molecules from the extracellular space to the intracellular space where movement of water molecules is restricted. This indicates cellular swelling and cytotoxic edema, which usually are considered irreversible injury and cell death, with few exceptions.

The exact mechanism of RD in DAI is still uncertain, and proposed mechanisms include excitotoxic edema due to release of a high concentration of glutamate and other neurotransmitters, associated hypotension and hypoxia leading to trauma induced ischemia or collapse of the cytoskeleton of injured axons [15, 27, 29, 30] (Fig. 17.11). There is increase in extracellular levels of amino acids glutamate and aspartate after TBI, and experiments have shown that N-methyl-D aspartate (NMDA) receptor antagonists have protective role. Glutamate receptor antagonists help the neurons to deal with the increased permeability of the cell membrane to ions as well as reduced efficacy of Na + extrusion [31, 32]. Damage at the node of Ranvier results in a traumatic defect in the axonal membrane. This defect causes excessive neurotransmitter release with increase in intracellular

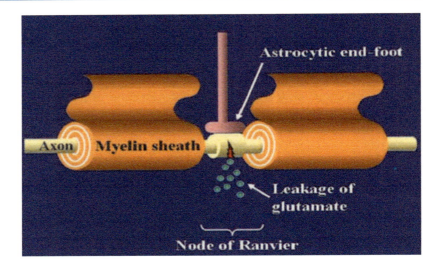

Fig. 17.11 Leakage of glutamate in diffuse axonal injury. Diffuse axonal injury is presumably due to the leakage of glutamate at the node of Ranvier. The astrocytic end-foot is located on the axon at the node of Ranvier and may protect the axons

calcium ions, as in brain ischemia, which leads to axonal and glial cell swelling (cytotoxic or neurotoxic edema). These changes can eventually lead to axonal degeneration or necrosis with microglial and astrocytic reactive changes. Accumulation of hemosiderin-laden macrophages is also seen in the chronic phase. Glutamate is the most important excitatory amino acid and is responsible for many neurological functions such as cognition, memory, movement, and sensation. Glutamate mediates neuronal death in pathological conditions through the activation of NMDA receptor subtypes [33].

Cytotoxic edema, which seems to be the cause of reduced ADC in ischemic brain injury, can also occur in the early phase of DAI. However, reduced ADC is presumably due to the development of retraction balls and concomitant cytoskeletal collapse along the severed axons [25]. The time course of the ADC abnormality seems to be different from that of ischemic brain injury. Prolonged decrease in ADC, over 2 weeks, has occasionally been observed in DAI [26], and cytotoxic edema in the corpus callosum can be partially reversible on follow-up imaging using T2-weighted sequences. Axonal and glial cell swelling in DAI is thought to be mainly due to excitotoxic mechanisms that essentially propagates through the white matter tracts. It can also be a slower or reversible form of cellular swelling than that seen in ischemic brain injuries [18, 27, 28]. Hemorrhagic components, which often accompany these brain injuries, will affect the signal intensity on DW images.

The lesions with RD are usually not reversible; however, lesions with increased diffusion are partially reversible. A few isolated case reports of reversible intramyelinic white matter cytotoxic edema have been reported in traumatic brain injury patients [29].

DWI can also detect some hemorrhagic lesions but is not as sensitive as GRE or SWI (Fig. 17.9). The acute hemorrhagic foci which contain oxyhemoglobin are bright on DWI but dark on ADC and have a surrounding halo of increased diffusion because of vasogenic edema (Fig. 17.12 and 17.13). The hemorrhagic lesions then turn hypointense on DWI when they have deoxyhemoglobin, intracellular methemoglobin, or hemosiderin. Analysis of DWI and ADC data are less reliable in the presence of blood products [34, 35]. Moreover, the areas of the brain near the skull base, petrous pyramids, sphenoid, and frontal sinuses usually generate susceptibility artifact and may lead to false-positive or false-negative detection of lesions.

DWI images are helpful in predicting enlargement of the areas of hemorrhage seen on the initial CT scan after mild to moderate TBI. A study conducted by Kin et al. in Japan on trauma patients comparing CT and DWI MRI done in the acute phase of trauma patients found that the

17 Trauma 497

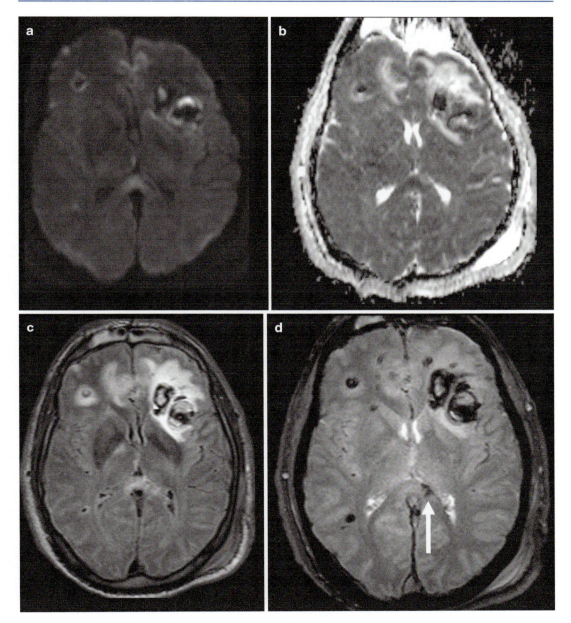

Fig. 17.12 (**a–d**) 22-year-old female with high-speed MVA shows multiple hemorrhagic contusions in bilateral frontal and right temporal lobes and DAI involving the splenium of corpus callosum. DWI (**a**) shows RD in the splenium of corpus callosum and multiple hemorrhagic contusions. ADC (**b**) shows dark SI in the splenium suggestive of RD. FLAIR (**c**) and GRE (**d**) images show the DAI lesion in the splenium of corpus callosum has both hemorrhagic (*arrow* on **d**) and nonhemorrhagic components. The hemorrhagic component on the left side is better seen on GRE and nonhemorrhagic component in the midline is better perceived on the DWI (**a**)

patients having a larger region of diffusion restriction compared to the size of initial hemorrhage on the CT scan have a 71.4% chance of increase in the size of hemorrhagic lesions on the follow-up CT scans. Only 3% of the patients without a mismatch showed increase in the size of the hemorrhagic lesions. The fact that CT and MRI were performed at the same time makes this

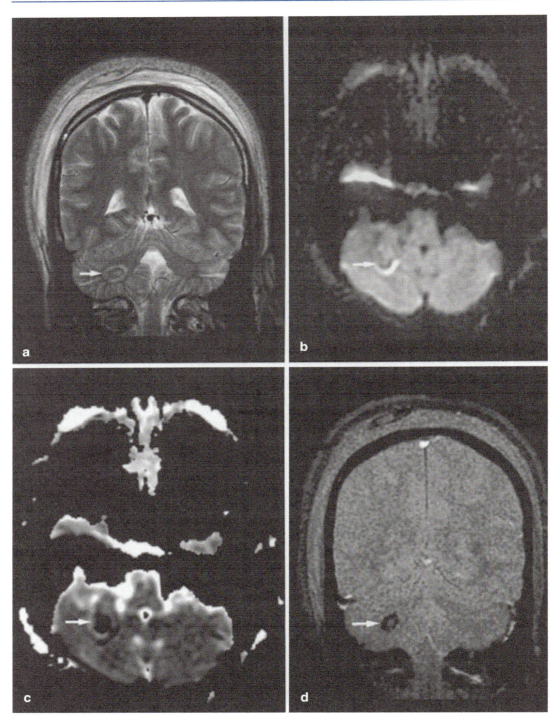

Fig. 17.13 (**a**–**d**) Diffuse axonal injury in the cerebellum of an 18-year-old male patient after a motor vehicle accident. (**a**) T2-weighted image shows a hypointense lesion in the right middle cerebellar peduncle (*arrow*), (**b**) DW image shows a hypointense lesion with a hyperintense rim, representing a hemorrhagic lesion (*arrow*). (**c**) ADC map reveals decreased ADC in this lesion (*arrow*). This may be due to a paramagnetic susceptibility artifact. (**d**) Coronal GRE image clearly demonstrates hemorrhagic lesions as hypointense (*arrow*)

study unique. The authors called this finding CT-DWI mismatch and hypothesized that these patients developed cytotoxic edema at the time of injury, and subsequent vasodilation increased the areas of hemorrhage. Therefore, the DWI may have an impact in management of the patients and decision-making during treatment [36].

Moen et al. conducted a longitudinal study to see the evolution of the DAI lesions in patients with moderate and severe TBI. They found that many nonhemorrhagic DAI lesions seen on FLAIR decrease in size and number in the scans performed after three months when compared to initial scans. The hemorrhagic lesions on GRE attenuated at a slower pace and did so after three months. MRI is the modality of choice for evaluating sequelae of TBI in subacute to late phases. However, MRI when performed earlier after injury provides better prognostic information and outcome. They found more lesions on FLAIR images as compared to DWI in the initial MRI scans, probably because half of the MRI scans were performed after 7 days of trauma [37]. However, more lesions were detected on the DWI as compared to FLAIR/T2 when MRI was performed within 48 hours of trauma in a different study [20]. They detected 310 shear lesions on DWI and only 248 shear lesions on FLAIR/T2. 65% of the lesions seen on DWI had restricted diffusion.

DWI is excellent in detecting the nonhemorrhagic lesions of DAI and the lesion load correlates well with the initial GCS and duration of coma in these patients. Multiple lesions are predictive of poorer outcome and lesion load in the corpus callosum has been confirmed by multiple studies to correlate with poorer outcome. However, the timing of the scan is important, as the lesion conspicuity and number on DWI decreases as time passes.

DWI is comparable to FLAIR in the detection of nonhemorrhagic DAI lesions [38, 39]. However, the GRE sequence is better in detecting the hemorrhagic lesions and SWI is even more sensitive and can detect a greater number of hemorrhagic lesions (Fig. 17.9). In a study conducted by Bansal et al., they detected a mean number of 7.47 lesions on DWI, 13.27 lesions on GRE, and 22.13 lesions on SWI. SWI has been found to detect 3–6 times more lesions as compared to GRE because it uses the magnetic susceptibility difference in the tissues resulting in phase difference between the paramagnetic deoxygenated blood products and surrounding normal tissues [22, 23]. However, there was no difference in the grading of DAI between the three sequences. Specifically, the grade of injury including involvement of the brainstem carries a poorer prognosis as compared to number of lesions in the hemispheric white matter [38, 40].

Huisman et al. found that DWI found the maximum number and overall volume of lesions in the brain in patients with DAI as compared to T2, FLAIR, and GRE sequences [20]. Schaefer et al. found that the larger volume of the DWI abnormalities in the brain in DAI cases have the highest correlation with GCS score at admission and with subacute Rankin scale score [27]. They also found a statistically significant correlation between reduction in the FA values in the posterior limb of the internal capsule and splenium of the corpus callosum and the severity of head injury measured by GCS score and Frankin score at discharge [20].

The modified Rankin scale measures the degree of disability and dependency in daily life after neurological injuries. The overall volume of the abnormal signal intensities on the DWI images has been found to have the strongest correlation with the modified Rankin scale at discharge in one study. A study found that lesion numbers seen on all sequences also strongly correlated with the modified Rankin scale. They found that location of lesions in the corpus callosum also had a strong correlation with this scale [27].

Hou et al. concluded that quantitative ADC measurements in different parts of the brain can be used to detect non-visible DAI and this information can be used to predict severity of injury and long-term outcome in trauma patients. They compared 37 trauma patients with 35 controls who had no brain injury. Mean ADC values in areas without visible DAI lesions were significantly different from the normal controls. The patients with unfavorable outcomes had significantly higher ADC values as compared to patients with favorable outcomes and normal controls. They concluded, therefore, that ADC maps can be used to detect non-visible lesions [41].

MR has a value in prognostication as a larger number of DAI lesions seen on DWI predicts poorer outcome and more disability. The initial GCS, age, number of DAI lesions, and ADC scores can predict the duration of a coma according to a study conducted on 74 trauma patients. They found that advanced age, higher number of lesions, higher ADC values, and lower GCS scores predict longer periods of unconsciousness and poor prognosis [42].

17.6 Pediatric Patients

A study was conducted to evaluate the role of DWI in infants and toddlers with shaken baby syndrome (SBS), also called nonaccidental trauma. All 26 children enrolled in the study had SDHs, 18 cases of which were confirmed to have SBS. All of these 18 cases had DWI abnormalities in the brain and the lesions were larger on DWI compared to other MR pulse sequences. Most of these patients had SDHs, retinal hemorrhages, and fractures. Traumatic axonal injuries are also seen in these patients which are much better seen on MRI as compared to CT. Hence, the American Association of Pediatrics recommends an MRI when the medical condition is not explained by the CT findings alone (Fig. 17.14) [43].

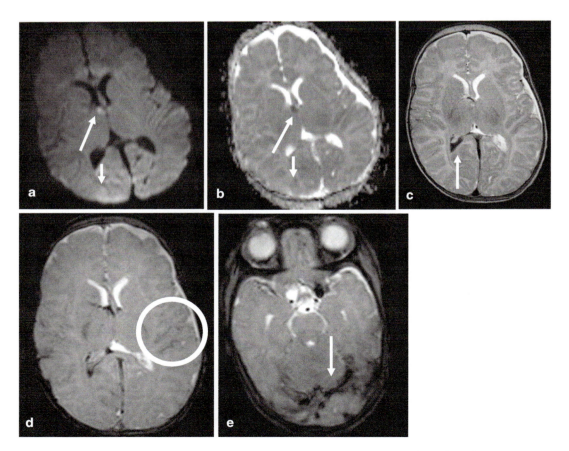

Fig. 17.14 (a–e) Four-month-old male child after nonaccidental trauma shows DAI with RD in the fornix (**a** is DWI and **b** is ADC) and IVH (**c** is T2 and **d** is GRE) and SDH (**e** is GRE) along the tentorium due to shaken baby syndrome. Mild RD in right occipital lobe is also seen (short arrow in **a**). Very subtle SAH is seen on the GRE in temporal lobes (circle in **d**)

A study was conducted on pediatric trauma patients and found that ADC values have prognostic significance in that lower ADC values in the peripheral white matter predict poorer outcome. The peripheral white matter had reduced ADC values in patients with severe TBI and poor outcomes when compared to patients with severe injury who experienced a relatively good outcome. They also concluded that average whole brain ADC values can predict clinical outcome in the trauma patients [40].

17.7 Hypoxic Ischemic Injuries

Hypoxic ischemic injuries (HII) in neonates can also cause RD on DWI in the brain. Areas of RD can be seen in the corpus callosum, basal ganglia, ventrolateral thalami, periventricular white matter, and/or peri-rolandic cortex depending on the gestational age, severity, and duration of the ischemic insult. Epelman et al. found that RD in the corpus callosum is more common than previously thought when neonates with suspected HII are scanned within the first week of age as pseudonormalization of RD happens earlier in the neonates [44].

17.8 Cerebral Fat Embolism (CFE)

Fat emboli to the brain is a rare entity which occurs after severe trauma when multiple long bone fractures lead to transfer of bone marrow fat into the systemic and pulmonary circulation by an unknown mechanism. This may lead to either generalized encephalopathy or focal neurological symptoms. This process should be suspected when there is altered mental status after a period of post-traumatic normal mental function in a patient with long bone fractures or after orthopedic fixation of long bone fractures [45]. CT is very insensitive and usually misses the findings. MRI generally shows patchy or confluent areas of vasogenic and cytotoxic edema in the deep white matter, basal ganglia,

cerebellum, and corpus callosum. This is better seen on GRE or SWI as a diffuse pattern of multiple lesions with micro-susceptibility artifacts because of vascular stasis, deoxygenated blood, and microthrombi formation, as well as larger areas of restricted diffusion (Fig. 17.15) [2, 46, 47].

Appearance of lesions 2–3 days after injury in a diffuse and symmetrical manner in addition to involvement of the cerebellum favors fat emboli over TAI. The DWI and T2* are helpful to distinguish fat embolism from DAI. Diffuse confluent larger lesions with restricted diffusion and a greater number of small hemorrhages are seen in CFE, while larger or more linear hemorrhages and fewer number of scattered foci of RD are more typical of DAI [46]. The prognosis is generally worse for DAI.

17.9 Traumatic Optic Neuropathy (TON)

DWI has high specificity for diagnosing traumatic optic neuropathy in patients with the appropriate clinical setting. TON is usually a clinical diagnosis, but in some comatose or otherwise difficult to examine patients, MRI can be very helpful. Specifically, identification of RD in the optic nerve can indicate traumatic contusion and ischemia and has been shown to have 27.6% sensitivity and 100% specificity in the diagnosis TON (Fig. 17.16) [48]. One of the reasons for low sensitivity in their study may be the use of 5 mm slices for DWI; use of 3 mm slices may increase the sensitivity of MR for TON. The presence of high signal intensity on DWI is useful to diagnose TON, but absence of RD in the optic nerve has lesser negative predictive value, in that the optic nerves may not be well seen because of motion or susceptibility artifacts. RD tended to be seen in the posterior segment of the optic nerves in this study which may be due to increased vulnerability of the nerve in or near the optic canal and the potential for compartment syndrome.

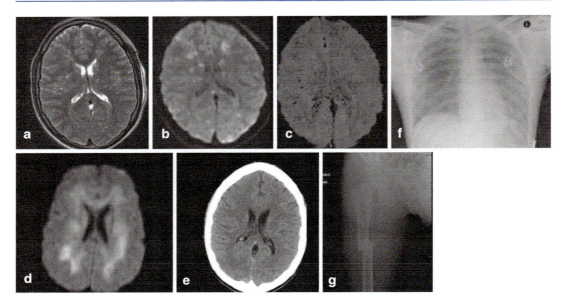

Fig. 17.15 (a–g) 19-year-old man with MVA. T2WI (a) and DWI (b) show starfield pattern of lesions associated with numerous micro-hemorrhages on susceptibility-weighted image (c). 7-day follow-up DWI (d) shows diffuse white matter changes. 2 months follow-up CT (e) demonstrates reversibility of the edema. Cerebral fat embolism syndrome occurs in 2–5% of long bone fractures (g). It is also associated with sickle cell disease, pancreatitis, and liposuction. Fat emboli and/or toxic free fatty acids which disrupt capillary endothelium are the cause of the syndrome and pulmonary edema (f). Reversible diffuse white matter changes can be seen during the course of the syndrome

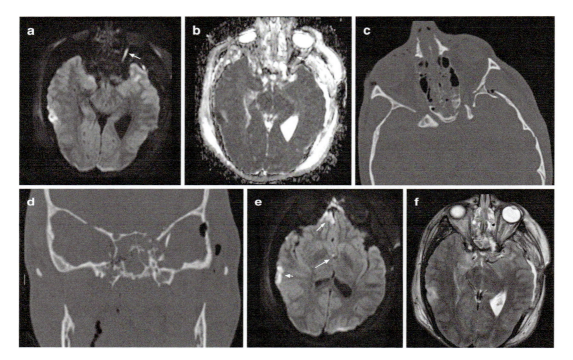

Fig. 17.16 (a–f) 18-year-old male after MVC and loss of vision in left eye. DWI (Image a) shows RD in the left optic nerve and shows hypointensity on the ADC maps (b) suggestive of optic nerve injury which was due to multiple fractures around the left orbital apex and optic nerve canal (c, d). DAI in the fornix (arrow in e) with multiple contusions in frontal and temporal lobes (e) are also seen. T2 (f) shows subtle hyperintensity and swelling of the left optic nerve

17.10 DWI in Mild Traumatic Brain Injuries (mTBI)

70–90% of all hospital-treated injuries are mild with an incidence of approximately 300 in 100,000 [33]. These lesions are greatly underdiagnosed as they are not seen on the CT scan and even on routine MRI pulse sequences. Very few trauma patients with mild injuries receive MRI of the head. Many of these patients will suffer long-term cognitive deficits. Common issues of cognitive impairment suffered by these patients after mTBI are memory, information processing speed, attention, and executive function. DWI and DTI have been shown to detect cases of mTBI [49, 50].

DWI is a sensitive technique to detect DAI as it can evaluate structural integrity of the white matter tracts [25, 51], even in patients with mild traumatic brain injuries (mTBI). mTBI is defined as patients with GCS > or equal to 13. 70 to 90% of the patients with traumatic brain injuries have only mTBI [2, 52]. Many studies have been performed confirming structural damage to the white matter tracts in some patients after mTBI which is not seen on conventional MRI.

17.11 Diffusion Tensor Imaging (DTI) and Fractional Anisotropy (FA)

Diffusion tensor imaging (DTI) is a robust tool to detect mild DAI and is superior to conventional MRI. DTI is derived from directionally encoded diffusion-weighted data by obtaining diffusion parameters in multiple (minimum six but usually many more) non-collinear planes and post processing the data set to produce three-dimensional white matter tracts. DTI measures directional diffusion of water molecules in the white matter tracts. The diffusivity of water in CSF and in the gray matter is isotropic, as it can equally move in all directions without any hindrance or preference. The diffusivity of the water molecules in the white matter tracts is anisotropic, which means that water molecules cannot move equally in all directions. The diffusivity is maximum along the direction of the white matter tract and this phe-

nomenon is called fractional anisotropy (FA), which can be measured. The FA of CSF in the ventricles and FA of gray matter is close to zero and FA of large white matter tracts in the corpus callosum is close to one. DTI data when combined with post-processing techniques can generate diffusion tensor tractography maps which show the three-dimensional anatomy of the white matter tracts [53–55].

Fractional anisotropy is the main quantitative metric obtained from DTI and measures anisotropic diffusion. Higher FA means homogeneity in fiber orientation, increased fiber density and axonal diameter. Reduced FA in white matter indicates damage to myelin, damage to axon membranes, a reduced number of axons, increased edema, or decreased axonal coherence [33, 56, 57]. DTI imaging can show two different patterns of the early phase of DAI: (1) decreased FA with decreased or isointense ADC which represents mixed intra- and extracellular edema and broken fibers, and (2) normal FA with decreased ADC which represents pure cytotoxic edema and presumably preserved fiber connectivity (Figs. 17.17 and 17.18). In the late phase of DAI, decreased FA and increased ADC are observed. DT imaging is thought to be useful in the early detection of DAI and a prognostic measure of subsequent brain damage [56].

Many studies have found changes in FA in patients with mTBI in both acute and chronic phases. Most reports are consistent in the finding of reduced FA during the chronic phase (>2 weeks) [33, 58]. However, the literature varies in the FA values in the acute phase after mTBI and they may be increased or decreased. Eierud and colleagues published a meta-analysis in 2014 after reviewing 122 publications on DTI and mTBI and found that increased FA was reported more frequently than decreased FA in acute settings [59]. This increased FA in acute settings may be due to axonal injury in areas of crossing fibers and markedly reduced extracellular diffusivity in the setting of cytotoxic edema [33].

The FA is reduced, and diffusivity is increased in cases of moderate to severe TBI and several studies have validated this observation in adult and pediatric patients [11, 25, 60]. The degree of reduction of FA also correlates with TBI severity [61].

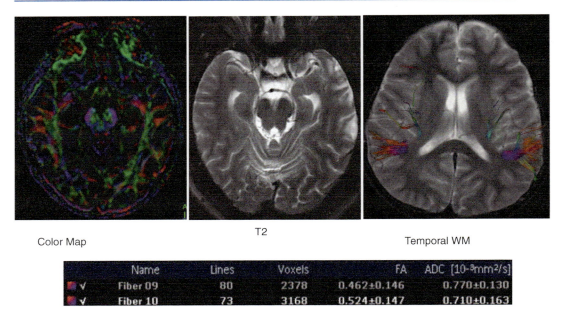

Fig. 17.17 16-year-old male suffering from Post-Concussion syndrome after TBI after MVA shows decreased FA and increased diffusivity in the left temporal lobe. (Case Courtesy by Dr. Gaurang Shah)

Axial diffusivity (AD) and radial diffusivity (RD) are other DTI metrics. AD, also called longitudinal diffusivity, is the diffusivity along the fastest direction of diffusion which is invariably along the long axis of the fiber tract and is affected by the pathologies of the axons. RD, also called transverse diffusivity, measures the diffusivity perpendicular to the fiber tract and is affected by the pathologies of the myelin [62]. The AD and RD show different patterns of increased or decreased values based on the severity of injury and time since injury.

Those patients who suffer from post-concussion syndrome (PCS) after mTBI have more structural impairment as compared to the patients of mTBI without PCS. A study was conducted on 53 patients with mTBI and 40 healthy volunteers. The DWI was performed on a 3 T magnet in 50 non-collinear gradient directions in the subacute and late phases of the injury. They discovered that patients with PCS had decreased fractional anisotropy (FA) and increased mean and axial diffusivity in association, projection, and commissural white matter tracts [63].

Many studies have cross-validated DTI detection of DAI by using microdialysis of CSF, where reduction in the FA correlated to interstitial fluid tau levels. Tau is a structural protein of axons and increased levels in CSF are seen after TBI [11, 64].

The deterioration of white matter tracts continues for up to 2 years after initial injury according to numerous investigations [60, 65]. Many studies have seen continuous measurable deterioration in the white matter integrity parameters after the initial insult and linked this to ongoing microstructural changes which continue after initial injury. The authors suggested that there is delayed activation of complex intracellular biochemical cascades after initial injury which lead to axonal transection called secondary axotomy and may be the cause of progressive clinical decline after initial trauma [11].

DTI evaluation of the corpus callosum is superior to smaller white matter tracts because of the large size of the bundle and unidirectional orientation of tracts in the corpus callosum. However, DTI cannot resolve crossing fibers as well, and FA is usually decreased in regions of crossing

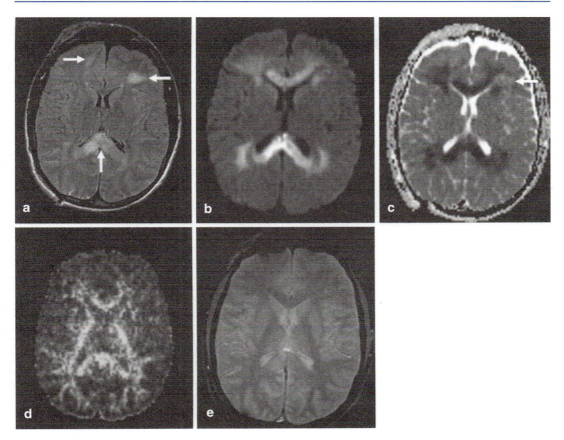

Fig. 17.18 (a–e) Diffuse axonal injury in a 24-year-old man after a motor vehicle accident. (a) FLAIR image shows multiple asymmetric hyperintense lesions in the bilateral frontal white matter and the corpus callosum (*arrows*). (b) DW image shows diffuse hyperintense lesion in the deep white matter and the corpus callosum. (c) ADC map reveals decreased ADC in the deep white matter and the corpus callosum. The left frontal lesion seen on FLAIR image has iso- to slightly increased ADC (*arrow*). (d) FA is preserved in most of the diffuse white matter abnormalities suggestive of a pure cytotoxic edema. Decreased FAs are observed in the lesions in the bilateral frontal white matter and splenium of the corpus callosum seen on the FLAIR image. (e) GRE image demonstrates hemorrhagic foci in the frontal white matter

fibers which makes it difficult to evaluate the areas of brain where white matter tracts are crossing [66]. The changes in the metrics of DTI and FA are not specific to DAI and can be seen in a wide variety of white matter disorders.

Multiple studies have documented that many patients of mTBI who had no radiological evidence of trauma in the brain, and who then died from other causes, had microscopic diffuse axonal injuries on autopsy [6, 62]. Yuh and colleagues conducted a study on mTBI patients and concluded that the prognostic utility of DTI is better than CT, clinical, or demographic socioeconomic variables in the prediction of 3- and 6-month outcome [67].

However, there are many limitations including high cost, MRI safety issues, medical stability of the polytraumatism patients, variable protocols, lack of standardized metrics, post-processing techniques, and lack of correlation with clinical findings which impede routine use of DTI for TBI patients [11].

17.12 Diffusion Kurtosis Imaging (DKI)

Diffusion kurtosis imaging uses multishell imaging with numerous b-values of more than 1000 s/mm² to quantify the non-Gaussian behavior of diffusion. The diffusion images have a Gaussian behavior when b values are equal or less than 1000 s/mm² and it becomes non-Gaussian at values above b-1000. Kurtosis is a measure of the deviation from a Gaussian distribution and depicts tissue microstructure complexity. This technique can detect subtle injuries even in areas where FA is low [62, 66, 68].

17.13 DWI Thermometry

DWI thermometry is a novel research technique which can measure brain core temperature using DWI data, calculations, and the principles of kinetic theory. The diffusion coefficient of the non-restricted water molecules in the lateral ventricles can be measured which can help to calculate the temperature [69]. Tazoe et al. conducted a study in 2014 which measured brain core temperatures in patients with mTBI and found that they were reduced, which may be due to a global decrease in metabolism or perfusion or both [70]. However, brain temperature increased after moderate to severe TBI due to increased intracranial pressure and higher resistance to blood flow.

17.14 DWI and Cognition

Conventional imaging findings in mTBI do not predict the neurocognitive outcome. However, Miles and colleagues found a positive correlation between low FA and poor executive functions [71]. In a different study, global burden of the injuries in mTBI as measured by DTI correlated with a decline in executive function and cognitive processing speed [51]. The volume and total number of traumatic lesions on DWI (whether facilitated or restricted diffusion) in the acute phase of head injury has shown strong correlation with memory deficits in patients with mild trau-matic injuries and with modified Rankin scale in moderate to severe trauma [27, 72].

17.15 DWI in Focal Traumatic Lesions

CT is excellent in the initial evaluation of extra-dural and subdural hematomas, traumatic sub-arachnoid hemorrhage, parenchymal hematomas, brain contusions, fractures, and complications such as midline shift and herniation. However, MRI has its own advantages in certain situations and is more sensitive for subtle lesions.

17.16 Contusions

Brain contusions are defined as traumatic injuries to the cortical surface of the brain and are caused by direct impact by the skull to the brain and can be coup and/or countercoup injuries. They are most commonly seen in the inferior surface of the frontal lobes, anterior and inferior aspect of the temporal lobes, and lateral aspects of the brain due to impact from hard bony ridges of the skull base. Contusions are large, multiple, bilateral, more ill-defined, more likely to be hemorrhagic, and are seen in the superficial aspect of the brain (Figs. 17.12, 17.16, 17.19, 17.20, and 17.21). Cytotoxic edema in brain contusions is also related to excitotoxic mechanisms [73–75].

CT scan underestimates contusions especially when they are smaller and nonhemorrhagic. MRI is more sensitive in detecting these contusions and DWI shows that they are heterogeneous and have mixed areas of cytotoxic and vasogenic edema. Brain contusions can show an interesting appearance on DWI, with a core of low SI on diffusion and increased ADC surrounded by a rim of high SI on diffusion with decreased ADC. This happens because of disintegration and homogenization of the intra- and extracellular components in the central area, whereas cellular swelling is predominant in the peripheral areas [74].

Occasionally MR may be performed in such patients when there is unexplained neurological deficit and a mismatch between CT findings and

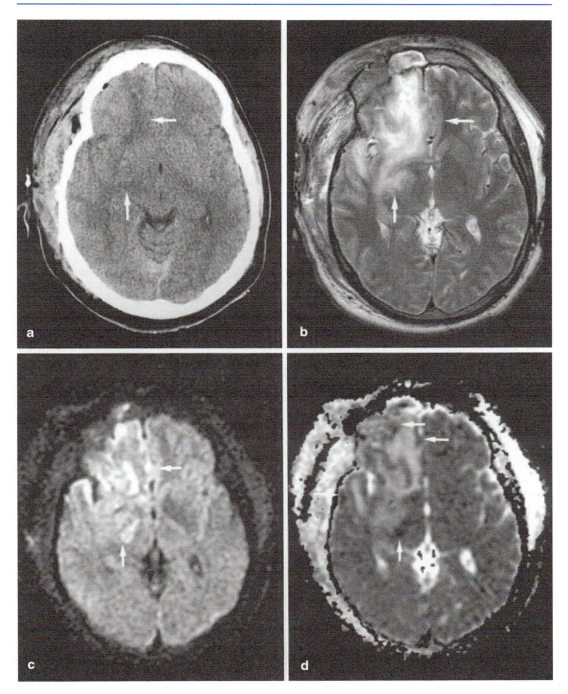

Fig. 17.19 (**a–d**) Brain contusion in the frontal lobe in a 37-year-old man after a motor vehicle accident. (**a**) On CT obtained after evacuation of epidural hematoma, it is difficult to delineate the extent of contusion in the right frontal lobe (*arrows*). (**b**) T2-weighted image delineates the extent of the edematous brain contusion (*arrows*). (**c**) DW image shows heterogeneous signal intensity in these lesions, representing mixed vasogenic and cytotoxic edema with hemorrhagic necrotic tissues (*arrows*). (**d**) ADC map reveals mixed increase and relative decrease of ADC (*arrows*) in these lesions

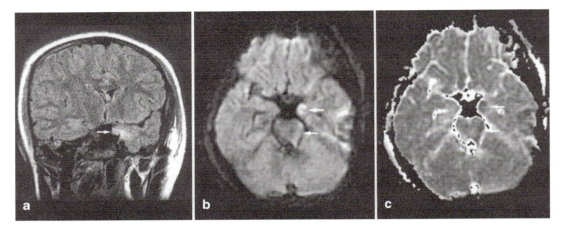

Fig. 17.20 (a–c) Brain contusion in the hippocampus in an 11-year-old girl after a motor vehicle accident. (a) FLAIR image shows a hyperintense lesion in the left hippocampus (*arrow*). (b) DW image shows this lesion as hyperintense. (c) ADC is decreased in the left hippocampus and left side of the brain stem (*arrows*), representing mainly cytotoxic edema

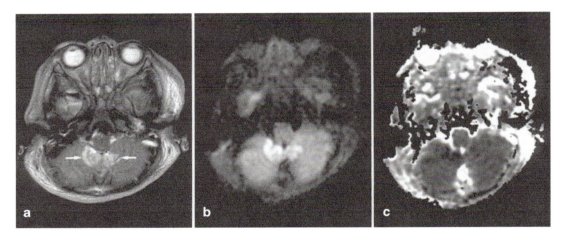

Fig. 17.21 (a–c) Brain contusion in the cerebellar tonsil in an 11-year-old girl after a motor vehicle accident. (a) T2-weighted image shows hyperintense lesions in the cerebellar tonsils (*arrows*). (b) DW image shows this lesion as hyperintense. (c) ADC is partially decreased

clinical examination. MR is more sensitive for detection of nonhemorrhagic contusions, especially when they are small. FLAIR and DWI will depict them as foci of abnormal signal intensity. DWI may show them as restricted or facilitated diffusion depending on various factors. Small hemorrhagic contusions are better seen on GRE and SWI sequences, with SWI 3–6 times more sensitive. Most institutions perform either GRE or SWI, as they serve the same purpose.

17.17 Extra-axial Hematoma

Traumatic hemorrhages result from injury to a cerebral vessel (artery, vein or capillary) [4]. Subdural hematomas originate from disruption of the bridging cortical veins, which are vulnerable to rapid stretching. Epidural hematoma can have either an arterial or a venous sinus origin, typically associated with a skull fracture. MR imaging is extremely helpful to detect hematomas, especially along the vertex and skull base, and can in certain questionable cases differentiate between subdural and epidural hematomas [4, 76–79] (Figs. 17.22, 17.23, 17.24, and 17.27).

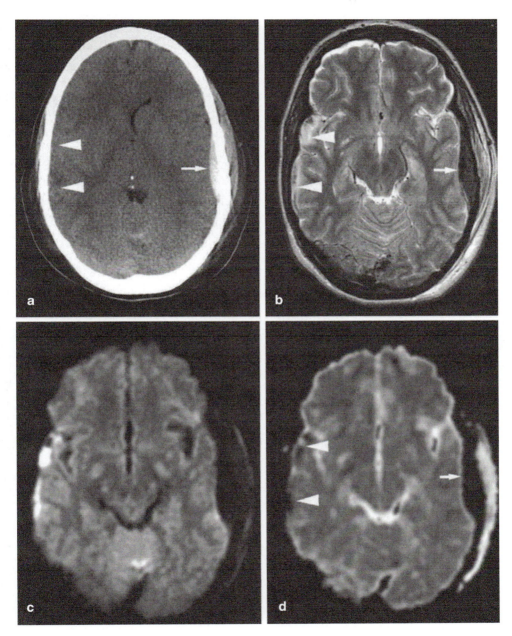

Fig. 17.22 (a–d) Epidural and subdural hematoma in a 26-year-old man after a motor vehicle accident. (**a**) CT shows a left epidural hematoma (*arrow*) but it is difficult to depict the isodense small subdural hematoma in the right side (*arrowheads*). (**b**) T2-weighted image shows the left epidural hematoma (*arrow*) as a hypointense lesion and the right subdural hematoma as partially hypointense lesions (*arrowheads*). (**c**) DW image shows the epidural hematoma as very hypointense due to deoxy-hemoglobin, and the subdural hematoma as very hyperintense presumably due to high viscosity or hypercellularity of hematoma. (**d**) ADC map shows hypointensity due to loss of pixels with background masking in the left epidural hematoma (*arrow*). ADC map also shows decreased ADC in the right subdural hematoma (*arrowheads*)

Very thin (1–2 mm thickness) SDH are better seen on MRI on T1-weighted images as thin curvilinear areas of hyperintensity due to methemoglobin formation. These can also be seen on FLAIR, DWI, T2, or GRE and will have different signal intensities based on the age of hemorrhage and other factors. MRI is more sensitive than CT for detecting these thin SDH because of high imaging contrast between hematoma and signal void of bone. However, subdural hematomas that are missed on CT are almost always very thin and of doubtful clinical significance. MRI can also help to predict the approximate age of the hematoma [2, 4, 8, 80] (Figs. 17.22, 17.23, and 17.27).

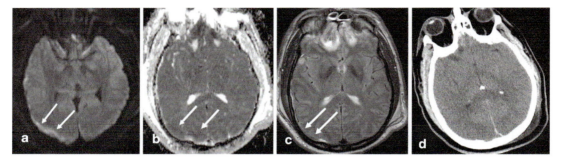

Fig. 17.23 (a–d) Acute subdural hematoma. 38-year-old male patient after fall from roof shows thin right convexity SDH as RD on DWI (a) and is difficult to see on the CT scan (d). DWI and other MR sequences (b is ADC and c is T2) are more sensitive for thin SDH because of better contrast resolution and signal void of the adjacent bone

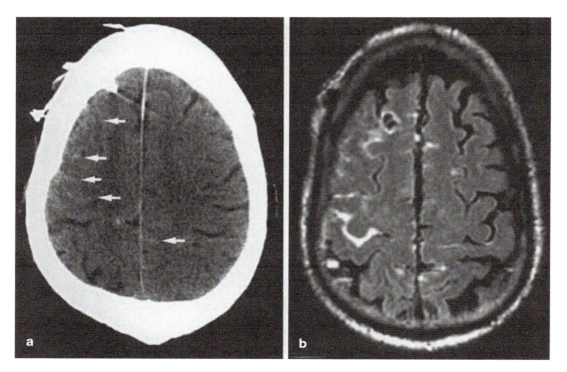

Fig. 17.24 (a–d) Subarachnoid hemorrhage in a 68-year-old man with ruptured aneurysm of the right middle cerebral artery bifurcation. (a) Postoperative CT shows subtle high density of subarachnoid space in the right frontoparietal area (*arrows*). (b) FLAIR image shows subarachnoid hemorrhage as hyperintensity. (c) DW image also shows subarachnoid hemorrhage as hyperintensity with mildly increased ADC (not shown). (d) Coronal GRE shows the hemorrhage as low signal intensity

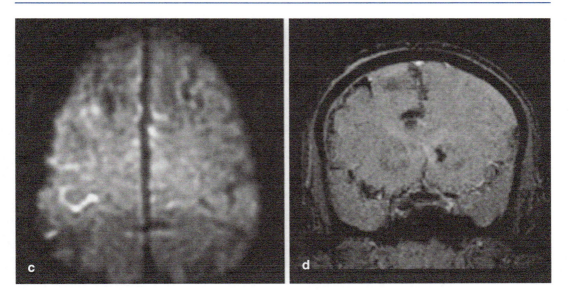

Fig. 17.24 (continued)

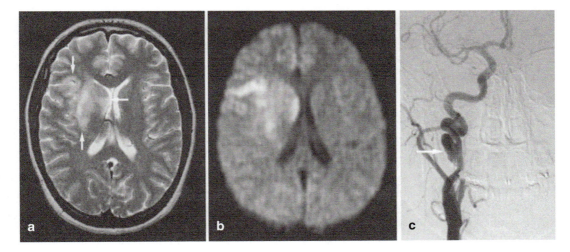

Fig. 17.25 (**a–c**) Cerebral infarction after carotid artery dissection with pseudoaneurysm in a 20-year-old female patient after a motor vehicle accident. (**a**) T2-weighted image shows hyperintense lesions in the right middle cerebral artery territory including the right basal ganglia (*arrows*). (**b**) DW image also shows these lesions as hyperintense with decreased ADC (not shown), representing acute infarction. (**c**) Conventional angiogram shows pseudoaneurysm of the right carotid artery (*arrow*)

17.18 Diffusion in Vascular Injuries and Infarcts

Traumatic arterial and venous injuries (dissections, lacerations, occlusions, pseudoaneurysm, arteriovenous fistulas) are more prevalent than generally believed. Many asymptomatic lesions probably escape detection, and others are recognized several days to months after the injury (Fig. 17.25). Vertebral artery injuries are more common after blunt trauma, mainly due to fractures of the cervical spine, LeFort II and III facial fractures and skull base fractures. Carotid artery injuries are more common with penetrating trauma. These injuries may cause dissection, occlusion, pseudoaneurysm, and other abnormalities which can lead to thromboembolism or obstruction of flow with resultant infarction. Fractures of the occipital and temporal bones and the skull vault may also predispose to dural sinus thrombosis leading to venous infarcts within a few days after the initial trauma [2, 31, 81].

CTA and CTV have high accuracy to detect vascular injuries and are the best initial tests to evaluate the arterial and venous structures whenever vascular injuries are suspected. MR head along with MRA or MRV can be performed for the evaluation of possible infarcts, or when iodinated contrast is contraindicated. Diffusion-weighted imaging is the most sensitive sequence for the detection of acute infarcts as it can show restricted diffusion within minutes of clinical onset.

Conventional angiography is still the gold standard in the diagnosis of vascular injuries but is usually reserved for neurointervention, problem-solving cases or in cases marred by metallic artifact after gunshot injury.

17.19 Diffusion in Secondary Injuries and Postoperative Complications

Prolonged and prominent midline shift because of large SDH or EDH can cause compression on the anterior and posterior cerebral arteries leading to infarcts. Descending transtentorial herniation can cause duret hemorrhages, contusions, and edema in the brainstem. DWI is extremely sensitive in picking up these findings of acute infarction and edema, if the patient is a candidate for an MRI [2, 4]. However, in many such cases, the patients are very sick and too unstable to undergo an MRI. CT head is then usually performed.

DWI is very sensitive and accurate for the diagnosis of hypoxic-ischemic brain injuries which may result from catastrophic cardiac or vascular problems. Restricted diffusion is seen in the affected areas which usually involve the cerebral cortex, cerebellar hemispheres, and basal ganglia [82].

Some patients develop intracranial infections after craniotomies and skull base fractures which cause persistent CSF leaks. These patients may develop subdural or extradural empyema, abscesses, or cerebritis. MRI brain with and without contrast is extremely valuable in such patients. Diffusion images show restricted diffusion within abscesses, as well as in empyema because of pus accumulation. However, hemorrhage in acute phases can also show restricted diffusion due to blood degradation products; hence these cases should be interpreted with caution. DWI has limitations in differentiating postoperative subdural empyema from hemorrhagic, noninfected fluid collections after intracranial surgeries and accuracy improves approximately three months after surgery [83]. One study found a 37% rate of false-positive DWI findings for infection in the postoperative period [84]. This was because noninfected hemorrhagic fluid collections due to craniotomies or subdural hematomas may show restricted diffusion in the acute to subacute stages. Evaluation of precontrast T1-weighted images is helpful as hemorrhagic fluid collections will be hyperintense. They also found that infections in extradural fluid collections are less likely to show restricted diffusion. The imaging appearance on all pulse sequences, comparison with all prior imaging studies, change in size and morphology with time, and clinical parameters should be carefully assessed to distinguish hemorrhagic fluid collections from empyema (Figs. 17.26 and 17.27).

17.20 Summary

TBI are very common and CT is the mainstay for the management and triage in the majority of these patients. However, MR plays a significant role in problem-solving cases when there is an unexplained neurological deficit not explained by the CT, or if certain complications are suspected. Injuries can be focal or diffuse and DAI is a diffuse injury which is often missed on CT. FLAIR,

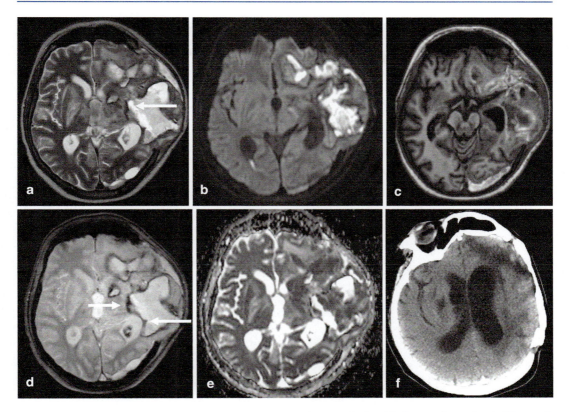

Fig. 17.26 (a–f) 46-year-old female patient with history of MVA and left-sided craniectomy for evacuation of left-sided hematoma shows a fluid collection in left temporal lobe on T2 (a) with some areas of RD on DWI (b). These areas are hypointense on ADC (e), hyperintense on DWI (b) and have some hyperintensity on T1WI (c) and hypointense rim on T2WI (a) and GRE (d) (arrow). This represents a hemorrhagic fluid collection and not an abscess as there was no supporting clinical features and patient remained stable for next 9 months. A CT scan (f) after 9 months shows interval resolution without any surgery or antibiotic treatment. The DWI has limitations after surgery to detect infection and both sensitivity and specificity are reduced. The presence of T1 hyperintensity due to methemoglobin as seen in c and T2 or T2* hypointense rim due to hemosiderin as seen in a and d are suggestive of hematoma rather than infection

DWI, GRE, and SWI are all very helpful in the evaluation of nonhemorrhagic and hemorrhagic DAI as well as other traumatic injuries on MRI.

Patients with moderate and severe DAI will have obvious findings on the DWI, FLAIR, GRE, and SWI sequences and many patients will even have some abnormalities on the CT to suggest damage to the brain. However, many patients with mild TBI will have a normal or near-normal CT and conventional MRI but will suffer from long-term cognitive problems. Both biomarkers and autopsies have shown that most such patients have microscopic injuries to the white matter tracts which are not revealed by conventional imaging. DTI is a promising tool to diagnose and prognosticate patients with mild TBI and is currently a topic of intense research. However, there is as yet insufficient evidence to support the routine clinical use of advanced neuroimaging studies such as DTI for diagnosis and/ or prognostication of individual patients [66].

17.21 Treatment of Head Injury

Hiroto Kawasaki

Head injury causes damage to the brain through two processes, primary brain injury, and secondary injury. The primary injury occurs at the time

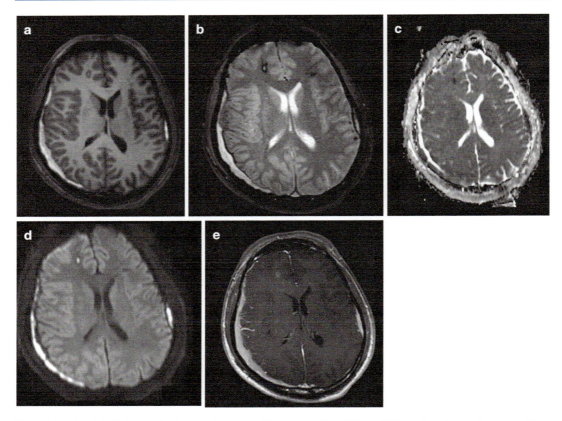

Fig. 17.27 (**a–e**) MR brain of 22-year-old male with MVC and ejection shows bilateral subacute SDH which are hyperintense on precontrast T1 (**a**) and show RD on DWI (**d**) and ADC (**c**). There is dural and leptomeningeal enhancement on postcontrast T1 (**e**) on the surface of brain on the right side near the larger SDH due to vascular congestion. RD on DWI and contrast enhancement in a subdural fluid collection may indicate empyema; however history of traumatic SDH and hyperintensity on precontrast T1 and clinical picture should discourage the misdiagnosis

of trauma that include contusion of cerebral cortex or brain stem, and diffuse axonal injury. The secondary injury develops subsequent to the initial injury, such as cerebral edema, intracranial hematoma, ischemia, anoxia, and infection [85]. Head trauma is often associated with other type of injuries in not only head and neck areas but also in other part of bodies which may contribute development of secondary injuries [86]. Treatment of head injury is aimed for controlling the secondary injury because the primary injury is already occurred [87]. The secondary injury develops over wide range of time lines. It is important to predict and find out evolution of the secondary injury in timely manner in order to address promptly to mitigating ongoing problems and preventing further progress of deterioration (Fig. 17.28).

17.21.1 Space-Occupying Lesion

Since the brain is confined in the rigid skull, any increasing volume of pathologic processes increase intracranial pressure, which results in decrease of cerebral perfusion pressure that would subsequently lead to temporary or permanent brain injuries. Such space-occupying lesion includes hematoma in subdural, epidural, and

17 Trauma

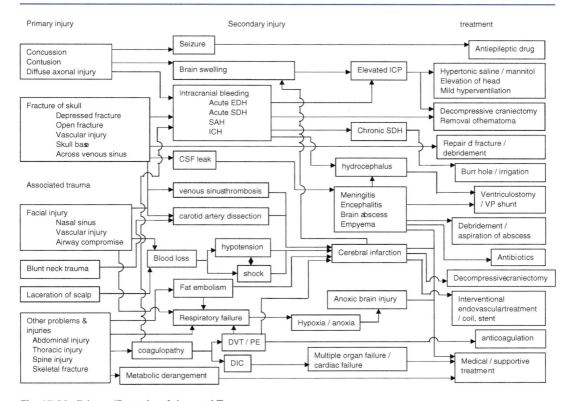

Fig. 17.28 Primary/Secondary Injury and Treatment

intracerebral space, hydrocephalus, depressed fracture, foreign bodies, and brain swelling due to contusion, infection, or infarction. Depending on the size, location, and speed of development, some of such lesions must be addressed surgically without delay [86, 88–90]. Goal of surgery is to reduce intracranial pressure. Decompressive craniectomy, removal of space-occupying lesion, and ventriculostomy are often performed.

Open skull fracture and leakage of cerebrospinal fluid render patients to high risk for intracranial infection. Debridement of open wound must be performed in timely manner and if there are free bone fragments they must be removed [91]. CSF leak indicate there are fracture of skull and laceration of dura matter. It may be addressed by placing CSF diversion by either lumbar drain or ventriculostomy. If there is a sizable displaced skull base fracture over the nasal sinus, it often has to be surgically repaired.

Blunt trauma to the head or neck may cause injury to the carotid artery and vertebral artery [92]. Dissection of major vessel walls may progress into occlusion of the blood vessel in delayed fashion, which could result in cerebral infarction [93]. Dural sinus thrombosis also could occur after head trauma, which may result in elevated ICP and venous infarction of the brain [94].

Patients of head trauma frequently have injuries to other part of body which may affect progression of the secondary brain injury, for example, excessive bleeding either internal or external may cause hypotension and hypoperfusion of the brain [85, 86]. Fractures of long bones or pelvis may cause fat embolism in the brain [95, 96]. Severe trauma regardless of head or body could causes coagulopathy which results in intracranial hemorrhagic disease [97]. Severe trauma also causes derangement of metabolism, for example, hyponatremia is frequently seen after head trauma, which would induce exacerbation of brain swelling and cognitive state [98].

References

1. Gennarelli TA (1993) Mechanisms of brain injury. J Emerg Med 11(Suppl 1):5–11
2. Mutch CA, Talbott JF, Gean A (2016) Imaging evaluation of acute traumatic brain injury. Neurosurg Clin N Am 27(4):409–439
3. Alsop DC, Murai H, Detre JA, McIntosh TK, Smith DH (1996) Detection of acute pathologic changes following experimental traumatic brain injury using diffusion-weighted magnetic resonance imaging. J Neurotrauma 13(9):515–521
4. Gentry LR (1994) Imaging of closed head injury. Radiology 191(1):1–17
5. Kelly AB, Zimmerman RD, Snow RB, Gandy SE, Heier LA, Deck MD (1988) Head trauma: comparison of MR and CT—experience in 100 patients. AJNR Am J Neuroradiol 9(4):699–708
6. Adams JH, Doyle D, Ford I, Gennarelli TA, Graham DI, McLellan DR (1989) Diffuse axonal injury in head injury: definition, diagnosis and grading. Histopathology 15(1):49–59
7. Strich SJ (1956) Diffuse degeneration of the cerebral white matter in severe dementia following head injury. J Neurol Neurosurg Psychiatry 19(3):163–185
8. Gentry LR, Thompson B, Godersky JC (1988) Trauma to the corpus callosum: MR features. AJNR Am J Neuroradiol 9(6):1129–1138
9. Mittl RL, Grossman RI, Hiehle JF, Hurst RW, Kauder DR, Gennarelli TA et al (1994) Prevalence of MR evidence of diffuse axonal injury in patients with mild head injury and normal head CT findings. AJNR Am J Neuroradiol 15(8):1583–1589
10. Abu Hamdeh S, Marklund N, Lannsjö M, Howells T, Raininko R, Wikström J et al (2017) Extended anatomical grading in diffuse axonal injury using MRI: Hemorrhagic lesions in the substantia Nigra and Mesencephalic Tegmentum indicate poor long-term outcome. J Neurotrauma 34(2):341–352
11. Tsitsopoulos PP, Abu Hamdeh S, Marklund N (2017) Current opportunities for clinical monitoring of axonal pathology in Traumatic brain injury. Front Neurol 8:599
12. Gennarelli TA, Graham DI (1998) Neuropathology of the head injuries. Semin Clin Neuropsychiatry 3(3):160–175
13. Hanstock CC, Faden AI, Bendall MR, Vink R (1994) Diffusion-weighted imaging differentiates ischemic tissue from traumatized tissue. Stroke 25(4):843–848
14. Ashikaga R, Araki Y, Ishida O (1997) MRI of head injury using FLAIR. Neuroradiology 39(4):239–242
15. Katayama Y, Becker DP, Tamura T, Tsubokawa T (1990) Cellular swelling during cerebral ischaemia demonstrated by microdialysis in vivo: preliminary data indicating the role of excitatory amino acids. Acta Neurochir Suppl (Wien) 51:183–185
16. Albensi BC, Knoblach SM, Chew BG, O'Reilly MP, Faden AI, Pekar JJ (2000) Diffusion and high resolution MRI of traumatic brain injury in rats: time course and correlation with histology. Exp Neurol 162(1):61–72
17. Assaf Y, Beit-Yannai E, Shohami E, Berman E, Cohen Y (1997) Diffusion- and T2-weighted MRI of closed-head injury in rats: a time course study and correlation with histology. Magn Reson Imaging 15(1):77–85
18. Barzó P, Marmarou A, Fatouros P, Hayasaki K, Corwin F (1997) Contribution of vasogenic and cellular edema to traumatic brain swelling measured by diffusion-weighted imaging. J Neurosurg 87(6):900–907
19. Ito J, Marmarou A, Barzó P, Fatouros P, Corwin F (1996) Characterization of edema by diffusion-weighted imaging in experimental traumatic brain injury. J Neurosurg 84(1):97–103
20. Huisman TAGM, Sorensen AG, Hergan K, Gonzalez RG, Schaefer PW (2003) Diffusion-weighted imaging for the evaluation of diffuse axonal injury in closed head injury. J Comput Assist Tomogr 27(1):5–11
21. Yanagawa Y, Tsushima Y, Tokumaru A, Un-no Y, Sakamoto T, Okada Y et al (2000) A quantitative analysis of head injury using T2*-weighted gradient-echo imaging. J Trauma 49(2):272–277
22. Babikian T, Freier MC, Tong KA, Nickerson JP, Wall CJ, Holshouser BA et al (2005) Susceptibility weighted imaging: neuropsychologic outcome and pediatric head injury. Pediatr Neurol 33(3):184–194
23. Tong KA, Ashwal S, Holshouser BA, Shutter LA, Herigault G, Haacke EM et al (2003) Hemorrhagic shearing lesions in children and adolescents with posttraumatic diffuse axonal injury: improved detection and initial results. Radiology 227(2):332–339
24. Mata-Mbemba D, Mugikura S, Nakagawa A, Murata T, Ishii K, Kushimoto S et al (2018) Traumatic midline subarachnoid hemorrhage on initial computed tomography as a marker of severe diffuse axonal injury. J Neurosurg 129(5):1317–1324
25. Arfanakis K, Haughton VM, Carew JD, Rogers BP, Dempsey RJ, Meyerand ME (2002) Diffusion tensor MR imaging in diffuse axonal injury. AJNR Am J Neuroradiol 23(5):794–802
26. Liu AY, Maldjian JA, Bagley LJ, Sinson GP, Grossman RI (1999) Traumatic brain injury: diffusion-weighted MR imaging findings. AJNR Am J Neuroradiol 20(9):1636–1641
27. Schaefer PW, Huisman TAGM, Sorensen AG, Gonzalez RG, Schwamm LH (2004) Diffusion-weighted MR imaging in closed head injury: high correlation with initial glasgow coma scale score and score on modified Rankin scale at discharge. Radiology 233(1):58–66
28. Takayama H, Kobayashi M, Sugishita M, Mihara B (2000) Diffusion-weighted imaging demonstrates transient cytotoxic edema involving the corpus callosum in a patient with diffuse brain injury. Clin Neurol Neurosurg 102(3):135–139
29. Al Brashdi YH, Albayram MS (2015) Reversible restricted-diffusion lesion representing transient intramyelinic cytotoxic edema in a patient with traumatic brain injury. Neuroradiol J 28(4):409–412

30. Faden AI, Demediuk P, Panter SS, Vink R (1989) The role of excitatory amino acids and NMDA receptors in traumatic brain injury. Science 244(4906):798–800

31. Moritani T, Smoker WRK, Sato Y, Numaguchi Y, Westesson P-LA (2005) Diffusion-weighted imaging of acute excitotoxic brain injury. AJNR Am J Neuroradiol 26(2):216–228

32. Obrenovitch TP, Urenjak J (1997) Is high extracellular glutamate the key to excitotoxicity in traumatic brain injury? J Neurotrauma 14(10):677–698

33. Borja MJ, Chung S, Lui YW (2018) Diffusion MR imaging in mild traumatic brain injury. Neuroimaging Clin N Am 28(1):117–126

34. Hergan K, Schaefer PW, Sorensen AG, Gonzalez RG, Huisman TAGM (2002) Diffusion-weighted MRI in diffuse axonal injury of the brain. Eur Radiol 12(10):2536–2541

35. Rugg-Gunn FJ, Symms MR, Barker GJ, Greenwood R, Duncan JS (2001) Diffusion imaging shows abnormalities after blunt head trauma when conventional magnetic resonance imaging is normal. J Neurol Neurosurg Psychiatry 70(4):530–533

36. Kin K, Ono Y, Fujimori T, Kuramoto S, Katsumata A, Goda Y et al (2016) The usefulness of CT-diffusion weighted image mismatch in patients with mild to moderate traumatic brain injury. Acta Med Okayama 70(4):237–242

37. Moen KG, Skandsen T, Folvik M, Brezova V, Kvistad KA, Rydland J et al (2012) A longitudinal MRI study of traumatic axonal injury in patients with moderate and severe traumatic brain injury. J Neurol Neurosurg Psychiatry 83(12):1193–1200

38. Bansal M, Sinha VD, Bansal J (2018) Diagnostic and prognostic capability of newer magnetic resonance imaging brain sequences in diffuse axonal injury patient. Asian J Neurosurg 13(2):348–356

39. Kinoshita T, Moritani T, Hiwatashi A, Wang HZ, Shrier DA, Numaguchi Y et al (2005) Conspicuity of diffuse axonal injury lesions on diffusion-weighted MR imaging. Eur J Radiol 56(1):5–11

40. Galloway NR, Tong KA, Ashwal S, Oyoyo U, Obenaus A (2008) Diffusion-weighted imaging improves outcome prediction in pediatric traumatic brain injury. J Neurotrauma 25(10):1153–1162

41. Hou DJ, Tong KA, Ashwal S, Oyoyo U, Joo E, Shutter L et al (2007) Diffusion-weighted magnetic resonance imaging improves outcome prediction in adult traumatic brain injury. J Neurotrauma 24(10):1558–1569

42. Zheng WB, Liu GR, Li LP, Wu RH (2007) Prediction of recovery from a post-traumatic coma state by diffusion-weighted imaging (DWI) in patients with diffuse axonal injury. Neuroradiology 49(3):271–279

43. Biousse V, Suh DY, Newman NJ, Davis PC, Mapstone T, Lambert SR (2002) Diffusion-weighted magnetic resonance imaging in Shaken Baby Syndrome. Am J Ophthalmol 133(2):249–255

44. Epelman M, Daneman A, Halliday W, Whyte H, Blaser SI (2012) Abnormal corpus callosum in neonates after hypoxic-ischemic injury. Pediatr Radiol 42(3):321–330

45. Decaminada N, Thaler M, Holler R, Salsa A, Ladiges C, Rammlmair G (2012) Brain fat embolism. A report of two cases and a brief review of neuroimaging findings. Neuroradiol J 25(2):193–199

46. Rutman AM, Rapp EJ, Hippe DS, Vu B, Mossa-Basha M (2017) T2*-Weighted and diffusion magnetic resonance imaging differentiation of cerebral fat embolism from diffuse axonal injury. J Comput Assist Tomogr 41(6):877–883

47. Stoeger A, Daniaux M, Felber S, Stockhammer G, Aichner F, zur Nedden D (1998) MRI findings in cerebral fat embolism. Eur Radiol 8(9):1590–1593

48. Bodanapally UK, Shanmuganathan K, Shin RK, Dreizin D, Katzman L, Reddy RP et al (2015) Hyperintense optic nerve due to diffusion restriction: diffusion-weighted imaging in traumatic optic neuropathy. Am J Neuroradiol 36(8):1536–1541

49. Budde MD, Skinner NP (2018) Diffusion MRI in acute nervous system injury. J Magn Reson San Diego Calif 1997 292:137–148

50. Irimia A, Wang B, Aylward SR, Prastawa MW, Pace DF, Gerig G et al (2012) Neuroimaging of structural pathology and connectomics in traumatic brain injury: toward personalized outcome prediction. NeuroImage Clin 1(1):1–17

51. Niogi SN, Mukherjee P (2010) Diffusion tensor imaging of mild traumatic brain injury. J Head Trauma Rehabil 25(4):241–255

52. Langlois JA, Rutland-Brown W, Wald MM (2006) The epidemiology and impact of traumatic brain injury: a brief overview. J Head Trauma Rehabil 21(5):375–378

53. Basser PJ, Pierpaoli C (2011) Microstructural and physiological features of tissues elucidated by quantitative-diffusion-tensor MRI. 1996. J Magn Reson San Diego Calif 1997 213(2):560–570

54. Ducreux D, Huynh I, Fillard P, Renoux J, Petit-Lacour MC, Marsot-Dupuch K et al (2005) Brain MR diffusion tensor imaging and fibre tracking to differentiate between two diffuse axonal injuries. Neuroradiology 47(8):604–608

55. Naganawa S, Sato C, Ishihra S, Kumada H, Ishigaki T, Miura S et al (2004) Serial evaluation of diffusion tensor brain fiber tracking in a patient with severe diffuse axonal injury. AJNR Am J Neuroradiol 25(9):1553–1556

56. Inglese M, Makani S, Johnson G, Cohen BA, Silver JA, Gonen O et al (2005) Diffuse axonal injury in mild traumatic brain injury: a diffusion tensor imaging study. J Neurosurg 103(2):298–303

57. Wilde EA, McCauley SR, Barnes A, Wu TC, Chu Z, Hunter JV et al (2012) Serial measurement of memory and diffusion tensor imaging changes within the first week following uncomplicated mild traumatic brain injury. Brain Imaging Behav 6(2):319–328

58. Grossman EJ, Inglese M, Bammer R (2010) Mild traumatic brain injury: is diffusion imaging ready for primetime in forensic medicine? Top Magn Reson Imaging TMRI 21(6):379–386

59. Eierud C, Craddock RC, Fletcher S, Aulakh M, King-Casas B, Kuehl D et al (2014) Neuroimaging after mild traumatic brain injury: review and meta-analysis. NeuroImage Clin. 4:283–294
60. Sidaros A, Engberg AW, Sidaros K, Liptrot MG, Herning M, Petersen P et al (2008) Diffusion tensor imaging during recovery from severe traumatic brain injury and relation to clinical outcome: a longitudinal study. Brain J Neurol 131(Pt 2):559–572
61. Rutgers DR, Fillard P, Paradot G, Tadié M, Lasjaunias P, Ducreux D (2008) Diffusion tensor imaging characteristics of the corpus callosum in mild, moderate, and severe traumatic brain injury. AJNR Am J Neuroradiol 29(9):1730–1735
62. Shenton ME, Hamoda HM, Schneiderman JS, Bouix S, Pasternak O, Rathi Y et al (2012) A review of magnetic resonance imaging and diffusion tensor imaging findings in mild traumatic brain injury. Brain Imaging Behav 6(2):137–192
63. Messé A, Caplain S, Pélégrini-Issac M, Blancho S, Montreuil M, Lévy R et al (2012) Structural integrity and postconcussion syndrome in mild traumatic brain injury patients. Brain Imaging Behav 6(2):283–292
64. Magnoni S, Mac Donald CL, Esparza TJ, Conte V, Sorrell J, Macrì M et al (2015) Quantitative assessments of traumatic axonal injury in human brain: concordance of microdialysis and advanced MRI. Brain J Neurol 138(Pt 8):2263–2277
65. Ljungqvist J, Nilsson D, Ljungberg M, Esbjörnsson E, Eriksson-Ritzén C, Skoglund T (2017) Longitudinal changes in diffusion tensor imaging parameters of the corpus callosum between 6 and 12 months after diffuse axonal injury. Brain Inj 31(3):344–350
66. Wintermark M, Sanelli PC, Anzai Y, Tsiouris AJ, Whitlow CT (2015) American College of Radiology Head Injury Institute. Imaging evidence and recommendations for traumatic brain injury: advanced neuro- and neurovascular imaging techniques. AJNR Am J Neuroradiol 36(2):E1–E11
67. Yuh EL, Cooper SR, Mukherjee P, Yue JK, Lingsma HF, Gordon WA et al (2014) Diffusion tensor imaging for outcome prediction in mild traumatic brain injury: a TRACK-TBI study. J Neurotrauma 31(17):1457–1477
68. Marrale M, Collura G, Brai M, Toschi N, Midiri F, La Tona G et al (2016) Physics, techniques and review of neuroradiological applications of diffusion kurtosis imaging (DKI). Clin Neuroradiol 26(4):391–403
69. Kozak LR, Bango M, Szabo M, Rudas G, Vidnyanszky Z, Nagy Z (2010) Using diffusion MRI for measuring the temperature of cerebrospinal fluid within the lateral ventricles. Acta Paediatr Oslo Nor 1992 99(2):237–243
70. Tazoe J, Yamada K, Sakai K, Akazawa K, Mineura K (2014) Brain core temperature of patients with mild traumatic brain injury as assessed by DWI-thermometry. Neuroradiology 56(10):809–815
71. Miles L, Grossman RI, Johnson G, Babb JS, Diller L, Inglese M (2008) Short-term DTI predictors of cognitive dysfunction in mild traumatic brain injury. Brain Inj 22(2):115–122
72. Kurca E, Sivák S, Kucera P (2006) Impaired cognitive functions in mild traumatic brain injury patients with normal and pathologic magnetic resonance imaging. Neuroradiology 48(9):661–669
73. Kawamata T, Katayama Y, Mori T, Aoyama N, Tsubokawa T (2002) Mechanisms of the mass effect of cerebral contusion: ICP monitoring and diffusion MRI study. Acta Neurochir Suppl 81:281–283
74. Kawamata T, Katayama Y, Aoyama N, Mori T (2000) Heterogeneous mechanisms of early edema formation in cerebral contusion: diffusion MRI and ADC mapping study. Acta Neurochir Suppl 76:9–12
75. Maeda T, Katayama Y, Kawamata T, Yamamoto T (1998) Mechanisms of excitatory amino acid release in contused brain tissue: effects of hypothermia and in situ administration of Co2+ on extracellular levels of glutamate. J Neurotrauma 15(9):655–664
76. Dechambre SD, Duprez T, Grandin CB, Lecouvet FE, Peeters A, Cosnard G (2000) High signal in cerebrospinal fluid mimicking subarachnoid haemorrhage on FLAIR following acute stroke and intravenous contrast medium. Neuroradiology 42(8):608–611
77. Melhem ER, Jara H, Eustace S (1997) Fluid-attenuated inversion recovery MR imaging: identification of protein concentration thresholds for CSF hyperintensity. AJR Am J Roentgenol 169(3):859–862
78. Singer MB, Atlas SW, Drayer BP (1998) Subarachnoid space disease: diagnosis with fluid-attenuated inversion-recovery MR imaging and comparison with gadolinium-enhanced spin-echo MR imaging—blinded reader study. Radiology 208(2):417–422
79. Taoka T, Yuh WT, White ML, Quets JP, Maley JE, Ueda T (2001) Sulcal hyperintensity on fluid-attenuated inversion recovery mr images in patients without apparent cerebrospinal fluid abnormality. AJR Am J Roentgenol 176(2):519–524
80. Wiesmann M, Mayer TE, Yousry I, Medele R, Hamann GF, Brückmann H (2002) Detection of hyperacute subarachnoid hemorrhage of the brain by using magnetic resonance imaging. J Neurosurg 96(4):684–689
81. Kohler R, Vargas MI, Masterson K, Lovblad KO, Pereira VM, Becker M (2011) CT and MR angiography features of traumatic vascular injuries of the neck. AJR Am J Roentgenol 196(6):W800–W809
82. Arbelaez A, Castillo M, Mukherji SK (1999) Diffusion-weighted MR imaging of global cerebral anoxia. AJNR Am J Neuroradiol 20(6):999–1007
83. Berndt M, Lange N, Ryang Y-M, Meyer B, Zimmer C, Hapfelmeier A et al (2018) Value of diffusion-weighted imaging in the diagnosis of postoperative intracranial infections. World Neurosurg 118:e245–e253
84. Farrell CJ, Hoh BL, Pisculli ML, Henson JW, Barker FG, Curry WT (2008) Limitations of diffusion-weighted imaging in the diagnosis of postoperative infections. Neurosurgery 62(3):577–583; discussion 577–583
85. Chesnut RM et al (1993) The role of secondary brain injury in determining outcome from severe head injury. J Trauma 34(2):216–222

86. Bullock MR et al (2006) Surgical management of traumatic parenchymal lesions. Neurosurgery 58(3 Suppl):S25–S46; discussion Si–iv
87. The Brain Trauma Foundation (2000) The American Association of Neurological Surgeons. The Joint Section on Neurotrauma and Critical Care. Initial management. J Neurotrauma 17(6–7):463–469
88. Bullock MR et al (2006) Surgical management of acute subdural hematomas. Neurosurgery 58(3 Suppl):S16–S24; discussion Si–iv
89. Bullock MR et al (2006) Surgical management of acute epidural hematomas. Neurosurgery 58(3 Suppl):S7–S15; discussion Si–iv
90. Bullock MR et al (2006) Surgical management of posterior fossa mass lesions. Neurosurgery 58(3 Suppl):S47–S55; discussion Si–iv
91. Bullock MR et al (2006) Surgical management of depressed cranial fractures. Neurosurgery 58(3 Suppl):S56–S60; discussion Si–iv
92. Stein DM et al (2009) Blunt cerebrovascular injuries: does treatment always matter? J Trauma 66(1):132–143; discussion 143–4
93. Anson J, Crowell RM (1991) Cervicocranial arterial dissection. Neurosurgery 29(1):89–96
94. Ferrera PC, Pauze DR, Chan L (1998) Sagittal sinus thrombosis after closed head injury. Am J Emerg Med 16(4):382–385
95. Riska EB, Myllynen P (1982) Fat embolism in patients with multiple injuries. J Trauma 22(11):891–894
96. Fabian TC et al (1990) Fat embolism syndrome: prospective evaluation in 92 fracture patients. Crit Care Med 18(1):42–46
97. Kaufman HH et al (1984) Clinicopathological correlations of disseminated intravascular coagulation in patients with head injury. Neurosurgery 15(1):34–42
98. Harrigan MR (1996) Cerebral salt wasting syndrome: a review. Neurosurgery 38(1):152–160

Brain Neoplasm

18

Jayapalli Rajiv Bapuraj, Toshio Moritani, Shotaro Naganawa, and Akio Hiwatashi

Christopher Becker, Yoshie Umemura, and Michelle M. Kim

18.1 Introduction

Conventional MRI sequences are the mainstay in the detection and diagnoses of brain neoplasms. Advances in MR imaging techniques have resulted in increased specificity in determining the histological diagnosis of brain tumors. Routine MR imaging is the sensitive method of detecting tumors of the brain. It is, however, not specific enough to determine the histologic nature of most tumors. This chapter will demonstrate diffusion-weighted (DW) imaging characteristics of intracranial tumors. DW imaging is one of the most important aspects in the characterization and grading of brain tumors and offers the added alternative to distinguish neoplastic processes from close mimics such as parenchymal infections. This chapter will focus on an overview of the DW imaging characteristics of intracranial tumors.

The 2016 revision of the WHO classification of brain tumors (Table 18.1) [1] presents the most comprehensive classification of brain neoplasms which is an update on the 2007 version (Table 18.2) [2]. The focus of this revision is to integrate conventional and advanced imaging techniques with molecular and genetic markers to present an objective diagnosis of brain tumors which till date were based primarily on histopathological evaluation. The aim of this classification is to correlate the pathology with tumor behavior and tumorigenesis. Previous systems of classifications and grading of tumors were divided by astrocytic, oligodendroglial, or ependymal lineage based on histopathology alone. However, tumors may exhibit features one or more lineages which makes classifications difficult at times. In prior WHO classifications the prognosis of tumors was not accurately reflected on the histological type and hence grade of tumors. With the advent of refined genetic and molecular features a clearer picture of tumor behavior has been observed and these have been incorporated into the revised WHO classification [3].

J. R. Bapuraj (✉)
Division of Neuroradiology, University of Michigan, Ann Arbor, MI, USA
e-mail: jrajiv@med.umich.edu

T. Moritani
Department of Radiology, Division of Neuroradiology, Clinical Neuroradiology Research, University of Michigan, Ann Arbor, MI, USA
e-mail: tmoritan@med.umich.edu

S. Naganawa
Department of Radiology, University of Michigan, Ann Arbor, MI, USA
e-mail: snaganaw@umich.edu

A. Hiwatashi
Department of Clinical Radiology, Kyushu University, Fukuoka, Japan
e-mail: hiwatasi@radiol.med.kyushu-u.ac.jp

C. Becker
Department of Neurology, University of Michigan, Ann Arbor, MI, USA
e-mail: cbec@umich.edu

Y. Umemura · M. M. Kim
University of Michigan, Ann Arbor, MI, USA
e-mail: yoshie@umich.edu; michekim@med.umich.edu

© Springer Nature Switzerland AG 2021
T. Moritani, A. A. Capizzano (eds.), *Diffusion-Weighted MR Imaging of the Brain, Head and Neck, and Spine*, https://doi.org/10.1007/978-3-030-62120-9_18

Table 18.1 The 2016 WHO classification of tumors of the central nervous system [1]

Diffuse astrocytic and oligodendroglial tumou
Diffuse astrocytoma, IDH-mutant
  Gemistocytic astrocytoma, IDH-mutant
Diffuse astrocytoma, IDH-wildtype
Diffuse astrocytoma, NOS
 	
Anaplastic astrocytoma, IDH-mutant
Anaplastic astrocytoma, IDH-wildtype
Anaplastic astrocytoma, NOS
 	
Glioblastoma, IDH-wildtype
  Giant cell glioblastoma
  Gliosarcoma
  Epithelioid glioblastoma
Glioblastoma, IDH-mutant
Glioblastoma, NOS
 	
Diffuse midline glioma, H3 K27M–mutant
 	
Oligodendroglioma, IDH-mutant and
  1p/19q-codeleted
Oligodendroglioma, NOS
 	
Anaplastic oligodendroglioma, IDH-mutant
  and 1p/19q-codeleted
Anaplastic oligodendroglioma, NOS
 	
Oligoastrocytoma, NOS
Anaplastic oligoastrocytoma, NOS
 	
Other astrocytic tumours
Pilocytic astrocytoma
  Pilomyxoid astrocytoma
Subependymal giant cell astrocytoma
Pleomorphic xanthoastrocytoma
Anaplastic pleomorphic xanthoastrocytoma
 	
Ependymal tumours
Subependymoma
Myxopapillary ependymoma
Ependymoma
  Papillary ependymoma
  Clear cell ependymoma
  Tanycytic ependymoma
Ependymoma, *RELA* fusion–positive
Anaplastic ependymoma
 	
Other gliomas
Chordoid glioma of the third ventricle
Angiocentric glioma
Astroblastoma
 	
Choroid plexus tumours
Choroid plexus papilloma
Atypical choroid plexus papilloma
Choroid plexus carcinoma
	Neuronal and mixed neuronal-glial tumours
	Dysembryoplastic neuroepithelial tumour
	Gangliocytoma
	Ganglioglioma
	Anaplastic ganglioglioma
	  Dysplastic cerebellar gangliocytoma
	  (Lhermitte–Duclos disease)
	Desmoplastic infantile astrocytoma and
	  ganglioglioma
	Papillary glioneuronal tumour
	Rosette-forming glioneuronal tumour
	Diffuse leptomeningeal glioneuronal tumour
	Central neurocytoma
	Extraventricular neurocytoma
	Cerebellar liponeurocytoma
	Paraganglioma
	
	Tumours of the pineal region
	Pineocytoma
	Pineal parenchymal tumour of intermediate
	  differentiation
	Pineoblastoma
	Papillary tumour of the pineal region
	
	Embryonal tumours
	Medulloblastomas, genetically defined
	  Medulloblastoma, WNT-activated
	  Medulloblastoma, SHH-activated and
	    TP53-mutant
	  Medulloblastoma, SHH-activated and
	    TP53-wildtype
	  Medulloblastoma, non-WNT/non-SHH
	    Medulloblastoma, group 3
	    Medulloblastoma, group 4
	Medulloblastomas, histologically defined
	  Medulloblastoma, classic
	  Medulloblastoma, desmoplastic/nodular
	  Medulloblastoma with extensive nodularity
	  Medulloblastoma, large cell / anaplastic
	Medulloblastoma, NOS
	
	Embryonal tumour with multilayered rosettes,
	  C19MC-altered
	Embryonal tumour with multilayered
	  rosettes, NOS
	Medulloepithelioma
	CNS neuroblastoma
	CNS ganglioneuroblastoma
	CNS embryonal tumour, NOS
	Atypical teratoid/rhabdoid tumour
	CNS embryonal tumour with rhabdoid features

18 Brain Neoplasm

Table 18.1 (continued)

Tumours of the cranial and paraspinal nerves
Schwannoma
    Cellular schwannoma
    Plexiform schwannoma

Melanotic schwannoma
Neurofibroma
    Atypical neurofibroma
    Plexiform neurofibroma
Perineurioma
Hybrid nerve sheath tumours
Malignant peripheral nerve sheath tumour
    Epithelioid MPNST
    MPNST with perineurial differentiation

Meningiomas
Meningioma
Meningothelial meningioma
Fibrous meningioma
Transitional meningioma
Psammomatous meningioma
Angiomatous meningioma
Microcystic meningioma
Secretory meningioma
Lymphoplasmacyte-rich meningioma
Metaplastic meningioma
Chordoid meningioma
Clear cell meningioma
Atypical meningioma
Papillary meningioma
Rhabdoid meningioma
Anaplastic (malignant) meningioma

Mesenchymal, non-meningothelial tumours
Solitary fibrous tumour / haemangiopericytoma**
    Grade 1
    Grade 2
    Grade 3
Haemangioblastoma
Haemangioma
Epithelioid haemangioendothelioma
Angiosarcoma
Kaposi sarcoma
Ewing sarcoma / PNET
Lipoma
Angiolipoma
Hibernoma
Liposarcoma
Desmoid-type fibromatosis
Myofibroblastoma
Inflammatory myofibroblastic tumour
Benign fibrous histiocytoma
Fibrosarcoma
Undifferentiated pleomorphic sarcoma /
    malignant fibrous histiocytoma
Leiomyoma
Leiomyosarcoma

Rhabdomyoma
Rhabdomyosarcoma
Chondroma
Chondrosarcoma
Osteoma
Osteochondroma
Osteosarcoma

Melanocytic tumours
Meningeal melanocytosis
Meningeal melanocytoma
Meningeal melanoma
Meningeal melanomatosis

Lymphomas
Diffuse large B-cell lymphoma of the CNS
Immunodeficiency-associated CNS lymphomas
    AIDS-related diffuse large B-cell lymphoma
    EBV-positive diffuse large B-cell lymphoma, NOS
    Lymphomatoid granulomatosis
Intravascular large B-cell lymphoma
Low-grade B-cell lymphomas of the CNS
T-cell and NK/T-cell lymphomas of the CNS
Anaplastic large cell lymphoma, ALK-positive
Anaplastic large cell lymphoma, ALK-negative
MALT lymphoma of the dura

Histiocytic tumours
Langerhans cell histiocytosis
Erdheim–Chester disease
Rosai–Dorfman disease
Juvenile xanthogranuloma
Histiocytic sarcoma

Germ cell tumours
Germinoma
Embryonal carcinoma
Yolk sac tumour
Choriocarcinoma
Teratoma
    Mature teratoma
    Immature teratoma
Teratoma with malignant transformation
Mixed germ cell tumour

Tumours of the sellar region
Craniopharyngioma
    Adamantinomatous craniopharyngioma
    Papillary craniopharyngioma
Granular cell tumour of the sellar region
Pituicytoma
Spindle cell oncocytoma

Table 18.2 The 2007 WHO classification of tumors of the central nervous system and of grade 1–4 (modified from [2])

Tumors of neuroepithelial tissue
Astrocytic tumors
Pilocytic astrocytoma 1
Pilomyxoid astrocytoma 2
Subependymal giant cell astrocytoma 1
Pleomorphic xanthoastrocytoma 2
Diffuse astrocytoma 2
Fibrillary astrocytoma
Gemistocytic astrocytoma
Protoplasmic astrocytoma
Anaplastic astrocytoma 3
Glioblastoma 4
Giant cell glioblastoma
Gliosarcoma
Gliomatosis cerebri
Oligodendroglial Tumors
Oligodendroglioma 2
Anaplastic oligodendroglioma 3
Oligoastrocytic tumors
Oligoastrocytoma 2
Anaplastic oligoastrocytoma 3
Ependymal tumors
Subependymoma 1
Myxopapillary ependymoma 1
Ependymoma 2
– Cellular
– Papillary
– Clear cell
– Tanycytic
Anaplastic ependymoma 3
Choroid plexus tumors
Choroid plexus papilloma 1
Atypical choroid plexus papilloma 2
Choroid plexus carcinoma 3
Other neuroepithelial tumors
Astroblastoma
Chordoid glioma of the third ventricle 2
Angiocentric glioma 1
Neuronal and mixed neuroglial tumors
Dysplastic gangliocytoma of cerebellum (Lhermitte-Duclos)
Desmoplastic infantile astrocytoma/ganglioglioma 1
Dysembryoplastic neuroepithelial tumor 1
Gangliocytoma 1
Ganglioglioma 1
Anaplastic ganglioglioma 3
Central neurocytoma 2
Extraventricular neurocytoma 2
Cerebellar liponeurocytoma 2
Papillary glioneuronal tumor 1

Table 18.2 (continued)

Tumors of neuroepithelial tissue
Rosette-forming glioneuronal tumor of the fourth ventricle 1
Paraganglioma
Tumors of the pineal region
Pineocytoma 1
Pineal parenchymal tumor of intermediate differentiation 2, 3
Pineoblastoma 4
Papillary tumor of the pineal Region 2, 3
Embryonal tumors
Medulloblastoma 4
– Desmoplastic/nodular medulloblastoma
– Medulloblastoma with extensive nodularity
– Anaplastic medulloblastoma
– Large cell medulloblastoma
CNS primitive neuroectodermal tumor 4
CNS Neuroblastoma
CNS Ganglioneuroblastoma
Medulloepithelioma
Ependymoblastoma
Atypical teratoid/rhabdoid tumor 4
Tumors of cranial and paraspinal nerves
Schwannoma (neurilemoma, neurinoma) 1
– Cellular
– Plexiform
– Melanotic
– Neurofibroma 1
– Plexiform
Perineurioma 1–3
Malignant perineurioma
Malignant peripheral nerve sheath tumor (MPNST) 2–4
– Epithelioid MPNST
– MPNST with mesenchymal differentiation
– Melanotic MPNST
– MPNST with glandular differentiation
Tumors of the meninges
Tumors of meningothelial cells
Meningioma
– Meningothelial 1
– Fibrous (fibroblastic) 1
– Transitional (mixed) 1
– Psammomatous 1
– Angiomatous 1
– Microcystic 1
– Secretory 1
– Lymphoplasmacyte-rich 1
– Metaplastic 1
– Chordoid 2
– Clear cell 2
– Atypical 2
– Papillary 3

18 Brain Neoplasm

Table 18.2 (continued)

Tumors of neuroepithelial tissue
– Rhabdoid 3
– Anaplastic (malignant) 3
Mesenchymal tumors
Lipoma
Angiolipoma
Hibernoma
Liposarcoma
Solitary fibrous tumor
Fibrosarcoma
Malignant fibrous histiocytoma
Leiomyoma
Leiomyosarcoma
Rhabdomyoma
Rhabdomyosarcoma
Chondroma
Chondrosarcoma
Osteoma
Osteosarcoma
Osteochondroma
Hemangioma
Epithelioid hemangioendothelioma
Hemangiopericytoma 2
Anaplastic hemangiopericytoma 3
Angiosarcoma
Kaposi sarcoma
Ewing sarcoma—PNET
Primary melanocytic lesions
Diffuse melanocytosis
Melanocytoma
Malignant melanoma
Meningeal melanomatosis
Other neoplasms related to the meninges
Hemangioblastoma 1
Lymphomas and hemopoietic neoplasms
Malignant lymphomas
Plasmacytoma
Granulocytic sarcoma
Germ cell tumors
Germinoma
Embryonal carcinoma
Yolk sac tumor
Choriocarcinoma
Teratoma
– Mature
– Immature
– Teratoma with malignant transformation
Mixed germ cell tumor
Tumors of the sellar region
Craniopharyngioma 1
– Adamantinomatous
– Papillary

Table 18.2 (continued)

Tumors of neuroepithelial tissue
Granular cell tumor 1
Pituicytoma 1
Spindle cell oncocytoma of the adenohypophysis 1
Metastatic tumors

The first reported genetic alterations which influence this revised classification is the discovery of 1p and 19q co-deletions in oligodendrogliomas. This was followed by the differentiation of tumors based on the gene mutations of isocitrate dehydrogenase 1 and 2 (IDH1 and IDH2). These genetic mutations were found exclusively in infiltrating gliomas (astrocytoma and oligodendrogliomas) but not in well-circumscribed gliomas. The presence of these mutations was noted to be significantly correlated with better prognosis of the gliomas. The classifier "Gliomatosis cerebri" has been discarded and replaced by the concept of multifocal infiltration by any subset of gliomas.

The second major revision is in the classification of histologically proven astrocytoma. All IDH1 and IDH2 mutant gliomas without 1p19q co-deletions are classified as astrocytoma. If ATRX and TP53 mutations are present in the presence of IDH mutant gliomas, the diagnosis of oligodendroglioma is again excluded. The terms oligoastrocytoma, anaplastic oligoastrocytoma, and glioblastoma with an oligodendroglial component are deleted. Pediatric patients presenting without 1DH mutations or 1p19q co-deletions are now categorized as diffuse or anaplastic astrocytomas, IDH wild type.

The third major revision is the classification of glioblastoma with and without IDH mutations. GBMs with IDH mutations (GBM, IDH mutant) is the term used for most glioblastomas which were classified as secondary GBMs and GBM without mutations (GBM wild type) is the term now given to primary GBMs. The term epithelioid glioblastoma is a newer variant listed in the revised classification. These tumors without INI1 or BRG1 mutations (associated with atypical teratoid/rhabdoid tumor (ATRT) often show BRAFV 600E mutations.

The fourth major revision is the inclusion of new entities described in light of their unique histopathological features and molecular markers. The most noteworthy of these lesions are the infiltrative high-grade astrocytomas which occur in the brainstem, spinal cord, or thalamus containing mutations at position K27M in the gene for Histone H3 (most of at the H3F3A or HIST1H3B/C locus) are a new entity and have been termed as diffuse midline gliomas. These tumors are classified as WHO grade 4 and are predominantly seen in the pediatric age group but can present in adults as well. It is reported that H3 K27M mutation was found in 15% of pediatric patients and 24% of adult patients with brain tumor of midline localization initially diagnosed as diffuse astrocytomas, oligodendrogliomas, pilocytic astrocytomas, subependymomas, ependymomas, and medulloblastomas [4].

The second new entity described in this revision is the diffuse leptomeningeal glioneuronal tumor (DLGNT) which is leptomeninges. These tumors are predominantly seen in children and are relatively rare [5]. They have not been designated a distinct WHO grade till date. These tumors are associated with chromosome 1p deletions and BRAF fusions. The third new entity, again of uncertain class assignment, is the multinodular and vacuolating neuronal tumor which are nearly always located in the subcortical white matter of the temporal lobe. The origin of these lesions is debatable; however, they contain characteristic vacuolated and dysplastic neurons. The lesions are well circumscribed and are thought to be benign hamartomatous lesions [6].

The fourth major revision is in the categorization of embryonal tumors. Medulloblastoma which are the quintessential lesion in this group of tumors has been be re-designated based on distinct molecular signatures [7]. The new transcriptome-based classification contains four entities: medulloblastoma WNT activated with somatic mutations of CTNNB1 encoding b-catenin with WNT signaling; medulloblastoma SHH (sonic hedgehog) activated with and without TP53 mutations; medulloblastoma non-WNT, non-SHH group 3; and medulloblastoma non-WNT, non-SHH group 4. All medulloblastomas are now classified as WHO grade 4 tumors regardless of their histology/genetics. In addition, embryonal tumors also encompass atypical teratoid tumors, and embryonal tumor with multilayered rosettes (C19MC altered), apart from medulloepitheliomas, neuroblastomas, ganglioneuroblastoma, and embryonal tumors not otherwise specified which do not have genetic markers.

18.2 Tumors of Neuroepithelial Tissue

The WHO revised its classification of CNS tumors in 2016 and presented a more nuanced approach to the diagnosis of neuroepithelial tumors. This layered approach comprises 4 elements: molecular information, WHO grade, histological classification, and a final integrated diagnosis [9]. The current classification strategy rest on specific genetic markers, the primary being presence or absence of isocitrate dehydrogenase (IDH) mutation status which is an integral part of the citric acid cycle. Two homodimers IDH1 and IDH2 are identifiable. Isocitrate is converted to alpha-ketoglutarate in the presence of IDH. D 2-hydroxyglutarate (2HG) is the product of conversion of alpha ketoglutarate by mutated IDH. 2HG can be detected by advanced MRS technique and acts as a surrogate imaging biomarker to detect the presence of IDH (Fig. 18.1). The cascade of differentiation of glial progenitor cells into various tumor pathways is as follows (Fig. 18.2) [8].

All IDH mutated tumors with 1p19q codeletions with class defining loss of function mutations of ATRX and TP53 will result in diffuse astrocytomas which are generally classified as WHO grade II with further de-differentiation to WHO grade III (anaplastic astrocytomas) and WHO grade IV (secondary GBM). These tumors with IDH mutation and 1p19q deletions with intact ATRX are categorized as oligodendrogliomas WHO grade II and may undergo dedifferentiation to Grade III anaplastic oligodendrogliomas.

18 Brain Neoplasm

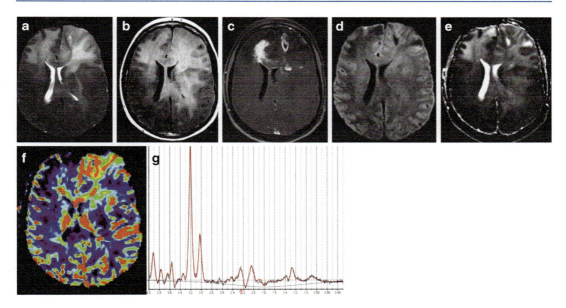

Fig. 18.1 (**a–g**) Anaplastic astrocytoma WHO grade III (IDH1-mutant, 1p/19q-intact) in a 25-year-old female with Lynch syndrome (MSH6 mutation). (**a**) Fat-saturated T2-weighted image and (**b**) FLAIR show hyperintensity in the bilateral frontal lobes and anterior corpus callosum. (**c**) Gadolinium-enhanced T1-weighted image shows areas of necrosis in the lesion. (**d**) DWI and e ADC show no diffusion restriction. (**f**) DSC-perfusion shows decreased perfusion rCBV in the right frontal lobe and increased perfusion in the left frontal lobe. (**g**) MR-spectroscopy with TE = 97 msec shows a small peak of 2-hydroxyglutarate (2HG) at 2.25 ppm, indicating IDH mutation. Estimated amount by LC-model is 1.36 mM (%SD 13%)

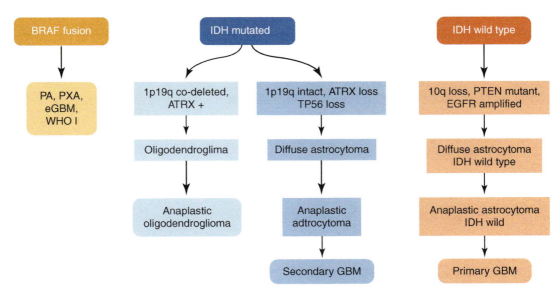

Fig. 18.2 The cascade of differentiation of glial progenitor cells into various tumor pathways modified from reference [8]

IDH wild-type tumors with EGR amplification, 10q loss and PTEN mutations are classified as diffuse astrocytoma (IDH wild type) and may further progress to their grade III (anaplastic astrocytoma IDH wild type) and grade IV (GBM) successors as shown in the flow chart above.

Additionally, infiltrative lesions which occur in the midline within the brainstem, thalami, and spinal cord which lack the IDH mutation but contain mutations in histone H3 gene are categorized as midline gliomas and occur usually in the pediatric age group.

Representative tumors which are grade I include pilocytic astrocytomas and subependymal giant cell astrocytomas. All infiltrative astrocytomas are at least Grade II and are defined by cellular atypia alone. Grade III tumors show a degree of anaplasia and mitotic figures. These two feature together with microvascular proliferation and/or necrosis are classified as grade IV. Ki67 proliferative index is often used as measure to differentiate and referee the grade in case of ambivalence on histopathological examination.

Gliomas are classified as tumors of neuroepithelial tissue, including localized astrocytomas, diffuse astrocytic and oligodendroglial tumors, ependymal tumors, and other gliomas. The signal intensity of gliomas on DW images is variable and depends mainly on their T2 and apparent diffusion coefficient (ADC) values [10–31]. Some gliomas are hyperintense on DW images with decreased ADC, which generally reflects high tumor cellularity and reduced volume of the extracellular space. Other gliomas have normal or increased ADC, and if the DW signal is high, it is due to a T2 shine-through effect. However, calculation of the ADC values is more important and more specific for the diagnosis of the brain tumor. High ADC values of low-grade gliomas reflect relatively lower cellularity, a lower nuclear-to-cytoplasm ratio, but also reflect abundant tumor-cell-associated extracellular matrix that includes glycosaminoglycans and fibrous proteins (collagen, elastin, fibronectin, laminin), myxoid degenerative changes, and microcystic changes [32] (Fig. 18.3).

18.2.1 Localized Astrocytomas (Other Astrocytomas)

Pilocytic astrocytomas (Fig. 18.4) and subependymal giant cell astrocytomas appear as well-

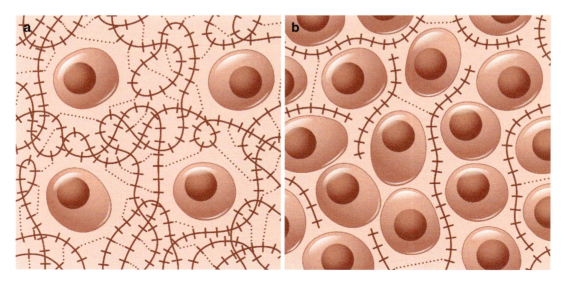

Fig. 18.3 (**a**, **b**) Diffusion of water movement in tumors reflects its (1) cellularity and (2) extracellular matrix composition. (**a**) Low-grade tumor: low cellularity and high hydrophilic extracellular materials (jagged lines). (**b**) High-grade tumor: high cellularity and low hydrophilic extracellular materials (jagged lines)

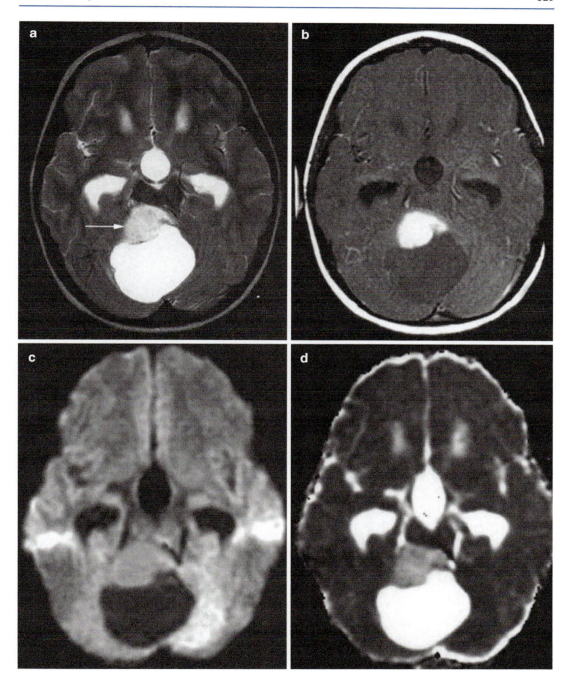

Fig. 18.4 (**a–e**) Juvenile pilocytic astrocytoma in a 10-year-old boy. (**a**) T2-weighted image shows a hyperintense cystic mass in the cerebellum and hydrocephalus. There is a mural nodule (*arrow*) in the tumor. (**b**) Gadolinium-enhanced T1-weighted image shows enhancement in the nodule. (**c**) DW image shows hypointensity in the cystic component and isointensity in the nodule. (**d**) ADC map shows hyperintensity in the cystic component and hyperintensity in the nodule (1.41–1.67 × 10^{-3} mm^2/s) of the mass. (**e**) A high choline/NAA ratio and lactate peak are observed despite the benign histology of this tumor

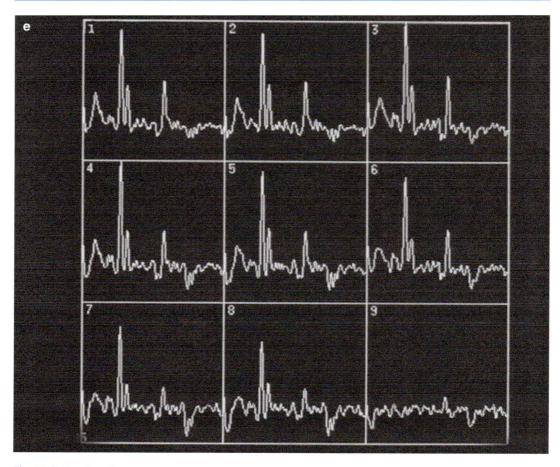

Fig. 18.4 (continued)

defined lesions without infiltrative margins. The pilocytic astrocytoma often occurs as a cystic lesion with an eccentric peripheral nodule in the posterior fossa. Subependymal giant cell tumors are seen as a syndromic constituent of tuberous sclerosis and as the name implies are almost exclusively located in the lateral ventricles in the vicinity of the foramen of Monro. Pilomyxoid astrocytoma is a recently described entity which is a variant of pilocytic astrocytoma. It appears as solid-appearing mass most commonly in the suprasellar region with contiguous involvement of the hypothalamus and medial portions of the temporal lobe. These are bulky masses which often contain areas of hemorrhage and disseminate cross CSF pathways. The ADC values in pilocytic and pilomyxoid astrocytomas are often higher than 1.4 or 1.5×10^{-3} mm^2/s (Figs. 18.4 and 18.5) [33, 34] which reflect abundant extracellular myxoid matrix and microcystic changes. This finding is useful in the differential diagnosis because MR spectroscopy can show a high choline/NAA and lactate peak despite the benign histology of pilocytic astrocytomas [35]. Pleomorphic xanthoastrocytoma (Fig. 18.6) are well-defined cortical partially cystic lesions frequently presenting as seizures. DWI shows hyperintense with relatively low ADC values (0.70–0.94×10^{-3} mm^2/s) reflecting intermediate hypercellularity.

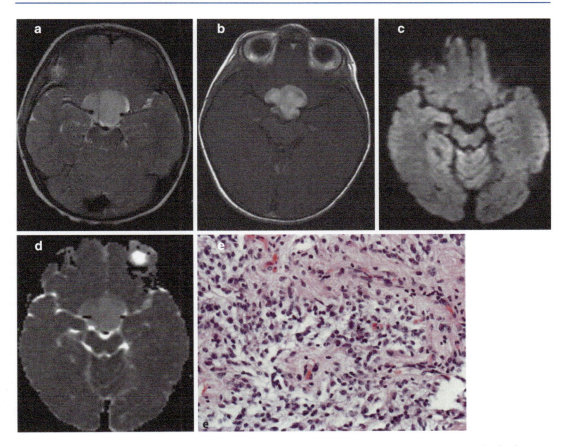

Fig. 18.5 (a–e) Hypothalamic pilocytic astrocytoma in a 5-year-old boy with headache. (**a**) T2-weighted image shows a hyperintense mass in the hypothalamus. (**b**) Gadolinium-enhanced T1-weighted image shows enhancement in the mass. (**c**) DW image shows isointensity. (**d**) ADC map shows hyperintensity in the mass (1.53×10^{-3} mm^2/s). (**e**) Pathology shows intermediate cellularity and abundant extracellular matrix (Rosenthal fibers and microcystic changes)

18.2.2 Diffuse Astrocytic and Oligodendroglial Tumors

On conventional MR sequences most infiltrative gliomas are hypointense on T1-weighted images with ill-defined margins and hyperintense on T2 and FLAIR sequences. Presence of hemorrhage will result in shortening of T1 relaxation times resulting in hyperintense signals, which in turn will appear hypointense on SWI and T2* sequences. Enhancement in lower-grade lesions is absent. In higher-grade lesions patchy enhancement is present. Enhancement, Frankly aggressive GBMs appear as solitary rim-enhanced masses with hypointense cores and heterogeneous hyperintense signals on the T2 and FLAIR sequence. Hemorrhage is sine qua non in GBMs and a feature which invariably prompts caution. Conventional scans have proven to be of limited use in predicting the grade of infiltrative gliomas [36, 37].

The basic premise of using diffusion techniques is based on ADC which are a measure of the combination of both cellularity and extracellular matrix on conventional DWI sequences. Low-grade astrocytomas and oligodendrogliomas have a high concentration of glycosaminoglycans, which is highly hydrophilic causing

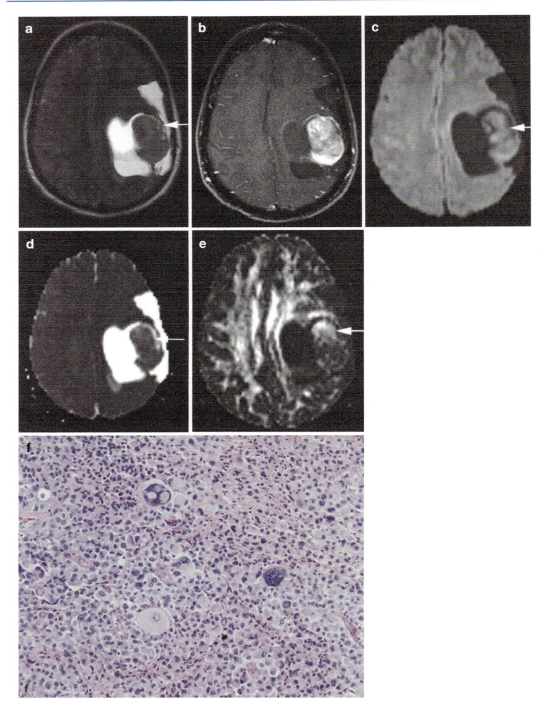

Fig. 18.6 (**a–f**) Pleomorphic xanthoastrocytoma in a 36-year-old woman. (**a**) T2-weighted image shows a hypointense solid mass (*arrow*) with surrounding cystic components in the left frontoparietal region. (**b**) Gadolinium-enhanced T1-weighted image with fat saturation shows intense enhancement in the solid component. (**c**) DW image shows slight hyperintensity in the solid mass (arrow) and hypointensity in the cystic components. (**d**) ADC map shows isointensity in the solid component ($0.70–0.94 \times 10^{-3}$ mm^2/s). (**e**) FA is partially increased in the solid component (arrow). (**f**) Pathology shows cellular pleomorphism and hypercellularity

the shift of water molecules in the extracellular matrix [32]. Significant differences have been reported between the ADC values of low- and high-grade gliomas [17, 21]. The solid components of low-grade astrocytomas (Figs. 18.3, 18.4, 18.5, and 18.7) and oligodendrogliomas (Figs. 18.8 and 18.9) generally show slightly low, iso-, or slightly high signal intensity on DW images associated with increased ADC.

The measurements of fractional anisotropy and diffusivity on diffusion tensor imaging (DTI) sequences are indicative of the integrity of the white matter tracts [33]. The periphery of low-grade gliomas contains preserved white matter fiber tracts, while these fiber tracts are disarranged and displaced in high-grade gliomas [39] (Figs. 18.9, 18.10, and 18.11).

The application of diffusion techniques can be divided into the following categories:

1. Grading gliomas and prediction of histology and identifying molecular fingerprint.
2. Treatment planning and assessment of treatment response.

The compactness and higher cellular density with higher grades of gliomas have been linked to increase in restricted diffusion, which are in turn linked with lower ADC values [21, 40]. However, given the presence of necrosis and hemorrhage in tumors such as GBMs this feature may not be specific to predict a higher grade [41]. As a corollary

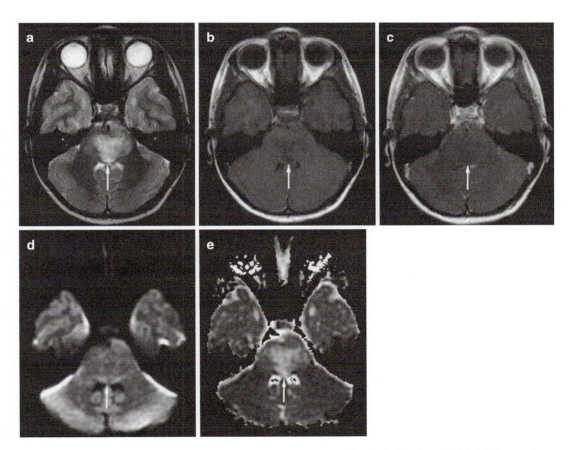

Fig. 18.7 (a–e) Brainstem glioma in an 8-year-old girl with headache. (a) T2-weighted image shows a hyperintense lesion (*arrow*) with surrounding edema in pons. (b) T1-weighted image shows the hypointense lesion (*arrow*), (c) gadolinium-enhanced T1-weighted image shows no significant enhancement. (d) DW image shows isointensity in the lesion (*arrow*). (e) ADC map shows hyperintensity in the lesion (0.85–1.17 × 10^{-3} mm^2/s; *arrow*). The isointensity on the DW image is caused by a balance between increased T2 and ADC. This case is an old case suggesting histologically low grade. H3K27M is not examined

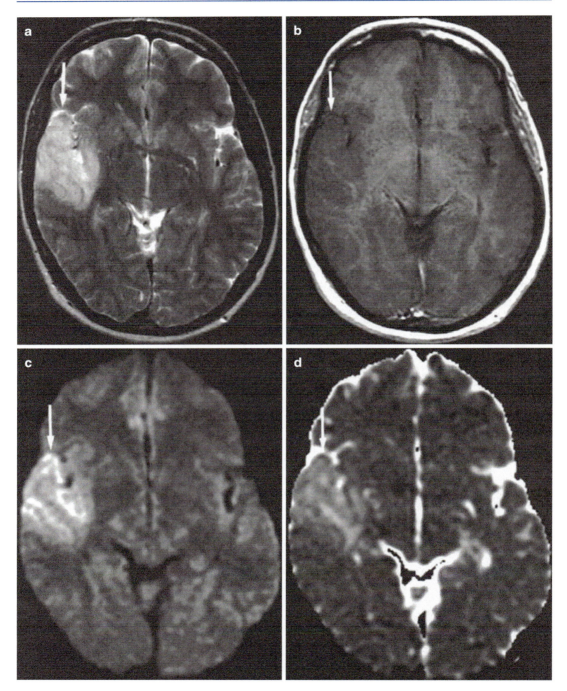

Fig. 18.8 (**a–d**) Low-grade oligoastrocytoma in a 48-year-old woman with seizures. (**a**) T2-weighted image shows a hyperintense lesion in the right temporal lobe (*arrow*). (**b**) Gadolinium-enhanced T1-weighted image shows a slightly hypointense lesion and no enhancement (*arrow*). (**c**) DW image shows hyperintensity (*arrow*). (**d**) ADC map shows hyperintensity in the lesion (0.98–1.19 × 10^{-3} mm^2/s; *arrow*)

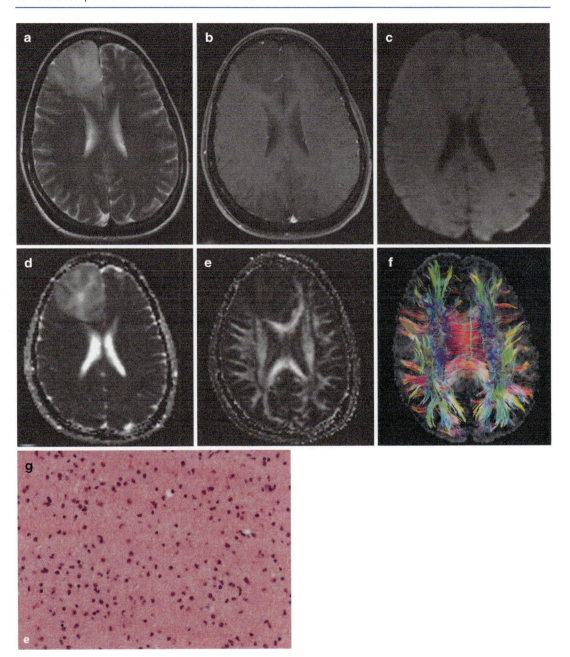

Fig. 18.9 (**a–g**) Low-grade oligodendroglioma in a 40-year-old woman. (**a**) T2-weighted image shows a hyperintense mass lesion in the right frontal lobe. (**b**) Gadolinium-enhanced T1-weighted image with fat saturation shows a slight hypointense lesion and no enhancement. (**c**) DW image shows iso- and slight hypointensity. (**d**) ADC map shows hyperintensity in the lesion (0.82–1.53 × 10^{-3} mm^2/s). (**e**) Pathology shows low cellularity and fibrillary background. (**f**) FA map shows decreased anisotropy in the right frontal mass but white matter structure is identified in the mass. (**g**) White matter fiber tracts in the tumor are relatively preserved on the DT fiber tractography (Courtesy of Jinsuh Kim MD, The University of Iowa Hospitals and Clinics, USA)

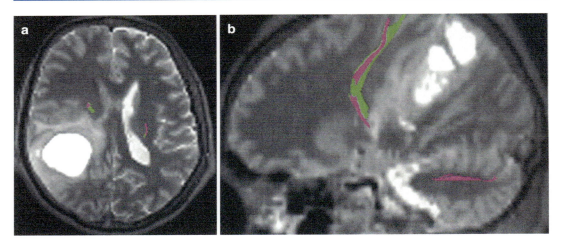

Fig. 18.10 (**a, b**) Glioblastoma in a 58-year-old woman. (**a, b**) Diffusion tensor fiber tractography shows the displacement of the corticospinal tract (motor; *red*) and the corticothalamic tract (sensory; *green*) (Courtesy of Yamada K MD, Kyoto Prefectural University of Medicine, Japan)

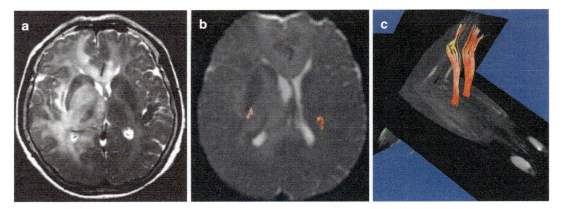

Fig. 18.11 (**a–c**) Gliomatosis cerebri in a 73-year-old woman. (**a**) T2-weighted image shows extensive, asymmetric white matter hyperintensity bilaterally. (**b, c**) Diffusion tensor fiber tractography shows only minimal shift of the pyramidal tracts. (Courtesy of Aoki S MD, University of Tokyo, Japan) (From [38]). In the WHO 2016 classification, "Gliomatosis cerebri" has been discarded and replaced by the concept of multifocal infiltration by any subset of gliomas

areas of restricted diffusion in an otherwise heterogeneous appearing tumor may indicate the presence of an aggressive higher-grade component within a lesion. Diffusion sequences alone may be sufficient to build a preoperative profile of a tumor, but combine with other advanced techniques such as perfusion imaging and MRS holds great promise in the detection and management of higher-grade gliomas [28, 42]. In the prediction of the molecular fingerprint of a given lesion the focus has been on detection of 2HG peaks as a surrogate marker on MRS for 1p19q deletions. This cannot be convincingly demonstrated by diffusion techniques, however, in a narrowly defined attempt to define the MGMT promoter status in GBM. ADC histogram analyzes by performing a 2-Gaussian curve fit of the histogram data from the enhancing component of GBM. This technique showed that the low median ADC was linked to MGMT status which predicted better outcomes [43, 44]. This was not replicated on subsequent studies based on overall median ADC values [45].

18.2.3 High-Grade Gliomas

High-grade gliomas include anaplastic glioma (anaplastic astrocytoma, oligodendroglioma, oligoastrocytoma and ependymoma) and glioblastoma (GBM) (Figs. 18.6, 18.10, 18.11, 18.12, 18.13, 18.14, 18.15, 18.17 and 18.18). It has been reported that high-grade gliomas typically are hyperintense on DW images with decreased ADC [12, 17–19, 21, 22, 28]. High tumor cellularity is probably the major determinant of the decreased ADC values in high-grade brain tumors [12, 17, 21, 27]. Other studies have suggested that ADC correlates not only with tumor cellularity, but also with total nuclear area and tumor grade [17, 21, 22, 26, 28], with high-grade tumors having high cellular density and decreased ADC. Other studies have correlated areas of decreased ADC and found it to be associated with increased choline on MR spectroscopy. Choline is a marker for cell membrane turnover [16, 18]. Minimal ADC values in high-grade astrocytomas are negatively correlated with the Ki-67 labeling index and related to posttreatment prognosis [46]. FA may be better than ADC for assessment and delineation of the different degrees of pathologic changes in gliomas [47].

Although there is a general principle of high-grade gliomas having high DW signal with decreased ADC, there are still controversies regarding how well DWI can differentiate between high-grade primary brain tumors, lymphoma, and metastasis. Krabbe et al. reported that both the contrast-enhancing portions and the peritumoral edema of metastasis have higher ADC than high-grade gliomas [15]. In the individual case the distinction between metastasis and high-grade glioma is often difficult to make, as some high-grade gliomas also have high ADC [27, 48]. For lymphomas, Guo et al. reported that ADC was generally lower than in high-grade gliomas. This could be useful to differentiate the two [25], but in the clinical situation there is often overlap between lymphoma and high-grade glioma. In our experience, the ADC of lymphoma ranges between 0.51 and 0.71 $\times$ 10^{-3} mm^2/s, whereas that of high-grade gliomas ranges between 0.58 and 0.89 $\times$ 10^{-3} mm^2/s. Lymphomas tend to have lower ADC values because of a higher nuclear-to-cytoplasmic ratio [25]. The FA and ADC values of primary cerebral lymphoma are significantly lower than those of GBM [49] These are general principles, but in practical clinical work it is sometimes difficult to distinguish between lymphomas, metastasis, and high-grade gliomas, even with the most sophisticated ADC maps [13, 19–22, 27].

Glioblastoma (GBM) is the most common primary brain tumor in adults. Despite advances in microneurosurgery, radiation therapy, chemotherapy, and advances in imaging, only 10% of patients will survive 3 years following diagnosis [50]. Recent molecular and genetic approaches have provided dramatic insights into glioma biology, including genetic alterations in tumorigenesis and molecular mechanisms of angiogenesis.

Solid components of GBM are typically hyperintense on DW images with slightly decreased or slightly increased ADC (Figs. 18.12, 18.13, 18.14, 18.15, 18.16, and 18.17). Cystic necrotic components of GBM are usually hypointense on DW images with increased ADC (Fig. 18.14). One of the important differential diagnoses is brain abscess in which cystic components are usually hyperintense on DW images with decreased ADC. Background vasogenic edema and micronecrosis affect the DW imaging signal intensity and ADC values. Decreased ADC can be observed in the cystic component or non-enhancing portion of GBM. The causes of the decreased ADC are: (1) tumor cell infiltration with hypercellularity (Figs. 18.12 and 18.13), (2) tumoral hemorrhage, (3) coagulative necrosis resulting from tumoral ischemia (Fig. 18.14), (4) cytotoxic edema due to glutamate excitotoxicity released by infiltrating GBM cells (Figs. 18.15, 18.17, and 18.18), and (5) neutrophil infiltration due to immune-mediated reaction to GBM and tumor necrosis (Fig. 18.19) [51, 52].

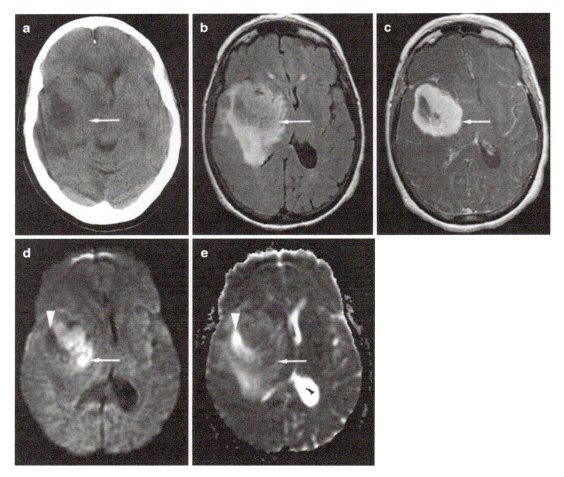

Fig. 18.12 (**a–e**) Glioblastoma in a 69-year-old woman with left-side weakness. (**a**) unenhanced CT image shows a heterogeneous iso- to hypodense lesion in the right temporal lobe (*arrow*). (**b**) Fluid-attenuated inversion-recovery image shows the heterogeneous hyperintense lesion in the right temporal lobe (*arrow*). (**c**) Gadolinium-enhanced T1-weighted image shows heterogeneous enhancement in the mass (*arrow*). (**d**) DW image shows hyperintensity in the enhancing portion of the mass (*arrow*) and hypointensity in the cystic/necrotic portion of the mass (*arrowhead*). (**e**) ADC map shows heterogeneous hypointensity ($0.74–0.85 \times 10^{-3}$ mm^2/s; *arrow*) in the enhancing portion of the mass compared to the surrounding vasogenic edema. Cystic/necrotic portion of the mass (*arrowhead*) is hyperintense. These findings may correspond to the high cellularity of the enhancing tumor and increased diffusivity of the cystic/necrotic portion

18.2.4 Peritumoral Infiltration

The value of DWI for the delineation of peritumoral invasion in primary brain tumors is controversial. Some authors have suggested that ADC is useful to determine the extent of tumor invasion [12, 28], but most of the recent studies have shown that it is not possible to determine accurately the degree of peritumoral infiltration by DWI and ADC mapping [13, 19–21, 27, 28]. The poor delineation is probably due to the conjoined effects of T2 and ADC on DW images. For tumors that are biologically different, such as glioblastomas and meningiomas, it has been reported that ADC, T1, and fractional anisotropy of the enhancing tumor and its peritumoral edema are markedly different [24]. In GBM, tumor cells produce proteases and infiltrate into

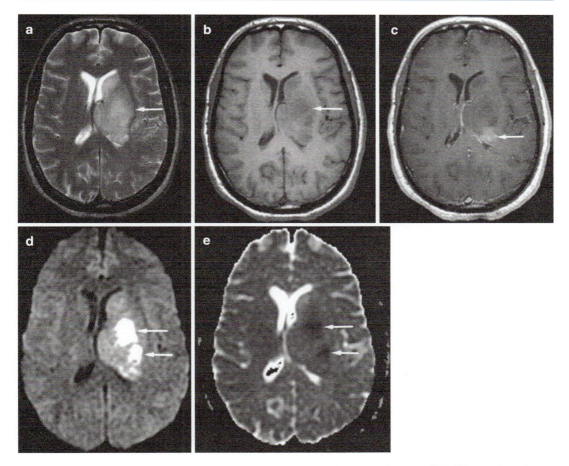

Fig. 18.13 (a–e) Glioblastoma in a 51-year-old woman with right-side weakness. (a) T2-weighted image shows a hyperintense mass in the left basal ganglia and thalamus (*arrow*). (b) T1-weighted image shows hypointensity in the lesion (*arrow*). (c) Gadolinium-enhanced T1-weighted image shows heterogeneous enhancement in the posterior portion of the tumor (*arrow*). (d) DW image shows hyperintensities (*arrows*). The areas of marked hyperintensity on the DW image does not show contrast enhancement in this patient. (e) ADC map shows heterogeneous hypointensity in the lesion (0.58–0.89 × 10^{-3} mm^2/s; *arrows*)

the extracellular space in the white matter. Tumor cells produce vascular endothelial growth factor (VEGF) resulting in increased vascular permeability and vasogenic edema. Tumor cells also release glutamate resulting in surrounding neurotoxicity that facilitates infiltration by the tumor cells. This may cause cytotoxic edema in peritumoral areas and in white matter infiltrations (Figs. 18.17 and 18.18).

DTI may distinguish presumed tumor-infiltrated edema from purely vasogenic edema [47, 53, 54]. However, reliable differentiation between infiltration and vasogenic edema is not yet possible on the basis of DTI [55]. The narrow rim of increased FA and decreased ADC observed at the edge of GBM is caused by compressed white matter fibers or peripheral cellular infiltration and associated cytotoxic edema [53, 55]. FA values in peritumoral normal-appearing white matter are higher in meningiomas than in gliomas [53]. The axiomatic concept is that tumor extension in the white matter tracts beyond the margins of the tumor and the surrounding vasogenic edema as not defined on conventional MRI sequences. This is especially

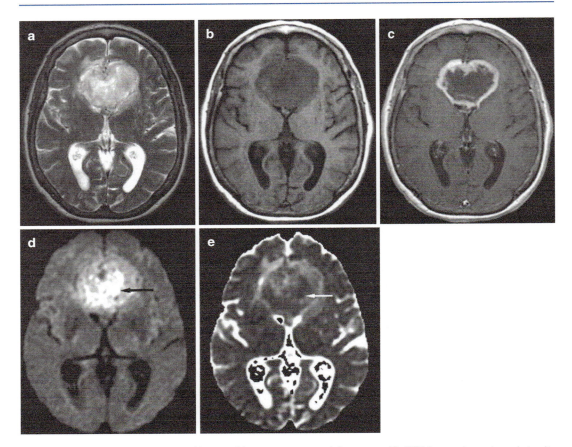

Fig. 18.14 (a–e) Glioblastoma in an 80-year-old woman with personality changes. (a) T2-weighted image shows a hyperintense mass, which involves the genu of corpus callosum (butterfly tumor). (b) T1-weighted image shows hypointensity in the lesion. (c) Gadolinium-enhanced T1-weighted image shows irregular ring-like enhancement of the tumor. (d) DW image shows hyperintensity (*arrow*). (e) ADC map shows heterogeneous intensity in the mass. Note the hypointensity in the center of the lesion (0.65×10^{-3} mm^2/s; *arrow*). These findings may correspond to the cellularity of the tumor

so when combined with parameters derived from perfusion and spectroscopy [56]. In the referenced study which showed three multimodal patterns to indicate presence of tumor which included a combination of lower ADC, abnormal Cho/NAA ratio and higher rCBV in the solid-appearing "tumor" portion of the lesion, higher ADC, normal Cho/NAA ratio and lower CBV in the "edema" portion of the lesion and intermediate ADC, abnormal Cho/NAA ratio and rCBV in the tumor/edema portion of the lesion.

Another important tool of functional MRI is, with assistance with DTI based tractography, one can facilitate an accurate surgical approach to plan resection of a lesion. This can reduce operative time by delineating eloquent areas and minimizing adverse patient outcomes. Tumor cells invade and change white matter fiber structures by widening, displacing, and disrupting the fiber bundles [57, 58] (Figs. 18.10). Fiber tractography can be useful for preoperative planning and intraoperative image-guided surgery [59, 60].

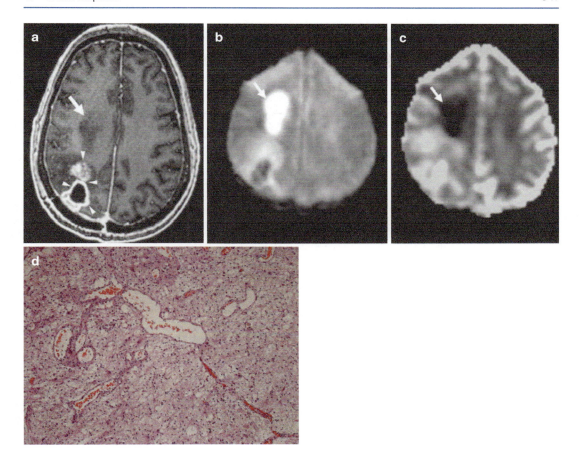

Fig. 18.15 (**a–d**) Glioblastoma in a 65-year-old man. (**a**) Gadolinium-enhanced T1-weighted image shows a necrotic enhancing mass in the right parietal area (*arrowhead*) and non-enhancing lesion in the right frontal area (*arrow*). (**b**) DW image shows strong hyperintensity in the non-enhancing lesion (*arrow*). (**c**) ADC map shows strong hypointensity in this lesion (0.34×10^{-3} mm^2/s). This finding is rare but may represent cytotoxic edema associated with tumor invasion in the white matter. A 3-month follow-up MR image revealed an enhancing tumor in this area (not shown). (**d**) Pathology (another case) shows cytotoxic edema associated with tumor cell infiltration

18.2.5 Gliomatosis Cerebri

Despite its initial recognition in 1938, gliomatosis cerebri remains a controversial entity with little consensus in its definition, histology, or treatment [61]. In the WHO 2007 (Table 18.2) define gliomatosis cerebri as a diffuse glioma growth pattern, infiltrating at least three lobes. However, in the WHO 2016 classification, "Gliomatosis cerebri" has been discarded as a distinct pathological entity, and replaced by the concept of multifocal infiltration by any subset of gliomas (Table 18.1). Although no longer considered a distinct pathologic entity, GC represents a disease with a unique phenotype. Despite aggressive treatment, patients have a uniformly poor outcome with 26–52% surviving less than a year from symptom onset [61]. Pathologically, myelin sheaths are destroyed but axons and neurons are relatively preserved. If GBM occurs in gliomato-

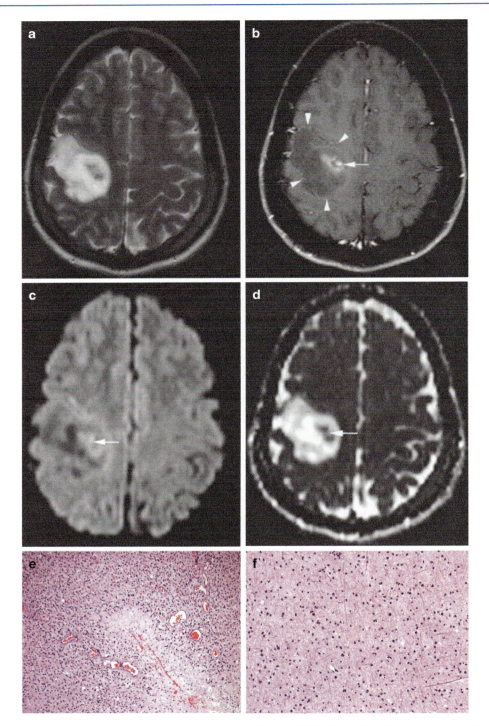

Fig. 18.16 (a–f) Glioblastoma secondary to anaplastic astrocytoma in a 37-year-old man. (**a**) T2-weighted image shows a hyperintense mass in the right frontal lobe. (**b**) Gadolinium-enhanced T1-weighted image with fat saturation shows a necrotic enhancing lesion (*arrow*) within a non-enhancing mass (*arrowheads*). (**c**) DW image shows mild hyperintensity in the enhancing lesion (*arrow*). (**d**) The enhancing lesion has a lower ADC (0.97×10^{-3} mm^2/s) than the surrounding non-enhancing mass (1.20×10^{-3} mm^2/s) (*arrow*). (**e**) Pathology of the enhancing lesion shows hypercellularity, pleomorphism, endothelial proliferation, and necrosis consistent with glioblastoma multiforme, (**f**) pathology of surrounding non-enhancing mass shows intermediate cellularity and pleomorphism consistent with anaplastic astrocytoma

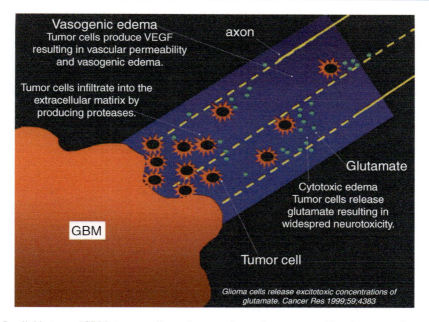

Fig. 18.17 In glioblastoma (*GBM*), tumor cells produce proteases and infiltrate into the extracellular space in the white matter. Tumor cells produce vascular endothelial growth factor (*VEGF*) resulting in increased vascular permeability and in vasogenic edema. Tumor cells also release glutamate resulting in surrounding neurotoxicity that facilitates infiltration of the tumor cells. This may cause the cytotoxic edema in peritumoral areas and rarely in the white matter tumor infiltration

sis cerebri, it can present as multiple enhancing mass lesions (Fig. 18.20). It is often difficult to differentiate multicentric GBMs from multifocal GBMs associated with gliomatosis cerebri based on MR imaging [62]. Diffusion tensor fiber tractography shows the fiber tracking passing through the tumor (Fig. 18.11) [38].

18.2.6 Pseudoprogression and Pseudoresponse

DW imaging has been attempted to follow response to treatment and disease progress. For example, animal studies have shown a tendency to an increase in ADC during treatment, followed by a return to the pretreatment level during recurrent tumor growth [29–31]. DWI and microvascular characteristics early in the course of radiotherapy can be used to generate parametric response map which can predict progression or pseudoprogression [63, 64] (Fig. 18.20). "Pseudoprogression" is a term that is used to describe the imaging feature on MRI studies when chemoradiation results in abnormal contrast uptake and enlargement of the residual tumor mass. Pseudoprogression is an important condition to recognize because it is managed differently than the primary glioma. This led to the change in the response evaluation criteria: Response evaluation in Neuro Oncology (RANO) criteria with a recommendation "not to enroll patients relapsing within 3 months from the end of radiotherapy trials on recurrent glioblastoma, unless the recurrence is histologically proven or progressive abnormalities lie outside the radiation field" [65].

ADC values have been the mainstay in the evaluation and prediction of pseudoprogression with trends to indicate greater sensitivity than specificity [65]. Pooled specificity and sensitivity of ADC maps in detection of pseudoprogression range from 78–87% and 71–82%, respectively [66–68]. A combination of MRI perfusion and diffusion studies is reported to be marginally accurate but does not necessarily appear to be "superior." Dynamic susceptibility contrast (DSC)

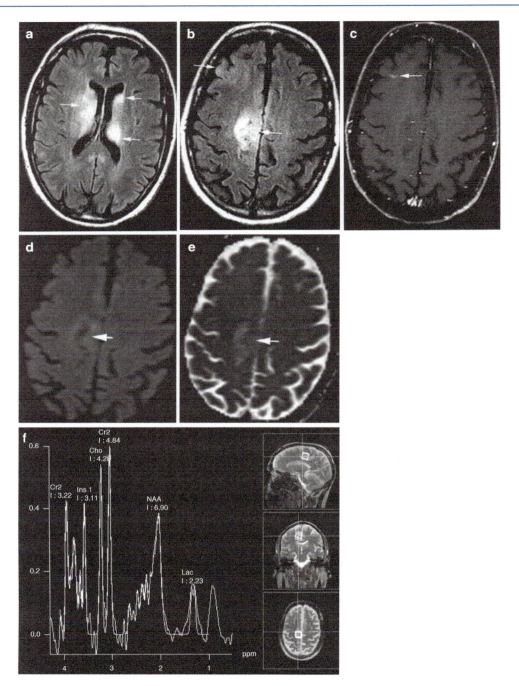

Fig. 18.18 (a–j) Glioblastoma secondary to diffuse infiltrating astrocytoma (gliomatosis cerebri) in a 70-year-old man with seizures. (**a, b**) FLAIR imaging shows multiple hyperintense lesions in the bilateral basal ganglia and right frontal lobe (*arrows*). (**c**) Gadolinium-enhanced T1-weighted image with fat saturation shows minimal enhancement in the frontal lesion (*arrow*). (**d, e**) DW images show mild hyperintensity and increased ADC (*arrow*), (**f**) MR spectroscopy shows a high lactate peak but no high choline peak (Courtesy of Kim J MD, The University of Iowa Hospitals and Clinics, USA). (**g**) One-month follow-up MR image shows multiple enhancing masses in the right frontal area. (**h, i**) DW imaging shows peripheral and peritumoral hyperintensity associated with decreased ADC (*arrowheads*). (**j**) MR spectroscopy shows not only a high lactate peak but also high choline and glutamate/glutamine peaks (*arrow*)

18 Brain Neoplasm

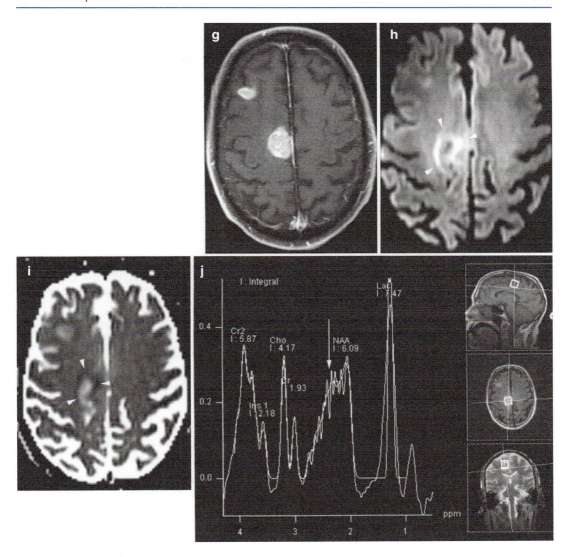

Fig. 18.18 (continued)

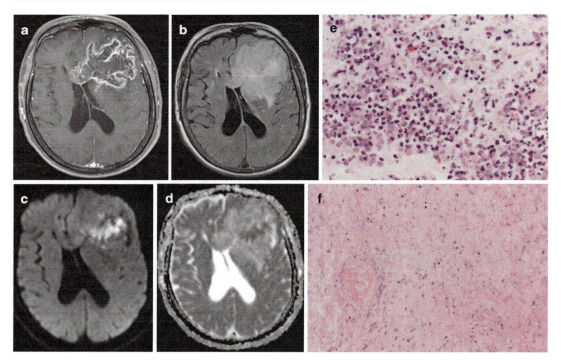

Fig. 18.19 (**a–f**) Glioblastoma with numerous polymorphonuclear leukocytes (PMNs) infiltration in a 76-year-old female. He complained of confusion, memory loss, and personality changes. (**a**) FLAIR shows a hyperintense lesion with mass effect in the left frontal lobe. (**b**) Gadolinium-enhanced T1-weighted image shows peripheral enhancement. (**c**) DWI and (**d**) ADC show central areas of diffusion restriction. (**e**) HE stain in the diffusion restriction shows necrosis with PMNs likely immune-mediated reactive changes to GBM and tumor necrosis. (**f**) HE stain in less diffusion restricted area shows necrosis with thrombosed vessels

MR-perfusion is becoming a standard of care for the monitoring of glioblastoma. The pooled sensitivity and specificity are 89% and 88%, if use "corrected rBV" (uncorrected, rBV specificity 41%) [69, 70]. For dynamic contrast-enhanced (DCE) perfusion, the pooled sensitivity was 89% and the specificity was 85%. It is pertinent to note that mean ADC values may not be accurate in determining if there is indeed recurrence or residual tumor because of coexisting treatment-related necrosis, presence of cytotoxic edema, and liquefaction of the treated tumor/brain [71]. Voxelwise mapping may define focal areas of developing changes in evolving pseudoprogression but is labor intensive and requires technical finesse [65, 72, 73]. The application of DTI is promising but not widely used [74]. Multiband imaging is a technique which uses multiple b values to acquire images in quick succession and holds some promise with advanced processing techniques such as neurite orientation and dispersion imaging (NODDI) [75]. An additional technique is intravoxel incoherent motion (IVIM) which has features of both diffusion and perfusion imaging but is largely experimental [76].

On the other hand, the term "pseudoresponse" refers to the phenomenon in which a tumor appears to be responding to a particular treatment on imaging, but in fact the lesion remains stable or has progressed. Pseudoresponse is known to occur following administration of angiogenesis inhibitor such as monoclonal antibody against vascular endothelial growth factor (VEGF) (bevacizumab) or VEGF receptor inhibitor (cediranib). After initial treatment with bevacizumab, areas of contrast enhancement and T2 hyperintensity can be rapidly decreased due to reduced BBB permeability independent of real tumor response, while DWI often shows local hyperintensity with reduced ADC values, reflect-

18 Brain Neoplasm

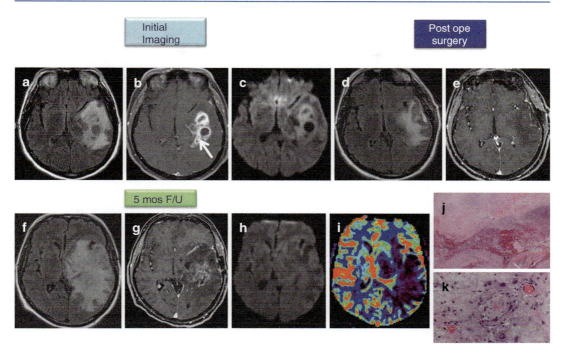

Fig. 18.20 (**a–h**) Pseudoprogression after postoperative chemoradiation for GBM in a 64-year-old male. (**a**) Preoperative FLAIR shows a hyperintense lesion in the left temporal lobe. (**b**) Gadolinium-enhanced T1-weighted image shows areas of ring-like enhancement with a cystic component (*arrow*) in the lesion. (**c**) DWI shows hyperintensity corresponding to the enhancement. (**d**) Postoperative FLAIR and (**e**) Gadolinium-enhanced T1-weighted image show decreased FLAIR hyperintensity in the left temporal lobe and no enhancement around the surgical cavity. Five months after postoperative chemoradiation (temozolomide), (**f**) FLAIR and (**g**) gadolinium-enhanced T1-weighted image show increased FLAIR hyperintensity with mass effect and dot and curvilinear enhancement with surrounding hypointensity. (**h**) DWI shows no hyperintensity with associated increased ADC (not shown), and (**i**) DSC perfusion shows decreased rCBV, suggesting most likely pseudoprogression or radiation necrosis. He had reoperation and the pathology shows extensive necrosis (**j**) and scattered areas of cellular atypia (**k**)

ing coagulation necrosis on pathology. In such case, it is important to watch the size of diffusion restriction carefully because stable diffusion restriction indicates local necrosis due to treatment, while progressive diffusion restriction may suggest less necrosis surrounded by expanding tumor (Fig. 18.21).

18.2.7 Gliosarcoma

Gliosarcoma is a subtype of GBM characterized by neoplastic glial cells and sarcomatous components. It is rare (1.8–8.0% of GBMs, M > F). The age distribution and survival characteristics of gliosarcomas are similar to typical GBMs. The exact origin of the sarcoma cells in gliosarcomas remains obscure. Macroscopically, gliosarcomas tend to have a hard consistency and are usually well delineated from the surrounding tissue. In contrast, the typical GBM usually infiltrates surrounding white and gray matter. Gliosarcomas can either arise de novo (Fig. 18.22) or secondary to irradiation of GBM or anaplastic gliomas. Dwyer et al. reported that gliosarcomas tend to abut a dural surface but they may be indistinguishable from the typical GBM on MR imaging including DW imaging [77].

18.2.8 Ependymal Tumors

Ependymoma and oligodendroglioma together constitute the largest subgroup in the non-

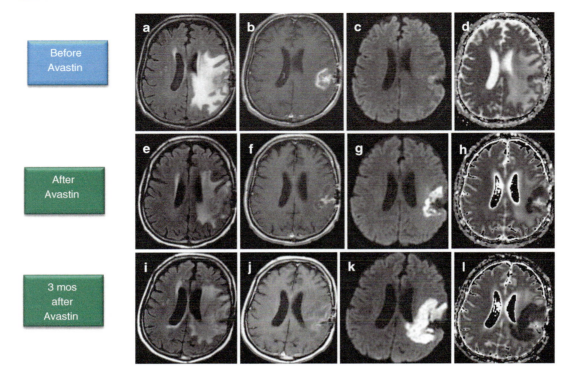

Fig. 18.21 (**a–k**) Pseudoresponse with the use of bevacizumab (anti-VEGF monoclonal antibody, Avastin) for the recurrence of GBM in a 64-year-old male. Courtesy of Aaron Berg MD. He had a surgical resection of GBM in the left temporal lobe and postoperative chemoradiation 2 years ago. (**a**) FLAIR shows a hyperintense lesion around the surgical cavity, and (**b**) gadolinium-enhanced T1-weighted image shows mass-forming avid enhancement in the surgical cavity and linear enhancement in the adjacent white matter. (**c**) DWI and (**d**) ADC show diffusion restriction corresponding to the mass-forming enhancement, indicating recurrence of GBM. After the use of bevacizumab, (**e**) FLAIR hyperintensity has mildly decreased and (**f**) gadolinium-enhanced T1-weighted image shows decreased enhancement, but (**g**) DWI and (**h**) ADC show an enlargement of area of restricted diffusion. Three months after the use of bevacizumab, (**i**) FLAIR hyperintensity has mildly increased with mass effect, and (**j**) gadolinium-enhanced T1-weighted image shows decreased enhancement with subtle linear enhancement contouring the DWI hyperintensity. (**k**) DWI and (**l**) ADC show enlarged area of diffusion restriction surrounding resection cavity, consistent with pseudoresponse (tumor recurrence)

astrocytic gliomas. Ependymomas can occur in the brain and spinal cord. These are very unique lesions in that the tumors found in the posterior fossa differ from those in the supratentorial compartment in their genetic and molecular make-up. In the 2016 WHO classification there are 4 distinct intracranial ependymomas: subependymomas (Fig. 18.23), ependymomas, RELA fusion positive ependymomas, and anaplastic ependymomas (Fig. 18.24).

The subependymoma is slow-growing intraventricular, WHO grade 1 tumor most commonly encountered in middle age and elderly individuals, males more frequently than females. They are described as composed of bland to mildly pleomorphic mitotically inactive cells embedded in an abundant fibrillary matrix with frequent microcystic change. They are most commonly encountered in the fourth ventricle followed by the lateral ventricles. They are sharply demarcated, nodular, non-enhancing masses with rare associated hemorrhage or calcification. They are iso-hypointense on T1-weighted images and heterogeneously hyperintense on T2-weighted images. They do not restrict diffusion (Fig. 18.23). Specific reports on diffusion features are limited to case reports and small series [78–80].

18 Brain Neoplasm

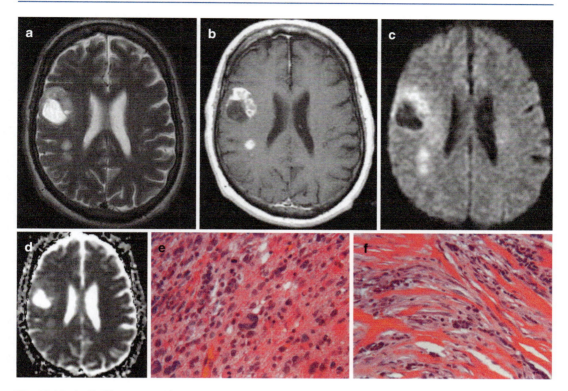

Fig. 18.22 (**a–f**) Gliosarcoma (de novo). A 74-year-old man presenting with a focal motor seizure. (**a**) T2-weighted image shows a cystic/necrotic tumor in the right frontal lobe. (**b**) On gadolinium-enhanced T1-weighted image, the tumor shows peripheral and irregular solid enhancement. A solid part is attached to a dural surface. There is another smaller enhancing nodule posterior to this mass. (**c, d**) On DW imaging, the solid part of the tumor shows increased signal intensity with mildly elevated ADC (**e, f**) The tumor has a biphasic histologic pattern with areas displaying astrocytic (**e**) and sarcomatous (**f**) differentiation. (Courtesy of Oka M MD, University of Rochester Medical Center, USA)

"Classic" ependymomas are the most common subtype of all subependymomas. Their incidence is influenced by their location, histological variations, and molecular group. Posterior fossa ependymomas constitute approximately 60% of all ependymomas whereas the rest occur in the supratentorial compartment. Of the posterior fossa lesions 95% occur in the fourth ventricle and the remainder in the cerebellopontine angle cistern. These are WHO grade II tumors; however, there is not validate correlation between the grade, histology, and survival related to this tumor. The posterior fossa ependymomas are further classified as PF-EPN-A and PF-EPN-B subgroups; the former occurs in young children with male preponderance while the latter occurs in adolescent and young adults with a slight female preponderance. These are the classical WHO grade II "plastic ependymomas" which enlarge the fourth ventricle and insinuate into the lateral recess and foramen of Magendie, and then, in advanced cases, extend into the adjacent posterior fossa cisterns involving the exiting cranial nerves. Supratentorial ependymomas exhibit almost exclusively RELA fusion and appear as large bulky aggressive masses with large cystic spaces and associated hemorrhage. These are classified as WHO grade II or III. Ependymomas generally appears as heterogeneously hyperintense on the T2-weighted images and FLAIR sequence and mixed intensity on T1-weighted images. Hemorrhagic areas appear as hypointense signals on the T2* or SWI sequence. All tumors show heterogeneous enhancement, with the cystic portions appearing as non-enhancing

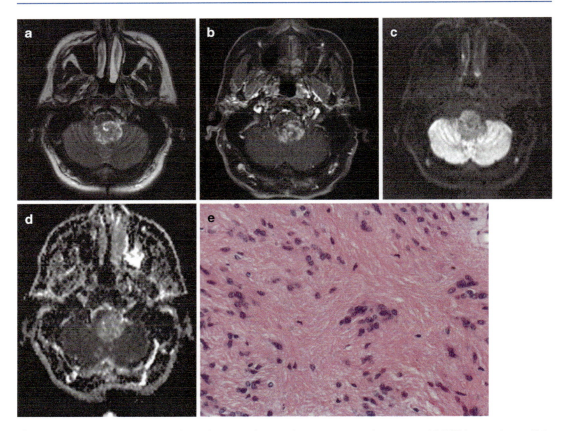

Fig. 18.23 (a–e) Low-grade subependymoma in a 49-year-old man. (**a**) T2-weighted image shows a hyperintense mass lesion in the fourth ventricle. (**b**) Gadolinium-enhanced T1-weighted image with fat saturation shows heterogeneous enhancement. (**c**) DW image shows slight hypointensity. (**d**) ADC map shows hyperintensity in the lesion ($0.96–1.30 \times 10^{-3}$ mm^2/s). (**e**) Pathology specimen shows low cellularity and abundant fibrillary background

fluid signal spaces. Both of the varieties of the tumor do not exhibit impeded diffusion.

DWI serves an important tool in distinguishing these tumors from other posterior fossa masses which occur primarily in children. Based on histology tumors graded as high grade and low grade showed significant variations in mean ADC and mean ADC ratios with values of 1.3 and 1.5 for low-grade tumors and 0.9 and 1.2 for high-grade lesions [81] (Fig. 18.26). Voxelwise volumetric ADC histogram analysis has been performed in a group of primary fourth ventricular tumors 71% to 82% sensitivity, 91% to 95% specificity, 75% to 78% positive predictive value, and 89% to 95% negative predictive value for differentiation of ependymoma, medulloblastoma, and pilocytic astrocytoma [82]. Aspects of machine learning based on support vector based classifiers have yielded good discriminators using ADC histogram features [83, 84].

18.2.9 Other Gliomas

Chordoid glioma of the third ventricle is a rare neuroepithelial tumor arising from the anterior wall or roof of the third ventricle. In the 2016 revision of the WHO classification of CNS tumors, it is classified grade II, and defined as follows: "A slow-growing, non-invasive glial tumor located in the third ventricle." Microscopically, it consists of solid neoplasms composed of tumor cells within a variably mucinous stroma with a lymphoplasmacytic infiltrate. MRI typically demonstrates a well-defined, T1 isointense,

18 Brain Neoplasm

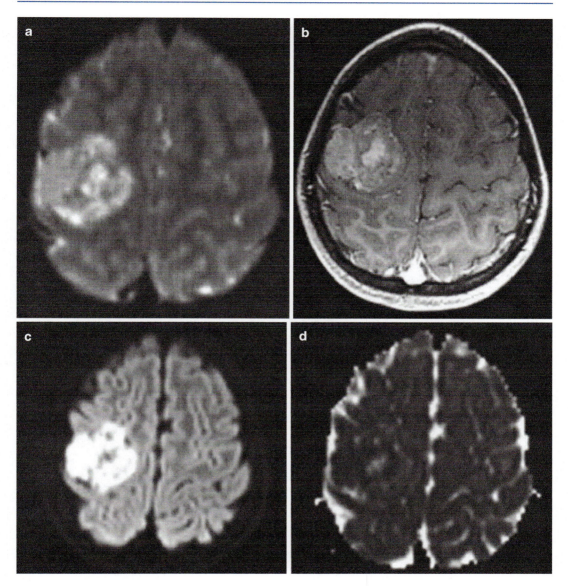

Fig. 18.24 (**a–d**) Anaplastic ependymoma in a 7-year-old boy. (**a**) T2-weighted (b0) image shows a hyperintense solid mass in the right frontal area. (**b**) Gadolinium-enhanced T1-weighted image shows heterogeneous enhancement. (**c**) DW image shows hyperintensity in the solid mass. (**d**) ADC map shows hypointensity ($0.50–0.64 \times 10^{-3}$ mm^2/s) with hyperintensity (1.44×10^{-3} mm^2/s) in a central necrotic area

T2 hyperintense mass with avid post-contrast enhancement, often mimicking intraventricular meningiomas [84]. DWI usually shows no diffusion restriction (Fig. 18.25).

Angiocentric glioma is an uncommon, low-grade neoplasm of the brain, most commonly centered in the cerebral cortex of the frontal, temporal, or parietal lobes. It is classified as a grade I tumor by the World Health Organization (WHO), but it typically presented with refractory seizures in children and young adults. Microscopically, angiocentric gliomas are characterized by elongate glial cells arranged in perivascular pseudorosettes, and the neoplastic cells infiltrate surrounding neural parenchyma with predilection for perivascular spread, form nodules comprised of spindled tumor

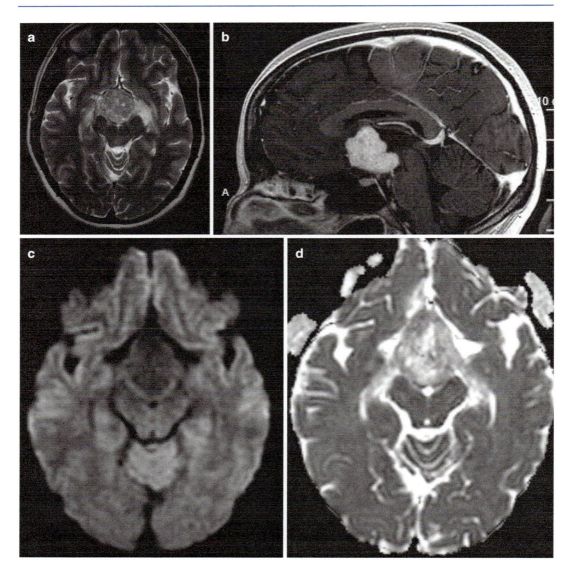

Fig. 18.25 (**a–d**) Choroid glioma of the third ventricle WHO grade II in a 38-year-old female. She complained of blurred vision in both eyes. (**a**) T2-weighted image shows a heterogeneous, mildly hyperintense mass in the third ventricle. (**b**) Gadolinium-enhanced T1-weighted image shows avid homogenous enhancement. (**c**) DWI shows hypointensity, probably due to low T2 signal. (**d**) ADC value is relatively increased, representing myxoid stroma

cells, and aggregate underneath the pia mater. MRI demonstrates a T1 hypointense, T2 hyperintense mass without post-contrast enhancement, sometimes accompanied by cystic component with ring-like T1 hyperintensity and surrounding T2 hyperintensity, mimicking encephalomalacia [85]. DWI shows no restricted diffusion (Fig. 18.26).

Astroblastoma is an extremely rare glial tumor occurring in persons of any age, with a bimodal age distribution, with one peak in infancy (between 5 and 10 years) and the other one in young adults (between 21 and 30 years), commonly arising in cerebral hemispheres. It is classified as a high-grade neuroepithelial tumor (Grade IV) with unknown origin. On macroscopic examination, it is described as superficial, well-demarcated, lobulated, solid, or cystic masses. Microscopically, it is defined by the pres-

18 Brain Neoplasm

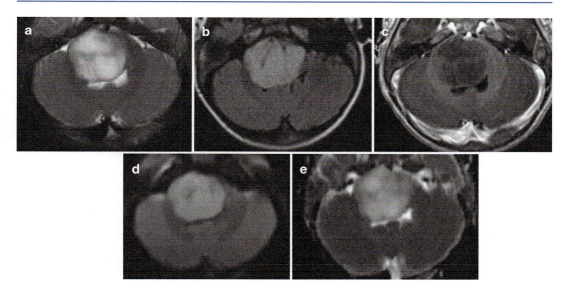

Fig. 18.26 (**a–e**) Angiocentric glioma, WHO grade 1 in a 2-year-old male. Tumor DNA sequencing revealed the presence of an MYB-QKI gene fusion. (**a**) T2-weighted image shows an expansile, hyperintense mass in the pons, associated with band-like hypointensities within the mass. (**b**) FLAIR image shows hyperintensity. (**c**) Gadolinium-enhanced T1-weighted image shows no enhancement. (**d**) DWI shows mostly homogeneous hyperintensity. (**e**) Mean ADC value is increased at 1.4×10^{-3} mm^2/s, representing myxoid component

ence of perivascular pseudorosettes and prominent perivascular hyalinization and the lack of fibrillary background. CT often shows punctate calcification. MRI demonstrates heterogeneously T2 hyperintense, T1 hypo/isointense, heterogeneously enhancing mass consisted with mixture of cystic and solid components. DWI shows restricted diffusion in the solid component (Chap. 19, Fig. 19.37).

18.2.10 Choroid Plexus Tumors

Choroid plexus tumors are classified into three categories: choroid plexus papilloma, atypical choroid plexus papilloma, and choroid plexus carcinomas. Choroid plexus papilloma (CPP) is histologically classified as WHO grade I tumors, atypical choroid plexus (aCPP) tumors are classified as WHO grade II, and choroid plexus carcinoma are graded as WHO grade III lesions. Choroid plexus papilloma are benign intraventricular papillary neoplasms derived from the choroid plexus epithelium. They are frequently located in the lateral ventricles followed by the fourth and third ventricles. They are isodense or hypodense on CT studies. They are T1 isointense and T2 hyperintense intraventricular masses associated with hydrocephalus. They typically have a frond-like morphology and enhance following contrast administration. Associated speckled calcification has been described. Atypical choroid plexus papilloma are difficult to identify on imaging studies and are classified solely on the basis of histology. These tumors exhibit ≥2 mitoses per 10 high power fields compared to ≥5 mitoses per 10 high powered fields for choroid plexus carcinomas. Choroid plexus carcinomas (CPC) are WHO grade III tumors most commonly seen in children and located within the lateral ventricles. These tumors are also associated with Aicardi and Li-Fraumeni syndromes. They are characterized by nuclear pleomorphism, increased cellular density, blurred papillary pattern with poorly demarcated sheets of tumor cells showing frequent mitoses. The tumors frequently express mutations of the TP53 (p53 tumor suppression gene). They are characteristically T1 iso- to hypointense on T1-weighted sequence and show hypointense susceptibility signals on the T2-GRE sequence due to associated calcification and hemorrhage. All tumors show intense heterogeneous enhancement.

Choroid plexus carcinomas have a higher cellular density compared to CPPs and aCPPs, and therefore show decreased water diffusivity and exhibit a lower ADC compared to CPP. The aCPPs show intermediate ADC values compared to CPC and CPP (see Chap. 19, Figs. 19.41, 19.42, and 19.43). Given the heterogeneous cellular composition of these tumors reports of higher values of the ADCs in these tumors compared to other pediatric brain tumors has been highlighted in the literature [86]. Recent research specific to these intraventricular tumors has suggested that there is correlation between the ADC values and the tumor volume to differentiate CPP from its malignant counterpart. Sasaki T et al. have reported a mean ADC value of ($1.734 \pm 0.390 \times 10^3$ mm^2/s) for CPP, 1.319 ± 0.344 for aCPP, and 1.128 ± 0.466 for CPC and concluded that a mean ADC value of ≤ 1.397 and tumor volume of 21.05 mL predicted significantly poorer outcomes with a positive correlation with higher grades of these subsets of tumors [87].

18.3 Neuronal and Mixed Neuronal-Glial Tumors

Neuronal and mixed neuronal-glial tumors are a group of slow-growing usually cortical-based well-circumscribed low-grade tumors which show neuronal as well as glial differentiation. These are typically grouped as "long-term epilepsy associated tumors" [88]. Dysembryoplastic neuroepithelial tumors (DNET) and ganglioglioma are the most commonly encountered tumors in this group. Lhermitte-Duclos disease or dysplastic gangliocytoma remains the sine qua non of these tumors. There are two new additions to this group of lesions in the 2016 WHO revision: multinodular and vacuolating neuronal tumors (MVNT) and diffuse leptomeningeal glioneuronal tumor.

18.3.1 Dysplastic Cerebellar Gangliocytoma (DCG)/ Lhermitte-Duclos Disease

Dysplastic cerebellar gangliocytoma (DCG), also known as Lhermitte-Duclos disease, is a benign WHO grade I neoplasm of the cerebellum characterized by dysplastic ganglion cells which remain conformed with the normal cortical cytoarchitecture of the cerebellum [88]. Adult with DCG show mutations of the PTEN gene as do several entities within the domain of Cowden syndrome. This association with the syndrome is also termed as the COLD syndrome (Cowden-Lhermitte-Duclos syndrome). Cowden syndrome is an autosomal dominant disorder consisting of hamartomatous lesions derived from all three germ cell layers including mucocutaneous lesions such as facial trichilemmomas, acral keratosis and mucocutaneous papillomatous papules. Patients carry an increased risk of breast thyroid, endometrial, renal, and colon cancers. DCG appear as areas of abnormal thickened folia in the affected portions of the cerebellum. Some tumors may show cystic areas. The histopathological characteristics include widening of molecular layers occupied by abnormal ganglion cells, absence of the Purkinje cell layer and hypertrophy of the granular cell with associated atrophy of the cerebellar white matter.

MRI features are typically described as tigroid given the thickened and distorted appearance of the cerebellar folia. Alternating bands of variable T1 iso-hypointensity and T2 hyperintensity are noted [89, 90]. The lesions do not typically enhance; however recent studies have suggested that this is relatively common and, if present, may reflect vascular (venous) proliferation [90, 91]. DWI typically shows slight increase in ADC compared to the normal cerebellum (Fig. 18.27). The hyperintense signals seen on DWI is secondary to a T2-shine-through effect. The range of ADC values encountered in a recent study was 967.8 ± 115.7 vs. $770.4 \pm 47.3 \times 10^{-6}$ mm^2/s. The ADC value reflects the intermediate cellularity, showing increased number and size of ganglion cells replacing the granular and Purkinje cell lay-

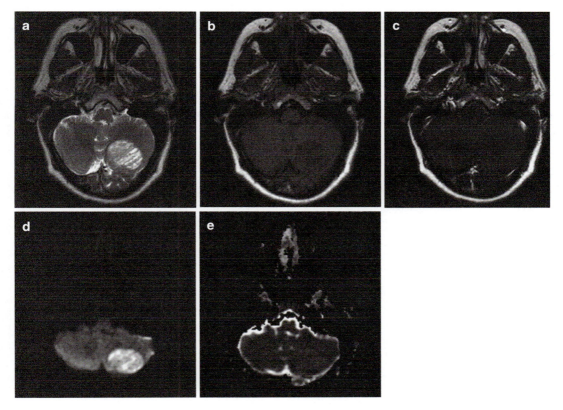

Fig. 18.27 (a–e) Lhermitte-Duclos disease in a 48-year-old woman, (a, b) T1- and T2-wighted images show a well-circumscribed mass with a striated pattern. (c) Gadolinium-enhanced T1-weighted image shows minimal vascular enhancement in the mass. (d, e) DW imaging shows a hyperintense mass associated with slightly increased ADC that may reflect an increased number and size of ganglion cells replacing the granular and Purkinje cell layers. (Courtesy of Nakamura H MD, Kitanosono T MD, University of Rochester Medical Center, USA)

ers. MR spectroscopy characteristically shows elevated lactate and slightly reduced NAA and choline peaks [92].

18.3.2 Dysembryoplastic Neuroepithelial Tumor (DNET)

Dysembryoplastic neuroepithelial tumor (DNET or DNT) is benign WHO grade 1 tumor most commonly (over 65%) located in the cortex of the temporal lobe. These childhood tumors are often detected in imaging studies carried out during investigations for intractable seizures. Histopathological features include a multinodular architecture of so-called glioneuronal elements characterized by columns of axon bundles oriented perpendicular to the cortical surface [1]. Oligodendroglial-like cells, thin vasculature, hanging neurons, and myxoid matrix are also required features. DNET often has adjacent cortical involvement that is responsible for the epileptogenic activity. Although it is not common, DNET can be histologically coexistent with oligodendroglial-like nodules, ganglioglioma, astrocytoma, or cortical dysplasia.

On conventional MR sequences the lesions are composed of T2 hyperintense cysts or pseudocysts. Non-cystic, solid-appearing areas are characterized by T1 hypointense signals which are relatively hyperintense of FLAIR and T2 sequences. The lesions tend to encompass the entire cortex and characteristically demonstrated gently excavated deformations of the adjacent portion of the inner table of skull. Calcification is uncommon in these tumors. Enhancement is seen in 20–33% of the lesions.

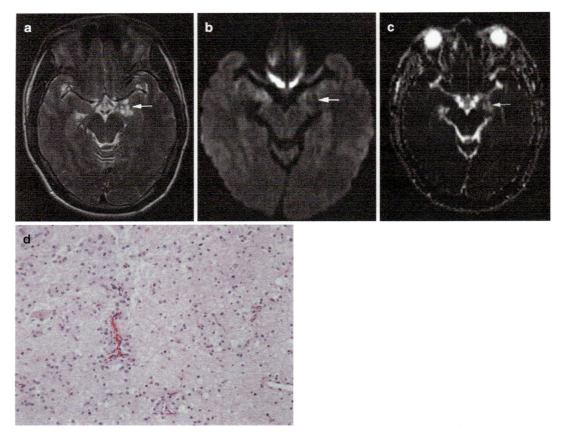

Fig. 18.28 (a–d) Dysembryoplastic neuroepithelial tumor in 32-year-old man with seizures. (**a**) T2-weighted image shows multicystic lesions in the medial temporal lobe with no edema (*arrow*). (**b, c**) DW imaging shows hypointense lesions with high ADC values (1.87–2.34 × 10^{-3} mm^2/s) (*arrow*). (**d**) Pathology shows oligodendroglial-like cells, thin vessels, scattered neurons, and myxoid matrix

DWI shows DNET as a hypointense lesion with significantly higher ADC values (>2 × 10^{-3} mm^2/s) compared with those of low-grade glial tumors (0.96 × 10^{-3} mm^2/s to 1.92 × 10^{-3} mm^2/s) (Fig. 18.28) [28]. Yamasaki F et al. have described a range of 2.354–2.722 × 10^{-3} mm^2/s [93]. Since ganglioglioma and focal cortical dysplasia (FCD) are the principle differential diagnosis of these tumors, an attempt has been made to differentiate these benign entities based on their diffusion characteristics. Diffusion image can differentiate between these epileptogenic entities and the perilesional normal-appearing white matter which may be part of the focus which needs to be resected during epilepsy surgery. Rau A et al. have shown that DNET could be differentiated from FCD on the basis of mean diffusivity and FCD could be differentiated on the basis of radial diffusivity [94]. Both glioneuronal tumors could be differentiated from the perilesional normal-appearing white matter on the basis of fractional anisotropy (FA) and radial diffusivity. A threshold values for FA of ≤0.32 or a radial diffusivity of ≥0.56.10^3 mm/s^2 was considered to be statistically significant.

18.3.3 Ganglioglioma

Ganglioglioma is WHO grade I tumors frequently seen in the temporal lobes [95]. These slow-growing tumors are characterized by dysplastic ganglion cells and neoplastic glial cells in varying proportions [96]. The ganglion cells in these tumors lack specific architectural arrangements or cytological characteristics of cortical neurons. Although these tumors are commonly found in the cerebrum, they can be located in the brainstem, cerebellum, spinal cord, optic nerves, pituitary gland, and the pineal gland. Cerebral lesions frequently present as seizures. Classical MRI appearances include well-circumscribed tumor with solid- and cystic-appearing components. The solid components are T1 hypointense or isointense, and hyperintense on the T2 sequences [88]. The cystic component shows variable signals depending upon the presence of hemorrhage and the proteinaceous material. Remodeling of the inner table of the skull is frequently demonstrated which is secondary to the slow-growing nature of the tumor. Calcification is seen in approximately 35% of tumors and these areas demonstrated amorphous hypointense signals on the T2*/GRE sequences. Variable enhancement has been described in the solid component of the tumor. Differential diagnosis includes DNET, pleomorphic xanthoastrocytoma, oligodendroglioma, and desmoplastic infantile astrocytoma.

DWI has shown that these lesions show ADC values comparable to the cellularity of the tumors (Figs. 18.29 and 18.30). In a comparative estimation of the minimum ADC (minADC) of these lesions and astrocytoma, Kikuchi, T et al. have indicated that mean cutoff of the minADC for ganglioglioma in their series was $1.45 \pm 0.20 \times 10^3$ mm^2/s, which was significantly higher than astrocytoma [97]. They also concluded that the minADC is inversely correlated with tumor cellularity.

18.3.4 Central Neurocytoma

Central neurocytoma are uncommon WHO grade II intraventricular tumors typically arising from the neuronal cells of the septum pellucidum. Central neurocytoma occurs predominantly in young adults. These tumors consist of small, round, uniform neoplastic cells with neuronal phenotype. The cells stain positive for syaptophysin, NeuN, and neuron-specific enolase and do not stain for GFAP. IDH mutations and 1p19q deletions are not seen which is helpful in differ-

entiating this tumor from oligodendroglioma. The tumors can also arise in the extraventricular location, without an associated intraventricular component.

Cystic components and calcifications are common. The tumors are isointense to gray matter, and show numerous T2 and FLAIR hyperintense cystic areas. Vascular flow voids can be demonstrated especially on the post-contrast T1 sequence. The tumor shows heterogeneous enhancement on this this sequence. Calcification, if present, is punctate and appears as hypointense signals on the T2*/GRE sequence. Calcification is variously described as clumped, amorphous, and globular [88]. Since these lesions may be indistinguishable from other intraventricular tumors such as ependymomas, high-grade gliomas, and intraventricular meningioma, attempts have been made to utilize DWI for objective differentiation of these lesions from other similar lesions as mentioned above. DWI shows a hyperintense lesion with lower ADC values ($0.65–0.95 \times 10^{-3}$ mm^2/s) which is lower than those of astrocytomas and non-astrocytic gliomas (Fig. 18.31) [54, 55]. The decreased ADC values reflect hypercellularity of the central neurocytoma. Yu Y et al. have demonstrated the relative minADC in the enhancing solid portions of the lesions not containing calcifications or hemorrhage was lower than other image intraventricular lesions [98]. The range in their series was 0.77 ± 0.16 compared to, for example, ependymomas which had a range of 1.16 ± 0.19.

Diffuse leptomeningeal glioneuronal tumor is a new entity included in the WHO 2016 revision [1] and is described as tumor with a oligodendroglial-like cytology having a predominant leptomeningeal component. The lesion has been described to be IDH mutant negative, with solitary 1p or 1p19q co-deletions and a high rate of concurrent KIAA1549-BRAF gene fusions [1]. Originally described as a tumor involving the spinal cord leptomeninges, it does involve the intracranial compartment with primary involvement of the leptomeninges of the brain stem, cerebellum, and the base of the brain.

MRI shows widespread diffuse enhancement of the leptomeninges. Small subpial cysts

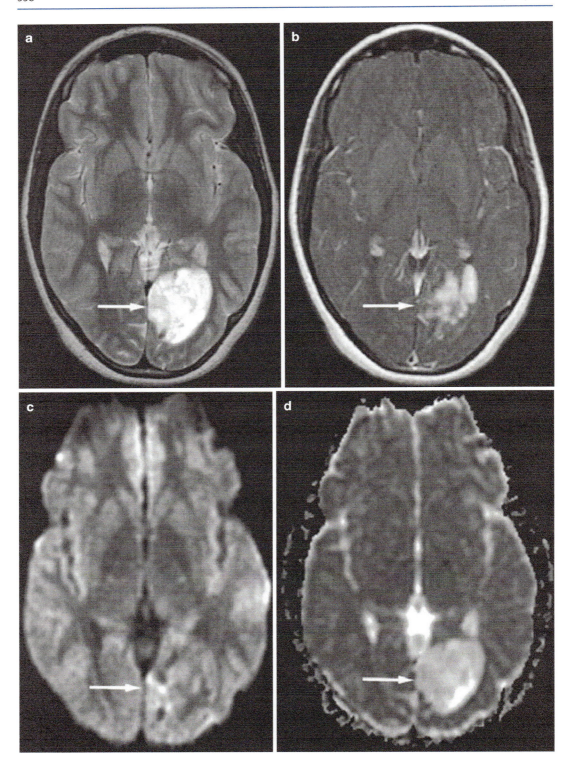

Fig. 18.29 (**a–d**) Ganglioglioma in a 12-year-old girl with seizures. (**a**) T2-weighted image shows a hyperintense lesion in the right occipital lobe (*arrow*). (**b**) Gadolinium-enhanced T1-weighted image shows heterogeneous enhancement (*arrow*). (**c**) DW image shows heterogeneous mild hyperintensity in the lesion (arrow). (**d**) ADC map shows hyperintensity in the lesion (0.98–1.35 × 10^{-3} mm^2/s; *arrow*)

18 Brain Neoplasm

Fig. 18.30 (a–e) Ganglioglioma in a 31-year-old man with seizures. (a) T2-weighted image shows a well-defined mildly hyperintense lesion in the right parietal cortex (*arrow*). (b) Gadolinium-enhanced T1-weighted image with fat saturation shows heterogeneous enhancement (*arrow*). (c) DW image shows hyperintensity in the lesion. (d) ADC map shows isointensity in the lesion (0.76–0.88 × 10^{-3} mm^2/s; *arrow*). (e) Pathology shows intermediate cellularity composed of ganglion cells and neoplastic astrocytes

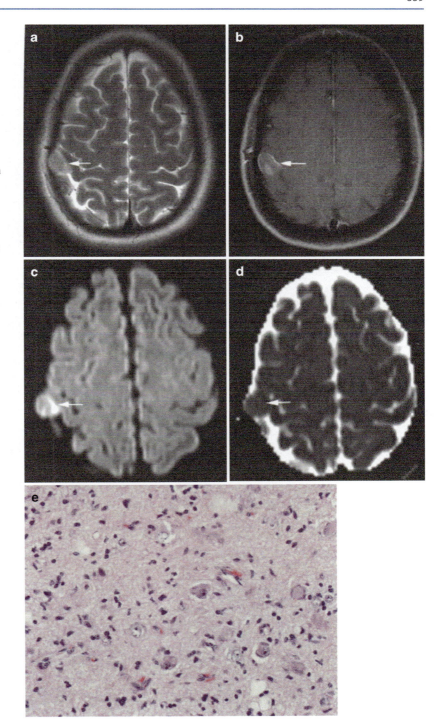

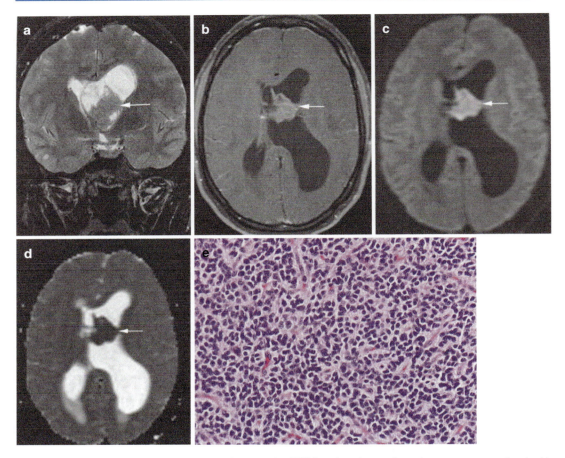

Fig. 18.31 (a–e) Central neurocytoma in 32-year-old woman. (**a**) Coronal T2-weighted image shows isointense intraventricular mass with cystic components involving the septum pellucidum (*arrow*). (**b**) Gadolinium-enhanced T1-weighted image with fat saturation shows heterogeneous enhancement in the mass (*arrow*). (**c, d**) DW imaging shows a hyperintense mass associated with decreased ADC (0.54×10^{-3} mm^2/s) that may reflect the hypercellularity of the central neurocytoma (*arrow*). (**e**) Pathology shows hypercellularity composed of small well-differentiated neurons with uniform nuclei

and T2 hyperintense cysts have been described in the spinal cord and brain [99]. Discrete intraparenchymal lesions are present in the spinal cord in 81% of cases in the largest reported series of this tumor [100] (Chap. 19, Fig. 19.45). Illustrated examples of this tumor have shown areas of low ADC signals, although quantified measurements of the diffuse parameters have been described in the literature, possibly because of the diffuse nature of the enhancing components of the lesion without a sizeable parenchymal lesion [99, 101]. The subpial cystic lesions have been presumed to represent dilated perivascular spaces.

Multifocal vacuolating neuronal tumor of the cerebrum is the second new entity which has been included in 2016 revision of the WHO Classification of CNS tumors. Because there are fewer than 100 cases described in the literature, the authors of the revision have included this tumor as an entity provisionally included as an appendix to gangliocytoma. The histopathological features of these well-circumscribed lesions include small to medium sized neuroepithelial cells with globose amphophilic cytoplasm and large nuclei with vesicular chromatin resembling small neurons. The cells are arranged in nodules involving the deep half of the cortex and/or the superficial white matter [1]. Imaging features suggest benignity with well-circumscribed T2 and FLAIR hyperintense lesions without evidence of restricted diffusion [102, 103].

18.4 Tumors of Pineal Region

Pineocytoma, pineoblastoma, and papillary tumor of the pineal region together with the pineal tumors of intermediate differentiation constitute the four major primary tumors of the pineal region. Pineal region tumors characteristically result in obstructive hydrocephalus resulting signs and symptoms of raised intracranial pressure such as papilledema. Additional involvement of the adjacent superior colliculus results in restriction of upward gaze; the constellation of these signs and symptoms is termed as Parinaud's syndrome. The association of pinealoblastomas and retinoblastoma (trilateral retinoblastoma syndrome) is well known and related to RBI gene abnormalities shared between the tumors. The other tumors frequently encountered in the pineal region are germ cell tumors and tumors arising from the midbrain tectum adjacent to the pineal gland.

Of the primary pineal region tumors, the pineal parenchymal tumor of intermediate differentiation comprises 45% of all pineal parenchymal tumors followed by pineoblastoma at 35% and pinealocytomas at 25% [1]. Histologically pineocytomas are the most well differentiate of

the primary tumors (WHO grade I) containing uniform cells forming well-circumscribed pineocytomatous rosettes together with pleomorphic cells with gangliocytic components.

Pineoblastoma, on the other hand, is a WHO grade IV tumor composed of highly cellular embryonal neoplasm comprising small round cells which resemble primitive neuroectodermal tumors of the CNS arranged dense patternless sheets lacking in the pinealocytic rosette formation. Pineoblastomas tend to have a lobular pattern and occupy the quadrigeminal cistern [104]. T1-weighted imaging shows pinealoblastoma as hypointense with homogeneous or heterogeneous enhancement (Table 18.3). DW imaging usually shows it as hyperintense associated with iso- or slightly decreased ADC, probably reflecting the cellularity (Fig. 18.32).

Pineal parenchymal tumors of intermediate differentiation [PPTID] (WHO grade II or III) are composed of, as the name suggests, monomorphic cells that appear to more differentiated than those seen in pinealoblastomas arranged in large lobules and sheets.

Papillary tumors of the pineal region [PTPR] (WHO grade II or III) are composed of cells thought to originate from the remnants of ependymal precursors in the subcommisural organ. Papillary tumors of the pineal region are well-circumscribed masses of the pineal region, commonly with a cystic component (Fig. 18.33). The prognosis of papillary tumors of the pineal region is usually worse and less sensitive to treatment than pineoblastoma. T1-hyperintensity in the tumor has been reported due to protein, glycoprotein, or other T1-shortening substances produced by tumor cells [105, 106] (Table 18.3). These tumors are indistinguishable from PPTID on imaging studies.

The role of diffusion imaging has been two-fold, one to differentiate between each of the

Table 18.3 Summarizes the MRI features of the primary pineal parenchymal tumors

	T1	T2/FLAIR	T2*/GRE	T1 post-contrast
Pineocytoma	Iso-hypointense	hyperintense	Hypointense	Avid/heterogeneous
PPTID	Iso-hypointense	Isointense/hyperintense	Hypointense	Avid/heterogeneous
Pineoblastoma	Iso-hypointense	Iso-hypointense	Hypointense	Avid/heterogeneous
PTPR	Iso-hypointense	Isointense/hyperintense	Hypointense	Avid/heterogeneous

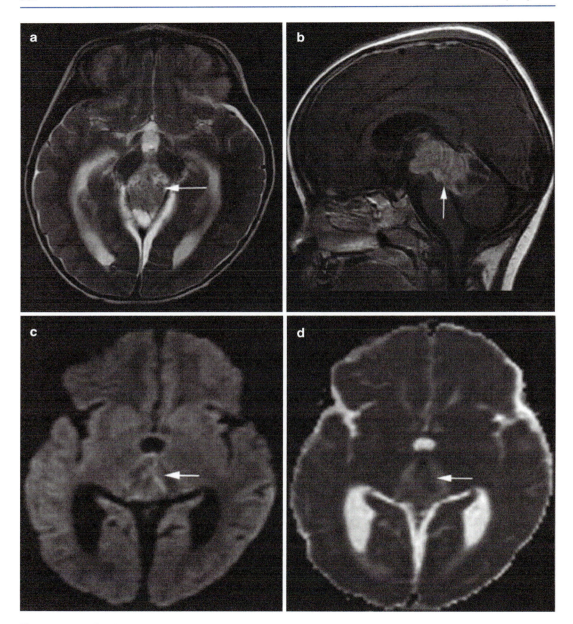

Fig. 18.32 (**a**–**d**) Pinealoblastoma in a 4-year-old boy. (**a**) T2-weighted image shows a mildly hyperintense lesion in the pineal region (*arrow*). (**b**) Gadolinium-enhanced sagittal T1-weighted image shows a heterogeneously enhancing mass with cystic components in the pineal region (*arrow*). (**c**) DW image shows isointensity or mild hyperintensity in the solid portion of the lesion (*arrow*). (**d**) ADC map shows isointensity or slight hyperintensity in the solid portion of the lesion (0.74–1.05×10^{-3} mm^2/s; *arrow*)

primary pineal tumors and the second to investigate the role in the differentiation between these primary tumors from other tumors in this region such as germinomas and gliomas. In a retrospective study of histopathological proven primary pineal tumors, Zhu l et al. have described evaluation of minADC values in a small cohort of primary pineal tumors and compared them to the percentage of Ki67-positive cell density [107]. They found that mean minADC values for pine-

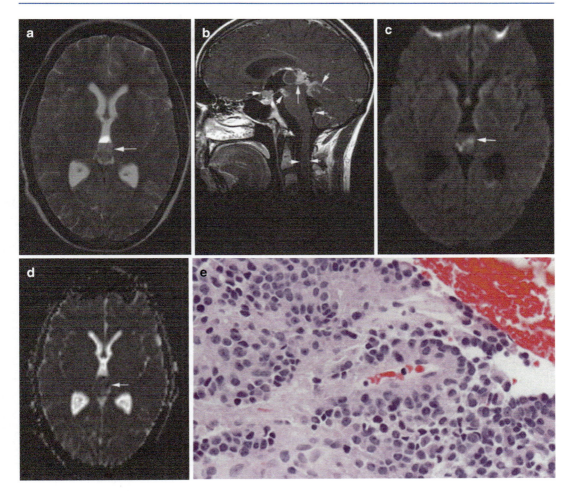

Fig. 18.33 (a–e) Papillary tumor of the pineal region in an 18-year-old male patient. (a) T2-weighted image shows a well-defined mildly hyperintense lesion with a cystic component and fluid–fluid level (*arrow*). (b) Gadolinium-enhanced sagittal T1-weighted image shows heterogeneously enhancing lesions in the pineal and suprasellar regions and leptomeningeal enhancement along the cerebellum and spinal cord due to tumor dissemination (*arrows*). (c) DW image shows a hyperintense lesion (*arrow*). (d) ADC map shows isointensity in the lesion (0.70–0.85×10^{-3} mm^2/s; *arrow*). (e) Micropathology specimen shows hypercellularity with a papillary growth pattern of plump epithelial-like cells and hemorrhage. Nuclei were uniform, (Courtesy of Sato TS, University of Iowa Carver College of Medicine, USA)

alocytomas was $0.911 \pm 0.044 \times 10^3$ mm^2/sec compared to $0.0701 \pm 0.032 \times 10^3$ mm^2/sec and $0.465 \pm 0.036 \times 10^3$ mm^2/sec for pineal parenchymal tumors of intermediate differentiation and pinealoblastomas, respectively. They concluded that there was persistent higher mean minADC values for pinealocytomas compared to the other two types of tumors in their series, and the values for the intermediate-grade tumors as higher than the pinealoblastomas. This may reflect the increased cellularity seen in pinealoblastomas [108].

As a corollary, in a short case series, diffusion characteristic were used to predict tumor cellularity and histology in a cohort of 20 patients with pineal tumors [109]. Authors in this series found that the mean apparent diffusion coefficient (ADC) values in pineoblastoma ($544 \pm 65 \times 10^{-6}$ mm²/s) and pineoblastoma/PNET ($595 \pm 144 \times 10^{-6}$ mm²/s) was lower than that of the germ cell tumors ($1284 \pm 334 \times 10^{-6}$ mm²/s; p < 0.0001 vs. pineoblastoma). Similar results were reported by Gasparetto EL et al. [110].

18.5 Embryonal Tumors

The 2016 revised WHO classification of embryonal tumors of the central nervous system can be simplified into three major categories [1]. Medulloblastoma is the commonest of the embryonal tumors. The second group of tumors are the non-medulloblastoma embryonal tumors which include embryonal tumors with multilayered rosettes (ETMR), medulloepitheliomas, CNS neuroblastomas, and CNS ganglioneuroblastomas. Atypical teratoid/rhabdoid tumors (AT/RT) are the third major constituent of this group of tumors. The previously described primitive neuroectodermal tumor (PNET) is no longer included in this current revision (Fig. 18.34).

Medulloblastomas have been classified traditionally into 4 histological types, which have been retained in the 2016 WHO iteration. Additionally, these tumors have also been classified into 4 distinct types based on the genetic definitions [1]. The histologically defined tumors are termed classical medulloblastomas, desmoplastic medulloblastoma, medulloblastoma with extensive nodularity, and large cell/anaplastic medulloblastoma. The genetically defined medulloblastomas include the WNT (wingless-integrated)-activated medulloblastomas, the SHH (sonic hedgehog)-activated medulloblastomas, and non-WNT/non-SHH (group 3 and group 4) tumor. Medulloblastomas are extremely cellular, WHO grade IV malignant tumors encountered primarily in children. They are commonly located in the midline posterior fossa and present as masses arising in the roof of the fourth ventricle or in the region of the lateral recess of the fourth ventricle. They are rapidly growing lesions often presenting with hydrocephalus. Location of the tumors in the cerebellum can be correlated with the genetic subtypes with the more laterally located, cerebellar peduncular masses most commonly associated with WNT subgroup and the off-center cerebellar lesions associated with SHH molecular signature. Midline centrally located tumors are most frequently associated with group 3 group 4 or SHH. Additionally, these tumors may show features of desmoplastic medulloblastoma, nodular medulloblastoma, or medulloblastoma with extensive nodular.

On conventional MR sequences they are predominantly hypointense to gray matter on the T1 and iso-hyperintense on the T2-weighted sequence. Necrosis and cyst formation within the tumor has been described. Hypercellularity of medulloblastomas predictably associated with restricted diffusion and low ADC values. Applications of diffusion imaging have led to differentiation of medulloblastomas from other posterior fossa tumors [111, 112], differentiation of the subtypes of medulloblastomas [113], delineating non-infiltrating and infiltrating planes in the surrounding cerebellar parenchyma to assist in surgical planning and resection [114], and for early detection of recurrent medulloblastoma [115] (Fig. 18.35, see Chap. 19, Figs. 19.25, 19.26, 19.27, and 19.28). MR spectroscopy reveals an elevated choline peak and an accompanying creased NAA peak. Detection of a taurine peak is also considered to be diagnostic [116].

Embryonal tumors are generally undifferentiated tumors histologically characterized by small blue round cells (SBRC) which show diffusion restriction. DW typically hyperintense with decreased ADC due to the high cellular density with high nuclear-to-cytoplasmic ratio [93, 117–120] in embryonal tumors such as ETMR (see Chap. 19, Fig. 19.31) and ATRT (see Chap. 19, Figs. 19.29 and 19.30). ATRT in children has more malignant biological behavior and is less sensitive to therapy than medulloblastoma [121]. Cerebellopontine angle involvement and intratumoral hemorrhage are more common than in medulloblastoma. The range of ADC values in AT/RT has been reported to be $0.47–0.83 \times 10^{-3}$ mm²/s [93, 121].

18 Brain Neoplasm

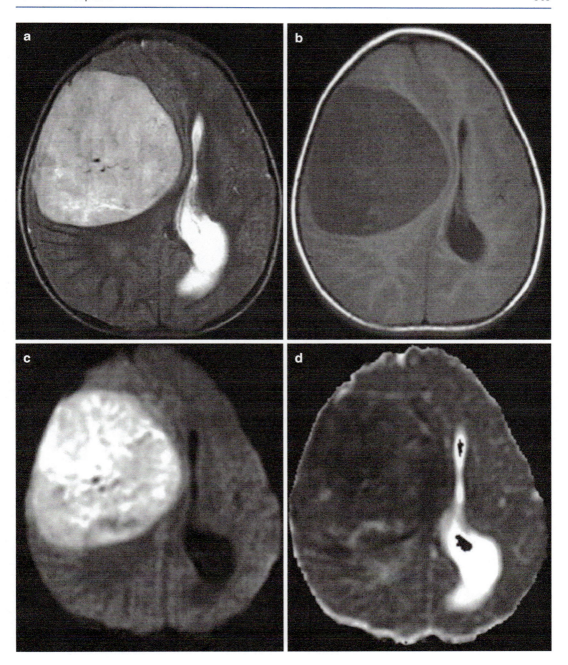

Fig. 18.34 (a–d) Previously diagnosed as primitive neuroectodermal tumor (PNET) in a 20-month-old girl with lethargy and nausea. (**a**) T2-weighted image shows a well-demarcated and heterogeneous intense mass in the right frontal lobe. (**b**) T1-weighted image shows heterogeneous hypointensity in the lesion. (**c**) DW image shows hyperintensity. (**d**) ADC map shows heterogeneous hypointensity (0.54–0.74×10^{-3} mm^2/s) in the lesion, which may represent hypercellularity. PNET is no longer included in this current revision, WHO 2016 classification

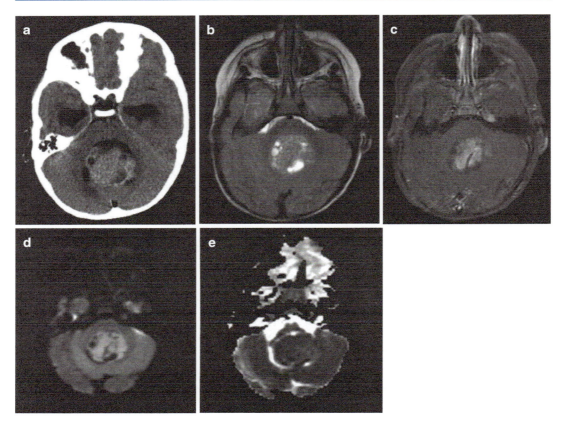

Fig. 18.35 (**a–e**) Medulloblastoma in a 10-year-old boy. (**a**) Precontrast CT shows a hyperdense mass. (**b**) T2-weighted image shows a mildly hyperintense mass. (**c**) Gadolinium-enhanced T1-weighted image with fat saturation shows a solid mass with enhancement in the cerebellar vermis. (**d**) DW image shows this solid mass as hyperintense. (**e**) ADC map shows decreased ADC of this mass. This is due to high cellular density causing restricted diffusion

18.6 Tumors of Cranial and Spinal Nerves

These are ubiquitous lesions with schwannoma, neurofibroma, and the malignant peripheral nerve sheath tumor being the most common representative tumors of this group of lesions.

Schwannomas comprise approximately 8% of all intracranial tumors. Cystic degeneration is common (5.7–24%), and may be accompanied by hemorrhage (5%). Intracranial schwannomas are typically well-encapsulated WHO grade 1 lesions encountered primarily in middle age and elderly adult patients, although they can be detected across all age groups. They are associated with the stems of the cranial nerves, most commonly the vestibular nerve, followed in decreasing incidence in relation to the trigeminal, facial, and lower cranial nerves (IX, X, and XI) in the jugular foramen. They are an essential component of Neurofibromatosis Type 2, where bilateral vestibular schwannomas are considered to be diagnostic. Involvement of other cranial nerves is rare as are the intraparenchymal tumors [1].

On histopathological evaluation, these tumors are composed entirely of neoplastic Schwann cells which are arranged in two distinct architectural patterns: Antoni Type A in which the cells are more numerous and compact with nuclear palisading; and Antoni Type B in which cells are sparsely arranged with indistinct processes and lipidization.

On conventional MRI sequences, the lesions are iso-hypointense to gray matter on the T1 sequence with low intensity areas seen in cystic areas. The tumors are hyperintense to gray matter on the T2-weighted images. The lesions show avid enhancement following administration of gadolinium contrast.

DW imaging can be useful for the differential diagnosis of cerebellopontine angle tumors [122]. Schwannomas do not show typical diffusion restriction and are hyperintense on DWI exhibiting a typical T2 shine-through effect. Vestibular schwannomas showed significantly higher mean and median ADC values compared to meningiomas [93, 123], reflecting the cellularity and histological types (Fig. 18.36). Attempts have been made to correlate the Antoni type with diffusion imaging in cases of vestibular schwannomas [124]. Higher ADC values were associated with Antoni Type B compared to Antoni Type A, given the sparse cellularity encountered in the former than the latter although this has been convincingly demonstrated and is at best controversial [125]. Whole tumor histogram analyses of the ADC values have been used to distinguish vestibular schwannomas in the cerebellopontine angle cistern and meningiomas in cases where the MRI morphology remains indeterminate. Assessment of the diffusion characteristics of extra-cranial schwannomas in the head and neck also has shown a distinct pattern of restricted diffusion in the peripheral aspect of tumors compared to a lesser impedance to diffusion in the central portion of the lesions [126].

Identifying the compressed facial nerve in cases of vestibular schwannoma is important so as to avoid complications during surgical removal. Diffusion tensor fiber tractography and its combination with contrast-enhanced high-resolution conventional (FIESTA) sequence have been used to assess the relationship of the facial and vestibular cochlear nerves in relation to large vestibular schwannomas as an adjunct for assessment of these nerves prior to surgical resection (Fig. 18.37) [127–129].

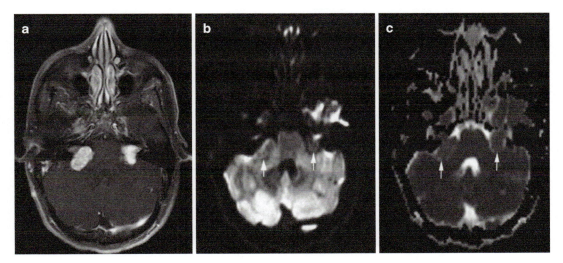

Fig. 18.36 (**a–c**) Bilateral vestibular schwannomas with neurofibromatosis type 2 in an 18-year-old male patient. (**a**) Gadolinium-enhanced T1-weighted image with fat saturation shows homogeneously enhancing masses in bilateral cerebellopontine angles. (**b, c**) DW image shows isointensity with increased ADCs (0.96–1.22 × 10^{-3} mm^2/s; *arrows*)

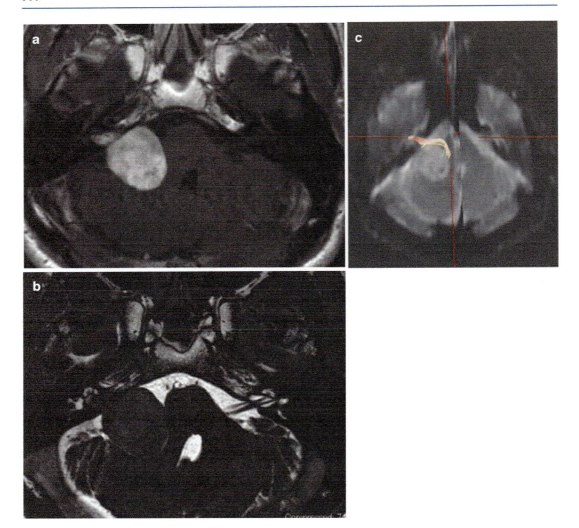

Fig. 18.37 (**a–c**) Vestibular schwannoma in a 39-year-old man. (**a**) Gadolinium-enhanced T1-weighted image shows a homogeneously enhancing mass in the right cerebellopontine angle and internal auditory canal. (**b**) CISS image cannot separate a hypointense tumor and the facial nerve. (**c**) DTI fiber tractography clearly shows the facial nerve located anterior to the vestibular schwannoma, which provides important preoperative information. (Courtesy of Dr. Toshiaki Taoka, Nagoya University, Japan)

18.7 Mesenchymal Meningothelial Tumors

18.7.1 Meningioma and Its Variants

Meningiomas are ubiquitous tumors arising from meningothelial cells and are seen throughout the intracranial compartments, within the orbits and in the spinal canal. They are rarely seen within the ventricles or in the extradural space. Meningioma is the most common extra-axial brain tumor, comprising 15% of all intracranial tumors. Histologically, 10% are atypical or malignant. Tumor recurrence is 20%–40% in atypical/malignant meningioma, while it is 5% in grade I meningioma. There are distinct histological variants of meningiomas which are grouped according to the WHO grades. Grade I meningiomas include the meningothelial (Fig. 18.38), fibrous (Fig. 18.39), transitional, psammomatous (Fig. 18.40), angiomatous, microcystic (Fig. 18.41),

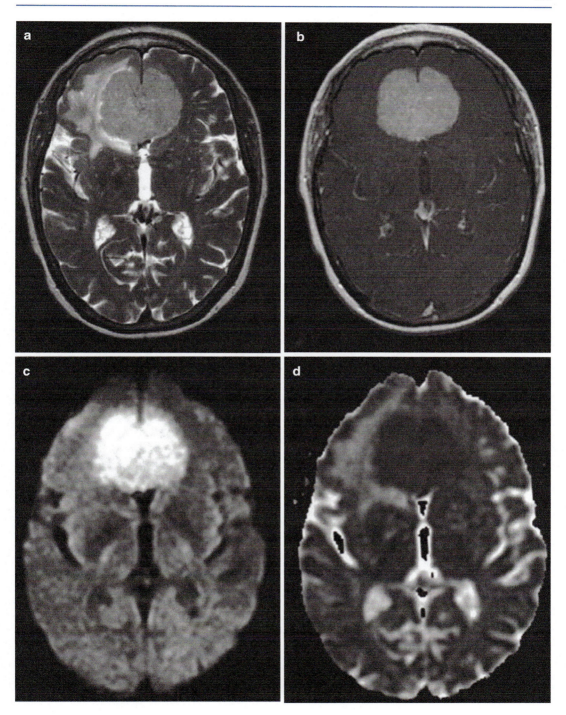

Fig. 18.38 (**a–d**) Meningothelial meningioma in a 72-year-old woman with a visual disturbance. (**a**) T2-weighted image shows a slightly hyperintense mass near the frontal aspect of the falx. (**b**) Gadolinium-enhanced T1-weighted image shows homogeneous enhancement. (**c**) DW image shows hyperintensity in the lesion. (**d**) ADC map shows mild hypointensity $(0.73–0.78 \times 10^{-3}$ mm^2/s)

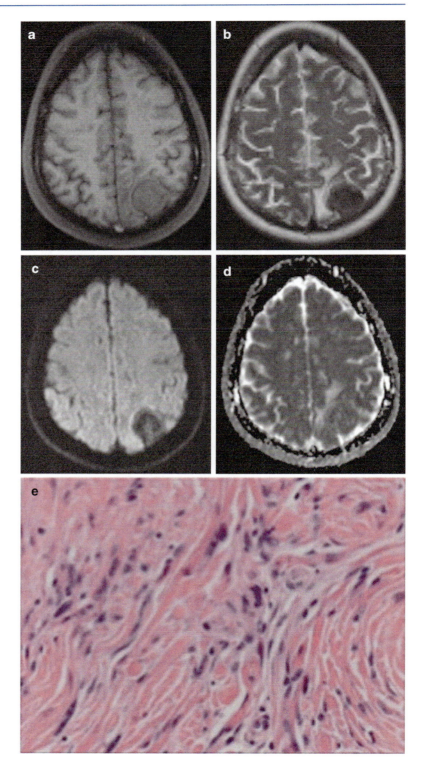

Fig. 18.39 (**a**–**e**) Fibrous meningioma in a 47-year-old woman. (**a**) T1-weighted image shows an isointense mass in the left parietal area. T2-weighted image shows a hypointense mass with vasogenic edema. (**b**, **c**) DW image shows hypointensity in the lesion (T2 dark through). (**d**) ADC map shows isointense (0.82–0.98 × 10^{-3} mm^2/s). (**e**) Pathology shows intermediate cellularity and dense fibrous extracellular matrix

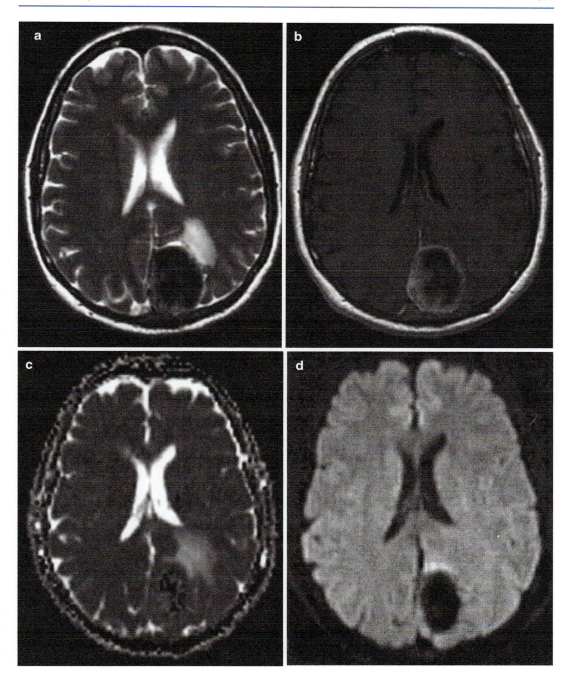

Fig. 18.40 (**a–d**) Psammomatous meningioma in a 56-year-old woman. (**a**) T2-weighted image shows a hypointense mass in the left medial occipital region with vasogenic edema. (**b**) Gadolinium-enhanced T1-weighted image also shows a dark signal mass with peripheral enhancement. (**c**) DW image shows hypointensity in the lesion (T2 blackout). (**d**) ADC map is not calculated accurately due to prominent diamagnetic susceptibility artifacts from the dense calcification

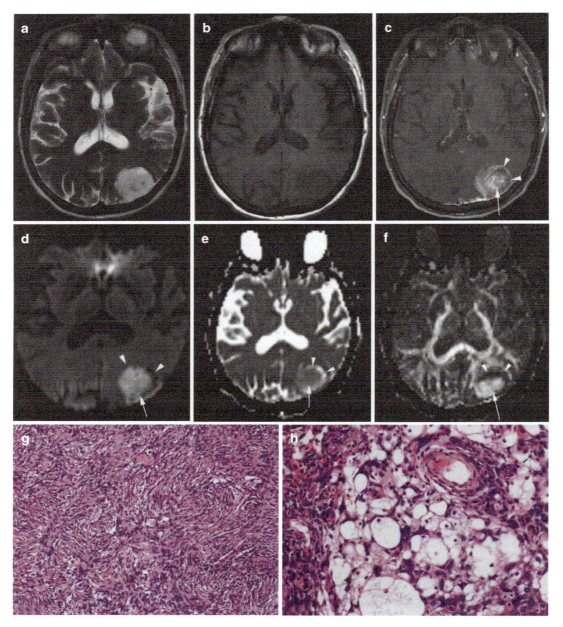

Fig. 18.41 (**a–h**) Microcystic meningioma in a 68-year-old woman. (**a**) T2-weighted image shows a hyperintense mass in the left occipital region with no vasogenic edema. (**b**) T1-weighted image shows a hypointense mass in the left occipital region. (**c**) Gadolinium-enhanced T1-weighted image with fat saturation shows a central heterogeneously enhancing mass (*arrow*) and peripheral microcystic components (*arrowheads*). (**d**) DW image shows a hypointense mass (*arrow*) with peripheral hypointensity (*arrowheads*), (**e**) ADC map shows iso- or slight hypointensity centrally (*arrow*) with peripheral hyperintensity in the microcystic components (*arrowheads*). (**f**) FA map shows increased anisotropy in the central solid portion (*arrow*) and decreased anisotropy in the peripheral microcystic areas (*arrowheads*). (**g**) Pathology of the central portion shows spindle-shaped tumor cells. (**h**) Pathology of the peripheral portion shows microcystic components

secretory, metaplastic, and lymphoplasmocyte-rich variants. Grade II meningiomas include the choroid (Fig. 18.42), clear cell, and atypical variants (Fig. 18.43). Grade III meningiomas are the papillary, rhabdoid, and anaplastic variants. Grade I meningiomas have a very low risk of recurrence or aggressive behavior whereas Grade II and grade III tumors have a high risk for recurrence and aggressive behavior as do any variant with high proliferative (Ki67) index.

Cysts associated with meningioma are seen in 4%–10% of all meningiomas [130]. There are different types of cysts associated with meningiomas. Based on Nauta classification, cysts are classified into Type I: intratumoral, Type II: peripheral, Type III: intracerebral cysts surround by glial reaction, and Type IV: evagination of arachnoid (Figs. 18.41 and 18.42). Peritumoral edema is seen in 40–60% of cases, presumably related to vasogenic edema substances such as vascular endothelial growth factor (VEGF) or vascular permeability factor with intratumoral congestion [131]. Typical MR imaging findings, including extra-axial T1 and T2 isointense solid mass with homogeneous enhancement and dural tail sign, are seen in 85% of cases. Elster AD et al. were the first to comprehensively correlate the MR imaging features to the histological type of meningiomas [132]. The signal characteristics of meningiomas on DW images are variable [20, 21, 27, 133, 134]. Most benign meningiomas are isointense on DW images and ADC maps, but some are slightly hyperintense on both DW images and ADC maps (Fig. 18.38). In meningioma, mixed histological subtypes are often observed in the same tumor. Fibroblastic, transitional, and calcified psammomatous meningioma can be hypointense on both T2-weighted [135] and DW images (Figs. 18.39 and 18.40). Microcystic meningiomas or components can be hypodense on CT images, hypointense on T1-weighted images, and hyperintense on T2-weighted images [136]. Microcystic menin-

gioma and chordoid meningioma can have high ADC values (Figs. 18.41 and 18.42). FA values in fibroblastic-type meningioma or fibrous components in meningiomas are higher than other histological subtypes presumably due to the fascicular arrangement of long spindle-shaped tumor cells [137].

Atypical and malignant meningioma usually has increased signal intensity on DW images and lower intratumoral ADC values than typical meningioma due to the higher tumor cellularity [21, 27, 91, 133, 138]. However, other factors such as multifocal areas of necrosis, numerous abnormal mitoses, and cytologic pleomorphism may also cause the high DW signal in atypical and malignant meningiomas (Fig. 18.43). The ADC values are similar in most of the histological subtypes [21, 91].

The role of diffusion imaging in the preoperative prediction of the histological grade of the tumors is at best only low to modest based on the technique using commonly used b values of 0 and 800 s/mm^2 or 1000 s/mm^2 in studies performed on 1 T systems [139] and 1.5 T systems [140]. On 3 T systems however the results are contradictory with small series reporting lower intra-tumoral FA, higher ADC, and greater proportion of spherical tensors in classic (WHO 2007 Grade1) meningiomas compared to WHO 2007 Grade 2 meningiomas. Significant inverse correlation of low minADC values and high-grade meningiomas has been reported in a series of cases performed at 3 T using b values of 4000 s/mm^2 in a retrospective study of 77 histopathological proven meningiomas [141]. An interesting application of diffusion imaging has been reported in the preoperative assessment of the consistency of meningiomas. Researchers were able to distinguish between "hard" and "soft" meningiomas based on ADC values alone or a combination of ADC values and visual analog scores derived from images of conventional MRI sequences [142, 143].

Fig. 18.42 (**a**–**e**) Chordoid meningioma in a 36-year-old woman. (**a**) Gadolinium-enhanced T1-weighted image shows a homogeneously enhancing mass with a dural tail and small type 2 and type 4 cysts in the right frontal region (*arrows*). (**b**) T2-weighted image shows a hyperintense mass with vasogenic edema. (**c**) DW image shows isointensity in the lesion (T2 washout). (**d**) ADC map shows isointense $(1.25–2.10 \times 10^{-3}\ mm^2/s)$. (**e**) Pathology shows meningothelial cells within abundant mucious extracellular matrix (Alcian blue stain)

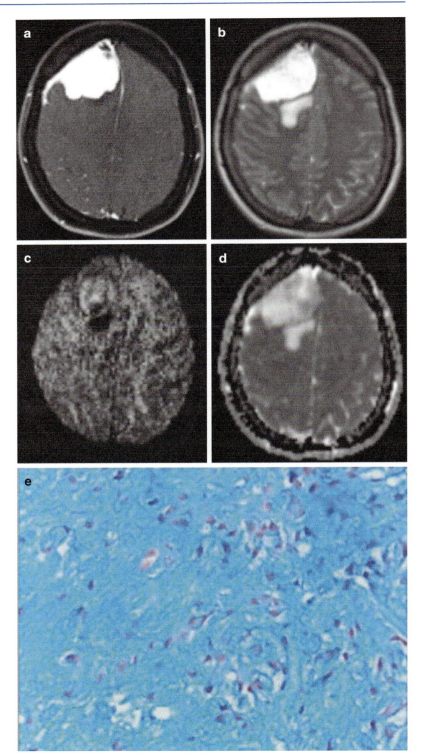

18 Brain Neoplasm

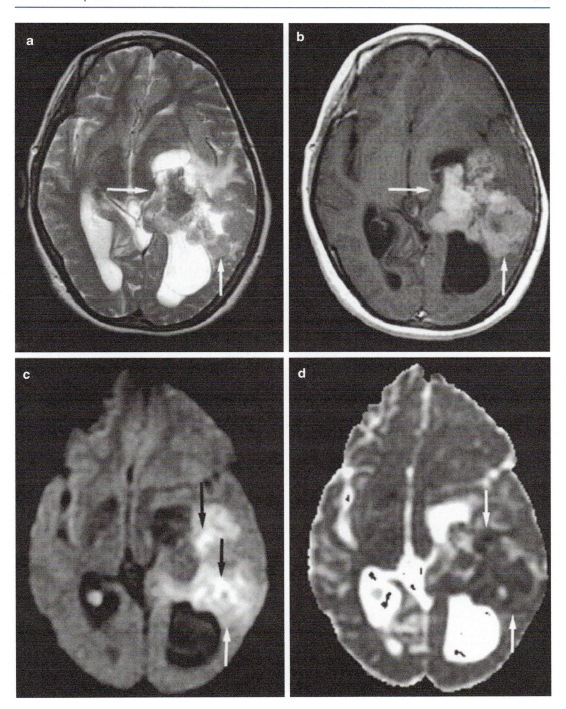

Fig. 18.43 (a–d) Atypical meningioma in a 45-year-old female patient with headache. (a) T2-weighted image shows a heterogeneous intense mass in the temporal lobe (*arrows*). (b) Gadolinium-enhanced T1-weighted image shows heterogeneous enhancement (*arrows*). (c) DW image shows heterogeneous hyperintensity (*arrows*). (d) ADC map shows hypointensity, especially in the right side of the mass (0.51×10^{-3} mm^2/s; *arrows*)

18.8 Mesenchymal Non-meningothelial Tumors

These tumors comprise a range of lesion from the benign mundane lesions (e.g., lipoma and osteoma) to the rare and aggressive (e.g., hemangiopericytoma). The low-grade (WHO grade I) lesions in this group include angiolipoma, chondroma, desmoid-type fibromatosis, hemangioblastoma, hemangioma, hibernoma, leiomyoma, lipoma, myofibroblastoma, osteochondroma, osteoma, and rhabdomyomas. Hemangiopericytomas, which can be either WHO grade I, II, or II, are now classified as variant of solitary fibrous tumor. Grade III tumors in this group include the angiosarcoma, chondrosarcoma, epithelioid hemagioendothelioma, Ewing's sarcoma, fibrosarcoma, Kaposi sarcoma, leiomyosarcoma, intracranial liposarcoma, osteosarcoma, rhabdomyosarcoma, and the undifferentiated pleomorphic sarcoma/malignant fibrous histiocytoma.

Among the benign WHO grade I tumors the best known is the intracranial lipoma. These lesions are thought to be remnants or maldevelopment of the menix premitiva [144] and the earliest of the tumors described my MR imaging [145]. These lesions are commonly seen in the pericallosal region followed by the quadrigeminal cistern, suprasellar cistern, cerebellopontine angle, Sylvian fissure, and rarely in the choroid plexus. The lesions are typically hyperintense on the T1 and T2 sequences and do not enhance following administration of gadolinium contrast. The lesions are suppressed on fat suppressed sequences. Diffusion sequences use the same chemical fat-suppression technique employed in fat-saturated T1-weighted sequences. Therefore, the lesions appear intensely hypointense on these images.

18.8.1 Hemangiopericytoma

Hemangiopericytoma was previously considered to be "angioblastic" meningiomas now been classified as a solitary fibrous tumor/hemangiopericytoma (SFT/HPC) derived from vascular pericytes based on the phenotype seen on histopathological evaluation [146]. Intracranial SFT/HPCs are rare, 2 to 4% of meningeal tumors in large series and < 1% of all intracranial tumors. The peak incidence is at 30–50 years. Men and women are roughly similarly affected. Recent genetic analysis. SFT/HPCs show NAB2-STAT6 fusion gene suggestive of true counterpart of soft tissue SFT. The SFT phenotype has been described as having a patternless architecture or short fascicular pattern of hypocellular and hypercellular areas separated by collagen bands. These tumors are Grade I lesions whereas HPCs have a phenotype of high cellularity with a rich reticulin network investing individual cells. There are typical staghorn vessels seen in both type of tumors which are considered to be pathognomonic.

CT shows mildly or moderately hyperdense, extra-axial mass with homogeneous or heterogeneous enhancement. Calcifications are not common. Underlying calvarium may show lytic bony changes but no hyperostosis like a meningioma. On conventional MRI sequences the lesions are isointense to gray matter on the T1 and T2 sequences with avid enhancement following administration of gadolinium contrast. Narrow dural-base and large deep intracranial component of the tumor are the findings to differentiate SFT/HPCs from meningiomas. DW signal characteristics are usually similar to meningioma (Fig. 18.44). The tumors share many common features with meningiomas; therefore, the chief aim of diffusion imaging has been to distinguish these lesions from the angiomatous and anaplastic meningiomas. In a single institution study performed on a 3 T magnet, it has been reported that diffusion parameter scan be employed in differentiating intracranial SFT/HPCs from meningiomas. In this study a normalized ADC (nADC) of $>1.3 \times 10^3$ mm^2/s was found to be 93% specific but with a low sensitivity of 35% in comparison to meningiomas having overlapping imaging characteristics with these tumors. On MR spectroscopy a prominent myoinositol peak with an absent alanine peak has been described [147].

18 Brain Neoplasm

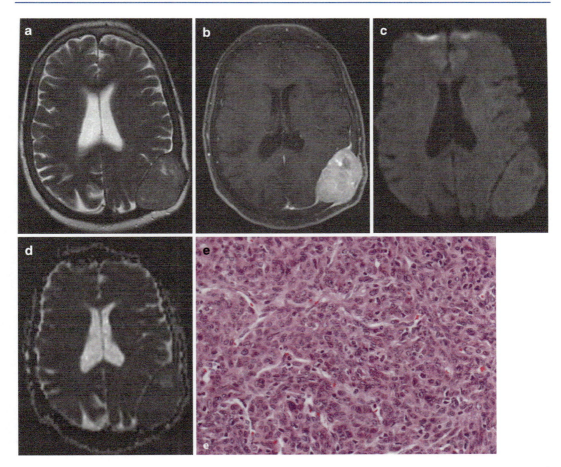

Fig. 18.44 (a–e) Hemangiopericytoma in a 50-year-old man. (**a**) T2-weighted image shows an extra-axial hyperintense mass involving the left parietal skull and scalp. (**b**) Gadolinium-enhanced T1-weighted image with fat saturation shows homogeneous enhancement with the dural tail. No adjacent hyperostosis or sclerotic changes are noted. (**c**) DW image shows mild hyperintensity. (**d**) ADC map shows decreased ADC of this mass, (**e**) micropathology specimen shows hypercellularity, dense interstitium, and dilated thin-walled vessels

18.8.2 Hemangioblastoma

Hemangioblastoma is a WHO grade I tumor which is the most common posterior fossa mass in adults of middle age, although in the overall spectrum of tumors it is relatively rare. It can occur sporadically (70%) or be an integral part of syndromes such as von Hipple Lindau disease (30%). Associations with multifocal renal cell carcinomas and pheochromocytoma have been described. Histologically, it is characterized by a network of capillary-like channels, separated by trabeculae or islands of stromal cells. On histological evaluation the tumor consists of two components: stroma cells and an abundance of vascular cells. There are two variants described: cellular and reticular based on the preponderance of either of the cell types.

The tumors are extremely vascular best demonstrated by cerebral angiography. On CT and MRI, the tumor typically consists of a cyst with a solid, enhancing mural nodule in 60% of cases, the rest appear as solid enhancing masses. Solid tumors in the posterior fossa often need to be distinguished from metastases or medullobalstomas. Vascular flow voids in and around the tumor can be a clue to the diagnosis.

DWI usually shows the solid portion of hemangioblastoma as low signal with increased ADC, presumably due to rich vascular spaces (Fig. 18.45) [80]. Metastatic renal cell carcinoma is an important differential diagnosis which is usually hyperintense on DW images with lower ADC values. A combination of ADC histogram analyses and structural imaging features has been used to achieve this goal [148]. Hemangioblastomas have a reportedly higher ADC values compared to metastases with a 90th percentile ADC of >2000 × 10^6 mm²/sec being the most sensitive value in resolving the presence of these tumors (AUC = 0.82 ($p < 0.001$)) in a study comprising 142 patients of posterior fossa lesions [148]. Further advancement by using high b values ($b = 4000$) on a 3 T imaging system compared to a lower b value ($b = 1000$) showed a positive predictive value of 100% for a cutoff value of 0.6×10^3 mm²/sec to distinguish between metastases and hemangioblastomas [149].

18.8.3 Lipoma

Lipoma is a congenital abnormality associated with persistence of the meninx primitiva. Locations of lipoma include the corpus callosum, pericallosal interhemispheric fissure, quadrigeminal plate, suprasellar cistern, cerebellopontine cistern, sylvian fissure, cerebellar vermis, and lamina terminalis. Lipoma is hyperintense on T1-weighted images, and is suppressed on fat-saturation images. DW imaging uses the same chemical fat-saturation technique as fat-saturated T1-weighted images (Fig. 18.46).

18.9 Lymphoma and Hematopoietic Neoplasm

18.9.1 Primary CNS Lymphoma

Primary CNS lymphomas are rare neoplasms and constitute approximately 2.5% of all brain tumors. The 2016 WHO classification groups primary CNS lymphomas into three broad cat-

egories. The most common histologic subtype of primary CNS lymphoma is the diffuse large B cell lymphoma (DLBCL) which accounts for approximately 95% of all primary CNS lymphomas. T-cell, NK/T-cell, low-grade B cell (MALT) lymphomas, and marginal zone B cell lymphomas constitute the rest.

Immunodeficiency-associated CNS lymphomas are the next important group of lymphomas seen in the CNS. AIDS-related diffuse B cell lymphoma, EBV-positive DLBC, lymphomatoid granulomatosis, and monomorphic or polymorphic posttransplant lymphoproliferative disorders are the representative histologically defined entities in this group. Intravascular (angiotropic) lymphomas constitute the third unique entity in the spectrum of lymphomas of the CNS.

On histopathological evaluation of the primary CNS lymphoma show masses of lymphocytes without a particular growth pattern. Extensive areas of geographical necrosis are common with frequent angiocentric/angioinvasive infiltrations. Perivascular cuffing is often seen with infiltration of the surrounding brain by the tumor cells. Rings of reticulin are seen in and around the affected vessels. Morphologically most primary CNS lymphoma is composed of mature B cells. The cells show round, oval, or irregular nuclei with distinct nucleoli. There is no genetic predisposition for primary CNS lymphoma. Unlike intracranial gliomas there are no driver mutations identified which are indicative of these tumors; however, protein changing mutations related to the CNS tumors are located on 8 specific changes including PTEN, CTNNB1, ATN, and TP53.

In the neuraxis, lymphomas are most commonly observed within the cerebral hemispheres. The lesions are often located in the periventricular white matter especially in the corpus callosum. The thalami and basal ganglia are the next common locations. Tumor spread along the ventricular ependyma is common as is the involvement of the choroid plexus. Approximately 15% of the cases primarily involve the cerebellum or the spinal cord. Ocular involvement is also noteworthy.

Classical descriptor for primary CNS lymphoma on CT is a hyperdense enhancing mass

18 Brain Neoplasm

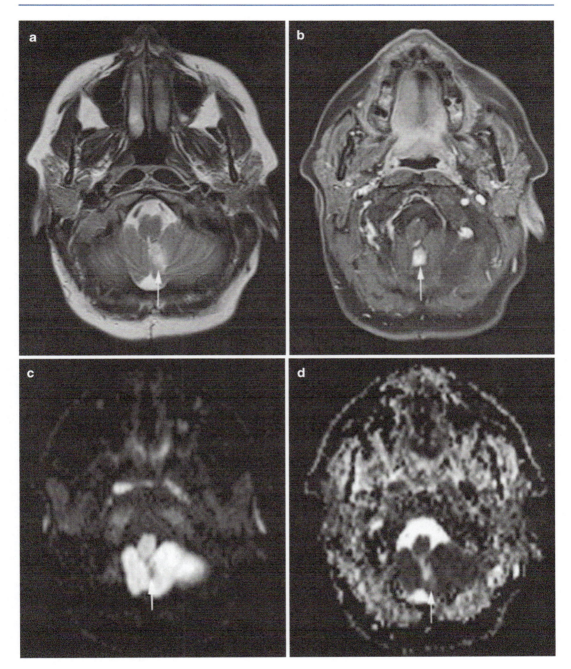

Fig. 18.45 (**a–d**) Hemangioblastoma in a 41-year-old woman. (**a**) T2-weighted image shows a hyperintense mass in the cerebellar vermis (*arrow*). (**b**) Gadolinium-enhanced T1-weighted image with fat saturation shows intense homogeneous enhancement (*arrow*). (**c**) DW image shows hyperintensity of the lesion (*arrow*). (**d**) ADC map shows increased ADC of the lesion presumably due to rich vascular spaces (*arrow*)

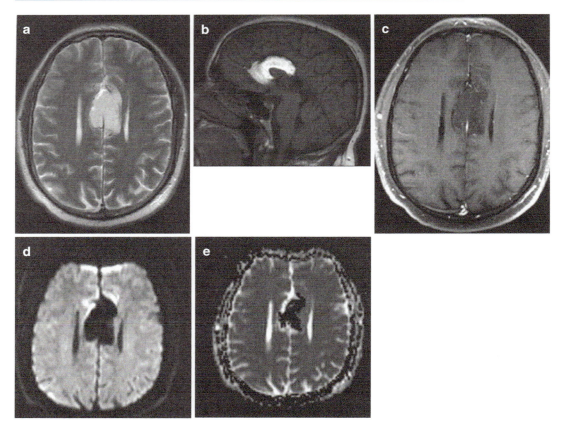

Fig. 18.46 (a–e) Lipoma in a 43-year-old woman, (**a**) T2-weighted image shows a hyperintense mass in the corpus callosum. (**b**) Sagittal T1-weighted image shows a well-demarcated very hyperintense mass along the corpus callosum. (**c**) Gadolinium-enhanced T1-weighted image with fat saturation shows a suppression of T1 hyperintensity of fat signals with no enhancement. (**d**) DW image shows the lipoma as hypointense due to the inherent fat saturation. (**e**) Accurate calculation of ADC values is difficult because of the fat saturation on both the DW and b0 images

within the basal ganglia or in the periventricular white matter. Primary CNS lymphoma appear iso- to slightly hypointense to gray matter on conventional T1-weighted images. They are isointense on the T2-weighted and FLAIR images. Following administration of intravenous contrast tumors show uniform solid homogenous or mildly heterogeneous enhancement. In immunosuppressed patients a rim enhancement is a more common finding, which is associated with angioinvasive distribution of lymphoma cells [27, 150–152]. If there are microhemorrhages, they show typical susceptibility blooming on the GRE/T2 star sequences. Gross hemorrhages are uncommon. MR spectroscopy often demonstrates typical elevated choline and high lipid peaks.

Given their high cellularity, 95% of the primary CNS lymphoma show impeded diffusion with iso to low ADC values [153, 154]. The enhancing components of lymphomas are generally hyperintense on DW images (Figs. 18.47 and 18.48) [25, 27, 155]. The ADC of lymphomas is

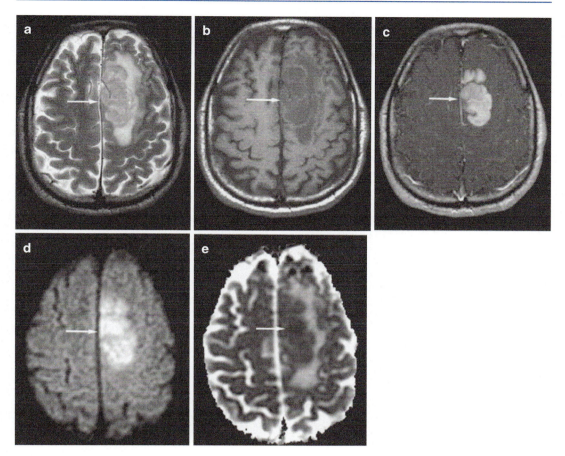

Fig. 18.47 (a–e) Lymphoma (diffuse large B cell type) in a 64-year-old male patient with seizure. (**a**) T2-weighted image shows a slightly hyperintense mass (*arrow*) with surrounding edema in the left frontal lobe. (**b**) T1-weighted image shows the hypointense mass (*arrow*) in the left fron- tal lobe. (**c**) Gadolinium-enhanced T1-weighted image shows the heterogeneously enhancing mass (*arrow*) in the left frontal lobe. (**d**) DW image shows hyperintensity in the lesion (*arrow*). (**e**) ADC map shows hypointensity in the lesion (0.51–0.71 × 10^{-3} mm^2/s; *arrow*)

often lower than that in high-grade gliomas [25]. As mentioned above, this corresponds to the hypercellularity and might help in differentiating between lymphomas and high-grade gliomas.

ADC estimations in the solid enhancing masses are in the periphery of rim-enhancing lesions and have ranged widely from approximately 0.167 to 1.067 × 10^3/mm^2/sec. Variations in the ADC values described in the literature arise from variations in the ADC parameters (mean ADC, minimum ADC and the 25th percentile ADC values) and also in the technique of placement of the region of interest, e.g., in the solid-appearing portions of the tumor versus averaged ADC values across entire sections of tumors regardless of tumor morphology. Comparisons have been made between the mean ADC values of the peritumoral region, the central portion of the lesion, and the contralateral normal-appearing white matter with ambiguous results [156].

Applications of diffusion techniques in recent times have been focused on the utility of diffusion techniques in differentiating primary CNS lymphoma from glioblastoma and metastases which are common in the age group patients where these tumors are generally encountered. In those instances where these tumors present as a solitary enhancing mass, the current literature

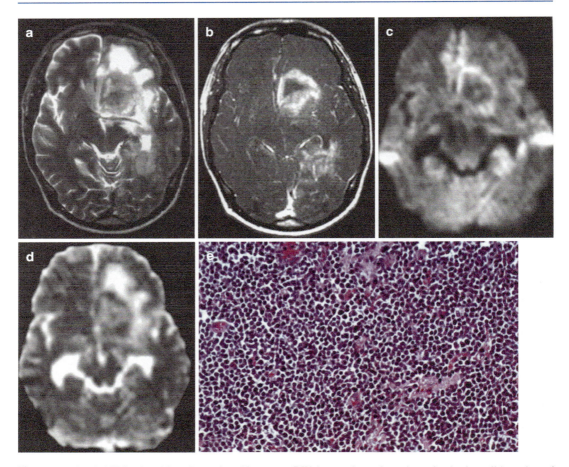

Fig. 18.48 (**a–e**) AIDS-related lymphoma in a 23-year-old man. (**a**) T2-weighted image shows iso- or mildly hyperintense masses in the left periventricular region with vasogenic edema. (**b**) Gadolinium-enhanced T1-weighted image shows ring or heterogeneous enhancement. (**c**) DW image shows hyperintensity in the solid portion of the lesions. (**d**) ADC map shows partially decreased ADC of the solid portion of the mass. (**e**) Pathology shows a diffuse infiltrate of fairly uniform, large cells with little cytoplasm

favors a multiparametric approach for resolving these differential diagnoses [157, 158]. The rCBV and ADC values were significantly lower in lymphomas compared to glioblastomas in both studies.

A combination of demographics, conventional MRI appearances, and diffusion/perfusion-weighted sequence has been applied to differentiate lymphomas in immunocompetent and immunocompromised individuals [159]. PCNSL associated with AIDS presents as multiple lesions in a younger age group of patient. Lesions are associated with confluent areas of necrosis with hemorrhage. Most lesions present as mildly enhanced ring lesions, the central core showing no enhancement. This morphology is shared by toxoplasmosis and progressive multifocal leukoencephalopathy both of which can coexist with lymphoma in this subset of patients. Application of diffusion-weighted imaging techniques has been reported with toxoplasmosis exhibiting a significantly higher diffusion than lymphoma. A proposed mean ADC ratio of 1.63 ± 0.41 was considered to be consistent with toxoplasmosis compared to 1.14 ± 0.25 for lymphoma in this study [160]. Although this ratio was replicated, it was considered to be relatively low specificity, with an overlap of a range of values for both conditions [161].

18.9.2 Posttransplant Lymphoproliferative Disorder (PTLD)

PTLD is the third most common disorder encountered in clinical practice in patients receiving transplants affecting the CNS [162]. CNS-PTLD is seen in the brain of 2–7% of posttransplant patients in autopsy series. The vast majority of CNS lesions comprise monomorphic B cells similar to PCNSL. Imaging morphology of lesions resembles those seen in AIDS-related CNS lymphoma with multifocal masses with central areas of necrosis. Transmural invasion of blood vessel walls by tumor cells (anigiocenteric/angioinvasive) and necrosis are common features. Polymorphic PTLD and PTLD associated with plasmacytic hyperplasia are reportedly less common in the CNS compared to the periphery.

Imaging features of these lesions include multifocal ring-enhancing masses. Multiple necrotic ring-enhancing lesions are the most common findings on CT and MR imaging. DW images show hypointensity in the central core necrosis of the lesions with relative hyperintense signals in the enhancing rims of the lesions (Fig. 18.49).

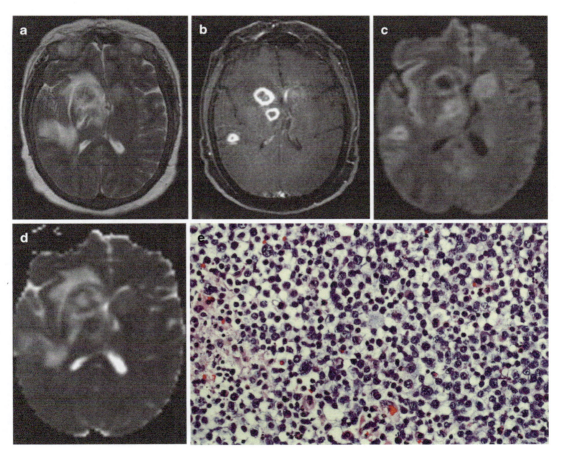

Fig. 18.49 (**a**–**e**) Posttransplant lymphoproliferative disease in a 54-year-old man after renal transplantation. (**a**) T2-weighted image shows iso- or mildly hyperintense masses in the left periventricular region with vasogenic edema. (**b**) Gadolinium-enhanced T1-weighted image shows ring or heterogeneous enhancement. (**c**) DW image shows hyperintense in the ring-enhancing solid portion and hypointense in the central necrosis. (**d**) ADC map shows partially decreased ADC of the solid portion of the mass. (**e**) Pathology shows a hypercellular mixed lymphoid infiltrate with mitosis and nuclear pleomorphism. (Courtesy of Sergei S MD, PhD, Department of Pathology, The University of Iowa Hospitals and Clinics, USA)

DW imaging has also been used for assessment response to treatment and to differentiate monomorphic B cell posttransplant lymphoproliferative disorder with primary B cell CNS lymphoma. In a series of pathology-proven monomorphic posttransplant lymphoproliferative disease, the reported pretreatment ADC values and ratios were 0.892×10^{-3} mm²/s (standard deviation 0.082×10^{-3} mm²/sec) and 1.19 (standard deviation of 0.15) compared to 0.721×10^{-3} mm²/s (standard deviation 0.0939×10^{-3} mm²/s) [163].

18.9.3 Histiocytic Tumors

Histiocytic tumors result from aggregated proliferation of Langerhans-type of cells which are characterized by expression of langerin (CD207) CD1a and S100 protein. The biological behavior of these multisystem tumors is variable; however, they are considered to be a malignancy. No WHO grade has been assigned to these tumors. The quintessential condition for this subset of hematopoietic tumors is Langerhans cell histiocytosis (LCH) which is a multisystem disease. The disease is primarily seen in children. Isolated involvement of the CNS is rare in this condition. The hallmark involvement of the skeletal system including the calvarium, spine, and the appendicular skeleton is well known. The CNS-specific osseous lesions include well-circumscribed lytic lesions without a sclerotic margin within the calvarium and a vertebra plana in the spine. Involvement of the skull base with and without soft tissue extension has been described. Intracranial extra-axial masses involving the hypothalamic pituitary region, meningitis, and choroid plexus are well known. There is a leukoencephalopathy-like pattern without involvement of the dental nucleus or basal ganglia. Isolated intraparenchymal involvement of the cerebral hemispheres is fair. Three distinct clinical presentations have been described including diabetes insipidus, neurodegeneration characterized by psychomotor degeneration and ataxia together with obstructive hydrocephalus [164]. Conventional MR images show correlative features for each of these clinical manifestations. Absence of the posterior pitu-

itary hyperintense signals on the T1-weighted images and the thickened enhanced appearance of its infundibulum. Lesions which are most commonly associated with neurodegeneration include symmetric appearing signal alterations within the dentate nucleus on the basal ganglia. Images are reportedly hyperintense on the T1-weighted sequence with variable signal alterations on the T2-weighted sequence. Later in the disease process, the lesions appear to be T2 hyperintense [165].

The diagnosis of LCH is primarily based on conventional CT and MRI imaging techniques. The role of diffusion imaging is limited. There are isolated reports of application of diffusion techniques in distinguishing the osseous lesions associated with this condition from other benign and malignant known processes, including LCH. It has been reported that lesions of Langerhans cell histiocytosis exhibit a range of ADC values from 0.96–1.55 with a mean value of 1.29 ± 0.18. In this study, the ADC cutoff value of more than or equal to 1.1×10^{-3} mm² per second was considered to be an exclusion criterion for malignant bone disease with a sensitivity of 89.7% and a specificity of 84.5% together with the positive predictive value of 82.6% and a negative predictive value of 95.3% [166].

The other important histiocytic tumors which affect the CNS include Erdheim-Chester disease, Rosai-Dorfman disease, and juvenile xanthogranuloma. Erdheim-Chester disease is a disease of middle age adults presenting with dural or parenchymal lesions. The extra-axial dural lesions may resemble meningiomas on imaging. The intraparenchymal lesions appear to be infiltrative enhancing lesions. Rosai-Dorfman disease is principally a disease of young adults and is characterized by solitary or multiple dural masses especially over the cerebral convexity, cranial base with involvement of the cavernous sinuses. The disease commonly involves lymph nodes. Occasional reports indicate involvement of the cerebral parenchyma or lesions within the sella. Juvenile xanthogranuloma is primarily a disease of young children and the lesions are localized to the brain or the spine. Involvement of the spinal nerve roots has also been described.

The malignant counterpart of histiocytic tumors is histiocytic sarcoma which is a rare, aggressive malignancy involving the brain parenchyma and the dura matter. The scope of diffusion-weighted imaging is limited in these conditions.

18.9.4 CNS Manifestations of Leukemia

The CNS manifestations of leukemia include a spectrum of disorders involving meninges as well as the parenchyma. Acute lymphoblastic leukemia accounts for nearly 80% of cases followed by acute myeloid leukemia with 20% of cases. Chronic myelocytic leukemia and chronic lymphocytic leukemia are primarily diseases of adults. The characteristic CNS lesion of leukemia is a localized mass containing primitive myeloblasts, promyelocytes, or myelocytes which was in the past termed as chloromas. The term chloroma was descriptive for the greenish tinge to these tumors on gross inspection, secondary to high levels of myeloperoxidase in the immature cells within these lesions. Not all of these tumors are green in color given that approximately 30% of the cells do not contain myeloperoxidase and may appear as tan, gray, or white-colored lesions. The term chloroma therefore has been abandoned and replaced by the term granulocytic (myeloid) sarcoma [167]. Granulocytic sarcoma can also be associated with other myeloproliferative disorders such as myelofibrosis with myeloid metaplasia, hypereosinophilic syndrome, or polycythemia vera [168, 169].

In the setting of leukemia granulocytic sarcoma represent focal tumor-like masses of the disease process as opposed to meningeal disease dominant as "carcinomatous meningitis" and diffuse intracranial intravascular tumor aggregates termed as "carcinomatous encephalitis."

Leukemic cells predominantly involve the orbits, paranasal sinuses, calvarium, and skull base. Parenchymal involvement is rare. However, leukemic cells in the bone marrow of the cranium invades traversing Haversian canals through the periosteum, dura and subarachnoid spaces through the arachnoidal vein, and breached pial-glial barrier, which results in the encephalitic and meningitic forms of the disease. Multifocal involvement is the norm. The lesions appear as focal isoechoic to slightly hypointense T1 and hyperintense T2 mass like lesions showing homogenous intense enhancement. Lesions restricted diffusion and appear to be hypointense on the ADC maps and hyperintense on the DWI sequence (Fig. 18.50) [170, 171]. DW techniques and morphological features have also been employed to assess treatment response in these tumors. Comparisons of mean, minimum, and

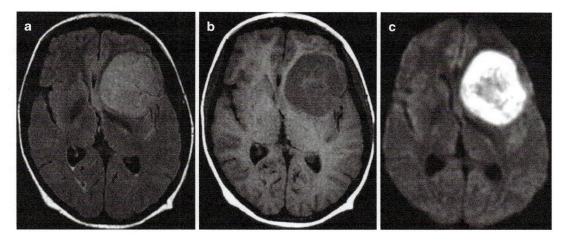

Fig. 18.50 (a–c) Granulocytic sarcoma in a 42-year-old man with acute myelogenous leukemia. (a) FLAIR image shows a mildly hyperintense mass in the left frontal region. (b) T1-weighted image shows a hypointense mass, (c) DW image shows a markedly hyperintense mass with decreased ADC (not shown)

maximum ADC values of these tumors have been reported to be significantly lower than that of normal brain. Together with arterial spin labelling and conventional sequences, diffusion-weighted sequences were reportedly helpful in the assessment and prediction of treatment response [172].

18.10 Germ Cell Tumor

Germ cell tumors of the central nervous system include the following entities: germinoma, embryonal carcinoma, yolk sac tumor, choriocarcinoma, teratoma, and mixed germ cell tumor. Germinomas are by far the most common tumors encountered in this group; therefore, for the sake of convenience the tumors are sometimes classified as germinomas and non-germinomatous germ cell tumors [173]. These tumors are commonly encountered in the pediatric age group and are frequently encountered in eastern Asian populations. An incidence ranging from 0.3% to 15% of pediatric cases has been described in the literature. These tumors have a predilection for prepubertal males and are localized to diencephalic centers regulating gonadal activity with a reported increased incidence in Klinefelter syndrome. This suggests that the development of these tumors is related to increased circulating gonadotropin levels. The most commonly used markers for detection of these tumors include alpha fetoproteins and human chorionic gonadotropin which serve as useful biomarkers along with imaging features to differentiate the subtypes of theses group of tumors [174]. The most common site for these tumors is the pineal gland followed by suprasellar region (pituitary infundibulum and neurohypophysis). Pineal and neurohypophyseal synchronous occurrence has been reported. Other locations include the intraventricular/periventricular regions, thalamostriate, bulbar intrasellar, intramedullary and bulbar locations. Cerebral hemispheric and congenital holocranial tumors have also been described [175]. Preoperative characterization of germ cell tumors by conventional imaging is a challenge.

Germ cell tumors typically present as solid contrast-enhanced masses on CT and MR studies.

Germinomas are thought to enhance more homogenously than other subtypes [176]. Germinomas are iso- to hypointense on T1-weighted images and iso-hyperintense on T2-weighted images. Calcification and cysts are common in the tumors, especially at the thalamic and basal ganglia locations. Teratomas are characteristically identified by the presence of fat, calcifications, and cysts. Hemorrhage is seen in choriocarcinoma but is rarely in germinoma. Congenital teratomas can be diagnosed by ultrasound or by fetal MRI techniques [177].

The solid portions of the tumors exhibit restricted diffusion possibly reflecting the hypercellularity of these tumors. DWI has been employed to aid in the differential diagnosis of these lesions. In a Study by Wu C-C, it was reported that mean ADC values ($\times 10^{-3}$ mm2/s) were significantly lower in germinomas (1.113 ± 0.415) than in NGGCTs (2.011 ± 0.694, $P = 0.001$). Combined a lack of T1 hyperintense foci and a mean ADC threshold value (1.143×10^{-3} mm2/s) had the highest specificity (91.3%) and positive predictive value (92.3%), while the combination of lack of a T1 hyperintense foci, no/mild enhancement, and a mean ADC threshold value had 100% sensitivity and 100% negative-predictive value for discriminating germinomas from NGGCTs [178]. Ipsilateral cerebral, brain stem, and basal ganglia atrophy has been reported in patients with basal ganglia germinoma, probably due to tumor involvement of fiber tracts and secondary Wallerian, retrograde, and transsynaptic degenerations [179–181]. DW imaging shows the solid portion as hyperintense with decreased ADC probably due to the hypercellularity (Fig. 18.51).

18.11 Epidermoid Cysts and Arachnoid Cysts

18.11.1 Epidermoid Cyst

Epidermoid cysts are benign neoplasms of ectodermal origin with stratified squamous epithelium and keratinaceous debris [22, 182–189]. Intracranial epidermoid cysts are relatively common congenital lesions which are present

18 Brain Neoplasm

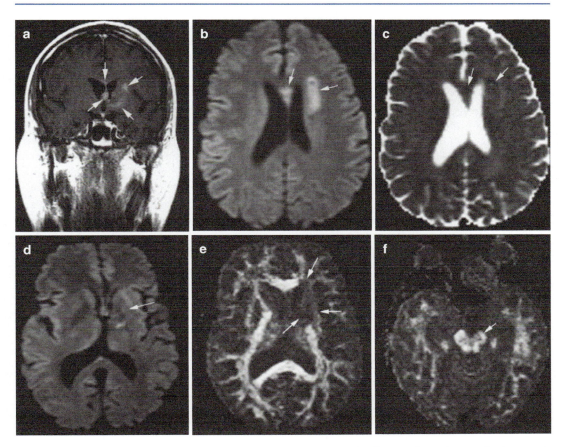

Fig. 18.51 (**a–f**) Germinoma in a 32-year-old man. (**a**) Gadolinium-enhanced coronal T1-weighted image shows enhancing lesions in the left basal ganglia, septum pellucidum, and corpus callosum (*arrows*). (**b, c**) DW image shows hyperintensity in the lesions with decreased ADC (*arrows*). (**d**) The left basal ganglia appears atrophic (*arrow*) compared to the other side, presumably due to the tumor involvement of fiber tracts and secondary degeneration. (**e**) FA map shows decreased anisotropy in the anterior limb and genu of internal capsules (*arrows*). Corticostriatal fibers (external capsule, subcallosal fasciculus of Muratoff) may also be involved (*arrows*). (**f**) Fractional anisotropy in the left cerebral peduncle is decreased, which represents Wallerian degeneration (*arrow*)

as extra-axial masses and are located preferentially within the basal cisterns. The lesions are believed to arise from inclusions of ectodermal elements (epiblasts) during neural tube closure [190]. Congenital cerebellopontine angle epidermoid cysts are thought to arise from the first branchial cleft. They are commonly encountered in the second to the fourth decades with a relative increased prevalence in males. They are slow-growing tumors and have a typical frond-like morphology. They have a propensity to grow around the cranial nerves especially within the cisterns of the posterior fossa. Therefore, the presenting symptoms include headaches, cranial nerve deficits, seizures, and cerebellar symptoms. They are similar in histology to cholesteatomas encountered in the middle ear and petrous apex. They are differentiated from dermoid cysts by the lack of skin appendages, and from teratomas which have representation of endoderm, ectoderm, and mesodermal elements. They are encapsulated lesions with a thin layer of squamous epithelium and may exhibit lobulated or nodular margins. Macroscopically they appear as pearly white masses containing cystic components which are filled with desquamated, flaky keratin ("dry" keratin), cholesterol crystals, and lined with stratified squamous epithelium.

On CT studies, the tumors have nearly identical attenuation values to CSF and do not enhance. On MR studies, they are indistinguishable from an arachnoid cyst or dilated CSF spaces with uniform appearing T1 hypointense signals and T2 hyperintense signals. On the FLAIR sequences they are inhomogeneously hyperintense relative to CSF [191].

DW imaging is highly sensitive in detecting intracranial epidermoids. The distinguishing feature of these lesions is on DW sequences where they show hyperintense signals on the DW images. The ADC values of these tumors are lower than that of CSF and equal to or higher than that of the brain parenchyma (Figs. 18.52 and 18.53) [182–184, 186–189, 192]. Therefore, the hyperintense signals on the DW images are associated with a T2 shine-through effect [193]. DW imaging is therefore very important in delineating residual tumor on postsurgical evaluation. The margins of the tumor are very well defined on these sequences and are helpful in determining plane of cleavage from the surrounding vital brain structures. Diffusion tensor imaging may show increased anisotropy on the FA maps.

18.11.2 Arachnoid Cyst

Arachnoid cysts are similar in signal characteristics to an epidermoid cyst on conventional MR sequences. Therefore, they are an important differential diagnosis for epidermoid cysts. There are also termed as meningeal cysts because they arise from the congenital cleavage of the arachnoid membrane resulting in loculation of the CSF within the potential space created by this cleavage. The common sites of arachnoid cysts include the suprasellar cistern, within the posterior fossa, within the ventricles, and in the spinal subarachnoid space. The cysts are slow-growing lesions and are often discovered incidentally. They appear as well-demarcated, featureless lesions especially in the posterior fossa, without a clear discernable limiting membrane. The signal intensity of these cysts is similar to CSF. All cysts are hypointense on the T1-weighted sequence and hyperintense on the T2-weighted sequence. They

do not show hyperintense signals on the DWI which is the differentiating feature from epidermoid cysts which also arise at locations similar to an arachnoid cyst (Fig. 18.54) [190].

18.12 Tumors of the Sellar Region

The 2016 WHO classification recognizes the following primary tumors of the sellar region: craniopharyngioma, granular cell tumor of the sellar region, pituicytoma, and spindle cell oncocytoma. Additionally, the WHO released a new classification of pituitary adenomas in 2017 [194]. In this section we will primarily review the applications for diffusion imaging related to craniopharyngioma and pituitary adenomas.

18.12.1 Craniopharyngioma

Craniopharyngiomas are benign sellar tumors, comprising 3% of all intracranial tumors, which arise from the remnants of the Rathke's pouch epithelium along the craniopharyngeal duct. Pathologically, squamoid foci can be seen and the pattern of keratinization with ghostlike nests of keratinocytes is known as "wet" keratin, in contrast to "dry" keratin seen in epidermoid cysts. Microscopic finger-like extensions into surrounding tissue are common. There are 2 clinical pathological varieties of the tumor, namely the adamantinomatous and papillary variety. The adamantinomatous variety of the tumor has a bimodal distribution; it is seen in children between the ages of 5 and 15 years and in adults in the age range of 45–60 years. The papillary craniopharyngioma is primarily seen in adults, in the age range of 40–55 years. The craniopharyngioma is primarily a suprasellar tumor with no apparent extension into the sella. Ectopic locations include the sphenoid sinus, the cerebellopontine angle cistern, and within the third ventricle. These tumors present as lobulated masses within both cystic and solid components.

The solid components of the tumor enhance both on CT and MR studies as do the walls of the cystic component. Calcification is present in the solid portions of the adamantinomatous vari-

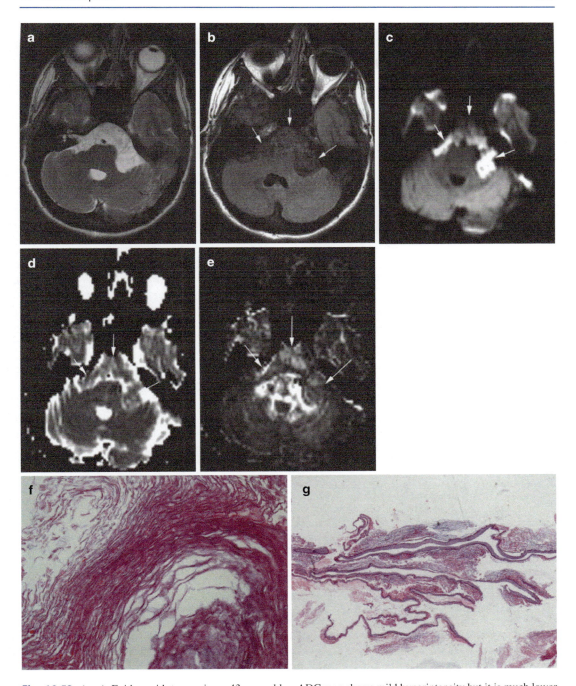

Fig. 18.52 (**a–g**) Epidermoid tumor in a 43-year-old woman. (**a**) T2-weighted image shows hyperintensity in the cerebellopontine angles and the prepontine cistern. (**b**) FLAIR image shows these areas as inhomogeneously hyperintense relative to the cerebrospinal fluid (*arrows*). (**c**) DW image shows hyperintensity in the lesions. (**d**) ADC map shows mild hyperintensity but it is much lower than that of the CSF (*arrows*). (**e**) FA map shows increased anisotropy in the lesions (*arrows*). (**f**, **g**) Pathology specimen shows keratinaceous materials (**f**) and stratified squamous epithelium (**g**)

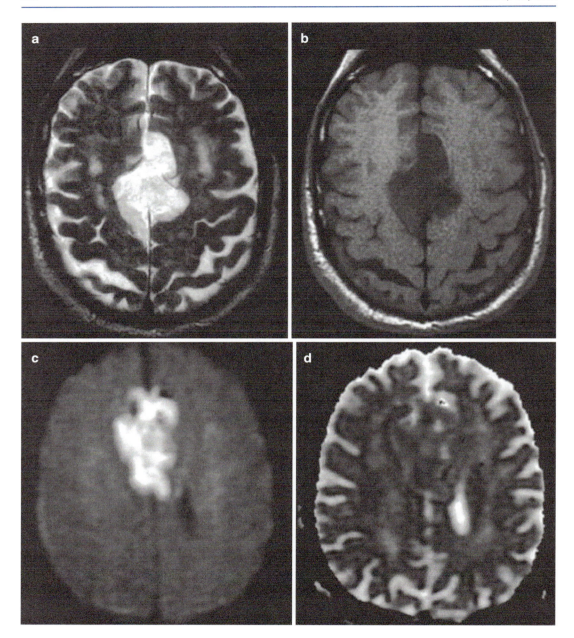

Fig. 18.53 (a–d) Epidermoid tumor in a 9-year-old girl without symptoms. (**a**) T2-weighted image shows a hyperintense mass near the falx. (**b**) T1-weighted image shows the hypointense lesion. (**c**) DW image shows hyperintensity in the lesion, which is caused by both increased T2 and restricted diffusivity. (**d**) ADC map shows heterogeneous iso- or hypointensity in the lesion, consistent with restricted diffusion similar to that of the brain parenchyma

ants of the tumor. The papillary variant does not show calcification and is commonly solid with no cystic component. The adamantinomatous variant shows infiltration of the surrounding brain structures and are noted to encase the vessels and nerves in the vicinity of the tumor. Dissemination of the tumor via the subarachnoid space or implantation along the surgical track is also encountered. On conventional MR sequences, the cystic component of the craniopharyngioma

18 Brain Neoplasm

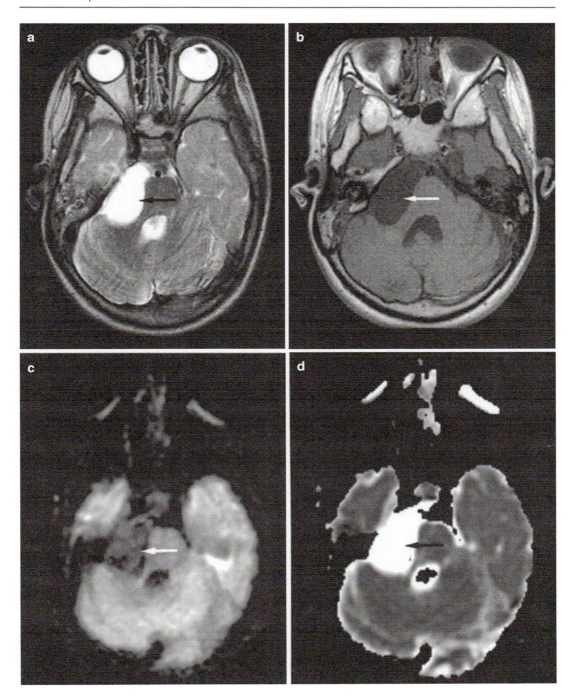

Fig. 18.54 (**a–d**) Arachnoid cyst in a 9-year-old girl with developmental delay. (**a**) T2-weighted image shows a large hyperintense lesion in the right cerebellopontine angle (*arrow*). (**b**) T1-weighted image shows hypointensity in the lesion (*arrow*). (**c**) DW image shows hypointensity (*arrow*). (**d**) ADC map shows hyperintensity in the lesion due to increased diffusivity (3.07–3.12 × 10^{-3} mm^2/s; *arrow*)

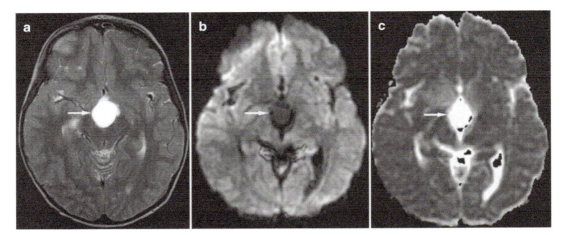

Fig. 18.55 (a–c) Craniopharyngioma in an 8-year-old boy with panhypopituitarism. (a) T2-weighted image shows a hyperintense mass (*arrow*) in the suprasellar region. (b) DW image shows hypointensity in the mass (*arrow*). (c) ADC map shows hyperintensity (2.25–2.38 × 10^{-3} mm^2/s; *arrow*)

is T1 hyperintense or hypointense and T2 hyperintense. This signal alteration is possibly dependent on the protein content of the fluid [195]. MR imaging shows the cystic components of craniopharyngioma as T1 hyper- or hypointense and T2 hyperintense, probably depending on the protein concentrations (4000–12,000 mg/dl) [195].

DW imaging usually shows a hypointense mass lesion with increased ADC (Fig. 18.55). Sener et al. reported hyperintensity on DW images, with increased ADC, corresponding to an increased diffusivity in the tumor and a T2 shine-through effect [196]. Variations of signal intensity have been described; Sener et al. reported hyperintensity on the DW images with increased ADC corresponding to an infused to facility in the tumor and a T2 shine-through effect in a large suprasellar craniopharyngioma. The study was carried out on a 1.5 T unit with a b value of 1000 mm^2/sec. The tumor was hyperintense on the diffusion sequence and had shown a high ADC value compared to the normal cerebellar parenchyma [196].

18.12.2 Rathke's Cleft Cyst

Rathke's cleft cyst are benign epithelial filled intrasellar cysts arising from the remnants of the Rathke's pouch. MR imaging shows various signals in Rathke's cleft cysts depending on the protein concentration [195]. The intensity can vary depending on the protein content in the cyst fluid. T1 hypo- and T2 hyperintense cysts contain CSF-like fluids. T1 hyper- and T2 hypointense cysts contain creamy yellow or white gelatinous fluid. Fluids with a protein concentration of more than 8000 mg/dL appear hyperintense on T1-weighted sequences whereas cysts containing more than 15,000 mg/dL exhibit T2 hypointense signals. DW sequences have also been employed to differentiate craniopharyngiomas from other lesions commonly seen in the suprasellar cyst region, namely Rathke's cleft cyst and germ cell tumors. The cysts do not impede diffusion and appear hypointense on DWI [195]. DW imaging usually shows a hypointense lesion (Fig. 18.56) [197].

18 Brain Neoplasm

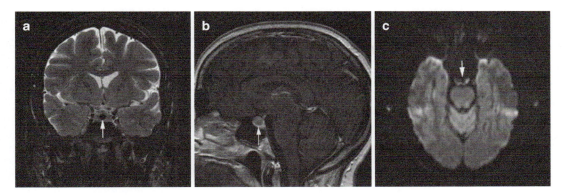

Fig. 18.56 (a–c) Rathke's cleft cyst in a 35-year-old woman. (a) Coronal T2-weighted image with fat saturation shows a hypointense lesion in the pituitary gland (*arrow*). (b) Post-contrast sagittal T1-weighted image shows a non-enhancing hyperintense lesion in the pituitary fossa (*arrow*). (c) DW image shows hypointensity in the lesion (*arrow*)

18.12.3 Germ Cell Tumor

Germ cell tumors arising in the suprasellar cistern may present as a diagnostic challenge since they share similar MRI demographic and morphological features as craniopharyngiomas. An attempt has been made to distinguish the two lesions based on diffusion techniques.

ADCs have been used to distinguish between craniopharyngiomas and germ cell tumors in the suprasellar lesion. Studies performed on both lower and high b values (1000 and 4000 s/mm^2) on 3 Tesla unit revealed that craniopharyngioma showed lower signal intensity on the DWI at $b = 1000$ and $b = 4000$ than in germ cell tumors. They showed high ADC values in comparisons to germ cell tumors on the logistic discriminant analysis which found the ADCmin at 4000 s/mm^2 was the best discriminator to differentiate between the two tumors [198].

18.12.4 Pituitary Adenoma

Pituitary adenomas account for 10–15% of all intracranial tumors, being five times more common than craniopharyngioma and Rathke's cleft cysts. Pituitary adenomas and benign tumors of the adenohypophyses are traditionally classified as tumors of endocrine organs under the WHO classification. The revised classification by the WHO in 2017 is more focused on the cell lineage of the adenohypophysis and immunohistochemical markers such as transcription factors. Three main pathways have been described: (1) corticotrophs determined by the t-box pituitary transcription factor (Tpit); (2) somatotrophs/lactotroph/mammosomatotroph/thyrotrophs determined by the pituitary transcriptions factor 1 (Pit-1), and (3) gonadotrophs determined by steroidogenic Factor-1 (SF-1) and/or GATA-2 in the presence of Estrogen Receptor-α [194, 199, 200]. In the present system of classification, pituitary adenomas are classified as Grade 0 with the rare malignant pituitary carcinomas and pituitary blastomas labelled as Grade 3. The term atypical adenoma is no longer included together with a lowered emphasis on the correlation of tumor behavior based on Ki67 and mitotic indices.

Pituitary adenomas are primarily intrasellar tumors and have long been classified as microadenomas which are less than 10 mm and macroadenomas which are larger than 1 cm. They can occur sporadically as well as constituents of syndromes such as MEN1, MaCune-Albright syndrome, and familial isolated pituitary adenomas (FIPA) syndrome.

On conventional MRI sequences macroadenomas are isointense to gray matter on T1- and T2-weighted images. All macroadenomas are solid masses. In cases of pituitary apoplexy, the signal alterations are altered due to the contained hemorrhage. Fluid–fluid levels can be identified

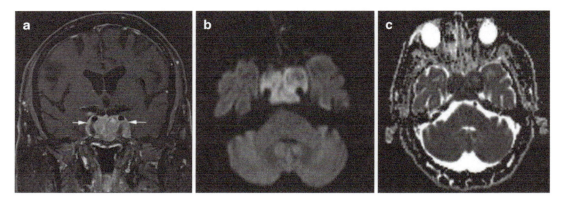

Fig. 18.57 (**a**–**c**) Pituitary adenoma in a 62-year-old female patient. (**a**) Gadolinium-enhanced coronal T1-weighted image shows a homogeneously enhancing mass in the pituitary fossa involving the bilateral cavernous sinuses (*arrows*). (**b, c**) DW image shows hypointensity in the lesion and decreased ADC (0.46–0.77×10^{-3} mm^2/s)

on all sequences especially the most sensitive for detection of hemorrhage (SWI or T2-star). Macroadenomas enhance avidly following administration of gadolinium-based contrast. Microadenomas are best visualized on dynamic imaging following administration of intravenous contrast and appear as a relatively hypointense lesions on today's background of the normally enhanced pituitary parenchyma.

DW imaging shows a hyperintense mass with ADC values ($0.84 \pm 0.3 \times 10^{-3}$ mm^2/s) (Fig. 18.57) [201]. There is a significant correlation between ADC values and tumor consistency of pituitary adenomas. Pituitary apoplexy results from hemorrhage and/or infarction of the pituitary gland. The DW signals and ADC values probably depend on the phase of hemorrhage and/or infarction in the pituitary gland or the pituitary adenoma (Fig. 18.58) [197, 202]. DW imaging has been effectively employed in the assessment of the consistency of the pituitary adenoma which has direct implications on the surgical technique and outcomes. Both objective assessment, based of ADC values, and subjective assessment of diffusion characteristics, based on the observed intensity of the tumors, have been made [203, 204]. Primarily the impedance of diffusion is based on the proportion of collagen or reticulin in the tumor given the texture described as hard or soft. Preoperative assessment for tumors labelled as soft led to selection of or influenced the outcomes of transsphenoidal excision which is less traumatic than the transcranial frontal approach [205]. A systematic review and the deduced evidence based guidelines, however, has not made formal recommendations on the efficacy of diffusion imaging alone due to insufficient evidence based on reviews of numerous publications [206]. In passing, attempts have also been made to correlate the texture with the functional type of the adenoma where first- and second-degree histogram analyses were reportedly helpful in differentiating functioning and nonfunctioning tumors [207]. Diffusion parameters have been employed with assessment of MIB1 and Ki67 status of the tumors to prognosticate on the local aggression exhibited by some pituitary adenomas [208, 209].

18.13 Metastatic Tumors

Metastases to the brain are primarily via the hematogenous route. Direct loco-regional extension of malignant tumors of the head and neck via the skull base and perineural extension are less common. This section is focused on parenchymal metastases. Brain metastasis accounts for about one-third of all intracranial tumors. While most metastases are multiple, up to 30% are solitary. MR imaging shows hypointensity on T1-weighted images, variable signal intensity on T2-weighted images, and enhancement. T2 hypointensity in brain metastatic lesions is often seen in well-differentiated adenocarcinoma [210].

18 Brain Neoplasm

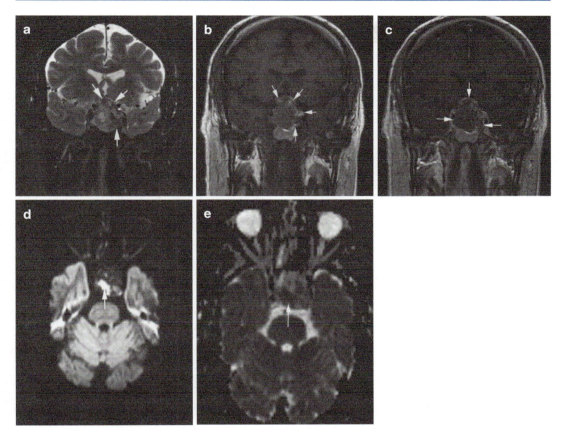

Fig. 18.58 (a–e) Pituitary apoplexy (pathologically proven) in a 29-year-old woman, (**a**) coronal T2-weighted image shows a large heterogeneous mass in the pituitary fossa. Hypointense areas represent hemorrhagic components (*arrows*). (**b**) Precontrast coronal T1-weighted image shows a hypointense mass in the pituitary fossa and cavernous sinuses with T1 hyperintense hemorrhagic components (*arrows*). (**c**) Gadolinium-enhanced coronal T1-weighted image shows a necrotic hypointense mass with partial enhancement (*arrows*). (**d, e**) DW image shows hypointensity with increased ADC in the necrosis and hyperintensity with decreased ADC in the hemorrhagic component (*arrow*)

Primary malignancies in the lung and gastrointestinal tract account for more than 60% of all brain metastases in adult men whereas breast cancer and lung account for approximately 60% of cases in adult females. Metastases are relatively uncommon in children and it has been reported that 6–10% of children with cancer will developed metastases to the CNS. Metastases in the CNS involve the brain, meninges, or spine. The majority of brain metastases (80%) are found in the cerebral hemisphere with 15% located in the cerebellum and 5% in the brain stem. Up to 30% of metastases in the brain are solitary and the rest are multiple. Lesions vary in size and number, solitary and multiple lesions occur in equal frequency. MRI has replaced CT in the detection of these lesions over the years. On conventional T1-weighted images lesions are iso- to hypointense; presence of hemorrhage can result in heterogeneous hyperintense and hypointense signal on this sequence. Melanoma secondaries are usually hyperintense given their melanin content. On the T2-weighted images and Flair sequence, lesions are predominantly hyperintense and occasionally hypointense if they are hypercellular. Perifocal edema is commonly seen around these lesions and appears hyperintense on FLAIR images and hypointense on T1-weighted images. Enhancement of lesions is variable depending on the presence or absence of hemorrhage; all lesions show some degree of enhancement. Most solid lesions appear as discs or spheres; central necrosis results in ring-like or geographic enhancement. Enhancement can vary from lesion to lesion in a given patient. Small, subcentimeter enhanced lesions can be detected using post-contrast volumetric T1-weighted spoiled gradient echo and magnetization-prepared rapid gradient echo sequences. Metastases from well-differentiated adenocarcinomas are hypointense on T2-weighted images [125].

The signal intensities on DW images of solid-appearing metastatic lesions are primarily dependent on the compact cellularity. The common signal abnormality of necrotic and cystic component of the parenchymal metastases may relate to an increase in free water resulting in hypointense signals on the DW images and increased ADC values. However, in the presence of extracellular methemoglobin and/or increased viscosity secondary to coagulative necrosis or presence of mucin, the DW images can appear hyperintense with decreased ADC. This situation is rare and specific to the conditions described above and is a differential diagnosis for pyogenic abscesses.

DWI provides two major surrogate biomarkers for assessment of the pathophysiology behind detection and management of metastatic tumors. Apparent diffusion coefficient has been correlated to cellularity, cytotoxic, and vasogenic edema. Disruption of the white matter tracts can be objectively measured using fractional anisotropy and mean diffusivity [211]. The application of diffusion imaging in the detection and assessment of parenchymal metastases falls into differentiation of metastatic lesions from malignant and benign conditions with similar morphology, assessment of treatment response, assessment of the primary source of the metastases and in the prognostication of treatment response. The signal intensity of non-necrotic components of metastases on DW images is variable and depends on their T2 and ADC [11, 15, 20, 21, 27, 28, 48, 188, 210, 212–219]. DW imaging findings of solid components of metastasis are similar to those of gliomas, probably reflecting the cellularity of the primary tumor. The cellularity is a major determinant of their DW signal intensity

[15, 20, 27, 188]. Brain metastasis from small-cell carcinoma often shows hyperintensity on DW images and decreased ADC probably due to the hypercellularity (Fig. 18.59). The common signal intensity of necrotic/cystic components of cerebral metastases may relate to an increase in free water, showing hypointensity on DW images and increased ADC. However, in the presence of extracellular met-hemoglobin and/or increased viscosity due to coagulative necrosis or mucin, DW images can show hyperintensity with decreased ADC (Figs. 18.60 and 18.61) [27, 212–219]. This situation is rare, but it should be considered as one differential diagnosis of pyogenic abscesses.

There are 4 major differential diagnoses which need to be considered when evaluating metastatic lesions, especially solitary metastases. They are glioblastoma, tumefactive demyelination, primary central nervous system lymphoma, and brain abscess. Conventional sequences can at the outset distinguish these lesions including the presence of lesions in the periventricular region in an immunocompetent patient (primary central nervous system lymphoma) with areas of impeded diffusion appearing in the solid portion of the lesion appearing hypointense on the ADC maps. The C-shaped enhancement facing the ventricle in cases of tumefactive demyelination may be accompanied by areas of decreased diffusion; however mass effect is significantly lacking in these patients as is the presence of significant perifocal edema. Ancillary imaging studies such as MR spectroscopy and perfusion scans have been the mainstay in aiding in the differential diagnosis of these lesions. It is important to note that irregular rim-enhancing lesions such as those of glioblastoma rarely show a central area of impeded diffusion which is supposedly the diagnostic feature of brain abscesses [220]. In a meta-analysis of 11 studies, the accuracy of DWI in differentiating abscesses from other ring-enhancing lesions was more than 50% [211, 221]. Differentiation of glioblastoma and metastases has been objectively assessed by using FA analyses of the enhancing rim with 100% accuracy [211, 222] although ADC measurements of the entire ADC for a specific lesion does not discriminate glioblastoma from metastases [91, 211]. Measurement of diffu-

18 Brain Neoplasm

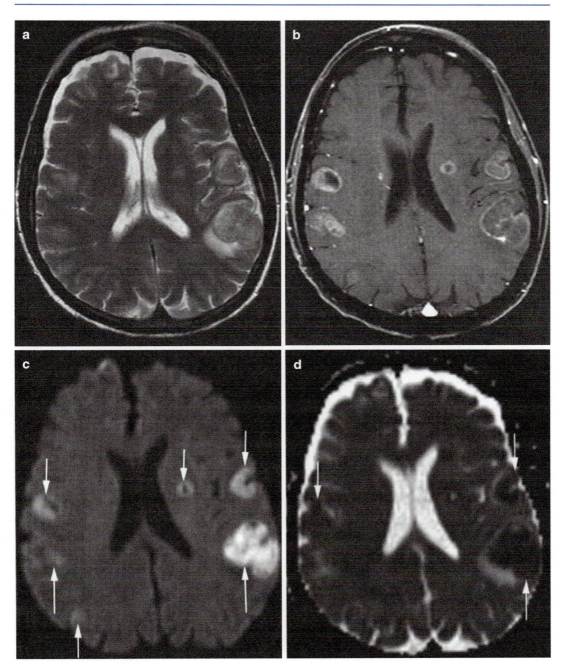

Fig. 18.59 (a–d) Metastasis (small-cell lung carcinoma) in a 65-year-old male patient. (a) T2-weighted image shows multiple hyperintense mass lesions and edema in the bilateral hemispheres. (b) Gadolinium-enhanced T1-weighted image shows multiple inhomogeneously enhancing mass lesions. (c) DW image shows hyperintensity in the solid enhancing portion of the mass lesions (*arrows*). (d) ADC map shows marked decreased ADC (0.32–0.59 × 10^{-3} mm^2/s) in the solid portion of the lesions (*arrows*)

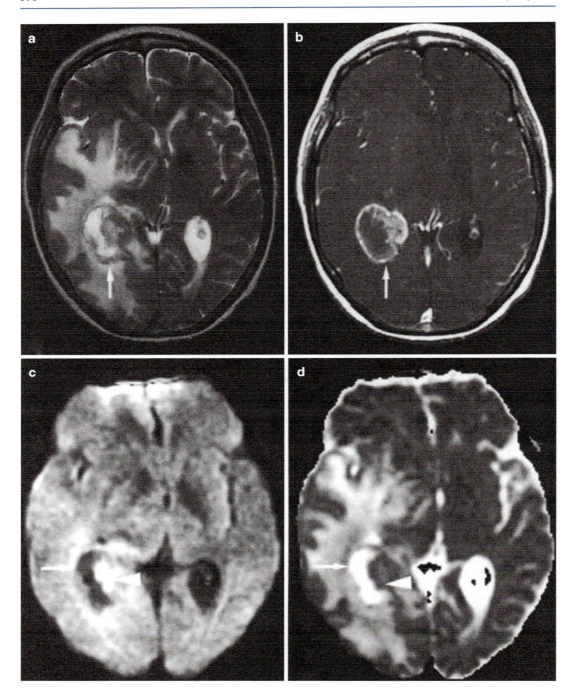

Fig. 18.60 (**a–d**) Metastasis (squamous cell lung carcinoma) in a 59-year-old female patient with adenocarcinoma of the lung. (**a**) T2-weighted image shows heterogeneous intensity of a mass (*arrow*) with surrounding edema in the right temporal lobe. (**b**) Gadolinium-enhanced T1-weighted image shows heterogeneous ring-like enhancement (*arrow*). (**c**) DW image shows hyperintensity in the solid portion (*arrowhead*) and hypointensity in the cystic/necrotic portion (*arrow*). (**d**) ADC map shows hypointensity in the solid portion (0.97–1.00 × 10^{-3} mm^2/s; *arrowhead*) and hyperintensity in the cystic portion (2.21–2.35 × 10^{-3} mm^2/s; *arrow*). Increased ADC is also seen in the surrounding vasogenic edema

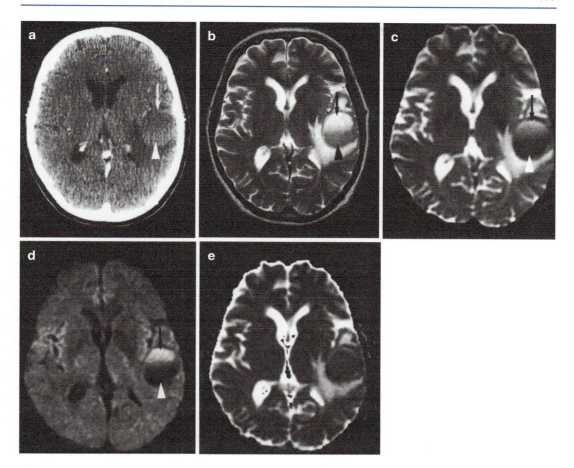

Fig. 18.61 (**a–e**) Metastasis (melanoma) in a 56-year-old man. (**a**) Post-contrast computed tomography shows a heterogeneous density mass, which shows hypodensity (*arrow*) in the anterior portions and hyperdensity (*arrowhead*) in the posterior portions. (**b**) T2-weighted image shows the heterogeneous intense mass, which contains anterior hyperintense portion (*arrow*) and posterior hypointense portion (*arrowhead*) with surrounding edema in the left temporal lobe. (**c**) b_0 image also shows anterior hyperintense portion (*arrow*) and posterior hypointense portion (*arrowhead*). (**d**) DW image again shows anterior hyperintense portion (*arrow*) and posterior hypointense portion (*arrowhead*). (**e**) ADC map shows iso- to hypointensity in the lesion. The accurate calculation of ADC in the hemorrhage is difficult

sion parameters in the peritumoral lesions has also been reported given that the high T2 signal is primarily related to edema in metastases but contain tumor infiltration and edema in cases of glioblastoma. Studies have included ADC values, mean diffusivity, and FA estimates as parameters to differentiate GBM and metastases with varying results [223–225].

Measurement of sequential variations in ADC has been used in the assessment of early response to treatment of metastases following stereotactic radiosurgery [226, 227]. The changes in ADC primarily reflect induction of cytotoxic edema and subsequent cell death, necrosis, and vasogenic edema which will lower and then increase the ADC as the treatment proceeds [211].

Diffusions techniques have been used to determine the underlying primary tumor in metastatic lesions with limited success. Although there are several conventional imaging and morphological characteristics which can be used for this purpose, the role of DWI techniques appears to be limited to measurement of ADC values with mixed results [228, 229].

Attempts have been made to utilize ADC values to predict survival following response to treatment in single brain metastases. Measurements of mean ADC values have shown higher values correlated with longer survival [211, 230, 231].

18.14 Radiation Necrosis

Radiation necrosis may occur several weeks to years after radiation, most commonly seen after 6–24 months. The early detection of recurrent tumors and the identification of radiation necrosis are important for adequate treatment. With conventional CT and MR imaging it is often difficult to differentiate between residual/recurrent tumors and radiation necrosis.

MRI perfusion has been widely used for the diagnosis radiation necrosis from tumor progression. The sensitivity and specificity in distinguishing between tumor recurrence and treatment changes/radiation necrosis are valuable in the reports [232–245]. DSC MR perfusion (74–90%, 86–92%, especially more reliable if use corrected rBV with cutoff 1.5–2.2) and DCE perfusion (89%, 85%, if use VE, VP, and Ktrans). The Cho/NAA and Cho/Cr ratios are higher in tumor recurrence than in radiation necrosis on MR spectroscopy (83–91%, 64–95%, cutoff of Cho/NAA > 2.3 for recurrence and < 1.1 for radiation necrosis) [238, 239, 244]. [18]FDG-PET (81–94%, 73%), [118]FFET-PET (93%, 86%), [1]C methionine-PET (88–95%, 90–100%), [201]T1 SPECT (40–92%, 69–93%), and CT perfusion (91–94%, 82–87%) also have been reported for the differentiation [244]. DW imaging of radiation necrosis has been reported. ADC values are significantly higher in radiation necrosis than in tumor recurrence or normal brain tissue [232, 240, 241, 245]. ROC curve analysis showed that the diagnostic sensitivity, specificity, and accuracy were 85%, 86.7%, and 85.7% when the ADC ratio was <1.65 and (or) FA ratio was >0.36 [245]. The maximum ADC has been reported higher in radiation necrosis than in tumor recurrence [242]. However, in some cases, radiation necrosis has shown restricted diffusion on ADC maps, which is not surprising given the potential role of ischemia in the occurrence of radiation necrosis (Fig. 18.62) [243]. Amide proton trans-

fer (APT) imaging is a new MRI technique that detects endogenous mobile proteins and peptides in tissue via saturation of the amide protons in the peptide bonds [245].

18.15 Conclusion

Diffusion-weighted imaging can provide valuable information about tumor cellularity and the extracellular matrix, and help in the characterization and grading of tumors of the brain. Diffusion-tensor imaging adds some information about the tumor characteristics and peritumoral infiltration. In most situations, it is difficult to differentiate between specific tumors and to determine tumor infiltration. Fiber tractography can be useful for preoperative planning and intraoperative image-guided surgery.

18.16 Treatment of Brain Neoplasm 1: Medical Management of Primary Brain Tumors in Adult

Christopher Becker and Yoshie Umemura

18.16.1 Introduction

The 2016 update to the WHO classification of central nervous system tumors introduced molecular characteristics in addition to histology for the diagnosis of glioma [246, 266]. There are multiple additional molecular markers with diagnostic and prognostic significance (see Table 18.4), and in many cases, genotype trumps the histologic phenotype in the updated criteria. For example, glioblastomas (WHO grade IV) are diagnosed based on histology, and the tumors are divided into *IDH* mutant and *IDH* wild-type. Diffuse astrocytomas can be low grade (WHO grade II) or anaplastic (WHO grade III), and the key molecular characteristic of these tumors are *ATRX* and *TP53* mutations, and lack of 1p/19q codeletion. These tumors are often *IDH* mutant, and *IDH* wild-type diffuse astrocytomas are

18 Brain Neoplasm

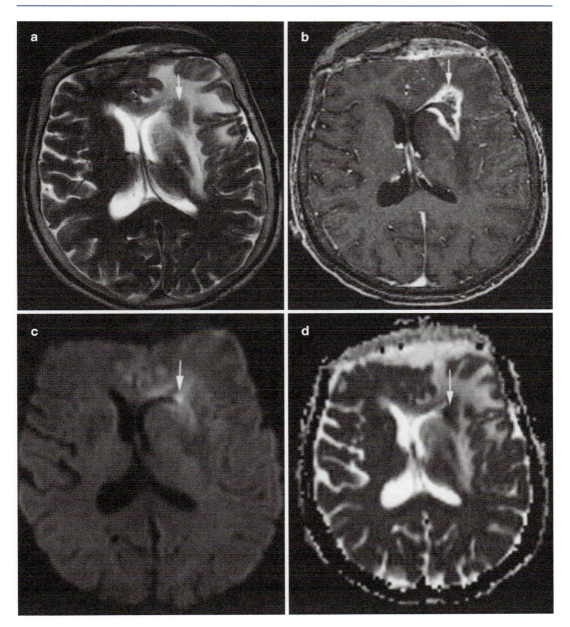

Fig. 18.62 (a–f) Radiation necrosis after the resection of olfactory neuroblastoma in a 65-year-old man. (**a**) T2-weighted image shows a mildly hyperintense necrotic area with surrounding edema in the left frontal deep white matter (*arrow*). Postoperative changes are seen in the frontal skull. (**b**) Gadolinium-enhanced T1-weighted image shows a necrotic enhancing mass lesion in the left frontal deep white matter (*arrow*). (**c**) DW image shows a central hyperintensity in the necrotic portion of the lesion (*arrow*). (**d**) ADC map shows iso- or hypointensity (0.51–0.82 × 10^{-3} mm^1/s) in the necrotic portion of the lesion (*arrow*). (**e**) MR spectroscopy (TE 135) shows a large lipid peak. A Cho/NAA ratio is less than 2.0. (**f**) Pathology shows a coagulative necrosis

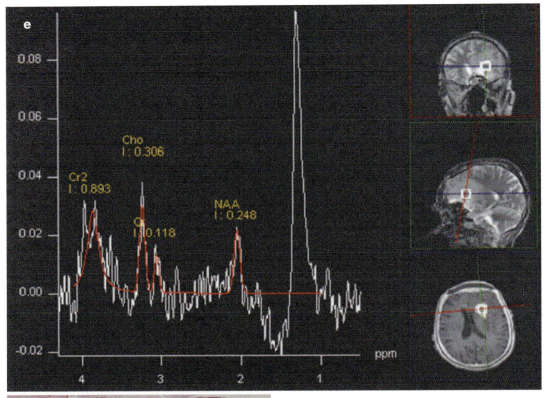

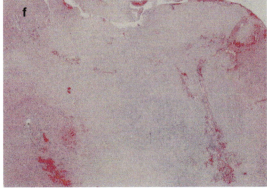

Fig. 18.62 (continued)

18 Brain Neoplasm

Table 18.4 Molecular markers in primary CNS malignancies

Molecular marker	Description	Significance
1p/19q codeletion	Loss of short arm of chromosome 1 and long arm of chromosome 19	Differentiates oligodendrogliomas (codeleted) from astrocytomas (non-codeleted) [246]. Associated with favorable prognosis and response to treatment [247–250].
IDH1/2 mutation	Isocitrate dehydrogenase; key enzyme in the Krebs cycle	One of the driver oncogenic mutation in low-grade infiltrating gliomas, and favorable prognosis compared to *IDH* wild-type diffuse gliomas [251–253]. In GBM, suggests secondary rather than primary GBM, with favorable prognosis [251, 254–256]. Epileptogenic [257, 258]
MGMT promoter methylation	Methylation of the O^6-methylguanine–DNA methyltransferase promoter; encodes a DNA damage repair enzyme	Improved prognosis overall and improved efficacy of alkylating agents [247, 250, 259–265].
ATRX mutation	Alpha-thalassemia/mental retardation syndrome X-linked gene	Characteristic but not required for diagnosis of astrocytoma [246].
H3 K27M mutation	K27M mutation in histone 3	Defines a subset of midline gliomas [246, 266] with aggressive nature with poor prognosis [267–270]
CIMP phenotype	CpG island hypermethylated phenotype	Improved survival in oligodendrogliomas [264].
TP53 mutation	Tumor suppressor	Characteristic but not necessary for diagnosis of astrocytoma [246]

known to behave more aggressively and associated with poorer prognosis. Low-grade and anaplastic oligodendrogliomas, in contrast to astrocytomas, must demonstrate the 1p/19q codeletion and *IDH* mutation. This chapter will focus on primary brain tumors that are usually treated with medical management with or without surgical resection and radiation therapy.

18.16.2 Treatment of Infiltrating Gliomas

The role of surgical resection has long been established for high-grade gliomas, both to establish a histologic diagnosis and for treatment. The aim is maximal surgical resection with preservation of neurologic function, and greater degrees of resection are associated with improved survival [271–273]. Similarly, the efficacy of adjuvant radiation therapy (RT) for high-grade gliomas is well established [274–276]. Adjuvant chemotherapy can be beneficial particularly in MGMT promotor methylated glioblastomas and *IDH* mutated diffuse gliomas. Optimization of chemotherapy regimens remains an active area of research, particularly for grade III gliomas [277]. A sum-

Table 18.5 Treatment summary for high-grade CNS neoplasms

Malignancy	Treatment
Glioblastoma	Maximal safe resection, RT, concurrent and adjuvant TMZ
High-risk low-grade/anaplastic astrocytoma	Maximal safe resection, RT, concurrent and adjuvant TMZ
High-risk low-grade/anaplastic oligodendroglioma	Maximal safe resection, RT, concurrent and adjuvant TMZ or adjuvant PCV
Diffuse midline glioma, H3 K27M–mutant	Maximal safe resection (usually biopsy), radiation ± medical therapy
Primary CNS lymphoma	Biopsy, HD-MTX-based multi-drug chemotherapy regimen, ± RT

mary of chemotherapy regimens for various CNS malignancies can be found in Table 18.5. This section will focus on upfront treatment of infiltrating gliomas.

18.16.2.1 Glioblastoma

The current standard of care for adjuvant therapy in glioblastoma is the so-called Stupp protocol [278]. This was established in 2005 based on a large randomized trial, and consists of six weeks of radiation therapy with concurrent administration of the oral alkylating agent temozolamide (TMZ; 75 mg/m²/day), followed by six cycles of adjuvant TMZ (150–200 mg/m²/day) on days 1–5 of 28 day cycles [278]. Compared to patients who received only radiation therapy, treatment with this protocol led to improvement in median survival from 12.1 to 14.6 months, two-year survival from 10.4% to 26.4%, and five-year survival of 1.9% to 9.8% [259, 278]. Attempts to modify the Stupp protocol by increasing the dose density of TMZ (i.e., dosing on days 1–21 rather 1–5) have shown no benefit [260, 279]. Similarly, increasing the duration of treatment beyond 6 cycles has shown no clear benefit in prospective [280] or retrospective studies [261, 281]. Temozolomide is relatively well tolerated compared to other chemotherapy regimens, with the primary adverse effects including nausea, fatigue, and hematologic toxicity that are generally well controlled [282, 283].

Tumor treating fields (TFields) deliver intermediate-frequency (200 kHz) alternating electric fields to the tumor site via electrodes applied to the shaved scalp, which are thought to interfere with microtubule function, leading to apoptosis in dividing cells [284, 285]. In an unblinded, multicenter, international clinical trial, addition of TTFields to the Stupp protocol led to significant improvements in progression-free and overall survival [286]. Treatment with the device was generally safe, with the most common adverse effects being minor local skin reactions at the electrode site, though questions have been raised about the lack of a placebo arm in the clinical trial [287] and the cost-effectiveness of the treatment [288].

18.16.2.2 Astrocytoma

Astrocytomas are divided into *IDH* mutant and *IDH* wild-type, with *IDH* wild-type tumors tending to be more aggressive and follow a course comparable to glioblastoma [251]. The treatment of anaplastic astrocytomas has generally involved regimens based on the Stupp protocol, though variability exists in clinical practice [277]. Recently published preliminary data from the ongoing CATNON trial supports this practice, demonstrating improvement in patients receiving 12 cycles of adjuvant TMZ following radiation compared to radiation alone [289]. This result is consistent with retrospective data showing that various chemotherapy regimens lead to improved survival in *IDH* mutant, 1p/19q non-codeleted gliomas [290], and prospective data showing survival benefit for PCV (procarbazine, lomustine, vincristine) in a mixed population of 1p/19q codeleted and non-codeleted high-grade gliomas [247]. When comparing various chemotherapy regimens, there is prospective data demonstrating no difference in survival for TMZ compared to nitrosurea therapy [252], and retrospective data finding no difference in survival for TMZ vs. PCV [291]. In both comparison studies, TMZ was better tolerated, further supporting the use of TMZ-based adjuvant chemotherapy regimens in these patients.

18.16.2.3 Oligodendroglioma

Oligodendrogliomas tend to be more responsive to chemotherapy and carry a more favorable prognosis than astrocytomas. A number of trials have shown that chemotherapy in addition to RT for patients with high-grade oligodendrogliomas is beneficial [247, 248]. Two commonly used regimens are PCV and TMZ. PCV has demonstrated survival benefit in two phase III trials in oligodendrogliomas [247, 248]. There are also evidence supporting the use of TMZ as it has been shown to be effective in recurrent anaplastic oligodendrogliomas [249, 292], and in gliomas without 1p19q co-deletion [289]. There have been no completed head-to-head comparisons to date, and there is an ongoing trial comparing TMZ and PCV in oligodendrogliomas (CODEL trial; NCT00887146). Currently, no consensus exists on the optimal regimen, though TMZ is more commonly used due to ease of administration (oral) and superior tolerability compared to PCV [252, 277, 291].

18.16.2.4 Diffuse Midline Glioma, *H3 K27M* Mutant

Midline gliomas are often associated with *H3 K27M* mutations and a diffuse growth pattern, affecting midline structures such as the thala-

18 Brain Neoplasm

mus, brainstem, and spinal cord [246, 266]. Adult diffuse midline gliomas with H3 K27M mutation are WHO grade IV, and typically occur in younger patients [246, 266]. They are aggressive and generally associated with a poor prognosis [267–270]. These tumors are generally in unfavorable location for maximal safe resection, and the tumor surgery is often limited to biopsy prior to definitive radiotherapy. The role of chemotherapy is still unclear; however there are many promising treatment specifically for this rare tumor, including ONC 201, a novel agent that antagonizes the D2 dopamine receptor and induces apoptosis in tumor cells. Administration of ONC 201 has led to clinical and radiographic improvement in these patients, and is currently being studied in clinical trials [293, 294].

18.16.3 Treatment of Primary CNS Lymphoma

In contrast to other types of primary CNS malignancies, primary CNS lymphoma (PCNSL) is very responsive to chemotherapy and diseased brain parenchyma can normalize after a successful treatment with chemotherapy alone. To minimize longstanding neurological deficit, initial surgery should be biopsy rather than resection when CNS lymphoma is the leading differential. The backbone of chemotherapy for PCNSL is high dose methotrexate (HD-MTX). The efficacy of HD-MTX has been demonstrated in a number of trials [295–302]. While HD-MTX is has some efficacy as a monotherapy [295, 300–302], outcomes are further improved when HD-MTX is combined with other agents such as cytarabine [303], or thiotepa and rituximab [304]. Most commonly used efficacious multi-drug HD-MTX regimen are R-MT (rituximab, HD-MTX, temozolomide) [305] and R-MPV (rituximab, HD-MTX, procarbazine, vincristine) [306, 307]. There is currently no consensus regarding the optimal regimen, though there is consensus that it should contain HD-MTX [308]. In elderly PCNSL patients, MTX monotherapy may be reasonable [300]. Radiation therapy has a role in PCNSL treatment as well, though it is associated with increased neurotoxicity [309, 310].

18.16.4 Future Directions

18.16.4.1 Targeted Therapy

Tumor genome sequencing and targeted molecular therapies have revolutionized the treatment of genomically defined subtypes of various types of cancer [311]. As previously discussed, numerous individual genetic and molecular markers with diagnostic, prognostic, and therapeutic implications have been identified (see Table 18.4). The identification of these molecular features has led to interest in the development of targeted therapies for high-grade gliomas.

One such potential target is *BRAF*, an oncogene that has been successfully targeted in the treatment of melanoma [312, 313], non-smallcell lung cancer [314], anaplastic thyroid cancer [315], and colorectal cancer [316]. *BRAF* mutations are present in up to 15% of low-grade gliomas [317], and are detected in a small minority of glioblastomas [318]. In open-label trials, BRAF inhibitors have shown antitumor effects in patients with *BRAF*-mutant gliomas [319]. This is an area of ongoing investigation.

Another potential target is *IDH*. *IDH1* inhibitors have been shown to impair the growth of *IDH*-mutant glioma cells in vitro [320], and vaccination against mutant *IDH* peptides led to an immune response with significantly reduced tumor size in vivo in mouse models [321]. Clinical trials are ongoing for small-molecule *IDH* inhibitors in patients with *IDH*-mutant gliomas [322, 323].

Molecular markers can have implications for non-targeted therapies as well. For example, a recent phase III trial involving glioblastoma patients with MGMT promotor methylation demonstrated survival benefit when adding lomustine to a standard TMZ-based chemotherapy regimen [324].

Further, combined analysis of multiple genetic and molecular markers through The Cancer Genome Atlas (TCGA) has enabled more detailed classification of gliomas into subgroups based on multiple molecular markers, which may have further implications for targeted therapies, prognosis, and response to treatment [318, 325–328].

18.16.4.2 Heterogeneity

Complicating the implementation of targeted therapies is the observation that, in addition to genetic heterogeneity between patients, there is also genetic heterogeneity within individual tumors [329]. Tumors are constantly evolving, resulting in the existence of multiple clonal populations within a single tumor that have differential molecular, genetic, and phenotypic characteristics [330–335], which can result in differential response to treatment [336, 337]. This has significant clinical implications, such as limiting the utility of single biopsy analysis in the initiation of targeted therapies [328], and complicating the use of targeted therapies, which in the setting of intra-tumor heterogeneity may simply lead to expansion of non-targeted clones via Darwinian selection [328, 329, 331, 335, 338] (Fig. 18.63).

18.17 Treatment of Brain Neoplasm 2: Radiation Therapy for Brain Tumors: Brain Metastases and Malignant Glioma

Michelle M. Kim

18.17.1 Brain Metastases

18.17.1.1 Background

Brain metastases are the most common intracranial malignancy affecting more than 100,000 patients per year [339]. Radiation therapy (RT) is the primary treatment for the majority of patients with a diagnosis of brain metastasis, with select patients undergoing surgery with diagnostic intent, or to address resectable, larger lesions with significant mass effect. Historically, systemic therapy has not been used as primary management, but newer agents with penetrance across the blood brain barrier and activity in the

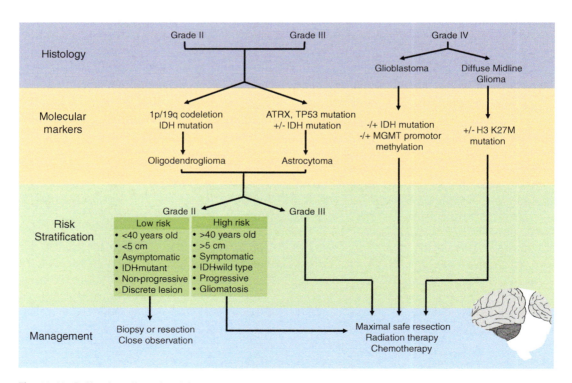

Fig. 18.63 Infiltrating glioma in adult

central nervous system (CNS) are increasingly used to treat small, asymptomatic lesions, such as immune checkpoint inhibitors and BRAF inhibitors for subsets of patients with malignant melanoma, or small molecule inhibitors with anti-HER2 activity in HER2-positive breast cancer patients, for example [340–343].

18.17.1.2 Radiation Treatment Techniques

Whole brain radiation therapy (WBRT) was the historical standard of care, but with advancements in technology and imaging, stereotactic radiosurgery (SRS) is now the standard treatment for patients with limited brain metastases after multiple phase III randomized trials demonstrated worse neurocognitive outcomes in patients receiving SRS plus WBRT compared with SRS alone, with no improvement in overall survival [344–347]. Using high-resolution T1-gadolinium-enhanced MR imaging, stereotactic radiosurgery involves the delivery of high doses of conformal radiotherapy in a single session of treatment, with relative sparing of the surrounding normal brain. Such precise technologies rely heavily on high-quality MR imaging as a component of accurate treatment delivery.

18.17.1.3 Diagnosis and Imaging Assessment

For diagnosis, an accurate assessment of the number and location of visible contrast-enhancing lesions is a first step in determining the optimal management of the patient. Randomized trials support the use of SRS for patients with up to 3–4 brain metastases, with increasing consideration of SRS patients for select patients with up to 10 or sometimes more metastases [348]. In addition to 3-dimensional (3D) volumetric gradient echo (GRE) T1 post-contrast images, the use of 3D volumetric fast spin echo (FSE) T1-weighted images ((Fig. 18.64) may assist the radiologist and the radiation oncologist in

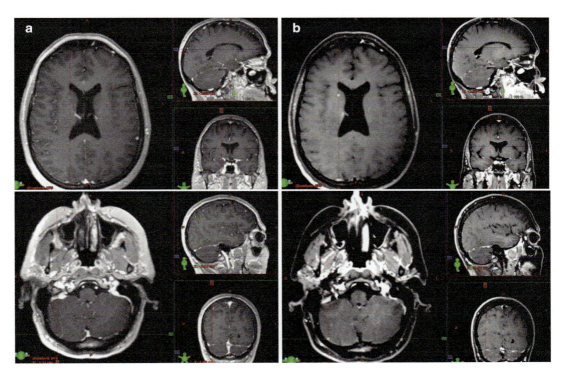

Fig. 18.64 Three-dimensional, T1-weighted gradient-echo images (column A) demonstrating subtle, enhancing punctate brain metastases (noted by cross-hairs) that are more clearly visible on corresponding three-dimensional, T1-weighted fast spin echo images (column B) from a single patient

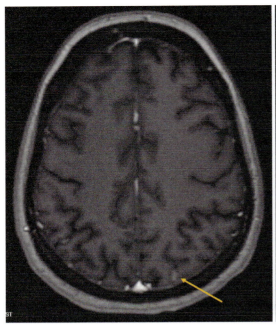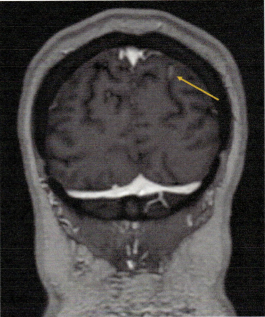

Fig. 18.65 Subtle finding of an enhancing leptomeningeal plaque in a patient with metastatic melanoma with 2 additional subcentimeter parenchymal brain metastases. This finding significantly alters additional management, prognosis, and therapeutic options. Rather than single-session radiosurgery for limited parenchymal brain metastases, diagnostic and treatment considerations will now include MR imaging of the entire neuro-axis, potential lumbar puncture, comprehensive whole brain rather than focal radiation, and may impact clinical trial eligibility and prognosis

detecting even small, asymptomatic lesions that may impact the radiation treatment plan, anticipated side effect profile, clinical trial eligibility, and overall management of a patient with brain metastases [349–351]. Importantly, determination of the presence or absence of leptomeningeal dissemination on the diagnostic MRI is a critical determination by the neuroradiologist which may influence the clinician's understanding of the patient's prognosis and optimal treatment strategies, and should be an integral part of the imaging assessment (Fig. 18.65).

18.17.1.4 Surveillance

In imaging surveillance following treatment, it is important for the neuroradiologist to be aware of the patient's history of brain tumor directed therapy in order to make informed determinations of the patient's imaging. The timing and history of radiation therapy and surgery relative to MR image acquisition is critical. As patient survival improves and patients undergo multiple courses of SRS or focal high dose radiotherapy, imaging interpretation becomes increasingly complex as the determination of response in treated lesions and the development of new enhancing lesions is monitored over time. At present, because neuroradiologists do not have ready access to radiation plans, careful monitoring must be undertaken with the radiation oncologist knowledgeable about the patient's radiation history. This is particularly important when the imaging demonstrates worsening contrast enhancement suspected to represent treatment effect, or tumor

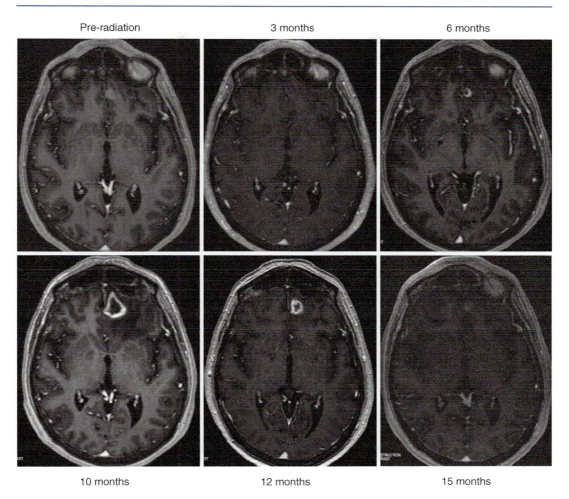

Fig. 18.66 A patient with ALK-rearranged non-small-cell lung cancer who demonstrated response of a single left frontal metastases 3 months postradiation but subsequent enlargement of the contrast-enhancing lesion at 6 months which peaked at 10 months postradiation with associated edema. It subsequently spontaneously improved. The patient was asymptomatic and did not require any steroids. Interestingly, the patient also developed radiation pneumonitis after a course of thoracic radiation, potentially indicating an inflammatory phenotype susceptible to treatment effect after radiation therapy

progression, or possibly the combination of both (Fig. 18.66). This perennial clinical conundrum affects up to 5–15% of patients received high-dose focal RT with increasing rates >30% observed with long-term follow-up after treating larger tumor volumes, and requires not just imaging evaluation, but clinical history, examination, knowledge of tumor-directed or supportive therapies received, and longitudinal assessment to help ascertain the underlying diagnosis which may only be conclusively determined with surgical resection, an option for only a select minority of patients [352, 353]. Increasingly, with the use of systemic therapies with CNS activity such as immune checkpoint inhibitors, immune-related imaging changes after high-dose focal RT for brain metastases, akin to that seen after treatment for gliomas, may be visualized on surveillance imaging and also mimic tumor progression [354–357]. Guidelines based on limited clinical experience and expert opinion are in continued evolution in the ever-changing landscape of oncology, and will require continued multidisciplinary cross talk between neuroradiologists, radiation oncologists, neuro-oncologists, and medical oncologists for optimal patient care and clinical research [358].

18.17.1.5 Malignant Glioma

The most common primary intracranial malignancy is glioblastoma, and advances in the molecular understanding of gliomas have altered the understanding of prognosis and natural history, pathogenesis, and potential therapy on or off clinical trials for the various types of glioma. For glioblastoma, the standard treatment is maximal safe resection followed by radiation and chemotherapy with concurrent and adjuvant temozolomide [278]. In unresectable cases including tumors in eloquent locations or multifocal tumors, biopsy followed by definitive radiation therapy with temozolomide is standard.

Imaging interpretation for diagnosis of a suspected glioma and initial tumor extent is important for determination of whether the tumor is unifocal or multifocal, or uncommonly, if gliomatosis cerebri is suspected based on the imaging characteristics. Centers with less experience with brain tumor patients may not be as aware of uncommon entities such as gliomatosis cerebri, and imaging appearance may be variable or not as appreciable on various imaging platforms. However, determination of visible tumor extent

may impact recommended therapy including whether diagnostic biopsy versus craniotomy and maximal tumor resection is pursued, the extent of the radiotherapy treatment fields, as well as the associated side effect profile of treatment and prognosis of the patient.

Radiation treatment of glioblastoma includes targeting the grossly visible extent of enhancing or sometimes non-enhancing tumor volume (known as gross tumor volume or GTV), a 2–3 cm isotropic margin around the GTV confined by anatomic boundaries to encompass the microscopic extension of tumor (known as clinical target volume or CTV), and a 3–5 mm margin for daily positioning and setup error (known as planning target volume or PTV). Targeting microscopic tumor extent within the 2–3 cm CTV derives from autopsy and pathologic biopsy series in which infiltrating glioma cells were observed within several cm from the index contrast-enhancing tumor on CT or MRI, as well as patterns of failure analyses demonstrating most recurrences within the high-dose region. The standard radiation dose is 60 Gy in 30 fractions that includes the high-risk, contrast-enhancing region [359, 360]. (Fig. 18.67). Varying protocols may treat the T2-FLAIR abnormality beyond the enhancing tumor region, presumed to contain a lower concentration of tumor cells, to the same or lower dose. In addition, various research efforts using advanced imaging techniques including diffusion-weighted MRI, dynamic contrast-enhanced perfusion MRI, proton MRI spectroscopy, and amino acid positron emission tomography (PET) imaging to better define biologically significant tumor regions for radiation target delineation are underway.

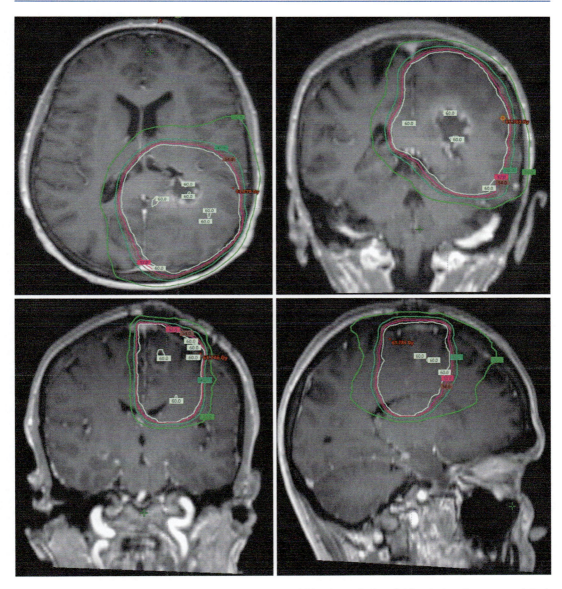

Fig. 18.67 Two representative radiation therapy plans from 2 patients with glioblastoma. A sizeable region beyond the enhancing tumor component is encompassed within the radiation fields, designed to targeted both the grossly visible and microscopic regions of tumor involvement

References

1. Louis DN, Perry A, Reifenberger G et al (2016) The 2016 World Health Organization classification of tumors of the central nervous system: a summary. Acta Neuropathol 131(6):803–820
2. Louis DN, Ohgaki H, Wiestler OD, Cavenee WK, Burger PC, Jouvet A, Scheithauer BW, Kleihues P (2007) The 2007 WHO classification of tumours of the central nervous system. Acta Neuropathol 114:97–109
3. Komori T (2017) The 2016 WHO classification of tumours of the central nervous system: the major points of revision. Neurol Med Chir (Tokyo) 57(7):301–311
4. Ebrahimi A, Skardelly M, Schuhmann MU et al (2019) High frequency of H3 K27M mutations in adult midline gliomas. J Cancer Res Clin Oncol 145(4):839–850
5. Lee JK, Ko HC, Choi JG, Lee YS, Son BC (2018) A case of diffuse leptomeningeal glioneuronal tumor misdiagnosed as chronic tuberculous meningitis without brain biopsy. Case Rep Neurol Med 2018: 1391943
6. Fukushima S, Yoshida A, Narita Y et al (2015) Multinodular and vacuolating neuronal tumor of the cerebrum. Brain Tumor Pathol 32(2):131–136
7. Ramaswamy V, Remke M, Bouffet E et al (2016) Risk stratification of childhood medulloblastoma in the molecular era: the current consensus. Acta Neuropathol 131(6):821–831
8. Osborn AG, Hedlund GL, Salzman KL (2018) Osborn's brain, 2nd edn. Elsevier
9. Johnson DR, Guerin JB, Giannini C, Morris JM, Eckel LJ, Kaufmann TJ (2017) 2016 Updates to the WHO brain tumor classification system: what the radiologist needs to know. Radiographics 37(7):2164–2180
10. LeBihan D, Breton E, Lallemand D, Grenier P, Cabanis E, Laval-Jeantet M (1986) MR imaging of intravoxel incoherent motions: application to diffusion and perfusion in neurologic disorders. Radiology 161:401–407
11. Hajnal JV, Doran M, Hall AS et al (1991) MR imaging of anisotropically restricted diffusion of water in the nervous system: technical, anatomic, and pathologic considerations. J Comput Assist Tomogr 15:1–18
12. Tien RD, Felsberg GJ, Friedman H, Brown M, MacFall J (1994) MR imaging of high-grade cerebral gliomas: value of diffusion-weighted echoplanar pulse sequences. AJR Am J Roentgenol 162:671–677
13. Eis M, Els T, Hoehn-Berlage M, Hossmann KA (1994) Quantitative diffusion MR imaging of cerebral tumor and edema. Acta Neurochir Suppl (Wien) 60:344–346
14. Brunberg JA, Chenevert TL, McKeever PE et al (1995) In vivo MR determination of water diffusion coefficients and diffusion anisotropy: correlation with structural alteration in gliomas of the cerebral hemispheres. AJNR Am J Neuroradiol 16:361–371
15. Krabbe K, Gideon P, Wagn P, Hansen U, Thomsen C, Madsen F (1997) MR diffusion imaging of human intracranial tumours. Neuroradiology 39:483–489
16. Gupta RK, Sinha U, Cloughesy TF, Alger JR (1999) Inverse correlation between choline magnetic resonance spectroscopy signal intensity and the apparent diffusion coefficient in human glioma. Magn Reson Med 41:2–7
17. Sugahara T, Korogi Y, Kochi M et al (1999) Usefulness of diffusion-weighted MRI with echo-planar technique in the evaluation of cellularity in gliomas. J Magn Reson Imaging 9:53–60
18. Gupta RK, Cloughesy TF, Sinha U et al (2000) Relationships between choline magnetic resonance spectroscopy, apparent diffusion coefficient and quantitative histopathology in human glioma. J Neuro-Oncol 50:215–226
19. Castillo M, Smith JK, Kwock L, Wilber K (2001) Apparent diffusion coefficients in the evaluation of high-grade cerebral gliomas. AJNR Am J Neuroradiol 22:60–64
20. Stadnik TW, Chaskis C, Michotte A et al (2001) Diffusion-weighted MR imaging of intracerebral masses: comparison with conventional MR imaging and histologic findings. AJNR Am J Neuroradiol 22:969–976
21. Kono K, Inoue Y, Nakayama K et al (2001) The role of diffusion-weighted imaging in patients with brain tumors. AJNR Am J Neuroradiol 22:1081–1088
22. Gauvain KM, McKinstry RC, Mukherjee P et al (2001) Evaluating pediatric brain tumor cellularity with diffusion tensor imaging. AJR Am J Roentgenol 177:449–454
23. Sinha S, Bastin ME, Whittle IR, Wardlaw JM (2002) Diffusion tensor MR imaging of high-grade cerebral gliomas. AJNR Am J Neuroradiol 23:520–527
24. Bastin ME, Sinha S, Whittle IR, Wardlaw JM (2002) Measurements of water diffusion and T1 values in peritumoural oedematous brain. Neuroreport 13:1335–1340
25. Guo AC, Cummings TJ, Dash RC, Provenzale JM (2002) Lymphomas and high-grade astrocytomas: comparison of water diffusibility and histologic characteristics. Radiology 224:177–183
26. Yang D, Korogi Y, Sugahara T et al (2002) Cerebral gliomas: prospective comparison of multivoxel 2D chemical shift imaging proton MR spectroscopy, echoplanar perfusion and diffusion-weighted MRI. Neuroradiology 44:656–666
27. Stadnik TW, Demaerel P, Luypaert RR et al (2003) Imaging tutorial: differential diagnosis of bright lesions on diffusion weighted MR images. Radiographics 23:E7–E7
28. Bulakbasi N, Kocaoglu M, Ors F, Tayfun C, Ucoz T (2003) Combination of single-voxel proton MR spectroscopy and apparent diffusion coefficient calculation in the evaluation of common brain tumors. AJNR Am J Neuroradiol 24:225–233
29. Chenevert TL, McKeever PE, Ross BD (1997) Monitoring early response of experimental brain

tumors to therapy using diffusion magnetic resonance imaging. Clin Cancer Res 3:1457–1466

30. Chenevert TL, Stegman LD, Taylor JM et al (2000) Diffusion magnetic resonance imaging: an early surrogate marker of therapeutic efficacy in brain tumors. J Natl Cancer Inst 92:2029–2036

31. Mardor Y, Roth Y, Lidar Z et al (2001) Monitoring response to convection-enhanced taxol delivery in brain tumor patients using diffusion-weighted magnetic resonance imaging. Cancer Res 61:4971–4973

32. Sadeghi N, Camby I, Goldman S, Gabius HJ, Balériaux D, Salmon I, Decaesteckere C, Kiss R, Metens T (2003) Effect of hydrophilic components of the extracellular matrix on quantifiable diffusion-weighted imaging of human gliomas: preliminary results of correlating apparent diffusion coefficient values and hyaluronan expression level. AJR Am J Roentgenol 181:235–241

33. Pope WB, Djoukhadar I, Jackson A (2016) Neuroimaging. Handb Clin Neurol 134:27–50

34. Murakami R, Hirai T, Kitajima M, Fukuoka H, Toya R, Nakamura H, Kuratsu J, Yamashita Y (2008) Magnetic resonance imaging of pilocytic astrocytomas: usefulness of the minimum apparent diffusion coefficient (ADC) value for differentiation from high-grade gliomas. Acta Radiol 49:462–467

35. Hwang JH, Egnaczyk GF, Ballard E, Dunn RS, Holland SK, Ball WS Jr (1998) Proton MR spectroscopic characteristics of pediatric pilocytic astrocytomas. AJNR Am J Neuroradiol 19:535–540

36. Scott JN, Brasher PM, Sevick RJ, Rewcastle NB, Forsyth PA (2002) How often are nonenhancing supratentorial gliomas malignant? A population study. Neurology 59(6):947–949

37. White ML, Zhang Y, Kirby P, Ryken TC (2005) Can tumor contrast enhancement be used as a criterion for differentiating tumor grades of oligodendrogliomas? AJNR Am J Neuroradiol 26(4):784–790

38. Akai H, Mori H, Aoki S, Masutani Y, Kawahara N, Shibahara J, Ohtomo K (2005) Diffusion tensor tractography of gliomatosis cerebri: fiber tracking through the tumor. J Comput Assist Tomogr 29:127–129

39. Goebell E, Paustenbach S, Vaeterlein O, Ding XQ, Heese O, Fiehler J, Kucinski T, Hagel C, Westphal M, Zeumer H (2006) Low grade and anaplastic gliomas: differences in architecture evaluated with diffusion-tensor MR imaging. Radiology 239:217–222

40. Kitis O, Altay H, Calli C, Yunten N, Akalin T, Yurtseven T (2005) Minimum apparent diffusion coefficients in the evaluation of brain tumors. Eur J Radiol 55(3):393–400

41. Lam WW, Poon WS, Metreweli C (2002) Diffusion MR imaging in glioma: does it have any role in the pre-operation determination of grading of glioma? Clin Radiol 57(3):219–225

42. Bulakbasi N, Guvenc I, Onguru O, Erdogan E, Tayfun C, Ucoz T (2004) The added value of the apparent diffusion coefficient calculation to magnetic resonance imaging in the differentiation and grading of malignant brain tumors. J Comput Assist Tomogr 28(6):735–746

43. Pope WB (2015) Genomics of brain tumor imaging. Neuroimaging Clin N Am 25(1):105–119

44. Pope WB, Lai A, Mehta R et al (2011) Apparent diffusion coefficient histogram analysis stratifies progression-free survival in newly diagnosed bevacizumab-treated glioblastoma. AJNR Am J Neuroradiol 32(5):882–889

45. Ahn SS, Shin NY, Chang JH et al (2014) Prediction of methylguanine methyltransferase promoter methylation in glioblastoma using dynamic contrast-enhanced magnetic resonance and diffusion tensor imaging. J Neurosurg 121(2):367–373

46. Higano S, Yun X, Kumabe T, Watanabe M, Mugikura S, Umetsu A, Sato A, Yamada T, Takahashi S (2006) Malignant astrocytic tumors: clinical importance of apparent diffusion coefficient in prediction of grade and prognosis. Radiology 241:839–846

47. Stadlbauer A, Ganslandt O, Buslei R, Hammen T, Gruber S, Moser E, Buchfelder M, Salomonowitz E, Nimsky C (2006) Gliomas: histopathologic evaluation of changes in directionality and magnitude of water diffusion at diffusion-tensor MR imaging. Radiology 240:803–810

48. Tung GA, Evangelista P, Rogg JM, Duncan JA 3rd (2001) Diffusion-weighted MR imaging of rim-enhancing brain masses: is markedly decreased water diffusion specific for brain abscess? AJR Am J Roentgenol 177:709–712

49. Toh CH, Castillo M, Wong AM, Wei KC, Wong HF, Ng SH, Wan YL (2008) Primary cerebral lymphoma and glioblastoma multiforme: differences in diffusion characteristics evaluated with diffusion tensor imaging. AJNR Am J Neuroradiol 29:471–475

50. Behin A, Hoang-Xuan K, Carpentier AF, Delattre JY (2003) Primary brain tumours in adults. Lancet 361:323–331

51. Ye ZC, Sontheimer H (1999) Glioma cells release excitotoxic concentrations of glutamate. Cancer Res 59:4383–4391

52. Moritani T, Smoker WR, Sato Y, Numaguchi Y, Westesson PL (2005) Diffusion-weighted imaging of acute excitotoxic brain injury. AJNR Am J Neuroradiol 26:216–228

53. Provenzale JM, McGraw P, Mhatre P, Guo AC, Delong D (2004) Peritumoral brain regions in gliomas and meningiomas: investigation with isotropic diffusion-weighted MR imaging and diffusion-tensor MR imaging. Radiology 232:451–460

54. Lu S, Ahn D, Johnson G, Law M, Zagzag D, Grossman RI (2004) Diffusion-tensor MR imaging of intracranial neoplasia and associated peritumoral edema: introduction of the tumor infiltration index. Radiology 232:221–228

55. Tropine A, Vucurevic G, Delani P, Boor S, Hopf N, Bohl J, Stoeter P (2004) Contribution of diffusion tensor imaging to delineation of gliomas and glioblastomas. J Magn Reson Imaging 20:905–912

56. Di Costanzo A, Scarabino T, Trojsi F et al (2006) Multiparametric 3T MR approach to the assessment of cerebral gliomas: tumor extent and malignancy. Neuroradiology 48(9):622–631

57. Yamada K, Kizu O, Mori S, Ito H, Nakamura H, Yuen S, Kubota T, Tanaka O, Akada W, Sasajima H, Mineura K, Nishimura T (2003) Brain fiber tracking with clinically feasible diffusion-tensor MR imaging: initial experience. Radiology 227:295–301

58. Stadlbauer A, Nimsky C, Buslei R, Salomonowitz E, Hammen T, Buchfelder M, Moser E, Ernst-Stecken A, Ganslandt O (2007) Diffusion tensor imaging and optimized fiber tracking in glioma patients: Histopathologic evaluation of tumor-invaded white matter structures. NeuroImage 34:949–956

59. Nimsky C, Ganslandt O, Hastreiter P, Wang R, Benner T, Sorensen AG, Fahlbusch R (2005) Preoperative and intraoperative diffusion tensor imaging-based fiber tracking in glioma surgery. Neurosurgery 56:130–137

60. Kinoshita M, Yamada K, Hashimoto N, Kato A, Izumoto S, Baba T, Maruno M, Nishimura T, Yoshimine T (2005) Fiber-tracking does not accurately estimate size of fiber bundle in pathological condition: initial neurosurgical experience using neuronavigation and subcortical white matter stimulation. NeuroImage 25:424–429

61. Yu A, Li K, Li H (2006) Value of diagnosis and differential diagnosis of MRI and MR spectroscopy in gliomatosis cerebri. Eur J Radiol 59:216–221

62. Lafitte F, Morel-Precetti S, Martin-Duverneuil N, Guermazi A, Brunet E, Heran F, Chiras J (2001) Multiple glioblastomas: CT and MR features. Eur Radiol 11:131–136

63. Tsien C, Galban CJ, Chenevert TL et al (2010) Parametric response map as an imaging biomarker to distinguish progression from pseudoprogression in high-grade glioma. J Clin Oncol 28(13):2293–2299

64. Wen PY, Macdonald DR, Reardon DA et al (2010) Updated response assessment criteria for high-grade gliomas: response assessment in neuro-oncology working group. J Clin Oncol 28(11):1963–1972

65. Thust SC, van den Bent MJ, Smits M (2018) Pseudoprogression of brain tumors. J Magn Reson Imaging 48(3):571–589

66. Park JE, Kim HS, Goh MJ, Kim SJ, Kim JH (2015) Pseudoprogression in patients with glioblastoma: assessment by using volume-weighted voxel-based multiparametric clustering of MR imaging data in an independent test set. Radiology 275(3):792–802

67. van Dijken BRJ, van Laar PJ, Holtman GA, van der Hoorn A (2017) Diagnostic accuracy of magnetic resonance imaging techniques for treatment response evaluation in patients with high-grade glioma, a systematic review and meta-analysis. Eur Radiol 27(10):4129–4144

68. Zhang H, Ma L, Shu C, Wang YB, Dong LQ (2015) Diagnostic accuracy of diffusion MRI with quantitative ADC measurements in differentiating glioma recurrence from radiation necrosis. J Neurol Sci 351(1–2):65–71

69. Steidl E, Müller M, Müller A, Herrlinger U, Hattingen E (2019) Longitudinal, leakage corrected and uncorrected rCBV during the first-line treatment of glioblastoma: a prospective study. J Neuro-Oncol 144(2):409–417. On text

70. Zikou A, Sioka C, Alexiou GA, Fotopoulos A, Voulgaris S, Argyropoulou MI (2018) Radiation necrosis, pseudoprogression, pseudoresponse, and tumor recurrence: imaging challenges for the evaluation of treated gliomas. Contrast Media Mol Imaging 2018:6828396

71. Cha J, Kim ST, Kim HJ et al (2013) Analysis of the layering pattern of the apparent diffusion coefficient (ADC) for differentiation of radiation necrosis from tumour progression. Eur Radiol 23(3):879–886

72. Reimer C, Deike K, Graf M et al (2017) Differentiation of pseudoprogression and real progression in glioblastoma using ADC parametric response maps. PLoS One 12(4):e0174620

73. Hamstra DA, Galban CJ, Meyer CR et al (2008) Functional diffusion map as an early imaging biomarker for high-grade glioma: correlation with conventional radiologic response and overall survival. J Clin Oncol 26(20):3387–3394

74. Wang S, Kim SJ, Poptani H et al (2014) Diagnostic utility of diffusion tensor imaging in differentiating glioblastomas from brain metastases. AJNR Am J Neuroradiol 35(5):928–934

75. Wen Q, Kelley DA, Banerjee S et al (2015) Clinically feasible NODDI characterization of glioma using multiband EPI at 7 T. Neuroimage Clin 9:291–299

76. Liu ZC, Yan LF, Hu YC et al (2017) Combination of IVIM-DWI and 3D-ASL for differentiating true progression from pseudoprogression of Glioblastoma multiforme after concurrent chemoradiotherapy: study protocol of a prospective diagnostic trial. BMC Med Imaging 17(1):10

77. Dwyer KW, Naul LG, Hise JH (1996) Gliosarcoma: MR features. J Comput Assist Tomogr 20:719–723

78. Fontenele GI, Okamoto K, Ito J et al (2001) Symptomatic child case of subependymoma in the fourth ventricle without hydrocephalus. Radiat Med 19(1):37–42

79. Koral K, Kedzierski RM, Gimi B, Gomez A, Rollins NK (2008) Subependymoma of the cerebellopontine angle and prepontine cistern in a 15-year-old adolescent boy. AJNR Am J Neuroradiol 29(1):190–191

80. Quadery FA, Okamoto K (2003) Diffusion-weighted MRI of haemangioblastomas and other cerebellar tumours. Neuroradiology 45(4):212–219

81. Dominguez-Pinilla N (2016) Martinez de Aragon A, Dieguez Tapias S, et al. Evaluating the apparent diffusion coefficient in MRI studies as a means of determining paediatric brain tumour stages. Neurologia 31(7):459–465

82. Payabvash S, Tihan T, Cha S (2018) Volumetric voxelwise apparent diffusion coefficient histogram analysis for differentiation of the fourth ventricular tumors. Neuroradiol J 31(6):554–564

83. Rodriguez Gutierrez D, Awwad A, Meijer L et al (2014) Metrics and textural features of MRI diffusion to improve classification of pediatric posterior fossa tumors. AJNR Am J Neuroradiol 35(5):1009–1015

84. Shinohara T, Inoue A, Kohno S et al (2018) Usefulness of neuroimaging and immunohistochemical study for accurate diagnosis of chordoid glioma of the third ventricle: a case report and review of the literature. Surg Neurol Int 9:226

85. Weaver KJ, Crawford LM, Bennett JA, Rivera-Zengotita ML, Pincus DW (2017) Brainstem angiocentric glioma: report of 2 cases. J Neurosurg Pediatr 20(4):347–351

86. Bull JG, Saunders DE, Clark CA (2012) Discrimination of paediatric brain tumours using apparent diffusion coefficient histograms. Eur Radiol 22(2):447–457

87. Sasaki T, Kim J, Moritani T et al (2018) Roles of the apparent diffusion coefficient and tumor volume in predicting tumor grade in patients with choroid plexus tumors. Neuroradiology 60(5):479–486

88. Shin JH, Lee HK, Khang SK et al (2002) Neuronal tumors of the central nervous system: radiologic findings and pathologic correlation. Radiographics 22(5):1177–1189

89. Moonis G, Ibrahim M, Melhem ER (2004) Diffusion weighted MRI in Lhermitte-Duclos disease: report of two cases. Neuroradiology 46:351–354

90. Thomas B, Krishnamoorthy T, Radhakrishnan VV, Kesavadas C (2007) Advanced MR imaging in Lhermitte-Duclos disease: moving closer to pathology and pathophysiology. Neuroradiology 49:733–738

91. Dhamija R, Wood CP, Porter AB, Hu LS, Weindling SM, Hoxworth JM (2019) Updated imaging features of dysplastic cerebellar gangliocytoma. J Comput Assist Tomogr 43(2):277–281

92. Gaballo A, Palma M, Dicuonzo F, Carella A (2005) Lhermitte-Duclos disease: MR diffusion and spectroscopy. Radiol Med 110(4):378–384

93. Yamasaki F, Kurisu K, Satoh K, Arita K, Sugiyama K, Ohtaki M, Takaba J, Tominaga A, Hanaya R, Yoshioka H, Hama S, Ito Y, Kajiwara Y, Yahara K, Saito T, Thohar MA (2005) Apparent diffusion coefficient of human brain tumors at MR imaging. Radiology 235:985–991

94. Rau A, Kellner E, Foit NA et al (2019) Discrimination of epileptogenic lesions and perilesional white matter using diffusion tensor magnetic resonance imaging. Neuroradiol J 32(1):10–16

95. Song JY, Kim JH, Cho YH, Kim CJ, Lee EJ (2014) Treatment and outcomes for gangliogliomas: a single-center review of 16 patients. Brain Tumor Res Treat 2(2):49–55

96. Zhang D, Henning TD, Zou LG, Hu LB, Wen L, Feng XY, Dai SH, Wang WX, Sun QR, Zhang ZG (2008) Intracranial ganglioglioma: clinicopathological and MRI findings in 16 patients. Clin Radiol 63:80–91

97. Kikuchi T, Kumabe T, Higano S, Watanabe M, Tominaga T (2009) Minimum apparent diffusion coefficient for the differential diagnosis of ganglioglioma. Neurol Res 31(10):1102–1107

98. Yu Y, Zhang H, Xiao Z et al (2018) Diffusion-weighted MRI combined with susceptibility-weighted MRI: added diagnostic value for four common lateral ventricular tumors. Acta Radiol 59(8):980–987

99. D'Arco F, Khan F, Mankad K, Ganau M, Caro-Dominguez P, Bisdas S (2018) Differential diagnosis of posterior fossa tumours in children: new insights. Pediatr Radiol 48(13):1955–1963

100. Rodriguez FJ, Perry A, Rosenblum MK et al (2012) Disseminated oligodendroglial-like leptomeningeal tumor of childhood: a distinctive clinicopathologic entity. Acta Neuropathol 124(5):627–641

101. Schwetye KE, Kansagra AP, McEachern J, Schmidt RE, Gauvain K, Dahiya S (2017) Unusual high-grade features in pediatric diffuse leptomeningeal glioneuronal tumor: comparison with a typical low-grade example. Hum Pathol 70:105–112

102. Nunes RH, Hsu CC, da Rocha AJ et al (2017) Multinodular and vacuolating neuronal tumor of the cerebrum: a new "leave me alone" lesion with a characteristic imaging pattern. AJNR Am J Neuroradiol 38(10):1899–1904

103. Nunes RH, Hsu CC, Osborn AG (2017) Presumptive diagnosis of multinodular vacuolating tumor: "more than meets the eye!". Neuroradiology 59(11):1067–1068

104. Cuccia V, Rodriguez F, Palma F, Zuccaro G (2006) Pinealoblastomas in children. Childs Nerv Syst 22:577–585

105. Chang AH, Fuller GN, Debnam JM, Karis JP, Coons SW, Ross JS, Dean BL (2008) MR imaging of papillary tumor of the pineal region. AJNR Am J Neuroradiol 29:187–189

106. Sato T, Kirby PA, Buatti JM, Moritani T (2009) Papillary tumor of the pineal region: report of a rapidly progressive tumor with possible multicentric origin. Pediatr Radiol 39:188–190

107. Zhu L, Ren G, Li K et al (2011) Pineal parenchymal tumours: minimum apparent diffusion coefficient in prediction of tumour grading. J Int Med Res 39(4):1456–1463

108. Tamrazi B, Nelson M, Bluml S (2017) Pineal region masses in pediatric patients. Neuroimaging Clin N Am 27(1):85–97

109. Choudhri AF, Whitehead MT, Siddiqui A, Klimo P Jr, Boop FA (2015) Diffusion characteristics of pediatric pineal tumors. Neuroradiol J 28(2):209–216

110. Gasparetto EL, Cruz LC Jr, Doring TM et al (2008) Diffusion-weighted MR images and pineoblastoma: diagnosis and follow-up. Arq Neuropsiquiatr 66(1):64–68

111. Pierce TT, Provenzale JM (2014) Evaluation of apparent diffusion coefficient thresholds for diagnosis of medulloblastoma using diffusion-weighted imaging. Neuroradiol J 27(1):63–74

112. Pierce T, Kranz PG, Roth C, Leong D, Wei P, Provenzale JM (2014) Use of apparent diffusion coefficient values for diagnosis of pediatric posterior fossa tumors. Neuroradiol J 27(2):233–244

113. Yeom KW, Mobley BC, Lober RM et al (2013) Distinctive MRI features of pediatric medulloblastoma subtypes. AJR Am J Roentgenol 200(4):895–903

114. Marupudi NI, Altinok D, Goncalves L, Ham SD, Sood S (2016) Apparent diffusion coefficient mapping in medulloblastoma predicts non-infiltrative surgical planes. Childs Nerv Syst 32(11):2183–2187

115. Aboian MS, Kline CN, Li Y et al (2018) Early detection of recurrent medulloblastoma: the critical role of diffusion-weighted imaging. Neurooncol Pract 5(4):234–240

116. Panigrahy A, Barnes PD, Robertson RL, Sleeper LA, Sayre JW (2005) Quantitative analysis of the corpus callosum in children with cerebral palsy and developmental delay: correlation with cerebral white matter volume. Pediatr Radiol 35(12):1199–1207

117. Kotsenas AL, Roth TC, Manness WK, Faerber EN (1999) Abnormal diffusion-weighted MRI in medulloblastoma: does it reflect small cell histology? Pediatr Radiol 29:524–526

118. Klisch J, Husstedt H, Hennings S, von Velthoven V, Pagenstecher A, Schumacher M (2000) Supratentorial primitive neuroectodermal tumours: diffusion-weighted MRI. Neuroradiology 42:393–398

119. Wilke M, Eidenschink A, Muller-Weihrich S, Auer DP (2001) MR diffusion imaging and 1H spectroscopy in a child with medulloblastoma. A case report. Acta Radiol 42:39–42

120. Erdem E, Zimmerman RA, Haselgrove JC, Bilaniuk LT, Hunter JV (2001) Diffusion-weighted imaging and fluid attenuated inversion recovery imaging in the evaluation of primitive neuroectodermal tumors. Neuroradiology 43:927–933

121. Koral K, Gargan L, Bowers DC, Gimi B, Timmons CF, Weprin B, Rollins NK (2008) Imaging characteristics of atypical teratoid-rhabdoid tumor in children compared with medulloblastoma. AJR Am J Roentgenol 190:809–814

122. Sener RN (2003) Diffusion magnetic resonance imaging of solid vestibular schwannomas. J Comput Assist Tomogr 27:249–252

123. Xu XQ, Li Y, Hong XN, Wu FY, Shi HB (2017) Radiological indeterminate vestibular schwannoma and meningioma in cerebellopontine angle area: differentiating using whole-tumor histogram analysis of apparent diffusion coefficient. Int J Neurosci 127(2):183–190

124. Chuang CC, Chang CS, Tyan YS, Chuang KS, Tu HT, Huang CF (2012) Use of apparent diffusion coefficients in evaluating the response of vestibular schwannomas to Gamma Knife surgery. J Neurosurg 117(Suppl):63–68

125. Park CK, Kim DC, Park SH et al (2006) Microhemorrhage, a possible mechanism for cyst formation in vestibular schwannomas. J Neurosurg 105(4):576–580

126. Das A, Bhalla AS, Sharma R, Kumar A, Thakar A, Goyal A (2016) Diffusion-weighted imaging in extracranial head and neck schwannomas: a distinctive appearance. Indian J Radiol Imaging 26(2):231–236

127. Taoka T, Hirabayashi H, Nakagawa H, Sakamoto M, Myochin K, Hirohashi S, Iwasaki S, Sakaki T, Kichikawa K (2006) Displacement of the facial nerve course by vestibular schwannoma: preoperative visualization using diffusion tensor tractography. J Magn Reson Imaging 24:1005–1010

128. Yoshino M, Kin T, Ito A et al (2015) Combined use of diffusion tensor tractography and multifused contrast-enhanced FIESTA for predicting facial and cochlear nerve positions in relation to vestibular schwannoma. J Neurosurg 123(6):1480–1488

129. Yoshino M, Kin T, Ito A et al (2015) Feasibility of diffusion tensor tractography for preoperative prediction of the location of the facial and vestibulocochlear nerves in relation to vestibular schwannoma. Acta Neurochir 157(6):939–946; discussion 946

130. Nauta HJ, Tucker WS, Horsey WJ, Bilbao JM, Gonsalves C (1979) Xanthochromic cysts associated with meningioma. J Neurol Neurosurg Psychiatry 42:529–535

131. Tanaka M, Imhof HG, Schucknecht B, Kollias S, Yonekawa Y, Valavanis A (2006) Correlation between the efferent venous drainage of the tumor and peritumoral edema in intracranial meningiomas: superselective angiographic analysis of 25 cases. J Neurosurg 104:382–388

132. Elster AD, Challa VR, Gilbert TH, Richardson DN, Contento JC (1989) Meningiomas: MR and histopathologic features. Radiology 170(3 Pt 1):857–862

133. Filippi CG, Edgar MA, Ulug AM, Prowda JC, Heier LA, Zimmerman RD (2001) Appearance of meningiomas on diffusion-weighted images: correlating diffusion constants with histopathologic findings. AJNR Am J Neuroradiol 22:65–72

134. Bitzer M, Klose U, Geist-Barth B (2002) Alterations in diffusion and perfusion in the pathogenesis of peritumoral brain edema in meningiomas. Eur Radiol 12:2062–2076

135. Maiuri F, Iaconetta G, de Divitiis O, Cirillo S, Di Salle F, De Caro ML (1999) Intracranial meningiomas: correlations between MR imaging and histology. Eur J Radiol 31:69–75

136. Paek SH, Kim SH, Chang KH, Park CK, Kim JE, Kim DG, Park SH, Jung HW (2005) Microcystic meningiomas: radiological characteristics of 16 cases. Acta Neurochir 147:965–972

137. Tropine A, Dellani PD, Glaser M, Bohl J, Plöner T, Vucurevic G, Perneczky A, Stoeter P (2007) Differentiation of fibroblastic meningiomas from other benign subtypes using diffusion tensor imaging. J Magn Reson Imaging 25:703–708

138. Hakyemez B, Yildirim N, Gokalp G, Erdogan C, Parlak M (2006) The contribution of diffusion-weighted MR imaging to distinguishing typical from atypical meningiomas. Neuroradiology 48: 513–520

139. Santelli L, Ramondo G, Della Puppa A et al (2010) Diffusion-weighted imaging does not predict histological grading in meningiomas. Acta Neurochir 152(8):1315–1319; discussion 1319

140. Surov A, Ginat DT, Sanverdi E et al (2016) Use of diffusion weighted imaging in differentiating between maligant and benign meningiomas. a multicenter analysis. World Neurosurg 88:598–602

141. Watanabe Y, Yamasaki F, Kajiwara Y et al (2013) Preoperative histological grading of meningiomas using apparent diffusion coefficient at 3T MRI. Eur J Radiol 82(4):658–663

142. Yogi A, Koga T, Azama K et al (2014) Usefulness of the apparent diffusion coefficient (ADC) for predicting the consistency of intracranial meningiomas. Clin Imaging 38(6):802–807

143. Watanabe K, Kakeda S, Yamamoto J et al (2016) Prediction of hard meningiomas: quantitative evaluation based on the magnetic resonance signal intensity. Acta Radiol 57(3):333–340

144. Kakita A, Inenaga C, Kameyama S et al (2005) Cerebral lipoma and the underlying cortex of the temporal lobe: pathological features associated with the malformation. Acta Neuropathol 109(3): 339–345

145. Truwit CL, Barkovich AJ (1990) Pathogenesis of intracranial lipoma: an MR study in 42 patients. AJNR Am J Neuroradiol 11(4):665–674

146. Schweizer L, Koelsche C, Sahm F et al (2013) Meningeal hemangiopericytoma and solitary fibrous tumors carry the NAB2-STAT6 fusion and can be diagnosed by nuclear expression of STAT6 protein. Acta Neuropathol 125(5):651–658

147. Smith AB, Horkanyne-Szakaly I, Schroeder JW, Rushing EJ (2014) From the radiologic pathology archives: mass lesions of the dura: beyond meningioma-radiologic-pathologic correlation. Radiographics 34(2):295–312

148. Payabvash S, Tihan T, Cha S (2018) Differentiation of cerebellar hemisphere tumors: combining apparent diffusion coefficient histogram analysis and structural MRI features. J Neuroimaging 28(6):656–665

149. Onishi S, Hirose T, Takayasu T et al (2017) Advantage of high b value diffusion-weighted imaging for differentiation of hemangioblastoma from brain metastases in posterior fossa. World Neurosurg 101:643–650

150. Jack CR Jr, Reese DF, Scheithauer BW (1986) Radiographic findings in 32 cases of primary CNS lymphoma. AJR Am J Roentgenol 146:271–276

151. Hochberg FH, Miller DC (1988) Primary central nervous system lymphoma. J Neurosurg 68:835–853

152. Poon T, Matoso I, Tchertkoff V, Weitzner I Jr, Gade M (1989) CT features of primary cerebral lymphoma in AIDS and non-AIDS patients. J Comput Assist Tomogr 13:6–9

153. Haldorsen IS, Krakenes J, Krossnes BK, Mella O, Espeland A (2009) CT and MR imaging features of primary central nervous system lymphoma in Norway, 1989–2003. AJNR Am J Neuroradiol 30(4):744–751

154. Ahn SJ, Shin HJ, Chang JH, Lee SK (2014) Differentiation between primary cerebral lymphoma and glioblastoma using the apparent diffusion coefficient: comparison of three different ROI methods. PLoS One 9(11):e112948

155. Chang L, Ernst T (1997) MR spectroscopy and diffusion weighted MR imaging in focal brain lesions in AIDS. Neuroimaging Clin N Am 7:409–426

156. Baehring JM, Fulbright RK (2012) Diffusion-weighted MRI in neuro-oncology. CNS Oncol 1(2):155–167

157. Neska-Matuszewska M, Bladowska J, Sasiadek M, Zimny A (2018) Differentiation of glioblastoma multiforme, metastases and primary central nervous system lymphomas using multiparametric perfusion and diffusion MR imaging of a tumor core and a peritumoral zone-Searching for a practical approach. PLoS One 13(1):e0191341

158. Makino K, Hirai T, Nakamura H et al (2018) Differentiating between primary central nervous system lymphomas and glioblastomas: combined use of perfusion-weighted and diffusion-weighted magnetic resonance imaging. World Neurosurg 112:e1–e6

159. Shin DJ, Lee EJ, Lee JE, Lee EK, Yang SY (2017) Common and uncommon features of central nervous system lymphoma on traditional and advanced imaging modalities. Neurographics 7(6):437–449

160. Camacho DL, Smith JK, Castillo M (2003) Differentiation of toxoplasmosis and lymphoma in AIDS patients by using apparent diffusion coefficients. AJNR Am J Neuroradiol 24(4): 633–637

161. Schroeder PC, Post MJ, Oschatz E, Stadler A, Bruce-Gregorios J, Thurnher MM (2006) Analysis of the utility of diffusion-weighted MRI and apparent diffusion coefficient values in distinguishing central nervous system toxoplasmosis from lymphoma. Neuroradiology 48(10):715–720

162. Castellano-Sanchez AA, Li S, Qian J, Lagoo A, Weir E, Brat DJ (2004) Primary central nervous system posttransplant lymphoproliferative disorders. Am J Clin Pathol 121(2):246–253

163. Ginat DT, Purakal A, Pytel P (2015) Susceptibility-weighted imaging and diffusion-weighted imaging findings in central nervous system monomorphic B cell post-transplant lymphoproliferative disorder before and after treatment and comparison with primary B cell central nervous system lymphoma. J Neuro-Oncol 125(2):297–305

164. D'Ambrosio N, Soohoo S, Warshall C, Johnson A, Karimi S (2008) Craniofacial and intracranial manifestations of langerhans cell histiocytosis: report

165. Prayer D, Grois N, Prosch H, Gadner H, Barkovich AJ (2004) MR imaging presentation of intracranial disease associated with Langerhans cell histiocytosis. AJNR Am J Neuroradiol 25(5):880–891

166. Wang T, Wu X, Cui Y, Chu C, Ren G, Li W (2014) Role of apparent diffusion coefficients with diffusion-weighted magnetic resonance imaging in differentiating between benign and malignant bone tumors. World J Surg Oncol 12:365

167. Arber DA, Orazi A, Hasserjian R et al (2016) The 2016 revision to the World Health Organization classification of myeloid neoplasms and acute leukemia. Blood 127(20):2391–2405

168. Ahn JY, Kwon SO, Shin MS, Kang SH, Kim YR (2002) Meningeal chloroma (granulocytic sarcoma) in acute lymphoblastic leukemia mimicking a falx meningioma. J Neuro-Oncol 60:31–35

169. Parker K, Hardjasudarma M, McClellan RL, Fowler MR, Milner JW (1996) MR features of an intracerebellar chloroma. AJNR 17:1592–1594

170. Hakyemez B, Yildirim N, Taskapilioglu O, Erdogan C, Aker S, Yilmazlar S, Parlak M (2007) Intracranial myeloid sarcoma: conventional and advanced MRI findings. Br J Radiol 80:e109–e112

171. Baba S, Matsuo T, Ishizaka S, Morikawa M, Suyama K, Nagata I (2010) Intracranial granulocytic sarcoma extending from the posterior fossa to the carotid space via the jugular foramen: a case report. No Shinkei Geka 38(1):53–59

172. Hou X, Du L, Yu H, Zhang X (2017) Use of magnetic resonance imaging for diagnosis and after treatment of patients with myeloid sarcoma of the brain. Oncotarget 8(60):102581–102589

173. Echevarria ME, Fangusaro J, Goldman S (2008) Pediatric central nervous system germ cell tumors: a review. Oncologist 13(6):690–699

174. Zhang S, Liang G, Ju Y, You C (2016) Clinical and radiologic features of pediatric basal ganglia germ cell tumors. World Neurosurg 95:516–524. e511

175. McCarthy BJ, Shibui S, Kayama T et al (2012) Primary CNS germ cell tumors in Japan and the United States: an analysis of 4 tumor registries. Neuro-Oncology 14(9):1194–1200

176. Liang L, Korogi Y, Sugahara T et al (2002) MRI of intracranial germ-cell tumours. Neuroradiology 44(5):382–388

177. Tonni G, Granese R, Martins Santana EF et al (2017) Prenatally diagnosed fetal tumors of the head and neck: a systematic review with antenatal and postnatal outcomes over the past 20 years. J Perinat Med 45(2):149–165

178. Wu CC, Guo WY, Chang FC et al (2017) MRI features of pediatric intracranial germ cell tumor subtypes. J Neuro-Oncol 134(1):221–230

179. Higano S, Takahashi S, Ishii K, Matsumoto K, Ikeda H, Sakamoto K (1994) Germinoma originating in the basal ganglia and thalamus: MR and CT evaluation. AJNR Am J Neuroradiol 15:1435–1441

180. Ozelame RV, Shroff M, Wood B, Bouffet E, Bartels U, Drake JM, Hawkins C, Blaser S (2006) Basal ganglia germinoma in children with associated ipsilateral cerebral and brain stem hemiatrophy. Pediatr Radiol 36:325–330

181. Okamoto K, Ito J, Ishikawa K, Morii K, Yamada M, Takahashi N, Tokiguchi S, Furusawa T, Sakai K (2002) Atrophy of the basal ganglia as the initial diagnostic sign of germinoma in the basal ganglia. Neuroradiology 44:389–394

182. Tsuruda JS, Chew WM, Moseley ME, Norman D (1990) Diffusion-weighted MR imaging of the brain: value of differentiating between extraaxial cysts and epidermoid tumors. AJNR Am J Neuroradiol 11:925–931

183. Tsuruda JS, Chew WM, Moseley ME, Norman D (1991) Diffusion-weighted MR imaging of extra-axial tumors. Magn Reson Med 19:316–320

184. Maeda M, Kawamura Y, Tamagawa Y (1992) Intravoxel incoherent motion (IVIM) MRI in intracranial, extraaxial tumors and cysts. J Comput Assist Tomogr 16:514–518

185. Laing AD, Mitchell PJ, Wallace D (1999) Diffusion-weighted magnetic resonance imaging of intracranial epidermoid tumours. Australas Radiol 43:16–19

186. Dechambre S, Duprez T, Lecouvet F, Raftopoulos C, Gosnard G (1999) Diffusion-weighted MRI postoperative assessment of an epidermoid tumour in the cerebellopontine angle. Neuroradiology 41:829–831

187. Chen S, Ikawa F, Kurisu K, Arita K, Takaba J, Kanou Y (2001) Quantitative MR evaluation of intracranial epidermoid tumors by fast fluid-attenuated inversion recovery imaging and echo-planar diffusion-weighted imaging. AJNR Am J Neuroradiol 22:1089–1096

188. Bergui M, Zhong J, Bradac GB, Sales S (2001) Diffusion-weighted images of intracranial cyst-like lesions. Neuroradiology 43:824–829

189. Annet L, Duprez T, Grandin C, Dooms G, Collard A, Cosnard G (2002) Apparent diffusion coefficient measurements within intracranial epidermoid cysts in six patients. Neuroradiology 44:326–328

190. Osborn AG, Preece MT (2006) Intracranial cysts: radiologic-pathologic correlation and imaging approach. Radiology 239(3):650–664

191. Hakyemez B, Aksoy U, Yildiz H, Ergin N (2005) Intracranial epidermoid cysts: diffusion-weighted, FLAIR and conventional MR findings. Eur J Radiol 54:214–220

192. Hu XY, Hu CH, Fang XM, Cui L, Zhang QH (2008) Intraparenchymal epidermoid cysts in the brain: diagnostic value of MR diffusion-weighted imaging. Clin Radiol 63:813–818

193. Okamoto K, Ito J, Ishikawa K, Sakai K, Tokiguchi S (2000) Diffusion-weighted echo-planar MR imaging in differential diagnosis of brain tumors and tumor-like conditions. Eur Radiol 10(8):1342–1350

194. Lopes MBS (2017) The 2017 World Health Organization classification of tumors of the pituitary gland: a summary. Acta Neuropathol 134(4): 521–535
195. Hayashi Y, Tachibana O, Muramatsu N et al (1999) Rathke cleft cyst: MR and biomedical analysis of cyst content. J Comput Assist Tomogr 23(1):34–38
196. Sener RN, Dzelzite S, Migals A (2002) Huge craniopharyngioma: diffusion MRI and contrast-enhanced FLAIR imaging. Comput Med Imaging Graph 26:199–203
197. Kunii N, Abe T, Kawamo M, Tanioka D, Izumiyama H, Moritani T (2007) Rathkes cleft cysts: differentiation from other cystic lesions in the pituitary fossa by use of singleshot fast spin-echo diffusion-weighted MR imaging. Acta Neurochir 149:759–769
198. Kinoshita Y, Yamasaki F, Tominaga A et al (2016) Diffusion-weighted imaging and the apparent diffusion coefficient on 3T MR imaging in the differentiation of craniopharyngiomas and germ cell tumors. Neurosurg Rev 39(2):207–213
199. Nishioka H, Inoshita N (2018) New WHO classification of pituitary adenomas (4th edition): assessment of pituitary transcription factors and the prognostic histological factors. Brain Tumor Pathol 35(2):57–61
200. Inoshita N, Nishioka H (2018) The 2017 WHO classification of pituitary adenoma: overview and comments. Brain Tumor Pathol 35(2):51–56
201. Pierallini A, Caramia F, Falcone C, Tinelli E, Paonessa A, Ciddio AB, Fiorelli M, Bianco F, Natalizi S, Ferrante L, Bozzao L (2006) Pituitary macroadenomas: preoperative evaluation of consistency with diffusion-weighted MR imaging-initial experience. Radiology 239:223–231
202. Rogg JM, Tung GA, Anderson G, Cortez S (2002) Pituitary apoplexy: early detection with diffusion-weighted MR imaging. AJNR Am J Neuroradiol 23:1240–1245
203. Yiping L, Ji X, Daoying G, Bo Y (2016) Prediction of the consistency of pituitary adenoma: a comparative study on diffusion-weighted imaging and pathological results. J Neuroradiol 43(3):186–194
204. Alimohamadi M, Sanjari R, Mortazavi A et al (2014) Predictive value of diffusion-weighted MRI for tumor consistency and resection rate of nonfunctional pituitary macroadenomas. Acta Neurochir 156(12):2245–2252
205. Boxerman JL, Rogg JM, Donahue JE, Machan JT, Goldman MA, Doberstein CE (2010) Preoperative MRI evaluation of pituitary macroadenoma: imaging features predictive of successful transsphenoidal surgery. AJR Am J Roentgenol 195(3):720–728
206. Chen CC, Carter BS, Wang R et al (2016) Congress of neurological surgeons systematic review and evidence-based guideline on preoperative imaging assessment of patients with suspected nonfunctioning pituitary adenomas. Neurosurgery 79(4): E524–E526
207. Sanei Taheri M, Kimia F, Mehrnahad M et al (2018) Accuracy of diffusion-weighted imaging-magnetic resonance in differentiating functional from nonfunctional pituitary macro-adenoma and classification of tumor consistency. Neuroradiol J 32(2):74–85. https://doi.org/10.1177/1971400918809825
208. Tamrazi B, Pekmezci M, Aboian M, Tihan T, Glastonbury CM (2017) Apparent diffusion coefficient and pituitary macroadenomas: pre-operative assessment of tumor atypia. Pituitary 20(2):195–200
209. Surov A, Meyer HJ, Wienke A (2017) Associations between apparent diffusion coefficient (ADC) and Ki 67 in different tumors: a meta-analysis. Part 1: ADCmean. Oncotarget 8(43):75434–75444
210. Hayashida Y, Hirai T, Morishita S, Kitajima M, Murakami R, Korogi Y, Makino K, Nakamura H, Ikushima I, Yamura M, Kochi M, Kuratsu JI, Yamashita Y (2006) Diffusion-weighted imaging of metastatic brain tumors: comparison with histologic type and tumor cellularity. AJNR Am J Neuroradiol 27:1419–1425
211. Pope WB (2018) Brain metastases: neuroimaging. Handb Clin Neurol 149:89–112
212. Noguchi K, Watanabe N, Nagayoshi T et al (1999) Role of diffusion-weighted echo-planar MRI in distinguishing between brain abscess and tumour: a preliminary report. Neuroradiology 41:171–174
213. Park SH, Chang KH, Song IC, Kim YJ, Kim SH, Han MH (2000) Diffusion-weighted MRI in cystic or necrotic intracranial lesions. Neuroradiology 42:716–721
214. Holtas S, Geijer B, Stromblad LG, Maly-Sundgren P, Burtscher IM (2000) A ring-enhancing metastasis with central high signal on diffusion-weighted imaging and low apparent diffusion coefficients. Neuroradiology 42:824–827
215. Hartmann M, Jansen O, Heiland S, Sommer C, Munkel K, Sartor K (2001) Restricted diffusion within ring enhancement is not pathognomonic for brain abscess. AJNR Am J Neuroradiol 22:1738–1742
216. Geijer B, Holtas S (2002) Diffusion-weighted imaging of brain metastases: their potential to be misinterpreted as focal ischaemic lesions. Neuroradiology 44:568–573
217. Chang SC, Lai PH, Chen WL et al (2002) Diffusion-weighted MRI features of brain abscess and cystic or necrotic brain tumors: comparison with conventional MRI. Clin Imaging 26:227–236
218. Lai PH, Ho JT, Chen WL, Hsu SS, Wang JS, Pan HB, Yang CF (2002) Brain abscess and necrotic brain tumor: discrimination with proton MR spectroscopy and diffusion-weighted imaging. AJNR Am J Neuroradiol 23:1369–1377
219. Guzman R, Barth A, Lovblad KO et al (2002) Use of diffusion-weighted magnetic resonance imaging in differentiating purulent brain processes from cystic brain tumors. J Neurosurg 97:1101–1107
220. Smirniotopoulos JG, Murphy FM, Rushing EJ, Rees JH, Schroeder JW (2007) Patterns of contrast enhancement in the brain and meninges. Radiographics 27(2):525–551

221. Xu XX, Li B, Yang HF et al (2014) Can diffusion-weighted imaging be used to differentiate brain abscess from other ring-enhancing brain lesions? A meta-analysis. Clin Radiol 69(9):909–915

222. Toh CH, Wei KC, Ng SH, Wan YL, Lin CP, Castillo M (2011) Differentiation of brain abscesses from necrotic glioblastomas and cystic metastatic brain tumors with diffusion tensor imaging. AJNR Am J Neuroradiol 32(9):1646–1651

223. Pavlisa G, Rados M, Pavlisa G, Pavic L, Potocki K, Mayer D (2009) The differences of water diffusion between brain tissue infiltrated by tumor and peritumoral vasogenic edema. Clin Imaging 33(2):96–101

224. Byrnes TJ, Barrick TR, Bell BA, Clark CA (2011) Diffusion tensor imaging discriminates between glioblastoma and cerebral metastases in vivo. NMR Biomed 24(1):54–60

225. Bette S, Huber T, Wiestler B et al (2016) Analysis of fractional anisotropy facilitates differentiation of glioblastoma and brain metastases in a clinical setting. Eur J Radiol 85(12):2182–2187

226. Jakubovic R, Zhou S, Heyn C et al (2016) The predictive capacity of apparent diffusion coefficient (ADC) in response assessment of brain metastases following radiation. Clin Exp Metastasis 33(3):277–284

227. Ruiz-Espana S, Jimenez-Moya A, Arana E, Moratal D (2015) Functional diffusion map: a biomarker of brain metastases response to treatment based on magnetic resonance image analysis. Conf Proc IEEE Eng Med Biol Soc 2015:4282–4285

228. Meyer HJ, Fiedler E, Kornhuber M, Spielmann RP, Surov A (2015) Comparison of diffusion-weighted imaging findings in brain metastases of different origin. Clin Imaging 39(6):965–969

229. Duygulu G, Ovali GY, Calli C et al (2010) Intracerebral metastasis showing restricted diffusion: correlation with histopathologic findings. Eur J Radiol 74(1):117–120

230. Berghoff AS, Spanberger T, Ilhan-Mutlu A et al (2013) Preoperative diffusion-weighted imaging of single brain metastases correlates with patient survival times. PLoS One 8(2):e55464

231. Zakaria R, Das K, Radon M et al (2014) Diffusion-weighted MRI characteristics of the cerebral metastasis to brain boundary predicts patient outcomes. BMC Med Imaging 14:26

232. Hein PA, Eskey CJ, Dunn JF, Hug EB (2004) Diffusion-weighted imaging in the follow-up of treated high-grade gliomas: tumor recurrence versus radiation injury. AJNR Am J Neuroradiol 25:201–209

233. Stokkel M, Stevens H, Taphoorn M, Van Rijk P (1999) Differentiation between recurrent brain tumour and postradiation necrosis: the value of 201Tl SPET versus 18FFDG PET using a dual-headed coincidence camera-a pilot study. Nucl Med Commun 20:411–417

234. Tsuyuguchi N, Takami T, Sunada I, Iwai Y, Yamanaka K, Tanaka K, Nishikawa M, Ohata K, Torii K, Morino M, Nishio A, Hara M (2004) Methionine positron emission tomography for differentiation of recurrent brain tumor and radiation necrosis after stereotactic radiosurgery-in malignant glioma. Ann Nucl Med 18:291–296

235. Jain R, Scarpace L, Ellika S, Schultz LR, Rock JP, Rosenblum ML, Patel SC, Lee TY, Mikkelsen T (2007) First-pass perfusion computed tomography: initial experience in differentiating recurrent brain tumors from radiation effects and radiation necrosis. Neurosurgery 61:778–786

236. Sugahara T, Korogi Y, Tomiguchi S, Shigematsu Y, Ikushima I, Kira T, Liang L, Ushio Y, Takahashi M (2000) Posttherapeutic intraaxial brain tumor: the value of perfusion-sensitive contrast-enhanced MR imaging for differentiating tumor recurrence from nonneoplastic contrastenhancing tissue. AJNR Am J Neuroradiol 21:901–909

237. Provenzale JM, Mukundan S, Barboriak DP (2006) Diffusion-weighted and perfusion MR imaging for brain tumor characterization and assessment of treatment response. Radiology 239:632–649

238. Rock JP, Scarpace L, Hearshen D, Gutierrez J, Fisher JL, Rosenblum M, Mikkelsen T (2004) Associations among magnetic resonance spectroscopy, apparent diffusion coefficients, and image-guided histopathology with special attention to radiation necrosis. Neurosurgery 54:1111–1117; discussion 1117–1119

239. Schlemmer HP, Bachert P, Henze M, Buslei R, Herfarth KK, Debus J, van Kaick G (2002) Differentiation of radiation necrosis from tumor progression using proton magnetic resonance spectroscopy. Neuroradiology 44:216–222

240. Zeng QS, Li CF, Liu H, Zhen JH, Feng DC (2007) Distinction between recurrent glioma and radiation injury using magnetic resonance spectroscopy in combination with diffusion-weighted imaging. Int J Radiat Oncol Biol Phys 68:151–158

241. Chan YL, Yeung DK, Leung SF, Chan PN (2003) Diffusion-weighted magnetic resonance imaging in radiation-induced cerebral necrosis. Apparent diffusion coefficient in lesion components. J Comput Assist Tomogr 27:674–680

242. Asao C, Korogi Y, Kitajima M, Hirai T, Baba Y, Makino K, Kochi M, Morishita S, Yamashita Y (2005) Diffusion-weighted imaging of radiation-induced brain injury for differentiation from tumor recurrence. AJNR Am J Neuroradiol 26:1455–1460

243. Biousse V, Newman NJ, Hunter SB, Hudgins PA (2003) Diffusion weighted imaging in radiation necrosis. J Neurol Neurosurg Psychiatry 74: 382–384

244. Furuse M, Nonoguchi N, Yamada K et al (2019) Radiological diagnosis of brain radiation necrosis after cranial irradiation for brain tumor: a systematic review. Radiat Oncol 14(1):28. Published 2019 Feb 6. https://doi.org/10.1186/s13014-019-1228-x

245. Li C, Gan Y, Chen H et al (2020) Advanced multimodal imaging in differentiating glioma recurrence from post-radiotherapy changes. Int Rev Neurobiol 151:281–297

246. Louis DN, Perry A, Reifenberger G, von Deimling A, Figarella-Branger D, Cavenee WK et al (2016) The 2016 World Health Organization classification of tumors of the central nervous system: a summary. Acta Neuropathol 131(6):803–820

247. van den Bent MJ, Brandes AA, Taphoorn MJ, Kros JM, Kouwenhoven MC, Delattre JY et al (2013) Adjuvant procarbazine, lomustine, and vincristine chemotherapy in newly diagnosed anaplastic oligodendroglioma: long-term follow-up of EORTC brain tumor group study 26951. J Clin Oncol 31(3):344–350

248. Cairncross G, Wang M, Shaw E, Jenkins R, Brachman D, Buckner J et al (2013) Phase III trial of chemoradiotherapy for anaplastic oligodendroglioma: long-term results of RTOG 9402. J Clin Oncol 31(3):337–343

249. Brandes AA, Tosoni A, Cavallo G, Reni M, Franceschi E, Bonaldi L et al (2006) Correlations between O6-methylguanine DNA methyltransferase promoter methylation status, 1p and 19q deletions, and response to temozolomide in anaplastic and recurrent oligodendroglioma: a prospective GICNO study. J Clin Oncol 24(29):4746–4753

250. Wick W, Roth P, Hartmann C, Hau P, Nakamura M, Stockhammer F et al (2016) Long-term analysis of the NOA-04 randomized phase III trial of sequential radiochemotherapy of anaplastic glioma with PCV or temozolomide. Neuro-Oncology 18(11):1529–1537

251. Yan H, Parsons W, Jin G, McLendon R, Rasheed BA, Yuan W et al (2009) IDH1 and IDH2 mutations in gliomas. N Engl J Med 360(8):765–773

252. Chang S, Zhang P, Cairncross JG, Gilbert MR, Bahary JP, Dolinskas CA et al (2017) Phase III randomized study of radiation and temozolomide versus radiation and nitrosourea therapy for anaplastic astrocytoma: results of NRG Oncology RTOG 9813. Neuro-Oncology 19(2):252–258

253. Wick W, Hartmann C, Engel C, Stoffels M, Felsberg J, Stockhammer F et al (2009) NOA-04 randomized phase III trial of sequential radiochemotherapy of anaplastic glioma with procarbazine, lomustine, and vincristine or temozolomide. J Clin Oncol 27(35):5874–5880

254. Ohgaki H, Kleihues P (2013) The definition of primary and secondary glioblastoma. Clin Cancer Res 19(4):764–772

255. Parsons DW, Jones S, Zhang X, Lin JC, Leary RJ, Angenendt P et al (2008) An integrated genomic analysis of human glioblastoma multiforme. Science 321(5897):1807–1812

256. Nobusawa S, Watanabe T, Kleihues P, Ohgaki H (2009) IDH1 mutations as molecular signature and predictive factor of secondary glioblastomas. Clin Cancer Res 15(19):6002–6007

257. Liubinas SV, D'Abaco GM, Moffat BM, Gonzales M, Feleppa F, Nowell CJ et al (2014) IDH1 mutation is associated with seizures and protoplasmic subtype in patients with low-grade gliomas. Epilepsia 55(9):1438–1443

258. Zhong Z, Wang Z, Wang Y, You G, Jiang T (2015) IDH1/2 mutation is associated with seizure as an initial symptom in low-grade glioma: a report of 311 Chinese adult glioma patients. Epilepsy Res 109:100–105

259. Stupp R, Hegi ME, Mason W, van den Bent M, Taphoorn JB, Janzer RC et al (2009) Effects of radiotherapy with concomitant and adjuvant temozolomide versus radiotherapy alone on survival in glioblastoma in a randomised phase III study- 5-year analysis of the EORTC-NCIC trial. Lancet Oncol 10(5):459–466

260. Gilbert MR, Wang M, Aldape KD, Stupp R, Hegi ME, Jaeckle KA et al (2013) Dose-dense temozolomide for newly diagnosed glioblastoma: a randomized phase III clinical trial. J Clin Oncol 31(32):4085–4091

261. Gramatzki D, Kickingereder P, Hentschel B, Feslberg J, Herrlinger U, Schackert G et al (2017) Limited role for extended maintenance temozolomide for newly diagnosed glioblastoma. Neurology 88(15):1422–1430

262. Hegi ME, D'iserens A, Gorila T, Hamous M, de Tribolet N, Weller M et al (2005) MGMT gene silencing and benefit from temozolomide in glioblastoma. N Engl J Med 352(10):997–1003

263. Esteller M, Garcia-Foncillas J, Andion E, Goodman SN, Hidalgo OF, Vanaclocha V et al (2000) Inactivation of the DNA-repair gene MGMT and the clinical response of gliomas to alkylating agents. N Engl J Med 343(19):1350–1354

264. van den Bent MJ, Erdem-Eraslan L, Idbaih A, de Rooi J, Eilers PH, Spliet WG et al (2013) MGMT-STP27 methylation status as predictive marker for response to PCV in anaplastic Oligodendrogliomas and Oligoastrocytomas. A report from EORTC study 26951. Clin Cancer Res 19(19):5513–5522

265. Lai A, Tran A, Nghiemphu PL, Pope WB, Solis OE, Selch M et al (2011) Phase II study of bevacizumab plus temozolomide during and after radiation therapy for patients with newly diagnosed glioblastoma multiforme. J Clin Oncol 29(2):142–148

266. Wen PY, Huse JT (2016) World Health Organization classification of central nervous system tumors. Continuum (Minneap Minn). 2017;23(6, Neuro-oncology):1531–1547

267. Khuong-Quang DA, Buczkowicz P, Rakopoulos P, Liu XY, Fontebasso AM, Bouffet E et al (2012) K27M mutation in histone H3.3 defines clinically and biologically distinct subgroups of pediatric diffuse intrinsic pontine gliomas. Acta Neuropathol 124(3):439–447

268. Korshunov A, Ryzhova M, Hovestadt V, Bender S, Sturm D, Capper D et al (2015) Integrated analysis of pediatric glioblastoma reveals a subset of biologically favorable tumors with associated molecular prognostic markers. Acta Neuropathol 129(5):669–678

269. Sturm D, Witt H, Hovestadt V, Khuong-Quang DA, Jones DT, Konermann C et al (2012) Hotspot muta-

tions in H3F3A and IDH1 define distinct epigenetic and biological subgroups of glioblastoma. Cancer Cell 22(4):425–437

270. Daoud EV, Rajaram V, Cai C, Oberle RJ, Martin GR, Raisanen JM et al (2018) Adult brainstem gliomas with H3K27M mutation: radiology, pathology, and prognosis. J Neuropathol Exp Neurol 77(4):302–311

271. Lacroix M, Abi-Said D, Fourney DR, Gokaslan ZL, Shi W, DeMonte F et al (2001) A multivariate analysis of 416 patients with glioblastoma multiforme: prognosis, extent of resection, and survival. J Neurosurg 95:190–198

272. Brown TJ, Brennan MC, Li M, Church EW, Brandmeir NJ, Rakszawski KL et al (2016) Association of the extent of resection with survival in glioblastoma: a systematic review and meta-analysis. JAMA Oncol 2(11):1460–1469

273. Oszvald A, Guresir E, Setzer M, Vatter H, Senft C, Seifert V et al (2012) Glioblastoma therapy in the elderly and the importance of the extent of resection regardless of age. J Neurosurg 116(2):357–364

274. Walker MD, Green SB, Byar DP, Alexander E, Batzdorf U, Brooks WH et al (1980) Randomized comparisons of radiotherapy and nitrosoureas for the treatment of malignant glioma after surgery. N Engl J Med 303(23):1323–1329

275. Andersen AP (1978) Postoperative irradiation of glioblastomas: results in a randomized series. Acta Radiol Oncol Radiat Phys Biol 17(6):475–484

276. Corso CD, Bindra RS, Mehta MP (2017) The role of radiation in treating glioblastoma: here to stay. J Neuro-Oncol 134(3):479–485

277. Nayak L, Reardon DA (2017) High-grade gliomas. Continuum (Minneap Minn). 23(6, Neuro-oncology):1548–1563

278. Stupp R, Mason W, van den Bent M, Weller M, Fisher B, Taphoorn JB et al (2005) Radiotherapy plus concomitant and adjuvant temozolomide for glioblastoma. N Engl J Med 352(10):987–996

279. Brada M, Stenning S, Gabe R, Thompson LC, Levy D, Rampling R et al (2010) Temozolomide versus procarbazine, lomustine, and vincristine in recurrent high-grade glioma. J Clin Oncol 28(30):4601–4608

280. Balana C, Barroso CM, Berron S, Losada E, Munoz-Langa J, Estival A et al (2019) Randomized phase IIb clinical trial of continuation or non-continuation with six cycles of temozolomide after the first six cycles of standard first-line treatment in patients with glioblastoma: A Spanish research group in neuro-oncology (GEINO) trial. J Clin Oncol 37(15_suppl):2001–2001

281. Blumenthal DT, Gorlia T, Gilbert MR, Kim MM, Burt Nabors L, Mason WP et al (2017) Is more better? The impact of extended adjuvant temozolomide in newly diagnosed glioblastoma: a secondary analysis of EORTC and NRG Oncology/RTOG. Neuro-Oncology 19(8):1119–1126

282. Gerber DE, Grossman SA, Zeltzman M, Parisi MA, Kleinberg L (2007) The impact of thrombocytopenia from temozolomide and radiation in newly diag-

nosed adults with high-grade gliomas. Neuro-Oncology 9(1):47–52

283. Grossman SA, Ye X, Lesser G, Sloan A, Carraway H, Desideri S et al (2011) Immunosuppression in patients with high-grade gliomas treated with radiation and temozolomide. Clin Cancer Res 17(16):5473–5480

284. Kirson ED, Gurvich Z, Schneiderman R, Dekel E, Itzhaki A, Wasserman Y et al (2004) Disruption of cancer cell replication by alternating electric fields. Cancer Res 64:3288–3295

285. Kirson ED, Dbaly V, Tovarys F, Vymazal J, Soustiel JF, Itzhaki A et al (2007) Alternating electric fields arrest cell proliferation in animal tumor models and human brain tumors. Proc Natl Acad Sci U S A 104(24):10152–10157

286. Stupp R, Taillibert S, Kanner AA, Kesari S, Steinberg DM, Toms SA et al (2015) Maintenance therapy with tumor-treating fields plus temozolomide vs temozolomide alone for glioblastoma: a randomized clinical trial. JAMA 314(23):2535–2543

287. Sampson JH (2015) Alternating electric fields for the treatment of glioblastoma. JAMA 314(23):2511–2513

288. Bernard-Arnoux F, Lamure M, Ducray F, Aulagner G, Honnorat J, Armoiry X (2016) The cost-effectiveness of tumor-treating fields therapy in patients with newly diagnosed glioblastoma. Neuro-Oncology 18(8):1129–1136

289. van den Bent MJ, Baumert B, Erridge SC, Vogelbaum MA, Nowak AK, Sanson M et al (2017) Interim results from the CATNON trial (EORTC study 26053-22054) of treatment with concurrent and adjuvant temozolomide for 1p/19q non-co-deleted anaplastic glioma: a phase 3, randomised, open-label intergroup study. Lancet 390(10103): 1645–1653

290. Juratli TA, Lautenschlager T, Geiger KD, Pinzer T, Krause M, Schackert G et al (2015) Radio-chemotherapy improves survival in IDH-mutant, 1p/19q non-codeleted secondary high-grade astrocytoma patients. J Neuro-Oncol 124(2):197–205

291. Brandes AA, Nicolardi L, Tosoni A, Gardiman M, Iuzzolino P, Ghimenton C et al (2006) Survival following adjuvant PCV or temozolomide for anaplastic astrocytoma. Neuro-Oncology 8(3): 253–260

292. van den Bent MJ, Taphoorn MJ, Brandes AA, Menten J, Stupp R, Frenay M et al (2003) Phase II study of first-line chemotherapy with temozolomide in recurrent oligodendroglial tumors: the European Organization for Research and Treatment of Cancer Brain Tumor Group Study 26971. J Clin Oncol 21(13):2525–2528

293. Arrillaga I, Kurz S, Sumrall A, Butowski NA, Harrison RA, De Groot JF et al (2019) Single agent ONC201 in adult recurrent H3 K27M-mutant glioma. J Clin Oncol 37(15_suppl):3005

294. Chi AS, Gardner SL, Arrillaga I, Wen PY, Batchelor T, Hall MD et al (2018) Integrated clinical experi-

ence with ONC201 in H3 K27M glioma. J Clin Oncol 36(15_suppl):2059

295. Batchelor T, Carson K, O'Neill A, Grossman SA, Alavi J, New P et al (2003) Treatment of primary CNS lymphoma with methotrexate and deferred radiotherapy: a report of NABTT 96-07. J Clin Oncol 21(6):1044–1049

296. Shibamoto Y, Ogino H, Takemoto M, Araki N, Isobe K, Tsuchida E et al (2008) Primary central nervous system lymphoma in Japan: changes in clinical features, treatment, and prognosis during 1985–2004. Neuro-Oncology 10(4):560–568

297. Ferreri AJ, Reni M, Villa E (2000) Therapeutic management of primary central nervous system lymphoma: lessons from prospective trials. Ann Oncol 11(8):927–937

298. Ferreri AJ, Reni M, Pasini F, Calderoni A, Tirelli U, Pivnik A et al (2002) A multicenter study of treatment of primary CNS lymphoma. Neurology 58(10):1513–1520

299. Pels H, Schmidt-Wolf IG, Glasmacher A, Schulz H, Engert A, Diehl V et al (2003) Primary central nervous system lymphoma: results of a pilot and phase II study of systemic and intraventricular chemotherapy with deferred radiotherapy. J Clin Oncol 21(24):4489–4495

300. Zhu JJ, Gerstner ER, Engler DA, Mrugala MM, Nugent W, Nierenberg K et al (2009) High-dose methotrexate for elderly patients with primary CNS lymphoma. Neuro-Oncology 11(2):211–215

301. Gerstner ER, Carson KA, Grossman SA, Batchelor TT (2008) Long-term outcome in PCNSL patients treated with high-dose methotrexate and deferred radiation. Neurology 70(5):401–402

302. Herrlinger U, Kuker W, Uhl M, Blaicher HP, Karnath HO, Kanz L et al (2005) NOA-03 trial of high-dose methotrexate in primary central nervous system lymphoma: final report. Ann Neurol 57(6): 843–847

303. Ferreri AJM, Reni M, Foppoli M, Martelli M, Pangalis GA, Frezzato M et al (2009) High-dose cytarabine plus high-dose methotrexate versus high-dose methotrexate alone in patients with primary CNS lymphoma: a randomised phase 2 trial. Lancet 374(9700):1512–1520

304. Ferreri AJM, Cwynarski K, Pulczynski E, Ponzoni M, Deckert M, Politi LS et al (2016) Chemoimmunotherapy with methotrexate, cytarabine, thiotepa, and rituximab (MATRix regimen) in patients with primary CNS lymphoma: results of the first randomisation of the International Extranodal Lymphoma Study Group-32 (IELSG32) phase 2 trial. Lancet Haematol 3(5):e217–ee27

305. Rubenstein JL, Hsi ED, Johnson JL, Jung SH, Nakashima MO, Grant B et al (2013) Intensive chemotherapy and immunotherapy in patients with newly diagnosed primary CNS lymphoma: CALGB 50202 (Alliance 50202). J Clin Oncol 31(25):3061–3068

306. Morris PG, Correa DD, Yahalom J, Raizer JJ, Schiff D, Grant B et al (2013) Rituximab, methotrexate, procarbazine, and vincristine followed by consolidation reduced-dose whole-brain radiotherapy and cytarabine in newly diagnosed primary CNS lymphoma: final results and long-term outcome. J Clin Oncol 31(31):3971–3979

307. Shah GD, Yahalom J, Correa DD, Lai RK, Raizer JJ, Schiff D et al (2007) Combined immunochemotherapy with reduced whole-brain radiotherapy for newly diagnosed primary CNS lymphoma. J Clin Oncol 25(30):4730–4735

308. Han CH, Batchelor TT (2017) Primary central nervous system lymphoma. Continuum (Minneap Minn). 23(6, Neuro-oncology):1601–1618

309. Korfel A, Thiel E, Martus P, Mohle R, Griesinger F, Rauch M et al (2015) Randomized phase III study of whole-brain radiotherapy for primary CNS lymphoma. Neurology 84(12):1242–1248

310. Thiel E, Korfel A, Martus P, Kanz L, Griesinger F, Rauch M et al (2010) High-dose methotrexate with or without whole brain radiotherapy for primary CNS lymphoma (G-PCNSL-SG-1): a phase 3, randomised, non-inferiority trial. Lancet Oncol 11(11):1036–1047

311. Hyman DM, Taylor BS, Baselga J (2017) Implementing genome-driven oncology. Cell 168(4):584–599

312. Ascierto PA, McArthur GA, Dréno B, Atkinson V, Liszkay G, Di Giacomo AM et al (2016) Cobimetinib combined with vemurafenib in advanced BRAFV600-mutant melanoma (coBRIM): updated efficacy results from a randomised, double-blind, phase 3 trial. Lancet Oncol 17(9):1248–1260

313. Robert C, Karaszewska B, Schachter J, Rutkowski P, Mackiewicz A, Stroiakovski D et al (2015) Improved overall survival in melanoma with combined dabrafenib and trametinib. N Engl J Med 372(1):30–39

314. Planchard D, Besse B, Groen HJM, Souquet P-J, Quoix E, Baik CS et al (2016) Dabrafenib plus trametinib in patients with previously treated BRAFV600E-mutant metastatic non-small cell lung cancer: an open-label, multicentre phase 2 trial. Lancet Oncol 17(7):984–993

315. Subbiah V, Kreitman RJ, Wainberg ZA, Cho JY, Schellens JHM, Soria JC et al (2018) Dabrafenib and trametinib treatment in patients with locally advanced or metastatic BRAF V600-mutant anaplastic thyroid cancer. J Clin Oncol 36(1):7–13

316. Corcoran RB, Atreya CE, Falchook GS, Kwak EL, Ryan DP, Bendell JC et al (2015) Combined BRAF and MEK inhibition with dabrafenib and trametinib in BRAF V600-mutant colorectal cancer. J Clin Oncol 33(34):4023–4031

317. Chi AS, Batchelor TT, Yang D, Dias-Santagata D, Borger DR, Ellisen LW et al (2013) BRAF V600E mutation identifies a subset of low-grade diffusely infiltrating gliomas in adults. J Clin Oncol 31(14):e233–e236

318. Brennan CW, Verhaak RG, McKenna A, Campos B, Noushmehr H, Salama SR et al (2013) The somatic genomic landscape of glioblastoma. Cell 155(2):462–477

319. Kaley T, Touat M, Subbiah V, Hollebecque A, Rodon J, Lockhart AC et al (2018) BRAF inhibition in BRAF(V600)-mutant gliomas: results From the VE-BASKET study. J Clin Oncol 36(35):3477–3484. https://doi.org/10.1200/JCO.2018.78.9990

320. Rohle D, Popovici-Muller J, Palaskas N, Turcan S, Grommes C, Campos C et al (2013) An inhibitor of mutant IDH1 delays growth and promotes differentiation of glioma cells. Science 340(6132):626–630

321. Schumacher T, Bunse L, Pusch S, Sahm F, Wiestler B, Quandt J et al (2014) A vaccine targeting mutant IDH1 induces antitumour immunity. Nature 512(7514):324–327

322. Mellinghoff IK, Penas-Prado M, Peters KB, Cloughesy TF, Burris HA, Maher EA et al (2018) Phase 1 study of AG-881, an inhibitor of mutant IDH1/IDH2, in patients with advanced IDH-mutant solid tumors, including glioma. J Clin Oncol 36(15_suppl):2002

323. Fan B, Mellinghoff IK, Wen PY, Lowery MA, Goyal L, Tap WD et al (2019) Clinical pharmacokinetics and pharmacodynamics of ivosidenib, an oral, targeted inhibitor of mutant IDH1, in patients with advanced solid tumors. Investig New Drugs 38(2):433–444

324. Herrlinger U, Tzaridis T, Mack F, Steinbach JP, Schlegel U, Sabel M et al (2019) Lomustine-temozolomide combination therapy versus standard temozolomide therapy in patients with newly diagnosed glioblastoma with methylated MGMT promoter (CeTeG/NOA–09): a randomised, open-label, phase 3 trial. Lancet 393(10172):678–688

325. Verhaak RG, Hoadley KA, Purdom E, Wang V, Qi Y, Wilkerson MD et al (2010) Integrated genomic analysis identifies clinically relevant subtypes of glioblastoma characterized by abnormalities in PDGFRA, IDH1, EGFR, and NF1. Cancer Cell 17(1):98–110

326. Phillips HS, Kharbanda S, Chen R, Forrest WF, Soriano RH, Wu TD et al (2006) Molecular subclasses of high-grade glioma predict prognosis, delineate a pattern of disease progression, and resemble stages in neurogenesis. Cancer Cell 9(3):157–173

327. Noushmehr H, Weisenberger DJ, Diefes K, Phillips HS, Pujara K, Berman BP et al (2010) Identification of a CpG island methylator phenotype that defines a distinct subgroup of glioma. Cancer Cell 17(5):510–522

328. Parker NR, Khong P, Parkinson JF, Howell VM, Wheeler HR (2015) Molecular heterogeneity in glioblastoma: potential clinical implications. Front Oncol 5:55

329. De Sousa EMF, Vermeulen L, Fessler E, Medema JP (2013) Cancer heterogeneity—a multifaceted view. EMBO Rep 14(8):686–695

330. Sottoriva A, Spiteri I, Piccirillo SG, Touloumis A, Collins VP, Marioni JC et al (2013) Intratumor heterogeneity in human glioblastoma reflects cancer evolutionary dynamics. Proc Natl Acad Sci U S A 110(10):4009–4014

331. Snuderl M, Fazlollahi L, Le LP, Nitta M, Zhelyazkova BH, Davidson CJ et al (2011) Mosaic amplification of multiple receptor tyrosine kinase genes in glioblastoma. Cancer Cell 20(6):810–817

332. Szerlip NJ, Pedraza A, Chakravarty D, Azim M, McGuire J, Fang Y et al (2012) Intratumoral heterogeneity of receptor tyrosine kinases EGFR and PDGFRA amplification in glioblastoma defines subpopulations with distinct growth factor response. Proc Natl Acad Sci U S A 109(8):3041–3046

333. Patel AP, Tirosh I, Trombetta JJ, Shalek AK, Gillespie SM, Wakimoto H et al (2014) Single-cell RNA-seq highlights intratumoral heterogeneity in primary glioblastoma. Science 344(6190):1396–1401

334. Gerlinger M, Rowan AJ, Horswell S, Math M, Larkin J, Endesfelder D et al (2012) Intratumor heterogeneity and branched evolution revealed by multiregion sequencing. N Engl J Med 366(10):883–892

335. Wang J, Cazzato E, Ladewig E, Frattini V, Rosenbloom DI, Zairis S et al (2016) Clonal evolution of glioblastoma under therapy. Nat Genet 48(7):768–776

336. Soeda A, Hara A, Kunisada T, Yoshimura S, Iwama T, Park DM (2015) The evidence of glioblastoma heterogeneity. Sci Rep 5:7979

337. Meyer M, Reimand J, Lan X, Head R, Zhu X, Kushida M et al (2015) Single cell-derived clonal analysis of human glioblastoma links functional and genomic heterogeneity. Proc Natl Acad Sci U S A 112(3):851–856

338. Bedard PL, Hansen AR, Ratain MJ, Siu LL (2013) Tumour heterogeneity in the clinic. Nature 501(7467):355–364

339. Stelzer KJ (2013) Epidemiology and prognosis of brain metastases. Surg Neurol Int 4(Suppl 4):S192–S202

340. Glitza Oliva IC, Schvartsman G, Tawbi H (2018) Advances in the systemic treatment of melanoma brain metastases. Ann Oncol 29(7):1509–1520

341. Tawbi HA, Forsyth PA, Algazi A, Hamid O, Hodi FS, Moschos SJ et al (2018) Combined nivolumab and ipilimumab in melanoma metastatic to the brain. N Engl J Med 379(8):722–730

342. Davies MA, Saiag P, Robert C, Grob JJ, Flaherty KT, Arance A et al (2017) Dabrafenib plus trametinib in patients with BRAF(V600)-mutant melanoma brain metastases (COMBI-MB): a multicentre, multicohort, open-label, phase 2 trial. Lancet Oncol 18(7):863–873

343. Kabraji S, Ni J, Lin NU, Xie S, Winer EP, Zhao JJ (2018) Drug resistance in HER2-positive breast cancer brain metastases: blame the barrier or the brain? Clin Cancer Res 24(8):1795–1804

344. Aoyama H, Shirato H, Tago M, Nakagawa K, Toyoda T, Hatano K et al (2006) Stereotactic radiosurgery plus whole-brain radiation therapy vs stereotactic radiosurgery alone for treatment of brain metastases: a randomized controlled trial. JAMA 295(21):2483–2491

345. Brown DR, Lanciano R, Heal C, Hanlon A, Yang J, Feng J et al (2017) The effect of whole-brain radiation (WBI) and Karnofsky performance status (KPS) on survival of patients receiving stereotactic radiosurgery (SRS) for second brain metastatic event. J Radiat Oncol 6(1):31–37

346. Chang EL, Wefel JS, Hess KR, Allen PK, Lang FF, Kornguth DG et al (2009) Neurocognition in patients with brain metastases treated with radiosurgery or radiosurgery plus whole-brain irradiation: a randomised controlled trial. Lancet Oncol 10(11):1037–1044

347. Kocher M, Soffietti R, Abacioglu U, Villa S, Fauchon F, Baumert BG et al (2011) Adjuvant whole-brain radiotherapy versus observation after radiosurgery or surgical resection of one to three cerebral metastases: results of the EORTC 22952-26001 study. J Clin Oncol 29(2):134–141

348. Yamamoto M, Serizawa T, Shuto T, Akabane A, Higuchi Y, Kawagishi J et al (2014) Stereotactic radiosurgery for patients with multiple brain metastases (JLGK0901): a multi-institutional prospective observational study. Lancet Oncol 15(4):387–395

349. Kim J, Kim MM, Starkey LJ (2018) A primer on secondary brain neoplasms: the essentials. Semin Roentgenol 53(1):101–111

350. Komada T, Naganawa S, Ogawa H, Matsushima M, Kubota S, Kawai H et al (2008) Contrast-enhanced MR imaging of metastatic brain tumor at 3 tesla: utility of T(1)-weighted SPACE compared with 2D spin echo and 3D gradient echo sequence. Magn Reson Med Sci 7(1):13–21

351. Reichert M, Morelli JN, Runge VM, Tao A, von Ritschl R, von Ritschl A et al (2013) Contrast-enhanced 3-dimensional SPACE versus MP-RAGE for the detection of brain metastases: consider-

ations with a 32-channel head coil. Investig Radiol 48(1):55–60

352. Sneed PK, Mendez J, Vemer-van den Hoek JG, Seymour ZA, Ma L, Molinaro AM et al (2015) Adverse radiation effect after stereotactic radiosurgery for brain metastases: incidence, time course, and risk factors. J Neurosurg 123(2):373–386

353. Kohutek ZA, Yamada Y, Chan TA, Brennan CW, Tabar V, Gutin PH et al (2015) Long-term risk of radionecrosis and imaging changes after stereotactic radiosurgery for brain metastases. J Neuro-Oncol 125(1):149–156

354. Okada H, Weller M, Huang R, Finocchiaro G, Gilbert MR, Wick W et al (2015) Immunotherapy response assessment in neuro-oncology: a report of the RANO working group. Lancet Oncol 16(15):e534–ee42

355. Reardon DA, Okada H (2015) Re-defining response and treatment effects for neuro-oncology immunotherapy clinical trials. J Neuro-Oncol 123(3):339–346

356. Colaco RJ, Martin P, Kluger HM, Yu JB, Chiang VL (2016) Does immunotherapy increase the rate of radiation necrosis after radiosurgical treatment of brain metastases? J Neurosurg 125(1):17–23

357. Kroeze SG, Fritz C, Hoyer M, Lo SS, Ricardi U, Sahgal A et al (2017) Toxicity of concurrent stereotactic radiotherapy and targeted therapy or immunotherapy: a systematic review. Cancer Treat Rev 53:25–37

358. Lin NU, Lee EQ, Aoyama H, Barani IJ, Barboriak DP, Baumert BG et al (2015) Response assessment criteria for brain metastases: proposal from the RANO group. Lancet Oncol 16(6):e270–e278

359. Bleehen NM, Girling DJ, Gregor A, Leonard RC, Machin D, McKenzie CG et al (1991) A Medical Research Council phase II trial of alternating chemotherapy and radiotherapy in small-cell lung cancer. The Medical Research Council Lung Cancer working party. Br J Cancer 64(4):775–779

360. Walker MD, Strike TA, Sheline GE (1979) An analysis of dose-effect relationship in the radiotherapy of malignant gliomas. Int J Radiat Oncol Biol Phys 5(10):1725–1731

Pediatrics

19

Lillian Lai, and Toshio Moritani

Satsuki Matsumoto, Mariko Sato,
Jeremy D. Greenlee, and John M. Buatti

19.1 Introduction

Diffusion-weighted imaging (DWI) is crucial in the evaluation of the pediatric brain, head and neck, and spine. Likewise, diffusion tensor imaging (DTI) can be a useful tool in evaluation of white matter structure. This chapter will cover the normal DWI and DTI imaging of the pediatric brain. It will also review different pathologies in which DWI and DTI are useful, including infarction/ischemia, hypoxic ischemic encephalopathy, accidental and nonaccidental trauma, infection, tumor, encephalopathy, demyelinating and toxic diseases, inborn errors of metabolism, and congenital anomalies. The major highlights of the chapter are tumors (brain, head/neck, and spine) and inborn errors of metabolism.

19.2 Water Content of the Pediatric Brain

The water content of the pediatric brain is considerably higher than that of the adult brain. This makes it more difficult to diagnose ischemic and other lesions in pediatric patients using computed tomography (CT) and MR imaging. Diffusion-weighted (DW) imaging is sensitive to alteration in diffusion of water molecules, and this technique can help overcome some of these difficulties [1]. DW imaging is primarily useful for detecting and characterizing ischemic lesions, but also for evaluation of myelination by demonstrating the anisotropy of the white matter earlier than conventional MR imaging [2, 3].

19.3 Normal Structures

Diffusion-weighted imaging characteristics of a normal brain in young infants are different from those in adults [4]. Apparent diffusion coefficient (ADC) values in both gray and white matter of newborns are considerably higher than in adults. This reflects the high water content of the pediatric brain [5]. For the same reason, the deep white matter in the newborn normally shows hypointensity on DW imaging associated with increased ADC (Fig. 19.1). With increasing age, there is a relative decrease in water content of the pediatric brain (Fig. 19.2). This is more evident in the white matter than in the gray matter. The decrease

---

L. Lai (✉)
Department of Radiology, Children's Hospital Los Angeles, Los Angeles, CA, USA

T. Moritani
Division of Neuroradiology, University of Michigan, Ann Arbor, MI, USA
e-mail: tmoritan@med.umich.edu

S. Matsumoto · M. Sato · J. D. Greenlee · J. M. Buatti
University of Iowa Hospitals and Clinics, Iowa City, IA, USA
e-mail: satsuki-matsumoto@uiowa.edu;
mariko-sato@uiowa.edu; jeremy-greenlee@uiowa.edu;
john-buatti@uiowa.edu

© Springer Nature Switzerland AG 2021
T. Moritani, A. A. Capizzano (eds.), *Diffusion-Weighted MR Imaging of the Brain, Head and Neck, and Spine*, https://doi.org/10.1007/978-3-030-62120-9_19

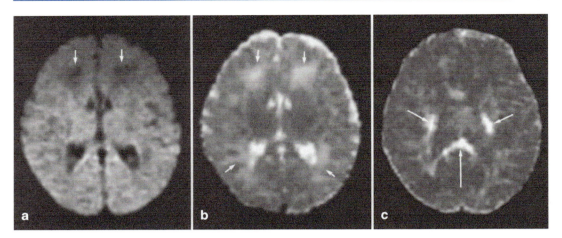

Fig. 19.1 (a–c) Normal pediatric DW imaging in a 2-day-old boy. (a) Low signal intensity and (b) increased ADC in the deep white matter are normal in this age group (*arrows*). (c) Fractional anisotropy map demonstrates high anisotropy along the anterior and posterior limbs of the internal capsules (*arrows*), the corpus callosum (*long arrow*), and the temporo-parieto-occipital white matter earlier than regular T1- and T2-weighted images

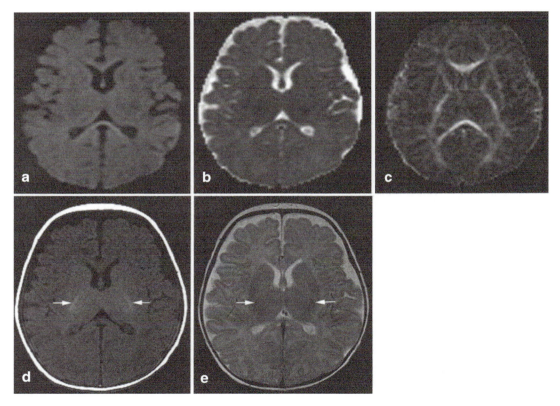

Fig. 19.2 (a–e) Normal MR image in a 2-month-old girl. (a, b) The low signal intensity on DW imaging and increased ADC in the deep white matter are no longer visualized in this age group. The ADC values in the gray matter and corpus callosum appear slightly lower than in the rest of the white matter. (c) Fractional anisotropy map demonstrates anisotropy noted not only in the corpus callosum and internal capsules but also the entire white matter including U-fibers. (d, e) T1- and T2-weighted images show myelination mainly in the posterior limb of the internal capsules (*arrows*)

in water content is caused by myelination with reduced water content during normal white matter development [2]. During the maturation period, the ADC histogram shifts from the large ADC values of the newborn brain ($>1.1 \times 10^{-3}$ mm^2/s) to more moderate ADC values, and eventually stabilizes in the adult period with peak ADC values of about 0.8×10^{-3} mm^2/s [6]. The optimum b-value to use in neonates depends on optimizing contrast to noise and the ADC differences between anisotropic and isotropic brain, but for neonates the b-value is often made shorter around 800 s/mm^2, about 200 s/mm^2 less than in adults [7].

19.4 Diffusion Tensor Imaging and Anisotropy

Normally anisotropy is much less evident in the immature brain than in the adult. One exception is the corpus callosum, where anisotropy is already visible by diffusion imaging as early as the 28th gestational week. This occurs although the corpus callosum is composed of non-myelinated fibers at that stage of development. The phenomenon has been called premyelination anisotropy [3]. The anisotropic effect in the immature brain is thought to be related to the structure of the axonal membrane. Anisotropy in the white matter of newborns and infants is lower than in adults (Figs. 19.1 and 19.2). The anisotropic pattern can vary depending on the irregularity of axonal orientation as well as the degree of myelination. Structural and functional alterations of the axons and oligodendrocytes that may affect diffusion anisotropy include an increase of the axonal diameter, increase in the concentration of the microtubule-associated proteins and microperoxysome, activity of Na$^+$/K$^+$-ATPase, and ion fluxes secondary to action potentials [8].

Diffusion tensor (DT) imaging is useful for evaluating the myelination and premyelination states of the infant brain. Data of fractional anisotropy (FA) and ADC values have been reported in utero, in newborns (preterm, term), infants, and early childhood [2, 9–16]. FA and ADC values dramatically change during the in utero period

in the pyramidal tract and the corpus callosum [9] and in the first 3 months of life. DT imaging allows earlier detection of specific anatomic microstructural abnormalities in infants at risk for neurological abnormalities and disability [10].

19.5 Infarction and Ischemia

Ischemic infarctions in children are uncommon when compared with adults and they have different etiologies. The reported incidence ranges from 2.3 to 13 per 100,000 children per year. In children strokes are more evenly divided between ischemic and hemorrhagic strokes, whereas in adults strokes are usually ischemic in 85% of cases [17]. Causes of ischemic strokes include thrombosis, embolism, arterial dissection, vasculitis, Moyamoya disease, sickle cell disease, child abuse, etc. (Figs. 19.3, 19.4, 19.5, and 19.6) [18, 19]. The most common etiologies are underlying cerebral arteriopathy (50% of cases) and cardioembolism (30% of cases) [20]. Hyperacute and acute infarctions are characterized by cytotoxic edema. Vasogenic edema occurs later and is typically seen in the subacute phase. DW imaging is useful for early detection of infarction in children, but also to differentiate between acute/subacute infarctions and chronic infarctions or ischemic gliosis.

19.5.1 Moyamoya Disease

Moyamoya disease is a chronic cerebrovascular occlusive disease of unknown origin that occurs predominantly in East Asia. In children it is characterized by progressive arterial stenosis with cerebral infarctions. The stenosis involves primarily the circle of Willis and the supraclinoid portion of the internal carotid arteries. Typically the internal carotid arteries are occluded bilaterally. In so-called "probable" Moyamoya disease, there is unilateral occlusion of one of the carotid arteries in its supraclinoid portion. DW imaging is useful for early detection of cerebral ischemia in this disease (Fig. 19.5) [17].

19.5.2 Sickle Cell Disease

About 5%–8% of patients with sickle cell disease develop symptomatic cerebrovascular disease [18]. The risk of stroke is greatest during thrombotic crises and during the first 15 years of life. Stenosis or occlusion of both large and small vessels can cause cerebral infarction. Sickle cell disease results in vasculopathy, which in many respects is similar to Moyamoya disease. Cortical and white matter watershed ischemia is common; however, patients with sickle cell disease often also demonstrate multiple ischemic white matter lesions. These lesions can occur in spite of normal MR angiography and conventional angiography (Fig. 19.6) [19]. They are thought to be due to small vessel ischemia similar to what is seen in small vessel disease of older patients.

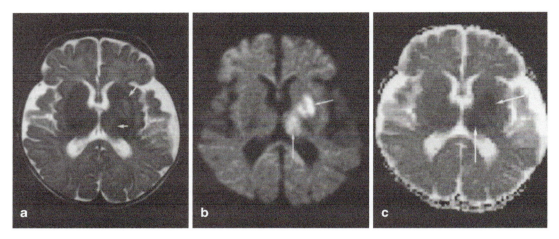

Fig. 19.3 (a–c) Cerebral infarction due to embolism in a 3-month-old boy with Down syndrome and ventricular septal defect. (a) T2-weighted image shows mild high signal lesions in the left putamen and thalamus (*arrows*). (b) DW image shows these lesions as high signal intensity (*arrows*). (c) ADC is decreased (*arrows*), consistent with acute infarcts

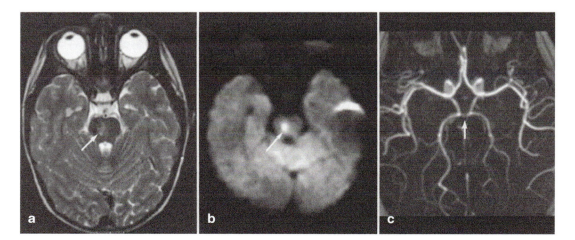

Fig. 19.4 (a–c) Dissection of the vertebrobasilar arteries and infarction in a 4-year-old girl. (a) T2-weighted image shows high signal lesion in the right paramedian pons (*arrow*). (b) DW image shows this lesion as hyperintense with decreased ADC (not shown), representing an acute infarct (*arrow*). (c) On MR angiography the vertebrobasilar arteries flow void are absent due to dissection (*arrow*). The posterior cerebral arteries are supplied from the anterior circulation

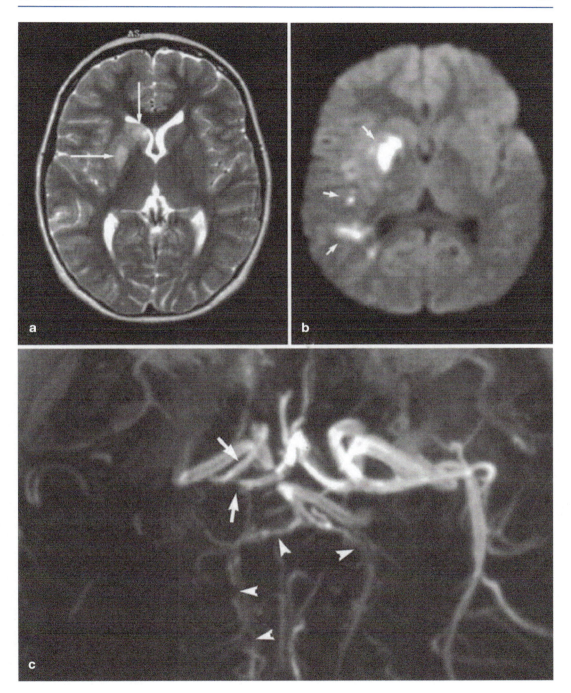

Fig. 19.5 (**a–c**) "Probable" Moyamoya disease in a 7-year-old girl. (**a**) T2-weighted image shows high signal lesions in the right basal ganglia. (**b**) DW image shows ischemic lesions not only in the basal ganglia but also in the right parieto-occipital region as high signal, representing acute infarcts (*arrows*). (**c**) MR angiography shows occlusion of the right middle cerebral artery and stenosis of the right internal carotid artery (*arrows*) and bilateral posterior cerebral arteries (*arrowheads*)

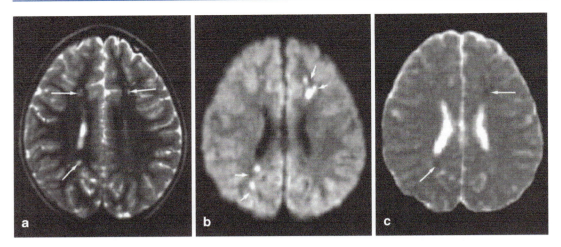

Fig. 19.6 (a–c) Sickle cell disease in a 4-year-old boy presenting with severe headache. (**a**) T2-weighted image shows multiple high signal spots in the white matter (*arrows*). (**b**) DW image shows some of these spots as very high signal intensity, representing small acute infarcts (*arrows*). (**c**) ADC map shows decreased ADC of these lesions consistent with small ischemic lesions (*arrows*)

Nontraumatic fat embolism is a rare but potentially lethal complication of sickle cell disease (Fig. 19.7). Fat embolism usually occurs as a complication of trauma such as long bone fractures, but in sickle cell disease, emboli arise from bone marrow infarcts and osteonecrosis [21]. Fat emboli from marrow are thought to enter osseous venous channels, and can ultimately reach the brain by traversing the pulmonary capillary bed or via a right-to-left cardiac shunt [21]. On MRI, fat emboli are characterized by multiple foci of restricted diffusion and microhemorrhages. The differential for these findings include diffuse axonal injury, cardiogenic, septic, or fat emboli; vasculitis; and tiny hemorrhagic metastases.

19.5.3 Cerebral Venous Sinus Thrombosis

Cerebral venous sinus thrombosis and venous infarction/hemorrhage are common in children, with an incidence of 0.4–0.7 per 100,000 children per year [20]. Risk factors include infections, perinatal complications, hematologic disorders, nephritic syndrome, malignancy, and collagen vascular disease among others. Parasagittal infarction/hemorrhage is seen in superior sagittal sinus thrombosis, temporal lobe involvement is associated with transverse sinus and vein of Labbe thrombosis, and thalamic or basal ganglia involvement is associated with deep vein thrombosis (Fig. 19.8). Reduced venous outflow due to venous sinus occlusion causes leakage of fluid (vasogenic edema) and hemorrhage into the extracellular space. If adequate venous collaterals are not established, subsequent venous infarction ensues. Gradient echo T2*-weighted imaging is very useful in the detection of acute- to subacute-phase thrombi as very low signal, especially before T1-weighted imaging shows high signal in the subacute-phase thrombi. DW imaging shows subacute-phase thrombi as high signal with decreased ADC. Accelerated myelination has been reported in association with cerebral venous thrombosis in neonates [22].

19.5.4 Vein of Galen Malformations

Vein of Galen malformation is thought to result from the development of an arteriovenous connection between the primitive choroidal vessels and median prosencephalic vein of Markowski. There are two main types: (1) the choroidal type (90%) characterized by numerous feeders occurring in neonates, (2) the mural type characterized by fewer feeders occurring in infants.

19 Pediatrics

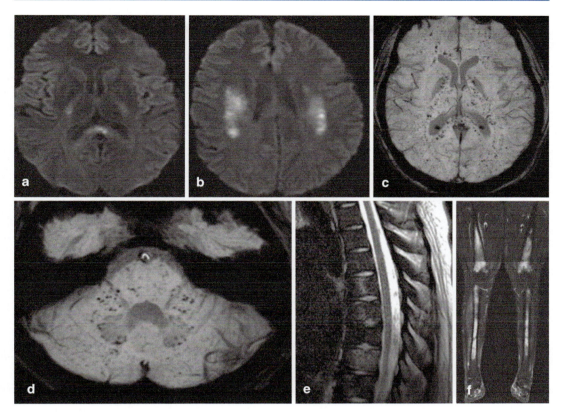

Fig. 19.7 (**a–f**) Nontraumatic fat-embolism due to osteonecrosis and sickle cell crisis in a 20-year-old female with sickle cell disease, who presented with waxing and waning mental status, confusion, and hallucinations two weeks after being treated for acute chest syndrome and spine pain. (**a, b**) Axial DWI sequences show foci of diffusion restriction in the splenium of the corpus callosum, posterior limbs of the internal capsules, and the periventricular white matter. (**c, d**) Susceptibility-weighted images (SWI) demonstrate multiple punctate foci of susceptibility throughout the supratentorial and infratentorial brain, consistent with microhemorrhagic emboli. (**e**) Sagittal STIR image of the thoracic spine show multilevel osteonecrosis and compression fractures. (**f**) Coronal STIR image of the lower extremities demonstrates extensive areas of osteonecrosis

Progressive stenosis of the jugular bulbs complicates the course in many cases. Ischemia can occur as arterial or venous type, associated with steal phenomenon of the arteriovenous shunt. Pre- and posttreatment evaluations of the extent of ischemic brain injury are important for providing information on likely neurological and developmental sequelae (Fig. 19.9) [23].

19.5.5 Hypoxic Ischemic Encephalopathy

Hypoxic ischemic encephalopathy is the result of decreased global perfusion or oxygenation. It is generally due to neonatal anoxia, suffocation, cardiac arrest, or child abuse. Regardless of its etiology, it is remarkably similar to infarcted brain in its histological appearance. The distribution of hypoxic ischemic encephalopathy varies according to the duration, degree, and abruptness of the hypoxic and/or ischemic insult, basal blood flow, and metabolic activity in the areas of ischemia, temperature, and serum glucose levels.

Diffusion-weighted imaging often depicts acute or subacute ischemic lesions when MR imaging and CT scans are normal or show only subtle abnormalities (Figs. 19.10 and 19.11) [24–28]. DWI findings may be subtle due to the high T2 signal of unmyelinated white matter, so it is

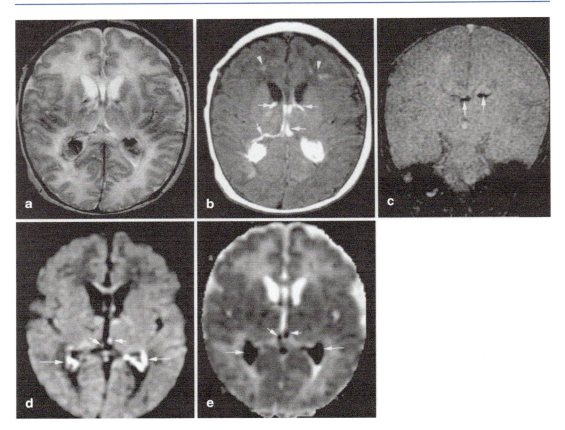

Fig. 19.8 (**a–e**) Cerebral venous sinus thrombosis in a 5-day-old boy with bacterial meningitis. (**a, b**) Hemorrhage in the choroid plexi is hyperintense on T1- and hypointense on T2-weighted image. Precontrast T1-weighted image shows thrombi in the bilateral internal cerebral veins and branches as hyperintense (*arrows*). Small T1 hyperintense petechial hemorrhage is seen in the bilateral frontal white matter related to venous ischemia (*arrowheads*). (**c**) Coronal gradient-echo image demonstrates the thrombi as hypointense (*arrows*). (**d, e**) DW imaging shows vasogenic edema in the bilateral frontal white matter as hypointense with increased ADC, and the venous thrombi and hemorrhage in the choroid plexi as hyperintense with decreased ADC (*arrows*)

essential to correlate with ADC values, which are decreased by approximately 30–50%. It has been suggested that ADC values $<0.8 \times 10^{-3}$ mm^2/s in the basal ganglia is associated with severe injury and poor prognosis [29]. DWI in conjunction with ADC maps are most useful in the first 1–5 days after hypoxic-ischemic event. DWI can "pseudo-normalize" about 1 week after [30]. The distribution of the lesions in the putamen, thalamus, and perirolandic cerebral cortex is related to intrinsic vulnerability of these areas to energy failure. One potentially important link among these areas is their interconnection by excitatory circuits. Thus, overactivity in excitatory pathways could propagate to other locations through synaptic connections. The corticospinal tract, corpus callosum, and deep gray matter can be secondarily involved through these pathways, also known as secondary Wallerian and transsynaptic degenerations [31]. Diffuse hyperintensity on DW imaging with decreased ADC in the corpus callosum, and along the pyramidal tract in the internal capsules and the brain stem is occasionally seen (Figs. 19.11 and 19.12). This is presumably due to cytotoxic edema of the glial cells, axons, and myelin sheaths [32].

The prognosis of hypoxic ischemic encephalopathy depends on the extension of the cytotoxic

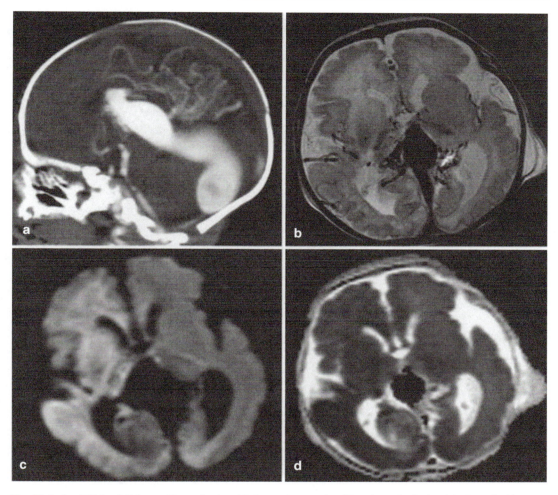

Fig. 19.9 (**a–d**) Vein of Galen malformation in a 10-day-old boy. (**a**) Post-contrast CT shows a dilated venous structure with multiple feeders. (**b**) T2-weighted image shows the vein of Galen malformation and dilated feeding arteries. Hyperintensity in the right frontal white matter suggests the presence of ischemia. (**c, d**) DW imaging shows cytotoxic edema in the entire right hemisphere and the left occipital lobe associated with decreased ADC

edema, which is seen as hyperintensity on DW imaging. Hypoxic ischemic injury with cytotoxic edema is usually irreversible. DW imaging is helpful in establishing both the diagnosis and the prognosis, but also in the management of hypoxic ischemic encephalopathy. Abnormal ADC and FA values may help in early and more accurate assessment of microstructural damage in hypoxic ischemic encephalopathy that may have predictive value for long-term functional outcome in neonates [33].

19.5.6 Hypoglycemic Encephalopathy

Hypoglycemia and hypoxic ischemic encephalopathy often coexist, as hypoxic ischemic encephalopathy can cause hypoglycemia. Neonatal hypoglycemia (blood glucose < 46 mg/dL) occurs in 5–15% of neonates, as they transition from an intrauterine to extrauterine environment [34, 35] (Fig. 19.13). Glucose is necessary for the smooth functioning of the brain and insufficient supply can lead to brain injury.

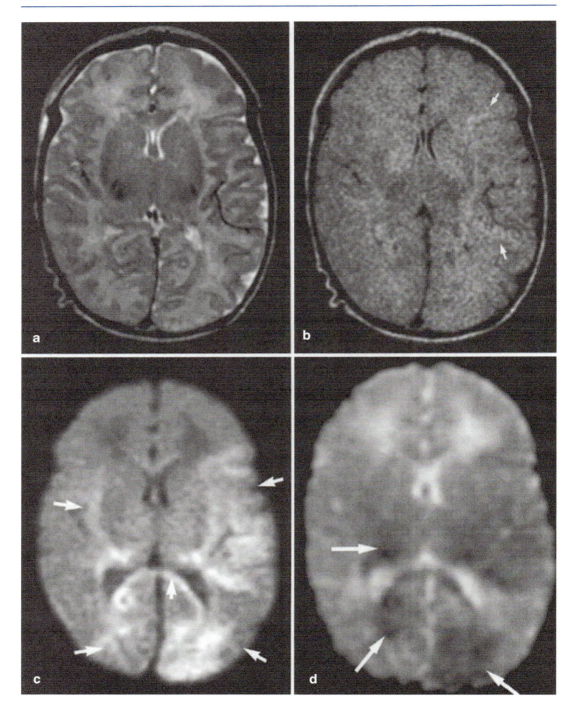

Fig. 19.10 (**a–d**) Hypoxic ischemic encephalopathy secondary to intrauterine cerebrovascular accident in a 2-day-old term girl. (**a**) T2-weighted image appears normal. (**b**) Fluid attenuated inversion-recovery (FLAIR) image shows slightly high signal in the white matter (*arrows*). (**c**) DW image shows bilateral hyperintense lesions in the temporo-occipital cortices, white matter, and corpus callosum (*arrows*), representing ischemic lesion and cytotoxic edema. (**d**) ADC map shows corresponding decreased ADC values

19 Pediatrics

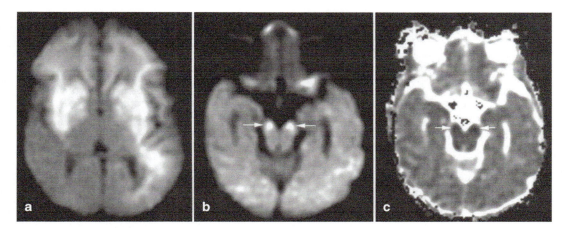

Fig. 19.11 (**a–c**) Hypoxic ischemic encephalopathy in a 10-day-old boy. (**a**) DW image shows extensive hyperintense lesions involving the fronto-temporo-parietal white matter, internal capsules, and basal ganglia bilaterally. (**b, c**) DW image shows hyperintense lesions with decreased ADC in the bilateral cerebral peduncles probably including both corticospinal tracts (*arrows*). These findings represent the early phase of Wallerian degeneration

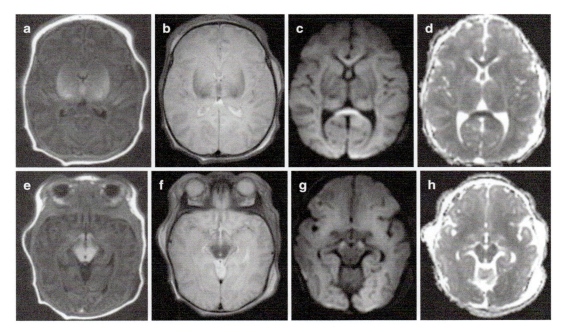

Fig. 19.12 (**a–h**) Severe hypoxic ischemic encephalopathy in a 7-day-old full-term girl born via emergent C-section for non-reassuring fetal heart tracings and low Agpar scores. (**a, b**) Axial T1- and T2-weighted images show increased T1 signal throughout the basal ganglia and thalami secondary to cell death and mineralization, as well as diffuse cerebral edema involving both gray and white matter (**c, d**) DWI and ADC show diffusion restriction throughout the supratentorial brain and especially the corpus callosum. (**e, f**) T1 and T2 images show myelination along the expected areas of the white matter tracts but also diffuse edema involving the corticospinal tracts and supratentorial brain parenchyma (**g, h**) DW image shows hyperintense lesions with decreased ADC in the bilateral cerebral peduncles and corticospinal tracts, as well as the brain parenchyma

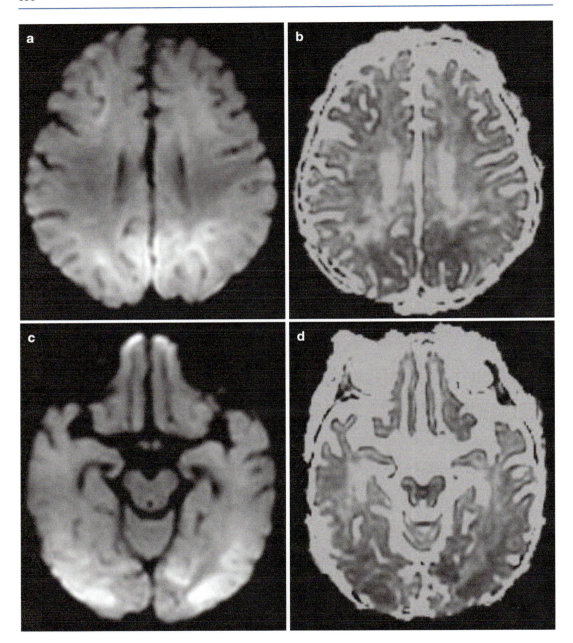

Fig. 19.13 (a–d) Hypoglycemia to 29 mg/dL in a 4 month-old male with rhinovirus, metabolic acidosis, and seizures. (**a, b**) DWI and ADC map show decreased diffusion in the bilateral parietal lobes and frontal lobe white matter. (**c, d**) DWI and ADC map show decreased diffusion in the bilateral occipital lobes

Patterns of injury caused by hypoglycemia include most commonly posterior white matter and pulvinar edema, with watershed pattern of injury and brainstem/basal ganglia involvement seen in more severe cases [35]. The imaging findings may appear similar to partial hypoxic ischemic injury, so correlation with history and injury pattern is important. DWI is the most sensitive imaging technique for identification of parieto-occipital injury especially in the first week after birth [36]. Injury due to hypoglycemia can cause visual impairment, epilepsy, and cognitive deficits [34, 35].

19.6 Trauma

19.6.1 Nonaccidental Head Injury

Nonaccidental head injury (NAHI) or abusive head trauma (AHT) is most commonly seen among children under 3 years of age with the majority of cases occurring during the first year of life. In the USA, there are an estimated 3,000 deaths per year from NAHI. Direct Blunt force and Shaken Baby syndrome are currently assumed to be the main etiologies of abusive head trauma [37].

Because of anatomic and developmental differences in the brain and skull of young children, the mechanisms and types of brain injury are distinctly different from those seen in older children and adults. Young infants have a relatively large head, weak neck muscles, and thin calvarial bones separated by soft membranous sutures and fontanelles, making them extremely vulnerable to traumatic injuries (deformation-mediated impact, shearing stress). Unmyelinated white matter is also vulnerable to such traumatic injuries and hypoxia [38].

In experimental studies of acute subdural hematomas in the infant rat, the glutamate concentration in the extracellular fluid of the cortex was increased more than seven times over the basal level [39]. The postnatal period of brain development is particularly vulnerable to excitotoxic injury. Excitatory amino acid receptors are abundant in the cortex during the first 2 years of life. The high rate of generation of synapses (synaptogenesis) results in an overexpression of glutamate receptors. NMDA receptors dominate in the immature brain when synaptic transmission is weak and extremely plastic. Experimental studies showed that too many or too few NMDA receptors can be threatening to developing neurons. During maturation, non-NMDA receptors, alpha-amino-3-hydroxy-5-methyl-5-isoxazolepropionate (AMPA) receptors and kainic receptors, predominate. This suggests that the primary increased release of glutamate from the presynaptic terminal following traumatic stimuli and the primary decreased reuptake of glutamate from the synapse following hypoxic or ischemic events are related to brain parenchymal injuries [31].

The clinical presentation of NAHI is nonspecific. NAHI is suspected when retinal hemorrhage is present (75%–90%), or when the magnitude of the injuries demonstrated clinically or on neuroimaging is discrepant with the history provided. Histologic similarities have been observed in child abuse victims and infants with hypoxic ischemic encephalopathy. However, a history of apnea suggesting hypoxic-ischemic injury was only found in 57% (16/28) of the child abuse cases [40]. In a neuropathology study it was noted that diffuse axonal injuries were rare among child abuse victims, only seen in three out of 53 cases [41].

Subdural hematomas are the most common associated intracranial pathology in NAHI. They result from defects in the cortical bridging veins from trauma. Trauma can also result in CSF-intensity subdural collections called subdural hygromas, which can form acutely or in a delayed fashion. Subdural hygromas can be difficult to distinguish from chronic subdural hematoma, which are rare, but nonetheless the presence of hygroma implies trauma and workup for abusive head trauma should be pursued. MRI can help distinguish subdural collections from benign enlargement of the subarachnoid spaces (BESS), as vessels course through the subarachnoid space in BESS but not the subdural space in subdural collections [37].

Other findings of AHT include parenchymal injuries. The distribution of parenchymal injuries is usually not related to the vascular territories. Some parenchymal lesions are located subjacent to subdural hematomas but other parenchymal lesions are not related to the location and size of subdural hematomas on CT and MR imaging (Figs. 19.14 and 19.15). It can be difficult to detect brain parenchyma injuries on CT as well as on routine MR imaging.

DWI has a significant role in recognizing the extent of brain parenchymal injury. The parenchymal lesions can be unexpectedly extensive and caution is needed to window DW imaging optimally (Fig. 19.16). Quantifying the ADC value is especially useful to detect extensive parenchyma abnormalities. The severity of abnormality in DW imaging correlates with the patient's outcome [42]. MR spectroscopy can also evaluate the severity of trauma, as this will show decreased N-acetyl aspartate (NAA), increased lactate (metabolic acidosis), and

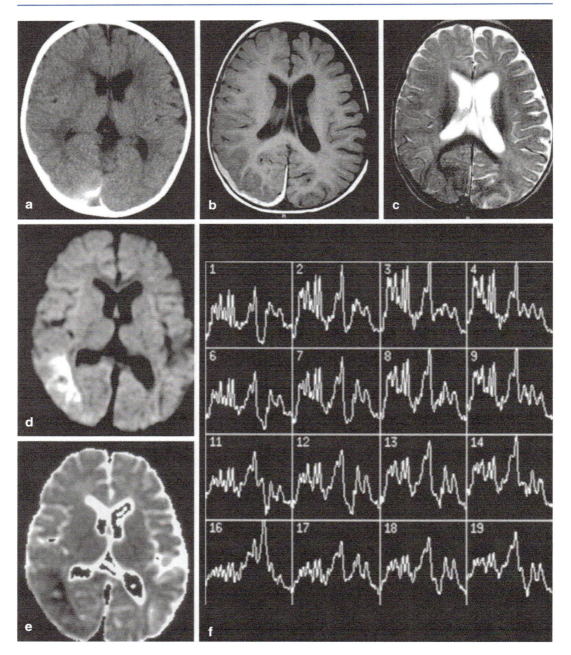

Fig. 19.14 (**a–f**) Nonaccidental head injury in a 9-month-old boy. (**a–c**) CT and T1- and T2-weighted images show an acute subdural hematoma in the right parieto-occipital region. CT and conventional MR images show no apparent parenchymal lesions. (**d, e**) DW image shows a hyperintense lesion in the right parieto-occipital region subjacent to the subdural hematoma. (**f**) Multivoxel MR spectroscopy (TE 30 ms) shows increased glutamate/glutamine and lipid/lactate peaks

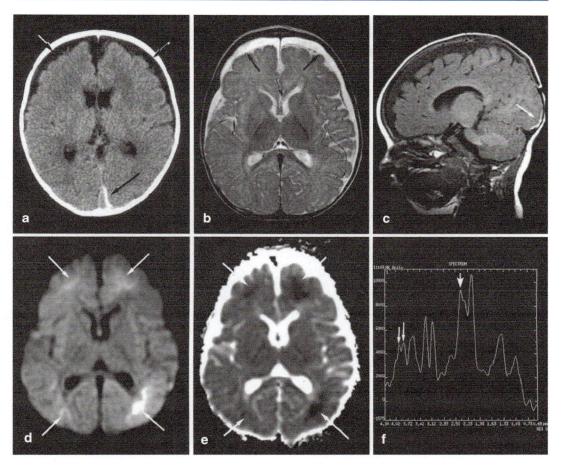

Fig. 19.15 (**a–f**) Nonaccidental head injury in a 6-month-old boy. (**a**) CT shows high density area representing acute subdural hematoma in the left occipital region (*long arrow*), and bilateral subdural fluid collections in the frontal region (*short arrows*). (**b**) T2-weighted image also shows bilateral subdural fluid collection and no apparent abnormalities in the brain parenchyma. (**c**) Sagittal T1-weighted image shows acute subdural hematoma as small linear hyperintensity in the occipital area (*arrow*). (**d, e**) DW image shows the extent of parenchymal abnormality as hyperintense lesions with decreased ADC in bilateral fronto-parieto-occipital white matter (*arrows*). The distribution of the parenchymal lesion is not related to that of the subdural hematomas and is rather similar to that of hypoxic-ischemic encephalopathy. (**f**) MR spectroscopy (TE 30 ms) shows an increased glutamate/glutamine peak (*arrow*)

increased glutamate/glutamine (Glx), the degree of these changes being related to the severity of brain damage (Figs. 19.14 and 19.15) [43]. Glx levels peak early after injury and then fall rapidly. This time course may become important in the future since neuroprotective effects have been reported with several kinds of selective glutamate receptor antagonists in animal studies [44–46].

A distinctive injury pattern of a "big black brain" response to acute subdural hematomas may be seen in infants. This is a pattern where cerebral edema/infarct may involve one or both cerebral hemispheres and the brain appears dark relative to a bright cerebellum giving the appearance of a big black brain [47] (Fig. 19.17). In children, the bilateral pattern is seen twice as

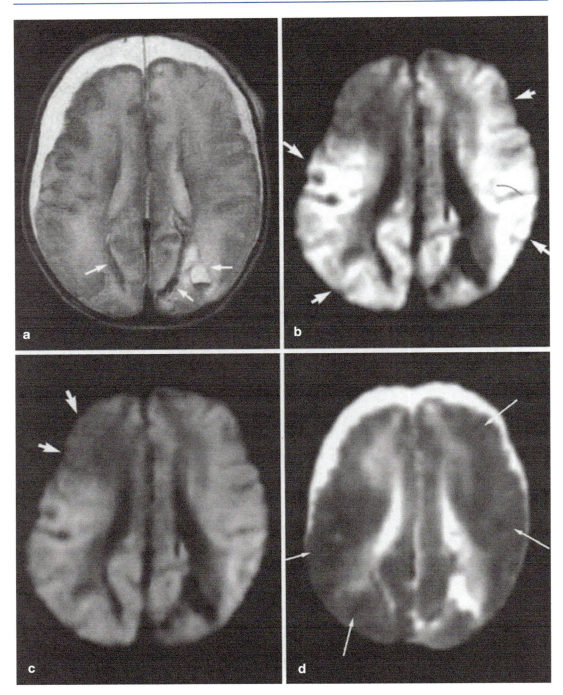

Fig. 19.16 (**a**–**d**) Nonaccidental head injury in a 2-month-old boy. (**a**) T2-weighted image shows intracranial hemorrhages with shearing injury (*arrows*) and bilateral chronic subdural hematomas in the bilateral occipital regions. (**b**) DW image shows diffusely increased signal in both hemispheres (*arrows*) with sparing of only the right frontal area. (**c**) DW image filmed with incorrect window and level setting, suggesting wrongly that the low signal in the right frontal area is abnormal (*arrows*), when indeed this is the only normal portion of the brain. Correct window and levels are critical, as is comparison with findings on other sequences. (**d**) ADC values are decreased (0.31×10^{-3}/mm^2/s) in the diffuse parenchymal abnormalities (*arrows*)

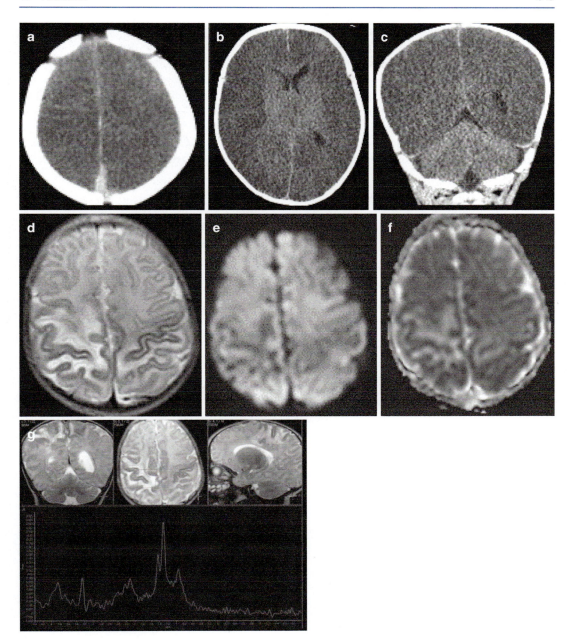

Fig. 19.17 (**a–g**) Big black brain injury. Nonaccidental trauma in a 1-month-old baby boy who presented with lethargy and bruises. (**a, b**) Axial noncontrast head CT shows a small amount of extra-axial blood along the superior falx and diffuse cerebral edema. (**c**) Coronal head CT highlights the "big black brain" of the supratentorium with contrasting hyperattenuation of the cerebellum. (**d**) Axial T2 image highlights the cerebral edema (**e, f**) DWI and ADC show cortical diffusion restriction within both cerebral hemispheres. (**g**) MRS showed elevated lipid/lactate with all other metabolites significantly decreased, consistent with brain damage

often as the unilateral pattern and usually in young infants, whereas older infants and toddlers usually develop the unilateral pattern [47]. Proposed mechanisms include microvessel spasm in response to hemorrhage, vulnerability of the young brain, apnea, seizures, hypotension, hypercarbia, etc. [47]. The results of "big black brain" are devastating, and timely hemicraniectomy can potentially save lives by averting herniation.

19.6.2 Diffuse Axonal Injury and Brain Contusion

It was once considered that edema following brain contusion or diffuse axonal injury (DAI) was vasogenic. Experimental studies using DWI have shown that edematous regions following injury consist of both vasogenic and cytotoxic edema [48, 49]. DAI usually occurs in older children. DAI is related to excitotoxic mechanisms, particularly glutamate and NMDA receptors. Axonal damage often occurs at the node of Ranvier (a short interval between processes of oligodendrocytes), resulting in a traumatic defect in the axonal membrane. DW imaging shows diffuse axonal injury as hyperintense, presumably due to cytotoxic edema (Fig. 19.18).

It should be noted, however, that hemorrhagic components often accompany these brain injuries, which will affect the signal intensity on DW imaging. Brain contusions near the skull base are also often overlooked on DWI due to susceptibility artifacts.

19.7 Infections

19.7.1 Encephalitis

DWI can detect early encephalitic changes [50] and is generally more sensitive than conventional MR imaging. Herpes encephalitis demonstrates pathologically severe edema including both cytotoxic and vasogenic edema and massive tissue necrosis with petechial or confluent hemorrhage. Herpes simplex type 1 encephalitis in older children and adults usually involves the limbic cortex in the medial temporal lobe, inferior frontal lobes, and insula (Fig. 19.19). Neonatal herpes simplex type 2 encephalitis involves the cortex and white matter extensively (Fig. 19.20). Widespread brain lesions in neonatal herpes encephalopathy are presumably related to the vulnerability to excitatory amines in the neonatal brain. The early detection by DW imaging is valuable for early institution of treatment.

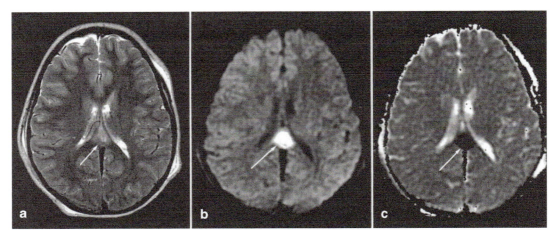

Fig. 19.18 (**a**–**c**) Diffuse axonal injury in an 11-year-old boy injured in a motor vehicle accident. (**a**) T2-weighted image shows a mildly hyperintense lesion in the corpus callosum (*arrow*). (**b**) DW image demonstrates this lesion as hyperintense (*arrow*). (**c**) ADC map shows decreased ADC of this lesion (*arrow*), probably representing cytotoxic edema associated with diffuse axonal injury

19 Pediatrics

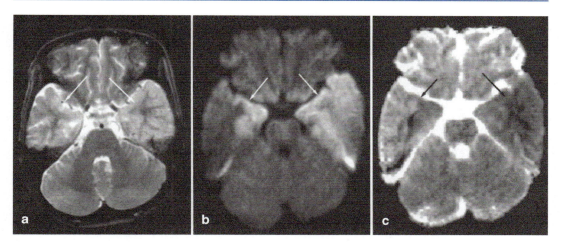

Fig. 19.19 (a–c) Herpes simplex type 1 encephalitis in an 11-year-old boy. (**a**) T2-weighted image shows hyperintense lesions in bilateral temporal lobes (*arrows*). (**b**) DW image clearly shows these lesions as hyperintense (*arrows*). (**c**) ADC map shows decreased ADC of these lesions (*arrows*)

Classic herpes simplex virus encephalitis is an acute viral infection that usually follows a monophasic disease course. However some patients, mainly children, may have a relapse of symptoms (choreoathetosis, behavioral changes and seizures) within weeks or months after the initial event. A postinfectious immune-mechanism has been postulated and recent studies have demonstrated that 7% of patients with herpes encephalitis harbor NR1 N-methyl-D-aspartate receptor IgG antibodies. Thus, a subgroup of post-herpes simplex virus encephalitis may actually represent anti-NMDAR encephalitis (Fig. 19.21) [51].

19.7.2 Brain Abscess

Abscesses in the brain are potentially fatal, but may be successfully treated by early medical or surgical intervention. DW imaging can discriminate a brain abscess from a cystic or necrotic tumor, which is often difficult with conventional MR imaging [52]. The brain abscess shows very high signal on DW imaging associated with decreased ADC (Fig. 19.22). Pus usually consists of both dead and still viable neutrophils, along with necrotic debris and bacteria, as well as exuded plasma. A possible explanation for the high signal on DW imaging is limited water mobility, presumably due to the high viscosity of continuous coagulative necrosis and hypercellularity of neutrophils in the pus. Systemic candida infection occurs in 3%–5% of very low-birth-weight neonates and infants and is often associated with high morbidity and mortality. Central nervous system candidiasis is a serious complication but it is often not identified until postmortem examination. Ultrasound and MR imaging are useful for the diagnosis [53]. DW imaging can show multiple candida microabscesses as hyperintense with decreased ADC (Fig. 19.23).

19.7.3 Acute Flaccid Myelitis

Acute flaccid myelitis (AFM) is a disease presenting with acute focal limb weakness and MRI findings of spinal cord lesion involving more than one spinal segment of gray matter or CSF pleocytosis of >5 WBCs/mm^3 [54] (Fig. 19.24). AFM has been on the uprise in the US in the last few years, with an outbreak in 2014 of enterovirus D68-related viruses. Other viruses including enterovirus 71 and poliovirus present with similar findings. Vigilant supportive care is the CDC recommendation for management [55]. The use of steroids, immunomodulating therapy, and antiviral medications is controversial [54]. On MRI, affected patients may show rhomboencephalitis affecting the dorsal pons and medulla,

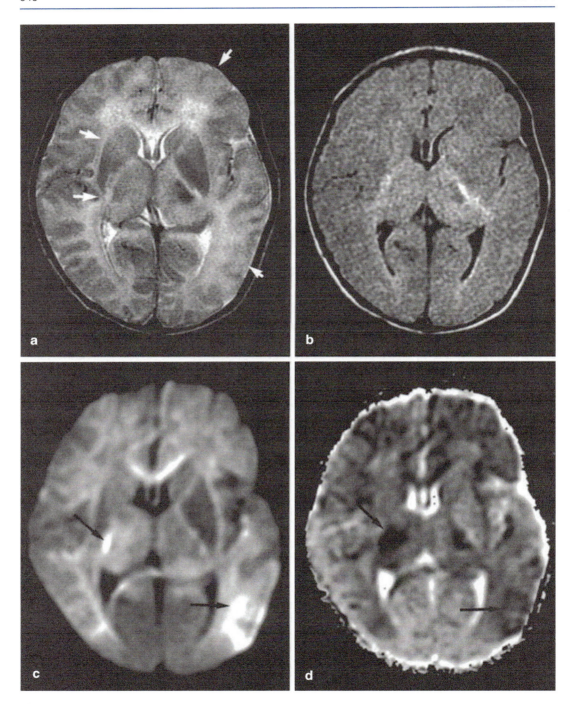

Fig. 19.20 (a–d) Herpes simplex type 2 encephalitis in a 2-week-old girl. (a) T2-weighted images show asymmetric hyperintense lesions in the thalami and right basal ganglia and cerebral cortices (*arrows*). The precise extent of the lesions is difficult to determine. (b) FLAIR image appears normal. (c, d) DW image shows asymmetric but extensive hyperintense lesions (*arrows*) with decreased ADC in the thalamus and gray and white matter of both hemispheres

19 Pediatrics

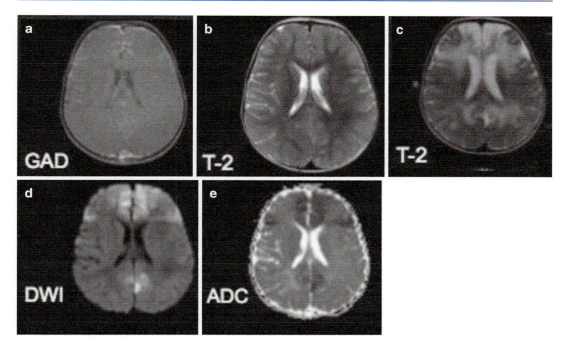

Fig. 19.21 (a–e) Herpes meningoencephalitis complicated by subsequent anti-NMDA encephalitis in an 11-month-old boy presenting with fever, lethargy, and seizures. 6 months after onset with completion of acyclovir treatment, he then presented with choreoathetosis and hypsarrhythmia on EEG. (**a**) T1 post-contrast images show diffuse leptomeningeal enhancement. (**b, c**) Axial T2 images show edematous changes within the cerebral cortex as well as throughout the deep and subcortical cerebral white matter. (**d, e**) DW image shows restricted diffusion and decreased ADC values involving multiple areas within the bilateral frontal and occipital cortices. (Courtesy of Dr Yutaka Sato)

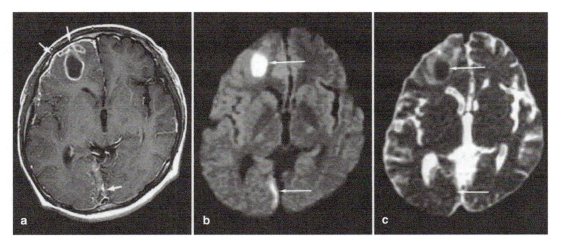

Fig. 19.22 (a–c) Brain abscess and subdural abscess in a 16-year-old boy with high fever and headache. (**a**) Gadolinium-enhanced T1-weighted image shows thin-walled ring or rim-enhancing lesions with pachymeningeal enhancement in the right frontal lobe and right medial occipital region (*arrows*). (**b**) DW image shows cystic components of the right frontal and occipital lesion as very hyperintense (*arrows*). (**c**) ADC map shows decreased ADC in these cystic components (*arrows*). (Courtesy of Morikawa M. MD, Nagasaki University, School of Medicine, Japan)

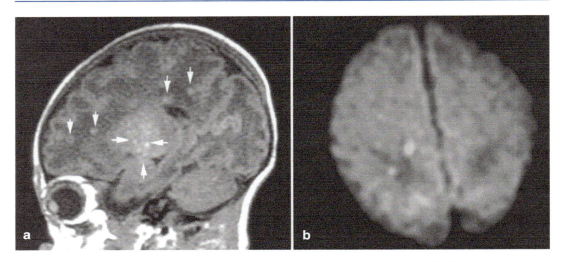

Fig. 19.23 (**a**, **b**) Central nervous system candidiasis in a 4-day-old very-low-birth-weight neonate. (**a**) Precontrast sagittal T1-weighted image shows multiple small nodular or ring-shaped lesions in the white matter and basal ganglia (*arrows*). (**b**) DW imaging shows multiple small hyperintense lesions consistent with candida microabscesses

and a radiculomyelitis with predilection for the anterior horn cells of the spinal cord and ventral nerve roots [54].

19.8 Tumors

19.8.1 Brain Tumors

The signal intensity on DW imaging and the ADC values of brain tumors are variable and related to the architecture of the tumor.

Medulloblastoma (Figs. 19.25, 19.26, 19.27, 19.28, 19.29, and 19.30), atypical teratoid-rhabdoid tumor (Figs. 19.31 and 19.32), embryonal tumor with multilayered rosettes (ETMR) (Fig. 19.33), anaplastic ependymoma (Figs. 19.34, 19.35, and 19.36), diffuse midline glioma (Fig. 19.37), desmoplastic infantile ganglioglioma (Fig. 19.41), choroid plexus carcinoma (Fig. 19.46), lymphoma, germ cell tumor, granulocytic sarcoma, and other primary and metastatic tumors can show high signal intensity on DW imaging associated with decreased ADC [56–62] (see Chap. 18). The decreased ADC values, in either benign or malignant tumors, are caused by increased intracellular water, hypercellularity, and/or decreased extracellular water in tumor interstitium.

On the other hand, brain tumors such as pilocytic and pilomyxoid astrocytoma (Fig. 19.38) and other low-grade gliomas show hypo-, iso-, or hyperintensity on DW imaging associated with increased ADC, indicating a T2 shine-through effect. The characteristics on DW imag-

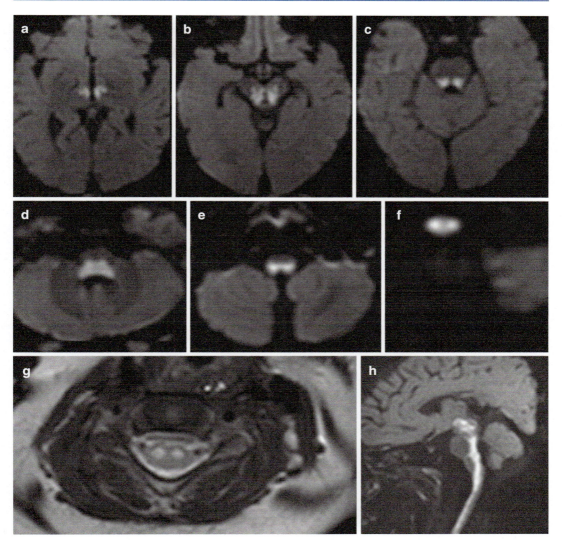

Fig. 19.24 (**a–j**) Acute flaccid myelitis due to Enterovirus 71 in a 6-month-old male who presented with increased secretions, vomiting, and concern for aspiration. (**a–f**) Axial DWI sequences show diffusion restriction affecting the dorsal brainstem and the gray matter of the spinal cord. (**g**) Axial T2 image shows high signal involving the anterior horn cells of the spinal cord. (**h**) Sagittal DWI image shows extensive diffusion restriction in the regions described. (**i, j**) Coronal DWI and ADC images redemonstrate these findings

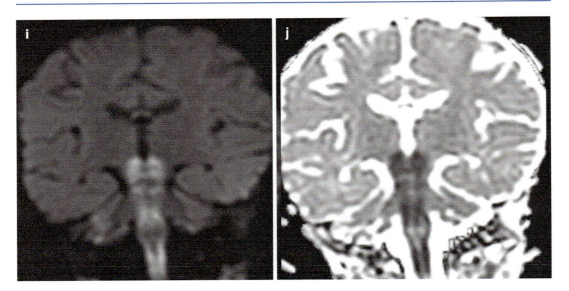

Fig. 19.24 (continued)

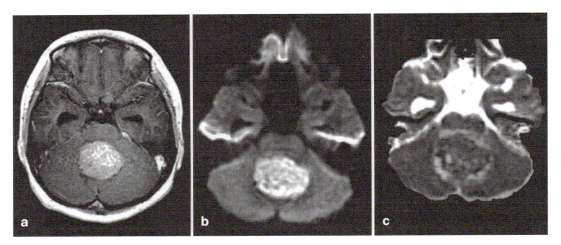

Fig. 19.25 (**a–c**) Medulloblastoma in a 10-year-old boy. (**a**) Gadolinium-enhanced T1-weighted image shows a solid mass with enhancement in the cerebellar vermis. (**b**) DW image shows this solid mass as hyperintense. (**c**) ADC map shows decreased ADC of this mass. This is due to high cellular density causing restricted diffusion. (Courtesy of Morikawa M., MD, Nagasaki University, School of Medicine, Japan)

ing and ADC maps have been reported to be correlated with the histological grade in pediatric brain tumors [63]. ADC values are useful in differentiating posterior fossa tumors in pediatric patients, separating pilocytic astrocytoma $>1.4 \times 10^{-3}$ mm²/s, ependymoma $1.0–1.3 \times 10^{-3}$ mm²/s, and medulloblastoma $<0.9 \times 10^{-3}$ mm²/s, with high specificity [64].

In the recently updated 2016 World Health Organization (WHO) classification of brain tumors, molecular genetics have been incorporated into the new classification system. This reflects new treatment options and prognostics for previously described tumors.

Several entities have been renamed according to genetics. For example, primitive neuroectoder-

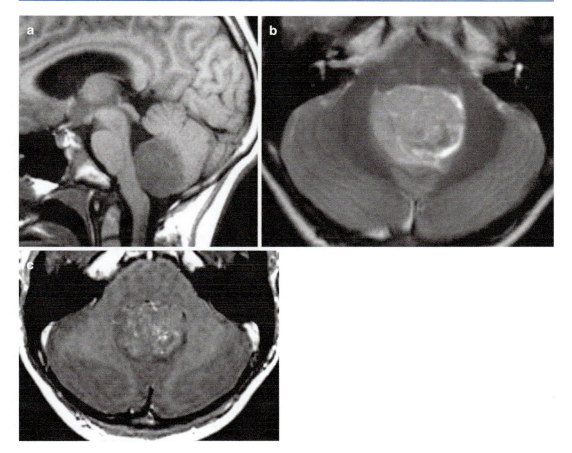

Fig. 19.26 (**a–d**) Medulloblastoma classic type (WNT) in a 14-year-old male with Turcot's syndrome (colorectal polyposis with CNS tumor). (**a**) Sagittal T1-weighted image shows a solid mass in the caudal midline cerebellar vermis. (**b**) T2 image shows this solid mass as hyperintense. (**c**) Gadolinium-enhanced T1-weighted image shows a solid mass with enhancement. (**d**) Colonic polyp biopsy showed low-grade adenomatous dysplasia on hematoxylin eosin stain × 100 (Courtesy of Dr Noriko Salamon)

mal tumor (PNET) previously used to encompass any highly malignant small round-blue cell tumor of neuroectodermal origin. Tumors of this category are now individually defined, including medulloblastoma; ATRT; and embryonal tumor with multilayer rosettes, CM19MC-altered [57]. Other high-grade tumors without genetic specification include medulloepithelioma, CNS neuroblastoma, CNS ganglioneuroblastoma, and CNS embryonal tumor NOS [57].

Medulloblastomas are now classified by both molecular subgroups and histological subtypes, which has implications on patient demographics and prognosis. WNT-activated have classic morphology, favorable prognosis, and occur in older children/younger adolescents (Figs. 19.26 and 19.29). Sonic hedgehog (SHH) have desmoplastic/nodular morphology, affects different age groups, and generally have a good prognosis (Figs. 19.27, 19.28, and 19.29) [57]. Group 3 and 4 medulloblastomas have classic or large cell/anaplastic histology, affect children, and have worse prognoses (Fig. 19.30) [57]. Medulloblastomas classified by genetics have a trend in localization of tumor subtypes: WNT-activated tumors are centered in the cerebellar peduncle or cerebellopontine angle, SHH (sonic hedgehog)-

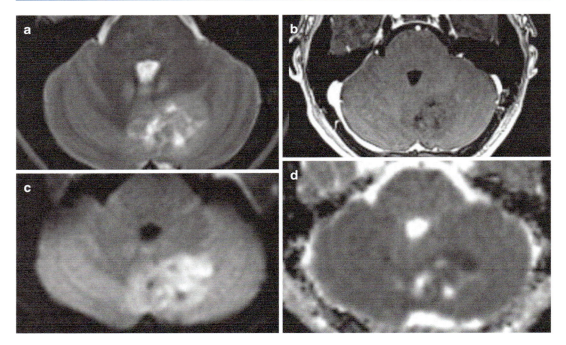

Fig. 19.27 (a–d) Medulloblastoma desmoplastic variant (SHH) in a 14-year-old male. (a) Axial T2-weighted image shows a nodular, hyperintense solid mass in the left hemispheric rostral region of the cerebellum. (b) Gadolinium-enhanced T1-weighted image demonstrates minimal enhancement. (c, d) Diffusion-weighted images show diffusion restriction within the lesion with associated low ADC values

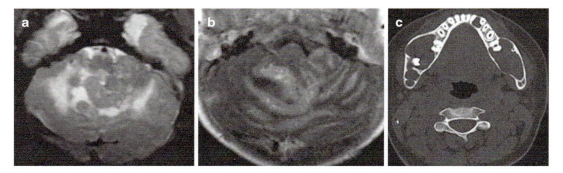

Fig. 19.28 (a–c) Medulloblastoma (SHH) with extensive nodularity in a 4-year-old female with Gorlin (basal-cell nevus) syndrome (a, b) Axial T2-weighted and gadolinium-enhanced T1 post-contrast images show extensive nodular and curvilinear enhancement along the foliae in the caudal cerebellar vermis extending to bilateral cerebellar hemispheres. (c) Axial CT of the mandible shows large cystic lesions by the mandibular molars, consistent with odontogenic keratocysts in the setting of Gorlin syndrome (Courtesy of Dr Kumiko Nozawa, Dr Aida Noriko)

activated tumors in the rostral cerebellar hemisphere, and group 3 and 4 tumors are located at the midline [57].

Certain medulloblastomas develop in association with genetic mutations. Classic type WNT medulloblastoma is seen in Turcot syndrome, due to a defect in APC (adenomatous polyposis coli) gene, a protein complex in WNT signaling pathway related to the pathogenesis of classic medulloblastoma (Fig. 19.26). Medulloblastoma with extensive nodularity (SHH) is seen with Gorlin (basal-cell-nevus) syndrome, which manifest with basal cell epitheliomas or carcinomas and odontogenic keratocysts (Fig. 19.28).

Fig. 19.29 Wnt and SHH pathways in medulloblastoma. Modified from reference [58]. *FZD* frizzled receptor protein, *PTCH* patched protein, *SMO* smoothened homolog

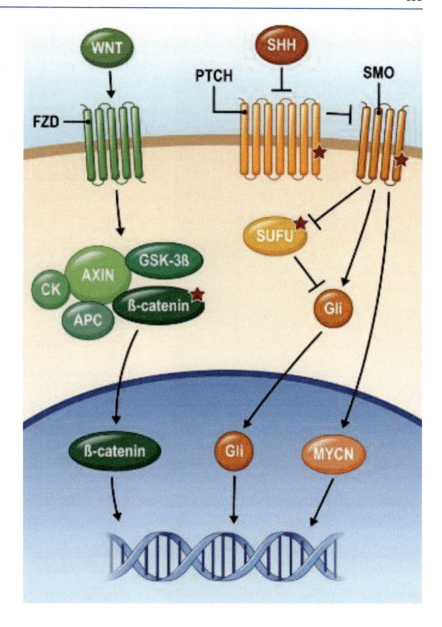

ATRT is an aggressive embryonal tumor in infants; it has a more malignant biological behavior and is less sensitive to therapy than meduloblastoma [62, 65] (Figs. 19.31 and 19.32). Cerebellopontine angle involvement and intratumoral hemorrhage are more common than in medulloblastoma. ATRT has been reported to be hyperintense on DW images with decreased ADC similar to medulloblastoma [62]. The diagnosis of ATRT is based on the mutation of tumor-suppressor gene on chromosome 22 such as SMARCB1 or INI1 mutation or inactivation of SMARCA4/BRG1 [57].

Embryonal tumor with multilayered rosettes (ETMR) has C19MC amplification in 93% of cases (Fig. 19.33). It encompasses previously described entities including ependymoblastoma, embryonal tumor with abundant neuropil and true rosettes (ETANTR), and medulloepithelioma.

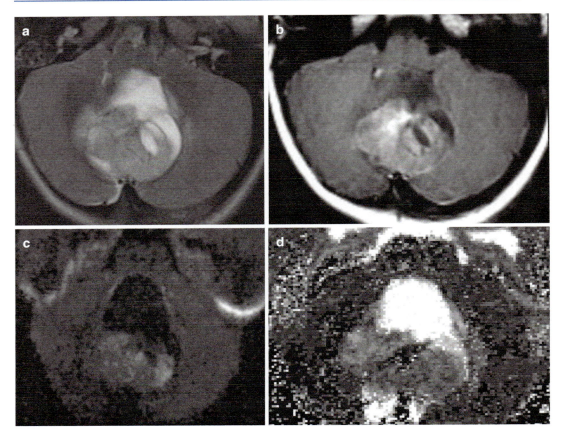

Fig. 19.30 (**a–d**) Medulloblastoma anaplastic type (group 3) in a 4-year-old boy with symptoms of being off-balance. (**a, b**) Axial T2-weighted and gadolinium-enhanced T1 images demonstrate a mildly enhancing mass with cystic/necrotic components centered in the caudal midline cerebellum extending to the rostral cerebellum, medulla oblongata and foramen of Magendie (**c, d**) Diffusion-weighted images show diffusion restriction and decreased ADC values (0.95–1.48×10^{-3} mm^2/s)

Ependymomas within the fourth ventricle do not always show reduced diffusion (Fig. 19.34), but supratentorial ependymomas tend to be anaplastic and may demonstrate diffusion restriction due to their high cellularity (Figs. 19.35 and 19.36). Within ependymomas, posterior fossa ependymomas are separated into EPN-A (younger, worse prognosis) and EPN-B (older, better prognosis). Among supratentorial ependymomas, RELA fusion positive are more aggressive and those with YAP1 fusion, which are found at a younger age and have a better prognosis [58].

Another entity that has been renamed is diffuse pontine glioma (DIPG) in which 60–80% of cases harbor mutations at position K27 in the gene for histone H3, which are now called diffuse midline glioma (DMG), H3 K27M-mutant (Fig. 19.37). H3K27M mutation confers a worse prognosis in brainstem midline gliomas, but overall survival may not be significantly different from wild-type thalamic gliomas [57].

Pediatric gliomas tend not to have common genetic alterations seen in adult infiltrating gliomas such as IDH mutation and 1p/19q codeletion, which

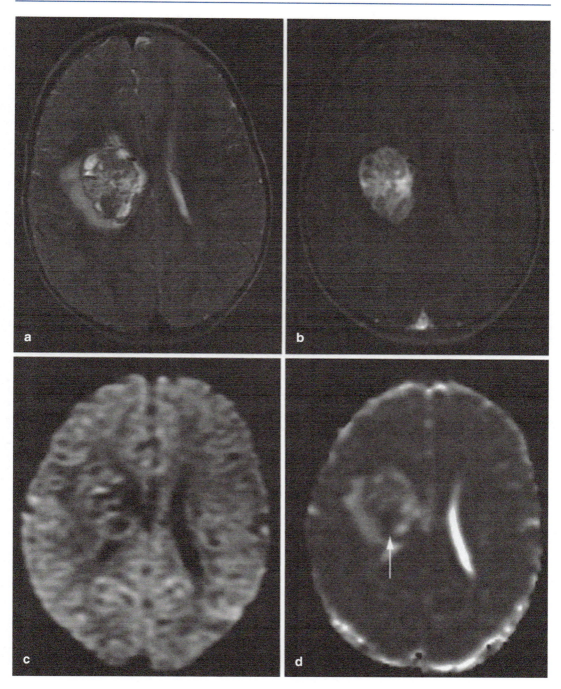

Fig. 19.31 (a–d) Atypical teratoid-rhabdoid tumor (ATRT) in a 14-month-old boy. (a) T2-weighted image shows a heterogeneous mass lesion with surrounding edema in the right frontal white matter. (b) Gadolinium-enhanced T1-weighted image shows a heterogeneously enhancing mass. (c) DW image shows an iso- or slightly hyperintense mass. (d) ADC map shows partially decreased ADC in this mass (*arrow*)

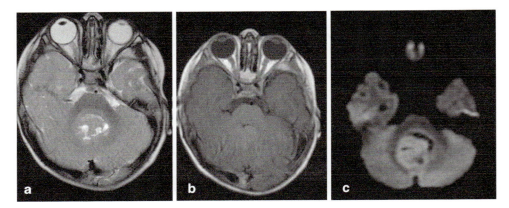

Fig. 19.32 (**a–c**) Atypical teratoid-rhabdoid tumor (ATRT) in a 15-month-old boy. (**a, b**) Axial T2 and T1 post-contrast images show a heterogeneously T2 hyperintense, minimally enhancing mass in the fourth ventricle. (**c**) DWI shows decreased diffusion in the mass

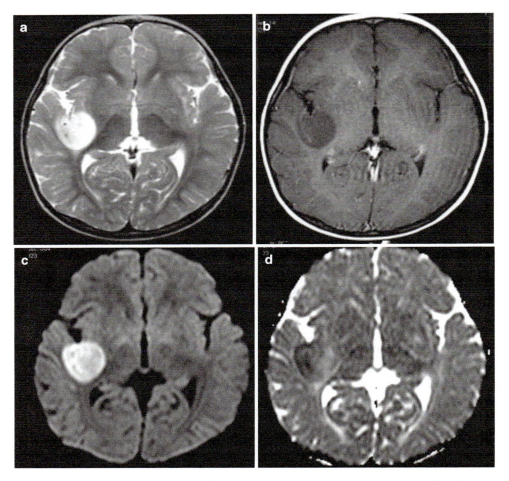

Fig. 19.33 (**a–d**) Embryonal tumor with multilayered rosettes (ETMR) in a 14-month-old boy with generalized seizure. (**a, b**) Axial T2-weighted and gadolinium-enhanced T1 images demonstrate a minimally enhancing mass centered in the right posterior subinsular region. (**c, d**) Diffusion-weighted images show diffusion restriction and low ADC values within the lesion

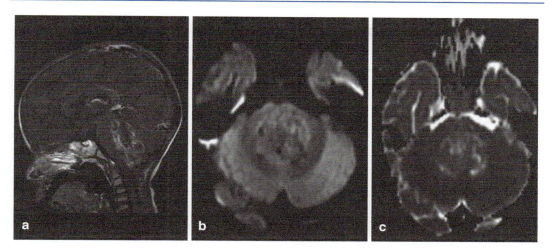

Fig. 19.34 (a–c) Ependymoma in a 3-year-old boy. (a) Gadolinium-enhanced T1-weighted image shows a heterogeneously enhancing mass in the fourth ventricle extending into the cisterns through the foramen of Magendie and Luschka (plastic ependymoma). (b, c) DW imaging shows isointensity with heterogeneously increased ADC in the mass

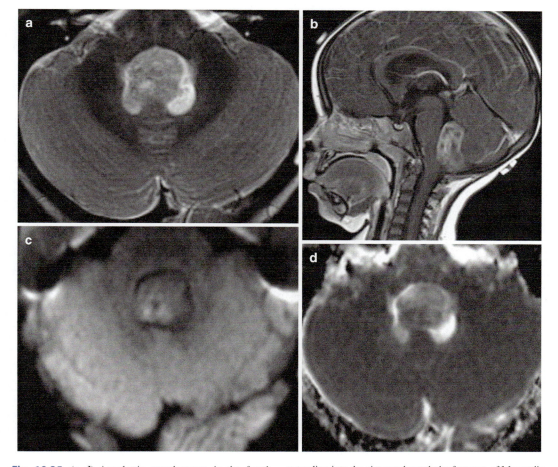

Fig. 19.35 (a–d) Anaplastic ependymoma in the fourth ventricle in a 1-year-old boy with headache. (a, b) Axial T2-weighted and sagittal T1 contrast-enhanced images show a T2 hyperintense, enhancing mass in the fourth ventricle extending into the cisterns through the foramen of Magendie. (c, d) DWI shows iso- to hyperintensity with heterogeneously decreased ADC in the mass (0.74–1.30 × 10^{-3} mm^2/s). On pathology, there was high cellularity and perivascular rosettes

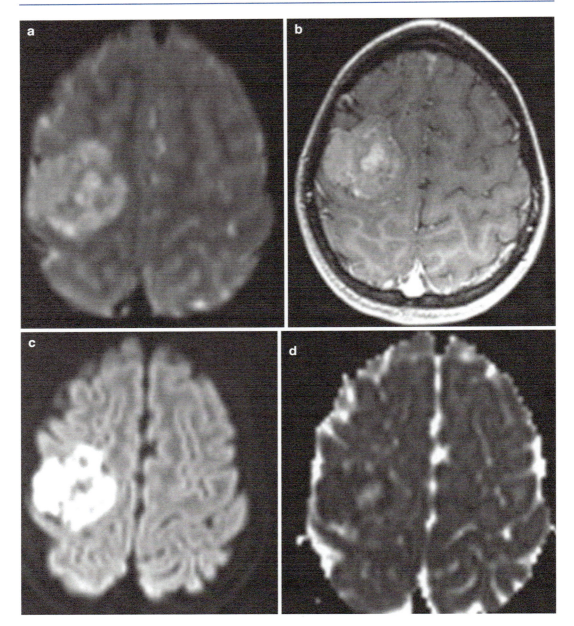

Fig. 19.36 (**a–d**) Supratentorial anaplastic ependymoma in a 7-year-old boy with headache. (**a, b**) Axial T2-weighted (b0) and gadolinium-enhanced T1-weighted image shows T2 hyperintense, enhancing, solid, right frontal lobe mass. (**c, d**) DW image demonstrates diffusion restriction with low ADC value (0.64×10^{-3} mm^2/s)

are rare in children, whereas other characteristic mutations are much more common (Fig. 19.38). In pediatric gliomas, mutations in Ras/RAF/MEK/ERK pathway or PI3K/PTEN/AKT/mTOR pathway are all factors in new treatments. MEK inhibitors, BRAFV600E inhibitors, mTOR and PI3K inhibitors are some of the new targeted therapies [58] (Fig. 19.39). In general, diffuse low-grade gliomas (i.e., diffuse astrocytomas grade II, gangliogliomas, and pleomorphic xanthroastrocytomas) confer a less favorable clinical outcome than non-diffuse gliomas (pilocytic or pilomyxoid astrocytoma).

19 Pediatrics

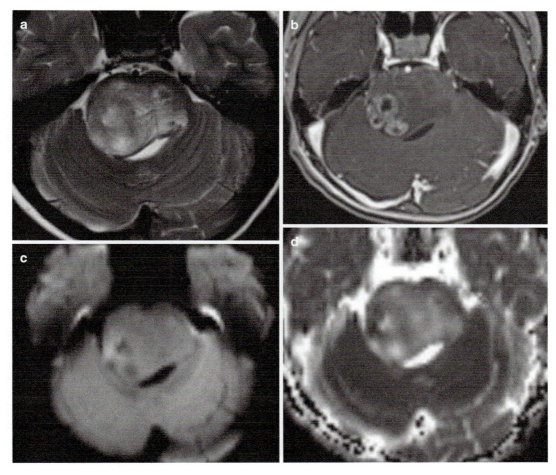

Fig. 19.37 (**a–d**) Diffuse midline glioma, H3-K27M mutant in a 5-year-old male with walking difficulty and tendency to fall towards left side. (**a**, **b**) Axial T2-weighted and gadolinium-enhanced T1 images demonstrate a large, minimally enhancing mass in the pons. (**c**, **d**) DW images show diffusion restriction and low ADC values in the right aspect of the mass

Astroblastoma is a rare glial neoplasm with perivascular pseudorosettes and variable biological behavior (Fig. 19.40). It is usually a supratentorial, circumscribed, solid-cystic mass, often with calcifications and heterogeneous enhancement. It can demonstrate diffusion restriction and can have a bubbly hyperintense T2 signal appearance [66].

Another less commonly seen tumor is desmoplastic infantile ganglioglioma (DIG) (Figs. 19.41 and 19.42). DIG is a large cystic tumor of infants involving the superficial cerebral cortex and leptomeninges, which presents with prominent desmoplastic stroma, neoplastic astrocytes, and neuronal component. It presents as a large, peripheral, supratentorial tumor with a large cyst and cortically based tumor nodule in an infant. The solid portion may demonstrate T2 hypointensity. It usually does not show reduced diffusion. It is a WHO grade 1 tumor, though often misdiagnosed as a higher grade tumor. It has a favorable prognosis and surgical resection is often curative. Ganglioglioma and pleomorphic xanthoastrocytoma may appear similar but are usually smaller and found in older patients [67].

Angiocentric glioma (Fig. 19.43) is another relatively recently described, rare, slow-growing WHO grade I tumor of the central nervous

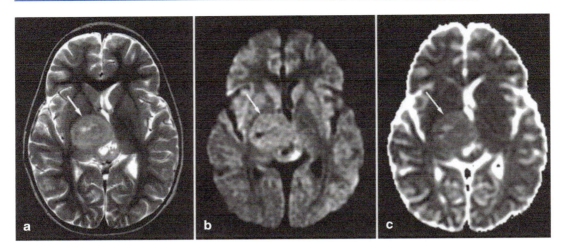

Fig. 19.38 (**a–c**) Pilocytic astrocytoma in a 4-year-old girl. (**a**) T2-weighted images show a hyperintense mass lesion in the right thalamus (*arrow*). (**b**) DW image shows this solid mass as hyperintense (*arrow*). (**c**) ADC map shows slightly increased ADC of this mass. Hyperintensity on DW imaging is due to T2 signal effect, i.e., T2 shine-through effect

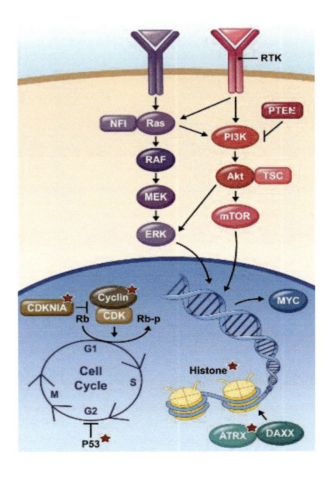

Fig. 19.39 Common signaling pathways involved in pediatric low and high-grade gliomas. Mutations in MAPK pathway, epigenetic regulators, cell-cycle pathway. Modified from reference [58]. *AKT* serine-threonine protein kinase, *GF* growth factor, *MEK* MAPK/extracellular signal-regulated kinase (ERK) kinase, *mToR* mammalian target of rapamycin, *MYC* Myc proto-oncogene protein, *NF1* neurofibromatosis type 1, *PI3K* phosphoinositide 3-kinase, *PTEN* phosphatase and tensin homolog, *RAS* Ras protein, *RTK* receptor tyrosine kinase, *M* mitotic phase, *Rb* retinoblastoma, *Rb-p* phosphorylated retinoblastoma, *S* S (synthesis) phase

19 Pediatrics

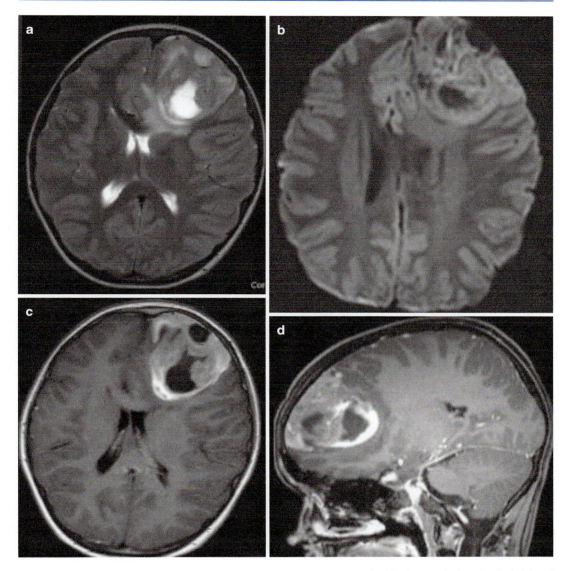

Fig. 19.40 (**a–d**) Anaplastic astroblastoma in a 12-year-old female with headache and one month of morning vomiting. (**a, b**) Axial T2 and axial DWI images show a cystic-solid, aggressive appearing left frontal lobe mass, but without much diffusion restriction. (**c, d**) Axial and sagittal post-contrast T1 images show avid enhancement within the mass

system mainly occurring in children and young adults. Histologically, angiocentric glioma cases reveal bipolar spindle-shaped cells with an angiocentric growth pattern [68]. However, atypically histology can occur with features similar to astroblastoma and ganglioglioma.

Choroid plexus papilloma (WHO grade 1) is a benign intraventricular papillary neoplasm derived from the choroid plexus epithelium and can be cured by surgery. The typical MR findings are of a homogeneous lobulated mass with papillary-appearance and with uniform intense enhance-

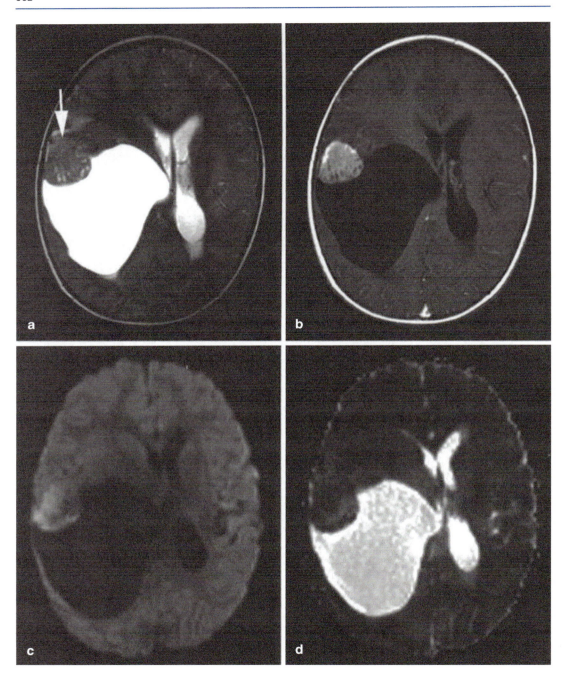

Fig. 19.41 (**a–d**) Desmoplastic infantile ganglioglioma in a 5-year-old girl. (**a**) T2-weighted image shows an isointense solid mass (*arrow*) with a large cystic component. (**b**) Gadolinium-enhanced T1-weighted image shows a homogeneous enhancement in the solid portion of the mass. (**c, d**) DW imaging shows hyperintensity with partially decreased ADC in the solid portion of the mass

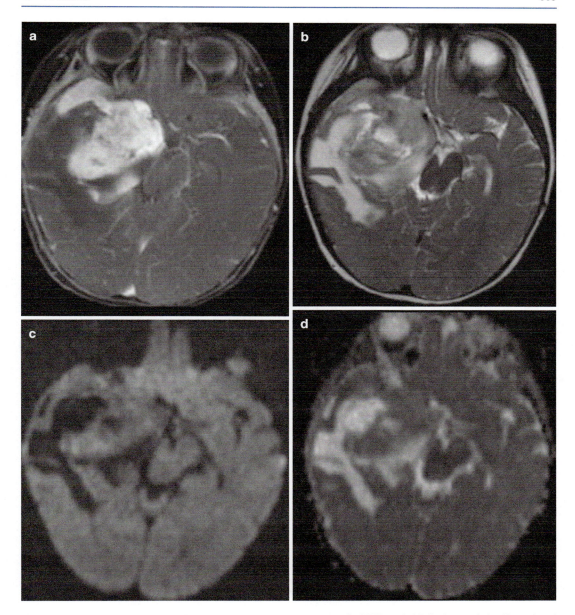

Fig. 19.42 (**a–d**) Desmoplastic infantile ganglioglioma (DIG) in a 7-year-old boy with multiple episodes of seizure. (**a, b**) Axial T2-weighted and gadolinium-enhanced T1-weighted image reveals a hemispheric cystic tumor with enhancing solid components with meningeal attachment. (**c, d**) DWI and ADC show minimally reduced diffusion in the lesion. Pathology showed desmoplastic elongated cell component and cellular neuroepithelial component with MIB-1 activity <2%

ment (Fig. 19.44). The WHO has introduced an additional entity with intermediate features, designated atypical choroid plexus papilloma (WHO grade 2), which is primarily distinguished from the choroid plexus papilloma by increased mitotic activity. Curative surgery is still possible but the probability of recurrence appears to be significantly higher. Choroid plexus carcinoma (WHO grade 3) is a malignant neoplasm with high mitotic activity, increased cellularity, blurring of the papillary pattern, necrosis, and frequent invasion of brain parenchyma (Fig. 19.45 and 19.46). Five-

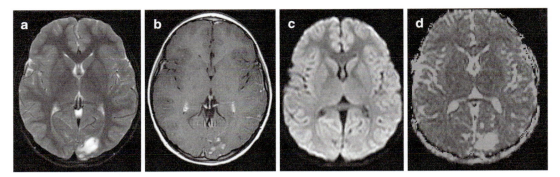

Fig. 19.43 (a–d) Angiocentric glioma in an 8-month-old boy. (a) T2-weighted image shows a T2 hyperintense cortically based tumor in the left occipital lobe. (b) Gadolinium-enhanced T1-weighted image demonstrates patchy rounded areas of enhancement in the lesion. (c, d) DWI and ADC images demonstrate facilitated diffusion within the lesion

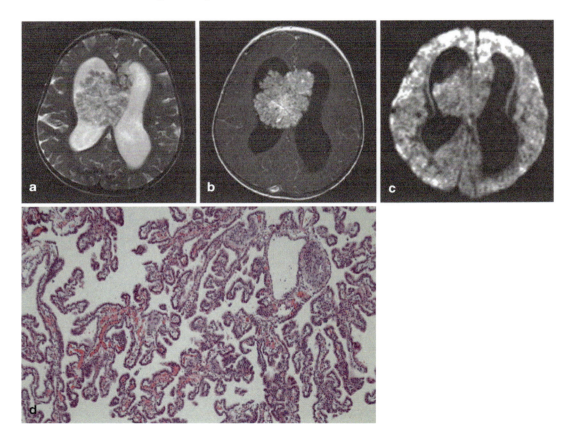

Fig. 19.44 (a–d) Choroid plexus papilloma in a 1-year-old boy. (a) T2-weighted image shows a lobulated hyperintense mass in the lateral ventricles with hydrocephalus. (b) Gadolinium-enhanced T1-weighted image shows a homogeneously enhancing mass with papillary appearance. (c) DW image shows an isointense mass with mildly increased ADC (not shown). (d) Pathology shows a papillary tumor which closely resembles normal choroid plexus

year survival rates have been reported to range between 26% and 43%. The typical MR findings are a more heterogeneous signal mass with irregular enhancing margins and edema in the adjacent brain [69]. DW imaging shows choroid plexus tumors as iso- or hyperintense with the slightly increased or decreased ADC values depending on the cellularity (Figs. 19.44, 19.45, and 19.46). Choroid plexus carcinomas may harbor INI1 mutation similar to ATRT [58].

Rosette-forming glioneuronal tumor (RGNT) is a recently described WHO I rare primary brain tumor which was recently included as a distinct glioneuronal neoplasm in 2007 [70] (Fig. 19.47). These usually occur in young adults (mean age ~31 years of age), are slow-growing, and gross total resection is usually curative [70]. The most common site is the fourth ventricle, followed by cerebellum, pineal region, cerebellopontine angle, and cerebral hemispheres. On imaging, they are well-circumscribed, have a mixed solid-cystic appearance, have variable calcification/hemorrhage, are hyperintense on T2, and demonstrate variable enhancement [70].

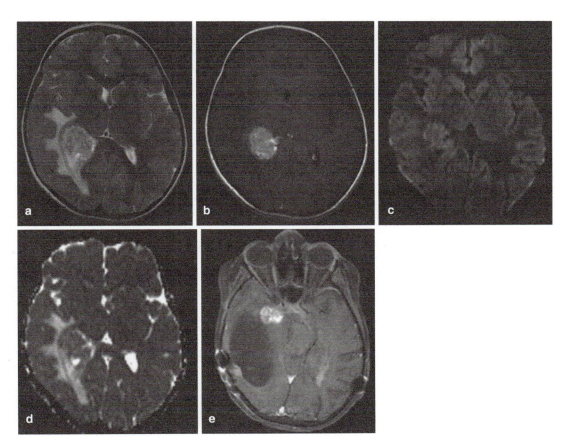

Fig. 19.45 (a–e) Atypical choroid plexus papilloma in a 6-year-old girl. (a) T2-weighted image shows a hyperintense mass in the occipital horn with surrounding edema suggesting brain parenchymal invasion. (b) Gadolinium-enhanced T1-weighted image shows heterogeneous enhancement of the mass. (c, d) DW image shows hyperintensity with slightly increased ADC in the mass. (e) Two-year follow-up MR image shows dissemination and recurrent tumor

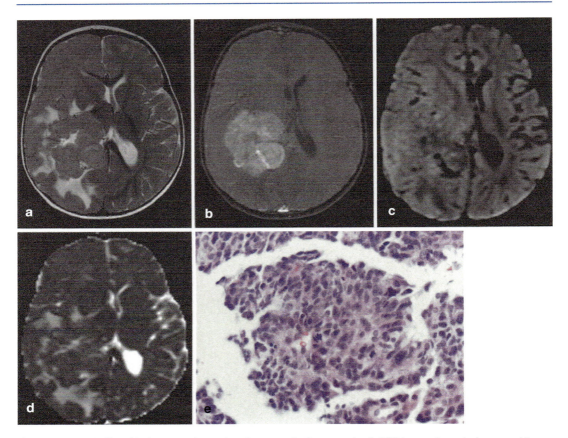

Fig. 19.46 (**a–e**) Choroid plexus carcinoma in a 2-year-old girl. (**a**) T2-weighted image shows an isointense solid mass with necrosis. (**b**) Gadolinium-enhanced T1-weighted image shows heterogeneous enhancement in the mass. (**c, d**) DW image shows isointense with partially decreased ADC in the mass. (**e**) Pathology shows increased pleomorphic cellularity, mitosis, and blurring of the papillary pattern

Another new, recently described entity is diffuse leptomeningeal glioneuronal tumor (DLGT), which is a rare tumor which presents with diffuse leptomeningeal enhancement and small nodular T2 hyperintense cystic lesions along the surfaces of the brain and spinal cord [71] (Fig. 19.48). Patients with DLGT present with hydrocephalus, and survival varies widely [72]. Imaging differentials include infectious leptomeningitis or leptomeningeal carcinomatosis/metastases.

19.9 Encephalopathies

19.9.1 Hypertensive Encephalopathy/Posterior Reversible Encephalopathy Syndrome (PRES)

Hypertensive encephalopathy, or posterior reversible encephalopathy syndrome (PRES), occurs most often secondary to renal diseases in children. It also occurs in children treated for myeloprolifer-

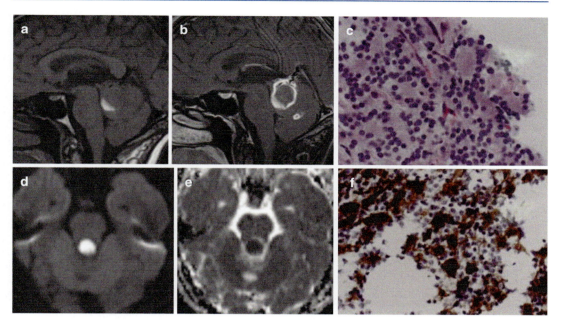

Fig. 19.47 (**a–f**) Rosette-forming glioneuronal tumor (RGNT) in a 19-year-old male with thunderclap headaches and diplopia and bilateral cranial nerve IV palsy. (**a, b**) Sagittal T1 and gadolinium-enhanced T1-weighted image reveals well-defined fourth ventricular tumor adherent to the ventricular wall with intratumoral hemorrhage and peripheral enhancement. (**c, d**) DWI and ADC show diffusely decreased ADC values in the hemorrhagic component. (**e**) Neurocyte-rich region contains well-defined neurocytic rosettes. (**f**) Synaptophysin highlights strong positivity in the neuropil-rich core of the rosettes

ative disorders possibly due to drug toxicity from chemotherapy agents [73]. In children, convulsions are often accompanied by severe headache and restlessness. The most common abnormality on MR imaging is bilateral high signal intensity in parieto-occipital subcortical white matter. These lesions can also occur in the frontal lobes and gray matter, including basal ganglia, thalamus, cerebellum, and brain stem. The mechanism of the disease is thought to be vasogenic edema from failure of autoregulation and/or a cytotoxic edema triggered by severe vasospasm. DW imaging can distinguish irreversible ischemic changes from reversible conditions with vasogenic edema (Fig. 19.49) [74].

19.9.2 Acute Necrotizing Encephalopathy

Acute necrotizing encephalopathy is acute encephalopathy with bilateral thalamotegmental involvement that occurs in infants and children. It is a clinicopathological entity recently separated from acute encephalopathy of unknown etiology. It may be associated with a cytokine storm after viral infections. It frequently occurs in East Asia but has also been identified in other parts of the world. The hallmark of acute necrotizing encephalopathy is multiple, bilateral symmetric brain lesions showing necrosis, pete-

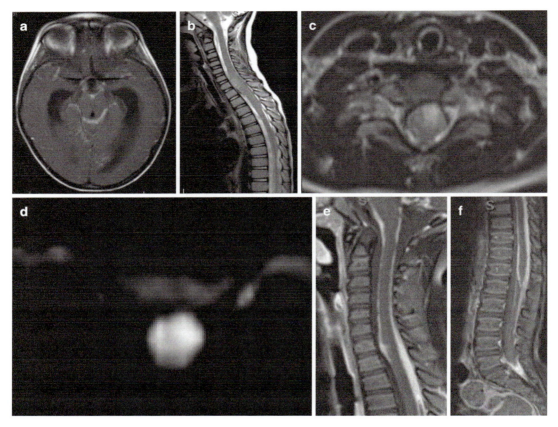

Fig. 19.48 (a–f) Diffuse leptomeningeal glioneuronal tumor (DLGT) in a 3-year-old boy with headaches for two months and a seizure episode. (a) Axial gadolinium-enhanced T1-weighted image shows diffuse leptomeningeal enhancement and hydrocephalus. (b, c) Sagittal and axial T2 images show a ventral spinal cord lesion at C7-T1 level. (d) Axial DWI shows diffusion restriction within this lesion. (e, f) Sagittal T1 post-contrast images show diffuse leptomeningeal enhancement throughout the spine

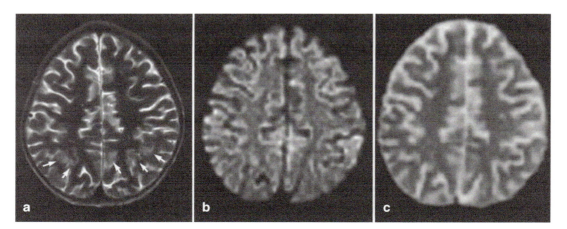

Fig. 19.49 (a–c) Hypertensive encephalopathy, or posterior reversible encephalopathy syndrome, in a 5-year-old girl with acute lymphoblastic leukemia during chemotherapy presenting with seizure. (a) T2-weighted image shows hyperintense lesions in bilateral parieto-occipital cortex (*arrows*). This high signal seems to be due to subtle vasogenic edema rather than frank ischemia. (b, c) DW image and ADC map show no apparent abnormal signal intensities

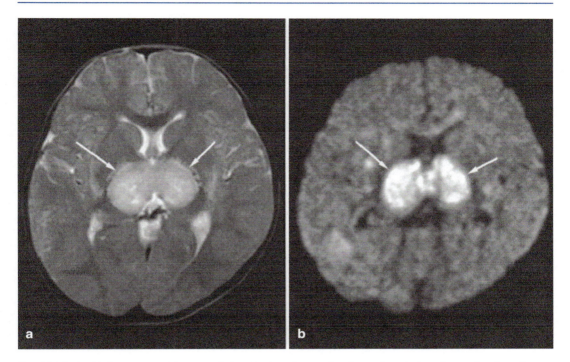

Fig. 19.50 (**a**, **b**) Acute necrotizing encephalopathy in a 1-year-old boy with seizure. (**a**) T2-weighted image shows multiple hyperintense lesions in bilateral thalami and right temporo-occipital region (*arrows*). (**b**) DW image also shows these lesions (*arrows*) as hyperintense associated with decreased ADC (not shown). (Courtesy of Ida M, MD, Ebara Municipal Hospital, Japan)

chial hemorrhage, and cytotoxic edema without inflammatory cell infiltration [75]. The prognosis is generally poor. DW imaging shows multiple symmetric hyperintense lesions with decreased ADC mainly seen in the bilateral thalami, the bilateral brain stem tegmenta, and the cerebral white matter (Fig. 19.50) [76].

19.10 Demyelinating Diseases

19.10.1 Acute Disseminated Encephalomyelitis and Multiple Sclerosis

Acute disseminated encephalomyelitis (ADEM) is more frequent than multiple sclerosis in children. ADEM is usually monophasic but relapses in patients initially diagnosed with ADEM, and conversion to multiple sclerosis has been reported [77, 78]. If these relapses represent part of the same acute monophasic immune process, the term "multiphasic ADEM" is used. If, however, relapses occur, with space and time dissemination, this supports the diagnosis of multiple sclerosis.

On MR images, ADEM lesions tend to be in the subcortical white matter, while multiple sclerosis lesions tend to be situated both in the subcortical and periventricular white matter. Cortical and deep gray matter lesions are more frequent in ADEM. ADEM lesions tend to be poorly marginated, whereas multiple sclerosis lesions have more clearly defined margins. ADEM lesions are characterized in the acute stage by restricted diffusion (ADC values: $0.56 \pm 0.16 \times 10^{-3}$ mm^2/s) and in the subacute stage by increased diffusion ($1.24 \pm 0.13 \times 10^{-3}$ mm^2/s) (Fig. 19.51) [79].

Multiple sclerosis in pediatric patients is relatively rare but may have been underreported. It is estimated that up to 10% of all patients with multiple sclerosis present during childhood [80]. The incidence of tumefactive plaques and posterior fossa plaques may be higher.

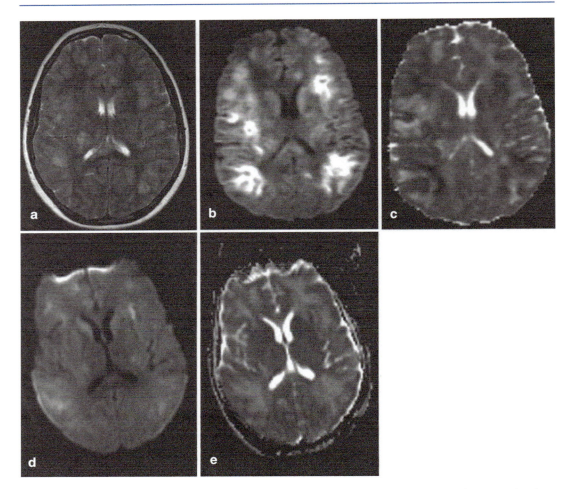

Fig. 19.51 (**a–e**) Acute disseminated encephalomyelitis in an 11-year-old boy with altered mental status. (**a**) T2-weighted image shows multiple ill-defined hyperintense lesions in the white matter, corpus callosum. (**b, c**) DW image shows multiple hyperintense lesions with mainly decreased ADC consistent with cytotoxic edema in the acute phase demyelination. (**d, e**) A 5-day follow-up DW image shows multiple mildly hyperintense lesions with mainly increased ADC consistent with vasogenic edema and the subacute-phase of demyelination

Hyperintense plaques on DW imaging with decreased ADC have been reported to be rare even in the active, enhancing multiple sclerosis plaques [81]. When present, a possible explanation for the hyperintense, cytotoxic multiple sclerosis plaques is intramyelinic edema (Fig. 19.52).

19.11 Metabolic and Toxic Diseases

19.11.1 Charcot-Marie-Tooth

Charcot-Marie-Tooth encompasses an heterogeneous group of primary hereditary motor sensory neuropathies, and is the most common genetic

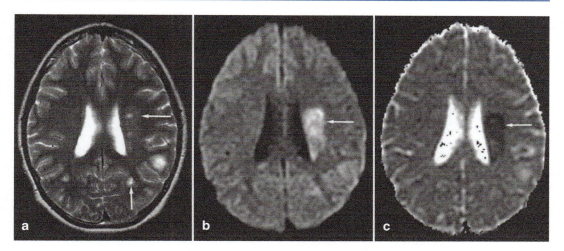

Fig. 19.52 (**a–c**) Acute multiple sclerosis in a 13-year-old girl. (**a**) T2-weighted image shows multiple hyperintense lesions in the periventricular and subcortical white matter (*arrows*). (**b, c**) DW image shows a hyperintense plaque with decreased ADC (*arrows*) in the left corona radiata. This is a cytotoxic plaque, presumably mainly composed of intramyelinic edema

neuromuscular disorder [82]. One disease subtype, X-linked Charcot-Marie-Tooth disease type I (CMTX1) is due to a mutation on the X chromosome in the GJB1 gene [82, 83]. The gene is expressed in myelinating Schwann cells and also in central oligodendrocytes and causes a loss of function. At pathology, axonal degeneration and myelin abnormalities are seen [82]. On MRI, characteristic findings of CMTX1 are reversible, bilaterally, non-enhancing white matter lesions with restricted diffusion [83] (Fig. 19.53). The disease mainly affects children and adolescents, who present with transient central nervous system phenomena including stroke-like episodes, transient paralysis, dysarthria, and ataxia [83].

19.11.2 Central Tegmental Tract Hyperintense Lesions

Cerebral central tegmental tract (CTT) lesions are bilateral DWI/T2-weighted hyperintense lesions along the CTT, which is the extrapyramidal tract connecting the red nucleus with the inferior olivary nucleus [84] (Fig. 19.54). It is seen in various conditions, including children with hypoxic ischemic brain injury with cerebral palsy, metabolic diseases, and those treated with vigabatrin for West syndrome [84–86]. The finding is not specific and can be seen in many other diseases. The pathogenesis is unclear but secondary degeneration after cerebral white matter injury or age-related selective vulnerability of the dorsal brain stem is suspected [84, 87].

Vigabatrin, an irreversible inhibitor of 4-aminobutyrate transaminase, the enzyme responsible for the catabolism of gamma-aminobutyric acid (GABA), has been suggested to cause central tegmental tract lesions in young infants treated for West syndrome [84] (Fig. 19.55). At pathology, there is white matter vacuolation and intramyelinic edema [88, 89]. Vigabatrin increases GABA leading to excitotoxicity in the immature brain since GABA is excitatory in early infants, but inhibitory in adults [90]. Vigabatrin-induced myelinopathy has a special distribution in chil-

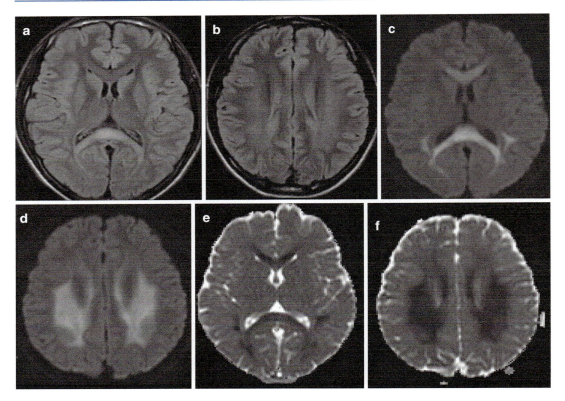

Fig. 19.53 (**a–f**) X-linked Charcot-Marie-Tooth neuropathy (CMTX1) due to GJB1 mutation in a 17-year-old male who presented with difficulty swallowing and dyspnea, who developed facial numbness in the setting of fevers. (**a, b**) Axial T2 FLAIR sequences show high signal in the periventricular and deep white matter and throughout the corpus callosum. (**c–f**) DWI and ADC demonstrate diffusion restriction and low ADC values in the involved white matter

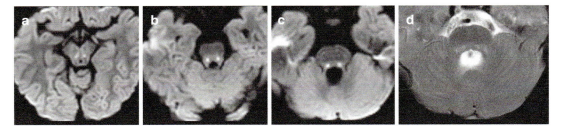

Fig. 19.54 (**a–d**) Central tegmental tract hyperintense lesions in a 2-year-old male with microcephaly, developmental delay, and hypotonia. (**a–c**) Axial DWI images show hyperintensity along the central tegmental tract. (**d**) Axial T2 image shows similar T2 hyperintensity in a similar area

dren. The distribution of the lesions corresponds to distribution of abundant areas of GABA receptors (globi pallidi and thalami) [91]. Distribution of GABA receptors evolves with brain maturation. In adults, vigabatrin may potentially cause a reversible corpus callosal lesion [92] but usually has no imaging changes [93].

19.11.3 Inborn Errors of Metabolism Including Leukodystrophies

Inborn errors of metabolism cover a broad spectrum of diseases, including leukodystrophies which affect only white matter, as well as mitochondrial disorders which affect both gray and

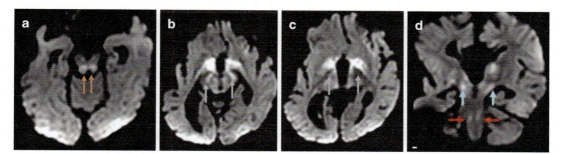

Fig. 19.55 (**a–d**) Central tegmental tract hyperintense lesions due to vigabatrin-induced myelinopathy in a 6-month-old female with refractory seizures treated with vigabatrin. (**a–c**) Axial DWI images show restricted diffusion along the central tegmental tract (red arrow) as well as diffusion restriction along the ascending tract connecting the reticular nuclei of the brainstem to the basal ganglia (blue arrows). (**d**) Coronal DWI also demonstrates similar findings, with reduced diffusion along the central tegmental tract (red arrow) and reticular nuclei of the brainstem (blue arrow)

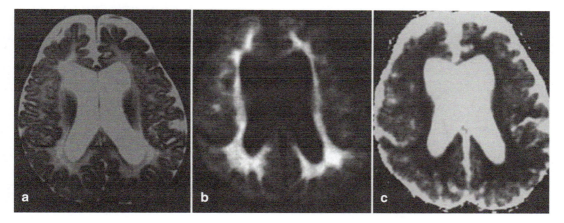

Fig. 19.56 (**a–c**) Metachromatic leukodystrophy in a 10-month-old boy with developmental delay. (**a**) T2-weighted image shows diffuse deep white matter hyperintensity. (**b, c**) DW imaging shows periventricular hyperintensity with decreased ADC in the active stage of the disease. Subcortical U-fibers are relatively spared. (Courtesy of Sener R N., MD, Department of Radiology, Ege University Hospital, Turkey). (From [78])

white matter. Leukodystrophies comprise a wide spectrum of inherited neurodegenerative disorders affecting white matter, while the term leukoencephalopathy is applied to all white matter disease [94]. Myelin is formed from the processes of oligodendrocytes and is composed of multiple layers of proteins (myelin basic protein and proteolipid protein) and lipids (cholesterol, phospholipids, and glycolipids: galactocerebroside and sulfatide).

19.11.4 Lysosomal Disorders

The lysosome is an organelle containing acid hydrolases responsible for digestion of degraded cellular constituents.

Metachromatic leukodystrophy is an autosomal recessive disorder caused by a deficiency of lysosomal enzyme arylsulfatase A (chromosome 22), resulting in the accumulation of sulfatides that are important constituents of the myelin sheath. A tigroid white matter pattern on MR imaging is due to the relative sparing of myelin around the medullary veins. Subcortical U-fibers are spared until late in the disease. DW imaging shows periventricular hyperintensity with decreased ADC in the active stage of the disease (Figs. 19.56 and 19.57) [95–97].

Krabbe disease (globoid cell leukodystrophy) is an autosomal recessive disorder caused by a deficiency of galactosylceramidase (14q21 to q31). The accumulation of galactocerebroside

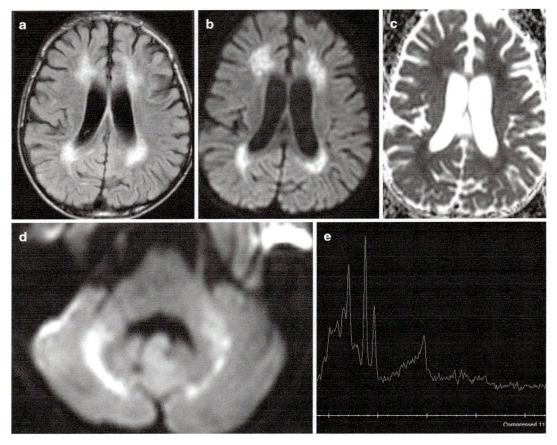

Fig. 19.57 (a–e) Metachromatic leukodystrophy in a 3-year-old female. (a) Axial T2 FLAIR image shows periventricular white matter hyperintensity with sparing of the subcortical U fibers. (b, c) DW imaging shows periventricular hyperintensity with decreased ADC in the active stage of the disease. (d) Restricted diffusion may involve the deep white matter of the cerebellum as well. (e) MR spectroscopy shows elevated lactate, severely depleted NAA, elevated choline and myo-inositol, and near normal creatine. Findings are consistent with considerable axonal damage and loss of the white matter

and galactosylsphingosine is toxic to oligodendrocytes. DW imaging may show hyperintensity in the subcortical white matter, caudate head, and internal capsule with decreased ADC in the early stage of the disease. As the disease progresses, the lesions show iso- or hypointensity with increased ADC [97] (Fig. 19.58). DT images are more sensitive than T2-weighted images for detecting white matter abnormalities [98].

Mucopolysaccharidoses are a genetically heterogeneous group of inborn errors of lysosomal glycosaminoglycan (dermatan, heparan, keratan, or chondroitin sulfate) metabolism. The major neuronal storage materials are a secondary accumulation of gangliosides. Multiple cystic areas in the white matter and basal ganglia correspond to enlarged perivascular spaces [99]. DW imaging shows the lesions as iso- or hypointense with increased ADC (Fig. 19.59).

In GM1 (beta-galactosidase, 3p21) and GM2 (Tay-Sachs hexosamidase A, 15q23-24, and Sandhoff diseases, hexosamidase A and B, 5q13) gangliosidoses, the accumulation of gangliosides in the cytoplasm of neurons results in extensive neuronal loss and white matter degeneration. Diffuse white matter T2 hyperintensity is seen. Thalamic T2 hypointensity with relatively reduced diffusion can be seen in Tay-Sachs disease [100].

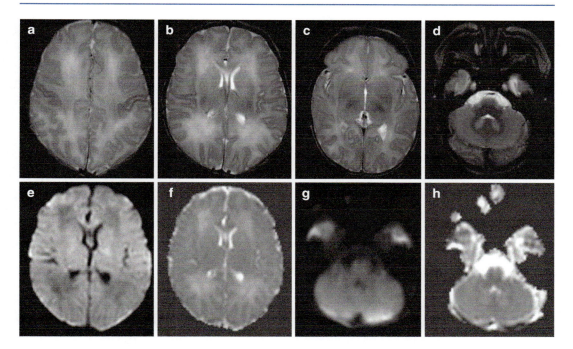

Fig. 19.58 (**a–h**) Krabbe disease in a 2-day-old female with heterozygous GALC gene and family history of Krabbe. (**a–d**) T2-weighted images demonstrate increased diffusivity and T2 signal within the deep and periventricular white matter. (**e–h**) Diffusion-weighted images with corresponding ADC maps show no significant restricted diffusion of the involved white matter

Salla disease is an extremely rare disease due to a defect in SLC17A5 (sialic acid transport protein), which results in accumulation of sialic acid in lysosomes [101]. It is autosomal recessive and most commonly seen in patients with Finnish descent. MRI findings include diffuse white matter signal abnormality involving U fibers, thinning of the corpus callosum, and basal ganglia susceptibility artifact related to iron deposition (Fig. 19.60) [101]. On MRS, free sialic acid has a peak at 2 ppm, which mimics NAA and can erroneously suggest Canavan disease [101].

19.11.5 Peroxisome Disorders

The peroxisome is an organelle that is largely located in oligodendrocytes and is involved in oxidation of very long-chain and branched-chain fatty acids. It is indispensable in myelin maintenance.

Zellweger syndrome (cerebrohepatorenal syndrome) is an autosomal recessive severe peroxisome disorder caused by multiple enzyme defects. MR imaging shows diffuse white matter hyperintensity with abnormal severe gyration in perisylvian and perirolandic regions. DW imaging shows extensive mild hypointensity with increased ADC corresponding to hypomyelination [97].

X-linked adrenoleukodystrophy (Xq28) is caused by a deficiency of acyl-CoA synthetase. MR imaging shows the white matter involvement with posterior predominance in 80% and frontal predominance in 15% of cases. The peripheral zone of the lesion enhances corresponding to the leading edge of demyelination. DW imaging can depict two or three different zones: (1) a central burn-out zone (gliosis) is hypointense; (2) an immune-mediated inflammatory zone may have relatively restricted diffusion; (3) the most peripheral demyelinating zone is minimally hyperintense with increased ADC (Figs. 19.61 and 19.62) [97, 102].

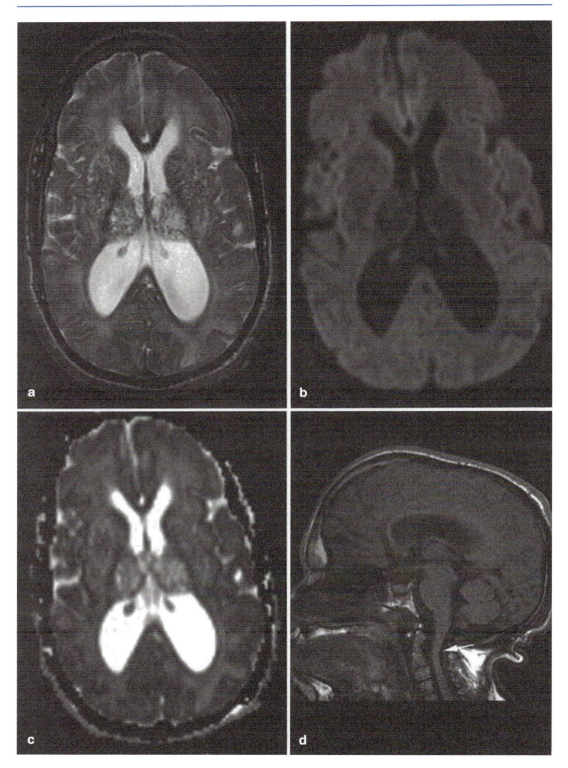

Fig. 19.59 (**a–d**) Mucopolysaccharidosis (Hurler-Sheie 1H/S) in an 18-year-old man. (**a**) T2-weighted image shows multiple cystic areas in the white matter, thalami, and basal ganglia corresponding to enlarged perivascular spaces. (**b**, **c**) DW imaging shows hypointensity with increased ADC in these lesions. (**d**) Sagittal T1-weighted image shows thickening of the dura causing a canal stenosis at the craniovertebral junction (*arrow*)

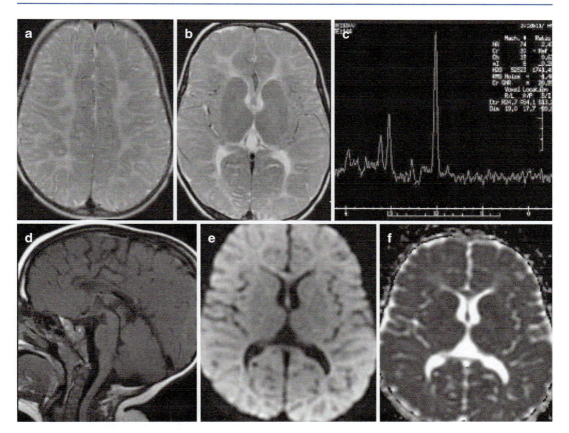

Fig. 19.60 (**a–f**) Salla disease in a 2-year-old male. (Case courtesy of Dr. Aaron Berg) (**a**, **b**) T2-weighted images show diffuse white matter hyperintensity involving U fibers. (**c**) Single voxel MRS (TE 144 msec) shows a large peak at 2 ppm due to free sialic acid. (**d**) Sagittal T1 image shows thinning of the corpus callosum. (**e**, **f**) DWI and ADC show no significant diffusion restriction

19.11.6 Mitochondrial Disorders

Mitochondria not only produce energy with the synthesis of adenosine triphosphate (ATP) through the electron transport chain (respiratory chain) but are also involved in oxidation of fatty acids, pyruvate, ketone, and amino acids. The associated diverse enzymes are encoded by the mitochondrial DNA (mtDNA) and/or the nuclear DNA (nDNA). The spectrum of mitochondrial diseases encompasses various mitochondrial syndromes and isolated enzymatic deficiencies: (1) mtDNA mutations (mitochondrial encephalomyopathy, mitochondrial myopathy, encephalopathy, lactic acidosis and stroke-like episodes: MELAS; myoclonic epilepsy with ragged-red fibers: MERRF; Leigh syndrome; Leber hereditary optic neuropathy: LHON; neuropathy, ataxia, retinitis pigmentosa: NARP; chronic progressive external ophthalmoplegia: CPEO; Kearns-Sayre syndrome, etc.), (2) nDNA mutations producing deletion or depletion of mtDNA (Leigh syndrome, Alpers disease, myo-neuro-gastrointestinal encephalopathy: MNGIE (Fig. 19.63), glutaric aciduria, pyruvate dehydrogenase or carboxylase deficiency, etc.) [103].

Mitochondrial encephalopathies can show various patterns of central nervous system involvement. These include multiple infarcts in the cortex, white matter, and basal ganglia, which do not usually follow vascular territories. Other features of mitochondrial encephalopathy are spongiform leukoencephalopathy due to splitting of the myelin lamellae, demyelination with intramyelinic edema, and atrophy [104, 105]. Either

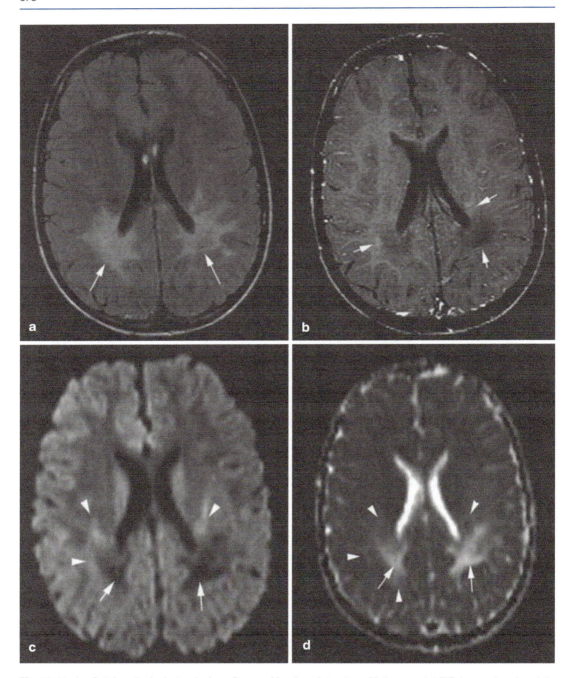

Fig. 19.61 (a–d) Adrenoleukodystrophy in an 8-year-old boy. (a) FLAIR image shows the posterior predominant white matter involvement (*arrows*). (b) Gadolinium-enhanced T1-weighted image shows minimal peripheral enhancement (*arrow*). (c, d) DW imaging shows a central hypointensity with increased ADC (*arrows*) and peripheral mild hyperintensity with mildly increased ADC (*arrowheads*). (Courtesy of Lee A MD The University of Iowa Hospitals and Clinics, USA)

19 Pediatrics 679

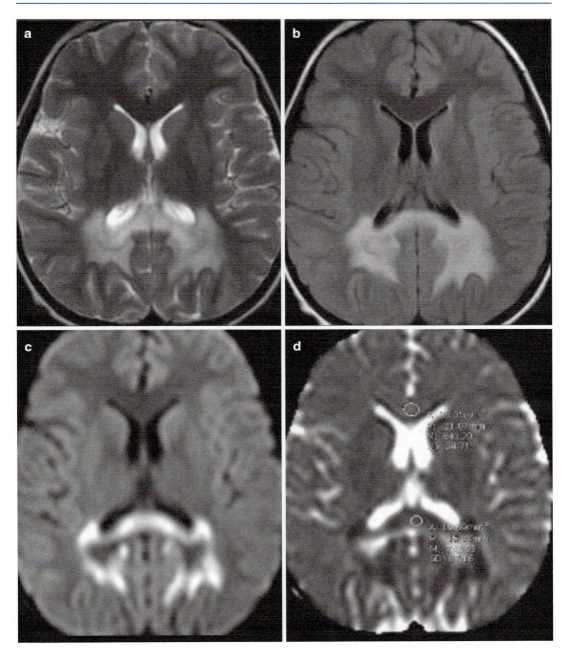

Fig. 19.62 (**a–d**) Adrenoleukodystrophy in a 7-year-old boy. (**a, b**) Axial T2 and T2 FLAIR images demonstrate peri-splenial distribution of signal abnormality in the white matter. (**c, d**) DWI shows restricted diffusion in the splenium and peripheral areas of the white matter lesions, which may be related to intramyelinic edema in the setting of acute demyelination and inflammation

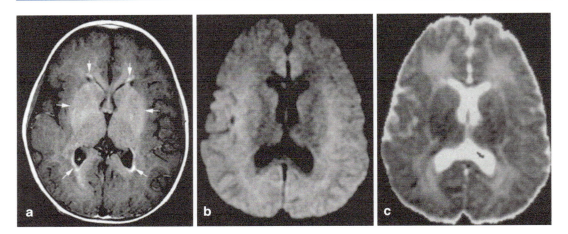

Fig. 19.63 (a–c) Myo-neuro-gastrointestinal encephalopathy (MNGIE) in an 11-year-old boy. (a) Gadolinium-enhanced T1-weighted image shows minimal enhancement in the basal ganglia and periventricular white matter (*arrows*). (b, c) DW imaging shows diffuse white matter isointensity with increased ADC

energy depletion or oxidative damage involves oligodendrocytes. DW imaging often shows the stroke-like lesions in MELAS as hyperintense. They have increased or normal ADC, which presumably represents vasogenic edema (Figs. 19.64 and 19.65) [106–109]. However, decreased ADC in the lesions representing cytotoxic edema can be observed in MELAS and other mitochondrial encephalopathies (Figs. 19.64, 19.65, 19.66, and 19.67) [110–112].

MELAS lesions do not follow vascular territories and angiography fails to demonstrate steno-occlusive disease, so the underlying mechanism is different from ischemic infarction. The main hypothesis of the pathophysiology of MELAS is angiopathy leading to ischemia or secondary energy failure from defective oxidative metabolic pathways or increased energy demand due to neuronal hyperexcitability [113]. The cytotoxic edema in MELAS may be reversible or can evolve to volume loss [113]. In patients with MELAS, there is predominant cortical involvement (occipital, parietal, and temporal lobes). T1 hyperintensity from cortical laminar necrosis and basal ganglia calcifications can also be seen.

Multiple Mitochondrial Dysfunction Syndrome (MMDS) is another type of mitochondrial disorder, also known as cavitating leukoencephalopathy with multiple mitochondrial dysfunction syndrome [114] (Fig. 19.68). MMDS is caused by iron-sulfur (Fe-S) cluster (ISC) gene mutations affecting essential for multiple processes critical for mitochondrial function, including: function of complexes I, II, and III of the electron transport chain, severe deficiency of pyruvate dehydrogenase complex (PDHc) and lipoic acid (required in the citric acid cycle) [114]. This results in marked impairment of neurologic development, non-ketotic hyperglycinemia, pulmonary hypertension, lactic acidosis, and severe regression leading to death usually before the age 15 months.

Alpers-Huttenlocher syndrome is an autosomal recessive hepatocerebral degenerative disorder, which is also called infantile diffuse cerebral degeneration with hepatic cirrhosis. It is found in with mutations in mitochondrial DNA polymerase-γ (POLG), which encodes the mitochondrial DNA replicase protein essential for maintaining the integrity of mitochondrial

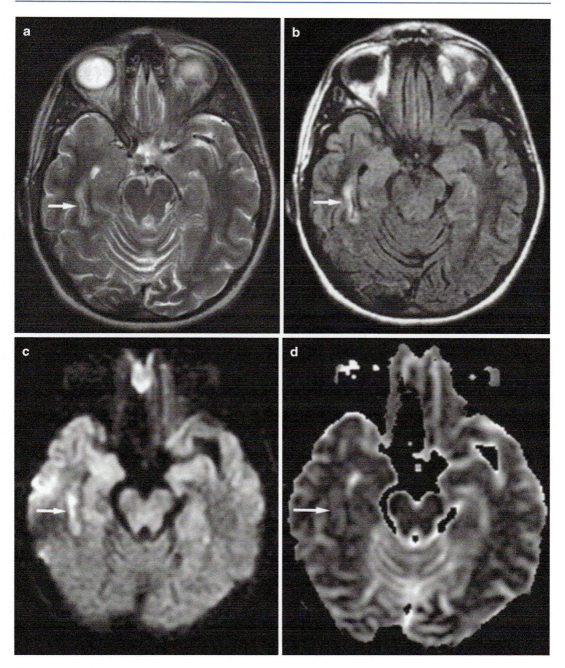

Fig. 19.64 (**a–d**) Mitochondrial encephalopathy with lactic acidosis and stroke (MELAS) in a 27-year-old woman. (**a, b**) T2-weighted and FLAIR images show a hyperintense lesion in the right temporal lobe (*arrow*). (**c, d**) DW image shows this lesion as hyperintense with increased ADC (*arrow*), mainly representing vasogenic edema

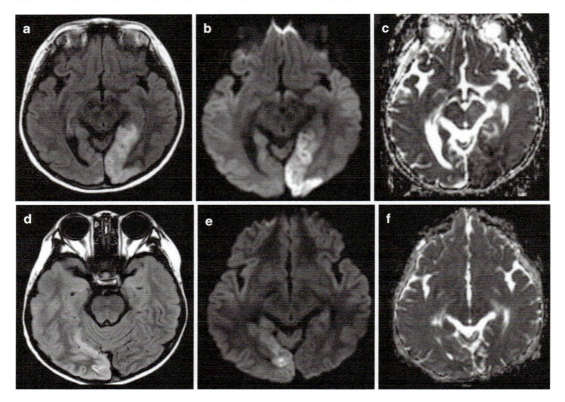

Fig. 19.65 (**a–f**) Mitochondrial encephalopathy, lactic acidosis, and stroke-like episodes (MELAS) in an 8-year-old boy with trouble seeing. (**a–c**) Axial T2 FLAIR, DWI, and ADC show diffusion restriction and edema in the left occipital cortex. (**d–f**) The same patient presented a year earlier with similar symptoms. Axial T2 FLAIR, DWI, and ADC show diffusion restriction and edema in the contralateral right occipital cortex

DNA [115]. Commonly seen findings are refractory myoclonic seizures, developmental delay, and liver dysfunction. Characteristic findings on imaging are initial occipital lobe involvement with diffusion restriction, then subsequent involvement of the basal ganglia, thalami, and deep gray nuclei of the brainstem [115] (Fig. 19.69).

In contradistinction to Alpers, Leigh syndrome (juvenile subacute necrotizing encephalopathy) first affects the brainstem, then followed by abnormalities in the deep gray nuclei and cerebral cortex, which is the reverse of Alpers. Leigh syndrome is a rapidly progressive neurologic disorder that manifests in infancy and early childhood. The defect can be either nuclear (80%) or mitochondrial DNA (20%), which disrupt the electron transport chain [116] (Fig. 19.70).

Glutaric acid is a five-carbon dicarboxylic acid, similar in structure to intermediates in the citric acid cycle, such as alpha ketoglutarate. Glutaric acid is predominantly formed by the catabolism of the amino acids lysine and tryptophan. Glutaric aciduria type-1 is an autosomal recessive disease caused by deficiency of the enzyme which catabolizes glutaric acid to crotonyl-CoA, glutaryl-CoA-dehydrogenase [117] (Fig. 19.71). One possible explanation for the central nervous system damage that occurs in glutaric acidurias is intramyelinic edema, which is one form of cytotoxic edema selectively occurring in myelin

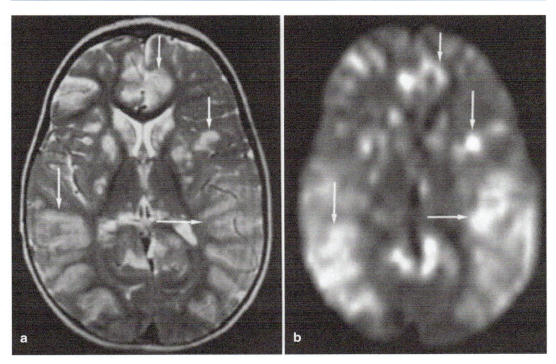

Fig. 19.66 (**a**, **b**) Mitochondrial encephalopathy (unknown enzyme abnormality) in a 20-month-old girl with seizures. (**a**) T2-weighted image shows multiple high signal lesions in bilateral basal ganglia and fronto-parieto-occipital cortex not corresponding to a vascular territory (*arrows*). (**b**) DW image shows multiple high signal intensity lesions associated with decreased ADC (*not shown*)

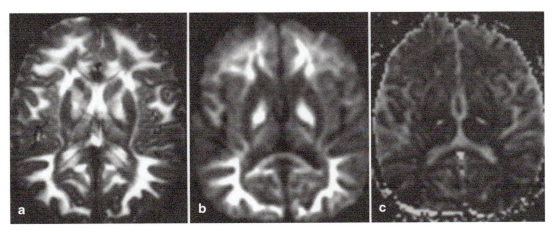

Fig. 19.67 (**a–c**) Kearns-Sayre syndrome in an 18-year-old woman. (**a**) T2-weighted image shows diffuse high signal intensity in bilateral basal ganglia, thalami, and the white matter. (**b**, **c**) DW image shows hyperintensity associated with decreased ADC. (Courtesy of Sacher M, MD, Department of Radiology, Mount Sinai Medical Center, USA). (From [93])

sheaths [118]. These organic acid disorders are characterized by accumulation of organic acids that share structural similarities to the excitotoxic amino acid glutamine. Similar to maple syrup urine disease (MSUD), glutaric acidurias can present with accelerated loss of motor function following an acute illness and fasting, as fasting increases lysine and tryptophan turnover [119].

19.11.7 Metabolic Leukoencephalopathies

Other metabolic encephalopathies/leukoencephalopathies can show hyperintense lesions associated with decreased ADC on DW imaging, which include phenylketonuria (Fig. 19.72), maple syrup urine disease (Figs. 19.73 and 19.74), L-2

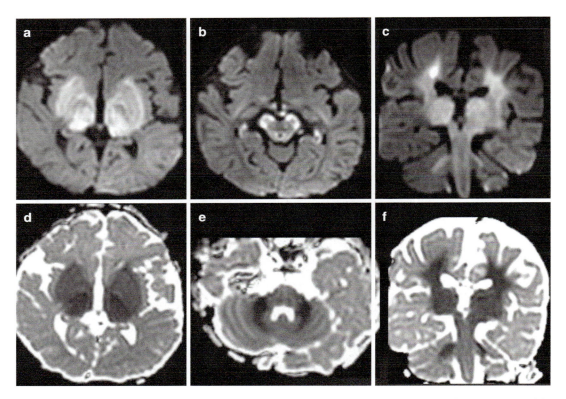

Fig. 19.68 (a–g) Multiple mitochondrial dysfunction syndrome with NFU1 mutation (MMDS1) in a 12-month-old female with neurologic development, failure to thrive with diffuse weakness, and respiratory failure (a–f) Restricted diffusion with low ADC values centered in the centrum semiovale, middle cerebellar peduncles, basal ganglia, thalamus, and dentate gyri. (g) MRS with increased lactate peak

19 Pediatrics

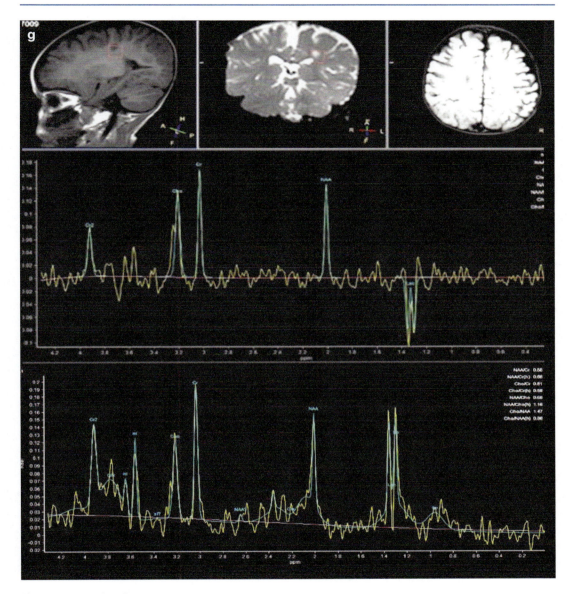

Fig. 19.68 (continued)

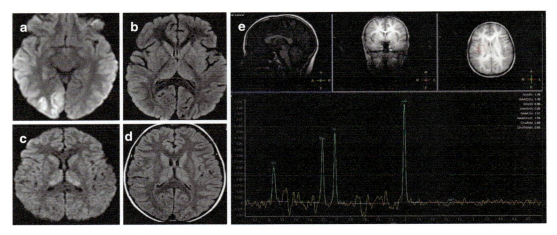

Fig. 19.69 (a–e) Alpers syndrome in an 8-year-old boy with developmental regression, and medication refractory focal epilepsy, cognitive decline. (a–b) Restricted diffusion seen initially within the right occipital lobe in 2015. (c–d) Restricted diffusion then seen in the bilateral thalami in 2017. (e) MRS shows a high lactate peak and reduced NAA:Creatine ratio

hydroxyglutaric aciduria (Fig. 19.75), HMG-coenzyme A lyase deficiency, Canavan's disease (Fig. 19.76), non-ketotic hyperglycinemia, hyperhomocysteinemia, tyrosinemia, citrullinemia, hyperammonemic encephalopathy secondary to urea cycle disorders (Fig. 19.77), propionic aciduria (Fig. 19.78), and infantile neuronal dystrophy [120–130].

One possible explanation for the hyperintense lesion is intramyelinic edema, which is one form of cytotoxic edema selectively occurring in myelin sheaths. Some organic acid disorders are characterized by an accumulation of organic acids that share structural similarities with the excitotoxic amino acid glutamate (D-2.1-2,3 hydroxyglutarate, glutarate) [31]. In urea cycle disorders, high levels of ammonia result in the conversion of large amounts of glutamate to glutamine by glutamine synthetase, which may cause astrocyte swelling and brain edema [129].

Phenylketonuria is an autosomal recessive disorder caused by a deficiency of phenylalanine hydroxylase. Accumulation of l-phenylalanine impairs glutamate receptor function and thus contributes to brain dysfunction in phenylketonuria. Pathologic findings include delayed or defective myelination, intramyelinic edema, diffuse white matter vacuolation, demyelination, and gliosis. DW imaging shows these lesions as hyperintense with decreased ADC, probably the result of intramyelinic edema and/or astrocytic swelling, presumably due to acute excitotoxic injury [31] (Fig. 19.70). With appropriate dietary control, these MR abnormalities can completely resolve.

Maple syrup urine disease (MSUD) is an inherited disorder of branched-chain amino acid metabolism that presents at 4–10 days of age with neurologic deterioration, ketoacidosis, and hyperammonemia. In the classic form of MSUD, diffusion restriction involves the basal ganglia, thalamus, brainstem, and cerebellum and usually affects the infratentorial greater than supratentorial brain (Fig. 19.73). In the intermittent form, diffusion restriction involves the supratentorial areas and cerebellum but spares the brainstem, thalami, and basal ganglia [131, 132] (Fig. 19.74).

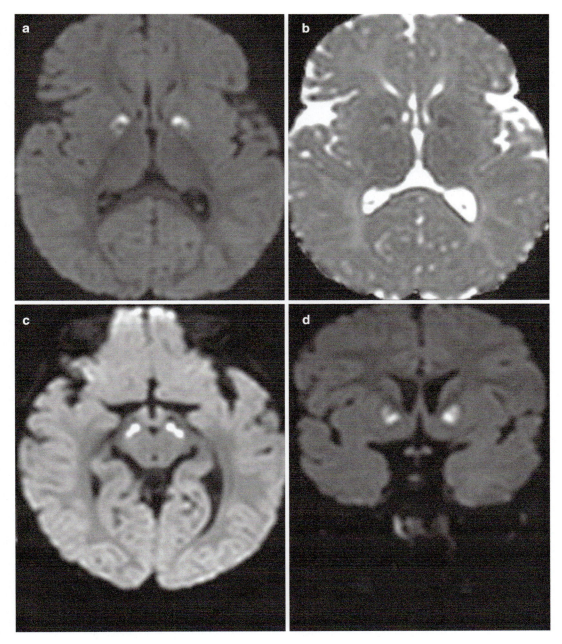

Fig. 19.70 (**a–d**) Leigh disease in a 3-year-old girl. (**a, b**) Axial DWI and ADC show diffusion restriction in the bilateral globi pallidi. (**c, d**) Axial and coronal DWI show diffusion restriction in the globi pallidi and extending into the cerebral peduncles of the midbrain

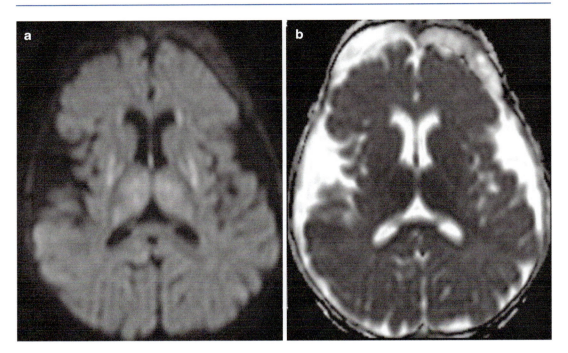

Fig. 19.71 (**a–b**) Glutaric Aciduria Type 1 in an 11-month-old female. (**a, b**) DWI and ADC show symmetric restricted diffusion in the bilateral putamina and thalami. There is also conspicuous widening of the Sylvian fissures/lateral sulci, characteristic of glutaric aciduria type 1

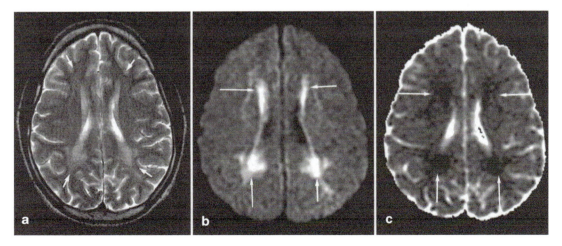

Fig. 19.72 (**a–c**) Phenylketonuria in a 36-year-old man. (**a**) T2-weighted image shows hyperintense lesions in the periventricular white matter (*arrows*). (**b**) DW image shows these lesions as hyperintense (*arrows*). (**c**) These hyperintense lesions have decreased ADC representing cytotoxic edema, especially intramyelinic edema (*arrows*)

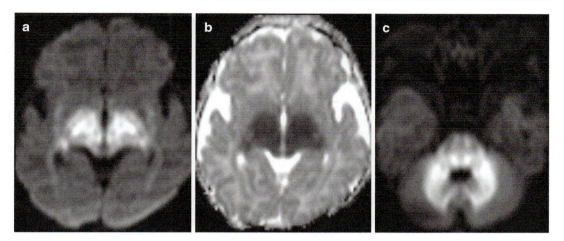

Fig. 19.73 (**a–c**) Maple syrup urine disease (MSUD) in a 1-year-old male. (**a, b**) DWI and ADC show symmetric restricted diffusion in the brainstem, posterior limb of the internal capsule, and regions of the cerebellum. (**c**) Restricted diffusion is also seen in the dentate nuclei and corticospinal tracts. This is the classic form of MSUD, caused by a defective BCKD-E1β subunit

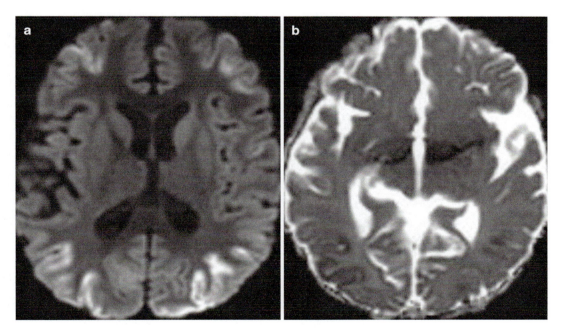

Fig. 19.74 (**a–b**) Maple syrup urine disease (MSUD) in a 2-year-old male. (**a, b**) DWI and ADC show cortical impeded diffusion in the bilateral occipital lobes. This patient had a defective DLD:E3 subunit deficiency causing MSUD. The pattern here is in contradistinction to the classic form as the brainstem, thalami, and basal ganglia are relatively spared

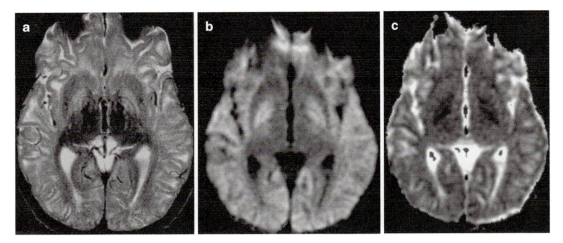

Fig. 19.75 (a–c) L-2 hydroxyglutaric aciduria in a 13-year-old male. (a, b) Symmetrically restricted diffusion in the globi pallidi and subcortical white matter (c) Additionally there is diffuse white matter signal hyperintensity evident on the T2-weighted images

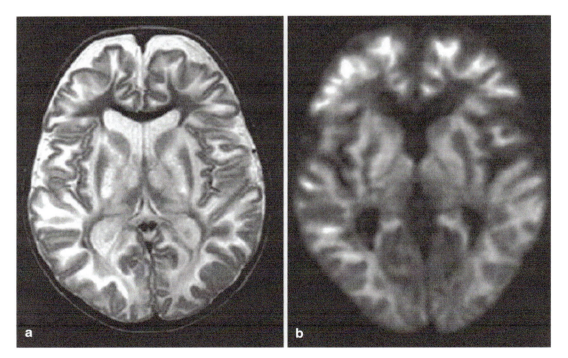

Fig. 19.76 (a, b) Canavan disease. A 15-month-old boy presented with delayed psychomotor development, seizures, and spasticity. (a) T2-weighted image reveals high signal in peripheral white matter, globi pallidi and thalami. Note diffuse atrophy and thinning of the cortex. (b) DW image shows high signal changes in the peripheral white matter and globi pallidi with mildly decreased ADC partially (not shown). (Courtesy of Sener RN, MD, Department of Radiology, Ege University Hospital, Turkey). (From [129])

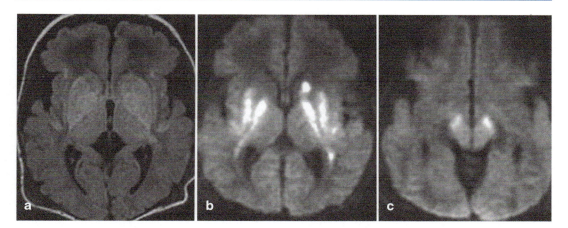

Fig. 19.77 (a–c) Hyperammonemic encephalopathy secondary to urea cycle disorders in a 9-day-old male infant. (a) FLAIR image reveals mild hyperintensity in the basal ganglia and internal capsules. (b, c) DW imaging shows symmetric hyperintense lesions in the basal ganglia, internal capsules, and cerebral peduncles with decreased ADC (not shown)

L-2 hydroxyglutaric aciduria is caused by deficiency of the enzyme L-2 hydroxyglutarate dehydrogenase, which results in the accumulation of L-2 hydroxyglutaric acid in urine, CSF, and plasma [125, 133] (Fig. 19.75). Imaging features include diffusely high T2 signal within the cerebral white matter and dentate nuclei, and hyperintense T2 signal in the basal ganglia with sparing of the thalami. There may be reduced diffusion in the basal ganglia, but often diffusion-weighted imaging is normal [133].

Canavan disease is an autosomal recessive disorder caused by mutations in the gene of aspartoacylase, which leads to an abnormal accumulation of N-acetyl-aspartate (NAA) in the brain, especially in oligodendrocytes, associated with macrocephaly. MRS shows a large peak at 2 ppm due to NAA. Pathology shows astroglial swelling, intramyelinic edema, and swollen mitochondria. Restricted diffusion may be seen in the white matter without any focal predominance (Fig. 19.76) [122–124]. Canavan is a rapidly progressive disease with death usually occurring in the first five years of life [119].

Urea cycle disorders result in abnormal accumulation of ammonia and nitrogen. Ammonia is directly toxic to the brain and causes cytokine release, as well as increased glutamate and excessive activation of N-methyl-D-aspartate receptors [118]. High levels of ammonia are also seen in hepatic encephalopathy. MRI findings include symmetrically restricted diffusion in the basal ganglia and sometimes cerebral cortex, as well as T1 shortening in the basal ganglia and cortex (Fig. 19.77) [134]. On MRS, there is decreased NAA, increased glutamate and glutamine, and decreased myo-inositol [134].

Propionic acidemia is an autosomal recessive disorder of deficiency in propionyl Co-A carboxylase, which is required in the processing of odd-numbered chained fatty acids. Imaging findings show restricted diffusion in the basal ganglia and cortex, and has been associated with intracranial hemorrhage (Fig. 19.78) [133].

Alexander disease (Fibrinoid leukodystrophy) is a sporadic leukodystrophy associated with macrocephaly. The cause appears to be mutations in the glial fibrillary acidic protein (GFAP) gene (chromosome 17q21). Rosenthal fibers, intracytoplasmic proteinaceous inclusions from aggregation of GFAP, are present. Pathologically, there is widespread myelin deficiency, cystic

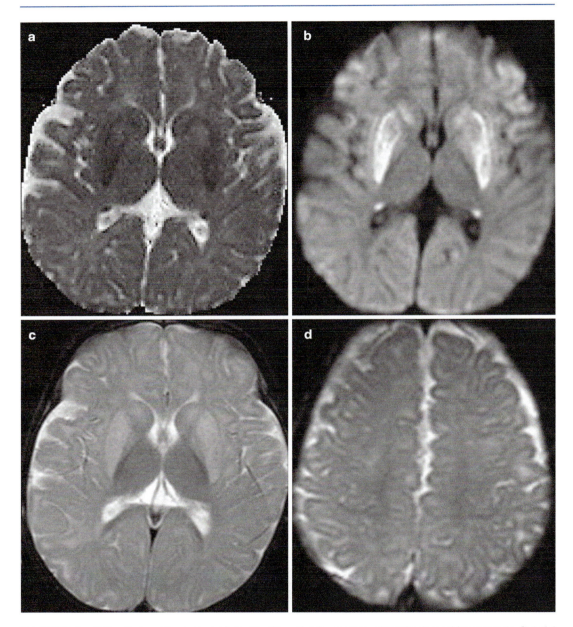

Fig. 19.78 (**a–d**) Propionic acidemia in an 18-month-old female. Case courtesy of Dr. Douglas Quint. (**a**, **b**) DWI and ADC show symmetric restricted diffusion of the bilateral striatum and fronto-parietal cortex. Facilitated diffusion is seen throughout the deep white matter. (**c**, **d**) Axial T2 images show hyperintensity in the striatum, cortex, and white matter

degeneration, and cavitation. MR imaging shows frontal predominant white matter changes with gadolinium enhancement in the deep white matter and basal ganglia. DW imaging shows diffuse hypointensity in the white matter and increased ADC [135] (Fig. 19.79).

Van der Knaap disease, also known as megalencephalic leukodystrophy with subcortical cysts or leukoencephalopathy with macrocephaly and mild clinical course, is an autosomal recessive disorder with its gene locus at the MLC 1 gene at chromosome 22q. It is clinically characterized

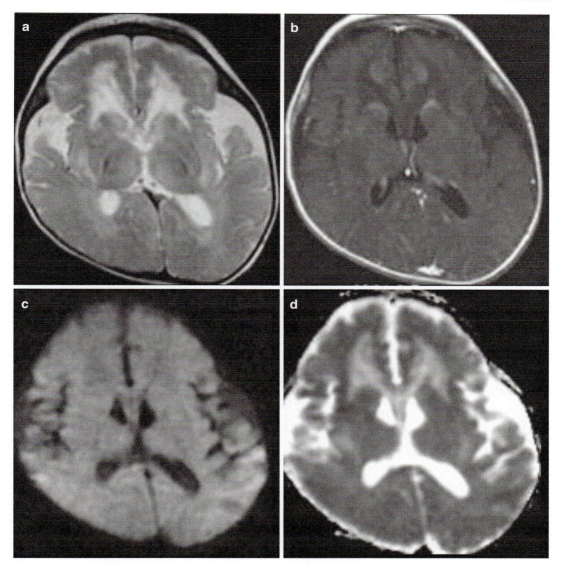

Fig. 19.79 (**a–d**) Alexander disease in a 5-month-old male. Case courtesy of Dr. Hiroshi Oba and Dr Mitsuru Matsuki. (**a, b**) Axial T2 and FLAIR sequences show extensive subcortical white matter T2/FLAIR hyperintensity, predominantly in the frontal lobes. (**c, d**) The T2 hyperintensity is related to facilitated diffusion

by early-onset macrocephaly, in combination with mild gross motor developmental delay, seizures, ataxia, spasticity, and extrapyramidal signs. Macrocephaly is observed in virtually all individuals, either at birth but more frequently develops during the first year of life. Pathology reveals a vacuolating myelinopathy in which the outer layer of myelin sheaths is affected. Subcortical cysts are seen in the frontal and temporal lobes. DW imaging shows diffuse hypointensity in the white matter and in the subcortical cysts associated with increased ADC (Fig. 19.80) [97].

Pelizaeus–Merzbacher disease is an X-linked leukodystrophy due to a defect of proteolipid protein (PLP gene Xq22), which is integral in the formation of myelin. It pathologically

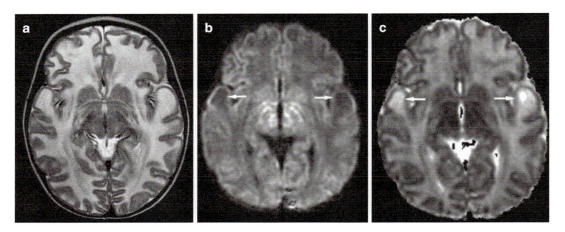

Fig. 19.80 (a–c) Van der Knaap disease in a 10-month-old boy with megalencephaly. (a) T2-weighted image shows diffuse hyperintensity in the white matter. (b, c) DW image shows diffuse hypointensity with increased ADC, especially prominent in symmetrical subcortical cysts in the temporal lobes (*arrows*)

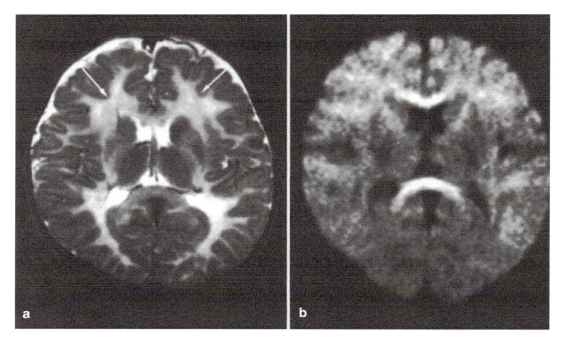

Fig. 19.81 (a, b) Pelizaeus–Merzbacher disease in a 7-month-old boy with developmental delay. (a) T2-weighted image shows diffuse white matter hyperintensity extending into the U-fibers due to hypomyelination (*arrows*). (b) DW image (*z axis*) demonstrates isointensity in the white matter and essentially normal anisotropy in the corpus callosum. ADC values are diffusely slightly increased in the white matter (not shown). (From [137])

shows hypomyelination and spares the axon. MR imaging shows total absence of myelination (connatal type) or arrested myelination (classical form). Despite hypomyelination in Pelizaeus–Merzbacher disease, DW imaging shows normal diffusional anisotropy in the white matter (Figs. 19.81 and 19.82) [136]. This finding suggests that anisotropy is primarily due to the axonal membrane in the immature brain.

Leukoencephalopathy with vanishing white matter (childhood ataxia with diffuse CNS hypomyelination) is an autosomal recessive disorder

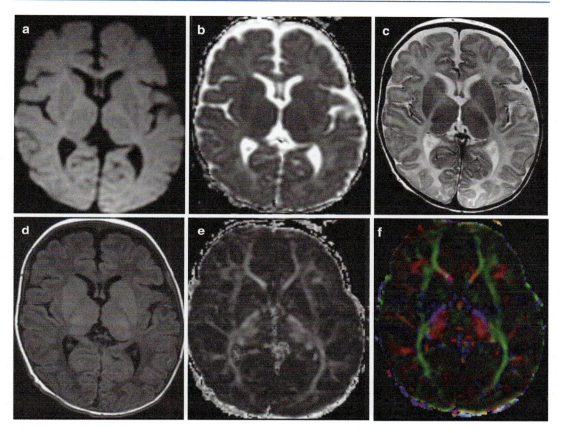

Fig. 19.82 (**a–f**) Pelizaeus–Merzbacher disease in a 3-month-old male. (**a**, **b**) Axial DWI and ADC do not show diffusion restriction (**c**, **d**) Axial T2 and T1 images show profoundly reduced myelination of the white matter, including the internal and external capsules. White matter abnormalities extend to the subcortical regions. (**e**, **f**) Fractional anisotropy is preserved suggesting preserved axonal membrane

with chronic progression and additional episodes of rapid deterioration, provoked by fever and minor head trauma. This leukoencephalopathy is a primary axonopathy, with myelin being secondarily affected. Mutations are identified in the eukaryotic translation initiation factor (eIF2B), which is essential for the initiation of translation of RNA into protein. Increased cerebrospinal glycine may be secondary to excitotoxic brain damage. Pathology shows axonal loss, hypomyelination, demyelination, and gliosis, primarily in subcortical white matter. In the late stage, there are extensive cystic degenerations of the white matter associated with reactive changes. Typical MR imaging findings are diffuse white matter signal hyperintensity on T2-weighted images similar to CSF intensity with additional lesions in the central tegmental tracts and basis pontis. MR spectroscopy shows mildly increased lactate and glucose peaks with decreased NAA, choline, and creatine peaks. DW imaging shows low signal intensity, presumably representing cystic degeneration (Fig. 19.83) [97].

19.12 Congenital Anomalies

19.12.1 Sturge–Weber Syndrome

Sturge–Weber syndrome (encephalotrigeminal angiomatosis) is a congenital, sporadic disorder of unknown cause. Impaired venous drainage, due to leptomeningeal angiomatosis, results in impaired arterial blood flow to the subjacent brain.

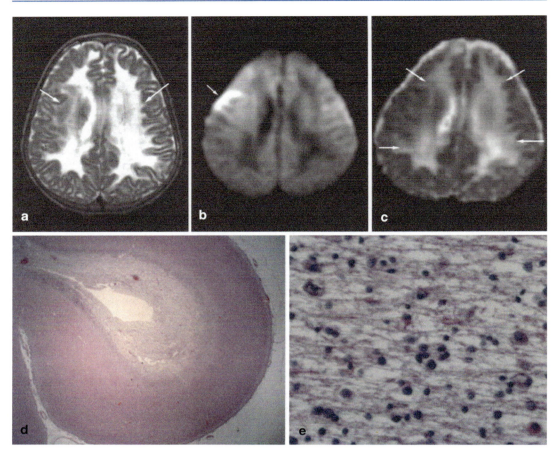

Fig. 19.83 (a–e) Vanishing white matter disease in an 8-year-old boy with progressive leukoencephalopathy. (**a**) T2-weighted image shows diffuse white matter hyperintensity extending into the U-fibers (*arrows*). (**b**) DW image demonstrates diffuse low signal intensity in the white matter. (**c**) ADC map shows diffusely increased ADC in the white matter due to cystic changes (*arrows*). (**d, e**) Pathology specimens show cystic degeneration and reactive astrogliosis involving in the subcortical white matter

The affected brain tissue is atrophic and displays neuronal loss, astrogliosis, dysgenetic cortex, and calcification in the cortical and subcortical white matter. MR imaging is the most sensitive imaging study demonstrating the precise extent and distribution of the leptomeningeal angiomatosis that is the hallmark of the diagnosis. Bilateral involvement occurs in 10%–20% of cases. Decreased T2 signal intensity in the subcortical white matter underlying the area of leptomeningeal angiomatosis reflects areas of calcification, cerebral blood oxygenation effect, and abnormal hypermyelination or accelerated myelination. The axon controls the formation and thickness of myelin. If ischemia occurs in the cortex, it could interfere with normal neuronal function and lead to premature axonal release of a myelinogenic trophic factor [138]. Increased FA and decreased ADC values in the white matter subjacent to the leptomeningeal angiomatosis in neonatal Sturge–Weber syndrome probably reflect such abnormal hypermyelination (Fig. 19.84) [139].

19.12.2 Hemimegalencephaly

Abnormally accelerated myelination has been reported in hemimegalencephaly [140]. Pathologically, neuronal maturation and increase in size of the axons occur earlier than in normal

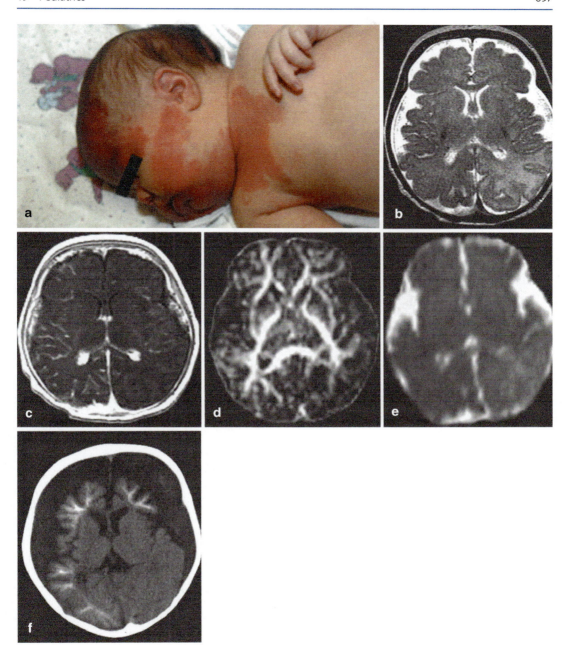

Fig. 19.84 (**a–f**) Sturge–Weber syndrome in a 7-day-old female infant. (**a**) Port wine stains are noted covering her entire head and extending onto her back and shoulders. (**b**) T2-weighted image shows hypointensity in the white matter of the right entire hemisphere and left fronto-temporo-parietal areas, compared to the left parieto-occipital white matter. (**c**) Post-contrast T1-weighted image shows extensive leptomeningeal enhancement in the right hemisphere and left fronto-temporo-parietal areas consistent with leptomeningeal angiomatosis. (**d**) Fractional anisotropy demonstrates homogeneously increased anisotropy in the entire right cerebral hemisphere and left fronto-temporo-parietal areas, compared to the left parieto-occipital white matter. (**e**) The ADC map shows decreased ADC in the white matter in the entire right hemisphere and left fronto-temporo-parietal areas, compared to the left parieto-occipital white matter. (**f**) A 6-month follow-up noncontrast CT shows diffuse cortical and subcortical calcifications and atrophy in the right hemisphere and left frontal lobe with sparing of the left temporo-occipital and parietal regions. (From [145])

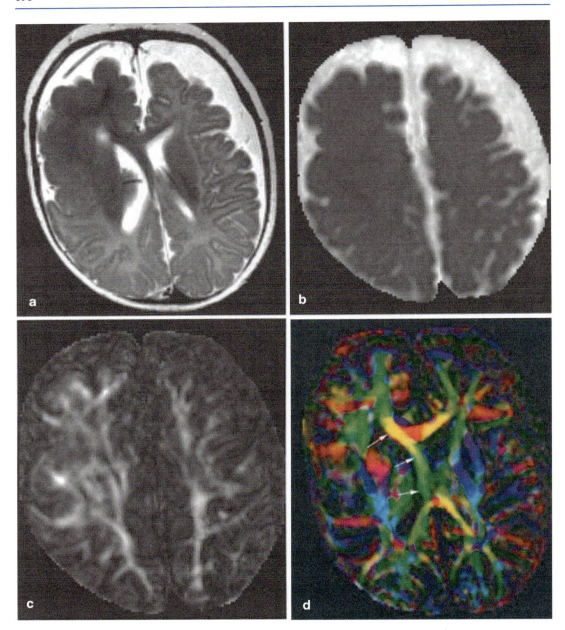

Fig. 19.85 (a–d) Hemimegalencephaly in a 4-month-old boy with infantile spasms. (**a**) T2-weighted image shows hypointense areas in the right frontal cortex and white matter which probably represents abnormally advanced myelination associated with hemimegalencephaly. (**b, c**) DT imaging shows increased FA and slightly decreased ADC suggesting accentuated myelination in the right hemisphere. (**d**) DT imaging color map shows aberrant midsagittal fiber tracts passing anteroposteriorly through between the two anterior horns of the lateral ventricles (*arrows*). (Courtesy of Salamon N, MD, The University of California, Los Angeles, USA)

brain, which may lead to advanced myelination. Restricted diffusion has been reported in hemimegalencephaly on prenatal DW imaging [141]. This finding probably results from a combination of abnormally advanced myelination and increased cellularity (immature neurons) related to excessive prenatal neurogenesis and heterotopia (Fig. 19.85) [142]. Increased FA values are also observed in the areas of abnormal advanced myelination. Aberrant midsagittal fiber tracts

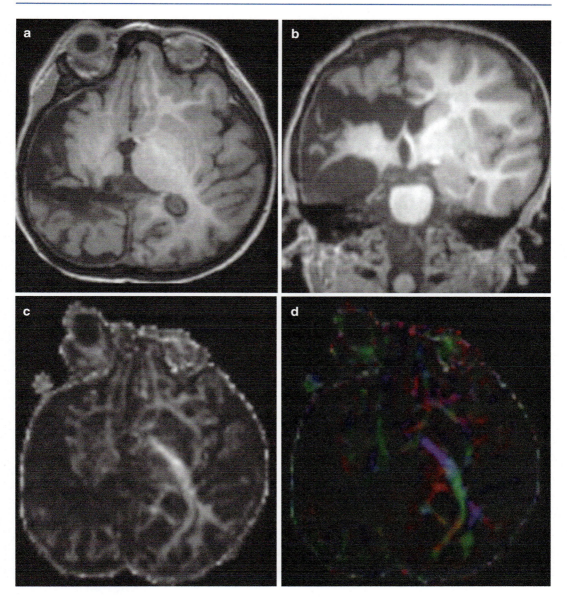

Fig. 19.86 (**a–d**) Failed hemispherotomy with recurrent seizures in a 4-year-old male with prior surgery for Sturge–Weber disease (**a, b**) axial and coronal T1 images show residual tracts connecting the two hemispheres through the anterior commissure. (**c, d**) FA and color DTI maps redemonstrate residual white matter connections through the anterior commissure

are observed in 57% of cases (15/26 patients) with hemimegalencephaly on MR and DT imaging [143]. DT imaging shows the fibers passing anteroposteriorly between the two anterior horns of the lateral ventricles (Fig. 19.85). DTI can also help evaluate for residual connections between the two hemispheres after functional hemispherectomy, which may require re-do surgery to complete the functional disconnection (Fig. 19.86).

19.12.3 Polymicrogyria, Focal Cortical Dysplasia, and Tuberous Sclerosis

Polymicrogyria is characterized by the abnormal arrangement of cortical layers and excessive folding of the cortical ribbon. Decreased FA and normal ADC are observed in the subcortical white matter underlying the polymicrogyric cortex [144].

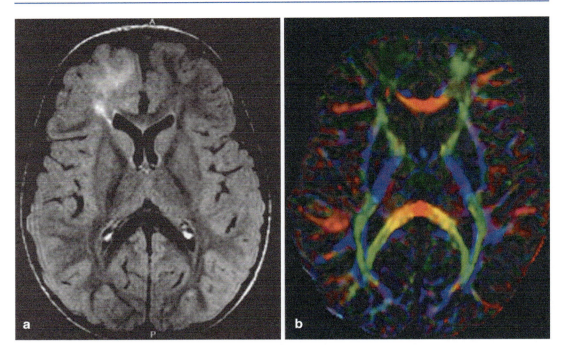

Fig. 19.87 (**a**, **b**) Cortical dysplasia in a 5-year-old boy with right frontal spikes. (**a**) FLAIR image shows cortical thickening and white matter hyperintensity in the right frontal lobe. (**b**) DT imaging color map shows decreased anisotropy in the right frontal abnormal area which may represent decreased fiber connection between deep white matter and dysplastic cortex. (Courtesy of Salamon N, MD, The University of California, Los Angeles, USA)

Focal cortical dysplasia was first described by Taylor and is characterized by the presence of cytomegalic neurons, balloon cells, and hypomyelination. DT imaging might show decreased FA and increased ADC within the region of dysplastic brain (Fig. 19.87) [145, 146]. Decreased fiber connections between the deep white matter and the dysplastic cortex and the aberrant white matter tract can be detected with fiber tractography.

In tuberous sclerosis, epileptogenic tubers may have a significant increase in ADC [147]. DT imaging demonstrates a decrease in anisotropy in normal-appearing white matter that may be associated with changes in myelin packing of axonal fibers disrupted by astrogliosis and myelination defects [148].

19.12.4 Corpus Callosum Agenesis/Dysgenesis

Corpus callosum agenesis/dysgenesis occurs as a result of the failure of commissural fibers to cross to the contralateral cerebral hemisphere via the callosal precursor due to a lack of induction by the massa commisuralis. Diffusion tensor fiber tractography demonstrates the arrangement of fiber tracts forming Probst bundles (Fig. 19.88), the rudimentary cingulum, and the dysplastic fornices [146, 149]. If the development of the commissural fibers is impaired by some insult such as cortical dysplasia, formation of the Probst bundle is impaired (Fig. 19.89). On DT imaging fiber tractography, the fibers from

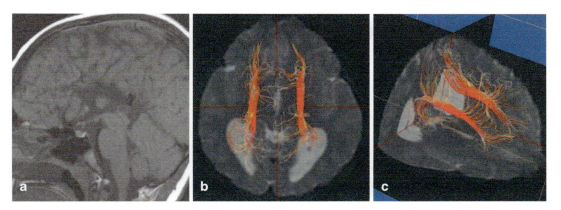

Fig. 19.88 (a–c) Corpus callosum agenesis in a 10-year-old boy. (a) Sagittal T1-weighted image shows agenesis of the corpus callosum. (b, c) DT imaging fiber tractography demonstrates the arrangement of fiber tracts forming Probst bundles (*orange*). (Courtesy of Mori H, MD, and Aoki S, MD, The University of Tokyo, Japan)

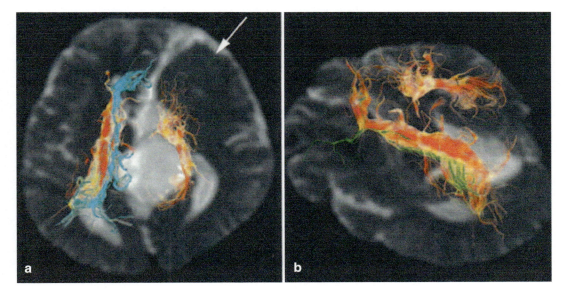

Fig. 19.89 (a, b) Complete callosal agenesis and cortical dysplasia in the left frontal lobe in a 34-year-old man. (a) DT imaging fiber tractography (Two-ROI method) shows that while the Probst bundle in the right hemisphere is well developed, that in the left hemisphere is poorly developed. Cortical dysplasia is shown in the left frontal lobe (*arrow*). The fibers from the right prefrontal area run along the innermost side of the Probst bundle (*blue lines*). (b) The fibers from the right orbital gyrus run along the outermost side in Probst bundle (*green lines*). (Courtesy of Utsunomiya H, MD, Fukuoka University, Japan). (From [149])

the prefrontal area run on the inner side of the Probst bundle and form the genu of the corpus callosum, while fibers from the caudal region of the frontal lobe run along the more lateral side and form the body of the corpus callosum. The fibers from the orbital gyri that form the rostrum of the corpus callosum run along the outermost side of the Probst bundle [149]. These findings support that the growth of the corpus callosum is primarily anteroposterior, with the genu forming first, followed by the body, splenium, and rostrum.

19.12.5 Other Anomalies

DT imaging fiber tractography findings have been reported in holoprosencephaly, lissencephaly, Joubert syndrome, and posterior fossa malformations [145, 146].

19.13 Conclusion

Diffusion-weighted imaging plays an important role in the diagnosis of various pathological conditions in the pediatric brain, which has a high water content. DW imaging can also depict acute or subacute ischemic changes in children when conventional MR imaging or CT is normal or shows only subtle abnormalities. DW imaging is useful in differentiating white matter diseases and in differentiating between tumor and abscess. The calculation of ADC maps or fractional anisotropy demonstrates the water content or more precisely than DW imaging. The recognition of imaging pitfalls is important for optimal interpretation of DW imaging. Diffusion tensor imaging (fractional anisotropy map, fiber tractography) is a useful tool for the evaluation of myelination and microstructural changes of the white matter, and for the demonstration of the white matter tract anatomy in various diseases in pediatric patients.

19.14 Treatment 1: Leukodystrophy

Satsuki Matsumoto

19.14.1 Definition

White matter disorders include acquired as well as genetic conditions. Examples of acquired causes include immune-mediated processes (such as acute disseminated encephalomyelitis, and multiple sclerosis), trauma, and vitamin deficiency (Vitamin B 12 deficiency). Leukodystrophies are heritable white matter disorders and it is defined as "genetic disorders affecting the white matter of the central nervous system (CNS) with or without peripheral nervous system involvement" [150].

Leukodystrophies are divided into two categories. Primary leukodystrophies are due to problems of glial cells, with resultant white matter changes. Genetic leukoencephalopathies are due to problems of neuronal, vascular, or systemic process, in which the white matter changes are felt to be secondary [151]. With more sophisticated genetic evaluation, the list of leukodystrophies is ever-expanding. Still leukodystrophies are relatively rare. Estimated combined incidence of leukodystrophies ranges from 1 in 50,000 to 1 in 7663 [152, 153].

19.14.2 Presentation

The most common presenting symptom for leukodystrophy is a motor symptom (developmental delay and regression). In infants or young children, developmental delay is more common in hypomyelinating disorders, whereas regression is more common in leukodystrophies with myelin destruction. Patients with vanishing white matter disease present with an acute deterioration of motor skills with an illness or a minor head trauma. Although gradual functional decline over time is the usual course with most leukodystrophies, some may have an apparently static course and even some improvement over time (*HEPACAM* and *EARS2* mutations) [154]. The age of onset ranges from neonatal period through adulthood. Though each leukodystrophy has a typical age of onset, such as infantile onset with Krabbe disease and early school age onset with adrenoleukodystrophy, clinicians need to recognize that there is a spectrum of presentation and that they may present outside of most-common or typical age range. Identifying non-neurological findings may help suspecting a specific diagnosis (Table 19.1). For an example, adrenal insufficiency is seen in X-linked adrenoleukodystrophy/adrenomyeloneuropathy and peroxisomal biogenesis disorders. Dental abnormalities such as hypodontia and oligodontia is seen in 4H leukodystrophy. Tendinous xanthomas is a sign of cerebrotendinous xanthomatosis.

Table 19.1 Examples of common leukodystrophies

	Gene Enzyme	Clinical features and other consideration
Metachromatic leukodystrophy	ARSA	Presentation ranges from late infantile to adult. Arylsulfatase A
Krabbe's disease	GALC	Patients with younger age of onset tend to do worse.
X-linked	ABCD1	Galactocerebrosidase
Adrenoleukodystrophy	ASPA	Adrenal dysfunction. Adult onset cases with myelopathy
Canavan's disease	GFAP	Infantile onset. Macrocephaly, irritability, hypotonia, nystagmus,
Alexander's disease		Macrocephaly, seizures, nystagmus, recurrent emesis

19.14.3 Diagnostic Evaluation

Brain MRI is the most crucial test in patients suspected of leukodystrophy and genetic leukoencephalopathies. Using a "pattern recognition" approach, it may be possible to determine a differential diagnosis [150] with MRI alone. In these cases, diagnosis can be confirmed by biochemical and single gene testing. Examples of biochemical testing include very long chain fatty acids for X-linked adrenoleukodystrophy/adrenomyeloneuropathy and peroxisomal biogenesis disorders. Lysosomal enzymes should be sent for suspected metachromatic leukodystrophy, Krabbe, and other lysosomal disorders (galactocerebrosidase for Krabbe). Diagnosis in these straightforward cases can be achieved in weeks.

However, when there is no definitive MRI pattern, diagnostic journey can take years. When there is no definite MRI pattern, gene panels, whole exome sequencing, or whole genome sequencing is the next step. Although the improved pattern recognition on MRI and the expansion of genetic testing have improved the diagnostic yield, at least 30–40% of primary leukodystrophies and genetic leukoencephalopathies, and 50% of hypomyelinating cases remain unresolved [150]. When diagnosis cannot be achieved, it is recommended to discuss an option to participate in research programs [154].

19.14.4 Treatment

Though there are no specific treatments for most leukodystrophies, there are a few treatable leukodystrophies. Bone marrow transplantation is used for pre-symptomatic and early stages of adrenoleukodystrophy, Krabbe disease, and metachromatic leukodystrophy. Cerebrotendinous xanthomatosis can be treated with both chenodeoxycholic acid and inhibitors of HMG-CoA reductase [155]. Gene therapies using viral vectors are investigated for X-linked adrenoleukodystrophy and metachromatic leukodystrophy [156].

Preventive and symptomatic care is important for health maintenance and quality of life. Patients are often faced with multiple medical issues such as respiratory, feeding, and muscle skeletal/skin problems. There is a consensus statement from Global Leukodystrophy Initiative (GLIA) Consortium [156], addressing multiple aspects of care.

19.15 Treatment 2: Pediatric Brain Tumors

Mariko Sato, Jeremy D. Greenlee, and John M. Buatti

19.15.1 Neurosurgery

Neurosurgery is the first and oftentimes most important intervention for the majority of children with brain tumors. The primary goal of surgery is to provide tissue to establish the histological diagnosis and therefore guide treatment. With recent advances in understanding tumor biology, tissue can now be tested for genomics that may facilitate directed and potentially patient-specific adjuvant therapies. Additional goals of surgery can include tumor debulking for relief of mass effect and related symptoms such as neurological deficits and cytoreduction to reduce tumor burden.

Surgical tissue sampling can be performed using several methods, and technological advances have added options to the armamentarium of surgeons. Image-guided (e.g., frameless stereotaxic) surgery provides millimetric accuracy that is helpful for small lesions. Real-time intraoperative imaging (e.g., ultrasound, CT, MRI) allow for confirmation and refinement of localization when necessary. The improvement of neurosurgical techniques now allow for the safe upfront biopsy of tumors not commonly biopsied in the past. For example, sampling of diffuse intrinsic pontine glioma has led to an evolving understanding of the biology and genomics of this tumor [157] although it is commonly diagnosed by imaging alone. Similarly, for certain deep-seated tumors, the risks imposed by a conventional surgical approach to them may be high, and for establishing a histological diagnosis, stereotactic biopsy techniques provide a reasonable alternative to open tumor debulking. CT- or MRI-guided stereotactic procedures are highly accurate in targeting deep-seated lesions and are associated with a morbidity of less than 5% and a mortality of less than 1% of patients [158, 159].

Tumor debulking is indicated when meaningful (based on tumor natural history and response to treatment) and/or to relieve neurological deficits. Benefits of maximal tumor resection must be weighed against potential surgery-induced neurological deficit. Truly complete tumor resection is feasible only for well-circumscribed benign tumors, such as pilocytic astrocytoma, ependymoma, oligodendroglioma, dysembryoplastic neuroepithelial tumor, and craniopharyngioma. In those patients who have high-grade tumors of any location, maximum tumor resection and adjuvant therapy are required, based on the high rate of mortality from the underlying tumor. In children who have deep-seated tumors (e.g., thalamic, basal ganglia, pineal, tectal, brain stem tumors), a biopsy is often the sufficient to achieve a diagnosis but in some cases resection surgery can be safely performed.

In cases of posterior fossa tumor (e.g., medulloblastoma, pilocytic astrocytoma, or ependymoma), complete macroscopic resection correlates with improved overall survival. Posterior fossa syndrome (PFS)/cerebellar mutism (CM) [160], defined as a constellation of mutism, hypotonia, and irritability, can occur in up to 25% of children with posterior fossa tumors, most notably, medulloblastoma. These symptoms occur at the immediate postoperative period and they can be completely or partially reversible over weeks to months. The pathogenesis of PFS/CM is unknown; however there are several proposed theories such as involvement of the vermis, brain stem, dentate, or transient impairment of the dentatothalamocortical pathways.

There are notable cases that surgery can be avoided to make diagnosis. In the case of CNS germinoma, the diagnosis can be made on the basis of elevation of serum or cerebrospinal fluid tumor markers (alpha-fetoprotein and beta-human chorionic gonadotropin) alone. Optic pathway glioma or low-grade glioma in children with neurofibromatosis type 1 can be treated without surgery. Diagnosis of diffuse intrinsic pontine glioma can be made sufficiently with imaging features, yet there has been a growing interest in performing biopsies at diagnosis following published data by Roujeau et al. [161].

19.15.2 Radiation Therapy

Radiation therapy is a mainstay of both curative and palliative treatment for pediatric brain tumors. The goal of radiation therapy is to deliver a prescribed tumoricidal dose of radiation to carefully identified gross target volumes while sparing normal tissues both through technical means and radiobiological factors such as fractionation. By combining advances in imaging with improved technology of radiation therapy delivery, pediatric brain tumors can now be treated with unprecedented precision. Despite this improvement, adverse effects of irradiation in the developing brain have also been increasingly well defined and quantified in the past 30 years. Due to these known sequelae and increasing recognition of pediatric brain tumor responsiveness to chemotherapy with acceptable toxicity, the current paradigm of delaying or avoiding irradiation in children at young age has become more common.

External beam radiation therapy (EBRT), using photon beams generated from a linear accelerator is the standard for radiation therapy delivery. Prior to treatment, a child receiving therapy will have detailed volumetric imaging in a well-defined and reproducible position for the definition of both the treatment targets and normal structures to be avoided. In addition, all dose calculations use the information to precisely calculate the dose that will be delivered. Smaller children may require anesthesia to assure stability and reproducibility. Once imaging is obtained, a plan is developed using the three-dimensional information. This most often involves placing numerous fields both in coplanar and non-coplanar configurations that define 3D-RT. These are often further modulated within the fields of delivery using multi-leaf collimators that selectively shape the dose using intensity modulated radiation therapy (IMRT).These techniques have revolutionized therapy and improved both target coverage and hence tumor control as well as reduced dose to normal tissue and hence decreased toxicities [162]. Most commonly, 3D-CRT and IMRT are delivered in fractions of 1.5–2.0 Gy/day for curative treatments. Palliative treatments often involve larger treatment fractions. Radiosurgery is a special application used for both palliative and curative treatments that employs high single-dose fractions. The time for a daily treatment is generally about 15 minutes.

A technique that is increasingly of keen interest is proton beam therapy. This requires a significantly larger and more expensive device to generate charged particles that have a dose deposition defined by the energy of the accelerated particles that then deposit the dose over a small range of depth and then stop. This enables sparing of tissues distant to the entering beam with lesser dose delivered proximally and the majority of dose delivered to the defined target structure. Protons have been used in cancer treatment since 1954 although the technology has been rapidly evolving to improve the uncertainties and quality of delivery. The potential of reduced mean dose to the normal tissues with application of protons is particularly appealing in children with cancers [162]. As of February of 2019, the number of currently operating proton therapy facilities worldwide is 92 [163]. In principle, proton therapy offers a substantial clinical advantage over the conventional photon therapy although full realization of this potential continues to evolve. Reduced incidence of severe late toxicities that include endocrine, neurological, IQ and QoL deficits has also reported with the use of proton therapy [164] although direct comparisons with modern advanced technology photon therapy is lacking. It is clear that the mean dose to normal tissues can be reduced with protons, hence making application to younger children with larger treatment targets such as craniospinal axis irradiation ideal candidates for this treatment. Both availability and expense currently limit broad use in all cases. The extensive follow-up of proton patient will still be required to determine incidences of late-onset toxicities and secondary malignancies [164].

It is essential for the use of craniospinal irradiation in order to cure certain brain tumors. The techniques and technologies for delivery have rapidly and continually evolved and improved both the tumor control and toxicity-related outcomes for children. Long-term consequences of cranial radiotherapy are related to both the dose and the volume of tissue treated and must always be considered and weighed against alternative approaches. These consequences include neuropsychological effects, endocrinopathies, and second malignancies but avoidance of radiotherapy has led to impaired disease control outcomes [165]. Acute side effect of radiation includes nausea, vomiting, fatigue, skin irritation, and hair loss. These generally occur during the course of radiation. Subacute reaction occurs weeks to a few months after radiation treatment. Common subacute effects include more prolonged nausea, vomiting, fatigue, somnolent syndrome (unexplained severe fatigue with excessive sleep generally with larger volume brain treatment), and Lehrmitte's syndrome (electroshock sensation down the spine on head flexion after craniospinal irradiation). Late effects occur beyond 6–12 months and may be permanent. Late effects include radiation necrosis, leukoencephalopathy, secondary neoplasms, endocrinopathies, and neurocognitive deficits.

19.15.3 Chemotherapy

The role of chemotherapy in the treatment of childhood brain tumors has become increasingly important over the past several decades particularly for some of the embryonal tumors in young children and low-grade gliomas.

Due to neurocognitive toxicity of radiation therapy for young children with unresectable low-grade glioma, systemic chemotherapy has been investigated as a first-line therapy or an adjuvant therapy since 1970s. Due to low mitotic activity of low-grade gliomas, the response rate varies as 13–70% [166], and event-free survival, defined as the need to consider another intervention to control tumor progression, has been consistently less than 50% at 5 years with several regimens. Prolonged stable disease with acceptable toxicities has been considered a "response" by most of investigators in cases of low-grade glioma. Though there is no standard first-line treatment, most of physicians use carboplatin and vincristine as a first line chemotherapy regimen based on Children's Oncology Group study [167]. Low-grade gliomas are thought to be a chronic condition for which several regimens of treatment may be required [168].

Systemic chemotherapy is also used as an adjuvant therapy of surgery plus radiation therapy for malignant brain tumors. Children with Medulloblastoma, the most common malignant brain tumor, are successfully treated with maximal surgical resection followed by radiation therapy with adjuvant chemotherapy as a radiation enhancer, followed by maintenance systemic chemotherapy. In 1983, a study was begun adding cisplatin to CCNU and vincristine chemotherapy regimen found to be of benefit in prospective randomized adjuvant chemotherapy trial and 5-year overall survival of 85% [169] was achieved. This chemotherapy regimen is now used as a backbone of current medulloblastoma study. Challenge lies that over 80% survival rate has not achieved without significant short-term and long-term toxicities, such as ototoxicity from Cisplatin, neurotoxicity from Vincristine in addition to neurocognitive, endocrine toxicities and secondary malignant neoplasms from craniospi-nal radiation therapy. Recently updated World Health Organization (WHO) classification of Tumors of the Central Nervous System, medulloblastoma consists of four molecularly distinct disease subgroups, which include WNT, SHH, Group 3 and Group 4 medulloblastoma. Among these subgroups, WNT-subgroup medulloblastoma accounts for approximately 10% of medulloblastoma patients, generally occurs in older patients (median age 10 years), is rarely metastatic and is associated with excellent survival using contemporary therapy, with a 5-year event-free survival of over 90% [170–172]. Recent cooperative clinical trial is investigating if children with WNT subgroup medulloblastoma can be cured with reduced dose of chemotherapy and radiation therapy.

High-dose systemic chemotherapy: tumor of the CNS may fail to respond to standard-dose chemotherapy as a result of inherent or acquired drug resistance or because of limited and/or heterogeneous drug exposure in the tumor tissue. In an attempt to overpower these resistance mechanisms and maximize the therapeutic potential for agents with a steep-dose response curve, the use of high-dose chemotherapy with autologous bone marrow or peripheral blood stem cell rescue has been explored by a number of investigators. High-dose systemic chemotherapy approaches in children with CNS tumors have been most widely evaluated in infants, for whom postponement of radiation therapy is desirable because of its potential late neurologic toxicities, and in patients with recurrent tumors. Feasibility has been clearly demonstrated and encouraging results have been seen in patients with medulloblastoma, atypical teratoid rhabdoid tumors, and germ cell tumors. High-dose chemotherapy experience in children with gliomas, including those of the brainstem, has been less promising.

The blood brain barriers (BBB) and blood-CSF barrier and blood-tumor barrier are important variable that may restrict the delivery of systemically administered chemotherapy to tumor tissue. In order to circumvent the limited penetration of most systemically administered agents across the blood-brain and blood-CSF barriers, regional therapy, such as intrathecal or intratumoral chemotherapy is developed and currently investigated in clinical trials.

19.15.4 Progress in Targeted Therapy and Immunotherapy

Clinical trials targeting molecular pathway are increasing in number to treat pediatric brain tumor patients. The molecular dissection of all oncology today has revealed significant insight into pathways that appear to play important roles in tumorigenesis.

The RAS/RAF/MEK/ERK pathway has been a particular focus in children with brain tumors as a result of our knowledge of neurofibromatosis type I (NF1), a disorder associated with a defect in RAS activation in which 15–20% of patients will develop a pediatric low-grade glioma [173], and tuberous sclerosis complex (TSC), in which subependymal giant cell astrocytomas (SEGAs) are common brain tumors. The recent discovery that the majority of sporadic pediatric low-grade gliomas have defects in BRAF has focused our efforts on understanding the biology related to this target [174]. BRAF is a major component of the RAS/ RAF/MEK/MAPK signaling pathway that functions to transmit extracellular signals from the cytoplasmic membrane to the nucleus. Cross-talk between this pathway and other important cellular signaling cascades, such as PI3K/AKT/mTOR, has been the focus of extensive research and had led to a detailed understanding of BRAF's role in cellular proliferation, differentiation, migration, and angiogenesis [175]. Various alterations in BRAF are associated with a number of pediatric tumors including brain tumors (low-grade, high-grade, ganglioglioma, pleomorphic xanthoastrocytoma, and craniopharyngiomas), Langerhans cell histiocytosis, and melanoma. Many tumors have a single nucleotide substitution that constitutively activates BRAF as a monomer; thus, these mutations are potential targets for BRAF inhibitors. Some pediatric low-grade gliomas have truncated fusion mutations of BRAF, which can be treated with combination of BRAF inhibitors and MEK inhibitors. Several case reports of successfully treated brain tumors with BRAF targeted therapy were published [174, 176–178] and well-designed clinical trials with Clinical Laboratory Improvement Amendments (CLIA)-certified confirmation of the BRAF mutation for eligibility are underway (Table 19.2).

Table 19.2 Current open clinical trials targeting BRAF alteration of pediatric brain tumor, as of July 2019

Identifier	Title of study
NCT01748149	Vemurafenib in Children With Recurrent/Refractory BRAF Gene V600E (BRAFV600E)-Mutant Gliomas
NCT02684058	Phase II Pediatric Study With Dabrafenib in Combination With Trametinib in Patients With HGG and LGG
NCT01677741	A Study to Determine Safety, Tolerability and Pharmacokinetics of Oral Dabrafenib In Children and Adolescent Subjects
NCT03698994	Ulixertinib in Treating Patients With Advanced Solid Tumors, Non-Hodgkin Lymphoma, or Histiocytic Disorders With MAPK Pathway Mutations (A Pediatric MATCH Treatment Trial)
NCT03213691	Selumetinib Sulfate in Treating Patients With Relapsed or Refractory Advanced Solid Tumors, Non-Hodgkin Lymphoma, or Histiocytic Disorders With Activating MAPK Pathway Mutations (A Pediatric MATCH Treatment Trial)
NCT03363217	Trametinib for Pediatric Neuro-oncology Patients With Refractory Tumor and Activation of the MAPK/ERK Pathway.

References

1. Rowley HA, Grant PE, Roberts TP (1999) Diffusion MR imaging. Theory and applications. Neuroimaging Clin N Am 9:343–361
2. Neil JJ et al (1998) Normal brain in human newborns: apparent diffusion coefficient and diffusion anisotropy measured by using diffusion tensor MR imaging. Radiology 209:57–66
3. Wimberger DM et al (1995) Identification of "pre-myelination" bydiffusion-weighted MRI. J Comput Assist Tomogr 19:28–33
4. Tanner SF et al (2000) Quantitative comparison of intrabrain diffusion in adults and preterm and

term neonates and infants. AJR Am J Roentgenol 174:1643–1649

5. Morriss MC et al (1999) Changes in brain water diffusion during childhood. Neuroradiology 41:929–934

6. Watanabe M et al (2013) Age-related apparent diffusion coefficient changes in the normal brain. Radiology 266:575–582

7. Kingsley PB, Monahan WG (2004) Selection of the optimum B factor for diffusion-weighted magnetic resonance imaging assessment of ischemic stroke. Magn Reson Med 51:996–1001

8. Prayer D et al (2001) Visualization of nonstructural changes in early white matter development on diffusion-weighted MR images: evidence supporting premyelination anisotropy. AJNR Am J Neuroradiol 22:1572–1576

9. Bui T et al (2006) Microstructural development of human brain assessed in utero by diffusion tensor imaging. Pediatr Radiol 36(11):1133–1140

10. Arzoumanian Y et al (2003) Diffusion tensor brain imaging findings at term-equivalent age may predict neurologic abnormalities in low birth weight preterm infants. AJNR Am J Neuroradiol 24:1646–1653

11. Forbes KPN, Pipe JG, Bird CR (2002) Changes in brain water diffusion during the 1st year of life. Radiology 222:405–409

12. McGraw P, Liang L, Provenzale JM (2002) Evaluation of normal age-related changes in anisotropy during infancy and childhood as shown by diffusion tensor imaging. AJR Am J Roentgenol 179:1515–1522

13. Hermoye L et al (2006) Pediatric diffusion tensor imaging: Normal database and observation of the white matter maturation in early childhood. NeuroImage 29:493–504

14. Boujraf S et al (2002) Study of pediatric brain development using magnetic resonance imaging of anisotropic diffusion. Magn Reson Imaging 20:327–336

15. Evans AC (2006) The NIH MRI study of normal brain development. NeuroImage 30:184–202

16. Filippi CG et al (2003) Diffusion-tensor MR imaging in children with developmental delay: preliminary findings. Radiology 229:44–50

17. Yamada I et al (1999) Moyamoya disease: evaluation with diffusion-weighted and perfusion echo-planar MR imaging. Radiology 212:340–347

18. Moran CJ, Siegel MJ, DeBaun MR (1998) Sickle cell disease: imaging of cerebrovascular complications. Radiology 206:311–321

19. Moritani T et al (2004) Sickle cell cerebrovascular disease: usual and unusual findings on MR imaging and MR angiography. Clin Imaging 204:173–186

20. Mirsky DM et al (2017) Pathways for neuroimaging of childhood stroke. Pediatr Neurol 69:11–23

21. Gibbs WN, Opatowsky MJ, Burton EC (2012) AIRP best cases in radiologic-pathologic correlation: cerebral fat embolism syndrome in sickle cell beta-thalassemia. Radiographics 32(5):1301–1306

22. Porto L et al (2006) Accelerated myelination associated with venous congestion. Eur Radiol 16(4):922–926

23. Meyers P, Halbach V, Barkovich AJ. (2011) Chapter 12: Anomalies of cerebral vasculature: diagnostic and endovascular considerations. In: Barkovich, A. J., Raybaud, C. Pediatric neuroimaging, 5th edition. Welters Kluwer Health, Philadelphia, pp. 1057–1067

24. Phillips MD, Zimmerman RA (1999) Diffusion imaging in pediatric hypoxic ischemia injury. Neuroimaging Clin N Am 9:41–52

25. Robertson RL et al (1999) MR line-scan diffusion-weighted imaging of term neonates with perinatal brain ischemia. AJNR Am J Neuroradiol 20:1658–1670

26. Johnson AJ, Lee BC, Lin W (1999) Echoplanar diffusion-weighted imaging in neonates and infants with suspected hypoxic-ischemic injury: correlation with patient outcome. AJR Am J Roentgenol 172:219–226

27. Forbes KP, Pipe JG, Bird R (2000) Neonatal hypoxic-ischemic encephalopathy: detection with diffusion-weighted MR imaging. AJNR Am J Neuroradiol 21:1490–1496

28. Wolf RL et al (2001) Quantitative apparent diffusion coefficient measurements in term neonates for early detection of hypoxic-ischemic brain injury: initial experience. Radiology 218:825–833

29. Rutherford M et al (2004) Diffusion-weighted magnetic resonance imaging in term perinatal brain injury: a comparison with site of lesion and time from birth. Pediatrics 114(4):1004–1014

30. Ghei SK et al (2014) MR imaging of hypoxic-ischemic injury in term neonates: pearls and pitfalls. Radiographics 34:1047–1061

31. Moritani T et al (2005) Diffusion-weighted imaging of acute excitotoxic brain injury. AJNR Am J Neuroradiol 26:216–228

32. Rumpel H et al (1997) Late glial swelling after acute cerebral hypoxia-ischemia in the neonatal rat: a combined magnetic resonance and histochemical study. Pediatr Res 42:54–59

33. Malik G et al (2006) Serial quantitative diffusion tensor MRI of the term neonates with hypoxic-ischemic encephalopathy (HIE). Neuropediatrics 37:337–343

34. Bathla G, Policeni B, Agarwal A (2014) Neuroimaging in patients with abnormal blood glucose levels. AJNR Am J Neuroradiol 35(5):833–840

35. Wong DS et al (2013) Brain injury patterns in hypoglycemia in neonatal encephalopathy. AJNR Am J Neuroradiol 34(7):1456–1461

36. Tam EW et al (2008) Occipital lobe injury and cortical visual outcomes after neonatal hypoglycemia. Pediatrics 122(3):507–512

37. Wittschieber D et al (2015) Subdural hygromas in abusive head trauma: pathogenesis, diagnosis, and forensic implications. AJNR Am J Neuroradiol 36(3):432–439

38. Chen CY, Zimmerman RA, Rorke LB (1999) Neuroimaging in child abuse: a mechanism-based approach. Neuroradiology 41:711–722

39. Bullock R et al (1991) Correlation of the extracellular glutamate concentration with extent of blood

flow reduction after subdural hematoma in the rat. J Neurosurg 74:794–802

40. Johnson DL, Boal D, Baule R (1995) Role of apnea in nonaccidental head injury. Pediatr Neurosurg 23:305–310

41. Geddes JF et al (2001) Neuropathology of inflicted head injury in children. I. Patterns of brain damage. Brain J Neurol 124:1290–1298

42. Suh DY et al (2001) Nonaccidental pediatric head injury: diffusion-weighted imaging findings. Neurosurgery 49:309–318; discussion 318–20

43. Holshouser BA et al (1997) Proton MR spectroscopy after acute central nervous system injury: outcome prediction in neonates, infants, and children. Radiology 202(2):487–496

44. Duhaime AC, Gennarelli LM, Boardman C (1996) Neuroprotection by dextromethorphan in acute experimental subdural hematoma in the rat. J Neurotrauma 13:79–84

45. Ikonomidou C et al (1996) Prevention of trauma-induced neurodegeneration in infant rat brain. Pediatr Res 39:1020–1027

46. Smith SL, Hall ED (1998) Tirilazad widens the therapeutic window for riluzole-induced attenuation of progressive cortical degeneration in an infant rat model of the shaken baby syndrome. J Neurotrauma 15:707–719

47. Duhaime AC, Durham S (2007) Traumatic brain injury in infants: the phenomenon of subdural hemorrhage with hemispheric hypodensity ("Big Black Brain"). Prog Brain Res 161:293–302

48. Barzó P et al (1997) Contribution of vasogenic and cellular edema to traumatic brain swelling measured by diffusion-weighted imaging. J Neurosurg 87:900–907

49. Liu AY et al (1999) Traumatic brain injury: diffusion-weighted MR imaging findings. AJNR Am J Neuroradiol 20:1636–1641

50. Tsuchiya K et al (1999) Diffusion-weighted MR imaging of encephalitis. AJR Am J Roentgenol 173:1097–1099

51. Hoftberger R et al (2013) Clinical neuropathology practice guide 4-2013: post-herpes simplex encephalitis: N-methyl-Daspartate receptor antibodies are part of the problem. Clin Neuropathol 32(4): 251–254

52. Ebisu T et al (1996) Discrimination of brain abscess from necrotic or cystic tumors by diffusion-weighted echo planar imaging. Magn Reson Imaging 14:1113–1116

53. Huang CC et al (1998) Central nervous system candidiasis in very low-birth-weight premature neonates and infants: US characteristics and histopathologic and MR imaging correlates in five patients. Radiology 209:49–56

54. Messacar K et al (2016) Acute flaccid myelitis: a clinical review of US cases 2012–2015. Ann Neurol 80(3):326–338

55. Maloney JA et al (2015) MRI findings in children with acute flaccid paralysis and cranial nerve dysfunction occurring during the 2014 enterovirus D68 outbreak. AJNR Am J Neuroradiol 36(2):245–250

56. Kotsenas AL et al (1999) Abnormal diffusion-weighted MRI in medulloblastoma: does it reflect small cell histology? Pediatr Radiol 29:524–526

57. Johnson DR et al (2017) 2016 updates to the WHO brain tumor classification system: what the radiologist needs to know. Radiographics 37:2164–2180

58. AlRayahi J et al (2018) Pediatric brain tumor genetics: what radiologists need to know. Radiographics 38:2102–2122

59. Klisch J et al (2000) Supratentorial primitive neuroectodermal tumours: diffusion-weighted MRI. Neuroradiology 42:393–398

60. Tien RD et al (1994) MR imaging of high-grade cerebral gliomas: value of diffusion-weighted echo-planar pulse sequences. AJR Am J Roentgenol 162: 671–677

61. Guo AC et al (2002) Lymphomas and high-grade astrocytomas: comparison of water diffusibility and histologic characteristics. Radiology 224:177–183

62. Koral K et al (2008) Imaging characteristics of atypical teratoid–rhabdoid tumor in children compared with medulloblastoma. AJR Am J Roentgenol 190:809–814

63. Kan P et al (2006) The role of diffusion-weighted magnetic resonance imaging in pediatric brain tumors. Childs Nerv Syst 22:1435–1439

64. Rumboldt Z et al (2006) Apparent diffusion coefficients for differentiation of cerebellar tumors in children. AJNR Am J Neuroradiol 27:1362–1369

65. Meyers SP et al (2006) Primary intracranial atypical teratoid/rhabdoid tumors of infancy and childhood: MRI features and patient outcomes. AJNR Am J Neuroradiol 27:962–971

66. Cunningham DA et al (2016) Neuroradiologic characteristics of astroblastoma and systematic review of the literature: 2 new cases and 125 cases reported in 59 publications. Pediatr Radiol 46(9):1301–1308

67. Shin JH et al (2002) Neuronal tumors of the central nervous system: radiologic findings and pathologic correlation. Radiographics 22(5):1177–1189

68. Ni HC et al (2015) Angiocentric glioma: a report of nine new cases, including four with atypical histological features. Neuropathol Appl Neurobiol 41(3):333–346

69. Meyers SP et al (2004) Choroid plexus carcinomas in children: MRI features and patient outcomes. Neuroradiology 46(9):770–780

70. Smith AB, Smirniotopoulos JG, Horkanyne-Szakaly I (2013) From the radiologic pathology archives: intraventricular neoplasms: radiologic-pathologic correlation. Radiographics 33(1):21–43

71. Gardiman MP et al (2010) Diffuse leptomeningeal glioneuronal tumors: a new entity? Brain Pathol 20(2):361–366

72. Louis DN et al (2016) The 2016 World Health Organization classification of tumors of the central nervous system: a summary. Acta Neuropathol 131(6):803–820

73. Cooney MJ et al (2000) Hypertensive encephalopathy: complication in children treated for myeloproliferative disorders—report of three cases. Radiology 214:711–716

74. Schwartz RB et al (1998) Diffusion-weighted MR imaging in hypertensive encephalopathy: clues to pathogenesis. AJNR Am J Neuroradiol 19:859–862

75. Yagishita A et al (1995) Acute encephalopathy with bilateral thalamotegmental involvement in infants and children: imaging and pathology findings. AJNR Am J Neuroradiol 16:439–447

76. Albayram S et al (2004) Diffusion-weighted MR imaging findings of acute necrotizing encephalopathy. AJNR Am J Neuroradiol 25:792–797

77. Mikaeloff Y et al (2004) MRI prognostic factors for relapse after acute CNS inflammatory demyelination in childhood. Brain 127:1942–1947

78. Dale RC et al (2000) Acute disseminated encephalomyelitis, multiphasic disseminated encephalomyelitis and multiple sclerosis in children. Brain 123:2407–2422

79. Balasubramanya KS et al (2007) Diffusion-weighted imaging and proton MR spectroscopy in the characterization of acute disseminated encephalomyelitis. Neuroradiology 49:177–183

80. Barkovich AJ, Patay Z (2011) Chapter 3: metabolic, toxic, and inflammatory brain disorders in: barkovich, A. J., Raybaud, C. Pediatric neuroimaging, 5th edition. Welters Kluwer Health, Philadelphia, pp. 133–136

81. Rovira A et al (2002) Serial diffusion-weighted MR imaging and proton MR spectroscopy of acute large demyelinating brain lesions: case report. AJNR Am J Neuroradiol 23:989–994

82. Ramchandren S (2017) Charcot-Marie-Tooth disease and other genetic polyneuropathies. Continuum (Minneap Minn) 23(5, Peripheral Nerve and Motor Neuron Disorders):1360–1377

83. Al-Mateen M, Craig AK, Chance PF (2014) The central nervous system phenotype of X-linked Charcot-Marie-tooth disease: a transient disorder of children and young adults. J Child Neurol 29(3):342–348

84. Yoshida S et al (2009) Symmetrical central tegmental tract (CTT) hyperintense lesions on magnetic resonance imaging in children. Eur Radiol 19(2):462–469

85. Aguilera-Albesa S et al (2012) T2 hyperintense signal of the central tegmental tracts in children: disease or normal maturational process? Neuroradiology 54(8):863–871

86. Singh P et al (2015) Symmetrical central tegmental tract hyperintensities on magnetic resonance imaging. J Pediatr Neurosci 10(3):235–236

87. Decramer T et al (2015) Wallerian degeneration of the superior cerebellar peduncle. JAMA Neurol 72(10):1206–1208

88. Horton M, Rafay M, Del Bigio MR (2009) Pathological evidence of vacuolar myelinopathy in a child following vigabatrin administration. J Child Neurol 24(12):1543–1546

89. Pearl PL et al (2018) White matter spongiosis with vigabatrin therapy for infantile spasms. Epilepsia 59(4):e40–e44

90. Ben-Ari Y (2006) Basic developmental rules and their implications for epilepsy in the immature brain. Epileptic Disord 8(2):91–102

91. Pearl PL et al (2009) Cerebral MRI abnormalities associated with vigabatrin therapy. Epilepsia 50(2):184–194

92. Kim SS et al (1999) Focal lesion in the splenium of the corpus callosum in epileptic patients: antiepileptic drug toxicity? AJNR Am J Neuroradiol 20(1):125–129

93. Cohen JA et al (2000) The potential for vigabatrin-induced intramyelinic edema in humans. Epilepsia 41(2):148–157

94. Vanderver A, Tonduti D, Schiffmann R, et al. (2014) Leukodystrophy Overview. In: Adam MP, Ardinger HH, Pagon RA, et al., editors. GeneReviews® [Internet]. Seattle (WA): University of Washington, Seattle; 1993–2020. Available from: https://www.ncbi.nlm.nih.gov/books/NBK184570/

95. Ono J et al (1997) Differentiation of dys- and demyelination using diffusional anisotropy. Pediatr Neurol 16:63–66

96. Sener RN (2002) Metachromatic leukodystrophy: diffusion MR imaging findings. AJNR Am J Neuroradiol 23:1424–1426

97. Patay Z (2005) Diffusion-weighted MR imaging in leukodystrophies. Eur Radiol 15:2284–2303

98. Guo AC et al (2001) Evaluation of white matter anisotropy in Krabbe disease with diffusion tensor MR imaging: initial experience. Radiology 218:809–815

99. Suzuki K, Suzuki K (2002) Lysosomal diseases. In: Lantos P, Graham DI (eds) Greenfield's neuropathology. Arnold, London; New York; New Delhi, pp 684–685

100. Takanashi J, Barkovich AJ, Cheng SF, Weisiger K, Zlatunich CO, Mudge C, Rosenthal P, Tuchman M, Packman S. (2003) Brain MR imaging in neonatal hyperammonemic encephalopathy resulting from proximal urea cycle disorders. AJNR Am J Neuroradiol. 24(6):1184–7. PMID: 12812952.

101. Morse RP et al (2005) Novel form of intermediate salla disease: clinical and neuroimaging features. J Child Neurol 20(10):814–816

102. Eichler FS et al (2002) Proton MR spectroscopic and diffusion tensor brain MR imaging in X-linked adrenoleukodystrophy: initial experience. Radiology 225:245–252

103. Chinnery PF, Lax NZ, Jaros E, Taylor RW, Turnbull DM, DiMauro S. (2015) Mitochondrial disorders. In: Love, S, Perry, A, Ironside, J, Budka, H (eds), Greenfields neuropathology, vol. I, London: CRC Press, pp 523–555

104. Ellison D et al (1998) Toxic injury of the CNS. In: Neuropathology. Mosby Ltd, London, p 25

105. Lerman-Sagie T et al (2005) White matter involvement in mitochondrial diseases. Mol Genet Metab 84:127–136
106. Ito H et al (2008) Serial brain imaging analysis of stroke-like episodes in MELAS. Brain Dev 30:483–488
107. Oppenheim C et al (2000) Can diffusion weighted magnetic resonance imaging help differentiate stroke from stroke-like events in MELAS? J Neurol Neurosurg Psychiatry 69:248–250
108. Yoneda M et al (1999) Vasogenic edema on MELAS: a serial study with diffusion-weighted MR imaging. Neurology 53:2182–2184
109. Yonemura K et al (2001) Diffusion-weighted MR imaging in a case of mitochondrial myopathy, encephalopathy, lactic acidosis, and strokelike episodes. AJNR Am J Neuroradiol 22:269–272
110. Sacher M et al (2005) MRI findings in an atypical case of Kearns-Sayre syndrome: a case report. Neuroradiology 47:241–244
111. Sakai Y et al (2006) Persistent diffusion abnormalities in the brain stem of three children with mitochondrial diseases. AJNR Am J Neuroradiol 27(9):1924–1926
112. Wang XY et al (2003) Serial diffusion-weighted imaging in a patient with MELAS and presumed cytotoxic oedema. Neuroradiology 45:640–643
113. Kim JH et al (2011) Diffusion and perfusion characteristics of MELAS (mitochondrial myopathy, encephalopathy, lactic acidosis, and stroke-like episode) in thirteen patients. Korean J Radiol 12(1):15–24
114. Invernizzi F et al (2014) Cavitating leukoencephalopathy with multiple mitochondrial dysfunction syndrome and NFU1 mutations. Front Genet 5:412
115. Wu J et al (2018) Case 250: Alpers-Huttenlocher syndrome. Radiology 286(2):720–725
116. Saneto RP, Friedman SD, Shaw DW (2008) Neuroimaging of mitochondrial disease. Mitochondrion 8(5–6):396–413
117. Twomey EL et al (2003) Neuroimaging findings in glutaric aciduria type 1. Pediatr Radiol 33(12):823–830
118. Starkey J et al (2017) Cytotoxic lesions of the corpus callosum that show restricted diffusion: mechanisms, causes, and manifestations. Radiographics 37(2):562–576
119. Cheon JE et al (2002) Leukodystrophy in children: a pictorial review of MR imaging features. Radiographics 22(3):461–476
120. Kono K et al (2005) Diffusion-weighted MR imaging in patients with phenylketonuria: relationship between serum phenylalanine levels and ADC values in cerebral white matter. Radiology 236:630–636
121. Sakai M et al (2005) Age dependence of diffusion-weighted magnetic resonance imaging findings in maple syrup urine disease encephalopathy. J Comput Assist Tomogr 29:524–527

122. Srikanth SG et al (2007) Restricted diffusion in Canavan disease. Child's Nerv Syst: ChNS: Official Journal of the International Society for Pediatric Neurosurgery 23:465–468
123. Sener RN (2003) Canavan disease: diffusion magnetic resonance imaging findings. J Comput Assist Tomogr 27:30–33
124. Janson CG et al (2006) Natural history of Canavan disease revealed by proton magnetic resonance spectroscopy (1H-MRS) and diffusion-weighted MRI. Neuropediatrics 37:209–221
125. Sener RN (2003) L-2 hydroxyglutaric aciduria: proton magnetic resonance spectroscopy and diffusion magnetic resonance imaging findings. J Comput Assist Tomogr 27:38–43
126. Sener RN (2005) Tyrosinemia: computed tomography, magnetic resonance imaging, diffusion magnetic resonance imaging, and proton spectroscopy findings in the brain. J Comput Assist Tomogr 29:323–325
127. Sener RN (2004) Diffusion magnetic resonance imaging patterns in metabolic and toxic brain disorders. Acta Radiol (Stockholm, Sweden: 1987) 45:561–570
128. Au WL et al (2003) Serial diffusion-weighted magnetic resonance imaging in adult-onset citrullinaemia. J Neurol Sci 209:101–104
129. Takanashi J-I et al (2003) Brain MR imaging in acute hyperammonemic encephalopathy arising from late-onset ornithine transcarbamylase deficiency. AJNR Am J Neuroradiol 24:390–393
130. Sener RN (2003) Diffusion magnetic resonance imaging in infantile neuroaxonal dystrophy. J Comput Assist Tomogr 27:34–37
131. Cheng A et al (2017) MRI and clinical features of maple syrup urine disease: preliminary results in 10 cases. Diagn Interv Radiol 23(5):398–402
132. Parmar H, Sitoh YY, Ho L (2004) Maple syrup urine disease: diffusion-weighted and diffusion-tensor magnetic resonance imaging findings. J Comput Assist Tomogr 28(1):93–97
133. Reddy N et al (2018) Neuroimaging findings of organic acidemias and aminoacidopathies. Radiographics 38(3):912–931
134. Yoon HJ et al (2014) Devastating metabolic brain disorders of newborns and young infants. Radiographics 34(5):1257–1272
135. Barkovich AJ, Messing A (2006). Alexander disease: not just a leukodystrophy anymore. Neurology, 66(4):468–469
136. Ono J et al (1994) MR diffusion imaging in Pelizaeus-Merzbacher disease. Brain Dev 16:219–223
137. Moritani T et al (2000) Diffusion-weighted echo-planar MR imaging: clinical applications and pitfalls—a pictorial essay. Clin Imaging 24: 181–192
138. Kennedy C et al (1970) Blood flow to white matter during maturation of the brain. Neurology 20:613–618

139. Moritani T et al (2008) Abnormal hypermyelination in a neonate with Sturge-Weber syndrome demonstrated on diffusion-tensor imaging. J Magn Reson Imaging 27(3):617–620

140. Yagishita A et al (1998) Hemimegalencephaly: signal changes suggesting abnormal myelination on MRI. Neuroradiology 40:734–738

141. Agid R et al (2006) Prenatal MR diffusion-weighted imaging in a fetus with hemimegalencephaly. Pediatr Radiol 36:138–140

142. Salamon N et al (2006) Contralateral hemimicrencephaly and clinical-pathological correlations in children with hemimegalencephaly. Brain J Neurol 129:352–365

143. Sato N et al (2008) Aberrant midsagittal fiber tracts in patients with hemimegalencephaly. AJNR Am J Neuroradiol 29(4):823–827

144. Trivedi R et al (2006) Diffusion tensor imaging in polymicrogyria: a report of three cases. Neuroradiology 48:422–427

145. Lee S-K et al (2005) Diffusion-tensor MR imaging and fiber tractography: a new method of describing aberrant fiber connections in developmental CNS anomalies. Radiographics: a review publication of the Radiological Society of North America, Inc 25:53–65; discussion 66–8

146. Rollins NK (2007) Clinical applications of diffusion tensor imaging and tractography in children. Pediatr Radiol 37:769–780

147. Jansen FE et al (2003) Diffusion-weighted magnetic resonance imaging and identification of the epileptogenic tuber in patients with tuberous sclerosis. Arch Neurol 60:1580–1584

148. Makki MI et al (2007) Characteristics of abnormal diffusivity in normal-appearing white matter investigated with diffusion tensor MR imaging in tuberous sclerosis complex. AJNR Am J Neuroradiol 28:1662–1667

149. Utsunomiya H et al (2006) Arrangement of fiber tracts forming Probst bundle in complete callosal agenesis: report of two cases with an evaluation by diffusion tensor tractography. Acta Radiol (Stockholm, Sweden: 1987) 47:1063–1066

150. Vanderver A (2014) Leukodystrophy overview. In: GeneReviews® [Internet]. https://www.ncbi.nlm. nih.gov/books/NBK184570/. Accessed 21 May 2019

151. Vanderver A, Prust M, Tonduti D, Mochel F, Hussey H, Helman G, Garbern J, Eichler F, Labauge P, Aubourg P, Rodriguez D, Patterson M, Van Hove J, Schmidt J, Wolf N, Boespflug-Tanguy O, Schiffmann R, van der Knaap M (2015) Case definition and classification of leukodystrophies and leukoencephalopathies. Mol Genet Metab 114:494–500

152. Heim P, Claussen M, Hoffmann B, Conzelmann E, Gärtner J, Harzer K, Hunneman DH, Köhler W, Kurlemann G, Kohlschütter A (1997) Leukodystrophy incidence in Germany. Am J Med Genet 71:475–478

153. Bonkowsky JL, Nelson C, Kingston JL, Filloux FM, Mundorff MB, Srivastava R (2010) The burden of inherited leukodystrophies in children. Neurology 75:718–725

154. Parikh S, Bernard G, Leventer RJ et al (2015) A clinical approach to the diagnosis of patients with leukodystrophies and genetic leukoencephelopathies. Mol Genet Metab 114:501–515

155. Yahalom G, Tsabari R, Molshatzki N, Ephraty L, Cohen H, Hassin-Baer S (2013) Neurological outcome in cerebrotendinous xanthomatosis treated with chenodeoxycholic acid: early versus late diagnosis. Clin Neuropharmacol. https://www.ncbi.nlm. nih.gov/pubmed/23673909. Accessed 21 May 2019

156. van der Knaap MS, Wolf NI, Heine VM (2016) Leukodystrophies: Five new things. Neurol Clin Practice. https://www.ncbi.nlm.nih.gov/pmc/articles/PMC5964825/. Accessed 22 May 2019

157. Cohen KJ, Jabado N, Grill J (2017) Diffuse intrinsic pontine gliomas-current management and new biologic insights. Is there a glimmer of hope? Neurooncology 19(8):1025–1034

158. Broggi G, Franzini A, Migliavacca F, Allegranza A (1983) Stereotactic biopsy of deep brain tumors in infancy and childhood. Childs Brain 10(2): 92–98

159. Lunsford LD (1987) Diagnosis of mass lesions using the Leksell system. Modern stereotactic surgery. Boston MA

160. Lanier JC, Abrams AN (2017) Posterior fossa syndrome: review of the behavioral and emotional aspects in pediatric cancer patients. Cancer 123(4):551–559

161. Roujeau T, Machado G, Garnett MR et al (2007) Stereotactic biopsy of diffuse pontine lesions in children. J Neurosurg 107(1 Suppl):1–4

162. WCL D (2016) Principles and practice of radiation therapy, 4th edn. Elsevier Mosby

163. Particle Therapy Co-Operative Group (2019) Particle therapy facilities in clinical operation; February. Available from https://www.ptcog.ch/index.php/facilities-in-operation

164. Huynh M, Marcu LG, Giles E, Short M, Matthews D, Bezak E (2018) Current status of proton therapy outcome for paediatric cancers of the central nervous system—analysis of the published literature. Cancer Treat Rev 70:272–288

165. Bouffet E, Bernard JL, Frappaz D et al (1992) M4 protocol for cerebellar medulloblastoma: supratentorial radiotherapy may not be avoided. Int J Radiat Oncol Biol Phys 24(1):79–85

166. Bouffet E, Jakacki R, Goldman S et al (2012) Phase II study of weekly vinblastine in recurrent or refractory pediatric low-grade glioma. J Clin Oncol: Official Journal of the American Society of Clinical Oncology 30(12):1358–1363

167. Ater JL, Zhou T, Holmes E et al (2012) Randomized study of two chemotherapy regimens for treatment of low-grade glioma in young children: a report

from the Children's Oncology Group. J Clin Oncol: Official Journal of the American Society of Clinical Oncology. 30(21):2641–2647

168. Qaddoumi I, Sultan I, Broniscer A (2009) Pediatric low-grade gliomas and the need for new options for therapy: why and how? Cancer Biol Ther 8(1):4–10

169. Packer RJ, Sutton LN, Elterman R et al (1994) Outcome for children with medulloblastoma treated with radiation and cisplatin, CCNU, and vincristine chemotherapy. J Neurosurg 81(5):690–698

170. Ellison DW, Onilude OE, Lindsey JC et al (2005) Beta-cCatenin status predicts a favorable outcome in childhood medulloblastoma: the United Kingdom Children's Cancer Study Group Brain Tumour Committee. J Clin Oncol: Official Journal of the American Society of Clinical Oncology 23(31):7951–7957

171. Schwalbe EC, Lindsey JC, Nakjang S et al (2017) Novel molecular subgroups for clinical classification and outcome prediction in childhood medulloblastoma: a cohort study. Lancet Oncol 18(7):958–971

172. Shih DJ, Northcott PA, Remke M et al (2014) Cytogenetic prognostication within medulloblastoma subgroups. J Clin Oncol: Official Journal of the American Society of Clinical Oncology. 32(9):886–896

173. Hirbe AC, Gutmann DH (2014) Neurofibromatosis type 1: a multidisciplinary approach to care. Lancet Neurol 13(8):834–843

174. Lassaletta A, Zapotocky M, Mistry M et al (2017) Therapeutic and prognostic implications of BRAF V600E in pediatric low-grade gliomas. J Clin Oncol: Official Journal of the American Society of Clinical Oncology. 35(25):2934–2941

175. Dent P (2014) Crosstalk between ERK, AKT, and cell survival. Cancer Biol Ther 15(3):245–246

176. Skrypek M, Foreman N, Guillaume D, Moertel C (2014) Pilomyxoid astrocytoma treated successfully with vemurafenib. Pediatr Blood Cancer 61(11):2099–2100

177. Fangusaro J, Onar-Thomas A, Young Poussaint T et al (2019) Selumetinib in paediatric patients with BRAF-aberrant or neurofibromatosis type 1–associated recurrent, refractory, or progressive low-grade glioma: a multicentre, phase 2 trial. Lancet Oncol 20(7):1011–1022

178. Robinson GW, Orr BA, Gajjar A (2014) Complete clinical regression of a BRAF V600E-mutant pediatric glioblastoma multiforme after BRAF inhibitor therapy. BMC Cancer 14:258

Head and Neck

20

Jerry M. Kovoor, Jack Kademian, and Toshio Moritani

Molly Heft Neal, Andrew C. Birkeland, and Matthew E. Spector

20.1 Introduction

Head and neck pathologies pose a challenge not only in making an initial diagnosis but also in follow-up imaging for malignancies following various treatment methods to differentiate tumor and nodal recurrence from tissue response to the treatment. Among the neuroradiologic diagnostic armamentarium, MRI is increasingly used for

---

J. M. Kovoor
Department of Clinical Radiology & Imaging Sciences, Indiana University School of Medicine, Indianapolis, IN, USA
e-mail: jkovoor@iu.edu

J. Kademian
Department of Radiology, University of Iowa Hospitals & Clinics, Iowa City, IA, USA
e-mail: jack-kademian@uiowa.edu

T. Moritani (✉)
Division of Neuroradiology, University of Michigan, Ann Arbor, MI, USA
e-mail: tmoritan@med.umich.edu

M. H. Neal
Department of Otolaryngology Head and Neck Surgery, University of Michigan, Ann Arbor, MI, USA
e-mail: mheftnea@umich.edu

A. C. Birkeland
University of California, Davis, Sacramento, CA, USA
e-mail: acbirkeland@ucdavis.edu

M. E. Spector
Division of Head and Neck Surgery, University of Michigan, Ann Arbor, MI, USA
e-mail: mspector@umich.edu

finding answers to these vexing problems because of its inherent radiation-free diagnostic capabilities and multiparametric imaging tools.

In head and neck pathologies, diffusion-weighted imaging (DWI) adds complementary information to routine sequences. Its benefits can be traced to the original work of Le Bihan and Turner, who attempted to use DWI to differentiate benign from malignant pathologies. DWI measures the diffusion at the tissue cellular level and has been used as a surrogate marker for tissue cellularity. It is influenced by cell density, membrane integrity, and microstructure [1, 2]. It often uses single-shot echoplanar technique due to its short acquisition time and unlike multi-shot echoplanar sequences, uses only one repetition time to fill the k-space. However, the former suffers from greater susceptibility effects, geometric distortion, and reduced spatial resolution, which are improved with multi-shot EPI technique. Non-echoplanar DWI techniques include single-shot spin-echo (SSTSE) sequences like Half-Fourier-Acquired Single-shot Turbo Spin Echo (HASTE) and Multishot Turbo Spin-Echo (MSTSE) sequences such as PROPELLER. Non-EPI DWI techniques have lesser susceptibility artifacts and higher spatial resolution, but at the cost of longer acquisition time and lower signal-to-noise ratio.

Advanced diffusion imaging analyses include assessment of structural anisotropy (diffusion tensor imaging-DTI), microvascularity (intravoxel incoherent motion-IVIM), and

---

© Springer Nature Switzerland AG 2021
T. Moritani, A. A. Capizzano (eds.), *Diffusion-Weighted MR Imaging of the Brain, Head and Neck, and Spine*, https://doi.org/10.1007/978-3-030-62120-9_20

microstructural complexity (diffusion kurtosis imaging-DKI). Diffusion tensor imaging is determined by tissue anisotropy and measures fractional anisotropy (FA) [3]. IVIM simultaneously assesses both tissue perfusion and diffusion by using different b values [1, 4]. IVIM parameters are perfusion fraction (f), pure diffusion coefficient (D), pseudo diffusion coefficient (D*), and apparent diffusion coefficient (ADC) [5]. DKI quantifies non-gaussianity (kurtosis) of water displacement distribution [6, 7]. The mean diffusion kurtosis is significantly higher in malignant tumors.

20.2 Cholesteatomas

Cholesteatomas are classified as congenital (2%–5%) or acquired (95%–98%), and represent a sac lined with stratified squamous epithelium with keratin debris [8–12]. The acquired forms of cholesteatoma arise at the pars flaccida of the tympanic membrane. The pars flaccida cholesteatoma extends into Prussak's space (bounded by the pars flaccida laterally, the lateral mallear ligament superiorly, the short process of the malleus inferiorly, and the neck of the malleus medially), with erosions primarily involving the scutum, middle ear ossicles, or lateral epitympanic wall [8, 10, 11, 13]. The pars tensa cholesteatoma erodes into the posterior tympanic cavity and can involve the sinus tympani, facial recess, ossicles, aditus ad antrum, or mastoid [10]. Histopathologically, cholesteatoma is identical to an epidermoid cyst [10].

In suspected cases of cholesteatoma, noncontrast high-resolution computed tomography (CT) is the initial test of choice to evaluate for a middle ear soft tissue density mass with associated bony erosions. MR imaging can be used in selected cases for further characterization [14]. On standard MR sequences, cholesteatomas are usually hypointense on T1-weighted images and hyperintense on T2-weighted images [10]. Some cholesteatomas may be of intermediate or high signal intensity on T1-weighted images [15]. Postcontrast gadolinium imaging demonstrates lack of enhancement except for a thin peripheral rim [10, 16, 17].

One of the major treatments for cholesteatoma is canal wall up tympanoplasty. However, a second-look surgery is often required 6–18 months after the original surgery to evaluate for residual cholesteatoma [17–19]. Nonenhancing residual cholesteatoma on postcontrast images can be confused with relatively poorly vascularized scar tissue. Improved specificity on postcontrast images can be obtained with delayed (30–45 min) imaging [17].

Several studies have shown the utility of DWI in the diagnosis of cholesteatoma [14, 16, 20–25] (Fig. 20.1). In a study by Fitzek et al., 13 of 15 patients with cholesteatomas demonstrated bright signal on single-shot spin echo echoplanar DWI [16]. Of the two false-negative findings in this study, one was an epitympanic retraction pocket (an early stage of the disease without production of significant cholesteatoma mass) and one in which the cholesteatoma mass spontaneously extruded into the external auditory canal. In a study by Vercruysse et al., 100 patients were evaluated with DWI to detect the presence of primary acquired cholesteatoma or residual cholesteatoma [14]. Increased signal on DWI was found in 89% of the cases of primary cholesteatoma, but only one of seven cases of residual cholesteatoma. The false-negatives seen with primary cholesteatomas demonstrated atelectatic retraction cholesteatoma or partially evacuated cholesteatoma with limited keratin accumulation. No false-positive results were found in the group of primary acquired cholesteatomas. In the second group of patients in which DW imaging was used to evaluate for residual cholesteatoma prior to second-look surgery, DW imaging was not found to be useful. However, all false-negative findings in this group of residual cholesteatomas were less than 4 mm in diameter. They concluded that the limitation in the detection of cholesteatoma on DWI was the size of lesion (4–5 mm) combined with low spatial resolution, thick slices, and air-bone artifacts. Other groups have also found size limitations in the 4–5 mm range [20, 24].

DWI has high specificity for diagnosis of cholesteatoma due to its high inherent keratin content. Due to the combined effect of restricted diffusion and the T2 shine-through effect, cholesteatomas demonstrate high signal on DWI. Its

20 Head and Neck

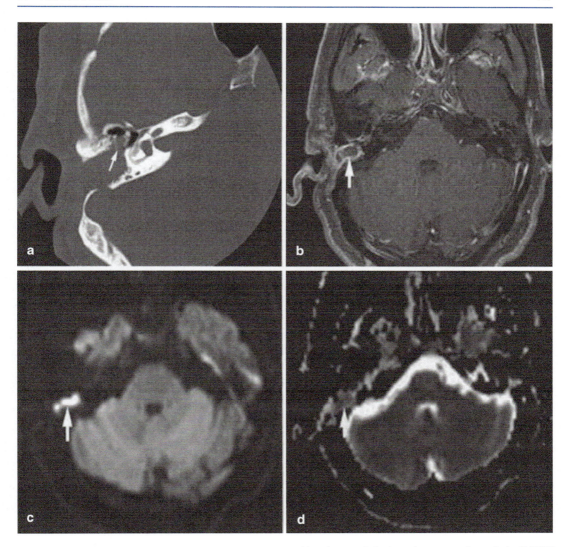

Fig. 20.1 (**a–d**) Recurrent cholesteatoma in a 45-year-old man. (**a**) CT shows right mastoidectomy and soft tissue density in the Prussak space with bony erosions (arrow). (**b**) Postcontrast T1-weighted image with fat saturation shows a recurrent cholesteatoma as hypointense with a characteristic rim enhancement (arrow). (**c, d**) DWI shows a hyperintense lesion with isointense ADC (0.82×10^{-3} mm^2/s) in the right mastoid representing a recurrent cholesteatoma (arrow)

major differential on routine MRI like granulation tissue, inflammation and fluid, show free diffusion [26]. Non-EPI DWI techniques are favored for detecting cholesteatomas. An advantage of echoplanar DWI over non-echoplanar DWI is its short acquisition time, but at the cost of artifacts at the air bone interface at the skull base and temporal bone [27, 28].

However, non-EPI DWI techniques include single-shot turbo spin-echo sequences (SSTSE) like half-Fourier acquisition single-shot turbo spin-echo (HASTE) DWI (Siemens Medical Solutions, Erlangen, Germany), HASTE and multishot turbo spin-echo (MSTSE) sequences such as PROPELLER DWI and BLADE DWI (Siemens Medical Solutions) (Fig. 20.2). They are superior to EPI DWI techniques due to the presence of less susceptibility artifact at the skull base and its ability to obtain thinner sections as thin as 2 mm, increasing sensitivity and resolution. Due to its high specificity, non-EPI DWI are indicated not only for postsurgical residual or

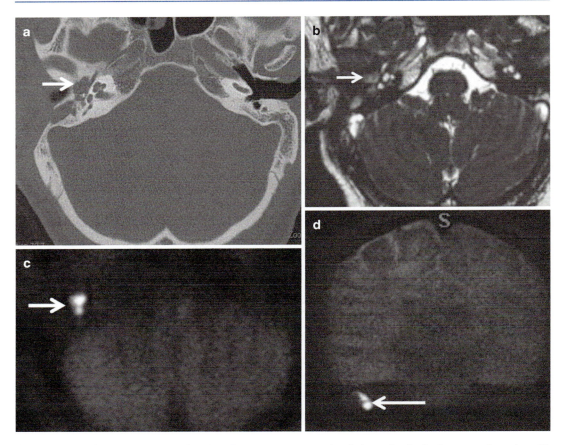

Fig. 20.2 (**a–d**) HASTE DWI in Recurrent Cholesteatoma. 21-year-old woman with a history of right ear surgery for cholesteatoma has a recurrence proven with cholesteatoma in the middle ear and granulation in the mastoidectomy site. (**a**) CT shows right mastoidectomy and soft tissue density in the tympanic cavity with bony erosions (arrow). (**b**) CISS-3D image showing recurrent cholesteatoma (arrow). (**c, d**) HASTE DWI bright signal represents recurrence (arrow)

recurrent middle ear cholesteatomas, but also for congenital or acquired de novo middle ear cholesteatomas [29, 30]. In a study by Fukuda et al., T1WI with DWI helped to increase the specificity and diagnostic accuracy in detecting cholesteatoma and differentiating it from cholesterol granuloma and fibrosis [31]. However, the limitation of non-echoplanar DWI includes decreased sensitivity for cholesteatomas less than 3 mm in size. Hence, serial follow-up with DWI is useful [32]. Causes for false-positive diagnosis include earwax, proteinaceous fluid, operative materials, tympanosclerosis, cholesterol granuloma, and squamous cell carcinoma of external auditory canal. Correlation with conventional MRI may avoid these pitfalls [33]. A large meta-analysis by Lingam et al., which included 26 studies and 1152 patient episodes, reported a sensitivity and specificity of 91% and 92%, respectively, in detecting middle-ear cholesteatoma [34].

In the study by Cavaliere M et al., the apparent diffusion coefficient median value of the cholesteatoma group (0.84×10^{-3} mm^2/s) significantly differed from the inflammatory granulation tissue (2.21×10^{-3} mm^2/s) group ($p < 2.2 \times 10^{-16}$) [35].

20.3 Subcutaneous and Intracranial Epidermoid Cysts

Subcutaneous epidermoid cysts are asymptomatic, slowly enlarging, dome-shaped lesions that are frequently seen in the neck and face and often arise from a ruptured pilosebaceous follicle [36]. Subcutaneous epidermoid cysts are also known as epidermal cysts, keratin cysts, epithelial cysts, or sebaceous cysts. Pathologically, subcutaneous epidermoid cysts and intracranial epidermoid cysts are thought to be identical. Intracranial epidermoid cysts are also known as primary cholesteatomas [37].

In a study of 24 patients by Hong et al., the signal intensities of ruptured and unruptured subcutaneous epidermal cysts were described as well in terms of enhancement patterns [38]. Unruptured cysts demonstrated thin, smooth rim cyst wall enhancement. Ruptured cysts had thick, irregular rim cyst wall enhancement, fuzzy enhancement in the surrounding subcutaneous tissue, and thin, smooth cyst wall enhancement (Fig. 20.3). In an MR imaging study of five cases of epidermoid cysts in the extremities by Shibata et al., the cysts had slightly high signal intensity on T1-weighted imaging in three of five cases and isointense signal intensity in two cases [39]. On T2-weighted images, all were of high signal intensity. Irregular areas of low signal intensity were seen on both T1- and T2-weighted images. There was no enhancement in the cysts.

In a study by Suzuki et al., using DWI, unruptured subcutaneous epidermal cysts in the head were compared with intracranial epidermoid cysts [40]. Signal intensity of subcutaneous epidermal cysts was low to mildly high on T1-weighted images (relative to muscle) and variable on T2-weighted images (nine high signal intensity, three low signal intensity, and two mixed signal intensity). This differed from intracranial epidermoid cysts, which were low on T1-weighted images and high on T2-weighted images. The subcutaneous epidermal cysts demonstrated no enhancement or thin and smooth rim enhancement. The measured ADC of intracranial epidermoid cysts was significantly higher than subcutaneous epidermal cysts (1.06×10^{-3} mm^2/s versus 0.81×10^{-3} mm^2/s). The authors hypothesize that the higher ADC for intracranial epidermoid cysts may be due to CSF extending into the cysts. The authors also noted the difficulty in measuring the ADC of head and neck lesions using echoplanar DWI because of the susceptibility artifacts. They proposed DWI techniques with decreased sensitivity to susceptibility artifacts should be used to evaluate head and neck lesions (Figs. 20.4 and 20.5).

20.4 Cholesterol Granuloma

Cholesterol granulomas have a characteristically high signal on T1-weighted images due to blood products (extracellular meth hemoglobin) and have a central high signal on T2-weighted images with peripheral decreased signal from hemosiderin deposition [10, 41, 42]. A case of cholesterol granuloma with increased signal on DWI has been reported [43]. DW signals are usually mildly hyperintense with a high ADC value. However, ADC maps can show a heterogeneous lesion, which presumably depends on the viscosity of blood products in a cholesterol granuloma (Figs. 20.6 and 20.7).

20.5 Mucocele

A mucocele is an opacified expanded gland that is the result of chronic ostial obstruction. MR signal characteristics depend on the concentration of protein. High water content results in low T1 signal and high T2 signal, whereas high protein content results in high T1 signal and low signal on T2 with inspissated mucus. White et al. reported a case of an ethmoid sinus mucocele with slightly low signal on DWI with increased ADC [44]. In a study by Hansen et al., of 40 patients who underwent frontal sinus obliteration, 6/40 showed potential postoperative frontal sinus mucocele [45]. MRI has a critical role in diagnosis mucoceles. Signal changes on T1 and T2 reflect the viscosity and fluid content. Fat graft can complicate evaluation of postoperative MRI and fat saturated signal can help. However, the fat graft with time can undergo fibrosis and or hemorrhage adding to difficulty in interpretation. DW signals and the ADC values in a mucocele are variable depending on the viscosity of the fluid in a mucocele (Figs. 20.8 and 20.9).

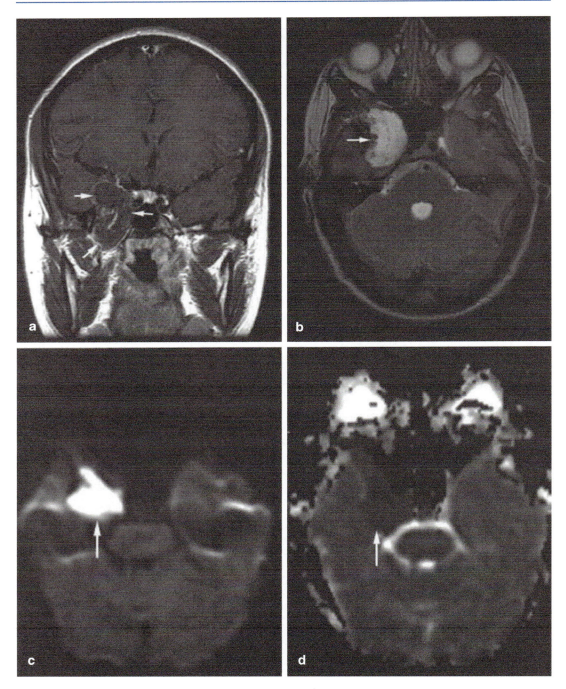

Fig. 20.3 (a–d) Epidermoid cyst in a 20-year-old woman. (a) Postcontrast coronal T1-weighted image shows a hypointense mass with rim enhancement in the right sphenoid bone and cavernous sinus (arrows). (b) T2-weighted image shows the mass as hyperintense (arrow). (c, d) DWI clearly shows an epidermoid as hyperintense with decreased ADC ($0.57–0.62 \times 10^{-3}$ mm^2/s) (arrow). (Courtesy of Vikas Jain MD, The University of Iowa, Hospitals and Clinics, USA)

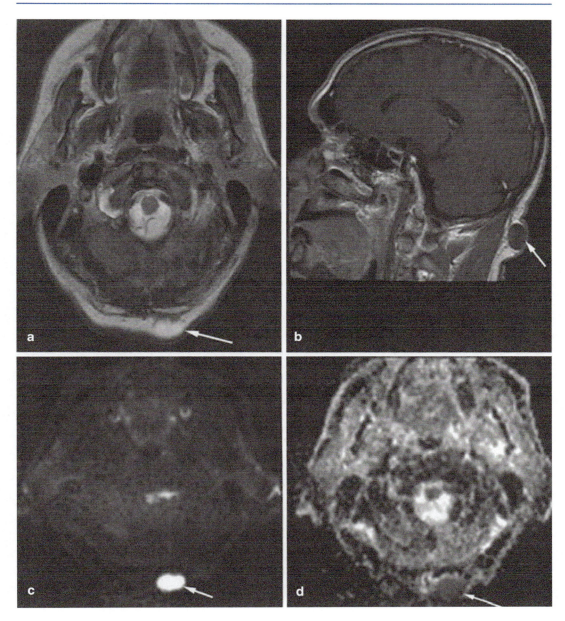

Fig. 20.4 (**a–d**) Epidermoid cyst in a 55-year-old man. (**a**) T2-weighted image shows an oval hyperintense lesion in the occipital scalp (arrow). (**b**) Postcontrast sagittal T1-weighted image shows a nonenhancing hypointense mass (arrow). (**c, d**) DWI clearly shows an epidermoid as a hyperintense lesion associated with isointense ADC $(0.97–1.10 \times 10^{-3}\ mm^2/s)$ (arrow), which may correspond to stratified keratinaceous debris and squamous epithelium

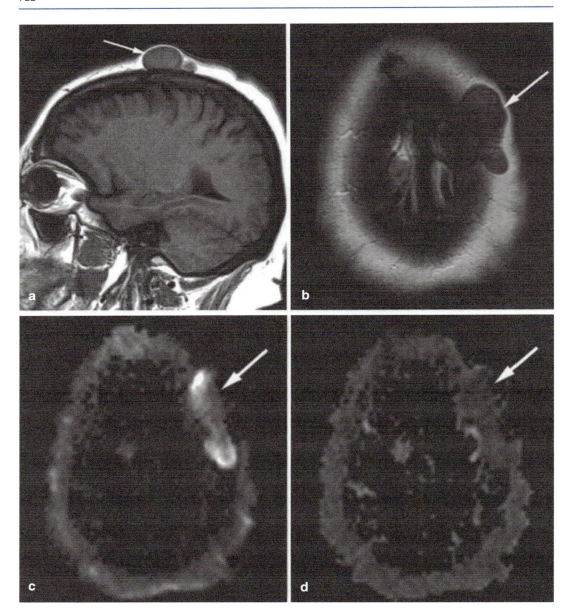

Fig. 20.5 (**a–d**) Epidermoid cyst in a 48-year-old woman. (**a**) Precontrast sagittal T1-weighted image shows an oval iso- or slightly hyperintense lesion in the frontoparietal scalp (arrow). (**b**) T2-weighted image shows this lesion as hypointense (arrow). (**c, d**) DWI shows the lesion as hyperintense associated with slightly low or isointense ADC (0.67–0.93×10^{-3} mm^2/s) (arrow), which may correspond to stratified keratinaceous debris and squamous epithelium

20.6 Fibrous Dysplasia, Paget's Disease, and Bone Marrow Hyperplasia

Fibrous dysplasia is a disorder of unknown etiology characterized by abnormal development of fibroblasts and replacement of normal bone by dysplastic fibro-osseous tissue. The radiologic findings are divided into three types: pagetoid, sclerotic, and cyst-like. CT demonstrates fibrous dysplasia best. CT findings include increased bone thickness, heterogeneous radiodensity, and loss of trabecular pattern (ground-glass appearance) [46]. On the other hand, MR imaging is

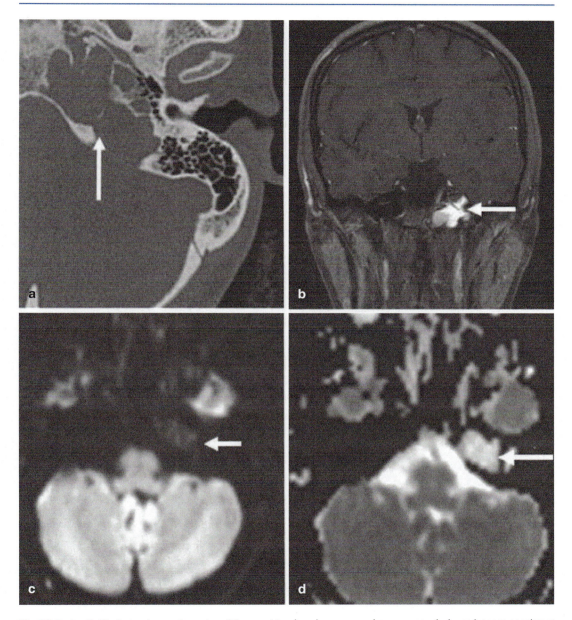

Fig. 20.6 (a–d) Cholesterol granuloma in a 35-year-old man. (a) CT shows a soft tissue density mass in the left petrous apex (arrow). (b) Postcontrast coronal T1-weighted image with fat saturation shows a nonenhancing mass as homogeneously hyperintense consistent with a cholesterol granuloma (arrow). (c, d) DWI shows a cholesterol granuloma as a mildly hyperintense lesion with increased ADC (2.32×10^{-3} mm^2/s) (arrow)

much less specific and shows a low-to-intermediate signal intensity with moderate to marked enhancement. Hayashida et al. used quantitative spin echo DW imaging to study 20 bone lesions (eight solitary bone cysts, five fibrous dysplasia, and seven chondrosarcomas) [47, 48]. DWI shows mild hyperintensity in fibrous dysplasia associated with increased ADC (Figs. 20.10 and 20.11). They found that the mean ADC values of benign tumors and chondrosarcomas were not significantly different, whereas the mean ADC value of simple bone cysts was significantly higher than either fibrous dysplasia or chondrosarcoma. DWI in fibrous

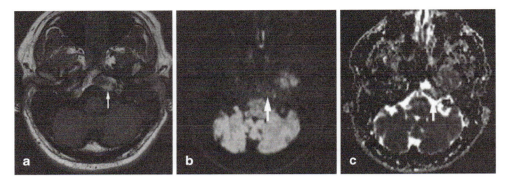

Fig. 20.7 (**a–c**) Cholesterol granuloma in a 55-year-old woman. (**a**) T1-weighted image shows the mass as partially hyperintense consistent with a cholesterol granuloma (arrow). (**b, c**) DWI shows a cholesterol granuloma as a mildly hyperintense lesion with high and low ADC values (0.82–2.45×10^{-3} mm^2/s) (arrows)

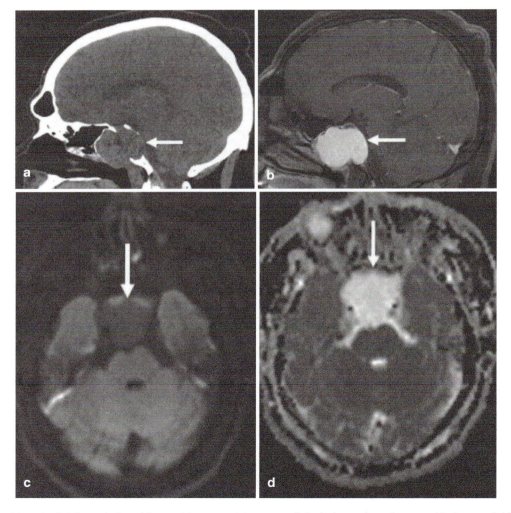

Fig. 20.8 (**a–d**) Mucocele in a 45-year-old woman. (**a**) CT shows an expansile slightly hyper- and isodense mass with calcifications of the wall originating from the frontal sinus (arrows). (**b**) Precontrast sagittal T1-weighted image shows the mass as hyperintense (arrow). (**c, d**) DWI shows most of the lesion as hyperintense with decreased ADC values (0.30–0.51×10^{-3} mm^2/s), which probably represents the high viscosity in a highly protein-containing mucocele (arrow). (Courtesy of Policeni B MD The University of Iowa Hospitals and Clinics)

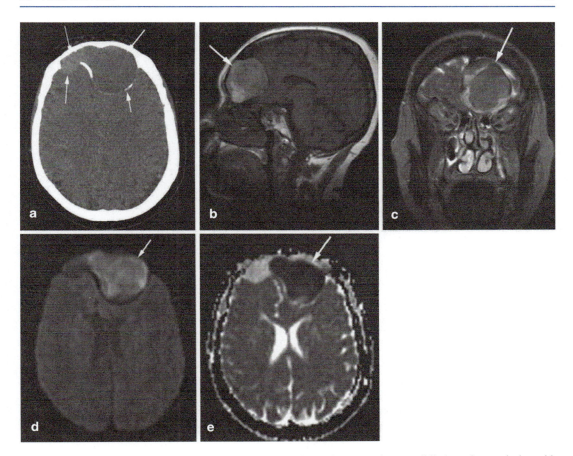

Fig. 20.9 (**a–d**) Mucocele in a 31-year-old man. (**a**) CT shows opacified and expanded sphenoid sinus (arrow). (**b**) Postcontrast sagittal T1-weighted image with fat saturation shows a nonenhancing mass as homogenously hyperintense, consistent with a mucocele (arrow). (**c, d**) DWI shows the mucocele as a mildly hyperintense lesion with increased ADC values (2.37×10^{-3} mm^2/s), which probably represents the high-water content and low viscosity in a protein-containing mucocele (arrow)

dysplasia usually shows higher ADC values than in malignant lesions, with mean ADC of 2×10^3 mm^2/s; however lower ADC values are also reported [49].

Paget's disease is a process of unknown cause in which osteoclastic activity is abnormal. The histopathology is divided into four phases: osteolytic, mixed, osteoblastic, and remodeled. The mixture of phases results in a heterogeneous lytic and sclerotic bone density (cotton-wool appearance) on CT. MR findings are variable. Contrast enhancement reflects the hypervascular nature of the process. DWI shows diffuse minimal hyperintensity in the skull associated with mildly increased ADC, which may reflect intermediate cellularity in the bone marrow spaces (Fig. 20.12).

Diffuse bone marrow disease is characterized by diffuse fat replacement in the bone marrow on MR imaging [50, 51]. Bone marrow hyperplasia is seen in hematologic disorders such as sickle cell disease, thalassemia, and aplastic anemia (Fig. 20.13).

20.7 Other Benign Lesions, Differential Diagnoses, and Artifacts

Mild hyperintense lesions on DWI associated with increased ADC include scalp or intraosseous hemangiomas (Fig. 20.14) and Langerhans' cell histiocytosis (Fig. 20.15) and neurogenic

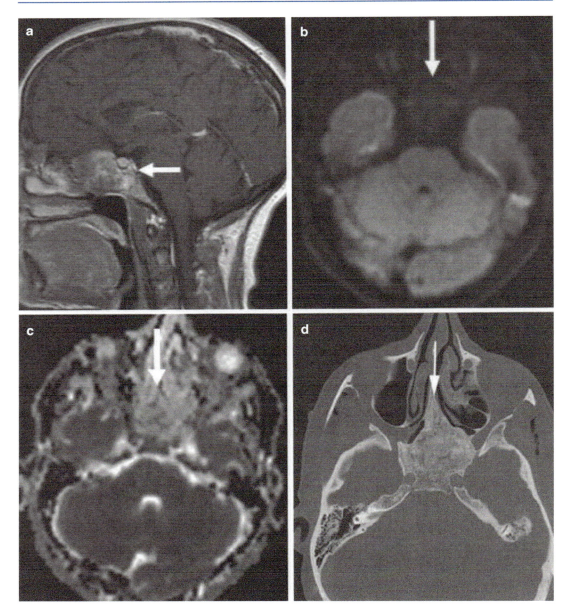

Fig. 20.10 (**a–d**) Fibrous dysplasia in 39-year-old woman. (**a**) Postcontrast sagittal T1-weighted image shows an inhomogeneously enhancing mass in the skull base similar to malignant tumor (arrow). (**b–c**) DWI reveals minimally hyperintense mass in the skull base with increased ADC ($1.320–1.970 \times 10^{-3}$ mm^2/s) (arrow) due to the presence of dysplastic fibro-osseous tissue. (**d**) Follow-up CT shows enlarged medullary space and typical ground-glass appearance of a fibrous dysplasia (arrow)

tumors: neurofibroma (Fig. 20.16) and schwannoma (Figs. 20.17, 20.18, and 20.19). Intraosseous meningioma can show DWI hyperintensity with decreased ADC (Fig. 20.20).

In a study by Sener using echo-planar DWI, six vestibular schwannomas were found to be isointense to brain parenchyma on b = 1,000 s/mm^2 images, but with ADC values significantly higher than parenchyma (schwannoma range $1.14–1.72 \times 10^{-3}$ mm^2/s with mean value $1.42 \pm 0.17 \times 10^{-3}$ mm^2/s; parenchyma range $0.64–0.98 \times 10^{-3}$ mm^2/s with average value

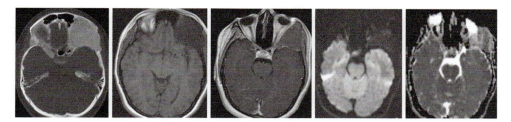

Fig. 20.11 (a–e) Fibrous dysplasia of the sphenoid wing in 29-year-old man. (a) CT bone window clearly demonstrates the classic ground glass appearance of left sphenoid wing fibrous dysplasia. (b, c) Pre- and postcontrast T1WI shows faint enhancement. (d, e) DWI shows hypointensity in fibrous dysplasia associated with increased ADC

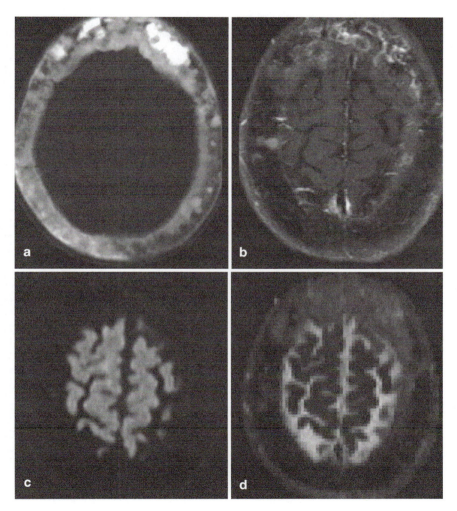

Fig. 20.12 (a–d) Paget's disease in a 45-year-old man. (a) CT shows diffuse bone thickening with a heterogeneous lytic and sclerotic bone density (cotton-wool appearance). (b) Postcontrast T1-weighted image with fat saturation shows a heterogeneous enhancement in the frontal skull. (c, d) DWI shows diffuse minimal hyperintensity in the skull associated with mildly increased ADC ($0.94–1.45 \times 10^{-3}$ mm^2/s) in the frontal thickened skull

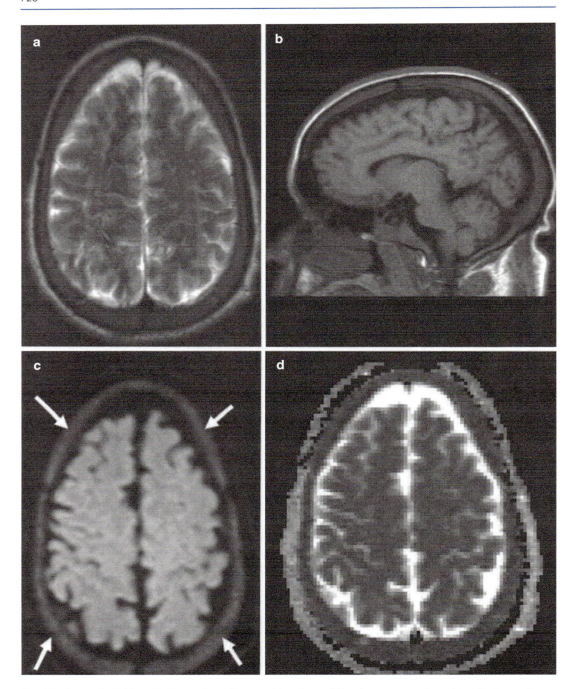

Fig. 20.13 (**a–d**) Sickle cell disease in a 22-year-old man. (**a**, **b**) Axial T2- and sagittal T1-weighted images show diffuse bone thickening of the skull. (**c**, **d**) DWI shows diffuse homogeneous hyperintensity (arrows) associated with mildly decreased ADC in the skull which corresponds to bone marrow hyperplasia

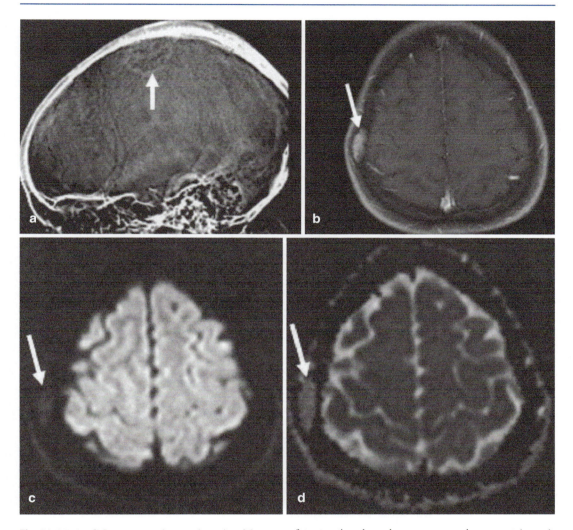

Fig. 20.14 (**a–d**) Intraosseous hemangioma in a 26-year-old man. (**a**) CT scanogram shows a calvarial lesion with sclerotic margins consistent with an intraosseous hemangioma (arrow). (**b**) Postcontrast T1-weighted image with fat saturation shows homogeneous enhancement (arrow). (**c, d**) DW imaging shows a slightly hyperintense lesion associated with slightly increased ADC (1.37–1.48 × 10^{-3} mm^2/s) in the right parietal skull (arrow)

0.80 ± 0.11 × 10^{-3} mm^2/s) [52]. The lesions studied were predominantly solid with minimal cystic degeneration. Srinivasan et al., using 3-T single-shot spin-echo echo-planar DW imaging, found a range of ADC values for six schwannomas of 0.74–2.1 × 10^{-3} mm^2/s [53]. They hypothesized differences could be due to differences in the internal architecture of the lesions. Maeda et al., using line-scan DW imaging, found that myxoid containing soft tissue tumors had significantly higher ADC values than non-myxoid soft tissue tumors [54]. Relatively low ADC values (0.45–0.60 × 10^{-3} mm^2/s) with increased signal on DW images were reported in a case of malignant oculomotor schwannoma [55]. In a study by Ahlawat et al., target sign was detected on T2-FSE and DWI in schwannomas and neurofi-

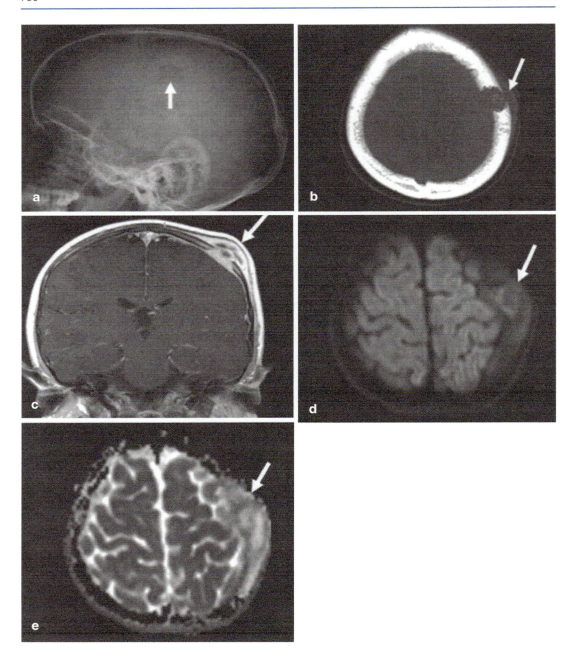

Fig. 20.15 (**a**–**e**) Langerhans' cell histiocytosis in a 3-year-old boy. (**a**) Skull X-ray shows a lytic bony defect without sclerotic margins (arrow). (**b**) CT shows a lytic lesion and soft tissue mass (arrow). (**c**) Postcontrast coronal T1-weighted image demonstrates an enhancing mass (arrow) and beveled edge bony erosions. (**d**, **e**) DWI shows a heterogeneous hyperintense mass with increased ADC (1.11–1.72×10^{-3} mm^2/s) involving the left frontoparietal skull and scalp (arrow)

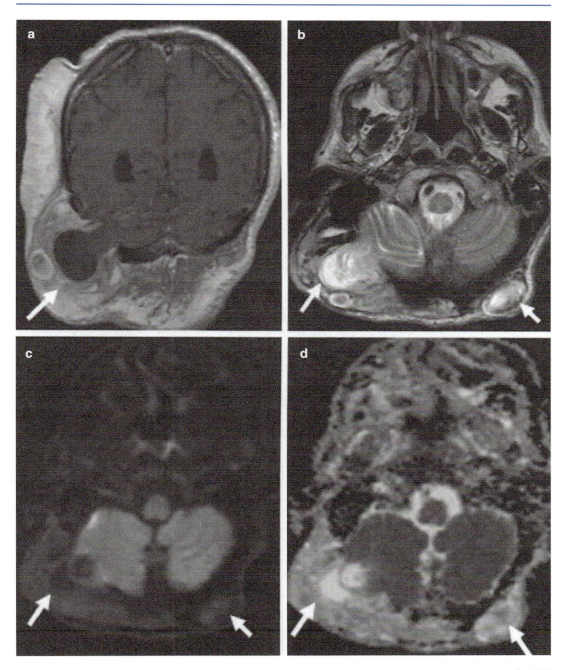

Fig. 20.16 (a–d) Neurofibromatosis type 1 in a 20-year-old man. (a, b) Postcontrast coronal T1- and axial T2-weighted images show multiple diffuse plexiform neurofibromatosis, a meningoencephalocele, and bony defect in the right occipital bone (arrows). (c, d) DWI shows multiple plexiform neurofibromas as slightly hyperintense with increased ADC (1.63–2.11 × 10^{-3} mm^2/s) (arrows)

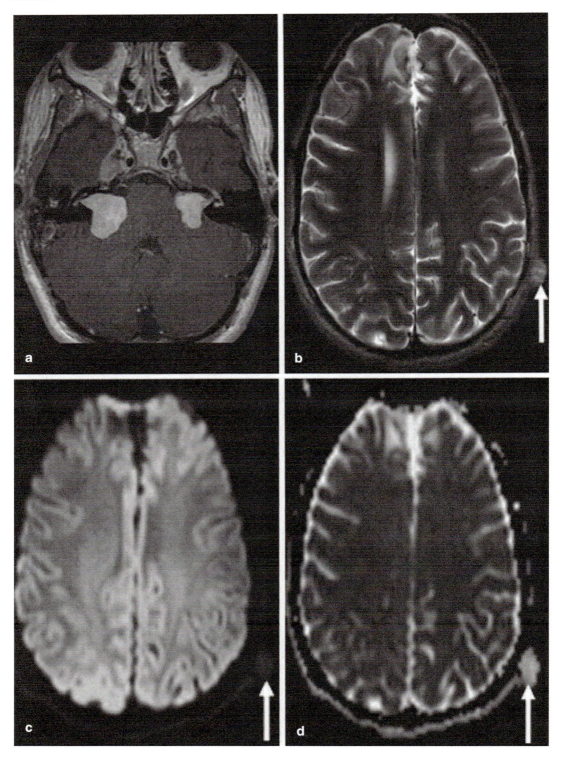

Fig. 20.17 (**a–d**) Neurofibromatosis type 2 and schwannoma in a 32-year-old woman. (**a**) Postcontrast T1-weighted image shows homogeneously enhancing vestibular schwannomas bilaterally. (**b**) T2-weighted image shows a round hyperintense lesion in the left parietal scalp (arrow). (**c, d**) DWI shows a subtle hyperintense lesion associated with increased ADC (1.82–2.02 × 10^{-3} mm^2/s) which may represent a mucoid degeneration of a schwannoma

20 Head and Neck

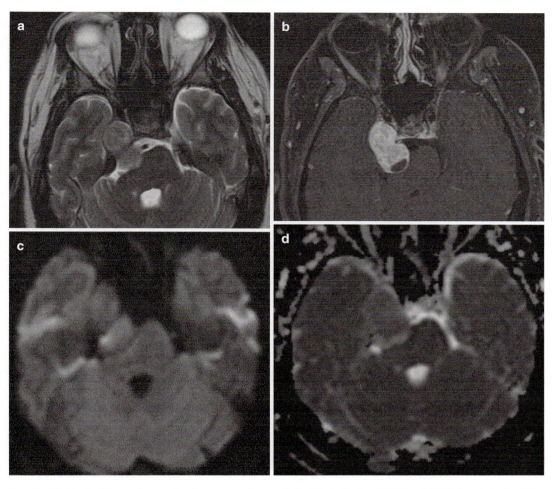

Fig. 20.18 (**a–d**) Right trigeminal schwannoma in a 44-year-old man, with (**a**) T2W image showing dumbbell configuration hyperintense mass extending across the petrous apex in the region of Meckel's cave. (**b**) Postcontrast T1W image shows enhancement of the mass in the Meckel's. (**c, d**) DWI and ADC show brighter diffusion than in normal surrounding parenchyma with slightly increased ADC ($1.0–1.5 \times 10^{-3}$ mm²/s) representing intermediate cellularity

bromas and was absent in malignant peripheral nerve sheath tumors [56]. Also the ADC values in malignant peripheral nerve sheath tumors (MPNST) were lower than that of benign PNST ($1.3 \pm 0.5 \times 10^{-3}$ mm²/s in benign PNSTs versus $0.7 \pm 0.3 \times 10^{-3}$ mm²/s in MPNSTs). Camargo et al. studied pretreatment ADC values of vestibular schwannomas in 20 patients who underwent radiosurgery and could find statistically significant difference in the responders and no responders using a cutoff pretreatment ADC value of 0.8×10^{-3} mm²/s [57].

Craniopharyngiomas are benign intracranial tumors that arise from Rathke cleft cyst epithelium. They can be located in the suprasellar, both supra and intrasellar, purely intrasellar location, or very rarely extracranial location. Of the two histologic subtypes, the adamantinomatous type is most common having lobulated contour with cystic and solid areas and calcification. The less common papillary variety is predominantly solid with less calcification. Unlike germ cell tumors, the craniopharyngiomas show high ADC values (See Chap. 18, Fig. 18.57) [58].

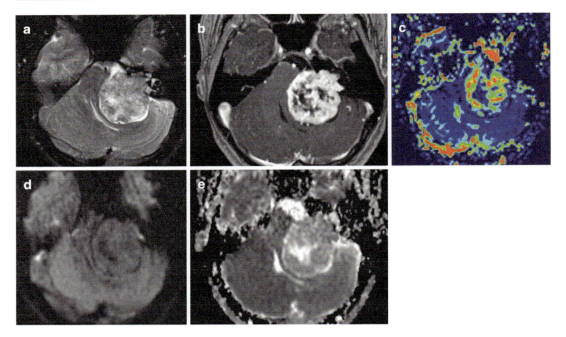

Fig. 20.19 (**a–e**) Left cerebellopontine angle growing schwannoma in a 37-year-old woman. (**a**) Fat-sat T2W image shows a large mixed signal intensity mass with microcystic components in the left cerebellopontine angle. (**b**) Postcontrast T1W image shows a heterogeneously enhancing mass. (**c**) Left cerebellopontine angle schwannoma shows increased perfusion. (**d, e**) DWI demonstrates an isointense mass with slightly increased ADC

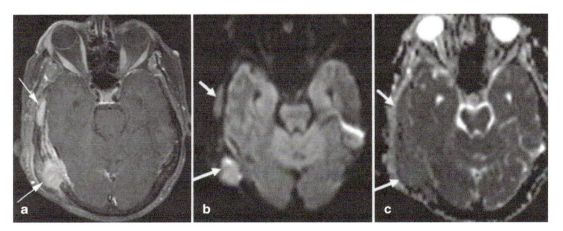

Fig. 20.20 (**a–c**) Intraosseous meningioma in a 57-year-old woman. (**a**) Postcontrast T1-weighted image with fat saturation demonstrates homogeneously enhancing masses with dural enhancement in the right temporo-occipital region (arrows). (**b, c**) DWI shows multiple hyperintense mass lesions with the isointense ADC (0.77–0.89 × 10^{-3} mm^2/s), related to cellularity of meningiomas (arrows)

Ecchordosis physaliphora (EP) consist of benign gelatinous lesions of notochordal origin. They are seen usually in the region of the clivus with a component in the intradural region in the prepontine cistern and are connected by a bony stalk to the clivus. They are hypointense on T1, hyperintense on T2WI, not enhancing with contrast and show high ADC values (Fig. 20.21) [59].

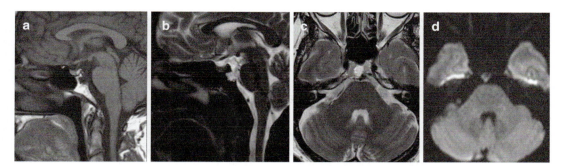

Fig 20.21 (**a–d**) Ecchordosis physaliphora (EP) in a 49-year-old man. There is a small T1 hypointense (**a**) and T2 hyperintense lesion (**b**, **c**) in the clivus protruded into the prepontine cistern. (**d**) DWI shows high signal intensity with increased ADC (not shown)

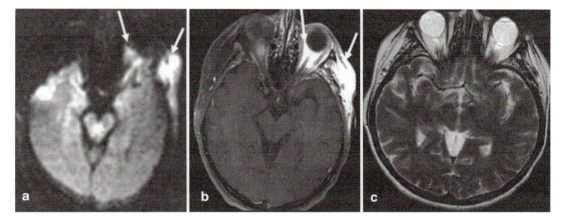

Fig. 20.22 (**a–c**) Artifacts similar to scalp mass lesion on DWI. (**a**) DWI shows high signals in the left periorbital and retro-orbital areas similar to lesions (arrows). (**b**) Postcontrast T1-weighted image with fat saturation shows an inadequate suppression of fat signals in exactly the same areas (arrows), which is due to susceptibility effects from metal of the tooth. (**c**) T2-weighted image shows no lesion in the areas

DWI uses a fat suppression technique (chemical fat saturation) that is used in conventional MR imaging (fat sat T1- and T2-weighted images). Inadequate fat suppression due to a susceptibility artifact causes a hyperintensity on DWI which is sometimes similar to a scalp lesion (Fig. 20.22). A scalp lipoma is seen as a very hypointense lesion because of suppressed fat signals on DW imaging (Fig. 20.23). Scalp or subgaleal hematomas can have various DW signals and ADC values depending on the phase of the hematomas (Fig. 20.24). Caution is needed when differentiating them from pus collection, abscess, or tumors.

20.8 Infection (Abscess and Pus Collection), Mastoiditis, Malignant Otitis Externa

Acute otomastoiditis and acute coalescent otomastoiditis are defined as acute infections of the middle ear and mastoid air cells. Acute otomastoiditis is without destruction of mastoid septations. Acute coalescent otomastoiditis is with destruction of septations and development of intramastoid empyema.

Figure 20.25 shows potential pathways for spread of mastoid infection. Spread of mastoid infection by osteoclastic breakdown of the mas-

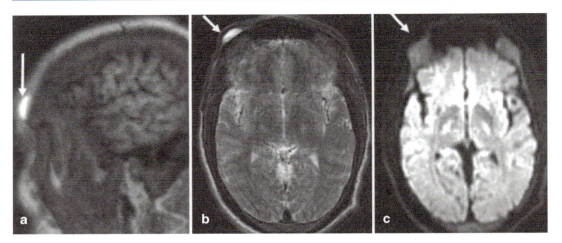

Fig. 20.23 (a–c) Lipoma in a 22-year-old man. (a, b) T1- and T2-weighted images show a hyperintense lesion in the right frontal scalp consistent with a lipoma (arrow). (c) DWI shows suppressed fat signals in the lipoma (arrow). This patient also has sickle cell disease. The thickened skull with increased DWI signals reflects red bone marrow hyperplasia

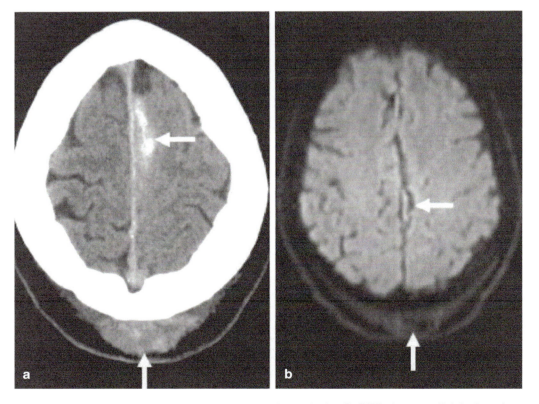

Fig. 20.24 (a–d) Subgaleal hematoma in a 35-year-old man. (a) CT shows an occipitoparietal subgaleal hematoma and a left parafalcine subdural hematoma (arrows). (b) T2-weighted image shows iso- and low signal areas in the subgaleal and subdural hematomas (arrows). (c, d) DWI shows a slightly hyperintense hematoma with a low signal in the center area of the subgaleal hematoma associated with decreased ADC values (arrows). DW signals of hematomas are variable depending on the phase

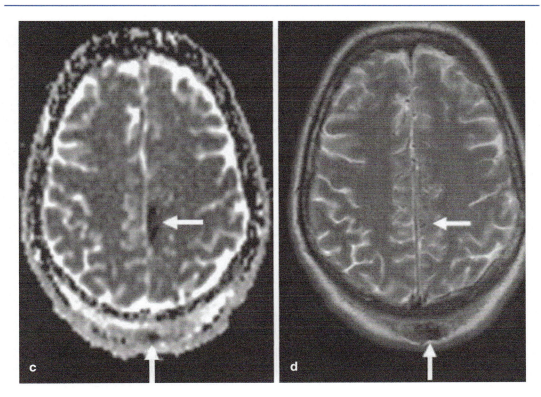

Fig. 20.24 (continued)

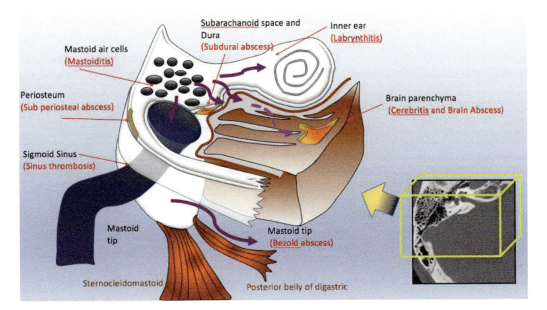

Fig. 20.25 Schematic diagram of potential pathways for spread of mastoid infection (Courtesy of Dr Umar Shafique Chaudhry and Dr Umber Shafique). Mastoid infection with osteoclastic breakdown of the mastoid or tegmen tympani leads to meningitis, subdural abscess, cerebritis, ventriculitis, and brain abscess. Inner ear involvement causes labyrinthitis. Infection propagates from the medial mastoid air cells to the adjacent sigmoid sinus through the sigmoid plate, causing venous sinus thrombosis/thrombophlebitis. Infection spreads under the periosteum causing subperiosteal abscess. Inferiorly the infections can spread beyond mastoid tip and extend anterior to sternocleidomastoid muscle causing Bezold's abscess

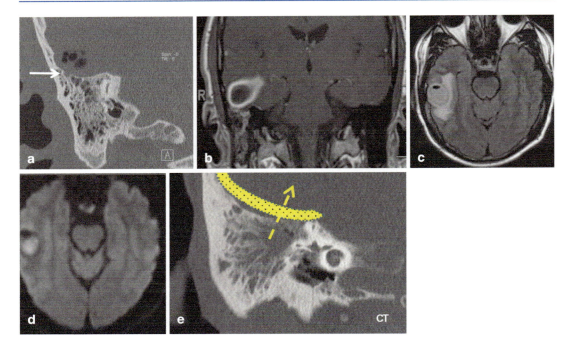

Fig. 20.26 (**a**–**e**) Coalescent mastoiditis with temporal lobe abscess in a 46-year-old male. (**a**) There is opacification of mastoid air cells with subtle superior cortical discontinuity of the mastoid bone (arrow) and pneumocephalus in right temporal lobe on coronal CT. (**b**) Ring enhancing lesion on postcontrast T1WI. (**c**) It is seen as air containing round lesion with surrounding edema in the right temporal lobe on FLAIR. (**d**) On DWI there is diffusion restriction consistent with an abscess. (**e**) Erosion of the mastoid or tegmen tympani by coalescent mastoiditis can lead to extension of infectious process in adjacent areas including meninges, temporal lobe. Uncontrolled mastoid inflammation causes local acidosis and ischemia leading to osteoclastic dissolution

toid or tegmen tympani can lead to meningitis, subdural abscess, cerebritis, ventriculitis, and brain abscess (Fig. 20.26). Uncontrolled mastoid inflammation causes local acidosis and ischemia, leading to osteoclastic dissolution. Infection spreads under the periosteum which can cause subperiosteal abscess (Fig. 20.27). Inferiorly the infections can spread beyond the mastoid tip and extend anterior to sternocleidomastoid muscle causing Bezold's abscess (Fig. 20.28). The mastoid communicates with the epitympanum portion of middle ear via the aditus ad antrum. Spread from mastoid to middle ear can potentially involve inner ear, which causes labyrinthitis. The medial mastoid air cells are separated from the adjacent sigmoid sinus by the sigmoid plate. The propagation of infection can be from small venules in the mastoid into the sigmoid sinus through blood, or direct spreading infection through a coalescent or cholesteatomatous bony erosion, resulting in the formation of venous sinus thrombosis/thrombophlebitis (Fig. 20.29).

Bezold's abscess, first described in 1908, is considered as a neck abscess spreading from the tip of the mastoid, extending deep to the sternocleidomastoid muscle, and may extend into the posterior cervical and perivertebral spaces. Unlike coalescent mastoiditis, Bezold's abscess lies inferior to the tip of the mastoid and does not extend superiorly to the lateral aspect of the mastoid [60, 61]. Coalescent mastoiditis with subperiosteal abscess is caused by an extension of infection via an eroded lateral mastoid cortex [60]. Distinguishing these entities is important because the surgical treatment is different (Bezold's abscess requires mastoidectomy and abscess drainage). DWI clearly shows the extent of the abscess (Figs. 20.27 and 20.28).

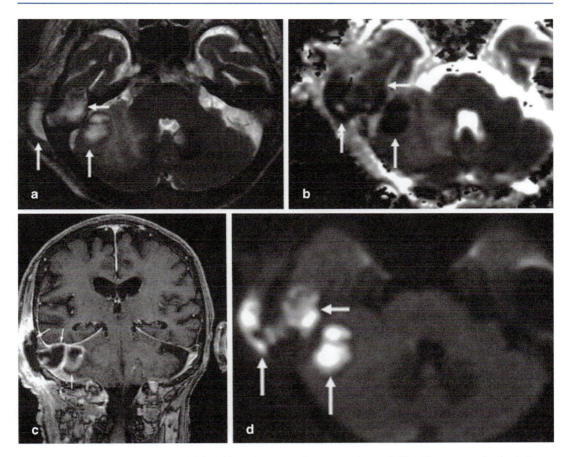

Fig. 20.27 (**a**–**d**) Coalescent mastoiditis with perimastoid (subperiosteal) abscess and brain abscess in a 50-year-old man. (**a**) T2-weighted image shows right mastoid, perimastoid, and brain abscesses as hyperintense lesions (arrows). (**b**) Postcontrast sagittal T1-weighted image shows these abscesses as hypointense with rim enhancement (arrows). There is a communication between the mastoid abscess and perimastoid abscess with an erosion of lateral wall of the mastoid and soft tissue swelling. (**c**, **d**) DWI shows the abscesses as very hyperintense with decreased ADC (0.35–0.46×10^{-3} mm^2/s) (arrows)

Malignant external otitis or necrotizing external otitis is an infection of the bony or cartilaginous external auditory canal with bone erosion and associated cellulitis or abscess formation. The adjacent soft tissue is also involved. On T2-weighted images, diffuse increased signal is seen with cellulitis and focal increased signal with abscess. Postcontrast T1-weighted images demonstrate diffuse enhancement with cellulitis and typical rim enhancement with abscess [62]. DWI shows the abscess or pus collection as hyperintense (Fig. 20.30).

Skull base osteomyelitis is difficult diagnosis to make clinically. It needs high suspicion in diabetic and other immunocompromised patients. They are life-threatening complications. Patients could have undergone treatment for other malignancy in these regions and MRI can pick up these subtle findings of altered signal intensity, enhancement, and bone marrow infiltration, which can mimic a primary neoplastic process. Evidence of increased T2 signal in adjacent soft tissues, lack of architectural distortion, and enhancement greater than or equal to mucosa are useful in differentiation from tumor [63]. DWI has a promising role in differentiation between both diagnoses. In a study by Ozgen et al., mean ADC values were 1.26×10^{-3} mm^2/s for 9 patients with skull base

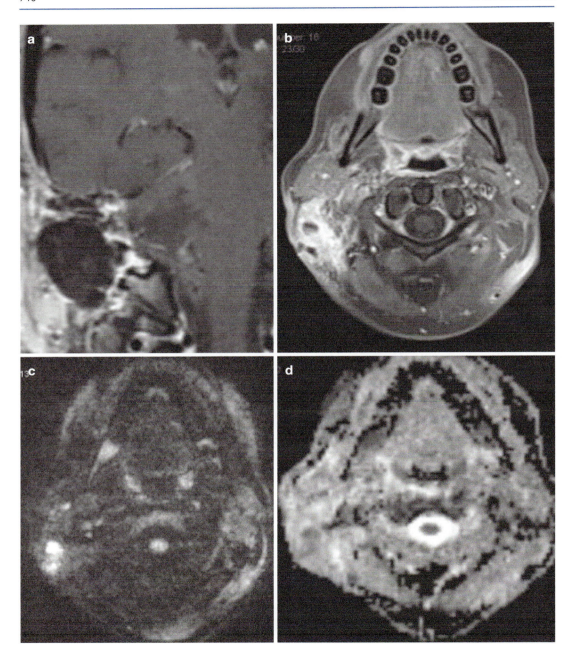

Fig. 20.28 (**a–d**) Bezold's abscess after mastoidectomy in a 46-year-old female with very high jugular bulb required decompression which resulted in intraoperative hemorrhage. (**a**) Postcontrast coronal T1WI shows operative bed hematoma, which presented with post auricular pain on right side. Redness in area developed over last two days. (**b**) Postcontrast T1WI shows peripherally enhancing collection spreading from the tip of the mastoid, extending into the posterior cervical space. (**c, d**) DWI demonstrates restricted diffusion with decreased ADC consistent with an abscess

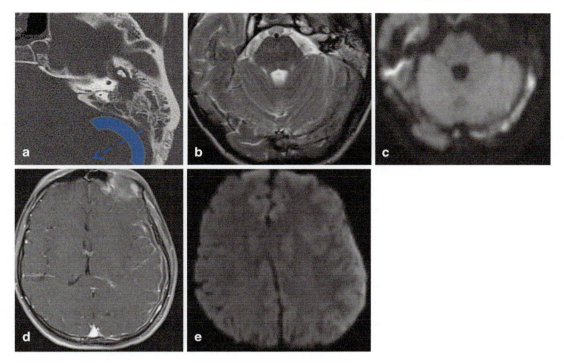

Fig. 20.29 (**a–e**) Mastoiditis with dural sinus thrombosis (subacute to chronic phase) and subdural empyema in a 22-year-old man. (**a**) CT shows otitis media and coalescent mastoiditis with erosion of the sigmoid plate. The propagation of infection can be direct spreading through a coalescent bony erosion resulting in the formation of venous sinus thrombosis/thrombophlebitis. (**b, c**) Subacute to chronic phase dural sinus thrombosis and mastoid fluid collection are seen on T2WI and DWI. (**d, e**) Left subdural empyema is noted with rim enhancing and DWI high signal in left subdural region

osteomyelitis, which was significantly higher than for skull base malignant cases of nasopharyngeal carcinoma, lymphoma, and metastasis. Using a cutoff value of 1.08×10^{-3} mm^2/s, the accuracy was 96% [64].

Pott's puffy tumor is a subperiosteal abscess with progressive frontal bone osteomyelitis. It is a potentially life-threatening complication of frontal sinusitis [65–67]. It was originally described by Sir Percival Pott around 1760. The subperiosteal abscess erodes the outer table of the frontal bone with associated soft tissue swelling, i.e., the puffy tumor. DW imaging shows the abscess as hyperintense with decreased ADC (Fig. 20.31). Surgical intervention (abscess drainage and debridement of the osteomyelitic bone) and antibiotic therapy prevent further suppurative complications. MRI with DWI clearly demonstrates the extension of bacterial abscesses in the head and neck area (Fig. 20.32).

Fungal infections like aspergillosis is often seen in immunocompromised individuals centered around the paranasal sinuses and can extend by eroding the skull base or orbits [68]. They present as mass lesions, which are hypointense on T1 and T2WI and enhancing with contrast. Fungal abscess can have higher ADC values when compared with pyogenic abscesses [69, 70].

20.9 Orbital Lesions

In cases of optic neuritis, studies have shown that acute and chronic optic neuritis differ in diameter, signal intensities, enhancement, and diffusion

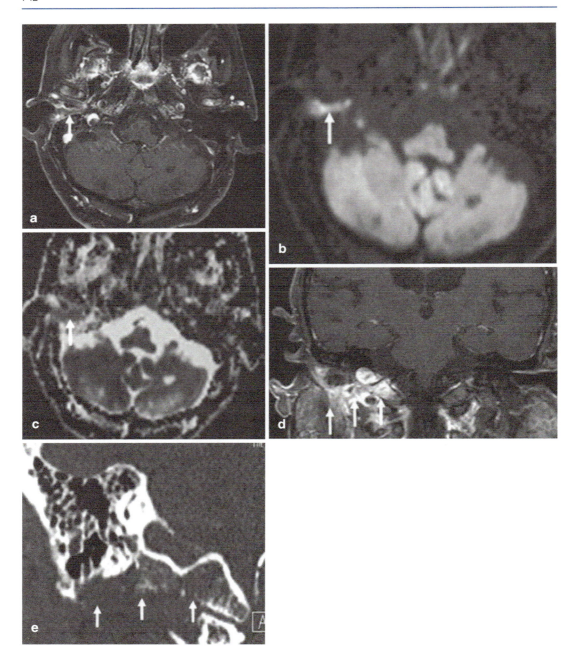

Fig. 20.30 (**a–e**) Malignant otitis externa in a 65-year-old man with type 2 diabetes mellitus. (**a**) Postcontrast axial T1-weighted image with fat saturation shows a rim enhancing fluid collection in the right external auditory canal (arrow). (**b, c**) DWI shows hyperintensity in the right external auditory canal with mildly decreased ADC representing pus collections (arrows). (**d**) Postcontrast coronal T1-weighted image with fat saturation shows extensive enhancement in the soft tissue and bone marrow consistent with cellulitis and osteomyelitis (arrows). (**e**) Coronal CT shows osseous destructions of the inferior aspect of the right petrous bone and clivus (arrows)

20 Head and Neck

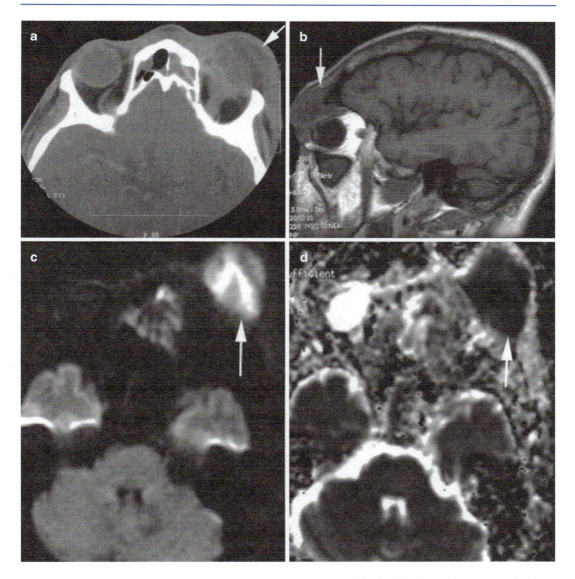

Fig. 20.31 (a–d) Pott's puffy tumor (subperiosteal abscess) in a 71-year-old man. (a) CT shows a left periorbital mass and soft tissue swelling (arrow). (b) Precontrast sagittal T1-weighted image demonstrates a heterogeneously hypointense mass located in the subperiosteal space (arrow). (c, d) DWI shows the subperiosteal abscess as very hyperintense lesion associated with very decreased ADC (0.26–0.48 × 10^{-3} mm^2/s), which is a characteristic of pus collections and abscess formations (arrow)

signal changes/ADC values [71] (Fig. 20.33). The orbit is a relatively common location for metastasis and other malignancies which will show diffusion abnormalities (Figs. 20.34 and 20.35). Orbital venous varix can be confounding due to blood products showing diffusion restriction with low ADC values and can thus be confused with tumors (Fig. 20.36).

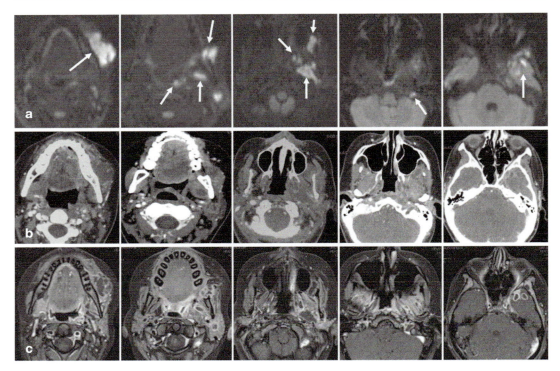

Fig. 20.32 (a–c) DWI (a) clearly demonstrates peritonsilar abscess extending into the parapharyngeal, masticator spaces, parotid gland, and anterior temporal lobe with an associated jugular vein thrombosis (arrows) in comparison with CT (b) and postcontrast T1WI. (c) ADC value in the abscess is very low (0.43–1.56 × 10^{-3} mm^2/s) (not shown)

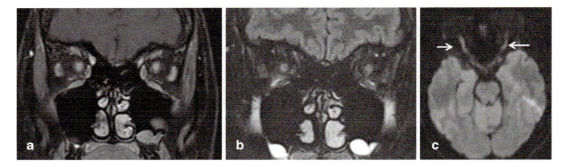

Fig. 20.33 (a–c) Optic neuritis in a 33-year-old woman with bilateral visual loss with raised intracranial pressure. (a) Postcontrast T1WI with fat saturation shows bilateral symmetric optic nerve enhancement and swelling, which are symmetric hyperintensity on FLAIR (b). (c) DWI clearly demonstrates the optic neuritis as high signal intensity

20.10 Salivary Gland Tumors

DWI can add information to imaging of salivary gland tumors. The mean ADC value of pleomorphic adenoma (1.5–2.2 × 10^{-3} mm^2/s) is significantly higher than those of both Warthin and malignant tumors [72, 73] (Figs. 20.37, 20.38, and 20.39). This is because of their heterogeneous composition containing epithelial, myoepithelial, and stromal cells with areas of fluid

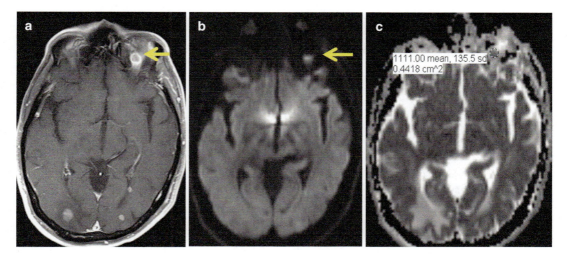

Fig. 20.34 (a–c) Orbital and brain metastasis from papillary thyroid carcinoma in a 62-year-old man. (a) Postcontrast T1WI shows a ring enhancing metastasis in the left orbit and multiple enhancing brain metastases in the occipital lobes. (b, c) DWI shows a hyperintense with intermediate ADC values (1.11×10^{-3} mm^2/s) suggestive of intermediate cellularity

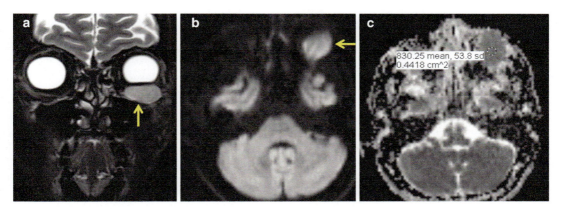

Fig. 20.35 (a–c) Spindle cell carcinoma of the left lower eyelid in a 59-year-old woman. (a) T2WI shows a homogeneous hyperintense mass lesion in the left lower eyelid. (b, c) DWI shows high signal with decreased ADC value measuring 0.83×10^{-3} mm^2/s, suggestive of relatively hypercellular malignant tumor

within the epithelial glandular tissue. Warthin tumors have low ADC values with a range of 0.72–0.96 × 10^{-3} mm^2/s (Fig. 20.38). This is due to the presence of epithelial and lymphoid stroma having protein-rich microcysts (74). Advanced diffusion methods like DTI can help to differentiate benign from malignant tumors with low FA values [74]. Both malignant salivary gland tumors and their recurrence will show low ADC values due to increased cellularity unlike post-treatment changes (Fig. 20.31). Higher ADC value of mucoepidermoid cancer has been linked to their increased mucus content [75].

20.11 Bone Metastases

Potentially, DWI provides information to allow better discrimination of soft tissue or osseous metastatic lesions in various locations of head and neck bony structures. However, DWI characteristics of benign and malignant lesions can

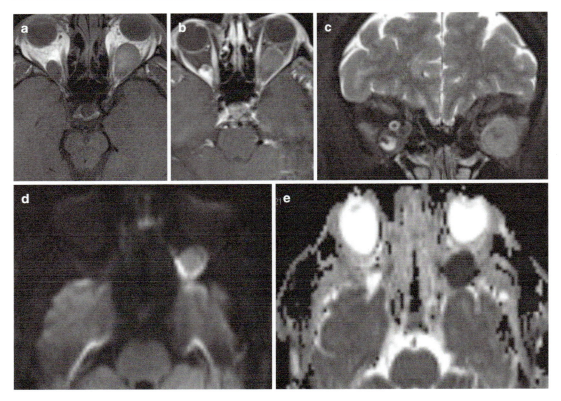

Fig. 20.36 (a–e) Bilateral orbital varices. A 58-year-old man woke up in the morning to find that he has double vision. (a, b) Pre- and postcontrast T1WI and (c) T2WI show bilateral orbital apical masses, right is enhancing with T2 hyperintense and left not enhancing with T2 isointense. (d, e) DWI shows a hyperintense mass with very low ADC values measuring 0.34×10^{-3} mm^2/s, which raised the possibility of malignancy as the patient was also known to have malignant melanoma and mastocytosis. Biopsy of the left mass revealed only blood clots consistent with a thrombosed varix

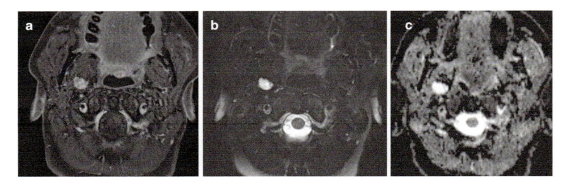

Fig. 20.37 (a–c) Pleomorphic adenoma. (a) Postcontrast T1WI shows enhancing lesion in the deep lobe of the right parotid gland. (b, c) Fat saturation T2WI shows hyperintensity of the lesion with increased ADC measuring 2.31×10^{-3} mm^2/s

20 Head and Neck

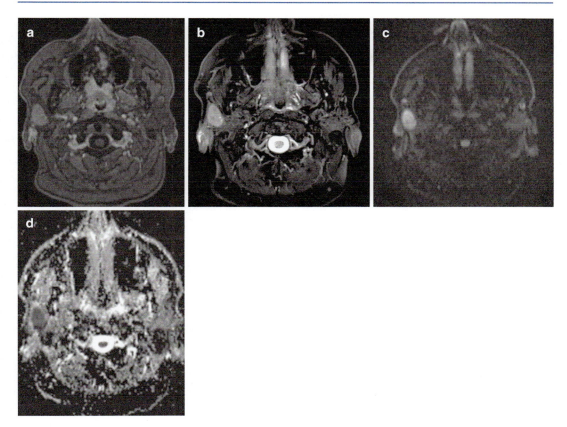

Fig. 20.38 (a–d) Warthin's tumor. (a) Postcontrast T1WI shows a homogeneously enhancing mass lesion in the superficial lobe of the right parotid gland. (b) Fat saturation T2WI shows mild hyperintensity of the lesion. (c) DWI shows hyperintense with decreased ADC measuring 0.71×10^{-3} mm^2/s (d)

overlap. Moon et al., using DWI with sensitivity encoding (SENSE), a parallel imaging technique that reduces susceptibility artifacts in the skull base, studied 13 patients with 20 cranial bone marrow metastases, and found that DWI of metastases demonstrated better lesion conspicuity than T1-weighted images and b0 images on a qualitative basis [76]. On a quantitative analysis, lesion contrast was best shown on b0 images. All metastatic lesions in the study demonstrated increased signal on DWI and b0 images compared to normal bone marrow.

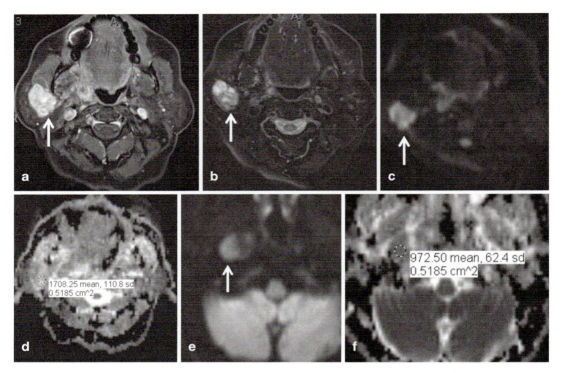

Fig. 20.39 (**a–f**) Pleomorphic adenoma with malignant transformation in deep lobe of the right parotid gland. (**a**) Postcontrast T1WI shows an enhancing mass lesion in the superficial lobe of the right parotid gland. (**b**) Fat saturation T2WI shows hyperintensity of the lesion. (**c, d**) DWI shows hyperintense of the mass in the superficial lobe of parotid with high ADC values of 1.7×10^{-3} mm^2/s which turned out to be benign pleomorphic adenoma. (**e, f**) The mass in the deep lobe has low ADC values of 0.9×10^{-3} mm^2/s which turned out to be carcinoma

In a study by Nemeth et al., the authors found that DWI improved the detection of skull metastatic disease over conventional MRI [77]. Detection of focal breast cancer and lung cancer metastatic disease was improved by 20% and 36.3%, respectively. However, the fat saturation technique was not used for conventional T2- and postcontrast T1-weighted images. Postcontrast T1-weighted images with fat saturation and DWI probably demonstrate better lesion conspicuity than other conventional MR sequences (Figs. 20.40, 20.41, 20.42, 20.43, 20.44, 20.45, 20.46, and 20.47). The signal intensity on DWI and the ADC values in bone metastases mainly depend on the tumor cellularity, extracellular matrix, and necrosis. Metastasis from hypercellular tumors such as Ewing sarcoma (Fig. 20.43), neuroblastoma (Fig. 20.44), and small cell carcinoma can show significant hyperintensity on DWI associated with decreased ADC. Intermediate cellular metastasis shows hyperintensity on DWI with mildly increased ADC (T2 shine-through) (Fig. 20.40, 20.41, and 20.46). The area of necrosis usually shows hypointensity on DWI with increased ADC (Fig. 20.41 and 20.43). The area of sclerotic bone metastasis may be difficult to detect on DWI because of the lack of mobile protons and diamagnetic susceptibility artifact from sclerotic osseous tissue mixed with the tumor cells. Some authors have advised caution when interpreting ADC values in the bone marrow because of the high lipid marrow component, especially if more than 30%, and its possible effect on DW signals and ADC values [78, 79].

20 Head and Neck

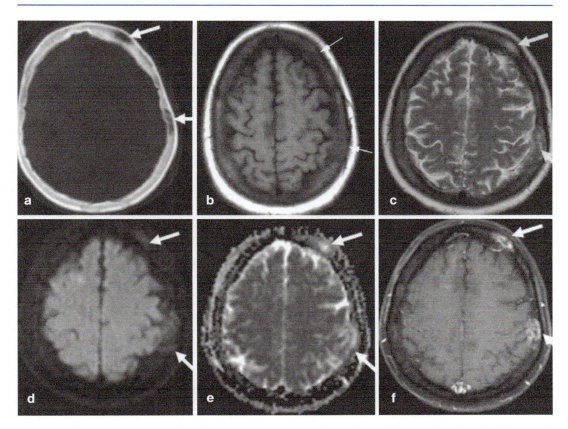

Fig. 20.40 (a–f) Bone metastasis from breast carcinoma in a 38-year-old woman. (a) CT shows permeative lytic lesions in the left calvarium (arrows). (b) Precontrast sagittal T1-weighted image shows the lesions as isointense (arrows). (c) T2-weighted image shows the lesions as slightly hyperintense (arrows). (d, e) DWI clearly shows the lesions as hyperintense and associated with increased ADC in the skull (intermediate cellularity and necrosis) (arrows). (f) Postcontrast with fat saturation T1-weighted image demonstrates necrotic enhancing bone metastases (arrows)

Since DWI is innately T2-weighted with fat saturation, T2 blackout can affect the signals as an artifact due to the presence of fat. DWI also shows scalp metastases as hyperintense signals.

DWI can be useful for evaluating the therapeutic response of leukemic infiltration (Fig. 20.46) [80, 81]. Moon et al. displayed the DWI in an inverted gray-white scale in the evaluation of bone metastasis or bone marrow infiltration, similar to that used in bone scans, for their qualitative analysis [76]. They felt this allowed easier comparison with bone scans and PET images.

Myeloma is a malignant bone marrow disorder due to excess proliferation of monoclonal plasma cells. Five different infiltrative patterns have been described on MRI, of which salt and pepper infiltrative pattern is the most common, although classic description on CT and radiographs is the punched out lytic lesion. DWI allows increased lesion conspicuity and ADC measurement allows detection of response to treatment with an initial rise followed by a fall. Initial increase is attributed to death of plasma cells with increased extracellular water, followed by sustained decrease in ADC [82].

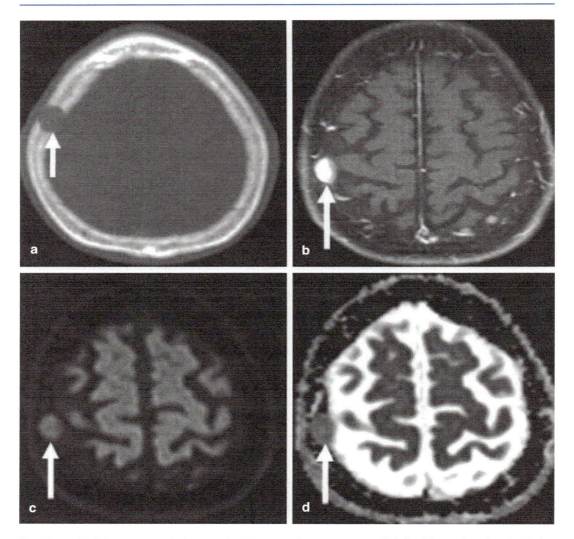

Fig. 20.41 (a–d) Bone metastasis from renal cell carcinoma in a 64-year-old man. (a) CT shows a lytic bone metastasis from renal cell carcinoma in the skull (arrow). (b) Postcontrast T1-weighted image with fat saturation demonstrates a well-defined intensely enhancing lesion (arrow). (c, d) DWI shows the lesion as hyperintense associated with slightly increased ADC values representing intermediate cellularity (arrow)

20.12 Squamous Cell Carcinoma (SCCA) and Lymphoma in Head and Neck Area

In a study using echo-planar DW imaging by Wang et al., the mean ADC of malignant lymphomas was lower than that of carcinomas (lymphoma $0.66 \pm 0.17 \times 10^{-3}$ mm²/s versus carcinomas $1.13 \pm 0.43 \times 10^{-3}$ mm²/s) (Figs. 20.48, 20.49, 20.50, 20.51, 20.52, 20.53, and 20.54) [83]. They also found the ADC of lymphoma and carcinoma to be significantly lower than that of benign solid tumors or benign cystic lesions (benign solid tumors $1.56 \pm 0.51 \times 10^{-3}$ mm²/s; mean ADC of benign cystic lesions $2.05 \pm 0.62 \times 10^{-3}$ mm²/s)

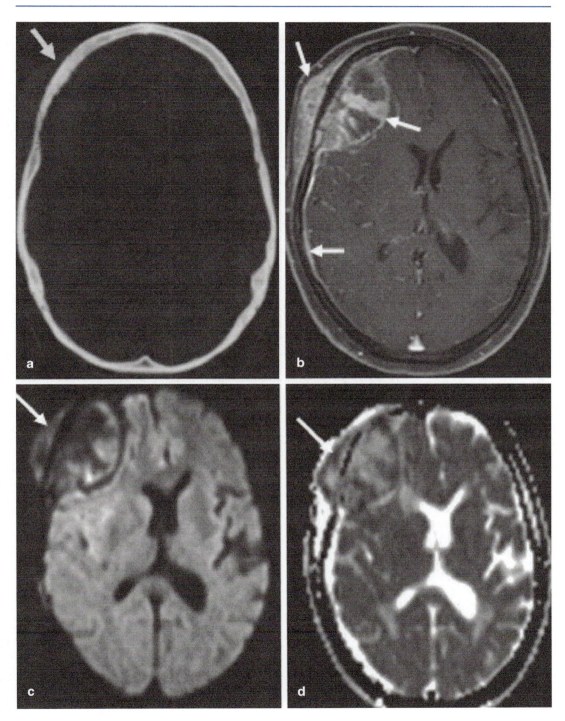

Fig. 20.42 (**a–d**) Bone metastasis from breast carcinoma in a 45-year-old woman. (**a**) CT shows a large soft tissue density mass involving the right frontal skull and scalp with underlying sclerotic bony changes (arrow). (**b**) Postcontrast T1-weighted image with fat saturation shows a heterogeneously enhancing necrotic mass and dural enhancement (arrows). (**c**) DWI shows a large mass with central low and peripheral iso- or high signal intensity associated with central high and peripheral low ADC values (arrow). (**d**) The area of sclerotic bone metastasis may be difficult to detect on DWI because of the lack of mobile protons in the sclerotic bone changes surrounding tumor cells

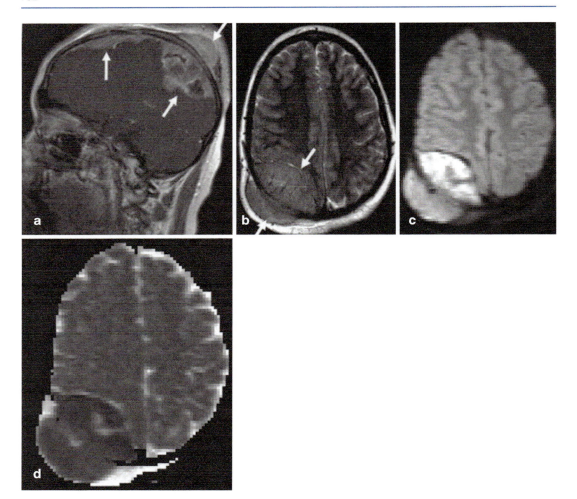

Fig. 20.43 (a–d) Bone metastasis from Ewing sarcoma in a 14-year-old boy. (**a**) Postcontrast T1-weighted image with fat saturation shows a heterogeneously enhancing mass and dural enhancement involving the right frontoparietal skull and scalp (arrows). (**b**) T2-weighted image shows a large isointense mass (arrows). (**c, d**) DWI reveals a homogeneously very hyperintense mass lesion associated with greatly decreased ADC (0.48–0.79 × 10^{-3} mm^2/s), which represents hypercellularity of the Ewing tumor. The DWI characteristics help differentiate such hypercellular small round cell tumors from other types of metastatic disease

(Fig. 20.55). In order to reduce susceptibility artifacts commonly seen with echo-planar DW imaging in the evaluation of head and neck lesions, Maeda et al. used line-scan DW imaging to study squamous cell carcinomas and malignant lymphomas [84]. They found ADC values to be significantly lower in lymphomas than in squamous cell carcinomas (lymphoma 0.65 ± 0.09 × 10^{-3} mm^2/s versus squamous cell carcinoma 0.96 ± 0.11 × 10^{-3} mm^2/s).

King et al. also found a threshold value that helped differentiate squamous cell carcinoma from lymphoma [85]. They found that an ADC value greater than 0.82 × 10^{-3} mm^2/s could identify and differentiate squamous cell carcinoma from lymphoma which has an ADC value less than 0.767 × 10^{-3} mm^2/s with a specificity of 100%. Sensitivity for squamous cell carcinoma was 94% and for lymphoma 88%.

The ADCs of skull base and sinus malignancies are significantly lower than those of benign lesions ($p = 0.012$) (Figs. 20.48, 20.49, and 20.50) [86]. ADC map can help to detect bone marrow infiltration of the skull base and helps in

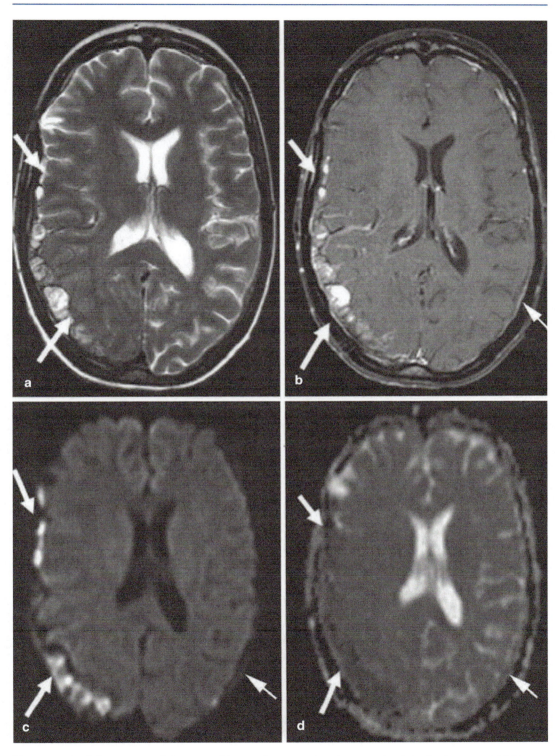

Fig. 20.44 (**a–d**) Bone metastasis from neuroblastoma in a 15-year-old boy. (**a**) T2-weighted image shows multiple hyperintense mass lesions along the right frontoparietooccipital skull and dura (arrows). (**b**) Postcontrast T1-weighted image with fat saturation shows heterogeneously enhancement and dural enhancement (right more than left) (arrows). (**c, d**) DWI reveals irregular dural based hyperintense mass in the right frontoparietal region with decreased ADC (0.52–0.89 × 10^{-3} mm^2/s) corresponding to the hypercellularity of neuroblastoma (arrows)

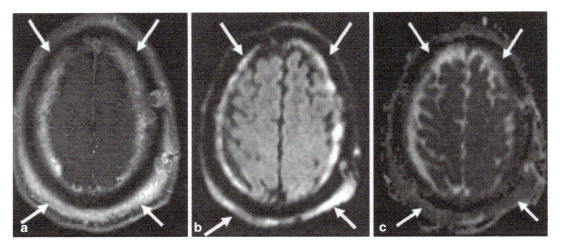

Fig. 20.45 (**a–c**) Diffuse bone, dural, and scalp metastasis from prostate carcinoma in an 89-year-old man. (**a**) Postcontrast T1-weighted image with fat saturation shows diffuse marked enhancement in the dura and scalp (arrows). Diffuse sclerotic bony changes are noted in the skull. (**b, c**) DWI shows diffuse hyperintense lesions in the dura and scalp associated with decreased ADC (arrows). Diffuse sclerotic bone metastases are seen as low signal intensity on DW images. It is difficult to calculate the ADC value of the bone marrow infiltration accurately

the differentiation between malignant and benign tumors [87]. The mean ADC value of nasal and paranasal sinus malignant lesions (1.10×10^{-3} mm^2/s) is significantly different ($P = 0.001$) from that of benign lesions (1.78×10^{-3} mm^2/s) [86] (Figs. 20.49, 20.55, 20.56, and 20.57).

However, when evaluated in conjunction with nasopharyngeal carcinoma (Fig. 20.54), the determination of a threshold value with high sensitivity and specificity was problematic because of overlapping ADC values. Using 3-T DW imaging, Srinivasan et al. found malignant head and neck lesions to have significantly lower ADC values than benign lesions [53]. White et al., despite moderately overlapping values, also found the mean ADC values for malignant lesions to be significantly lower than for benign lesions [44]. In pharyngeal squamous cell carcinoma, DWI did not add significantly to the negative predictive value obtained with conventional MRI in evaluation of the primary pathology although studies have shown that lower mean ADC values in malignant lesions compared to benign lesions [88]. According to Herman [89], in squamous cell cancer, DWI appears helpful in distinguishing radiotherapy-induced tissue changes from persistent or recurrent cancer.

In recurrent head and neck squamous cell carcinoma, it is often difficult to detect recurrence on routine MRI due to morphological changes induced by treatment like edema, fibrosis, ulceration, denervation atrophy, etc. In a study of 74 patients with head and neck squamous cell carcinoma, Becker M et al. report that using ADC mean ≤ 1.208, the sensitivity for the detection of recurrence was 80.5% and the specificity was 82.0%. Combining with PET SUV, they found that it improved sensitivity and specificity as DWI helped to discriminate false-positive findings on PET [90, 91] (Figs. 20.50 and 20.51).

In melanomas, low ADC values have also been described [92] (Fig. 20.55), as well as primary or metastatic hypercellular tumors such as rhabdomyosarcoma, olfactory neuroblastoma, and neuroblastoma (Fig. 20.56). Benign lymphoid tissues in tonsils and adenoids can show hyperintensity on DW imaging associated with relatively low ADC values (Fig. 20.57). Juvenile nasopharyngeal angiofibromas (JNA) is a rare benign neoplasm seen in young adolescents with male predilection. They are centered in the nasopharynx presenting commonly with nasal obstruction with or without epistaxis. On MRI, they appear as intensely enhancing mass lesions centered in

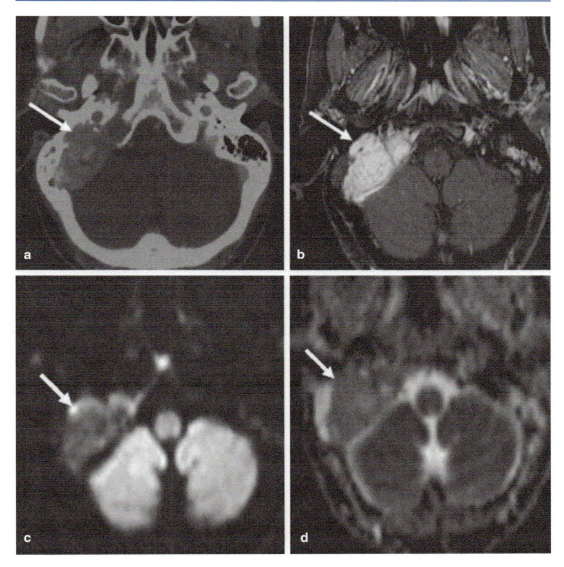

Fig. 20.46 (a–d) Mastoid bone metastasis from breast carcinoma in a 58-year-old woman. (**a**) CT shows a lytic bone destruction in the right petrous bone (arrows). (**b**) Postcontrast T1-weighted image with fat saturation shows intense homogeneous enhancement in the mass (arrows). (**c, d**) DWI shows a hyperintense mass with mildly increased ADC ($0.96–1.66 \times 10^{-3}$ mm^2/s) in the right mastoid (arrows), which probably corresponds to the intermediate cellularity of the tumor

the nasopharynx extending into pterygopalatine and infratemporal fossae. They are usually hypointense on T1 and heterogeneously hyperintense on T2WI. High ADC values have been reported in juvenile nasopharyngeal angiofibromas [93] (Fig. 20.57).

20.12.1 Lymph Node Metastasis

Benign lymph nodes can show hyperintensity on DW imaging associated with relatively low ADC values (Fig. 20.58) [94–97]. Sumi et al. found that metastatic lymph nodes with moderately dif-

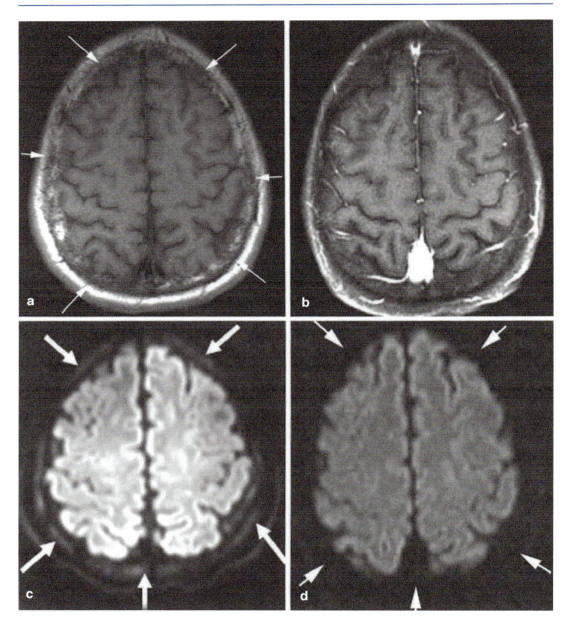

Fig. 20.47 (**a**–**d**) Leukemia in a 23-year-old woman. (**a**, **b**) Pre- and postcontrast T1-weighted images show diffuse heterogeneous signals in the bone marrow of the skull (arrows). (**c**) DW image shows diffuse hyperintense lesions in the skull which probably represents leukemic infiltrations (arrow). (**d**) After the course of chemotherapy, the DW imaging abnormalities have disappeared (arrow)

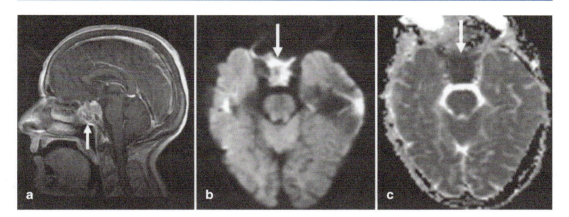

Fig. 20.48 (a–d) Malignant lymphoma in the skull base in a 74-year-old woman. (a) Postcontrast sagittal T1-weighted image shows an inhomogeneously enhancing mass in the skull base (arrow). (b, c) DWI reveals a homogeneously very hyperintense mass in the skull base with decreased ADC (0.46–0.62×10^{-3} mm^2/s) (arrow), (d) which corresponds to hypercellularity of the lymphoma

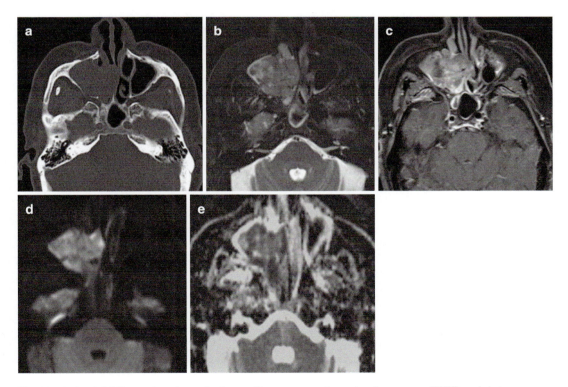

Fig. 20.49 (a–e) Malignant lymphoma in the maxillary sinus in a 69-year-old man. (a) CT shows a mass lesion in the right maxillary sinus extending into the right nostril with bony erosions. (b, c) MRI demonstrates heterogeneous low signal mass on T2WI and heterogeneous enhancement on fat-sat postcontrast T1WI. (d, e) DWI demonstrates hyperintensity with low ADC values (0.49–0.88×10^{-3} mm^2/s)

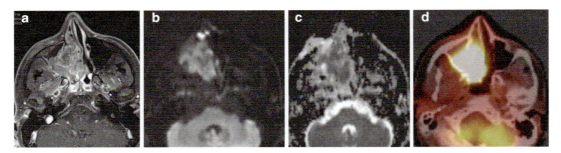

Fig. 20.50 (**a–d**) Sinonasal squamous cell carcinoma. (**a**) Postcontrast T1WI shows a heterogeneously enhancing sinonasal mass. (**b, c**) DWI demonstrates hyperintensity with low ADC values (0.70–1.12×10^{-3} mm^2/s.). (**d**) FDG-PET reveals an avid uptake in the tumor

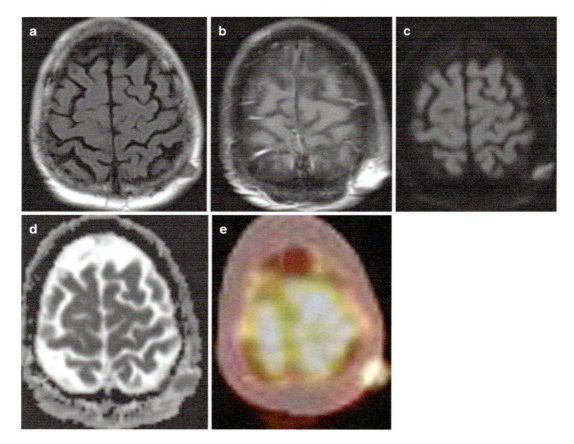

Fig. 20.51 (**a–e**) Scalp metastatic squamous cell carcinoma. (**a**) FLAIR, (**b**) Postcontrast T1WI, show a left parietal scalp enhancing lesions. (**c**) DWI clearly shows the scalp tumor due to nulling of the fat and free water in comparison with conventional MRIs. (**d**) The ADC value (1.01×10^{-3} mm^2/s) suggests an intermediate cellularity of the tumor. (**e**) FDG-PET reveals an avid uptake in the scalp tumor

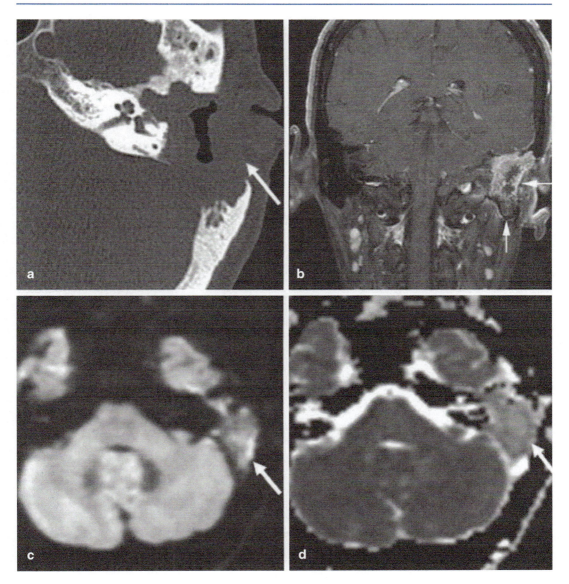

Fig. 20.52 (**a–d**) Primary squamous cell carcinoma in the middle ear in a 64-year-old man. (**a**) CT shows a soft tissue density mass with bone destruction in the left mastoid and middle ear cavity (arrow). (**b**) Postcontrast T1-weighted image with fat saturation shows heterogeneously enhancing necrotic mass (arrow). (**c, d**) DWI shows hyperintensity in the left mastoid and middle ear cavity with mildly increased ADC (1.03–1.46×10^{-3} mm^2/s) (arrow), which probably corresponds to the intermediate cellularity and necrosis in squamous cell carcinoma

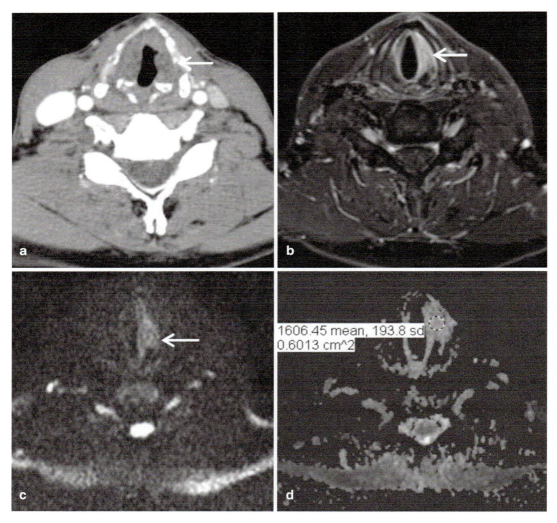

Fig. 20.53 (**a–d**) Laryngeal carcinoma (squamous cell carcinoma) in a 64-year-old man. (**a, b**) Contrast-enhanced CT and MRI showing mildly enhancing lesion in the left vocal cord (arrow). (**c, d**) DWI shows hyperintensity with increased ADC measuring 1.6×10^{-3} mm^2/s

ferentiated carcinomas had significantly higher ADC values than those of poorly differentiated carcinoma and approximated those of malignant lymphoma [96] (Figs. 20.59, 20.60, and 20.61). Abdel Razek et al. found the mean ADC of metastatic and lymphomatous nodes to be significantly lower than benign nodes [94]. Additionally, they found two patients with benign nodes (sarcoid and cat scratch disease) with relatively low ADC values. Castleman disease is a benign B cell lymphoproliferative disorder that can affect the neck. It is also called angiofollicular lymph node hyperplasia or giant lymph node hyperplasia. On DWI it can show decreased ADC values [98] (Fig. 20.62).

20.12.2 Perineural Tumor Spread

Perineural tumor spread is an important imaging feature to look for on MRI. Conventional MRI demonstrates neuroforaminal enlargement, oblit-

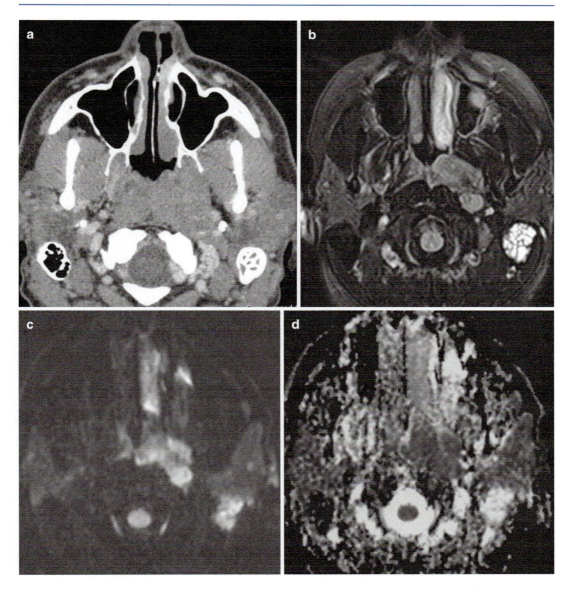

Fig. 20.54 (a–d) Nasopharyngeal carcinoma in a 31-year-old male with 16-year smoking history and HPV positive. (a) Contrast-enhanced CT of neck shows mildly enhancing mass in the left nasopharynx. (b) fat-sat T2WI shows left nasopharyngeal mass and left retropharyngeal lymphadenopathy. (c, d) DWI and ADC map demonstrate hyperintensity with low ADC measuring 0.5×10^{-3} mm^2/s

eration of the normal distribution of the fat pad, abnormal enhancement, or mass lesion along the nerve. DWI can clearly show the perineural tumor spread due to nulling of the fat and free water in comparison with conventional MRIs (Figs. 20.63 and 20.64). Rouchy RC et al. report that DTI is a potentially useful tool for the evaluation of perineural tumor spread. Average path-length on diffusion tractography was significantly higher with perineural tumor spread along with visualization of the changes on tractography map, although FA values did not differ [99].

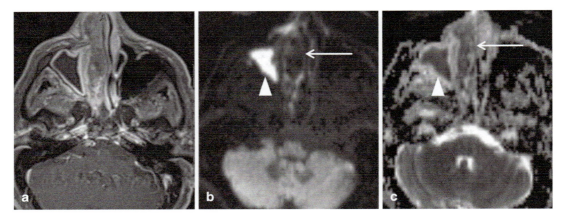

Fig. 20.55 (**a–c**) Nasal melanoma and right maxillary sinus viscus fluid. 82-year-old male who 2 months prior to initial consultation underwent surgery to remove a skin cancer from his left hand. When nasal cannula was placed, it was painful and his nose started to bleed. (**a**) Postcontrast T1WI shows a heterogeneous enhancing nostril mass. Mucosal thickening and fluid collection in the right maxillary sinus are seen. (**b**) DWI demonstrates very hyperintensity in the sinus fluid (arrowhead). DWI hypointensity in the nostril mass is likely due to T2 shortening of the presence of melanin (arrow). (**c**) ADC measurement revealed low ADC in right maxillary sinus due to viscosity of the retained mucous fluid (arrowhead). Right nostril mass shows low ADC values due to hypercellularity of melanoma (arrow)

20.13 Conclusion

DWI demonstrates benign and malignant head and neck lesions well, even if the lesion is very small or diffuse, because of the significant contrast in the surrounding scalp and skull structures with fat saturation techniques. DWI with ADC maps demonstrates characteristics unique to certain etiologies, particularly abscesses, hypercellular tumors, and epidermoids.

20.14 Treatment of Head and Neck Cancers

Molly Heft Neal, Andrew C. Birkeland, and Matthew E. Spector

Head and neck cancers are the sixth most common cancer worldwide [100, 101]. The vast majority of head and neck cancers are squamous cell carcinomas (HNSCC), and the most commonly affected sites include the oral cavity, larynx, and oropharynx [102]. Traditionally, tobacco and alcohol use have been the main causative agents for HNSCC, particularly of the oral cavity and larynx as well as the oropharynx [100]. However, over the past three decade there has been a decrease in tobacco use and an increase in high-risk HPV infections resulting in an increasing incidence of HPV-mediated oropharyngeal squamous cell carcinoma (OPSCC) with a subsequent decrease in HPV-negative OPSCC [102–104]. Due to this rising incidence, OPSCC now represents the most common site of HNSCC [102]. Overall patients with HPV-mediated disease have improved survival compared to patients with HPV-negative tumors and HPV has become one of the only predictive biomarkers in HNSCC [103]. HPV status is routinely tested, using p16 as a surrogate marker, for all patients presenting with oropharyngeal squamous cell carcinoma [105].

The improved prognosis of HPV-mediated disease is one of changes reflected in the recent update to the American Joint Committee on Cancer (AJCC) 8th edition for HNSCC. These changed were put into effect starting in 2018 [106]. The oral cavity, larynx, and oropharynx subsites each have separate primary tumor stag-

20 Head and Neck

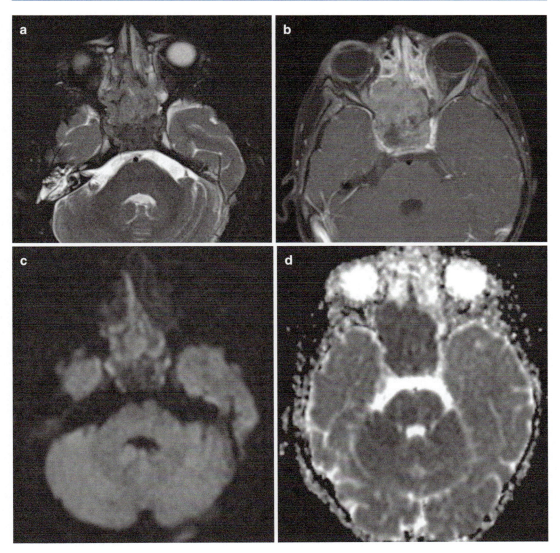

Fig. 20.56 (**a–d**) Metastatic neuroblastoma in a 5-year-old female with loss of vision. Stage IV neuroblastoma status post-surgery, chemotherapy, and autologous stem cell transplant. T2WI (**a**) and postcontrast T1WI (**b**) show a relatively T2 low and enhancing mass filling the naso- pharynx and posterior ethmoid sinus. DWI (**c**) demonstrates mildly mixed hypo- and hyperintensity with homogeneously decreased ADC (**d**) in the mass. The hypointensity on DWI in the mass is due to T2 dark through effect

ing criteria (T1-4) and nodal staging has been divided into clinical and pathologic staging (N1-3; Tables 20.1, 20.2, 20.3, and 20.4). HPV-mediated OPSCC has a separate T and N staging as well as overall staging criteria (Tables 20.1, 20.2, 20.3, and 20.4) to reflect the improved survival in this cohort. The AJCC 8th edition has also included notable changes to staging for oral cavity SCCs as discussed below. Radiologic imaging (in particular MR) is critical in determining the extent of disease and providing accurate staging of HNSCC which helps to guide appropriate treatment planning. Surgery, cytotoxic chemotherapy, and radiation therapy (XRT)

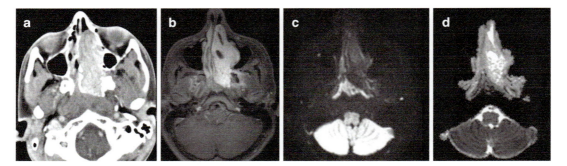

Fig. 20.57 (**a–d**) Juvenile nasopharyngeal angiofibroma, 15-year-old male with a 6-year history of nasal obstruction. (**a**) Contrast-enhanced CT of neck shows avidly enhancing mass in the left nasopharynx, nasal cavity, and left sphenopalatine foramen/pterygopalatine fossa. (**b**) Postcontrast T1WI shows homogeneous intense enhancement with flow voids. (**c, d**) DWI and ADC map demonstrate slight hyperintensity with increased ADC measuring $1.8–2.5 \times 10^{-3}$ mm^2/s. Enlarged nasopharyngeal tonsils shows DWI hyperintense with intermediate ADC values 0.9×10^{-3} mm^2/s

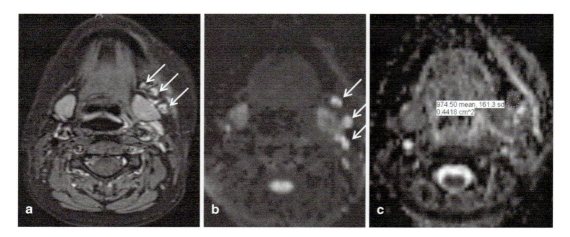

Fig. 20.58 (**a–c**) Reactive lymph node swelling to head and neck infection in an 18-year-old female. (**a**) Postcontrast T1WI shows multiple enhancing lymph nodes with a fatty hilum in the left neck. (**b, c**) DWI and ADC map demonstrate hyperintensity with intermediate ADC values 0.95×10^{-3} mm^2/s indicating a benign etiology

are the primary treatment modalities in HNSCC; these are used in different combinations based on tumor site and stage, among other characteristics. National Cancer Care Network (NCCN) guidelines are used to determine appropriate treatment for HNSCC based on site and stage [107]. Neck dissection is utilized for all patients with clinical or radiographic evidence of nodal disease and in select patients with advanced disease depending of the primary tumor site. Radiographic levels of the neck are important for staging purposes and include: level Ia (submental group) bounded by the anterior bellies of the digastric muscle, level Ib (submandibular group) bounded by the anterior and posterior bellies of the digastric muscle and the inferior border of the mandible, level II (upper jugular chain) bounded by the skull base superiorly, hyoid bone inferiorly, sternocleidomastoid muscle posteriorly and strap muscles anteriorly, level III (mid

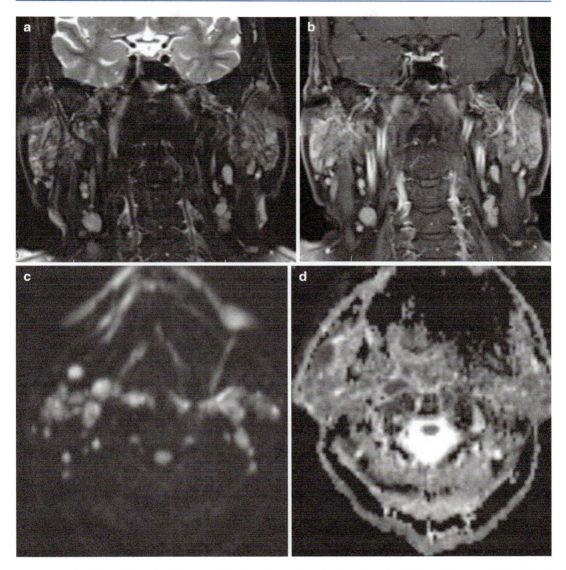

Fig. 20.59 (a–d) Lymphoma in a 50-year-old male, radiation worker presenting with enlarged painful parotid glands with extensive cervical lymphadenopathy. (**a, b**) Coronal T2WI and postcontrast T1WI show multiple enhancing lymph nodes in the swollen parotid glands and in the bilateral neck areas. (**c, d**) DWI shows restriction due to the high cellularity of the lymphoma with decreased ADC values ($0.5–0.7 \times 10^{-3}$ mm^2/s)

jugular chain) which extends from the hyoid bone superiorly to the cricoid cartilage inferiorly with the same anterior and posterior borders as those in level II and level IV (lower jugular chain) bounded superiorly by the cricoid and inferiorly by the clavicle (anterior and posterior borders remain SCM and strap musculature) [108]. Beyond surgery and CRT, novel therapies, such as immunotherapy targeting PD-1, are actively being investigated with encouraging initial results [109, 110], and are now approved as first line for recurrent/metastatic disease [111]. However, these treatment modalities are restricted to recurrent/metastatic setting and are not part of initial standard of care for curable disease.

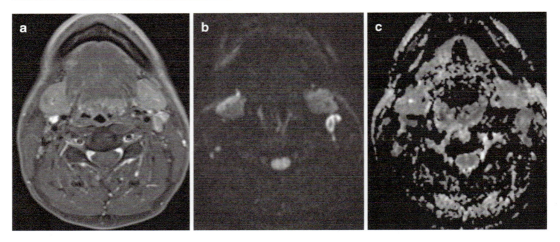

Fig. 20.60 (a–c) Metastatic necrotic lymph node from left vocal cord squamous cell carcinoma in 69-year-old man. (a) Postcontrast T1WI shows an 8 × 1.5 mm left level 2A enhancing necrotic lymph node. (b) DWI demonstrates the necrotic lymph node as hyperintense with the ADC value measuring 0.7×10^{-3} mm^2/s in the solid portion. (c) Lymph node metastasis was proven by a biopsy

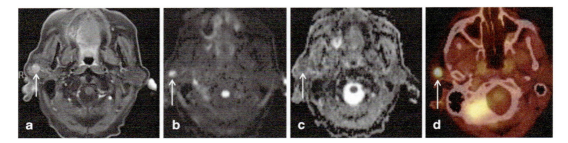

Fig. 20.61 (a–d) Metastatic intraparotid lymph node from scalp squamous cell carcinoma. (a) Postcontrast T1WI with fat saturation shows an enhancing intraparotid lymph node (arrows). (b) DWI clearly demonstrates the lymph node as a high signal lesion (arrow). (c) The ADC values were 0.8×10^{-3} mm^2/s due to the high cellularity of the lymph node metastasis (arrow). (d) PET scan shows a high uptake in the area

20.14.1 Staging and Treatment of Oral Cavity Squamous Cell Carcinoma

For the AJCC 8th edition staging for oral cavity SCC, radiographic evidence of a tumor greater than 2 cm in maximum dimension or greater than 5 mm depth of invasion upstages a tumor to T2, and a tumor greater than 4 cm or depth of invasion greater than 10 mm upstages a tumor to T3. Invasion through cortical bone upstages cancers to T4a. Tumors involving the pterygoid plates or skull base, internal artery encasement, and masticator space invasion are considered T4b, and surgically unresectable (Table 20.1). Nodal disease ranges from no clinical or radiographic evidence of disease (N0), to clinically evident disease with extranodal extension (N3b) (Table 20.3).

The gold standard for treatment of oral cavity SCCs is surgical resection, with adjuvant XRT or chemoradiation as dictated by final surgical stage and pathology (i.e., margin status, perineural invasion). Radiation and chemoradiation

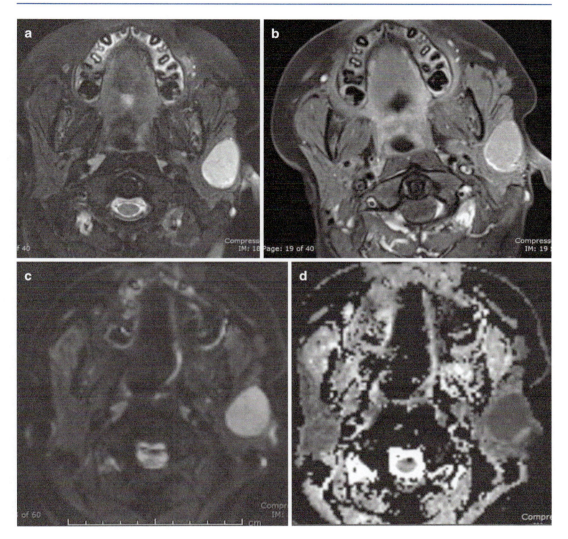

Fig. 20.62 (**a–d**) Castleman's disease involving parotid gland and neck lymph nodes in a 36-year-old woman. (**a**) T2WI with fat saturation shows a hyperintense mass in the left parotid. (**b**) Postcontrast T1WI with fat saturation shows homogeneous enhancing left parotid mass. (**c**) DWI shows bright signal and decreased ADC (0.5–0.6×10^{-3} mm^2/s) (**d**)

alone have been proven to be ineffective for oral cavity SCC, but may be utilized in surgically unresectable cases. Depending on the extent of resection in the oral cavity, reconstructive options are often considered, ranging from primary closure for small defects to soft tissue and bone free tissue transfers for extensive defects. Neck dissections are recommended for clinically or radiographically positive disease, generally including neck levels I-IV. Ipsilateral neck dissections are acceptable for lateralized tumors that do not approach midline, otherwise bilateral neck dissections are recommended. For N0 necks, advanced tumors (T3 or T4) and/or depth of invasion greater than 4 mm warrant a neck dissection [112].

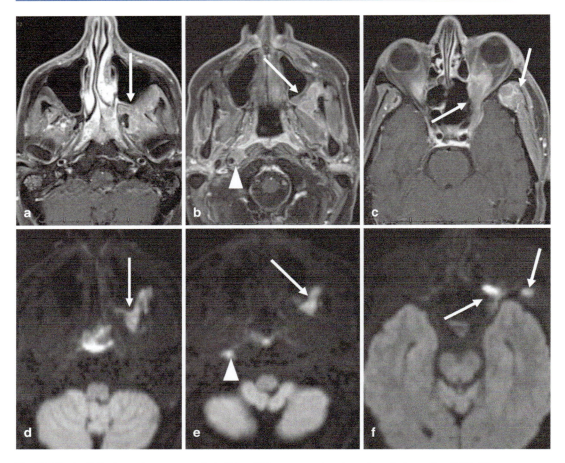

Fig. 20.63 (**a–f**) Perineural tumor spread via V2 and V3. 56-year-old man with nasopharyngeal carcinoma. (**a–c**) Postcontrast T1WIs with fat saturation show enhancing nasopharyngeal soft tissue mass extending into the left widening sphenopalatine foramen, pterygopalatine fossa, and pterygomaxillary fissure (arrows), and right retropharyngeal node metastasis (arrowhead) (**b**). There are superior and inferior extension along the left masticator space with involvement of the left foramen rotundum (arrow) (**c**). (**d–f**) DWI clearly demonstrates the perineural tumor spread (arrows), and right retropharyngeal node (arrowhead)

20.14.2 Staging and Treatment of Larynx Squamous Cell Carcinoma

For laryngeal SCC, imaging is critical for accurate tumor staging. Involvement of more than one laryngeal subsite makes a tumor at least T2. Tumor extension into the paraglottic or preepiglottic spaces upstages cancers to T3. Evidence of invasion through the outer cortex of the thyroid cartilage, outside the larynx, or to the extrinsic muscles of the tongue upstages cancers to T4a. Radiologic indicators of unresectability (T4b) include internal carotid artery encasement, involvement of the prevertebral fascia, and mediastinal structures (Table 20.1). Neck disease is staged similarly to oral cavity SCC (Table 20.3).

Laryngeal SCC, depending on stage and functionality of the larynx, may be treated with XRT with or without chemotherapy, or surgery with possible adjuvant treatment based upon pathology. Early stage laryngeal SCCs are often treated with endoscopic laryngeal conservation surgery or XRT alone. For advanced laryngeal SCCs, it has been established that organ preservation protocols (combinations of chemotherapy and XRT)

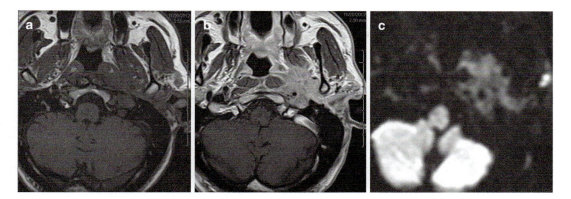

Fig. 20.64 (a–c) Perineural tumor spread via auriculo-temporal nerve. 67-year-old male with facial nerve palsy and a history of T4bNx squamous cell carcinoma of nasopharynx. (**a**, **b**) Pre- and postcontrast T1WIs show enhancing mass in the left parapharyngeal and masticator spaces extending along the auriculo-temporal nerve to the left parotid gland. Left retropharyngeal lymph node and petrous bone involvement are also seen. DWI (**c**) clearly demonstrates the perineural tumor spread and the extension of the tumor. Left periparotid lymph node metastasis is noted

Table 20.1 Primary tumor staging (oral cavity and larynx)

T stage	Oral cavity	Larynx
Tx	Cannot be assessed	Cannot be assessed
Tis	Carcinoma in situ	Carcinoma in situ
T1	Size ≤2 cm; depth of invasion (DOI) ≤5 mm	*Supraglottis*: Tumor limited to one supraglottic subsite *Glottis*: Tumor limited to the vocal cords with normal movement
T2	Size >2 cm, ≤4 cm, DOI ≤10 mm; *or* size ≤2 cm, DOI >5 mm, ≤10 mm	*Supraglottis*: Tumor involving more than one supraglottic subsite *Glottis*: Tumor involving supraglottis or subglottis and/or vocal cord paresis
T3	Size >4 cm and/or DOI >10 mm	Tumor involving paraglottic or pre-epiglottic spaces, inner cortex of the thyroid, and/or vocal cord paralysis
T4a	Invasion through cortical maxillary or mandibular bone, maxillary sinus, or involving facial skin	Tumor extension through outer cortex of thyroid, and/or extension into extralaryngeal tissues
T4b	Involvement of pterygoid plates, masticator space, skull base, and/or internal carotid artery encasement	Involvement of prevertebral space and/or mediastinal structures, internal carotid artery encasement

Table 20.2 Primary tumor staging (p16-positive and -negative oropharynx staging)

T stage	p16 positive	p16 negative
T0	No primary identified, with p16-positive nodal disease	No primary identified
T1	Size ≤2 cm	Size ≤2 cm
T2	Size >2 cm, ≤4 cm	Size >2 cm, ≤4 cm
T3	Size >4 cm, and/or extension to lingual surface of epiglottis	Size >4 cm, and/or extension to lingual surface of epiglottis
T4	Involvement of larynx, extrinsic tongue muscles, medial pterygoid, mandible, hard palate, and further	T4a: Moderately advanced local disease Tumor invades the larynx, deep/extrinsic muscle of the tongue, medial pterygoid, hard palate, or mandible T4b: Very advanced local disease Tumor invades the lateral pterygoid muscle, pterygoid plates, lateral nasopharynx, or skull base, or encases the carotid artery

Table 20.3 Oral cavity, larynx, and p16-negative oropharynx clinical nodal staging

N stage	Clinical (radiologic)	Pathologic
N0	No regional (cervical) lymph nodes	No regional (cervical) lymph nodes
N1	Single node ≤3 cm, no extranodal extension (ENE)	Single node ≤3 cm, ENE (−)
N2a	Single node >3 cm, ≤6 cm, ENE (−)	Single node >3 cm, ≤6 cm, ENE (−) or Single ipsilateral or contralateral lymph node ≤3 cm in size, ENE (+)
N2b	Two or more ipsilateral nodes, >3 cm, ≤6 cm, ENE (−)	Two or more ipsilateral nodes, >3 cm, ≤6 cm, no ENE
N2c	Bilateral or contralateral nodes, ≤6 cm, no ENE	Bilateral or contralateral nodes, ≤6 cm, no ENE
N3a	Node >6 cm, ENE (−)	Node >6 cm, no ENE
N3b	Clinically positive ENE	Metastasis in a lymph node larger than 3 cm with ENE (+) or multiple ipsilateral, bilateral or contralateral lymph nodes, ENE (+)

Table 20.4 p16-positive oropharynx nodal staging

N stage	Clinical (radiologic)	Pathologic
N0	No regional (cervical) lymph nodes	No regional (cervical) lymph nodes
N1	One or more ipsilateral nodes, ≤6 cm	Four or fewer nodes
N2	Bilateral or contralateral nodes, ≤6 cm	More than four nodes
N3	Node >6 cm	n/a

may be as effective as surgery [113, 114]. Thus, NCCN guidelines suggest both surgical (total laryngectomy with bilateral neck dissections of levels II-IV) and chemoradiation treatments are acceptable options [107]. Often, the choice of treatment is dictated by the function of the larynx (e.g., in a nonfunctional larynx, organ conservation therapies have less utility), patient choice, and overall health.

20.14.3 Staging and Treatment of p16-Positive Oropharyngeal Squamous Cell Carcinoma

As mentioned above, the etiology of oropharyngeal SCC generally is due to high-risk HPV infection, as opposed to tobacco and alcohol use as in other mucosal head and neck subsites. p16-positive SCCs carry an overall better prognosis compared to traditionally tobacco and alcohol-related HNSCCs. Notably, with the AJCC 8th edition staging system, T4a and T4b classification of p16-positive oropharyngeal SCCs are eliminated, in favor of a general T4 stage (Table 20.2). The updated nodal staging in the AJCC 8th edition is different for p16-positive oropharyngeal SCC than other mucosal SCC, with separate and unique clinical and pathologic staging (Table 20.4). Notably, for radiologic assessment, extranodal extension is not a criteria for upstaging, unlike oral cavity and laryngeal SCC nodal disease.

Treatment options depend on the primary tumor site stage and anatomy, as well as cervical nodal status. For early stage tumors, surgical and XRT options are both acceptable. Transoral robotic surgery or transoral laser approaches may be employed in cases with resectable, accessible tumors. In surgical cases, ipsilateral neck dissection of levels II-IV is performed for lateralized tumors, while bilateral necks must be addressed in midline tumors. After primary surgery, pathology dictates whether adjuvant radiation or chemoradiation is necessary [115–117]. Radiation alone is an alternative treatment option in early stage tumors without aggressive features. In a similar fashion, the primary site and nodal levels II-IV must be addressed. For advanced stage tumors chemoradiation with cytotoxic chemotherapy is often utilized. Given the good prognosis and response to therapy of p16-positive oropharyngeal SCCs, many de-escalation trials are currently being investigated to maintain successful treatment rates while decreasing treatment-related toxicities; however, definitive data for such de-escalation remains to be seen [118].

References

1. Connolly M, Srinivasan A (2018) Diffusion-weighted imaging in head and neck cancer: technique, limitations, and applications. Magn Reson Imaging Clin N Am 26(1):121–133
2. Thoeny HC, De Keyzer F, King AD (2012) Diffusion-weighted MR imaging in the head and neck. Radiology 263(1):19–32
3. Le Bihan D, Mangin JF, Poupon C, Clark CA, Pappata S, Molko N et al (2001) Diffusion tensor imaging: concepts and applications. J Magn Reson Imaging 13(4):534–546
4. Noij DP, Martens RM, Marcus JT, de Bree R, Leemans CR, Castelijns JA et al (2017) Intravoxel incoherent motion magnetic resonance imaging in head and neck cancer: a systematic review of the diagnostic and prognostic value. Oral Oncol 68:81–91
5. Iima M, Le Bihan D (2016) Clinical intravoxel incoherent motion and diffusion MR imaging: past, present, and future. Radiology 278(1):13–32
6. Marrale M, Collura G, Brai M, Toschi N, Midiri F, La Tona G et al (2016) Physics, techniques and review of neuroradiological applications of diffusion kurtosis imaging (DKI). Clin Neuroradiol 26(4):391–403
7. Steven AJ, Zhuo J, Melhem ER (2014) Diffusion kurtosis imaging: an emerging technique for evaluating the microstructural environment of the brain. AJR Am J Roentgenol 202(1):W26–W33
8. Som PM, Curtin HD (eds) (2011) Head and neck imaging. Mosby, St. Louis
9. Chakeres DW, Spiegel PK (1983) A systematic technique for comprehensive evaluation of the temporal bone by computed tomography. Radiology 146(1):97–106
10. Harnsberger HR (1990) Head and neck imaging. Year Book Medical Publishers, Chicago
11. Swartz JD (1998) In: HR Harnsberger (ed.) Imaging of the temporal bone. 3rd ed. Thieme, New York
12. Thompson LDR, Bishop JA (eds) (2019) Head and neck pathology. Third edition. Elsevier, Philadelphia, PA
13. Lingam RK, Kumar R, Vaidhyanath R (2019) Inflammation of the temporal bone. Neuroimaging Clin N Am 29(1):1–17
14. Vercruysse JP, De Foer B, Pouillon M, Somers T, Casselman J, Offeciers E (2006) The value of diffusion-weighted MR imaging in the diagnosis of primary acquired and residual cholesteatoma: a surgical verified study of 100 patients. Eur Radiol 16(7):1461–1467
15. Jackler RK, Parker DA (1992) Radiographic differential diagnosis of petrous apex lesions. Am J Otol 13(6):561–574
16. Fitzek C, Mewes T, Fitzek S, Mentzel HJ, Hunsche S, Stoeter P (2002) Diffusion-weighted MRI of cholesteatomas of the petrous bone. J Magn Reson Imaging 15(6):636–641
17. Williams MT, Ayache D, Alberti C, Heran F, Lafitte F, Elmaleh-Berges M et al (2003) Detection of postoperative residual cholesteatoma with delayed contrast-enhanced MR imaging: initial findings. Eur Radiol 13(1):169–174
18. Shelton C, Sheehy JL (1990) Tympanoplasty: review of 400 staged cases. Laryngoscope 100(7):679–681
19. Bennett M, Wanna G, Francis D, Murfee J, O'Connell B, Haynes D (2018) Clinical and cost utility of an intraoperative endoscopic second look in cholesteatoma surgery. Laryngoscope 128(12):2867–2871
20. Aikele P, Kittner T, Offergeld C, Kaftan H, Huttenbrink KB, Laniado M (2003) Diffusion-weighted MR imaging of cholesteatoma in pediatric and adult patients who have undergone middle ear surgery. AJR Am J Roentgenol 181(1):261–265
21. De Foer B, Vercruysse JP, Bernaerts A, Maes J, Deckers F, Michiels J et al (2007) The value of single-shot turbo spin-echo diffusion-weighted MR imaging in the detection of middle ear cholesteatoma. Neuroradiology 49(10):841–848
22. Dubrulle F, Souillard R, Chechin D, Vaneecloo FM, Desaulty A, Vincent C (2006) Diffusion-weighted MR imaging sequence in the detection of postoperative recurrent cholesteatoma. Radiology 238(2):604–610
23. Maheshwari S, Mukherji SK (2002) Diffusion-weighted imaging for differentiating recurrent cholesteatoma from granulation tissue after mastoidectomy: case report. AJNR Am J Neuroradiol 23(5):847–849
24. Stasolla A, Magliulo G, Parrotto D, Luppi G, Marini M (2004) Detection of postoperative relapsing/residual cholesteatomas with diffusion-weighted echo-planar magnetic resonance imaging. Otol Neurotol 25(6):879–884
25. Yoshida T, Ito K, Adachi N, Yamasoba T, Kondo K, Kaga K (2005) Cholesteatoma of the petrous bone: the crucial role of diffusion-weighted MRI. Eur Arch Otorhinolaryngol 262(5):440–441
26. Lingam RK, Nash R, Majithia A, Kalan A, Singh A (2016) Non-echoplanar diffusion weighted imaging in the detection of post-operative middle ear cholesteatoma: navigating beyond the pitfalls to find the pearl. Insights Imaging 7(5):669–678
27. Jindal M, Riskalla A, Jiang D, Connor S, O'Connor AF (2011) A systematic review of diffusion-weighted magnetic resonance imaging in the assessment of postoperative cholesteatoma. Otol Neurotol 32(8):1243–1249
28. Muzaffar J, Metcalfe C, Colley S, Coulson C (2017) Diffusion-weighted magnetic resonance imaging for residual and recurrent cholesteatoma: a systematic review and meta-analysis. Clin Otolaryngol 42(3):536–543
29. Mas-Estelles F, Mateos-Fernandez M, Carrascosa-Bisquert B, Facal de Castro F, Puchades-Roman I,

Morera-Perez C (2012) Contemporary non-echo-planar diffusion-weighted imaging of middle ear cholesteatomas. Radiographics 32(4):1197–1213

30. Schwartz KM, Lane JI, Bolster BD Jr, Neff BA (2011) The utility of diffusion-weighted imaging for cholesteatoma evaluation. AJNR Am J Neuroradiol 32(3):430–436

31. Fukuda A, Morita S, Harada T, Fujiwara K, Hoshino K, Nakamaru Y et al (2017) Value of T1-weighted magnetic resonance imaging in cholesteatoma detection. Otol Neurotol 38(10):1440–1444

32. Steens S, Venderink W, Kunst D, Meijer A, Mylanus E (2016) Repeated postoperative follow-up diffusion-weighted magnetic resonance imaging to detect residual or recurrent cholesteatoma. Otol Neurotol 37(4):356–361

33. Lingam RK, Connor SEJ, Casselman JW, Beale T (2018) MRI in otology: applications in cholesteatoma and Meniere's disease. Clin Radiol 73(1):35–44

34. Lingam RK, Bassett P (2017) A meta-analysis on the diagnostic performance of non-echoplanar diffusion-weighted imaging in detecting middle ear cholesteatoma: 10 years on. Otol Neurotol 38(4):521–528

35. Cavaliere M, Di Lullo AM, Cantone E, Scala G, Elefante A, Russo C et al (2018) Cholesteatoma vs granulation tissue: a differential diagnosis by DWI-MRI apparent diffusion coefficient. Eur Arch Otorhinolaryngol 275(9):2237–2243

36. Zuber TJ (2002) Minimal excision technique for epidermoid (sebaceous) cysts. Am Fam Physician 65(7):1409–1412, 17–8, 20

37. Warakaulle DR, Anslow P (2003) Differential diagnosis of intracranial lesions with high signal on T1 or low signal on T2-weighted MRI. Clin Radiol 58(12):922–933

38. Hong SH, Chung HW, Choi JY, Koh YH, Choi JA, Kang HS (2006) MRI findings of subcutaneous epidermal cysts: emphasis on the presence of rupture. AJR Am J Roentgenol 186(4):961–966

39. Shibata T, Hatori M, Satoh T, Ehara S, Kokubun S (2003) Magnetic resonance imaging features of epidermoid cyst in the extremities. Arch Orthop Trauma Surg 123(5):239–241

40. Suzuki C, Maeda M, Matsumine A, Matsubara T, Taki W, Maier SE et al (2007) Apparent diffusion coefficient of subcutaneous epidermal cysts in the head and neck comparison with intracranial epidermoid cysts. Acad Radiol 14(9):1020–1028

41. Isaacson B (2015) Cholesterol granuloma and other petrous apex lesions. Otolaryngol Clin N Am 48(2):361–373

42. Raghavan D, Lee TC, Curtin HD (2015) Cholesterol granuloma of the petrous apex: a 5-year review of radiology reports with follow-up of progression and treatment. J Neurol Surg B Skull Base 76(4):266–271

43. Kosling S, Bootz F (2001) CT and MR imaging after middle ear surgery. Eur J Radiol 40(2):113–118

44. White ML, Zhang Y, Robinson RA (2006) Evaluating tumors and tumorlike lesions of the nasal cavity, the paranasal sinuses, and the adjacent skull base with diffusion-weighted MRI. J Comput Assist Tomogr 30(3):490–495

45. Hansen LS, Allard RH (1984) Encysted parasitic larvae in the mouth. J Am Dent Assoc 108(4):632–636

46. Hanifi B, Samil KS, Yasar C, Cengiz C, Ercan A, Ramazan D (2013) Craniofacial fibrous dysplasia. Clin Imaging 37(6):1109–1115

47. Hayashida Y, Hirai T, Yakushiji T, Katahira K, Shimomura O, Imuta M et al (2006) Evaluation of diffusion-weighted imaging for the differential diagnosis of poorly contrast-enhanced and T2-prolonged bone masses: initial experience. J Magn Reson Imaging 23(3):377–382

48. Atalar MH, Salk I, Savas R, Uysal IO, Egilmez H (2015) CT and MR imaging in a large series of patients with craniofacial fibrous dysplasia. Pol J Radiol 80:232–240

49. Stefanelli S, Mundada P, Rougemont AL, Lenoir V, Scolozzi P, Merlini L et al (2018) Masses of developmental and genetic origin affecting the paediatric craniofacial skeleton. Insights Imaging 9:571–589

50. Katsuya T, Inoue T, Ishizaka H, Aoki J, Endo K (2000) Dynamic contrast-enhanced MR imaging of the water fraction of normal bone marrow and diffuse bone marrow disease. Radiat Med 18(5):291–297

51. Vanel D, Dromain C, Tardivon A (2000) MRI of bone marrow disorders. Eur Radiol 10(2):224–229

52. Sener RN (2003) Diffusion magnetic resonance imaging of solid vestibular schwannomas. J Comput Assist Tomogr 27(2):249–252

53. Srinivasan A, Dvorak R, Perni K, Rohrer S, Mukherji SK (2008) Differentiation of benign and malignant pathology in the head and neck using 3T apparent diffusion coefficient values: early experience. AJNR Am J Neuroradiol 29(1):40–44

54. Maeda M, Matsumine A, Kato H, Kusuzaki K, Maier SE, Uchida A et al (2007) Soft-tissue tumors evaluated by line-scan diffusion-weighted imaging: influence of myxoid matrix on the apparent diffusion coefficient. J Magn Reson Imaging 25(6):1199–1204

55. Sener RN (2006) Malignant oculomotor schwannoma: diffusion MR imaging. J Neuroradiol 33(4):270–272

56. Ahlawat S, Fayad LM (2018) Imaging cellularity in benign and malignant peripheral nerve sheath tumors: utility of the "target sign" by diffusion weighted imaging. Eur J Radiol 102:195–201

57. Camargo A, Schneider T, Liu L, Pakpoor J, Kleinberg L, Yousem DM (2017) Pretreatment ADC values predict response to radiosurgery in vestibular schwannomas. AJNR Am J Neuroradiol 38(6):1200–1205

58. Kinoshita Y, Yamasaki F, Tominaga A, Ohtaki M, Usui S, Arita K et al (2016) Diffusion-weighted imaging and the apparent diffusion coefficient on 3T MR imaging in the differentiation of craniopharyngiomas and germ cell tumors. Neurosurg Rev 39(2):207–213; discussion 13

59. Park HH, Lee KS, Ahn SJ, Suh SH, Hong CK (2017) Ecchordosis physaliphora: typical and atypical radiologic features. Neurosurg Rev 40(1):87–94
60. Castillo M, Albernaz VS, Mukherji SK, Smith MM, Weissman JL (1998) Imaging of Bezold's abscess. AJR Am J Roentgenol 171(6):1491–1495
61. Swartz JD, Loevner LA (2009) Imaging of the temporal bone. Thieme, New York
62. Karantanas AH, Karantzas G, Katsiva V, Proikas K, Sandris V (2003) CT and MRI in malignant external otitis: a report of four cases. Comput Med Imaging Graph 27(1):27–34
63. Goh JPN, Karandikar A, Loke SC, Tan TY (2017) Skull base osteomyelitis secondary to malignant otitis externa mimicking advanced nasopharyngeal cancer: MR imaging features at initial presentation. Am J Otolaryngol 38(4):466–471
64. Ozgen B, Oguz KK, Cila A (2011) Diffusion MR imaging features of skull base osteomyelitis compared with skull base malignancy. AJNR Am J Neuroradiol 32(1):179–184
65. Palabiyik FB, Yazici Z, Cetin B, Celebi S, Hacimustafaoglu M (2016) Pott puffy tumor in children: a rare emergency clinical entity. J Craniofac Surg 27(3):e313–e316
66. Tatsumi S, Ri M, Higashi N, Wakayama N, Matsune S, Tosa M (2016) Pott's puffy tumor in an adult: a case report and review of literature. J Nippon Med Sch = Nippon Ika Daigaku zasshi 83(5):211–214
67. Koltsidopoulos P, Papageorgiou E, Skoulakis C (2018) Pott's puffy tumor in children: a review of the literature. Laryngoscope 130:225–231
68. Hegde AN, Mohan S, Pandya A, Shah GV (2012) Imaging in infections of the head and neck. Neuroimaging Clin N Am 22(4):727–754
69. Gaviani P, Schwartz RB, Hedley-Whyte ET, Ligon KL, Robicsek A, Schaefer P et al (2005) Diffusion-weighted imaging of fungal cerebral infection. AJNR Am J Neuroradiol 26(5):1115–1121
70. Mueller-Mang C, Castillo M, Mang TG, Cartes-Zumelzu F, Weber M, Thurnher MM (2007) Fungal versus bacterial brain abscesses: is diffusion-weighted MR imaging a useful tool in the differential diagnosis? Neuroradiology 49(8):651–657
71. Fatima Z, Motosugi U, Muhi A, Hori M, Ishigame K, Araki T (2013) Diffusion-weighted imaging in optic neuritis. Can Assoc Radiol J = Journal l'Association canadienne des radiologistes 64(1):51–55
72. Habermann CR, Gossrau P, Graessner J, Arndt C, Cramer MC, Reitmeier F et al (2005) Diffusion-weighted echo-planar MRI: a valuable tool for differentiating primary parotid gland tumors? Rofo 177(7):940–945
73. Mikaszewski B, Markiet K, Smugala A, Stodulski D, Szurowska E, Stankiewicz C (2017) Diffusion-weighted MRI in the differential diagnosis of parotid malignancies and pleomorphic adenomas: can the accuracy of dynamic MRI be enhanced? Oral Surg Oral Med Oral Pathol Oral Radiol 124(1):95–103

74. Abdel Razek AAK (2018) Routine and advanced diffusion imaging modules of the salivary glands. Neuroimaging Clin N Am 28(2):245–254
75. Razek A (2019) Prediction of malignancy of submandibular gland tumors with apparent diffusion coefficient. Oral Radiol 35(1):11–15
76. Moon WJ, Lee MH, Chung EC (2007) Diffusion-weighted imaging with sensitivity encoding (SENSE) for detecting cranial bone marrow metastases: comparison with T1-weighted images. Korean J Radiol 8(3):185–191
77. Nemeth AJ, Henson JW, Mullins ME, Gonzalez RG, Schaefer PW (2007) Improved detection of skull metastasis with diffusion-weighted MR imaging. AJNR Am J Neuroradiol 28(6):1088–1092
78. Herneth AM, Friedrich K, Weidekamm C, Schibany N, Krestan C, Czerny C et al (2005) Diffusion weighted imaging of bone marrow pathologies. Eur J Radiol 55(1):74–83
79. Mulkern RV, Schwartz RB (2003) In re: characterization of benign and metastatic vertebral compression fractures with quantitative diffusion MR imaging. AJNR Am J Neuroradiol 24(7):1489–1490; author reply 90–1
80. Ballon D, Dyke J, Schwartz LH, Lis E, Schneider E, Lauto A et al (2000) Bone marrow segmentation in leukemia using diffusion and T (2) weighted echo planar magnetic resonance imaging. NMR Biomed 13(6):321–328
81. Ballon D, Watts R, Dyke JP, Lis E, Morris MJ, Scher HI et al (2004) Imaging therapeutic response in human bone marrow using rapid whole-body MRI. Magn Reson Med 52(6):1234–1238
82. Messiou C, Kaiser M (2015) Whole body diffusion weighted MRI—a new view of myeloma. Br J Haematol 171(1):29–37
83. Wang J, Takashima S, Takayama F, Kawakami S, Saito A, Matsushita T et al (2001) Head and neck lesions: characterization with diffusion-weighted echo-planar MR imaging. Radiology 220(3):621–630
84. Maeda M, Kato H, Sakuma H, Maier SE, Takeda K (2005) Usefulness of the apparent diffusion coefficient in line scan diffusion-weighted imaging for distinguishing between squamous cell carcinomas and malignant lymphomas of the head and neck. AJNR Am J Neuroradiol 26(5):1186–1192
85. King AD, Ahuja AT, Yeung DK, Fong DK, Lee YY, Lei KI et al (2007) Malignant cervical lymphadenopathy: diagnostic accuracy of diffusion-weighted MR imaging. Radiology 245(3):806–813
86. Sasaki M, Eida S, Sumi M, Nakamura T (2011) Apparent diffusion coefficient mapping for sinonasal disease: differentiation of benign and malignant lesions. AJNR Am J Neuroradiol 32:1100–1106
87. Abdel Razek A, Mossad A, Ghonim M (2011) Role of diffusion-weighted MR imaging in assessing malignant versus benign skull-base lesions. Radiol Med 116(1):125–132

88. Payabvash S (2018) Quantitative diffusion magnetic resonance imaging in head and neck tumors. Quant Imaging Med Surg 8(10):1052–1065

89. Hermans R (2010) Diffusion-weighted MRI in head and neck cancer. Curr Opin Otolaryngol Head Neck Surg 18(2):72–78

90. Becker M, Varoquaux AD, Combescure C, Rager O, Pusztaszeri M, Burkhardt K et al (2018) Local recurrence of squamous cell carcinoma of the head and neck after radio (chemo) therapy: diagnostic performance of FDG-PET/MRI with diffusion-weighted sequences. Eur Radiol 28(2):651–663

91. Driessen JP, Peltenburg B, Philippens MEP, Huijbregts JE, Pameijer FA, de Bree R et al (2019) Prospective comparative study of MRI including diffusion-weighted images versus FDG PET-CT for the detection of recurrent head and neck squamous cell carcinomas after (chemo) radiotherapy. Eur J Radiol 111:62–67

92. Seeger A, Batra M, Susskind D, Ernemann U, Hauser TK (2018) Assessment of uveal melanomas using advanced diffusion-weighted imaging techniques: value of reduced field of view DWI ("zoomed DWI") and readout-segmented DWI (RESOLVE). Acta Radiol 60:977–984

93. Szymanska A, Szymanski M, Czekajska-Chehab E, Szczerbo-Trojanowska M (2014) Invasive growth patterns of juvenile nasopharyngeal angiofibroma: radiological imaging and clinical implications. Acta Radiol 55(6):725–731

94. Abdel Razek AA, Soliman NY, Elkhamary S, Alsharaway MK, Tawfik A (2006) Role of diffusion-weighted MR imaging in cervical lymphadenopathy. Eur Radiol 16(7):1468–1477

95. Holzapfel K, Duetsch S, Fauser C, Eiber M, Rummeny EJ, Gaa J (2009) Value of diffusion-weighted MR imaging in the differentiation between benign and malignant cervical lymph nodes. Eur J Radiol 72(3):381–387

96. Sumi M, Sakihama N, Sumi T, Morikawa M, Uetani M, Kabasawa H et al (2003) Discrimination of metastatic cervical lymph nodes with diffusion-weighted MR imaging in patients with head and neck cancer. AJNR Am J Neuroradiol 24(8):1627–1634

97. Koc O, Paksoy Y, Erayman I, Kivrak AS, Arbag H (2007) Role of diffusion weighted MR in the discrimination diagnosis of the cystic and/or necrotic head and neck lesions. Eur J Radiol 62(2):205–213

98. Sakai K, Toudou M, Shimura Y, Teranishi R, Takaichi S, Son C et al (2017) A resected case of Castleman's disease that was difficult to diagnose preoperatively. Gan to kagaku ryoho Cancer & Chemotherapy 44(12):1841–1843

99. Rouchy RC, Attye A, Medici M, Renard F, Kastler A, Grand S et al (2018) Facial nerve tractography: a new tool for the detection of perineural spread in parotid cancers. Eur Radiol 28(9):3861–3871

100. Argiris A, Eng C (2003) Epidemiology, staging, and screening of head and neck cancer. Cancer Treat Res 114:15–60

101. Argiris A, Karamouzis MV, Raben D, Ferris RL (2008) Head and neck cancer. Lancet (London, England) 371:1695–1709

102. Chaturvedi AK, Engels EA, Pfeiffer RM et al (2011) Human papillomavirus and rising oropharyngeal cancer incidence in the United States. J Clin Oncol: Official Journal of the American Society of Clinical Oncology 29:4294–4301

103. Ang KK, Harris J, Wheeler R et al (2010) Human papillomavirus and survival of patients with oropharyngeal cancer. N Engl J Med 363:24–35

104. Chaturvedi AK, D'Souza G, Gillison ML, Katki HA (2016) Burden of HPV-positive oropharynx cancers among ever and never smokers in the U.S. population. Oral Oncol 60:61–67

105. Lewis JS Jr, Beadle B, Bishop JA et al (2018) Human Papillomavirus testing in head and neck carcinomas: guideline from the College of American Pathologists. Arch Pathol Lab Med 142:559–597

106. Lydiatt WM, Patel SG, O'Sullivan B et al (2017) Head and neck cancers-major changes in the American Joint Committee on cancer eighth edition cancer staging manual. CA Cancer J Clin 67:122–137

107. Colevas AD, Yom SS, Pfister DG et al (2018) NCCN guidelines insights: head and neck cancers, version 1.2018. J Natl Compr Canc Netw: JNCCN 16:479–490

108. Shah J (2020) Jatin Shah's head and neck surgery and oncology. Elsevier

109. Ferris RL, Blumenschein G Jr, Fayette J et al (2016) Nivolumab for recurrent squamous-cell carcinoma of the head and neck. N Engl J Med 375:1856–1867

110. Seiwert TY, Burtness B, Mehra R et al (2016) Safety and clinical activity of pembrolizumab for treatment of recurrent or metastatic squamous cell carcinoma of the head and neck (KEYNOTE-012): an open-label, multicentre, phase 1b trial. Lancet Oncol 17:956–965

111. US F. FDA approves pembrolizumab for first-line treatment of head and neck squamous cell carcinoma. Available at: https://www.fda.gov/drugs/resources-information-approved-drugs/fda-approves-pembrolizumab-first-line-treatment-head-and-neck-squamous-cell-carcinoma

112. D'Cruz AK, Vaish R, Kapre N et al (2015) Elective versus therapeutic neck dissection in node-negative oral cancer. N Engl J Med 373:521–529

113. Forastiere AA, Goepfert H, Maor M et al (2003) Concurrent chemotherapy and radiotherapy for organ preservation in advanced laryngeal cancer. N Engl J Med 349:2091–2098

114. Wolf GT, Fisher SG, Hong WK et al (1991) Induction chemotherapy plus radiation compared with surgery

plus radiation in patients with advanced laryngeal cancer. N Engl J Med 324:1685–1690

115. Da Mosto MC, Zanetti F, Boscolo-Rizzo P (2009) Pattern of lymph node metastases in squamous cell carcinoma of the tonsil: implication for selective neck dissection. Oral Oncol 45:212–217

116. Shah JP (1990) Patterns of cervical lymph node metastasis from squamous carcinomas of the upper aerodigestive tract. Am J Surg 160:405–409

117. Shimizu K, Inoue H, Saitoh M et al (2006) Distribution and impact of lymph node metastases in oropharyngeal cancer. Acta Otolaryngol 126:872–877

118. Mirghani H, Blanchard P (2018) Treatment de-escalation for HPV-driven oropharyngeal cancer: where do we stand? Clin Transl Radiat Oncol 8:4–11

Spine Infection

21

John Kim, Eiyu Matsumoto, and Toshio Moritani

21.1 Introduction

Spinal and paraspinal infections may result in significant morbidity and increased mortality, especially in the postoperative setting [1]. Spinal infections may also arise in patients without recent surgery in the increasing elderly population, immunocompromised and diabetic individuals, intravenous drug users, and those undergoing vascular access procedures [2–5]. Therefore, early diagnosis and proper treatment is essential. Despite advances in medical and imaging technology, the diagnosis of this entity is still challenging since the clinical features can sometimes be subtle and misleading. Although conventional MRI of the spine is considered the gold standard for diagnostic imaging with its relatively high sensitivity, specificity, and accuracy, there are still a significant number of challenging cases resulting in delays or misdiagnosis.

J. Kim (✉)
Division of Neuroradiology, University of Michigan, Ann Arbor, MI, USA
e-mail: johannk@med.umich.edu

E. Matsumoto
University of Iowa Hospitals and Clinics, Iowa City, IA, USA
e-mail: eiyu-matsumoto@uiowa.edu;

T. Moritani
Department of Internal Medicine, University of Michigan, Iowa City, IA, USA
e-mail: tmoritan@med.umich.edu

Table 21.1 Common spinal and paraspinal infections

1	Vertebral osteomyelitis-discitis
2	Infectious facet arthropathy
3	Epidural and subdural infections/abscesses
4	Meningitis
5	Myelitis
6	Infections of paraspinal soft tissue and musculature

In such cases, suboptimal diagnosis and management can result in irreversible paralysis, septic shock, and even death [6].

Diffusion-weighted imaging (DWI) is a useful tool for the diagnosis of central nervous system infections, especially in the detection of abscesses and pus collections involving the brain and spine [7–12]. In this chapter, we demonstrate DWI findings of the common pyogenic and also atypical spinal infections involving the vertebral bodies, intervertebral discs, posterior elements, epidural/subdural spaces, leptomeninges, spinal cord, and paraspinal soft tissues/muscles as well as other disseminated infections (Table 21.1). We also illustrate and discuss the differential diagnosis and imaging pitfalls.

21.2 MRI and Diffusion-Weighted Imaging

When it comes to diagnosis of spinal infections, conventional MRI has high diagnostic sensitivity, specificity, and accuracy of >90%, making it the diagnostic modality of choice [2, 4, 5, 13–17].

© Springer Nature Switzerland AG 2021
T. Moritani, A. A. Capizzano (eds.), *Diffusion-Weighted MR Imaging of the Brain, Head and Neck, and Spine*, https://doi.org/10.1007/978-3-030-62120-9_21

However, even with conventional MRI sequences including gadolinium-enhanced T1-weighted imaging, it is occasionally difficult to differentiate abscess/pus collection from other pathologies such as postsurgical fluid collection, cystic/necrotic tumor, hematoma, CSF leak and unusual patterns of degenerative disc and facet joint changes [6].

Diffusion-weighted imaging along with conventional MR sequences can help identify abscesses and pus collections with greater accuracy. Abscesses and pus collections are viscous fluid containing cellular debris and necrosis with dead or viable neutrophils. The increased viscosity and density of neutrophils in abscesses cause restricted movement of water molecules which results in hyperintense signal on DWI [11, 12]. If gadolinium contrast-enhanced imaging cannot be performed owing to significant acute renal failure, severe contrast allergy, or if other MR sequences are suboptimal in delineating abscesses because of motion artifacts, DWI can play a pivotal role in diagnosis. For example, Fig. 21.1 shows a patient who did not receive gadolinium contrast due to acute renal failure with GFR of 20. With initial MRI lacking gadolinium-enhanced sequences, the preliminary read was incorrectly interpreted as degenerative changes of the cervical spine. However, DWI clearly delineates the extension and multiplicity of abscesses and pus collections within the retropharyngeal, prevertebral, and epidural spaces (Fig. 21.1).

The most commonly used technique is spin-echo-type echoplanar DWI, which allows for fast acquisition times with less motion artifacts. For the appropriate detection and evaluation of abscesses and pus corrections, DWI is performed with *b values* of 0 and 1000 s mm^{-2} followed by the calculated ADC map. Parallel imaging factor of 2 is used to reduce distortion in images. Newer techniques by vendors include spin-echo type, turbo spin echo (TSE) DWI which has significantly less distortion or susceptibility artifacts but longer acquisition times. TSE DWI may be of most help in cases where metal hardware is present or where decreasing susceptibility artifacts is critical. Small field-of-view (FOV) DWI is also useful for imaging the spinal cord or deep small organs.

Acquisition of the DWI can be done in both axial and sagittal planes. The axial plane DWI allows for better evaluation of paraspinal soft tissue infections due to its larger FOV and axial coverage. The sagittal plane DWI helps in evaluation of the spinal cord. In the authors' opinion, if only one plane were to be acquired, it is best to

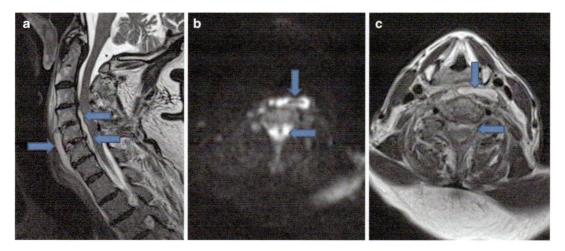

Fig. 21.1 (a–c) 75-year-old previously healthy male presented with neck pain and acute renal failure. No gadolinium contrast given due to severe renal dysfunction. *Staphylococcus aureus* was proven by blood culture. (**a**) Sagittal T2-weighted image reveals high signal intensities in the disc and vertebral bodies from C2 through C6, with epidural, prevertebral, and retropharyngeal abscesses. (**b**) Diffusion-weighted imaging clearly demonstrates the extension of the abscesses (arrows) better than the same slice axial T2-weighted image (**c**)

21 Spine Infection

acquire in the axial plane with 5 mm thick slices and reformat the images into sagittal plane as necessary to best demonstrate the extension and multiplicity of abscesses.

21.3 Typical Pyogenic Infections

The term pyogenic is defined as "involving or relating to production of pus." Majority or about two-thirds of causative organisms in pyogenic spinal infections are due to *Staphylococcus aureus*, including methicillin-resistant *S. aureus* (MRSA) and methicillin-susceptible *S. aureus* (MSSA) [2–5, 18]. MRSA is increasingly seen in both healthcare-associated and community-acquired infections and is associated with higher complication rates and prolonged treatment courses [19, 20]. Other less common infectious agents and their associations include *S. epidermis* (spine procedures), *Streptococcus* and *Enterococcus* (coexisting infective endocarditis), *Escherichia coli* (urinary tract infection), *Pseudomonas aeruginosa* (intravenous drug abuse), *Salmonella* (sickle cell disease), and anaerobic bacteria (abdominal and pelvic infections and gastrointestinal procedures). *Mycobacterium tuberculosis*, non-tuberculous mycobacteria, *Nocardia*, *Actinomyces,* and *Brucella* (endemic areas) are less common but can also be pyogenic (please see Sect. 21.6).

Organisms infect the spinal and paraspinal structures via two routes: hematogenous and non-hematogenous [2–5]. In approximately half of spinal infections, the source is hematogenous dissemination, one-third is contiguous spread (surgical intervention, trauma and direct inoculation) and in the remaining cases, the source of infection is unidentified. The dense region of arterial and venous channel networks is confined to bony end plates in adults, whereas in children, hyaline cartilage contains perforating vessels until 7 years of age with concomitant increased susceptibility to primary discitis [21–23]. However, disc revascularization can occur with degenerative disc changes and spondyloarthropathy [5]. Organisms that produce proteolytic enzymes quickly spread into the end plate and destroy the disc substance and then extend into the epidural or paraspinal spaces [5]. The valveless Batson's venous plexus may contribute to early extension and seeding of spinal and paraspinal infections [5, 16, 24–27]. The terminal branches of the same artery may supply the spinal and paraspinal area. Therefore, one site of spinal and paraspinal infections can extend locally or can disseminate hematogenously to other spinal/paraspinal areas or remote areas of the body.

The clinical features and laboratory findings of spinal infections can be subtle and misleading. Local back pain and fever are common but not always present. Elevated white blood cell count is detected in two-thirds of the cases. Elevated C-reactive protein and erythrocyte segmentation rate are useful screening laboratory tests. Mortality rates have been reported in the range of 2–20% for vertebral osteomyelitis and around 5% for epidural abscess, whereas in the pre-antibiotic era, they were much greater at 25–70% [3–5, 18, 25]. Paraplegia or tetraplegia may occur in 1% of patients, especially with cervical and thoracic spine infections secondary to cord compression or injury.

21.4 Common Patterns of Spinal Infection and Extension of Pyogenic Abscess

Pyogenic spinal and paraspinal infections can be categorized into five common patterns of extension (Table 21.2) [6].

Recognition of these patterns is helpful to identify abscess/pus collections and other spinal infections on MRI and DWI.

Table 21.2 Common patterns of spinal and paraspinal infections

1	Osteomyelitis/discitis
2	Epidural/paraspinal abscess with osteomyelitis/discitis
3	Epidural/paraspinal abscess with facet joint infection
4	Epidural/paraspinal abscess without concomitant osteomyelitis/discitis or facet joint infection
5	Intradural abscess (subdural abscess, purulent meningitis and spinal cord abscess)

21.4.1 Osteomyelitis/Discitis

The most common form of spinal infection is vertebral osteomyelitis, also referred to as osteomyelitis/discitis or spondylodiscitis, which involves the intervertebral disk and the adjacent vertebrae. The disease has a relatively insidious early clinical course, however if left untreated can have devastating consequences. Spondylodiscitis affects a bimodal age distribution, with peaks below 20 years of age and again between 50 and 70 years of age. For unknown reasons, males are twice as likely to be affected as females (2:1 male-to-female ratio). The most common causative agent of pyogenic infection is *Staphylococcus aureus*; however other organisms may be encountered, especially with immunocompromised patients or IV drug abusers. The infection is typically spread hematogenously to the vertebral endplate in adults, and it can continue to spread through the intervertebral disc to involve the contiguous vertebral body endplate. Other routes of transmission may also be encountered, including direct inoculation from spinal procedures, direct extension from nearby infection, and hematogenous spread to the facet joints (facet septic arthritis). The lumbar spine is the most commonly affected region. The typical presentation is nonspecific back pain, with fever present in half of patients. Neurological symptoms are rare. Laboratory findings such as leukocytosis and elevated ESR/CRP are also nonspecific but may help rule out infection if normal.

Unfortunately, early infection can often have a nonspecific appearance paralleling their nonspecific clinical symptoms. MR is the most sensitive and specific for diagnosis of spondylodiscitis; however due to the nonspecific clinical symptoms, there is generally a 4-month delay in obtaining MR imaging. MRI has also proven useful in follow-up imaging to evaluate treatment response in patients whose clinical symptoms have not improved. Plain radiographs are often the first imaging test obtained, yet are not adequate for diagnosis as imaging changes of infection often mimic degenerative changes early on and will not show the classic features of vertebral endplate destruction until late in the disease course. Gallium-67 SPECT and F-18 FDG PET studies have also provided useful information when the diagnosis is in doubt or when MRI is contraindicated.

On MRI, marrow edema (T1 hypointense, T2 hyperintense signal) is often the earliest abnormality encountered along the anterior aspects of a vertebral body endplate. Following involvement of the endplate, the infection spreads throughout the vertebral marrow and into the adjacent intervertebral disc resulting in discitis, which is demonstrated as fluid-like disc signal (T1 variable, T2 hyperintense signal). The infection will continue to spread locally through the disc to the neighboring vertebral endplate. Gadolinium enhancement is typically diffuse throughout the affected marrow and disc, although peripheral disc enhancement may be seen (Fig. 21.2). Multilevel involvement (greater than 2 levels) of vertebral bodies and discs can occur in pyogenic spinal infections but less commonly in tuberculosis. While the most well recognized imaging pattern involves two contiguous vertebrae and the intervening intervertebral disc, other atypical patterns of disc/vertebral involvement may be encountered including only one vertebral body, one vertebral body and one disc, or two vertebral bodies with a normal appearing intervertebral disc (Fig. 21.3). When diagnosis is in doubt, follow-up imaging may be obtained which can show advanced changes of infection in as little as 8 days.

As the infection progresses, erosions may occur in the vertebral endplates (Fig. 21.4). Vertebral body height loss and collapse may be seen later in the disease course. Surgical consult is often warranted at these later stages to determine if drainage, decompression, or stabilization is required.

21.4.2 Epidural/Paraspinal Abscess with Osteomyelitis/Discitis

In more extensive cases, enhancing phlegmon may begin to develop in the adjacent epidural and paraspinal areas, including the psoas mus-

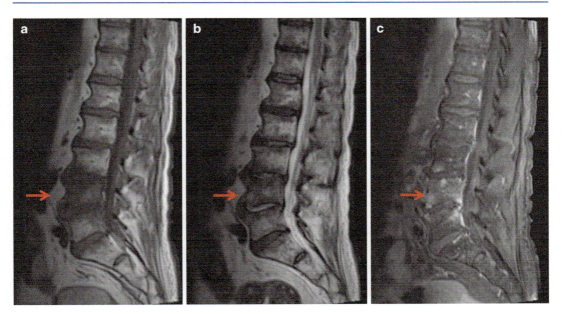

Fig. 21.2 (a–c) Sagittal T1- (a), T2- (b), and fat-saturated post-contrast T1 (c) images of the lumbar spine. There is T1 hypointense signal and patchy enhancement of the L4 vertebral body marrow (arrow), with early involvement of the superior endplate of L5 and anterior inferior endplate of L3. T2 images show edema within the L4-L5 greater than L3-L4 intervertebral discs, with mild marginal disc enhancement at L4-L5. There was no significant surrounding soft tissue or epidural enhancement at this time point

cle. These phlegmonous changes can evolve further to abscesses, which classically demonstrate fluid-like signal and peripheral enhancement (Fig. 21.4).

Spinal epidural abscess refers to a localized collection of pus between the dura mater and osseous spinal canal. Epidural/paraspinal abscess associated with osteomyelitis/discitis is the most common pattern of extension and is often seen in the anterior part of the epidural space. This pattern of extension more often occurs in the lumbar spine. Cervical spondylitis can progress anteriorly causing retropharyngeal abscess and inferiorly causing mediastinitis. Thoracic spondylitis can cause mediastinitis, empyema, and pericarditis, while lumbar spondylitis causes peritonitis, subdiaphragmatic abscess, and infection in the pelvis. Abscesses can also form within the vertebral body and disc [5]. Although epidural abscess usually extends over three to four vertebrae, it can involve the whole spine and is known as panspinal infection [3, 28, 29].

MRI findings of pyogenic osteomyelitis/discitis with large epidural abscesses on T2-weighted images may sometimes demonstrate spinal cord compression and abnormal cord signal [2, 11, 13, 16, 30, 31]. Gadolinium-enhanced T1-weighted images with fat saturation can differentiate infection from postsurgical changes, and pus collection from granulation/phlegmon, based on their enhancement patterns [13, 32, 33]. However, in cases where the abscesses are small and/or gadolinium-enhanced T1-weighted images are not available, DWI may prove to be crucial in detection of abscesses in the epidural space and paraspinal soft tissues (Figs. 21.1 and 21.5).

21.4.3 Epidural/Paraspinal Abscess with Facet Joint Infection

Facet joint infection (septic arthritis) is rare but has increased recently, owing to the increase in the elderly population, immunocompromised patients, and spine procedures [34–37]. This is another important route of infection resulting in epidural/paraspinal abscesses. Facet joint infection is often hematogenous but also caused by epidural anesthesia and spinal procedures. It is usually unilateral, and presents more acutely than does

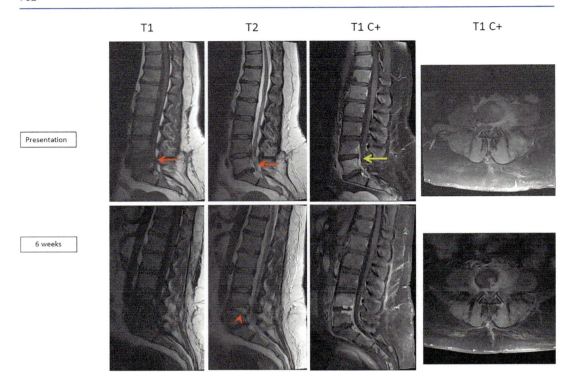

Fig. 21.3 Evolution of spondylodiscitis: The top row of images show initial presentation of L4 and L5 vertebral osteomyelitis, with sparing of the intervertebral disc (red arrow). The infection appears to have spread longitudinally as a ventral epidural phlegmon, extending from L4 to L5 (yellow arrow). The bottom row of images was obtained 6 weeks later after the patient complained of increasing back pain. These show increasing marrow signal abnormality with worsening endplate erosions along upper endplate of L5 posteriorly (red arrowhead). The intervertebral disc now demonstrates signs of infection with hyperintense T2 signal and peripheral enhancement. The epidural phlegmon and soft tissue enhancement are relatively unchanged. Findings suggest persistent, evolving infection

spondylodiscitis. It frequently involves the L4-L5 joints. Epidural abscess associated with facet joint infection tends to occur in the posterior part of the epidural space. Degenerative facet joints may constitute an increased risk for infection [35]. Infection of the facet joint often spreads contiguously to the epidural space and to the paraspinal musculature. Intradural extension associated with facet joint infection has also been reported [38]. If there is no evidence of spondylodiscitis, the facet joints should be evaluated very carefully.

The MRI findings of facet joint infection are sometimes very subtle and resemble degenerative joint disease. MRI shows swelling of the capsule and periarticular soft tissue of the facet joint. DWI is useful in the detection of small abscess or pus collection in the posterior paraspinal muscle adjacent to the facet joint (Fig. 21.5).

21.4.4 Epidural/Paraspinal Abscess Without Concomitant Osteomyelitis/Discitis or Facet Joint Infection

The route of this pattern of infection is variable: (1) isolated epidural or paraspinal abscess due to hematogenous spread, (2) direct extension from

21 Spine Infection

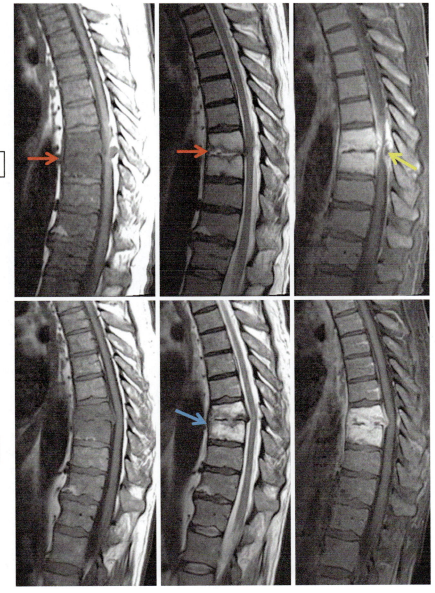

Fig. 21.4 The top row of images demonstrates abnormal marrow signal and enhancement at T8-T9 (red arrow) consistent with discitis/osteomyelitis. There is epidural enhancement with a small dorsal epidural abscess (yellow arrow). Follow-up MRI after 8 weeks of antibiotic therapy shows persistent discitis/osteomyelitis at T8-T9 with progression of endplate destructive changes and new T8 vertebral body height loss (blue arrow). The epidural abscess has resolved, with minimal residual epidural enhancement

wound infection after surgery or trauma, and (3) direct inoculation from spinal intervention such as epidural steroid injection or nerve block. Isolated epidural abscess is more commonly seen in the cervical spine [5, 18]. Isolated epidural abscess tends to occur posteriorly but can occur anteriorly. Diagnosis is often difficult clinically and radiologically. MRI with DWI is the key imaging technique in the diagnosis of isolated epidural abscess (Fig. 21.6).

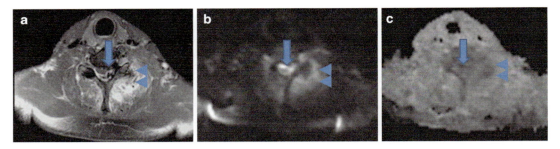

Fig. 21.5 (**a–c**) 43-year-old male with IV drug use. MSSA proven. Epidural and paraspinal abscesses with septic facet joint infection of the cervical spine. (**a**) Axial T1-weighted post-contrast with fat saturation, (**b**) DWI, and (**c**) ADC map demonstrate epidural abscesses (arrows) with left facet joint infection and paraspinal abscesses (arrowheads)

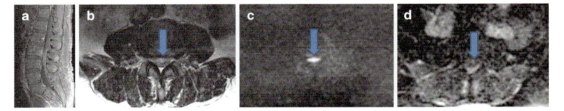

Fig. 21.6 (**a–d**) Isolated small ventral epidural abscess mimicking a disc herniation. *Streptococcus milleri* was proven by surgical drainage. (**a**) Sagittal post-contrast T1-weighted image shows a lesion at L3/4 ventrally with peripheral enhancement. There is no abnormal enhancement in the adjacent disc and vertebral body. (**b**) Axial T2-weighted image shows slightly hyperintense lesion on T2-weighted image. (**c, d**) Diffusion-weighted imaging (**c**) early reveals the lesion as hyperintense with decreased apparent diffusion coefficient (**d**) consistent with an epidural abscess (arrows). (Reprinted and adapted from Moritani and Kim et. al. BJR article)

21.4.5 Intradural Abscess (Subdural Abscess, Purulent Meningitis, and Spinal Cord Abscess)

Within the spinal canal, the epidural space is the most commonly affected but subdural involvement with meningitis and direct involvement of the spinal cord can occur [38–41]. Intradural abscess is a rare entity but it is a neurosurgical emergency associated with high morbidity and mortality. Progressive neurological deficits, severe pain, and fever suggest the diagnosis. Subdural abscess and purulent meningitis can be secondary to hematogenous spread, secondary infection after spine surgery and inoculation due to lumbar puncture, epidural steroid injection or nerve block (Fig. 21.7).

Extension of bacterial meningitis with spinal dysraphism is also an important etiology in children with this condition (Fig. 21.8). MRI with DWI is very useful for the diagnosis of intradural abscesses [41].

21.5 Management of Patients with Spinal and Paraspinal Infections

MRI, in particular DWI, may play an important role in defining burden of infection, treatment planning, site selection for biopsy, or decision-making of surgical drainage [6]. Optimal management of patients with spinal and paraspinal infections is crucial. Diagnostic delays and suboptimal management may potentially result in irreversible paralysis, worsening sepsis, and death.

21.5.1 Treatment of Osteomyelitis/Discitis

The most common sources of osteomyelitis/discitis include skin/soft tissue infection, genitourinary tract infection, infective endocarditis, intravenous drug abuse with contamination, respiratory tract infection, and intraabdominal infection. Although

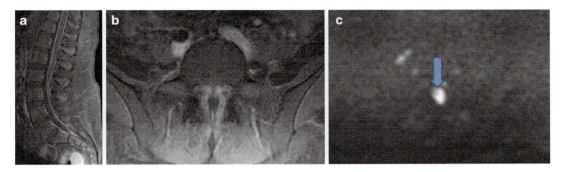

Fig. 21.7 (**a–c**) Purulent meningitis after steroid epidural injection at an outside hospital. Methicillin-susceptible *Staphylococcus aureus* was proven in the cerebrospinal fluid (CSF). (**a, b**) Sagittal (**a**) and axial (**b**) post-contrast T1-weighted image show extensive meningeal enhancement in the thecal sac. (**c**) Diffusion-weighted imaging demonstrates hyperintensity in the thecal sac consistent with purulent meningitis (arrow). Methicillin-resistant *Staphylococcus aureus* was proven in the CSF. (Reprinted and adapted from Moritani and Kim et. al. BJR article)

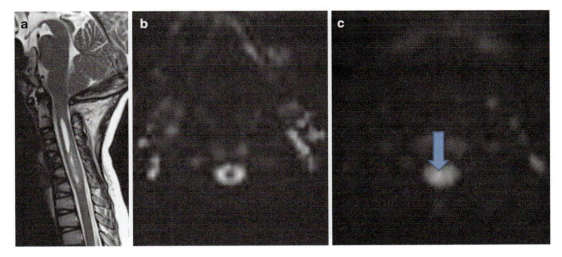

Fig. 21.8 (**a–c**) Spinal cord abscess with Chiari 1 malformation. (**a**) Sagittal T2-weighted image shows a syrinx as hyperintense lesions from C2 through C6. (**b, c**) Diffusion-weighted imaging demonstrates hypointensity in the syrinx (**b**) and hyperintensity in the spinal cord abscess (arrow) (**c**). (Reprinted and adapted from Moritani and Kim et. al. BJR article)

Staphylococcus aureus is the most common organism, other Gram-positive, Gram-negative, and even anaerobic bacteria can cause this disease entity. In addition, *Mycobacterium tuberculosis* and *Brucella* spp. are common in endemic regions. Therefore, no empiric treatment is recommended unless the patient is hemodynamically unstable [42]. Obtaining blood cultures followed by image-guided needle biopsy or surgical open biopsy should be pursued. Sensitivity of each procedure is 53% and 91%, respectively [43]. Preprocedural antibiotic greatly reduces the yield for needle biopsy, but not for open biopsy [43]. After confirming etiologic agent, 6 weeks of parenteral or highly bioavailable oral antimicrobial therapy are often curative for usual pyogenic infections [42]. Patient's symptoms and inflammatory markers (e.g., ESR, CRP) should be monitored. Repeat MRI for follow-up purpose has very limited value and may give an impression of clinical progression, even though there is otherwise clinical improvement.

Once treatment with IV antibiotics is begun, the adjacent epidural enhancement is often the first feature to improve on MR imaging. However, T2 hyperintensity and enhancement within the

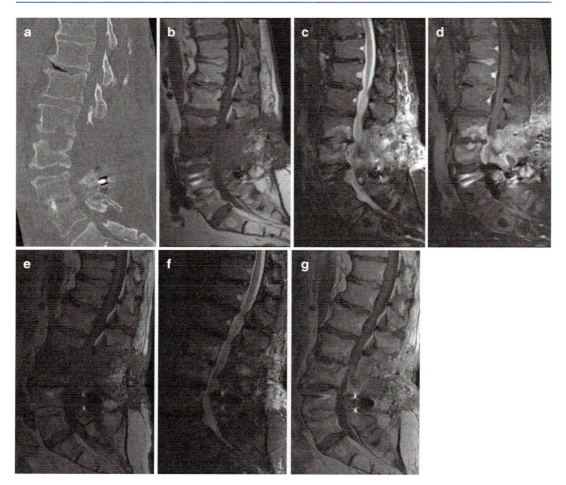

Fig. 21.9 (**a**–**g**) Sagittal CT (**a**) in a patient with recent L2-L3 laminectomy and discectomy and remote L4-L5 fusion demonstrates erosions involving the inferior endplate of L2 and superior endplate of L3. Sagittal T1 (**b**), STIR (**c**), and post-contrast fat-sat T1 (**d**) show the extent of infection involving the vertebral bodies, intervertebral disc, epidural space, and overlying soft tissues. A rim-enhancing abscess can be seen adjacent to the spinal hardware. Follow-up MRI after 6 weeks of antibiotic therapy with sagittal T1 (**e**), STIR (**f**), and post-contrast T1 (**g**) show persistent but improved marrow signal abnormalities and resolution of epidural enhancement. The patient was monitored clinically without further antibiotic therapy needed

marrow and intervertebral disc often persists after several weeks of antibiotics, and may even appear more extensive despite improving symptoms. This is postulated to represent granulation tissue and the effects of healing, and should not be taken as signs of treatment failure.

The recommended approach is to limit the use of follow-up MRI to patients with persistent elevation of inflammatory markers, in patients with persistent pain, or in those that develop new neurologic signs or symptoms. Routine repeat MRI images are no longer recommended [42]. If the patient is not improving clinically, follow-up MRI may be obtained after 4 weeks of treatment. As the endplates heal, fibrosis and sclerosis take the place of prior enhancing granulation tissue, leading to marrow hypointensity on all sequences and eventual lack of enhancement (Fig. 21.9).

21.5.2 Treatment of Spinal Epidural Abscess

The incidence of spinal epidural abscess has recently increased along with increased prevalence of intravenous drug use and healthcare-associated bacteremia. The infecting microorganism in most cases (50% to 90%) is *Staphylococcus aureus* with hematogenous dissemination. Concomitant osteomyelitis/discitis with or without psoas abscess is exceedingly common. Bacteremia is detected in 60% of cases [3].

Although the pathogenesis and microorganism are very similar to osteomyelitis/discitis, more urgent intervention is needed for the management of spinal epidural abscess as delay could lead to the future possibility of spinal cord injury. After blood cultures are obtained, empiric antibiotic with prompt surgical consultation should be obtained. Traditionally, surgical decompression along with drainage of the abscess followed by long-term antimicrobial therapy (4–8 weeks) has been the mandatory therapeutic principle [3–5, 18]. Since paralysis lasting more than 24–36 h is unlikely to reverse, urgent decompressive laminectomy is indicated for epidural abscess. However, there are a number of reports of success with a nonsurgical approach. Caution should be made in interpreting such data [3]. To date, there is no randomized trials performed for medical versus surgical management of spinal epidural abscess.

In regard to repeat MRI imaging, spinal epidural abscess differs from osteomyelitis/discitis. It is often recommended to obtain routine repeat MRI, especially in the case where the abscess was never surgically drained. Antibiotic duration is determined by a clinician with consideration of (1) patient symptoms, (2) inflammatory markers (ESR, CRP), and (3) MRI findings. The typical treatment duration is 6–8 weeks [3].

21.6 Tuberculosis and Atypical Infections

Tuberculosis is one of the more common infections in endemic regions of the world [4, 18, 44, 45]. Reactivation of tuberculosis has increased with HIV infection, recent chemotherapy and concurrent steroid use and the use of antitumor necrosis factor agents (infliximab). Among the 30 million people currently affected with tuberculosis worldwide, 1–3% have skeletal involvement.

Tuberculous spinal infections are more indolent than the typical bacterial pyogenic spinal infection with a more gradual onset of symptoms over months to years.

Tuberculous spondylitis, also known as Pott's disease, follows a slightly different course from the more typical bacterial pyogenic infection. Tuberculosis is more common in the thoracic spine than in the lumbar spine [4, 18]. Infection typically begins in the anterior vertebral body and spreads along the undersurface of the longitudinal ligaments (subligamentous spread) to involve multiple adjacent vertebrae and often form large paravertebral abscesses. Vertebral body collapse is much more common with tuberculosis than with typical bacterial pyogenic infections, creating the classic "gibbus deformity" of short segment kyphosis. Intervertebral discs are relatively preserved since *M. tuberculosis* does not have proteolytic enzymes that allow it to spread into the disc. Abscesses can grow to be quite large, without causing significant pain or pus formation, lending to the term "cold abscesses." Involvement of posterior elements of the spine and psoas abscess is another characteristic of tuberculosis. Paravertebral calcifications are a late finding, but help distinguish granulomatous from pyogenic infection. Evidence of pulmonary involvement is only seen in 50% of cases.

MRI typically demonstrates destruction of more than two consecutive vertebrae with relative sparing of the intervening disc and associated large paraspinal abscesses [4, 18, 44]. Epidural infection can be seen. DWI usually shows restricted diffusion in the abscess (Fig. 21.10). DWI can show partially hyper- and partially hypointense signal associated with high and low ADC values. The high ADC component may represent more serous fluid in a tuberculous cold abscess than in viscous pus formation. Routine surgery for spinal tuberculosis is not advocated. When necessary, the combined anterior and posterior approaches have been reported to be superior in lumbar and multilevel thoracic disease [46, 47].

Brucellosis is an important endemic infection commonly seen in Mediterranean countries or

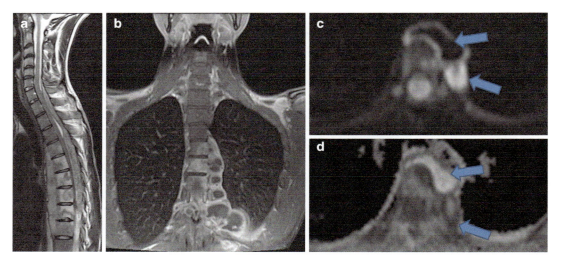

Fig. 21.10 (a–d) Tuberculosis. Epidural abscess and paraspinal abscesses with spondylodiscitis. Tuberculosis was proven by surgical drainage. (**a**, **b**) Sagittal T2-weighted image (**a**) and axial (B) post-contrast T1-weighted images with fat saturation show osteomyelitis from T4 through T9 with subligamentous extension, epidural abscess, and paraspinal abscesses. The discs are relatively spared. (**c**, **d**) Diffusion-weighted imaging (**c**) demonstrates partially hyper- and partially hypointensity with high and low apparent diffusion coefficient (ADC) values (arrows) (**d**). The high ADC component represents serous fluid in a cold abscess. (Reprinted and adapted from Moritani and Kim et. al. BJR article)

developing nations. *Brucella* spp. is a Gram-negative coccobacilli which is encountered most commonly from ingestion of unpasteurized milk or milk products. The organism has a predilection for the musculoskeletal system, particularly the spine where both focal and diffuse forms exist. Brucellar spondylitis is often difficult to distinguish from its tuberculous counterpart but is more likely to involve the lumbar spine [48]. Gibbus deformities and multilevel involvement are less commonly seen in brucellosis; however serological tests should be performed for both organisms for definitive diagnosis (Fig. 21.11). Paravertebral and epidural abscesses are also common in Brucellosis [48, 49].

Fungal spinal infections include candidiasis (Fig. 21.12), aspergillosis, blastomycosis, cryptococcosis, Sporothrix, histoplasmosis, and coccidioidomycosis [2, 3, 18, 40, 45]. Positive blood and tissue cultures are helpful in establishing the diagnosis but causative organisms are not proven in a significant number of cases. Therapy is often delayed because of the difficulty in making the diagnosis. The imaging findings of most fungal spinal infections are nonspecific. Vertebral body involvement with destruction can occur mimicking tuberculosis. Absence of T2 high signal in adjacent discs is suggestive of fungal spondylitis [11, 50–52]. Candida spondylitis may be a simultaneous occurrence or late manifestation of hematogenously disseminated candidiasis. The most common location of Candida spondylitis is the lumbar spine. The formation of epidural abscess is uncommon [51]. Echinococcosis, onchocerciasis, toxoplasmosis, and toxocariasis can also involve the spine [2, 53].

21.7 Mimics of Spinal Infection

21.7.1 Degenerative Disc Disease

Early changes often mimic degenerative disease, specifically Modic Type I degenerative endplate changes. Type I Modic changes represent edema within the vertebral endplates. The intervertebral disc may also demonstrate T2 hyperintensity and enhancement, although this is more common with infectious spondylitis. Vacuum phenomenon and lack of adjacent phlegmon/abscess are important findings that suggest degenerative changes as opposed to infection (Fig. 21.13).

21 Spine Infection

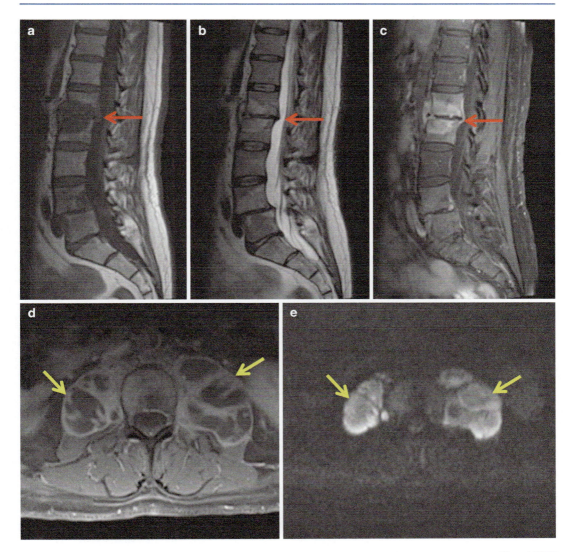

Fig. 21.11 (a–e) Patient is a 62-year-old recent immigrant from Mexico. Sagittal T1 (**a**), T2 (**b**), and fat-sat post-contrast T1 (**c**) show abnormal vertebral body marrow signal at L1-L2 and L4-L5 (red arrow). There is a small epidural phlegmon and pre-spinal soft tissue enhancement at L1-L2. Axial post-contrast (**d**) and DWI (**e**) show large, rim-enhancing fluid collections with diffusion restriction in both psoas muscles consistent with large abscesses (yellow arrow). Sampling of this fluid revealed Brucella as the causative organism

21.7.2 Schmorl's Nodes

Acute invagination of the vertebral body endplate by a portion of the intervertebral disc can also produce marrow edema and enhancement. This is usually confined to a concentric ring in the marrow around the abnormality, and will not involve the entire endplate or adjacent vertebral body. Additionally, surrounding soft tissues will be normal (Fig. 21.14).

21.7.3 Ankylosing Spondylitis

Early in its disease course, active inflammation and erosions at the corners of the endplates (Romanus lesions) may be indistinguishable from infection, although multiple levels of involvement provide a clue. A late manifestation of ankylosing spondylitis is pseudoarthrosis. This occurs after a traumatic event on the fused spine, creating a 3-column stress fracture that extends to

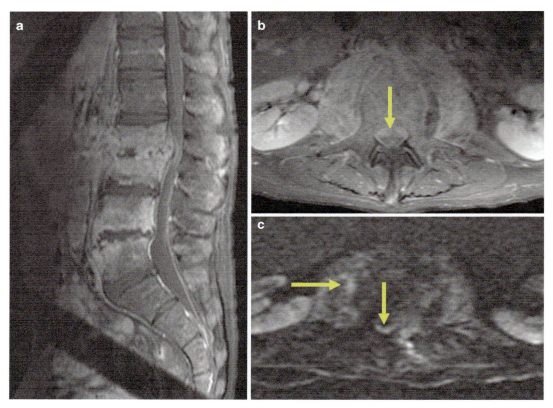

Fig. 21.12 (a–c) Candidiasis. Epidural and psoas infections with spondylodiscitis. Candida was proven by biopsy. (a, b) Sagittal (a) and axial (b) post-contrast T1-weighted image with fat saturation show spondylodiscitis at L2/3 and L4/5 with enhancing psoas and epidural lesions. (c) Diffusion-weighted imaging demonstrates hyperintensity in the epidural and psoas lesions suggestive of small pus collections (arrows)

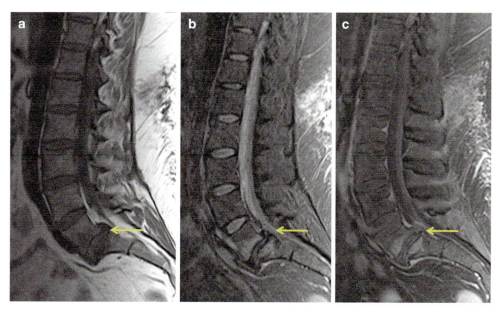

Fig. 21.13 (a–c) Sagittal T1 (a), STIR (b), and post-contrast fat-sat T1 (c) show Grade 1 spondylolisthesis at L5-S1 with Modic type I endplate changes (T1 hypointense, STIR hyperintense) and mild associated enhancement. There is loss of intervertebral disc height with decreased signal intensity on STIR, suggesting desiccation and degenerative disc disease

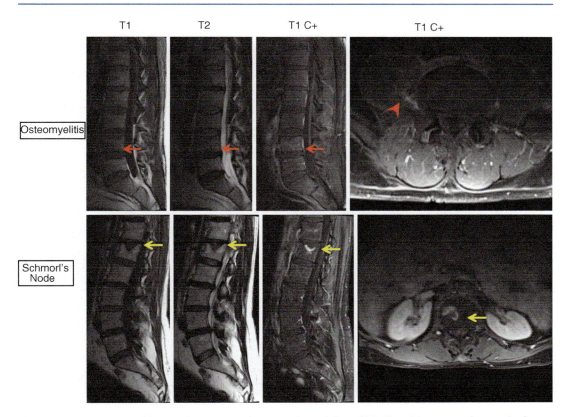

Fig. 21.14 The top row of images demonstrates irregularity of the inferior endplate of L4 with a small surrounding rim of edema and enhancement (red arrow). Axial post-contrast image shows a small abscess in the right psoas muscle confirming infectious spondylitis (short arrow). The bottom row shows an irregularity of the superior endplate of L1, also with marrow edema and enhancement (yellow arrow). There were no surrounding soft tissue abnormalities, and patient inflammatory markers were normal, making acute Schmorl's node the likely diagnosis

Table 21.3 Mimics of epidural and paraspinal abscesses: Differential diagnoses

Epidural, subdural, or subarachnoid hemorrhage
Cerebrospinal leak
Disc herniation
Synovial cyst
Granulation tissue
Tumor
Postsurgical fluid collections

the posterior elements. The fracture line provides a point of mobility in an otherwise fuse spine, and surrounding inflammation results (Andersson lesion). This should be distinguishable from infection given the clinical history, lack of widespread edema/enhancement, and involvement of the posterior processes (Table 21.3) (Fig. 21.15).

21.8 Mimics of Epidural/Paraspinal Abscesses

Disc herniation is extremely common and the diagnosis on MRI is usually straightforward. However, isolated epidural abscess (Fig. 21.6) can be similar to extruded or sequestrated disc herniation on MRI. DWI demonstrates facilitated diffusion in disc herniation (Fig. 21.16) while diffusion is restricted in an abscess.

Epidural/subdural hematoma (Fig. 21.17) and subarachnoid hemorrhage can show hyperintensity on DWI in the late subacute to early chronic phase and in the hyperacute phase. T1-weighted images usually show hyperintensity in the late subacute hematoma due to methemoglobin and can thus differentiate hematoma from abscess.

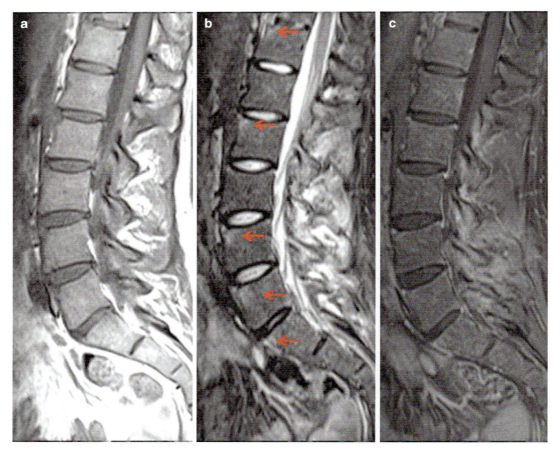

Fig. 21.15 (**a–c**) Sagittal T1 (**a**), STIR (**b**), and T1 post-contrast (**c**) images in a young patient with back pain demonstrate edema of the anterior superior endplates of T12, L2, L4, L5, and S1 without appreciable enhancement (best seen on STIR). Additionally, the patient was found to have bilateral sacroiliitis (not shown). Findings represent early inflammation of ankylosing spondylitis

However, the chronic phase of hematoma can show T1 iso- to hypointensity with restricted diffusion due to the high viscosity containing hemichrome.

CSF leaks can dissect through the epidural space associated with venous plexus engorgement and may appear similar to epidural abscess. However, DWI shows facilitated diffusion in the CSF collection in the epidural space and the venous plexus (Fig. 21.18).

Intraspinal epidermoid can have restricted diffusion that can mimic infection (Fig. 21.19).

Postsurgical wound infection (pus collection) has restricted diffusion while postsurgical fluid collection has facilitated diffusion (Fig. 21.20). However, postsurgical hematoma can have restricted diffusion with well-defined round shape at the postsurgical site (Fig. 21.21).

21.9 Limitation and Pitfalls on Diffusion-Weighted Imaging and Apparent Diffusion Coefficient Maps

Many kinds of echoplanar imaging (EPI) and non-EPI diffusion sequences with various b-values have been reported in the diagnosis of spine and spinal cord disease [54–56]. We routinely use spin-echo-type single-shot EPI

21 Spine Infection

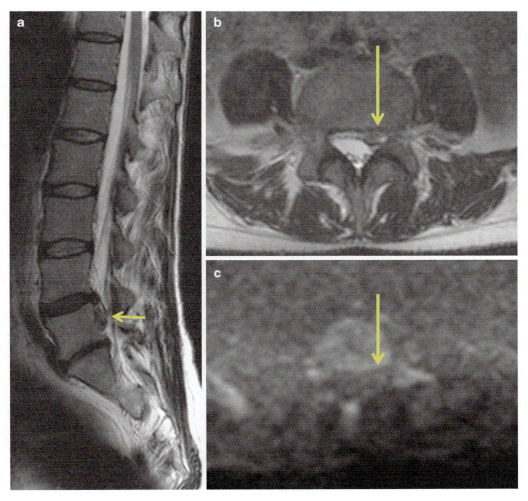

Fig. 21.16 (a–c) Extruded disc herniation. Sagittal (a) and axial (b) T2-weighted images show a left lateral recess extruded disc which demonstrated facilitated diffusion on DWI (c)

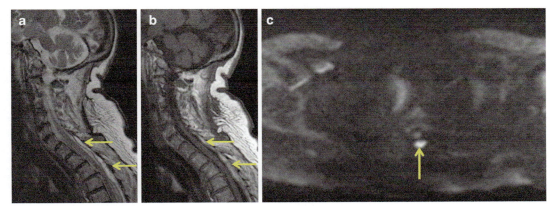

Fig. 21.17 (a–c) Epidural hematoma after trauma. (a, b) Sagittal T2- (a) and T1-weighted images (b) show hyperintense epidural hematoma from T2 through T6 posteriorly. (c) Diffusion-weighted imaging demonstrates hyperintensity in the epidural hematoma (arrow) similar to an epidural abscess

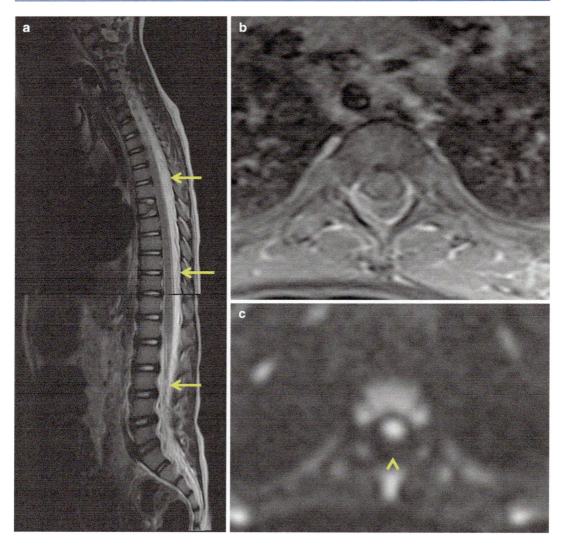

Fig. 21.18 (a–c) Cerebrospinal fluid leak after lumbar puncture in an infant. (**a**) Sagittal T2-weighted image shows hyperintensity in the posterior epidural space extending through the whole spine (arrows). (**b**) Axial post-contrast T1-weighted image with fat saturation shows epidural enhancement due to the prominent venous plexus. (**c**) Diffusion-weighted imaging demonstrates hypointensity in the posterior epidural space (arrowhead)

sequence with parallel imaging techniques in our spine protocols because of the general availability and short acquisition time. For the detection and differentiation of abscesses or pus collections, we use a b-value of 0 and 1000 s mm^{-2} with the ADC map. DWI with lower b-value can show the CSF as partially high signal intensity due to the intravoxel incoherent motion and T2 effect (Fig. 21.22) [57]. To acquire less distortion diffusion-weighted images with the appropriate diffusion weighting, we use a parallel imaging factor of two.

Since DWI is typically implemented with EPI with fat saturation, there are many artifacts (sus-

21 Spine Infection

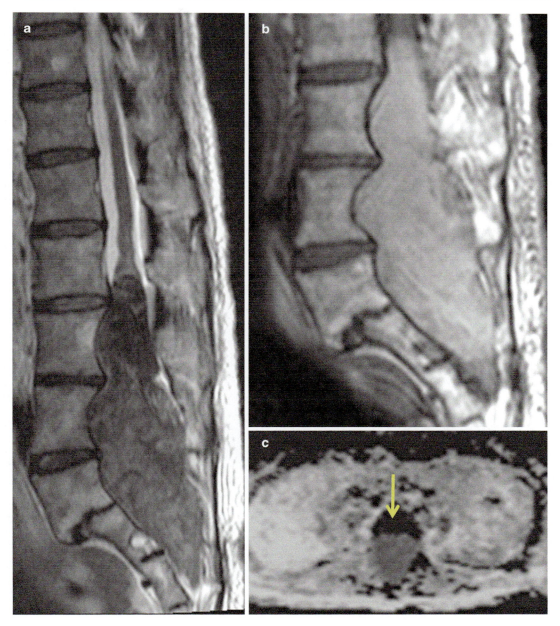

Fig. 21.19 (a–c) Ruptured epidermoid with chemical meningitis. (**a**, **b**) Sagittal MRI shows a large T2 hypointense (**a**) and T1 hyperintense (**b**) mass with posterior scalloping of the vertebral bodies. (**c**) Diffusion-weighted imaging demonstrates slight hyperintensity (not shown) in the mass with decreased apparent diffusion coefficient (arrow)

ceptibility artifact, incomplete fat suppression, N/2 ghosting artifact, eddy current artifact, and motion artifact) and imaging pitfalls on DWI and the ADC map. Paramagnetic susceptibility artifacts from surgical metallic devices cause significant image distortion on DWI (Fig. 21.23). Incomplete fat saturation also occurs related to paramagnetic and diamagnetic susceptibility artifacts.

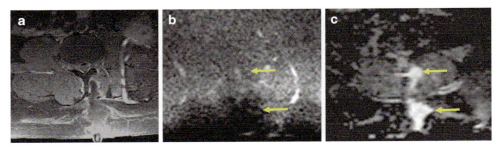

Fig. 21.20 (a–c) Postoperative fluid collection. (a) Axial post-contrast T1-weighted image with fat saturation shows fluid collections at the postoperative site with peripheral enhancement. (b, c) Diffusion-weighted imaging shows the fluid collections as hypointense (b) associated with increased apparent diffusion coefficient (c) consistent with seroma or pseudomeningocele (arrows)

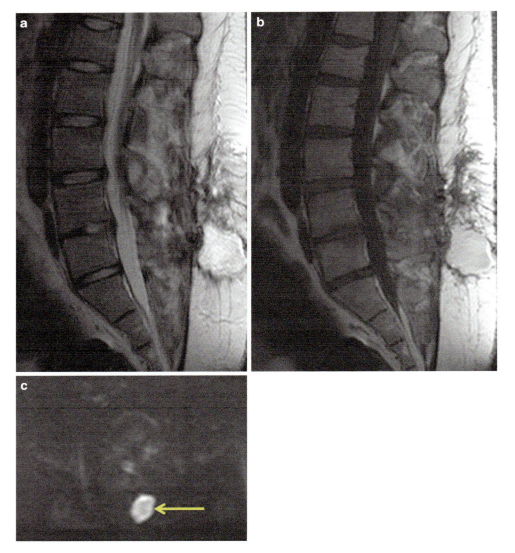

Fig. 21.21 (a–c) Postoperative hematoma. (a, b) Sagittal T2- (a) and T1-weighted images (b) show a hyperintense round lesion at the postoperative site. (c) Diffusion-weighted imaging shows hyperintense signal in the lesion (arrow) with decreased apparent diffusion coefficient (not shown) similar to an abscess. A few white blood cells with blood products were proven by drainage

21 Spine Infection

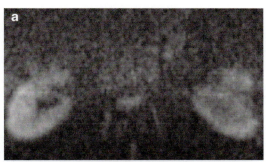

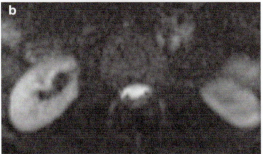

Fig. 21.22 (**a**, **b**) Diffusion-weighted imaging (DWI) with b-values of 500 vs. 1000 s mm^{-2}. (**a**) We routinely use DWI in spine protocols with a b-value of 1000 s mm^{-2} for the evaluation of abscess and pus collection. (**b**) DWI with a b-value of 500 s mm^{-2} shows partially hyperintense normal cerebrospinal fluid in the spinal canal, which is difficult to differentiate from pus collection. DWI use with low or intermediate b-value is not adequate for this purpose since the signal is more influenced by T2 effect and intravoxel incoherent motion

DWI usually shows hyperintensity in epidural and paraspinal abscesses associated with significantly lower ADC values than those in CSF collections, postoperative fluid collections, and muscles. However, ADC maps sometimes show mixed intensity and slightly higher values than those reported in brain abscesses. Mixed intensity and slightly higher ADC values have been reported in subdural, epidural abscess, purulent meningitis, and abdominopelvic abscesses than those in brain abscesses. The higher ADC values may be affected by prior antibiotic treatment, or may be diluted by exudates, CSF, or other fluid [8–10, 58]. If the abscess or pus collection is small, the ADC values can result in errors due to volume-averaging.

DWI has limited usefulness for the evaluation of vertebral body and disc. DWI usually shows slightly high signal intensity with increased ADC in vertebral osteomyelitis (Fig. 21.24). Pathologically, the signal abnormality corresponds to bone marrow necrosis and edema with inflammatory cell infiltration. ADC values of the bone marrow in spinal infection have been reported as significantly higher than those in malignancy. However, an overlap of ADC values is noted [11, 59–61]. DWI signals and the ADC values of the vertebral body are variable depending on the proportion between red and yellow bone marrow associated with aging, degenerative changes, and other conditions [56, 62]. The bone marrow fat (yellow bone marrow) causes signal void on DWI because DWI typically uses chemical fat saturation techniques. Moreover, bony trabeculae cause signal loss related to diamagnetic susceptibility artifacts. Thus, the calculated ADC values are affected by the chemical fat saturation and susceptibility artifacts. DWI signals and ADC values of the disc can also be different owing to the variable presence of water contents with aging and degenerative changes.

21.10 Conclusions

DWI with ADC maps is useful in early and accurate diagnosis of spinal and paraspinal infections, treatment planning and preoperative assessment for surgical drainage and biopsy. Important differential diagnoses include epidural, subdural, or subarachnoid hemorrhage, CSF leak, disc herniation, synovial cyst, granulation tissue, intra- or extradural tumor, and postsurgical fluid collections. Recognition of artifacts on DWI and ADC maps is essential when interpreting DWI of spinal and paraspinal infections.

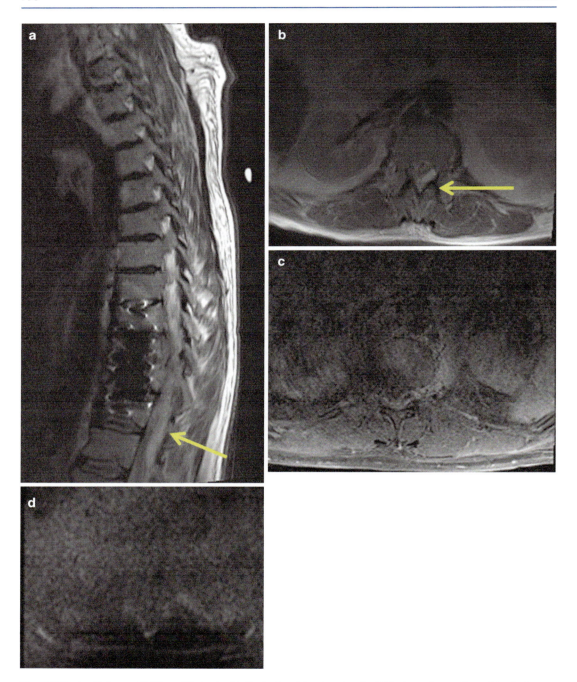

Fig. 21.23 (**a–d**) Susceptibility artifacts. (**a**, **b**) Sagittal (**a**) and axial (**b**) T2-weighted images show a hyperintense lesion in the epidural space posterolaterally (arrows) with relatively mild susceptibility artifacts from a fusion device. (**c**) Axial post-contrast T1-weighted image with fat saturation is difficult to detect the epidural abscess owing to motion artifacts. (**d**) Diffusion-weighted imaging shows no apparent hyperintensity owing to susceptibility artifacts from the fusion device, erroneously not identifying the epidural abscess

21 Spine Infection

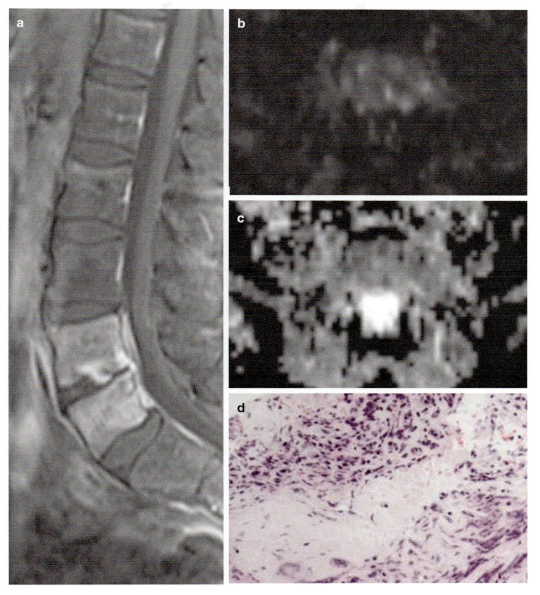

Fig. 21.24 (**a–d**) Vertebral osteomyelitis. (**a**) Sagittal post-contrast T1-weighted image with fat saturation shows enhancement in the disc and vertebral bodies at L4 and L5 consistent with discitis/osteomyelitis. (**b, c**) There is mild hyperintensity on diffusion-weighted imaging (**b**) with increased apparent diffusion coefficient (**c**) in the adjacent bone marrow. (**d**) Pathology demonstrates extensive bone necrosis and edema with patchy inflammatory cell infiltrations

References

1. Casper DS et al (2018) The effect of postoperative spinal infections on patient mortality. Spine (Phila Pa 1976) 43(3):223–227
2. Tali ET (2004) Spinal infections. Eur J Radiol 50(2):120–133
3. Darouiche RO (2006) Spinal epidural abscess. N Engl J Med 355(19):2012–2020
4. Kourbeti IS, Tsiodras S, Boumpas DT (2008) Spinal infections: evolving concepts. Curr Opin Rheumatol 20(4):471–479
5. Tins BJ, Cassar-Pullicino VN (2004) MR imaging of spinal infection. Semin Musculoskelet Radiol 8(3):215–229

6. Moritani T et al (2014) Pyogenic and non-pyogenic spinal infections: emphasis on diffusion-weighted imaging for the detection of abscesses and pus collections. Br J Radiol 87(1041):20140011
7. Fertikh D et al (2007) Discrimination of capsular stage brain abscesses from necrotic or cystic neoplasms using diffusion-weighted magnetic resonance imaging. J Neurosurg 106(1):76–81
8. Ferreira NP et al (2005) Imaging aspects of pyogenic infections of the central nervous system. Top Magn Reson Imaging 16(2):145–154
9. Abe M et al (2002) Purulent meningitis with unusual diffusion-weighted MRI findings. Eur J Radiol 44(1):1–4
10. Tsuchiya K et al (2003) Diffusion-weighted MRI of subdural and epidural empyemas. Neuroradiology 45(4):220–223
11. Thurnher MM, Bammer R (2006) Diffusion-weighted magnetic resonance imaging of the spine and spinal cord. Semin Roentgenol 41(4):294–311
12. Eastwood JD, Vollmer RT, Provenzale JM (2002) Diffusion-weighted imaging in a patient with vertebral and epidural abscesses. AJNR Am J Neuroradiol 23(3):496–498
13. Trombly R, Guest JD (2007) Acute central cord syndrome arising from a cervical epidural abscess: case report. Neurosurgery 61(2):E424–E425; discussion E425.
14. Palestro CJ, Love C, Miller TT (2006) Infection and musculoskeletal conditions: Imaging of musculoskeletal infections. Best Pract Res Clin Rheumatol 20(6):1197–1218
15. Butler JS et al (2006) Nontuberculous pyogenic spinal infection in adults: a 12-year experience from a tertiary referral center. Spine (Phila Pa 1976) 31(23):2695–2700
16. Boden SD et al (1992) Postoperative diskitis: distinguishing early MR imaging findings from normal postoperative disk space changes. Radiology 184(3):765–771
17. Modic MT et al (1985) Vertebral osteomyelitis: assessment using MR. Radiology 157(1):157–166
18. Lury K, Smith JK, Castillo M (2006) Imaging of spinal infections. Semin Roentgenol 41(4):363–379
19. Conaughty JM et al (2006) Efficacy of linezolid versus vancomycin in the treatment of methicillin-resistant Staphylococcus aureus discitis: a controlled animal model. Spine (Phila Pa 1976) 31(22):E830–E832
20. Stevens QE et al (2007) Reactivation of dormant lumbar methicillin-resistant Staphylococcus aureus osteomyelitis after 12 years. J Clin Neurosci 14(6):585–589
21. Mahboubi S, Morris MC (2001) Imaging of spinal infections in children. Radiol Clin N Am 39(2):215–222
22. Bair-Merritt MH, Chung C, Collier A (2000) Spinal epidural abscess in a young child. Pediatrics 106(3):E39
23. Glazer PA, Hu SS (1996) Pediatric spinal infections. Orthop Clin North Am 27(1):111–123
24. Wiley AM, Trueta J (1959) The vascular anatomy of the spine and its relationship to pyogenic vertebral osteomyelitis. J Bone Joint Surg (Br) 41-B:796–809
25. Ozuna RM, Delamarter RB (1996) Pyogenic vertebral osteomyelitis and postsurgical disc space infections. Orthop Clin North Am 27(1):87–94
26. Calderone RR, Larsen JM (1996) Overview and classification of spinal infections. Orthop Clin North Am 27(1):1–8
27. Uchida K et al (2010) Epidural abscess associated with pyogenic spondylodiscitis of the lumbar spine; evaluation of a new MRI staging classification and imaging findings as indicators of surgical management: a retrospective study of 37 patients. Arch Orthop Trauma Surg 130(1):111–118
28. Solomou E et al (2004) Multiple spinal epidural abscesses extending to the whole spinal canal. Magn Reson Imaging 22(5):747–750
29. Ghosh PS et al (2009) Holocord spinal epidural abscess. J Child Neurol 24(6):768–771
30. Ledermann HP et al (2003) MR imaging findings in spinal infections: rules or myths? Radiology 228(2):506–514
31. Wagner SC et al (2000) Can imaging findings help differentiate spinal neuropathic arthropathy from disk space infection? Initial experience. Radiology 214(3):693–699
32. Numaguchi Y et al (1993) Spinal epidural abscess: evaluation with gadolinium-enhanced MR imaging. Radiographics 13(3):545–559; discussion 559–60.
33. Longo M et al (2003) Contrast-enhanced MR imaging with fat suppression in adult-onset septic spondylodiscitis. Eur Radiol 13(3):626–637
34. Doita M et al (2007) Septic arthritis of lumbar facet joints without predisposing infection. J Spinal Disord Tech 20(4):290–295
35. Smida M et al (2004) Septic arthritis of a lumbar facet joint case report and review of the literature. Acta Orthop Belg 70(3):290–294
36. Mellado JM et al (2004) MR imaging of spinal infection: atypical features, interpretive pitfalls and potential mimickers. Eur Radiol 14(11):1980–1989
37. Muffoletto AJ et al (2001) Hematogenous pyogenic facet joint infection. Spine (Phila Pa 1976) 26(14):1570–1576
38. Coscia MF, Trammell TR (2002) Pyogenic lumbar facet joint arthritis with intradural extension: a case report. J Spinal Disord Tech 15(6):526–528
39. Velissaris D et al (2009) Spinal subdural staphylococcus aureus abscess: case report and review of the literature. World J Emerg Surg 4:31
40. Reihsaus E, Waldbaur H, Seeling W (2000) Spinal epidural abscess: a meta-analysis of 915 patients. Neurosurg Rev 23(4):175–204; discussion 205.
41. Dorflinger-Hejlek E et al (2010) Diffusion-weighted MR imaging of intramedullary spinal cord abscess. AJNR Am J Neuroradiol 31(9):1651–1652
42. Berbari EF et al (2015) 2015 Infectious Diseases Society of America (IDSA) clinical practice guide-

lines for the diagnosis and treatment of native vertebral osteomyelitis in adults. Clin Infect Dis 61(6):e26–e46

43. Marschall J et al (2011) The impact of prebiopsy antibiotics on pathogen recovery in hematogenous vertebral osteomyelitis. Clin Infect Dis 52(7):867–872

44. Harada Y, Tokuda O, Matsunaga N (2008) Magnetic resonance imaging characteristics of tuberculous spondylitis vs. pyogenic spondylitis. Clin Imaging 32(4):303–309

45. Skaf GS et al (2010) Non-pyogenic infections of the spine. Int J Antimicrob Agents 36(2):99–105

46. Karaeminogullari O et al (2007) Tuberculosis of the lumbar spine: outcomes after combined treatment of two-drug therapy and surgery. Orthopedics 30(1):55–59

47. Zhang HQ et al (2007) One-stage surgical management for multilevel tuberculous spondylitis of the upper thoracic region by anterior decompression, strut autografting, posterior instrumentation, and fusion. J Spinal Disord Tech 20(4):263–267

48. Oztekin O et al (2010) Brucellar spondylodiscitis: magnetic resonance imaging features with conventional sequences and diffusion-weighted imaging. Radiol Med 115(5):794–803

49. Al-Nakshabandi NA (2012) The spectrum of imaging findings of brucellosis: a pictorial essay. Can Assoc Radiol J 63(1):5–11

50. Chia SL et al (2005) Candida spondylodiscitis and epidural abscess: management with shorter courses of anti-fungal therapy in combination with surgical debridement. J Infect 51(1):17–23

51. Aganovic L, Hoda RS, Rumboldt Z (2004) Hyperintensity of spinal Cryptococcus infection on diffusion-weighted MR images. AJR Am J Roentgenol 183(4):1176–1177

52. Williams RL et al (1999) Fungal spinal osteomyelitis in the immunocompromised patient: MR findings in three cases. AJNR Am J Neuroradiol 20(3):381–385

53. Akhan O et al (1991) Spinal intradural hydatid cyst in a child. Br J Radiol 64(761):465–466

54. Andre JB, Bammer R (2010) Advanced diffusion-weighted magnetic resonance imaging techniques of the human spinal cord. Top Magn Reson Imaging 21(6):367–378

55. Hori M et al (2006) Line scan diffusion tensor MRI at low magnetic field strength: feasibility study of cervical spondylotic myelopathy in an early clinical stage. J Magn Reson Imaging 23(2):183–188

56. Raya JG et al (2006) Methods and applications of diffusion imaging of vertebral bone marrow. J Magn Reson Imaging 24(6):1207–1220

57. Le Bihan D et al (1986) MR imaging of intravoxel incoherent motions: application to diffusion and perfusion in neurologic disorders. Radiology 161(2):401–407

58. Oto A et al (2011) Diffusion-weighted MR imaging of abdominopelvic abscesses. Emerg Radiol 18(6):515–524

59. Castillo M et al (2000) Diffusion-weighted MR imaging offers no advantage over routine noncontrast MR imaging in the detection of vertebral metastases. AJNR Am J Neuroradiol 21(5):948–953

60. Pui MH et al (2005) Diffusion-weighted magnetic resonance imaging of spinal infection and malignancy. J Neuroimaging 15(2):164–170

61. Herneth AM et al (2005) Diffusion weighted imaging of bone marrow pathologies. Eur J Radiol 55(1):74–83

62. Padhani AR et al (2013) Assessing the relation between bone marrow signal intensity and apparent diffusion coefficient in diffusion-weighted MRI. AJR Am J Roentgenol 200(1):163–170

Primary and Metastatic Spine Tumors

22

Patrick W. Hitchon, Shotaro Naganawa, John Kim, Royce W. Woodroffe, Logan C. Helland, Mark C. Smith, and Toshio Moritani

22.1 Introduction

The presenting symptoms of night pain, pain at rest, or progressive neurologic deficit should prompt the clinician to entertain the diagnosis of primary or metastatic tumors of the spine. The primary complaint of most patients with spine tumors is pain, without an apparent difference between benign or malignant tumors. With the increased availability of MRI, the number of patients presenting with neurologic deficits will most likely decrease secondary to earlier diagno-

P. W. Hitchon · M. C. Smith
University of Iowa Carver College of Medicine, Iowa City, IA, USA
e-mail: patrick-hitchon@uiowa.edu;
mark-c-smith@uiowa.edu

S. Naganawa
Department of Radiology, University of Michigan, Ann Arbor, MI, USA
e-mail: snaganaw@umich.edu

J. Kim (⊠) · T. Moritani
Division of Neuroradiology, University of Michigan, Ann Arbor, MI, USA
e-mail: johannk@med.umich.edu;
tmoritan@med.umich.edu

R. W. Woodroffe · L. C. Helland
Department of Neurosurgery, University of Iowa Carver College of Medicine, Iowa City, IA, USA
e-mail: royce-woodroffe@uiowa.edu;
logan-helland@uiowa.edu

sis. Often, plain radiographs demonstrate the site of the lesion and in many cases can be diagnostic. However, a significant amount of destruction is necessary before plain radiographs show evidence of disease [1]. Hence, computed tomography (CT) and MRI are valuable for defining the extent and precise location of the lesion. The need for myelography to diagnose and define benign tumors of the spine has been nearly eliminated by these two imaging advances.

In the case of metastatic tumors, a CT of the chest, abdomen, and pelvis or positron emission tomography scan can help to identify any additional distant pathology. Ultimately, however, a tissue diagnosis by image-guided biopsy is required to aid in preoperative planning. Angiography can be an ancillary test in diagnosis, but mostly for preoperative embolization to decrease intraoperative blood loss and therefore the postoperative morbidity. Aneurysmal bone cysts, giant cell tumors, hemangiomas, and renal cell metastases should be considered for preoperative embolization.

22.2 DWI of Spinal Tumors

In this chapter, we address the utility of diffusion-weighted imaging (DWI) along with corresponding apparent diffusion coefficient (ADC) maps in addition to conventional MR sequences for

© Springer Nature Switzerland AG 2021
T. Moritani, A. A. Capizzano (eds.), *Diffusion-Weighted MR Imaging of the Brain, Head and Neck, and Spine*, https://doi.org/10.1007/978-3-030-62120-9_22

22.2.1 Technique

We routinely use DWI in spine protocols with b-value of 1000 sec/mm^2, spin-echo type echo-planar imaging, and a parallel imaging factor of 2 or 3. The ADC maps are calculated from b values of 0 and 1000 sec/mm^2. Lower b-values (e.g., 0–500) are not adequate for diffusion-weighted imaging due to influence by both slow perfusion (intravoxel incoherent motion) and T2 effect. A DWI image with b = 500 shows partially hyperintense normal CSF in the spinal canal, whereas this effect is absent in the b = 1000 image.

22.2.2 DWI Signal and ADC of the Spine

DW signal of the vertebral body is variable depending on the proportion between red and yellow bone marrow. The fat content of bone marrow causes a DWI signal void because DWI innately uses chemical fat saturation. Moreover, the bony trabeculae also cause signal loss due to diamagnetic susceptibility effects. The resulting calculated ADC values are thus affected by both chemical shift and susceptibility artifacts. DW signal and ADC values of the disc also vary secondary to degree of degenerative changes present.

22.3 Metastatic Tumors to the Spine

By far and away, the most common adult spine tumors are metastatic, with more than 90% of spinal tumors being metastatic [2, 3]. Most common cancers affecting the spine include breast, lung, prostate, and kidney [4]. The American Cancer Society predicts that in 2019 there will be an estimated 1,762,450 new cases of cancer in the USA, with 606,900 deaths. Thirty to seventy percent of patients who die from cancer have evidence of vertebral metastases visible on postmortem examination [1]. Even though only 10% of metastatic tumors will prove unstable requiring stabilization, accuracy in diagnosis and appropriate management are paramount.

The frequency of metastatic disease to the spine does vary with the type of the primary cancer. Prostate cancer is the most common cancer associated with spinal metastases. This is followed in frequency by breast, melanoma, lung, thyroid, and renal, lymphoma, myeloma, and pancreatic cancers [1, 4, 5]. However, some centers have developed areas of specialization dealing with one type of cancer over others. At the University of Iowa (UIHC), specialized care in neuroendocrine tumors has resulted in a significantly larger proportion of such tumors in our practice.

22.3.1 Imaging

As stated above, plain films are often inadequate except in advanced cases. On CT scan, the majority of metastatic tumors to the spine are lytic (Figs. 22.1, 22.2, 22.3, and 22.4). Bone scans can reveal the multiplicity of lesions, favoring metastatic disease rather than primary bone tumors. On MRI, expansion and compression of the spinal canal is better appreciated, with enhancement of the cancerous tissue. The enhancement reflects tumor extension into the canal as well as the paraspinal space (Fig. 22.5). The diagnosis can sometimes be surmised in the presence of other lesions noted in the kidney or lung. Prostate metastases can be mixed with lytic and sclerotic lesions (Fig. 22.6). The sclerotic or blastic appearance on CT associated with increased activity on bone scan is diagnostic of prostate metastases.

Metastatic tumors generally show DWI hyperintensity with reduced ADC values (Figs. 22.7, 22.8, 22.9, and 22.10). The ADC values depend on a combination of factors including the hypercellularity of the primary tumor, the degree of necrosis, and the makeup of the extracellular tumor matrix. Since DWI uses

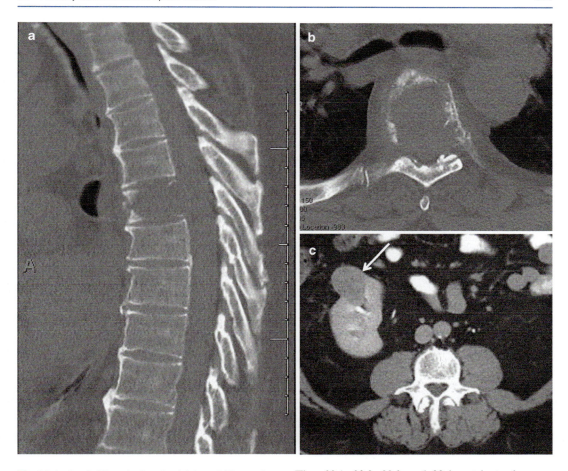

Fig. 22.1 (**a–c**) CT sagittal and axial (**a** and **b**) reveals a lytic lesion involving T6 vertebral body and pedicles bilaterally. Abdominal CT (**c**, arrow) also shows a mass involving the right kidney compatible with renal cell carcinoma (Figs. 22.1, 22.2, 22.3, and 22.4 pertain to the same patient. A middle-aged gentleman presents with a 2-month history of right interscapular pain without a history of weight loss or malignancy)

fat saturation and free water saturation techniques with a larger FOV than conventional MRI, the detection of primary tumors and other metastatic foci are often enhanced. Recently, whole-body DWI technique is used to detect primary and metastatic lesions [6]. A few studies show DWI can be of high diagnostic accuracy in detecting metastases, with comparable results to PET/CT [7, 8].

22.3.2 Management

In cases of pain from lymphoma, myeloma, or small cell lung cancer, radiation therapy with chemotherapy is obviously the treatment of choice [5]. Tumors that are moderately sensitive include breast, prostate, and thyroid. However, in the presence of neurological deficit interfering with mobility or pain unresponsive to radiation and chemotherapy, and in the absence of medical contraindications, surgery is indicated. Surgery is also recommended in cases of instability with kyphosis or subluxation. Less often, surgery can be appropriate where the diagnosis has been elusive in spite of multiple attempts at biopsy. There are extant guidelines for surgery in metastatic spinal disease, such as the Spinal Instability Neoplastic Score (SINS) [5, 9, 10]. As is often the case, the indications for surgery are often selected after

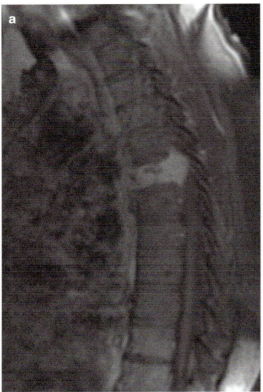

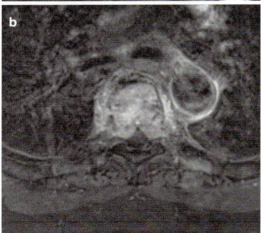

Fig. 22.2 (**a**, **b**) Contrast-enhanced T1-weighted sagittal (**a**) and axial (**b**) MRI shows a mass involving T6 with loss in height and extension of tumor into the spinal canal and paraspinal space

multidisciplinary discussions between the patient and the treating team. There are exceptions to every guideline, and it is the patient who bears the consequence of an ill-advised operation.

22.4 Primary Spine Tumors

The American Cancer Society estimates approximately 3,450 new cases of bone cancer will be diagnosed in 2018 [11]. The incidence of primary bony spinal neoplasms has been estimated at 2.5 to 8.5 per 100,000 people per year [12]. As a general rule, two important clinical features need to be considered in evaluating the potential malignancy of a lesion in the spine: age and location. More than 75% of lesions located in the vertebral body are malignant, compared to one-third of lesions in the posterior elements. Second, more than two-thirds of all lesions seen in children younger than age 18 are benign, whereas this figure is reversed in adults. In a recent review at the Mayo Clinic, of nearly 10,000 skeletal tumors distributed throughout the skeleton, 2,900 were benign, and 7,100 were malignant [13]. A further analysis of this group revealed that 1,100 tumors involving the spine were malignant and only 274 were benign.

22.5 Benign Tumors

22.5.1 Giant Cell Tumor

Giant cell tumors of the spine are locally aggressive, benign primary bone tumors that constitute about a third of benign spinal tumors [13]. The mean age of involvement is approximately 30 years, with a range of 13 to 62 years [14]. The incidence in women appears to outnumber that in men by a ratio of 2:1 [15]. Most patients present with pain localized to the site of the lesion, and occasionally with a neurologic deficit, depending on the location. Giant cell tumors primarily occur in the vertebral body, but may extend into the posterior elements [2]. Malignant transformation occurs in approximately 10% of cases. Some giant cell tumors are biologically aggressive lesions. In patients with these tumors, local recurrence is common after incomplete resection.

22.5.1.1 Imaging

The diagnosis of giant cell tumors may be made from MRI and CT scans (Figs. 22.11 and 22.12).

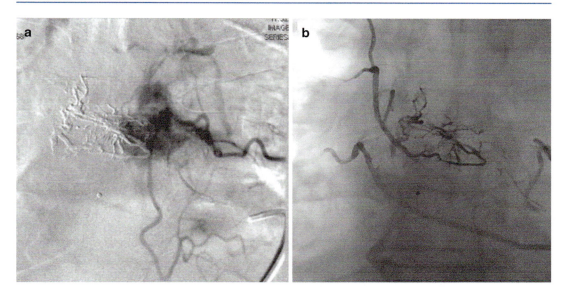

Fig. 22.3 (**a, b**) For the reduction of intraoperative blood loss in vascular tumors such as renal cell carcinoma, embolization with Onyx glue (ethylene-vinyl alcohol copolymer) was undertaken through T7 and T8 segmental arteries. Images before (**a**) and after (**b**) embolization are shown

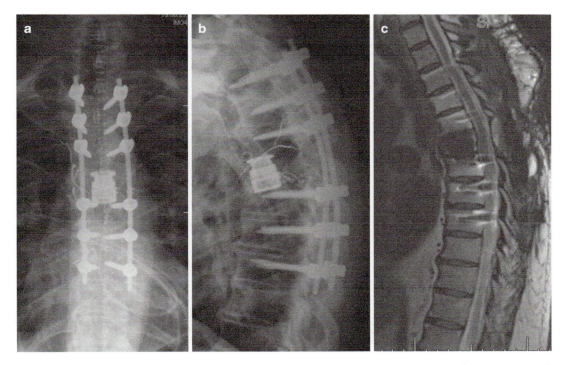

Fig. 22.4 (**a, b**) On account of the symptoms and unresponsive nature of renal cell cancer, the patient underwent corpectomy of T6, decompression of the spinal canal, and stabilization. Postoperative plain films in the anteroposterior (**a**) and lateral projection (**b**) are presented. Postoperative sagittal T2-weighted MRI (**c**) shows adequate decompression when compared to the preoperative images in Fig. 22.2

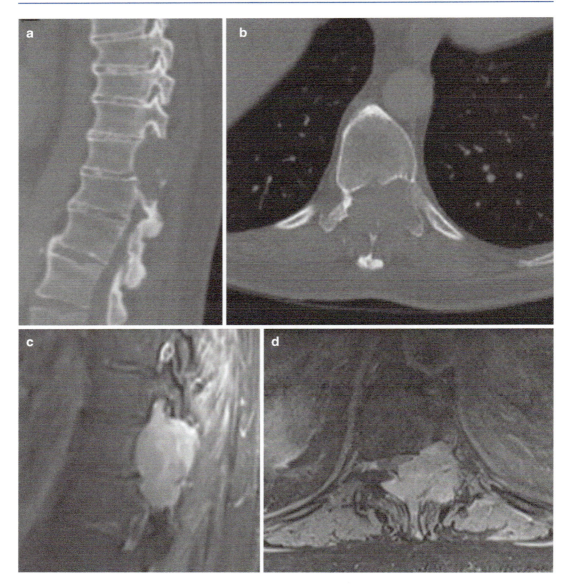

Fig. 22.5 (**a–d**) A middle-aged gentleman presents with 2-month history of worsening back pain and 20-pound weight loss. Endorses knees giving out while walking and numbness in legs for the past 2 weeks. Pathology was that of neuroendocrine tumor. CT scan sagittal (**a**) and axial (**b**) shows a large mass involving T11 with erosion of the left pedicle and bilateral lamina as well as the spinous process. There is some erosion of the posterior elements of T12 as well. Sagittal (**c**) and axial (**d**) enhanced MRI shows a large extradural lesion within the left pedicle and posterior elements of T11 resulting in severe cord compression. Multiplicity of spinal lesions seen on other images suggests metastatic disease

The lesion is characterized as a destructive, expansile enhancing mass that may contain blood degradation products. Pathologically, giant cell tumors consist of multinucleated osteoclastic giant cells and spindle cell stroma, occasionally with secondary "aneurysmal bone cystlike" change [16]. This pathologic feature of hypercellularity corresponds to lower ADC values [17].

22 Primary and Metastatic Spine Tumors

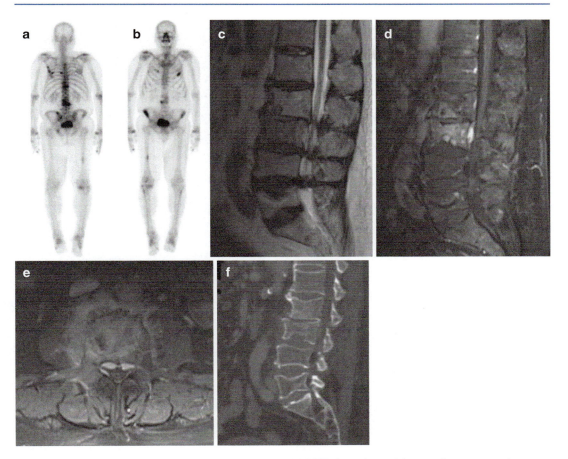

Fig. 22.6 (**a–f**) A gentleman with a 2-year history of prostate cancer presents with leg weakness, mild back pain, and the need to use a cane on one side and a crutch on the other for the past couple of months. Technetium-99 m methylene diphosphonate (Tc-99 m MDP) bone scan shows multiple foci of abnormal uptake consistent with multiple osseous metastases. (**a, b**) Sagittal T2 (**c**), sagittal T1 contrast-enhanced (**d**) and axial T1 contrast-enhanced (**e**) MRI shows interval increase in marrow replacement, most prominently at L3, with significant enhancement consistent with spread of metastatic disease. Interval reduction of vertebral body height at this level is suggestive of new pathologic fracture. Sagittal (**f**) CT scan shows pathologic compression fractures in the lumbar spine with lytic and sclerotic features characteristic of metastatic prostate cancer

22.5.1.2 Management

Giant cell tumors are large expansile masses that frequently result in the destruction of the vertebral body. The most acceptable treatment approach seems to be an attempted wide resection [18–20]. However, due to the vascular nature of these tumors, preoperative embolization is frequently performed [2]. Radiation therapy may be considered with subtotal surgical excision [21]. Giant cell tumors can recur relatively early after even the most radical surgical excision. In such cases, it may be reasonable to consider radiation therapy if it is believed that further excisional attempts will also be unsuccessful. The 10-year success rate of radiation alone was 69%, compared to 83% for postoperative radiation therapy [22]. Unfortunately, progression to a high-grade sarcoma occurs in 5–15% of cases following radiation treatment [22]. Therefore, radiation therapy should be reserved for patients with recurrent or residual disease after attempted resection [20]. In the spine, wide resection may cause destabilization and may necessitate instrumentation of the spine and fusion (Fig. 22.13).

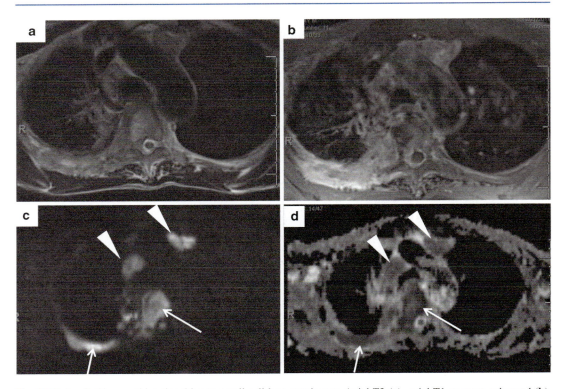

Fig. 22.7 (a–d) 64-year-old male with non-small cell lung carcinoma. Axial T2 (a), axial T1 contrast-enhanced (b), DWI (c), and ADC map (d) clearly shows vertebral, right rib, and mediastinal lymph node metastases

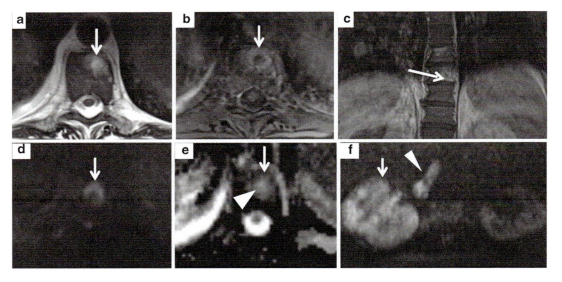

Fig. 22.8 (a–f) 57-year-old male with renal cell carcinoma. Bull's eye or halo pattern seen on T2 (a) contrast-enhanced T1 (b and c), DWI (d), and ADC (e) is due to necrotic tumor center, which is reported as characteristic for metastasis [98]. ADC value in the necrotic center is 1.52×10^{-3} mm²/s, significantly higher than solid outer ring, 0.65×10^{-3} mm²/s. In addition, DWI reveals right renal tumor and renal vein tumor thrombus (f)

22 Primary and Metastatic Spine Tumors

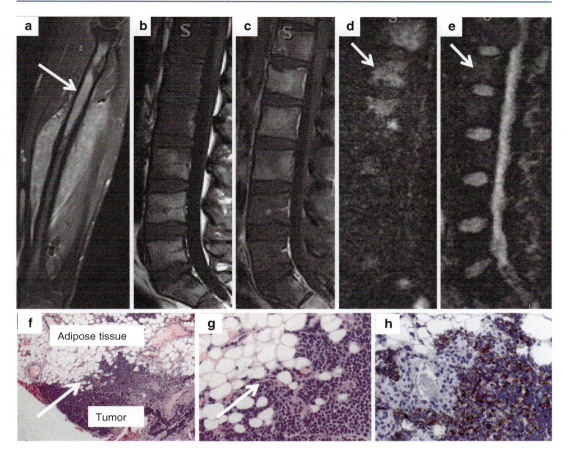

Fig. 22.9 (**a–h**) 25-year-old male with Primary Ewing Sarcoma in the radius (**a**). T1 (**b**) and contrast-enhanced T1 (**c**) shows multiple enhancing lesions. DWI (**d**) demonstrates homogeneous hyperintensity due to hypercellularity, indicating bone metastases. ADC map (**e**) shows low ADC values in the vertebral body (0.48–0.61 × 10^{-3} mm²/s) as markedly hypercellular tumor replaces the normal fatty bone marrow as seen on histology (**f–h**)

22.5.2 Hemangioma

Hemangioma is one of the common benign lesions involving the spinal axis. It is often discovered incidentally during evaluation of patients with back or neck pain. Of the 275 benign spinal tumors described by Unni et al. [13], the incidence of hemangioma was 15%, with less than 5% of patients with hemangiomas developing symptoms [12]. Vertebral hemangiomas most commonly occur in the thoracic and lumbar spine and can occur in the body, pedicle, or lamina [2]. These lesions can cause local pain, but spinal surgeons typically become involved with the treatment of hemangioma when the lesion causes spinal cord or nerve root compression, or when a pathologic fracture occurs.

22.5.2.1 Imaging

Plain radiography and CT can clearly demonstrate the typical coarsened trabeculae within the involved vertebrae, with a characteristic honeycombed appearance. Gadolinium enhancement and MRI evidence of a soft tissue component are often observed (Fig. 22.14).

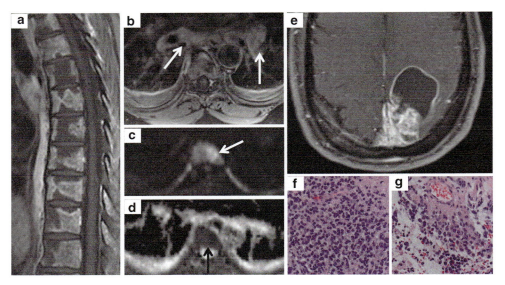

Fig. 22.10 (**a–g**) 52-year-old male with Glioblastoma as a primary tumor in the left frontoparietal lobes. Sagittal (**a**) and axial (**b**) contrast-enhanced T1 shows osseous and mediastinal metastases. DWI (**c**) demonstrates hyperintensity in the bone metastases with reduced ADC (**d**) due to hypercellularity of glioblastoma (ADC: 0.64×10^{-3} mm^2/s). Pathology of the primary GBM (**e**) and bone metastasis shows hypercellularity (**f**) and necrosis (**g**)

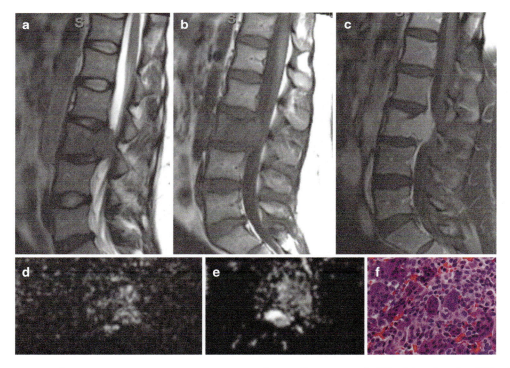

Fig. 22.11 (**a–f**) T2-weighted (**a**), T1 (**b**), T1 + Gd (**c**), DWI (**d**), and ACD map (**e**) magnetic resonance imaging scans reveal the bony tumor arising from L3 with extension anteriorly and posteriorly. DWI demonstrates mild hyperintensity in giant cell tumor (GCT) with reduced ADC due to hypercellularity (ADC: 0.84×10^{-3} mm^2/s). Differentiation from malignant tumor is difficult based on the ADC value. A needle biopsy revealed a giant cell rich hypercellular tumor (**f**) (Figs. 22.11, 22.12, and 22.13 pertain to the same patient: a young lady who has suffered with back, left hip, and left leg pain for the past 6 months. The intensity of the pain has increased with the passage of time)

22 Primary and Metastatic Spine Tumors

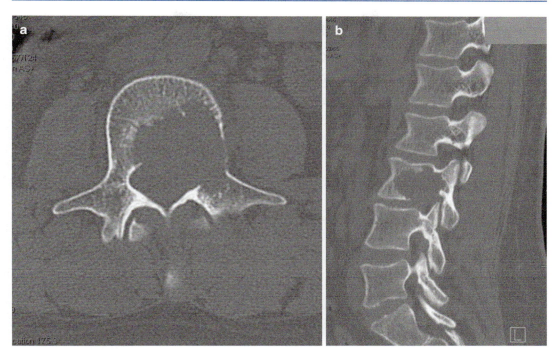

Fig. 22.12 (**a, b**) Axial (**a**) and sagittal (**b**) CT scans demonstrate the expansile intramedullary tumor with extension into the spinal canal

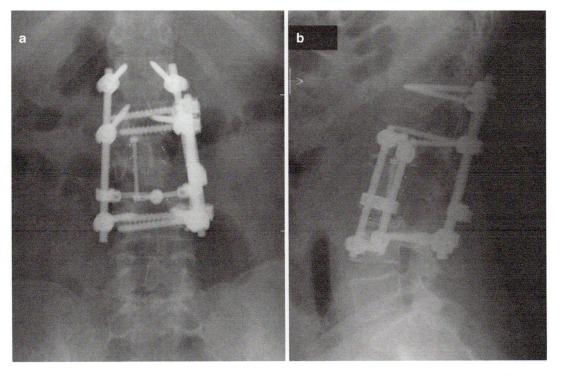

Fig. 22.13 (**a, b**) Three years following lateral corpectomy and posterior instrumentation, AP (**a**) and lateral (**b**) radiographs show satisfactory alignment with hardware in place

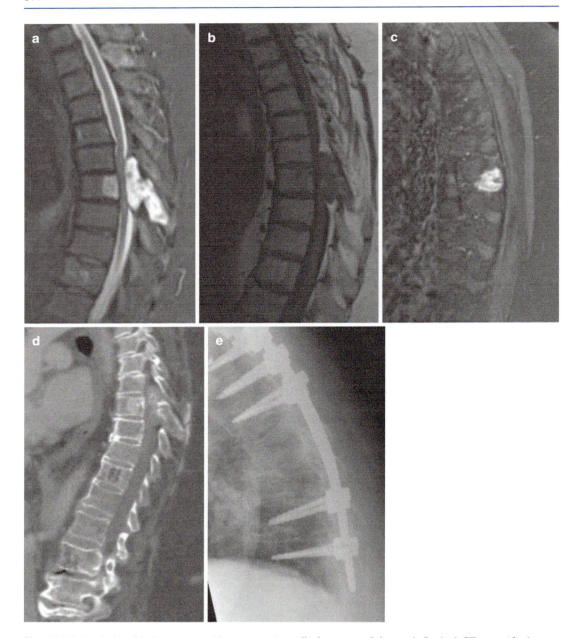

Fig. 22.14 (**a–e**) An elderly woman with paraparesis. MRI shows a thoracic hemangioma. T2 (**a**), T1 (**b**), and T1 + Gd (**c**) sequences show tumor involving body, pedicle, transverse process, and spinous process, with anterior displacement of the cord. Sagittal CT scan (**d**) demonstrates the trabeculated appearance of the hemangioma. The tumor mass was resected with the implantation of instrumentation (**e**)

Spinal hemangiomas often have varying fatty component, and MR signal intensity may be suppressed on fat-suppressed images such as DWI, depending on the amount of fat tissue. This signal loss should not be mistaken as low ADC values. Typical hemangiomas often show hyperintense appearance on T1- and T2-weighted images (Fig. 22.15), but some (atypical) hemangiomas show hypointense signal on T1-weighted image (Fig. 22.16), which can mimic malignancy

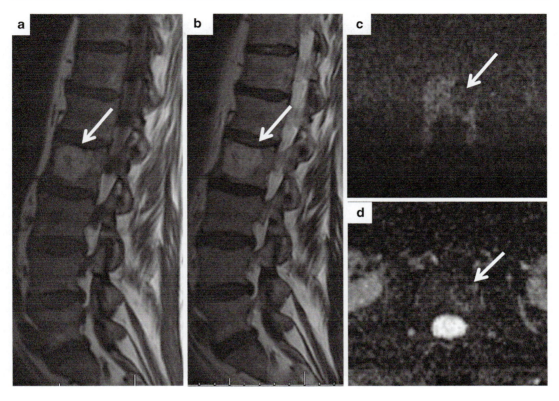

Fig. 22.15 61-year-old male. There is a well-defined round mass in the L1 vertebral body. Hyperintense appearance on T1- (**a**) and T2- (**b**) weighted images indicates typical hemangioma. DWI (**c**) demonstrates very low signal in fat-contained hemangioma with blackout on the ADC map (**d**) due to chemical fat saturation

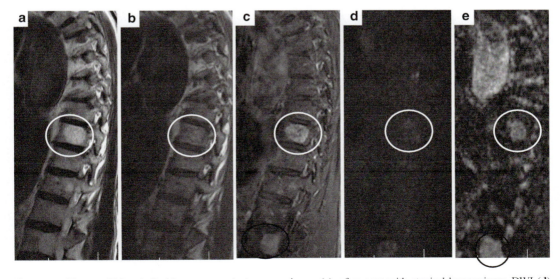

Fig. 22.16 83-year-old female. In this case, tumor in the vertebral body shows hyperintensity on T2-weighted image (**a**), iso- to hypointensity on T1-weighted image (**b**) with inhomogeneous enhancement on contrastenhanced T1-weighted image (**c**), often seen with atypical hemangioma. DWI (**d**) demonstrates mild hyperintensity in atypical hemangiomas with increased ADC (**e**) (1.35×10 mm /s), which is significantly higher than in metastasis and lymphoma

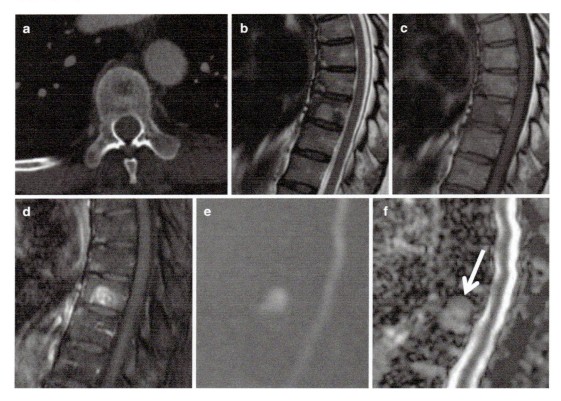

Fig. 22.17 (**a–f**) 62-year-old female with a history of breast cancer metastasis to the liver. She was found to have a growing lytic lesion in the T9 vertebral body on chest CT (**a**). The tumor demonstrated hyperintense signal on sagittal T2-weighted image (**b**) and hypointense signal on T1-weighted images (**c**) with homogeneous enhancement on T1-weighted contrast-enhanced image (**d**), mimicking a new bone metastasis. DWI (**e**) also shows hyperintensity and low ADC value (0.7×10^{-3} mm^2/s) (**f**) favoring metastatic disease

[23]. To differentiate atypical hemangiomas from malignancy, it has been reported that ADC values in metastatic lesions are lower than those in hemangiomas (Fig. 22.17) [24, 25].

22.5.2.2 Management

Surgical decompression is recommended if there is progressive neurologic decline. Because of the potential morbidity and relative lack of efficacy associated with radiation therapy, total lesion removal often should be attempted. Preoperative embolization may also be performed to reduce intraoperative blood loss [26]. When postoperative instability is suspected, instrumentation is implanted following excision (Fig. 22.14e).

At the UIHC, since 2005 we have evaluated 56 patients with vertebral hemangioma. Of these, only 7 have undergone surgery for decompression. As most of these lesions are chronic and extradural, complications have been nil. Vertebroplasty and kyphoplasty have also been advocated for the treatment of symptomatic hemangiomas. Studies have recently reported excellent pain relief with no evidence of post-treatment instability [27, 28]. This may be performed alone in patients who are not good surgical candidates, or as an adjunct to decompressive surgery [27, 28]. While radiotherapy is typically reserved for patients who undergo a subtotal resection, some advocate for its use as a standalone treatment [29, 30].

22.5.3 Eosinophilic Granuloma (Langerhans Cell Histiocytosis)

Most commonly, eosinophilic granulomas present in children in the first two decades of life and are identified in the cervical spine, with the vertebral body typically being involved [31, 32]. While these lesions can occur in any bone, spinal lesions comprise 6.5% to 25% of cases [33]. Eosinophilic granulomas involving the adult spine are less frequent, but do occur [31, 34]. These lesions may be identified incidentally, but patients often present with localized neck or back pain with restricted motion [22, 31, 32]. These self-limiting, benign lesions cause osteolytic damage secondary to the local proliferation of histiocytes [35].

22.5.3.1 Imaging

Radiographically, eosinophilic granulomas are identified as destructive bony lesions with well-demarcated borders and no evidence of a soft tissue mass (Fig. 22.18). Extensive bony destruction occasionally results in vertebra plana. The adjacent disc spaces are well preserved (Fig. 22.19 MRI). These findings differentiate eosinophilic granulomas from other lesions in the differential diagnosis, including infection, benign tumor, or malignancy.

22.5.3.2 Management

In many cases, symptoms will resolve over time, and a conservative approach should always be considered first. Bracing and non-steroidal anti-inflammatory drugs may provide symptomatic relief. In patients where the diagnosis is not clear, biopsy is recommended [36]. The vertebral body height can be restored spontaneously if the areas of endochondral ossification are preserved. Therefore, treatment is generally conservative with activity limitations and bracing. For symptomatic relief, vertebroplasty may occasionally be indicated [37]. In cases where bony destruction leads to instability that persists despite a course of conservative management, arthrodesis is required [35]. For patients deemed to be poor surgical candidates with progressive, intractable lesions, radiation therapy may be considered [38].

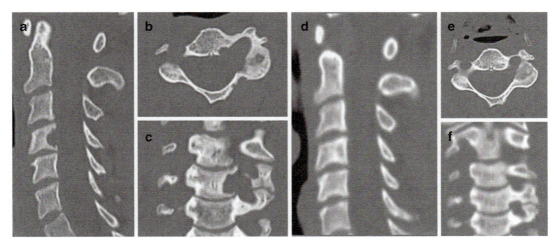

Fig. 22.18 (**a–f**) A young man complains of neck pain following a motor vehicle accident. The pain radiates into his left shoulder and sometimes into his head. His past medical history is unremarkable, and he continues to work as a cook. Sagittal (**a**), axial (**b**), and coronal (**c**) CT scans show a lytic process involving the C4 body, left pedicle, and lateral mass. The clear margins and sclerosis suggest a benign process such as eosinophilic granuloma. On follow-up 4 years later, sagittal (**d**), axial (**e**), and coronal (**f**) CT show resolution of the lytic process without treatment, confirming the diagnosis of eosinophilic granuloma

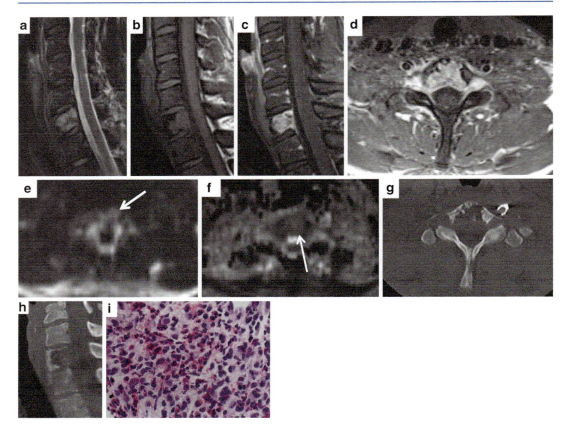

Fig. 22.19 (**a–i**) 24-year-old male with Langerhans cell histiocytosis (LCH). Sagittal T2 (**a**), T1 (**b**), and T1 contrast-enhanced (**c** and **d**) images demonstrate a C7 vertebral body lesion. DWI (**e**) demonstrates hyperintensity in LCH with intermediate ADC (**f**) due to the hypercellularity (ADC: 0.99×10^{-3} mm^2/s). Differentiation from malignant tumor is difficult based on the ADC value. Axial (**g**) and sagittal (**h**) CT demonstrate the lytic process. Pathology demonstrates intermediate cellularity of LCH (**i**).

22.5.4 Osteoid Osteoma and Osteoblastoma

Osteoid osteomas originate from cancellous bone and are a histologic continuum of osteoblastomas. Osteoid osteomas by definition are less than 2.0 cm in diameter, while osteoblastomas are lesions that are greater than 2.0 cm in diameter [39]. The most common presenting symptom is localized pain that is worse at night and relieved by salicylates or other non-steroidal anti-inflammatory drugs [40]. Osteoblastomas constitute about 16% of benign primary spinal tumors [13]. Patients are usually in their second or third decade at presentation [41]. Osteoblastomas are distributed throughout the spine, and in the series by Boriani et al. [42], 16 of 30 lesions occurred in the lumbar spine, 8 in the thoracic spine, and 6 in the cervical spine. Two-thirds of these lesions are confined to the dorsal elements. These tumors are also associated with scoliosis, and patients may present with neurologic deficit. It is important to remember that both osteoid osteoma and osteoblastoma should be considered in any young patient with back or neck pain, painful scoliosis, or radicular pain.

22.5.4.1 Imaging

These lesions often become symptomatic before they are visible on plain radiographs. MRI shows a heterogeneously enhancing mass arising from the posterior elements (Fig. 22.21).

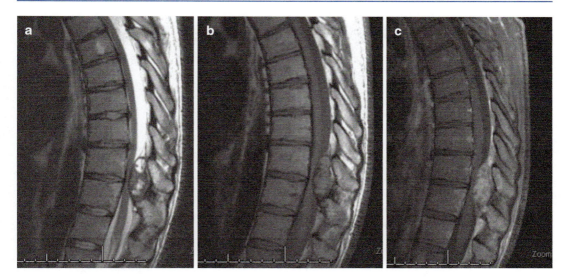

Fig. 22.20 (**a–c**) Sagittal T2 (**a**), T1 (**b**), and T1 + Gd (**c**) MRI show a 48 × 37 × 21 mm mass posterior to the cord at T10-T11. The mass contains fluid–fluid level cystic components and shows heterogeneous intense enhancement with pedicle and vertebral body involvement. The mass compresses and displaces the spinal cord anteriorly. Based on these findings, primary bone tumor, such as aneurysmal bone cyst, or osteoblastoma was entertained (Figs. 22.20 and 22.21 pertain to the same patient: a young man who presents with numbness and weakness in his legs. He has been using a cane in the last couple of weeks. He also endorses problems with bladder emptying)

Osteoblastomas can progressively enlarge, and on CT show a well-defined, lobulated, lytic, expansile mass that usually involves the neural arch structures (Fig. 22.22).

22.5.4.2 Management

The initial management of osteoid osteoma should be conservative with observation and treatment with salicylates or other non-steroidal anti-inflammatory drugs [40]. Patients with intractable pain or scoliotic deformity are indicated for excision [43]. Wide en bloc excision appears to be curative, while intralesional resection has been shown to have a 7% recurrence rate [44]. Osteoblastomas should initially be treated surgically with total resection [45, 46]. Again, wide en bloc excision is preferred, as there is a high recurrence rate with intralesional resection, 24% in one series [47]. With larger, aggressive lesions, radiation therapy and embolization may be considered as adjuncts to surgical resection, but the potential risks of radiation therapy must be considered, including the risk of sarcomatous transformation. Radiofrequency ablation of both osteoid osteoma and osteoblastoma has been shown to be effective for initial procedural intervention as well as in cases of recurrence [48].

22.5.5 Osteochondroma

Osteochondromas constitute about 9% of benign spinal tumors [13]. They consist of cartilage-covered cortical bone with underlying medullary bone. Histologically, the cartilaginous cap and underlying bone are identical to normal bone. Osteochondromas most commonly occur in the third decade, with a male/female predominance of 2:1. They tend to occur more commonly in the cervical spine and in the posterior elements [49, 50]. Patients usually have localized pain, although neurologic deficit, including cord or nerve root compression, can also occur [51]. Rarely, osteochondromas may also be a manifestation of hereditary multiple osteochondromas [52].

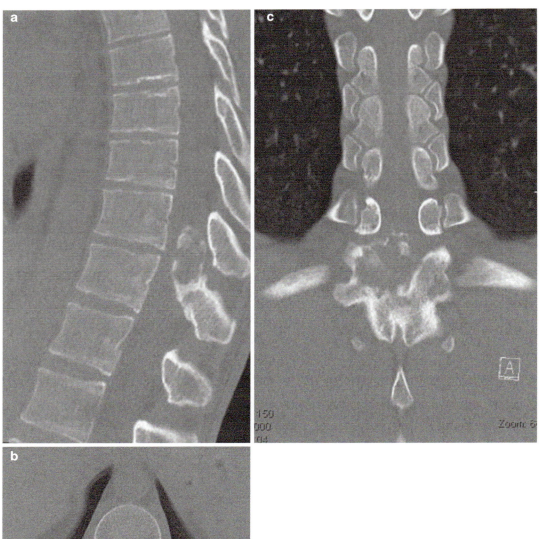
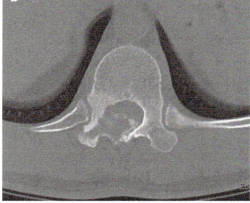

Fig. 22.21 (**a–c**) Sagittal (**a**), axial (**b**), and coronal (**c**) CT scan reveals a well-circumscribed expansile lesion containing calcifications and a sclerotic rim arising from the right posterior elements. Findings are most consistent with osteoblastoma or aneurysmal bone cyst. Patient underwent surgery with total excision of the mass, which was identified as osteoblastoma

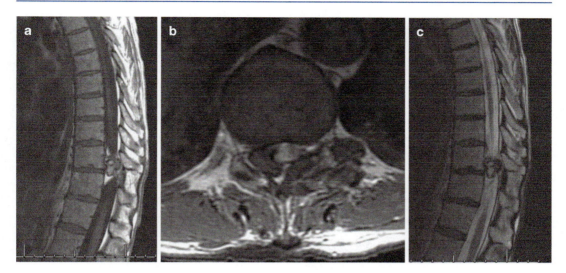

Fig. 22.22 (**a**–**c**) T1 sagittal MRI (**a**), T1 + Gd axial (**b**), and T2 sagittal (**c**) show a lobulated osteo-cartilaginous mass arising from the facet joint extending into the canal (Figs. 22.22, 22.23, and 22.24 pertain to the same patient. A middle-aged lady was referred to our clinic for evaluation of a spinal thoracic mass that was discovered incidentally during workup for hoarseness)

Additionally, radiation-induced osteochondroma has been reported in patients who have received radiation treatment [53].

22.5.5.1 Imaging

MRI of these lesions shows their lobulated, well-circumscribed enhancing masses involving the spinous and transverse processes (Fig. 22.22). CT scan confirms their well-circumscribed osteoid appearance (Fig. 22.23).

22.5.5.2 Management

For symptomatic lesions, surgical excision is the treatment of choice (Fig. 22.24) [54–56]. Wide surgical excision should be performed and should include the cartilaginous cap in order to prevent recurrence [52]. Radiation therapy is not recommended due to concern for transformation into secondary chondrosarcoma [57]. Given proper surgical resection, recurrence is generally rare [58].

22.5.6 Aneurysmal Bone Cysts

Aneurysmal bone cysts (ABCs) are rare, benign, proliferative non-neoplastic lesions that may occur in any part of the skeleton. Although this is not a tumor per se, its classical appearance and presentation should be familiar to clinicians dealing with spine lesions. ABCs of the spine typically affect the pediatric population, with a small female predominance [59, 60]. Approximately 40–45% involve the lumbar spine, with 30% involving the thoracic spine and 25–30% involving the cervical spine [61]. In one series, 75% of lesions arose in the neural arch and 40% extended into the body [59]. Lesions are often not confined to a single vertebra; instead, they bridge two or more levels in approximately 40% of cases [61]. Although primary aneurysmal bone cysts are of unknown cause, a secondary form of aneurysmal bone cyst has been described that arises within eosinophilic granulomas, simple bone cysts, osteosarcoma, chondroblastoma, or giant cell tumors [62].

Pain occurring especially at night and that is localized to the site of the mass is the most common presenting complaint [63]. The presence or absence of a neurologic deficit depends on the site of the tumor and on the degree of compression of adjacent neural elements. The clinical course is commonly progressive over several months because of the slow growth of these lesions, although rapid growth can also occur.

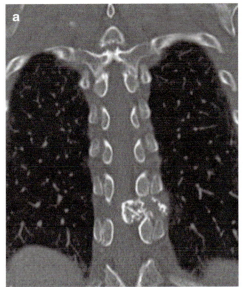

Fig. 22.23 (**a**, **b**) Coronal (**a**) and axial (**b**) CT scans show the calcified mass emanating from the facet joint extending into the canal

22.5.6.1 Imaging

Diagnosis is often best achieved with MRI in demonstrating the epidural extent of the mass. The classical appearance of the involved vertebra is that of a multiloculated, expansile, highly vascular mass with eggshell-like cortical bone and blood product fluid–fluid levels (Fig. 22.25a–c). Computed tomography demonstrates the bony scalloping and thinning of adjacent cortices without invasion favoring the benign nature of the tumor (Fig. 22.25d, e). The heterogeneity of cystic component is reflected by variety of ADC values (Fig. 22.26).

Selective spinal angiography has both diagnostic and, potentially, therapeutic value. Preoperative embolization is a useful adjunct that may decrease the intraoperative blood loss.

22.5.6.2 Management

Because of the destructive nature of ABCs and the risk of progressive instability coupled with the frequent presence of neurologic deficits secondary to compression of neural elements, complete surgical resection is often considered the treatment of choice, either with or without preoperative embolization [61, 64–67]. However, other options such as embolization alone, radiation therapy, sclerotherapy, or treatment with denosumab have also been reported [68–71]. In patients without instability or neural compression, bisphosphonate therapy may also serve as a definitive treatment [72]. The approach (ventral, dorsal, or dorsolateral) depends on the exact location and extent of the lesion. An eggshell-thin

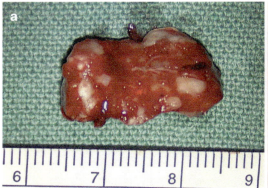
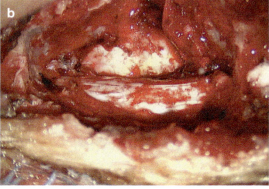

Fig. 22.24 (**a**, **b**) Intraoperative photographs show the mass removed from the canal (**a**) and the canal restored to its normal configuration (**b**) after removal of the mass. Pathology confirmed the diagnosis of osteochondroma

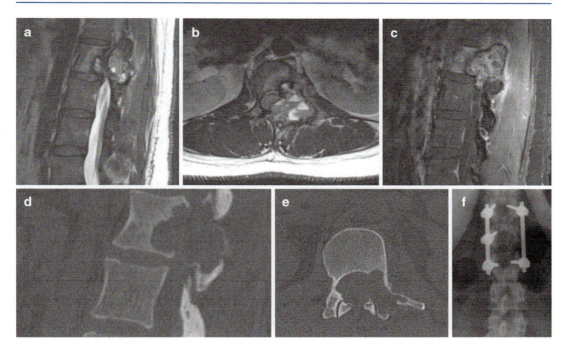

Fig. 22.25 (**a–f**) A young woman presents with severe back and leg pain on her left side. Sagittal T2 (**a**), T2 axial (**b**), and T1 + Gd (**c**) MRI scans show an enhancing lesion centered in the posterior elements of L1 vertebra with extension anteriorly involving the vertebral body, paraspinal soft tissue, and spinal canal with compression of the cord. A fluid/fluid level can be appreciated on the axial image. Sagittal (**d**) and axial (**e**) CT scan demonstrates the lytic lesion of the body, pedicle, and transverse process. Owing to symptoms and cord compression, the patient underwent resection with instrumentation as shown on the plain radiographs (**f**). Pathology was that of aneurysmal bone cyst

cyst of subperiosteal new bone that is continuous with adjacent cortex is observed at surgery. With complete excision, the prognosis is excellent and recurrence rates are rare in most series [61, 73]. En bloc resection should be the goal of surgical intervention. As with all resections of spinal neoplasms, postoperative spinal instability should always be considered and instrumented fusion performed when identified (Fig. 22.25f).

22.6 Malignant Spinal Tumors

22.6.1 Plasma Cell Tumors

Plasma cell tumors of the spine (multiple myeloma and solitary plasmacytoma) are the most common type of malignant primary spinal tumors, accounting for nearly one-third [13]. Half of patients diagnosed with plasmacytoma will ultimately develop multiple myeloma, most commonly within 2 years [74].

Plasma cell tumors of the spine usually present with pain, and in advanced cases with myelopathy. The duration of symptoms before diagnosis may vary; however, in general, symptoms worsen considerably in the 6 to 12 months before presentation. The diagnosis of solitary plasmacytoma is established histologically by either a needle biopsy or an open procedure. In plasmacytoma, the bone marrow is negative for plasma cell infiltrates, and serum-protein electrophoresis results are normal. Multiple myeloma is usually diagnosed definitively by a bone marrow biopsy, the presence of multiple bony lesions on bone survey, and an abnormal monoclonal immunoglobulin spike on serum or urine electrophoresis [74]. Most patients with multiple myeloma present with Bence-Jones proteinuria, reflecting the spillover of monoclonal immunoglobulin fragments into the urine.

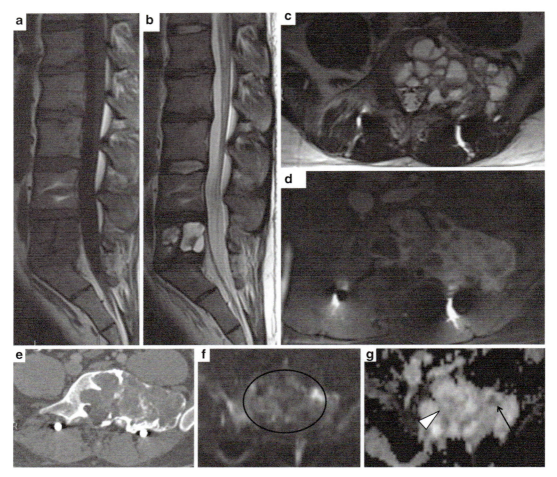

Fig. 22.26 (a–f) The patient is a 24-year-old male with aneurysmal bone cyst (ABC). Sagittal T1 (**a**), sagittal T2 (**b**), axial T2 (**c**), axial T1 postcontrast (**d**), axial CT (**e**), axial DWI (**f**), ADC (**g**). DWI demonstrates iso- to hypointensity with some hyperintense foci in ABC associated with increased ADC due to the cysts and hemorrhagic foci

22.6.1.1 Imaging

MRI and CT scan show the ill-defined enhancing lesions often associated with vertebral body collapse and destruction (Figs. 22.27 and 22.28). Bone involvement of these tumors is demonstrated by hyperintense DWI and range of mildly reduced to slightly elevated ADC due to hypercellularity (Fig. 22.29).

22.6.1.2 Management

The treatment of choice for solitary plasmacytoma in the absence of instability or rapid paralysis is radiation therapy [74–76]. It is recommended that patients with a diagnosis of solitary plasmacytoma be followed closely for the development of indexes characteristic of multiple myeloma. Chemotherapy is generally withheld until progression to multiple myeloma is documented. Vertebroplasty can help relieve pain and improve quality of life in patients without neurological deficit [77]. Because plasmacytomas are highly radiosensitive, surgical decompression and fusion is generally reserved for patients with progressive neurologic deficit and deformity.

22.6.2 Chordoma

Chordoma constitutes approximately a quarter of malignant tumors involving the spine [13]. The tumor originates from primitive remnants of the notochord. The vast majority of chordomas arise

22 Primary and Metastatic Spine Tumors

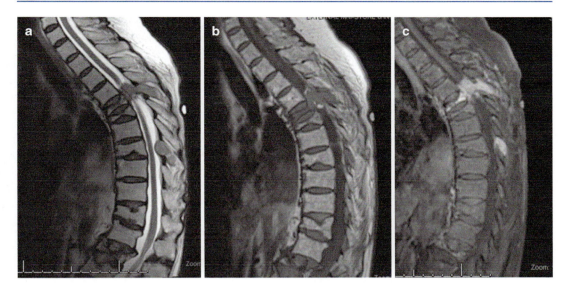

Fig. 22.27 (**a–c**) Sagittal T2 (**a**), T1 (**b**), and T1 + Gd (**c**) MRI now shows severe compression deformities of T5, T6, and L1. There is marrow replacement and displacement of the cord. Also noted is marrow replacement in the posterior elements of T8 (Figs. 22.27 and 22.28 pertain to the same patient. An elderly lady with multiple myeloma and bone marrow transplant 20 years ago presents with new onset right leg weakness and numbness in both legs since yesterday. She is known to have compression fractures of L1 and T5

in either the skull base or sacrococcygeal areas; those involving the mobile intermediate regions of the spine are rare [78]. These tumors, considered to be of low-grade malignancy, are extremely difficult to resect because of their proximity to the spinal cord and cauda equina. In addition, in 5% to 10% of cases, they tend to metastasize within 1 to 10 years of the diagnosis. Fifty percent of all chordomas occur in the fifth to seventh decades of life, with a mean age of onset of approximately 50 years. Men are twice as likely to be afflicted with this tumor as women [78, 79].

Chordomas arise from the vertebral body with ensuing ventral and dorsal extension. Pain is the presenting symptom in 75% of cases and a radicular component in 10% of patients. More than two-thirds of patients present with weakness or other neurologic deficits. Mean duration of symptoms at presentation is 14 months, with a range of 4–24 months. In chordomas arising from the sacrum, 40% complain of rectal dysfunction including constipation, tenesmus, or bleeding hemorrhoids (Figs. 22.30, 22.31, and 22.32). A palpable tumor on rectal exam can be identified in most patients [80]. These tumors can also affect two adjacent vertebral bodies while sparing the intervertebral disc.

Though a pseudocapsule separates the tumor from adjacent soft tissue, it is diffusely invasive within adjacent bone without clear margins [80].

22.6.2.1 Management

Percutaneous CT-guided biopsy is generally recommended to establish a definitive working diagnosis. The optimal treatment of chordomas is wide en bloc resection [81, 82]. The location of these lesions (close to neural structures) renders cure extremely unlikely. Some authors recommend a staged approach, where first a posterior approach is performed to mobilize the posterior elements, free the dura from the tumor pseudocapsule, and place posterior instrumentation, followed by an anterior approach to perform an en bloc vertebrectomy [80]. With involvement of the sacrococcygeal spine, resection can be accomplished by either ventral, dorsal, or combined approaches [83, 84]. These approaches are geared for the widest possible resection of tumor with sparing of as many nerves as possible [81]. Generally, sparing the S3 nerve root on either

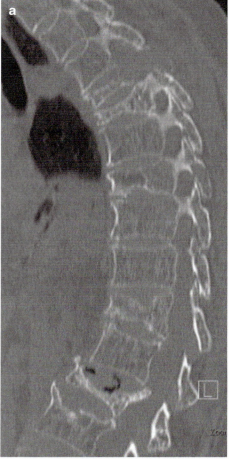
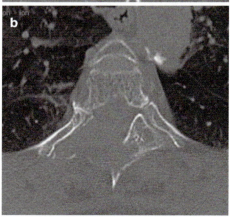

Fig. 22.28 (**a**, **b**) Sagittal (**a**) and axial (**b**) CT scan shows pathologic compression deformity at T5 with osteolysis extending into the posterior elements. Canal narrowing at this level is better appreciated on recent MRI. There is also osteolysis within the posterior elements of T8. Patient was treated with radiation therapy and steroids with recovery of function without surgery

side may be sufficient for bladder and fecal continence. Loss of sexual function also needs to be discussed with the patient preoperatively. Approximately 30% of spinal chordomas will develop metastases [79].

Chordomas are not generally radiosensitive. However, because of the high risk of recurrence—47% of patients will have either recurrence or progression [85]—postoperative radiation therapy is often recommended. The 40-year experience at MD Anderson from 1954 until 1994 yielded 27 patients [86]. The median Kaplan-Meier survival for the entire group was 7.4 years. The disease-free interval for patients undergoing radical resection was 2.3 years, compared to 8 months in those undergoing subtotal excision ($p < 0.0001$). The addition of radiation to the group undergoing subtotal resection increased survival from 8 months to 2 years ($p < 0.02$). Proton therapy has also been used as both adjuvant and definitive treatment with encouraging results [87, 88]. However, there is currently not sufficient evidence to demonstrate that proton therapy is superior to conventional radiation therapy [85]. The often-quoted 5-year survival has ranged, depending on the source, from 50% to 77%, with a 10-year survival of 50% [89, 90].

22.6.3 Primary Spinal Ewing's Sarcoma

Ewing's sarcoma constitutes 6% of all primary malignant bone tumors; however, primary spinal involvement occurs in only 3.5% of all patients with Ewing's sarcomas [13, 91]. This tumor afflicts males more commonly than females (2:1 ratio), and 88% of cases present in the first two decades of life [80, 91]. In terms of the level of involvement, frequency decreases in a caudal to rostral progression, with more than 50% of all cases occurring in the sacrum. The most common presenting feature is pain, with or without radicular involvement, depending on the level. In general, two of three patients present with a neurologic deficit. The duration of symptoms can range from 1 to 30 months; most symptoms are

22 Primary and Metastatic Spine Tumors

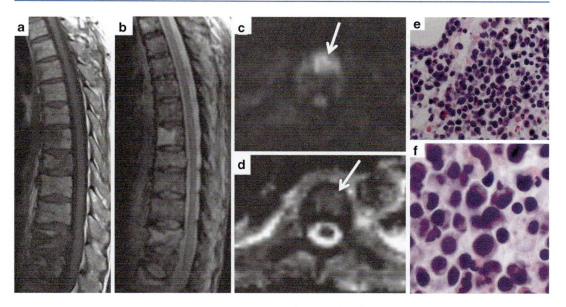

Fig. 22.29 The patient is a 71-year-old male with multiple myeloma. There are numerous T1 hypointense (**a**) and T2 hyperintense (**b**) lesions within the vertebral bodies. DWI (**c**) demonstrates homogeneous hyperintensity associated with mildly increased ADC (**d**) (1.25×10^{-3} mm2/s) in multiple myeloma infiltration. Bone marrow biopsy shows moderate hypercellularity of abnormal plasma cells (**e, f**)

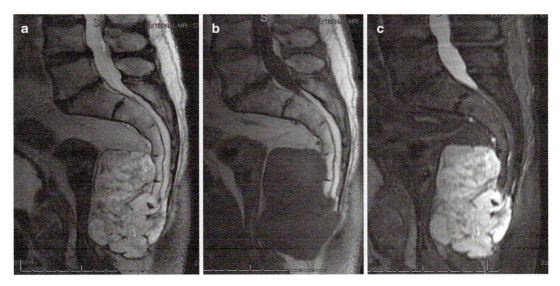

Fig. 22.30 (**a–c**) Sagittal T2 (**a**), T1 (**b**), and T1 + Gd (**c**) MRI shows a lobulated enhancing mass with well-defined margins arising from the sacrum with involvement of the coccyx. His mass displaces the sigmoid colon ventrally (Figs. 22.30, 22.31, and 22.32 pertain to the same patient. An elderly gentleman reports sacral pain for the last 3 years that has gotten worse in the last 6 months, especially when he sits down or while driving. He reports that his bowel movements are smaller in size, but no rectal bleeding. Rectal exam reveals a large presacral mass. CT-guided biopsy reveals chordoma)

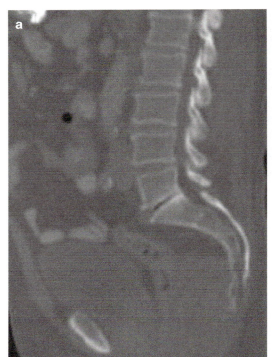

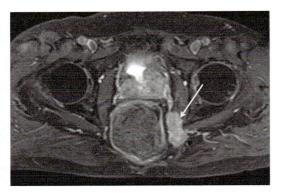

Fig. 22.32 MRI scan 1.5 years following surgery shows a heterogeneously enhancing mass medial to the left obturator internus/piriformis muscle and lateral to the rectum. This necessitated reoperation and radiation that unfortunately did not eradicate the chordoma, and the patient died 6 years later

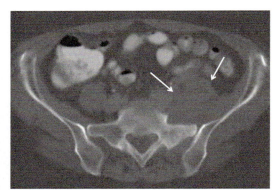

Fig. 22.33 CT scan shows an extraperitoneal pelvic, 4.8 × 5.0 × 2.8 cm soft tissue mass. This mass is displacing the left iliac vessels and extends to the S1 sacral foramina. It causes permeative bone destruction of the left sacral ala (Figs. 22.33 and 22.34 pertain to the same patient. A middle-aged, otherwise healthy lady presents with a 6-month history of low back pain. She denies any antecedent trauma or malignancy. These symptoms are localized to the lower back with radiation to the left posterior hip. She also describes left lower extremity weakness)

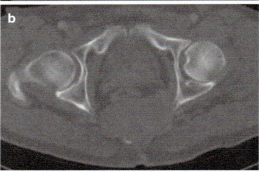

Fig. 22.31 (**a, b**) Sagittal (**a**) and axial (**b**) CT scan confirms the mass and erosive sacral changes, but does not add to the MRI. The patient underwent surgical excision through both anterior and posterior approaches. He did not have any radiation following surgery, but followed with sequential scans

1 year or less in duration. A rectal mass may be encountered on examination, considering that there is sacral involvement in one of four patients with primary spinal Ewing's sarcoma.

22.6.3.1 Imaging

In half of the cases, a lytic process is observed on plain radiographs, whereas other cases show blastic or mixed features. A paravertebral soft tissue mass may occur independently or concurrently with bony involvement. This may be best appreciated on CT or MRI scans (Figs. 22.33 and 22.34). DWI demonstrates homogeneous hyperintensity in the bone metastasis due to hypercellularity. There is loss of signal void on ADC because

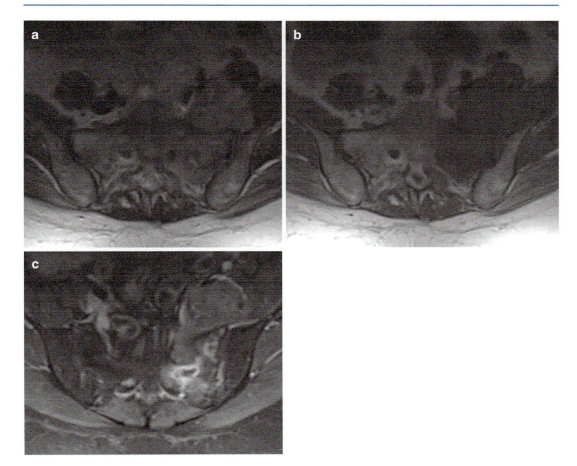

Fig. 22.34 (a–c) MRI T1 (a), T2 (b), and T1 + Gd (c) reveal a large soft tissue mass that involves the left sacral wing with extension into the pelvis. There is mild heterogeneous enhancement of the mass with high T2 and low T1 signal of the left sacral marrow consistent with bony infiltration. CT-guided biopsy yielded small cell blue cell tumor consistent with Ewing sarcoma. She was treated with 12 cycles of chemotherapy and radiation to the sacrum. She is tumor-free 8 years later

markedly hypercellular tumor is replacing the normal fatty bone marrow as seen on histology (Fig. 22.9).

22.6.3.2 Management

Surgery in the treatment of spinal Ewing's sarcoma is best performed after initial treatment with chemotherapy and radiation. Neoadjuvant therapy can reduce the size of the tumor and allow for adjacent bone to heal prior to surgical intervention. Indications for operation include high-grade epidural compression with symptomatic neurologic progression, stabilization, poor response to chemotherapy or radiotherapy, and radiographic residual tumor post-neoadjuvant treatment. When resection is attempted, an attempt at maximal resection should be undertaken. Evidence has shown that en bloc resection may improve local control, but does not significantly improve survival [92]. When surgical excision is attempted, preoperative embolization is recommended, followed by resection and instrumentation. In cases where an adequate surgical margin is not achievable, postoperative radiation should be added to the surgical bed [93].

Survival is improved in patients with local disease, tumors less than 500 ml in volume, peripheral involvement only, and gross total resection compared with patients who have metastatic involvement, tumor volume greater than 500 ml, central involvement, and no resection. This analysis suggested that aggressive surgery with radiation therapy might be an important prognostic factor. The best prognosis is provided by local irradiation and chemotherapy.

In summary, all patients with Ewing's sarcoma should initially be treated with chemotherapy. Surgical resection should be considered in all cases where the surgeon feels it is possible to achieve a complete resection. If the margins of the resection are <1 cm, as is often the case in spinal tumors, radiation therapy is added. Alternatively, chemotherapy and radiation treatment can be utilized alone in cases where an adequate resection is not possible [92].

22.6.4 Osteosarcoma

Osteosarcomas account for about 8% of malignant spine tumors [13]. Osteosarcomas occur most commonly in the fourth decade of life [94], have a slight predilection for males [95], and are the most common primary malignant bone tumor in the pediatric population. In addition, osteosarcoma has one of the lowest survival rates among pediatric cancers [92]. In adults, prognosis with this tumor is especially poor. Shives et al. reviewed 27 cases of spinal osteosarcoma and reported a median survival of 10 months from diagnosis [96].

Osteosarcomas can occur throughout the spine, though are more common in the thoracic spine and sacrum and typically arise in the posterior elements [94]. Osteosarcomas usually arise de novo or may occur secondarily in previously irradiated bone, usually several years later. Paget's disease is also a known risk factor for the development of osteosarcoma. Though as few as 1% of Paget's disease patients go on to develop

osteosarcoma, these patients make up as much as 50% of the patients in some registries [94].

Diagnosis is often delayed due to the nonspecific nature of the symptoms. Pain is the most common presenting feature and may be axial or radicular. Weakness is present in more than half of patients at the time of diagnosis, whereas loss of bowel and bladder function is generally seen only in advanced cases.

22.6.4.1 Imaging
Radiographically, these tumors can have a fairly diverse appearance. Plain radiographs and CT scans of osteosarcomas may demonstrate osteolytic or osteoblastic changes. MRI is superior for showing tumor extent within the bone marrow and associated soft tissue and for delineating epidural tumor extension. By far, osteosarcomas afflict long bones first, with involvement of the spine secondarily. The example shown in Figs. 22.35 and 22.36 is such a case.

22.6.4.2 Management
Based on the available information, the Spine Oncology Study Group recommends that all patients with osteosarcoma of the spine are treated with neoadjuvant chemotherapy. Surgical resection should be attempted when it is felt a complete resection can be achieved and is associated with an improvement in survival and local control [92].

22.6.5 Chondrosarcoma

Chondrosarcomas are primary malignant tumors arising from cartilaginous elements. They are rare tumors and make up about 8% of malignant primary tumors of the spine [13]. Like osteosarcomas, chondrosarcomas show a predilection for males; however, unlike osteosarcomas, they occur in middle-aged and older patients. Chondrosarcoma may arise de novo as a primary lesion or may occur as a secondary tumor from a preexisting solitary osteochon-

22 Primary and Metastatic Spine Tumors

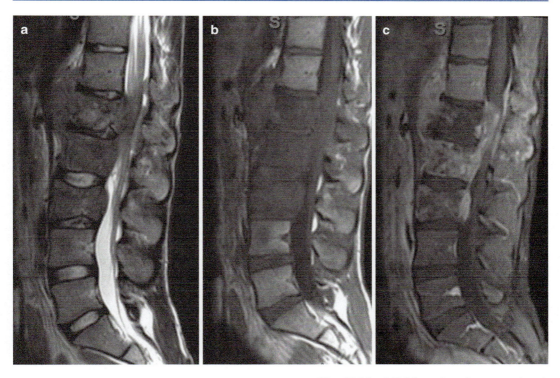

Fig. 22.35 (a–c) MRI images T2 (a), T1 (b), and T1 + Gd (c) show diffuse marrow replacement and enhancement of L1, L2, and L3 vertebral bodies. There is a large component of the mass encircling the conus medullaris at L1 and extending into the paravertebral space (Figs. 22.35 and 22.36 pertain to the same patient. A young man diagnosed with osteosarcoma of the right tibia 2 years earlier was treated with amputation and chemotherapy. Recently developed severe back pain with paraparesis)

droma (1%) or from hereditary multiple exostosis (20%) [96].

Pain, the most common presenting symptom, may be indolent, leading to a delay in diagnosis. Pathologically, chondrosarcomas do not demonstrate neoplastic osteoid tissue or bone evolving from a sarcomatous matrix. Instead, they display nuclear pleomorphism with numerous mitoses surrounded by a myxoid matrix. In addition to this conventional chondrosarcomatous appearance, variants may be subcategorized as predominantly myxoid, mesenchymal, or dedifferentiated.

22.6.5.1 Imaging

Plain radiographs and CT scans demonstrate osteolytic lesions with a calcified matrix. The amount of calcification correlates with the degree of differentiation. MRI is the study of choice for demonstrating the adjacent soft tissue and epidural extent of tumor spread. MRI also demonstrates the heterogeneity of the lesion (Fig. 22.37). Of note, lesions that are more malignant tend to have larger amounts of soft tissue components, more irregular calcification, and more extensive bone destruction.

22.6.5.2 Management

Although chondrosarcomas are slowly growing lesions, they have a relatively poor overall prognosis. Survival correlates with degree of malignancy. Because of the spinal location, resection is attempted but often is not possible (Fig. 22.38). This, combined with resistance of the tumor to chemotherapy and radiation therapy, predisposes to local recurrence of tumor (Fig. 22.39).

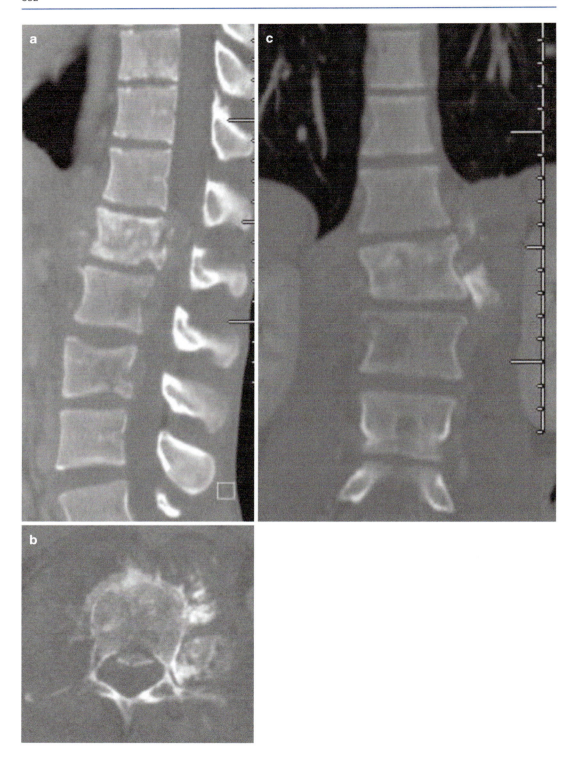

Fig. 22.36 (**a**–**c**) CT scan lateral (**a**), axial (**b**), and coronal (**c**) shows metastatic disease at L1-L3 with subtle irregularities at T10 and L4 corresponding to the recent MRI. There is also bony destruction and matrix formation at L1 resulting in severe spinal stenosis. Patient succumbed to his disease within 5 years of diagnosis

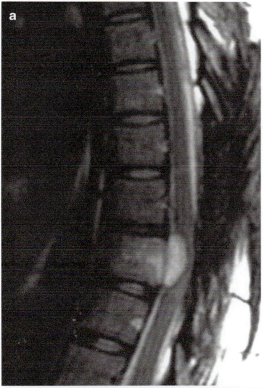
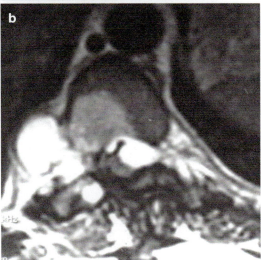

Fig. 22.37 (**a**, **b**) Sagittal (**a**) and axial (**b**) MRI scans with enhancement show a tumor arising from the body of T10 extending into the canal compressing the cord predominantly on the patient's left side. There is also tumor extension into the paravertebral space on the right side (Figs. 22.37, 22.38, and 22.39 pertain to the same patient. A young lady presents with pain and paraparesis of 5 months duration)

However, small numbers of long-term survivors with low-grade lesions have been observed. Such patients can be managed with multiple local excisions. Complete excision is the goal of surgery, considering the propensity of the tumor for local recurrence.

In a series of predominantly low-grade chondrosarcomas, Boriani et al. [97] showed improved local control with marginal or wide resections compared with intralesional resection. Despite the relative radioresistance of chondrosarcoma, treatment with high-dose 3-dimensional conformal radiotherapy (3D-CRT) or intensity modulated radiation therapy (IMRT) following resection with positive histologic margins is recommended.

22.7 Summary

Primary tumors that involve the spinal axis, although rare, are often best managed by surgery. It may be the only method to affect a cure in some patients. It is important for clinicians to recognize that they should be prepared to achieve total removal of this lesion if the potential gain justifies the morbidity. Subtotal removal may require early reoperation. Certainly, the best time to accomplish total tumor removal is at the first surgical procedure. Proper preoperative planning and, when appropriate, preoperative embolization often results in satisfactory patient outcomes.

Acknowledgement The authors acknowledge the invaluable assistance of Faith Vaughn in proofing and preparing this chapter for submission.

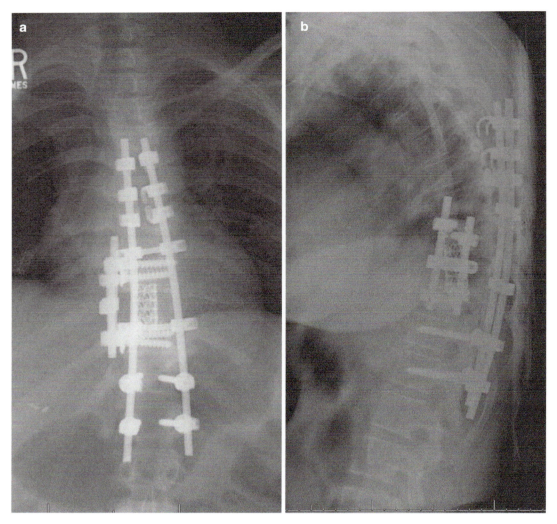

Fig. 22.38 (**a**, **b**) Through a right thoracotomy approach, the patient underwent a T10 corpectomy with tumor resection and anterior stabilization. Pathology confirmed chondrosarcoma. Figures (**a**) and (**b**) show the postoperative instrumentation in the anteroposterior and lateral planes, respectively

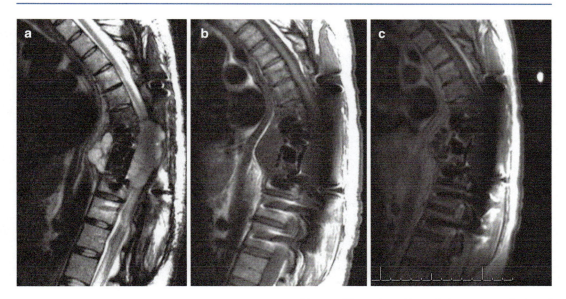

Fig. 22.39 (**a–c**) Five years later, after seven resections and radiation treatments, the patient shows recurrence of her tumor as seen on T2 (**a**), T1(**b**), and T1 + Gd (**c**) sagittal images. The patient ultimately became paraplegic and succumbed to her tumor

References

1. Wong DA, Fornasier VL, MacNab I (1990) Spinal metastases: the obvious, the occult, and the impostors. Spine (Phila Pa 1976) 15(1):1–4
2. Sansur CA et al (2007) Part II: spinal-cord neoplasms—primary tumours of the bony spine and adjacent soft tissues. Lancet Oncol 8(2):137–147
3. Simmons ED, Zheng Y (2006) Vertebral tumors: surgical versus nonsurgical treatment. Clin Orthop Relat Res 443:233–247
4. Yao A et al (2017) Contemporary spinal oncology treatment paradigms and outcomes for metastatic tumors to the spine: a systematic review of breast, prostate, renal, and lung metastases. J Clin Neurosci 41:11–23
5. Gibbs WN et al (2019) Spine oncology: imaging and intervention. Radiol Clin N Am 57(2):377–395
6. Li B et al (2014) Diagnostic value of whole-body diffusion-weighted magnetic resonance imaging for detection of primary and metastatic malignancies: a meta-analysis. Eur J Radiol 83(2):338–344
7. Ormond Filho AG et al (2019) Whole-body imaging of multiple myeloma: diagnostic criteria. Radiographics 39(4):1077–1097
8. Sung JK et al (2014) Differentiation of acute osteoporotic and malignant compression fractures of the spine: use of additive qualitative and quantitative axial diffusion-weighted MR imaging to conventional MR imaging at 3.0 T. Radiology 271(2):488–498
9. Barzilai O, Fisher CG, Bilsky MH (2018) State of the art treatment of spinal metastatic disease. Neurosurgery 82(6):757–769
10. Fisher CG et al (2010) A novel classification system for spinal instability in neoplastic disease: an evidence-based approach and expert consensus from the Spine Oncology Study Group. Spine (Phila Pa 1976) 35(22):E1221–E1229
11. Society, AC (2018) Key statistics about bone cancer. https://www.cancer.org/cancer/bone-cancer/about/key-statistics.html. Accessed 28 Dec, 2018
12. Chi JH et al (2008) Epidemiology and demographics for primary vertebral tumors. Neurosurg Clin N Am 19(1):1–4
13. Unni KK, Inwards CY, Mayo Foundation for Medical Education and Research (2010) Dahlin's bone tumors: general aspects and data on 10,165 cases, 6th edn. Wollters Kluwer Health/Lippincott Williams & Wilkins, Philadelphia, p 402
14. Weinstein JN (1989) Surgical approach to spine tumors. Orthopedics 12(6):897–905
15. Sanjay BK et al (1993) Giant-cell tumours of the spine. J Bone Joint Surg (Br) 75(1):148–154
16. Kwon JW et al (2007) MRI findings of giant cell tumors of the spine. AJR Am J Roentgenol 189(1):246–250
17. Patel KB et al (2014) Diffusion-weighted MRI "claw sign" improves differentiation of infectious from degenerative modic type 1 signal changes of the spine. AJNR Am J Neuroradiol 35(8):1647–1652
18. Luther N, Bilsky MH, Hartl R (2008) Giant cell tumor of the spine. Neurosurg Clin N Am 19(1):49–55

19. Junming M et al (2008) Giant cell tumor of the cervical spine: a series of 22 cases and outcomes. Spine (Phila Pa 1976) 33(3):280–288
20. Shikata J et al (1992) Surgical treatment of giant-cell tumors of the spine. Clin Orthop Relat Res 278:29–36
21. Leggon RE et al (2004) Giant cell tumor of the pelvis and sacrum: 17 cases and analysis of the literature. Clin Orthop Relat Res 423:196–207
22. Gasbarrini A et al. (2009) Management of benign tumors of the mobile spine. Orthop Clin North Am 40(1):9–19, v
23. Erlemann R (2006) Imaging and differential diagnosis of primary bone tumors and tumor-like lesions of the spine. Eur J Radiol 58(1):48–67
24. Shi YJ et al (2017) Differential diagnosis of hemangiomas from spinal osteolytic metastases using 3.0 T MRI: comparison of T1-weighted imaging, chemical-shift imaging, diffusion-weighted and contrast-enhanced imaging. Oncotarget 8(41):71095–71104
25. Winfield JM et al (2018) Apparent diffusion coefficient of vertebral haemangiomas allows differentiation from malignant focal deposits in whole-body diffusion-weighted MRI. Eur Radiol 28(4):1687–1691
26. Acosta FL Jr et al (2008) Comprehensive management of symptomatic and aggressive vertebral hemangiomas. Neurosurg Clin N Am 19(1):17–29
27. Gottfried ON, Dailey AT, Schmidt MH (2008) Adjunct and minimally invasive techniques for the diagnosis and treatment of vertebral tumors. Neurosurg Clin N Am 19(1):125–138
28. Wang B et al (2018) Intraoperative vertebroplasty during surgical decompression and instrumentation for aggressive vertebral hemangiomas: a retrospective study of 39 patients and review of the literature. Spine J 18(7):1128–1135
29. Bremnes RM, Hauge HN, Sagsveen R (1996) Radiotherapy in the treatment of symptomatic vertebral hemangiomas: technical case report. Neurosurgery 39(5):1054–1058
30. Mazonakis M et al (2016) Radiation dose and cancer risk to out-of-field and partially in-field organs from radiotherapy for symptomatic vertebral hemangiomas. Med Phys 43(4):1841
31. Huang WD et al (2013) Langerhans cell histiocytosis of spine: a comparative study of clinical, imaging features, and diagnosis in children, adolescents, and adults. Spine J 13(9):1108–1117
32. DiCaprio MR, Roberts TT (2014) Diagnosis and management of langerhans cell histiocytosis. J Am Acad Orthop Surg 22(10):643–652
33. Fenoy AJ et al (2006) Primary bone tumors of the spine in children. J Neurosurg 105(4 Suppl):252–260
34. Nakamura H, Nagayama R (2008) Eosinophilic granuloma presenting with local osteolysis in an adult lumbar spine. J Clin Neurosci 15(12):1398–1400
35. Greenlee JD et al (2007) Eosinophilic granuloma in the pediatric spine. Pediatr Neurosurg 43(4):285–292
36. Denaro L et al (2008) Eosinophilic granuloma of the pediatric cervical spine. Spine (Phila Pa 1976) 33(24):E936–E941
37. Tan HQ et al (2007) Percutaneous vertebroplasty for eosinophilic granuloma of the cervical spine in a child. Pediatr Radiol 37(10):1053–1057
38. Kriz J et al (2013) Radiotherapy in langerhans cell histiocytosis—a rare indication in a rare disease. Radiat Oncol 8:233
39. Winn HR (2017) Youmans and Winn neurological surgery, vol 3, 7th edn. Elsevier, Philadelphia, PA
40. Zileli M et al (2003) Osteoid osteomas and osteoblastomas of the spine. Neurosurg Focus 15(5):E5
41. Ozaki T et al (2002) Osteoid osteoma and osteoblastoma of the spine: experiences with 22 patients. Clin Orthop Relat Res 397:394–402
42. Boriani S et al (1992) Osteoblastoma of the spine. Clin Orthop Relat Res 278:37–45
43. Kneisl JS, Simon MA (1992) Medical management compared with operative treatment for osteoid-osteoma. J Bone Joint Surg Am 74(2):179–185
44. Quraishi NA et al (2017) A multicenter cohort study of spinal osteoid osteomas: results of surgical treatment and analysis of local recurrence. Spine J 17(3):401–408
45. Jiang L et al (2015) Surgical treatment options for aggressive osteoblastoma in the mobile spine. Eur Spine J 24(8):1778–1785
46. Boriani S et al (2012) Staging and treatment of osteoblastoma in the mobile spine: a review of 51 cases. Eur Spine J 21(10):2003–2010
47. Berry M et al (2008) Osteoblastoma: a 30-year study of 99 cases. J Surg Oncol 98(3):179–183
48. Rehnitz C et al (2012) CT-guided radiofrequency ablation of osteoid osteoma and osteoblastoma: clinical success and long-term follow up in 77 patients. Eur J Radiol 81(11):3426–3434
49. Albrecht S, Crutchfield JS, SeGall GK (1992) On spinal osteochondromas. J Neurosurg 77(2):247–252
50. Raswan US et al (2017) A solitary osteochondroma of the cervical spine: a case report and review of literature. Childs Nerv Syst 33(6):1019–1022
51. Song KJ, Lee KB (2007) Solitary osteochondroma of the thoracic spine causing myelopathy. Eur J Pediatr Surg 17(3):210–213
52. Yakkanti R et al (2018) Solitary osteochondroma of the spine-a case series: review of solitary osteochondroma with myelopathic symptoms. Global Spine J 8(4):323–339
53. Paulino AC, Fowler BZ (2005) Secondary neoplasms after radiotherapy for a childhood solid tumor. Pediatr Hematol Oncol 22(2):89–101
54. Gille O, Pointillart V, Vital JM (2005) Course of spinal solitary osteochondromas. Spine (Phila Pa 1976) 30(1):E13–E19
55. Srikantha U et al (2008) Spinal osteochondroma: spectrum of a rare disease. J Neurosurg Spine 8(6):561–566

56. Yagi M et al (2009) Symptomatic osteochondroma of the spine in elderly patients. Report of 3 cases. J Neurosurg Spine 11(1):64–70
57. Altay M et al (2007) Secondary chondrosarcoma in cartilage bone tumors: report of 32 patients. J Orthop Sci 12(5):415–423
58. Veeravagu A et al (2017) Cervical osteochondroma causing myelopathy in adults: management considerations and literature review. World Neurosurg 97:752, e5–752, e13
59. Sebaaly A et al (2015) Aneurysmal bone cyst of the cervical spine in children: a review and a focus on available treatment options. J Pediatr Orthop 35(7):693–702
60. Hay MC, Paterson D, Taylor TK (1978) Aneurysmal bone cysts of the spine. J Bone Joint Surg (Br) 60–B(3):406–411
61. Burch S, Hu S, Berven S (2008) Aneurysmal bone cysts of the spine. Neurosurg Clin N Am 19(1):41–47
62. Vandertop WP et al (1994) Aneurysmal bone cyst of the thoracic spine: radical excision with use of the cavitron. A case report. J Bone Joint Surg Am 76(4):608–611
63. Mohan V et al (1989) Aneurysmal bone cysts of the dorsal spine. Arch Orthop Trauma Surg 108(6):390–393
64. Dysart SH, Swengel RM, van Dam BE (1992) Aneurysmal bone cyst of a thoracic vertebra. Treatment by selective arterial embolization and excision. Spine (Phila Pa 1976) 17(7):846–848
65. Liu JK et al (2003) Surgical management of aneurysmal bone cysts of the spine. Neurosurg Focus 15(5):E4
66. Chuang VP et al (1981) Arterial occlusion: management of giant cell tumor and aneurysmal bone cyst. AJR Am J Roentgenol 136(6):1127–1130
67. DeRosa GP, Graziano GP, Scott J (1990) Arterial embolization of aneurysmal bone cyst of the lumbar spine. A report of two cases. J Bone Joint Surg Am 72(5):777–780
68. Boriani S et al (2001) Aneurysmal bone cyst of the mobile spine: report on 41 cases. Spine (Phila Pa 1976) 26(1):27–35
69. Papagelopoulos PJ et al (1998) Aneurysmal bone cyst of the spine. Management and outcome. Spine (Phila Pa 1976) 23(5):621–628
70. Patel RS et al (2018) Denosumab: a potential treatment option for aneurysmal bone cyst of the atlas. Eur Spine J 27(Suppl 3):494–500
71. Dubois J et al (2003) Sclerotherapy in aneurysmal bone cysts in children: a review of 17 cases. Pediatr Radiol 33(6):365–372
72. Kieser DC et al (2018) Bisphosphonate therapy for spinal aneurysmal bone cysts. Eur Spine J 27(4):851–858
73. Zileli M et al (2013) Aneurysmal bone cysts of the spine. Eur Spine J 22(3):593–601

74. Singh H, Meyer SA, Jenkins AL 3rd (2009) Treatment of primary vertebral tumors. Mt Sinai J Med 76(5):499–504
75. Caers J et al (2018) Diagnosis, treatment, and response assessment in solitary plasmacytoma: updated recommendations from a European Expert Panel. J Hematol Oncol 11(1):10
76. Poor MM, Hitchon PW, Riggs CE Jr (1988) Solitary spinal plasmacytomas: management and outcome. J Spinal Disord 1(4):295–300
77. McDonald RJ et al (2008) Vertebroplasty in multiple myeloma: outcomes in a large patient series. AJNR Am J Neuroradiol 29(4):642–648
78. Bakker SH et al (2018) Chordoma: a systematic review of the epidemiology and clinical prognostic factors predicting progression-free and overall survival. Eur Spine J 27(12):3043–3058
79. Bergh P et al (2000) Prognostic factors in chordoma of the sacrum and mobile spine: a study of 39 patients. Cancer 88(9):2122–2134
80. Sundaresan N, Rosen G, Boriani S (2009) Primary malignant tumors of the spine. Orthop Clin North Am 40(1):21–36
81. Samson IR et al (1993) Operative treatment of sacrococcygeal chordoma. A review of twenty-one cases. J Bone Joint Surg Am 75(10):1476–1484
82. D'Amore T, Boyce B, Mesfin A (2018) Chordoma of the mobile spine and sacrum: clinical management and prognosis. J Spine Surg 4(3):546–552
83. Ahmed R et al (2015) Disease outcomes for skull base and spinal chordomas: a single center experience. Clin Neurol Neurosurg 130:67–73
84. Jackson RJ, Gokaslan ZL (2000) Spinal-pelvic fixation in patients with lumbosacral neoplasms. J Neurosurg 92(1 Suppl):61–70
85. Zhou J et al (2017) Prognostic factors in patients with spinal chordoma: an integrative analysis of 682 patients. Neurosurgery 81(5):812–823
86. York JE et al (1999) Sacral chordoma: 40-year experience at a major cancer center. Neurosurgery 44(1):74–79; discussion 79–80
87. Aibe N et al (2018) Outcomes of patients with primary sacral chordoma treated with definitive proton beam therapy. Int J Radiat Oncol Biol Phys 100(4):972–979
88. Rotondo RL et al (2015) High-dose proton-based radiation therapy in the management of spine chordomas: outcomes and clinicopathological prognostic factors. J Neurosurg Spine 23(6):788–797
89. McMaster ML et al (2001) Chordoma: incidence and survival patterns in the United States, 1973–1995. Cancer Causes Control 12(1):1–11
90. Brada M, Pijls-Johannesma M, De Ruysscher D (2007) Proton therapy in clinical practice: current clinical evidence. J Clin Oncol 25(8):965–970
91. Grubb MR et al (1994) Primary Ewing's sarcoma of the spine. Spine (Phila Pa 1976) 19(3):309–313

92. Sciubba D et al (2009) Ewing and osteogenic sarcoma evidence for multidisciplinary management. Spine 34(22S):S58–S68
93. Sharafuddin MJ et al (1992) Treatment options in primary Ewing's sarcoma of the spine: report of seven cases and review of the literature. Neurosurgery. 30(4):610–618; discussion 618–9
94. Wang VY, Potts M, Chou D (2008) Sarcoma and the spinal column. Neurosurg Clin N Am 19(1):71–80
95. Dahlin DC, Coventry MB (1967) Osteogenic sarcoma. A study of six hundred cases. J Bone Joint Surg Am 49(1):101–110
96. Shives TC et al (1986) Osteosarcoma of the spine. J Bone Joint Surg Am 68(5):660–668
97. Boriani S et al (2000) Chondrosarcoma of the mobile spine: report on 22 cases. Spine (Phila Pa 1976) 25(7):804–812
98. Schweitzer ME et al (1993) Bull's-eyes and halos: useful MR discriminators of osseous metastases. Radiology 188(1):249–252

Spinal Cord Lesions

23

John Kim, Duy Q. Bui, Toshio Moritani,
Patrick W. Hitchon, Royce W. Woodroffe,
Jennifer L. Noeller, and Kirill V. Nourski

23.1 Introduction

Etiologies of spinal cord disease are extremely diverse, but can be grouped into the following most common 5 categories: vascular, inflammatory, infectious, mechanical, and neoplastic. Historically, MR imaging of these lesions has relied on the form and distribution of abnormal hyperintense signal on T2-weighted images, and

---

J. Kim (✉) · T. Moritani
Division of Neuroradiology, University of Michigan,
Ann Arbor, MI, USA
e-mail: johannk@med.umich.edu;
tmoritan@med.umich.edu

D. Q. Bui
Riverside Community Hospital, UC Riverside,
Riverside, CA, USA

P. W. Hitchon
University of Iowa Carver College of Medicine,
Iowa City, IA, USA
e-mail: patrick-hitchon@uiowa.edu

R. W. Woodroffe
Department of Neurosurgery, University of Iowa
Carver College of Medicine, Iowa City, IA, USA
e-mail: royce-woodroffe@uiowa.edu

J. L. Noeller
Department of Neurosurgery, University of Iowa
Hospitals and Clinics, Iowa City, IA, USA
e-mail: jennifer-noeller@uiowa.edu

K. V. Nourski
University of Iowa Hospitals and Clinics, Iowa City,
IA, USA
e-mail: kirill-nourski@uiowa.edu

on postcontrast T1-weighted images with attention to enhancement patterns, spatial distribution of lesions, and seldom unique characteristics of the known etiologies. In recent literature, there has been increased reports on the use of diffusion-weighted imaging (DWI) to evaluate spinal cord pathologies such as ischemia, infection, myelopathy, and inflammatory conditions [1–6].

The goal of this chapter is to discuss the combination of clinical information and MR imaging findings with emphasis on DWI and apparent diffusion coefficient (ADC) on spinal cord pathology to arrive at a specific diagnosis or to aid in limiting the differential diagnoses. We also demonstrate different kinds of diffusion techniques for the spinal cord including single-shot DWI with parallel imaging, multi-shot echo planar (RESOLVE-DWI), and BLADE-DWI [7].

23.2 MR Sequences of the Spinal Cord

Many kinds of echoplanar imaging (EPI) and non-EPI diffusion sequences with various b-values have been reported in the diagnosis of spine and spinal cord disease [7, 8]. Since DWI is typically implemented with EPI with fat saturation, there are many artifacts (susceptibility artifact, incomplete fat suppression, N/2 ghosting artifact, eddy current artifact, and motion artifact). Paramagnetic susceptibility artifacts from surgical

---

© Springer Nature Switzerland AG 2021
T. Moritani, A. A. Capizzano (eds.), *Diffusion-Weighted MR Imaging of the Brain, Head and Neck, and Spine*, https://doi.org/10.1007/978-3-030-62120-9_23

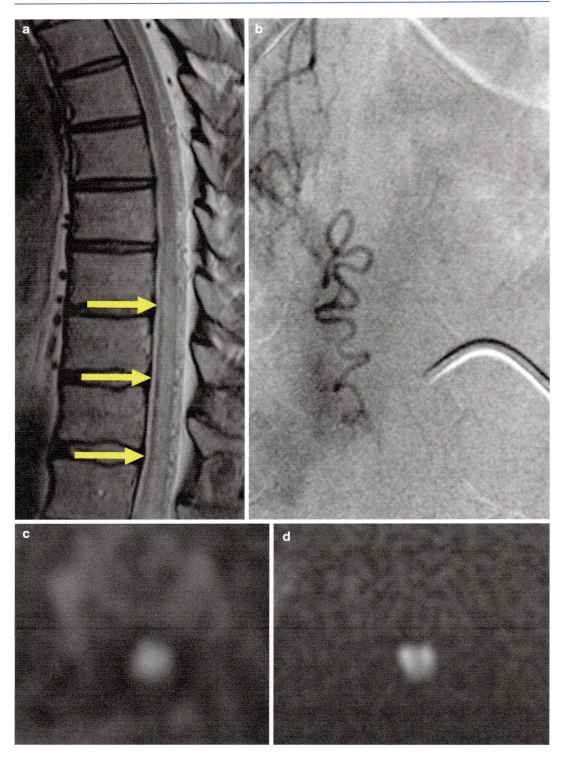

Fig. 23.1 (**a–d**) Type 2 intramedullary AVM and Foix-Alajouanine syndrome. Sagittal (**a**) T2-weighted image shows significant diffuse central cord edema in the thoracic spine (arrows). Conventional angiogram (**b**) shows an intramedullary AVM. Conventional single-shot EPI diffusion-weighted image (**c**) and multi-shot EPI diffusion-weighted imaging (**d**) show mildly high diffusion signal with ADC = 0.88×10^{-3} mm^2/s (not shown). Notice the improved resolution of multi-shot EPI DWI

23 Spinal Cord Lesions

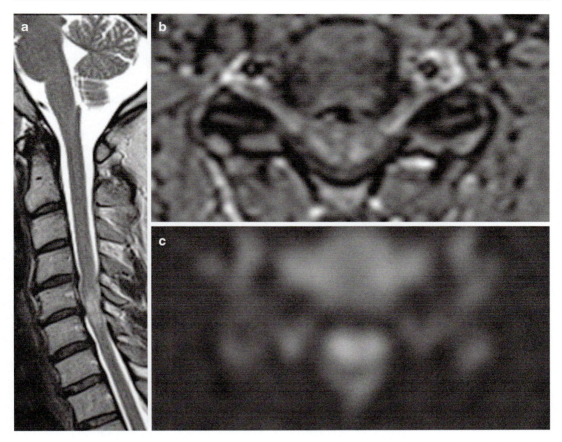

Fig. 23.2 (a–c) Compressive myelopathy. Patient presented with numbness and tingling in the left 4th and 5th digits. Sagittal (**a**) T2-weighted image shows a high signal lesion similar to demyelination or spinal cord tumor. The corresponding post-gadolinium T1-weighted axial (**b**) image shows multiple areas of enhancement in a scattering pattern with corresponding diffusion-weighted image (**c**). The ADC values are 1.34×10^{-3} mm^2/s (not shown)

metallic devices cause significant image distortion on DWI. We routinely use spin-echo-type single-shot EPI sequence with parallel imaging factor 2 or 3 in order to reduce distortion along with short acquisition time and general availability. For the evaluation of diffusion restriction in the spinal cord lesion, we use a b-value of 0 and 1000 sec/mm^2 with the ADC map since DWI with lower b-value can show high signal intensity due to the intravoxel incoherent motion and more T2 effect. New diffusion-weighted techniques including multi-shot echo planar DWI (RESOLVE DWI) (Fig. 23.1d), BLADE-DWI (Figs. 23.2b and 23.3b, c), turbo spin echo DWI (TSE-DWI), and reduced field of view single-shot echo planar DWI enable increased resolution and decreased magnetic susceptibility effects to help refine differential diagnoses [7, 8].

23.3 Vascular Etiologies
(Table 23.1)

23.3.1 Cord Infarction

The etiology of cord infarct is often multifactorial and most commonly attributed to systemic diseases such as atherosclerosis, aortic dissection, hypertension, diabetes, hypercoagulable states, and rarely associated with fibrocartilaginous embolization [8–10]. The mechanism of cord infarct is related to drop in perfusion pressure, which is determined by the difference between the mean arterial pressure and intraspinal canal pressure and is controlled through autoregulation [11–13].

The severity of clinical symptoms associated with spinal cord infarction varies greatly from minor weakness to paralysis. The onset of

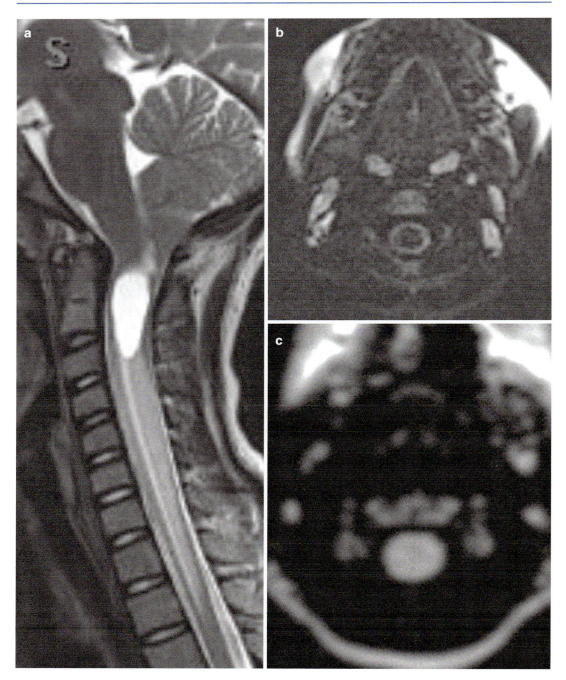

Fig. 23.3 (**a–c**) Pre-syrinx state. Sagittal T2-weighted image (**a**) of the cervical spine shows a hyperintense lesion involving a large portion of the cord secondary to Chiari I malformation. b,c BLADE DWIs at the level of syrinx (**b**) and just inferior to the syrinx (**c**) clearly demonstrate syrinx and pre-syrinx state without distortion. The ADC values are 3.61×10^{-3} mm^2/s in a syrinx and 1.76×10^{-3} mm^2/s in a pre-syrinx state representing interstitial edema

symptoms, however, is almost always abrupt whereas inflammatory etiologies may be acute or subacute. The neurologic presentation is specific to the cord level involved. The two most common infarction syndromes include the anterior spinal artery syndrome and the posterior spinal artery

23 Spinal Cord Lesions

Table 23.1 Vascular etiologies

	Infarct	AVM/AVF
Clinical picture	• Sudden onset and rapid progression of weakness. • Anterior spinal artery syndrome: loss of motor and pain/temperature sensation. • Pain/temperature sensation. • Posterior spinal artery syndrome: Loss of proprioception + vibratory sense.	• Slowly progressive to acute myeloradiculopathy. • Foix-Alajouanine: Subacute myelopathic necroses. Four types: • Type I: Dural AV fistula • Type II: Intramedullary glomus AVM[a] • Type III: Juvenile or combined AVM • Type IV: Intradural perimedullary AVF[b]
Intramedullary distribution	• Most commonly bilateral anterior cord.	• Central and diffuse cord involvement
Etiology	• Multifactorial most commonly atherosclerosis, hypertension, and diabetes	• AVF[b] or AVM leading to hemorrhage, venous hypertension, vascular steal or mass effect leading to cytotoxic vs. vasogenic edema.
Key MRI findings	• DWI: Hyperintense • Decreased ADC ($<0.9 \times 10^{-3}$ mm^2/s) in acute and subacute phase	• T2 flow voids. • Vasogenic edema: Increased ADC. • Cytotoxic edema: decreased ADC.

[a]AVM: Arteriovenous malformation
[b]Arteriovenous fistula

syndrome. Anterior spinal artery syndrome is characterized by loss of motor function and pain/temperature sensation, whereas posterior spinal artery syndrome is characterized by loss of proprioception and vibratory sense. Treatment entails a combination of blood pressure support and reduction of spinal canal pressure. Thrombolytic therapy has been reported but remains investigational.

Spinal cord infarct is classically characterized by central and well-defined hyperintense T2 signal with associated cord enlargement involving preferentially the gray matter [14]. Signal abnormality is most commonly found in the mid to lower thoracic spine due to the smaller caliber radicular arteries and watershed zone at the upper border of the artery of Adamkiewicz territory. Many patterns of abnormal signal distributions have been described, including unilateral anterior, bilateral anterior, central, total, transverse, bilateral posterior, and unilateral posterior; however, the most common distribution is bilateral anterior spinal cord infarct (the so-called snake eyes appearance), which account for approximately 56% of cases [8]. Postcontrast T1-weighted images show enhancement of the cord in the subacute phase.

Infarcts will be hyperintense on DWI with associated decreased ADC (Fig. 23.4). Literature review shows low ADC values in spinal cord infarct ranging between

$0.23–0.86 \times 10^{-3}$ mm^2/s [15–17]. ADC value of less than 0.90×10^{-3} mm^2/s is considered to be abnormal. Several studies have mapped out a rough time course for diffusion-related changes in spinal cord infarct [15, 16]. Generally, changes can be seen in the first several hours with normalization of diffusion and ADC signals within 1 week, whereas hyperintense T2 signal becomes more prominent over time; therefore diffusion is more sensitive than T2 images in the early stages.

23.3.2 Arteriovenous Malformations and Foix-Alajouanine Syndrome

The term spinal vascular malformations encompass a large group of vascular anomalies that include dural arteriovenous fistula (AVF), perimedullary AVF or arteriovenous malformation (AVM), and intramedullary AVF or AVM. A unique entity that may occur with spinal AVM is Foix-Alajouanine syndrome, a condition in which patients develop subacute myelopathic necrosis secondary to venous congestion, thrombosis of abnormal vascular channels or vascular steal with vasogenic edema and enhancement seen on imaging [18, 19]. Early diagnosis is mandatory, as congestive myelopathy may occur with both vasogenic edema and cytotoxic edema

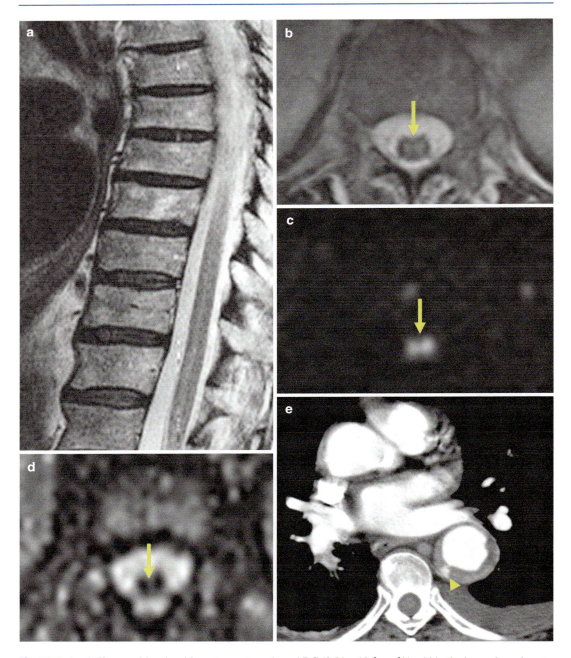

Fig. 23.4 (**a–e**) 60-year-old male with acute onset paralysis secondary to cord infarction. (**a**) Sagittal and (**b**) axial T2-weighted images along with (**c**) diffusion-weighted images show increased signal and (**d**) corresponding low ADC (0.54×10^{-3} mm^2/s) within the lower thoracic anterior horn of the spinal cord bilaterally (*arrows*). Cord infarction was secondary to descending aortic ulcer (**e**) (*arrowhead*)

[20, 21]. Multiple classification systems of spinal vascular malformations exist; however the most common is described by Spetzler as follows [22]:

- Type I: Dural AVF. The fistula is usually supplied by single arterial feeder in the subarachnoid space and drains into epidural veins distal to the AVF.

23 Spinal Cord Lesions

- Type II: Intramedullary glomus AVM (Fig. 23.1). An intramedullary nidus is fed by the anterior spinal artery and drains into the venous plexus on the cord surface, which in turn drains into epidural veins.
- Type III: Juvenile or combined AVM. Complex nidus with multiple feeding vessels.
- Type IV: Intradural perimedullary AVF. Direct communication between anterior spinal artery/posterior spinal artery and venous plexus without a nidus.

Depending on the results of a diagnostic angiography, embolization or surgical resection may be attempted for treatment.

Spinal AVMs may present with hyperintense intramedullary T2 signal due to edema of the cord with serpentine flow voids on spin echo images. These flow voids result from dilated and tortuous high flow veins which are best appreciated on sagittal views. Contrast-enhanced images show variable enhancement of the spinal cord, vessels, and nidus if present. The ADC value is helpful in prospectively evaluating reversibility and clinical recovery of patients [20, 23]. Vasogenic edema is characterized by higher ADC values, whereas cytotoxic edema will have lower ADC values [20]. Probability of reversibility potentially plays a major role in patient prognosis and treatment.

23.4 Inflammatory Etiologies (Table 23.2)

23.4.1 Idiopathic Transverse Myelitis (ITM)

Transverse myelitis occurs from various causes: autoimmune phenomenon after infection or vaccination, direct infection, systemic autoimmune disease, or acquired demyelinating disease such as multiple sclerosis or neuromyelitis optica. 15 to 30% of the cases of transverse myelitis are idiopathic [24, 25]. Idiopathic transverse myelitis (ITM) is immune-mediated inflammation in the spinal cord without any evidence of underlying CNS infection or other cause of acute myelopa-

thy affecting both halves of the cord (hence the term transverse). Symptoms may occur in an acute or subacute manner including bilateral motor weakness and pain. However, the most characteristic finding is a well-defined truncal (usually in the thoracic spine) sensory level loss in a band or transverse manner. There is usually some degree of sensory loss distal to this level. Autonomic abnormalities such as incontinence or sexual dysfunction have also been described. Treatment typically entails high dose intravenous glucocorticoid administration. Relapsing transverse myelitis is rare but can occur (Fig. 23.5) and currently lacks effective treatment [26].

Given the bilaterality of this disease, the most common imaging feature of ITM is a central hyperintense T2 signal that occupies more than 2/3 of the cord's cross-sectional area (88–100%) [27–29]. It is most commonly found in the thoracic spinal cord and typically spans three or more vertebral body segments (53–67%) [27–29]. As with other inflammatory pathologies, the contrast enhancement is variable depending on the activity of the lesion. In approximately half of patients, a central dot sign has been described whereby a dot of central gray matter is surrounded by high signal edema (47%) [28]. These conventional MRI findings have a large amount of overlap with acute cord infarct. Studies regarding diffusion and ITM are scarce. A single study with limited number of cases found increased ADC with reported values ranging from 0.90–1.18×10^{-3} mm²/s [30] (Fig. 23.5). Differentiation from acute cord infarct, which would show restricted diffusion, is of paramount value as treatment approaches are drastically different.

23.4.2 Acute Disseminated Encephalomyelitis (ADEM)

ADEM is usually the result of an environmental antigenic stimulus (post-infectious or post-vaccination) in a susceptible patient, and almost always leads to a monophasic abnormal inflammatory response that targets both the white and gray matter of the spinal cord. This differs from multiple sclerosis which is polyphasic. Clinical

Table 23.2 Inflammatory etiologies

	ITM[a]	ADEM[b]	MS[c]	NMO[d]	Sarcoidosis	SCD[e]
Clinical picture	• Pain and motor weakness. • Sensory loss below truncal level	• Prodrome --> neurologic deficits.	• Neurologic deficits separated by time and space.	• Optic neuropathy plus transverse myelitis	• Multiple organs affected.	• Decreased vibration sense, pyramidal signs and peripheral neuropathy.
Intramedullary distribution	• Central	• Central	• Peripheral -posterolateral			• Posterolateral and dorsal aspects. • Inverted V.
Etiology	• Idiopathic	• Post infectious or vaccination	• Demyelinating	• AQP4 antibodies	• Granulomatous disease	• B12 deficiency
Key MRI findings	• Central high T2. • >3 VB. • ADC possibly increased	• Central high T2 spanning >3-4 VB. • Acute: Diffusion restriction. • Subacute to chronic: Increased ADC	• <1 VB. • Acute plaque: Diffusion restriction. • Otherwise increased diffusion.	• Higher ADC than MS • >3 VB • MRI brain nondiagnostic for MS	• Nodular and peripheral CE+. • >3 VB.	• Acute phase: restricted diffusion in an inverted V pattern. • Hyperintense T2 in an inverted V pattern.

[a]ITM: Idiopathic transverse myelitis
[b]ADEM: Acute disseminated encephalomyelitis
[c]MS: Multiple sclerosis
[d]NMO: Neuromyelitis optica
[e]SCD: Subacute combined degeneration

23 Spinal Cord Lesions

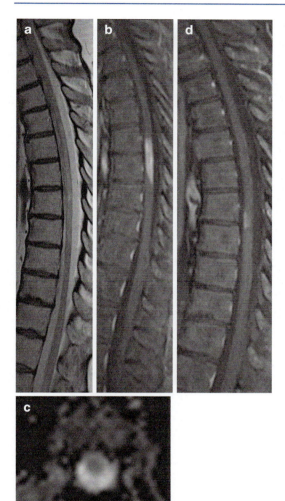

Fig. 23.5 (**a**–**d**) Recurrent idiopathic transverse myelitis in a 62-year-old female with bilateral lower extremity weakness. Sagittal T2-weighted (**a**) and gadolinium-enhanced T1-weighted (**b**) images show increased cord signal spanning four vertebral bodies with enhancement at T4 and T5. The increased ADC (1.36×10^{-3} mm^2/s) (**c**) suggests a subacute to chronic timeline. Follow-up sagittal gadolinium-enhanced T1-weighted image (**d**) shows interval decreased enhancement at T4 and T5 and new enhancement at T6/7

symptoms are usually preceded by a prodrome (71–74%) of febrile illness for up to 4 weeks. Patients may present with a prodrome of fever, headache, and vomiting that progresses to focal or multifocal neurologic deficits and encephalopathy [31–33]. Intravenous glucocorticoid therapy is considered first-line therapy followed by intravenous immunoglobulin and plasma exchange.

The cord lesion of ADEM is characterized by abnormal high T2 signal that is long, spanning three to four vertebral body levels. They have been classically described as vertical or flame-shaped lesions and may occur at any level of the spinal cord with no specific preference. On transverse views, lesions are typically centrally located overlapping with transverse myelitis and cord infarct. ADEM usually shows increased diffusion with hyperintense signal on DWI and increased ADC values (average of 1.35×10^{-3} mm^2/s) [34] in the subacute to chronic phases. In the acute setting, restricted diffusion may be seen with reported ADC values ranging from 0.37–0.68×10^{-3} mm^2/s [35]. Often these lesions are accompanied by vasogenic edema (increased ADC) representative of acute inflammation [36].

23.4.3 Multiple Sclerosis

Multiple sclerosis is a chronic demyelinating autoimmune disease that results from immune attack to myelin components. Under the microscope, an active plaque shows defined collections of foamy macrophages with preservation of the neurons. Conversely, an inactive plaque shows changes of gliosis. Clinicians look for a history of at least two separate episodes in which the patient suffered central nervous system deficits that have at least partially resolved. In the acute phase, intravenous glucocorticoids are recommended for treatment.

Typically, cord lesions in multiple sclerosis present in two varieties: (1) focal lesions which are well delineated with high T2 signal intensity or (2) poorly demarcated areas with slightly increased T2 signal intensity when compared to CSF. These lesions are usually peripherally located (most commonly posterolateral), predominantly in the cervical spinal cord, and span less than two vertebral body segments on sagittal views [37, 38] (Fig. 23.6).

DWI is typically hyperintense in subacute to chronic lesions, similar to other inflammatory

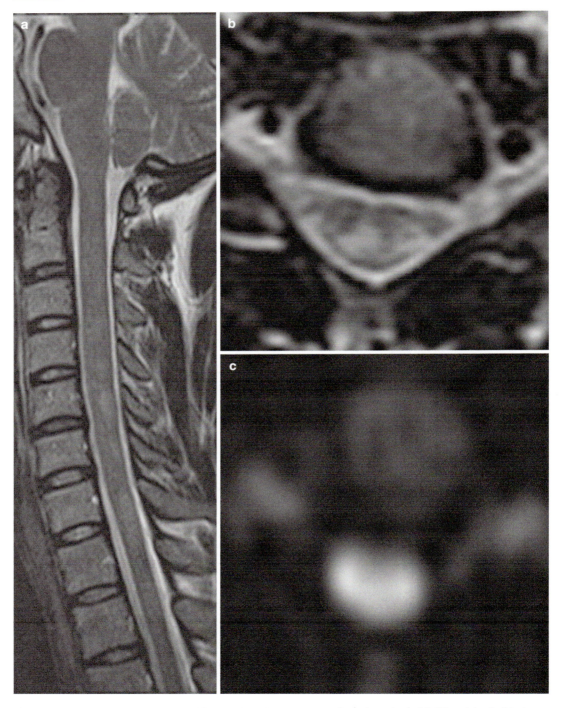

Fig. 23.6 (a–c) Multiple sclerosis in a 30-year-old male with resolving right-sided lower and upper extremity weakness but new generalized numbness. T2-weighted sagittal image (a) of the cervicothoracic spine shows multiple high signal plaques spanning approximately one vertebral body which enhance on the post-gadolinium sequence (not shown). Axial T2-weighted (b) image shows the corresponding lesions are located in the posterior and lateral white matter columns. These lesions have a round/ovoid morphology. There is high diffusion signal (c) and ADC (not shown) is slightly low to isointense ($0.85–0.93 \times 10^{-3}$ mm^2/s)

etiologies, and may likely be bright due to T2 shine through. Increased ADC values have been reported in a range from 1.06 to 1.82×10^{-3} mm^2/s with a mean of 1.36×10^{-3} mm^2/s, while the mean for healthy controls was 0.93×10^{-3} mm^2/s [34, 37, 39]. These higher ADC values are to be expected in subacute to chronic lesions given that components such as myelin sheaths, axons, and cellular membranes are damaged in MS [40]. Acute plaques may show restricted diffusion owing to cytotoxic edema [41].

23.4.4 Neuromyelitis Optica (NMO)

NMO involves both optic neuropathy (unilateral or bilateral) and transverse myelitis. Serum IgG autoantibodies against the water channel aquaporin-4(AQP4-Ab), are primarily found in astrocytes and mediate inflammatory attack targets. Positive AQP4-Ab antibody is thought to be pathogenic [40, 41]. However, some patients are seronegative for AQP4-Abs, which makes diagnosis more difficult. Some AQP4-Ab seronegative patients have antibodies against myelin-oligodendrocyte glycoprotein (MOG-Abs), which may have different pathogenic mechanisms [42]. Limited forms of the disease are known as NMO spectrum disorder (NMOSD). Pathologic findings typically show demyelination with progression to necrosis. Optic neuropathy and transverse myelitis may occur simultaneously but may also present at different times. NMO lesions commonly spare the brain in the early stages. Oral prednisone may be instituted for optic neuritis.

Winterchuk et al. used a number of varying diagnostic criteria for NMO. They found the following diagnostic criteria to have the highest combined sensitivity and specificity (99% and 90%, respectively): (1) a contiguous spinal cord lesion spanning three or more vertebral body lengths (Fig. 23.7) and (2) an initial brain MRI nondiagnostic for MS along with (3) positive AQP4 antibody titers [43]. Benedetti et al. found statistically significant increased diffusion (ADC values) in patients suffering from NMO versus those with MS, with average diffusion values of 1.40×10^{-3} mm^2/s for NMO and 1.24×10^{-3} mm^2/s for MS. They hypothesized that this may be due to decreased ability of NMO patients to recover from the severe demyelination and gray/white matter necrosis that develops leading to increased water diffusion [44].

23.4.5 Sarcoidosis

The pathogenesis of sarcoidosis is not well understood but may be pathologically described as a non-caseating granulomatous disorder likely initiated by CD4+ T cells, which affects multiple organs with no clearly implicated etiologic agent or genetic locus. Neurosarcoidosis is most commonly associated with granulomatous infiltrates involving the leptomeninges, dura, hypothalamus, pituitary gland, and cranial nerves and occurs in 5% to 16% of sarcoidosis patients [45]. Spinal cord neurosarcoidosis is rare with an incidence at 0.43% to 1% of all sarcoidosis patients. Spinal cord neurosarcoidosis is thought to be at high risk for severe neurological sequelae without prompt diagnosis and management. Spinal cord neurosarcoidosis is relatively refractory to corticosteroids and frequently requires corticosteroids plus additional immunosuppressant therapy including infliximab, cyclophosphamide, methotrexate, azathioprine, cyclosporine, leflunomide, mycophenolate mofetil, or adalimumab.

As many as 81% of spinal sarcoidosis patients present with intramedullary fusiform cord enlargement and almost always shows enhancement in a nodular and peripheral fashion (96%) [45] (Fig. 23.8). In addition to the peripheral enhancement, the radiologist should also look for leptomeningeal enhancement, which is seen in approximately half of the cases. These enhancing lesions may disappear with steroid treatment, but do not correlate well with clinical response. Sarcoidosis is most commonly found in the thoracic spine, followed by the cervical spine. The majority of cases span more than three vertebral body segments, which helps differentiate sarcoidosis from MS. There has been limited evaluation of intramedullary sarcoidosis using diffusion. Of the limited data available, the ADC values appear to vary widely ranging from 0.77×10^{-3} mm^2/s to 2.32×10^{-3} mm^2/s [30].

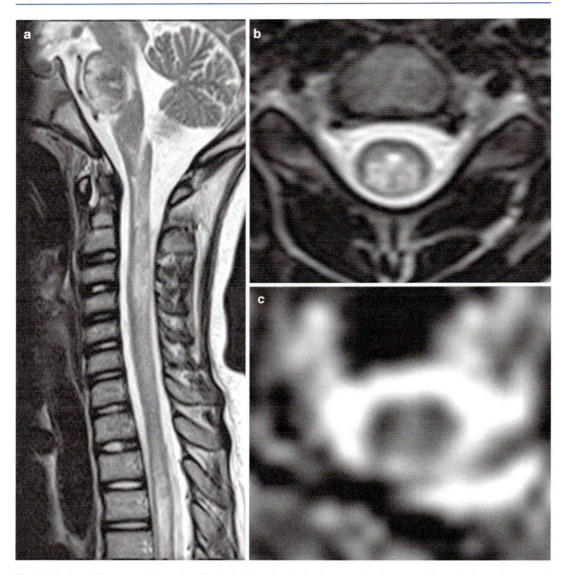

Fig. 23.7 (**a**–**c**) Neuromyelitis optica. Sagittal (**a**) and axial (**b**) T2-weighted images show multiple longitudinal heterogeneous high signals spanning more than 3 segments with central spinal cord distribution. There is brain stem involvement. These lesions show minimal enhancement. There is slightly increased ADC (**c**) (1.10×10^{-3} mm^2/s)

23.4.6 Subacute Combined Degeneration (SCD)

Although most accurately described as a demyelinating disease [46], SCD is placed under inflammatory etiology due to its many similarities. SCD can be caused by deficiencies in cobalamin (vitamin B12), nitrous oxide susceptibility, and copper deficiency. In the acute phase, SCD manifests pathologically as myelin sheath swelling. In the late stage, there is typically a combination of myelin sheath and axonal degeneration leading to Wallerian degeneration. Given that SCD is easily treated by vitamin B12 administration, it is imperative that radiologists are able to diagnose it. SCD is a well-known clinical syndrome characterized by symmetric diminished vibration sense, pyramidal signs, and peripheral neuropa-

23 Spinal Cord Lesions

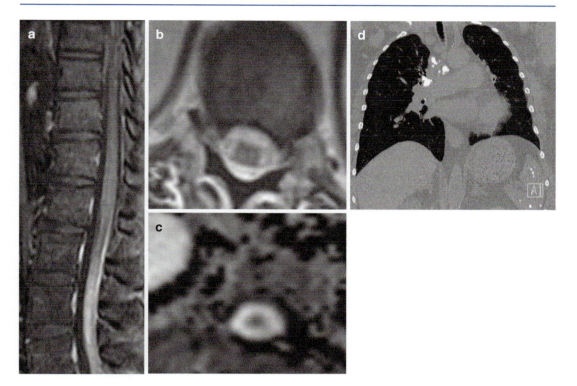

Fig. 23.8 (**a–d**) Sarcoidosis in a 70-year-old female with double vision, left 6th nerve palsy, and bladder and bowel incontinence. Sagittal (**a**) gadolinium-enhanced T1-weighted image shows moderate cauda equina enhancement. T2-weighted axial image (**b**) shows high signal within the cord associated with increased ADC (**c**) (1.29×10^{-3} mm^2/s). Chest CT (**d**) demonstrates hilar granulomatous calcifications

thy caused by "combined degeneration" of the posterior columns and/or lateral corticospinal tracts.

The classic MR finding of SCD is hyperintense T2 signal in the posterolateral and dorsal columns of the spinal cord, which has been described as an inverted V. Most cases do not show any enhancement [47–49]. Those cases that do enhance have been hypothesized to be an end stage lesion with breakdown of the blood-cord barrier. Three case reports showed restricted diffusion in the acute phase, which suggests cytotoxic edema of the myelin sheath [46, 50, 51]. DWI and ADC are useful in diagnosing and evaluating SCD (Fig. 23.9).

23.5 Infectious Etiologies
(Table 23.3)

23.5.1 Infectious Myelitis

Infectious myelitis can be further divided into bacterial, fungal, parasitic, and viral causes, with the latter being the most common. Examples of viral myelitis include polio, herpes, varicella zoster, influenza, and West Nile. Pathologies for each will vary depending on the organism. West Nile virus (WNV) typically targets gray matter of the spinal cord producing lower motor neuron disease. On the milder end of the spectrum, patients may suffer from fever, headache, and/or

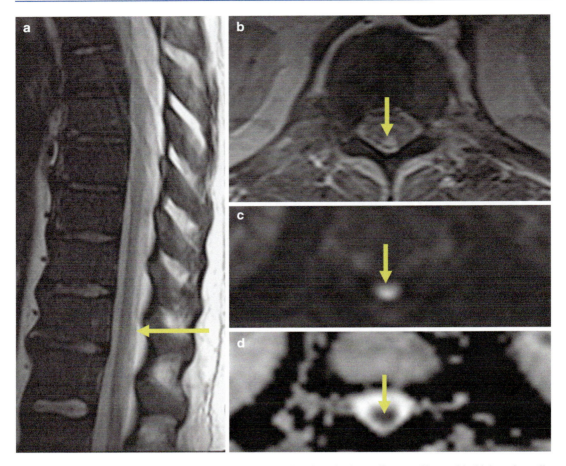

Fig. 23.9 (a–d) Symmetric T2 signals seen in the lateral and posterior columns are characteristic findings in subacute combined degeneration secondary to vitamin B12 deficiency (a, b). The demyelinating process selectively involves the large diameter fibers with thickened myelin sheath causing focal swelling of the myelin sheath without inflammatory reaction. DWI (c) can show restricted diffusion with low ADC (d) (0.81×10^{-3} mm^2/s)

generalized body aches. On the more severe end of the spectrum, patients will progress to meningoencephalitis (severe headache, fever, stupor, and muscle weakness), with risk of severe infection and death.

There are several spinal pathologies that may span multiple vertebral body segments. WNV myelitis is one of them and can easily span more than four vertebral body segments on sagittal T2-weighted images (Fig. 23.10). WNV may present with discrete foci of hyperintense T2 signal and therefore mimic transverse myelitis (clinical history and lab values can be key in making the differentiation). On contrast-enhanced images, leptomeningeal enhancement may be seen (possibly long segment). There is often thickening and enhancement of the cauda equina as well.

Enterovirus 71 (EV-71) is a major cause of hand-foot-mouth disease (HFMD) and has been associated with rhombencephalitis, acute flaccid paralysis, and myelitis. Characteristic MR imaging findings from EV-71 include non-enhancing dorsal brainstem and long segment anterior horn cell predominant spinal cord T2 hyperintensities. Enhancement of the ventral cauda equine nerve roots has been described [52]. Recent research suggests that there is retrograde axonal transport

23 Spinal Cord Lesions

Table 23.3 Mechanical and infectious etiologies

	Compressive myelopathy	Spinal cord contusion	West Nile virus	Intramedullary abscess
Clinical picture	• Progressive myelopathy	• Spinal cord bruise	• Meningoencephalitis	• Pain
Intramedullary distribution	• Variable	• Cervical spine	• Can be focal but can also span >4 vertebral bodies.	
Etiology	• Mass effect leading -> decreased perfusion-> infarct	• Young: High velocity trauma. • Old: Fall.	• Infectious myelitis	• Young: Spinal dysraphism or neural tube defect. • Adults: hematogenous or direct spread.
Key MRI findings	• Variable contrast enhancement. • ADC: Increased	• Acute: Restricted. • Chronic: Hyperintense T2/STIR	• Focal or long segment hyperintense T2 +/− leptomeningeal enhancement	• Well formed: Diffusion restriction. • Follows evolution of intracerebral abscess • Variable restriction.

of the EV-71 via the pharyngeal branch of the vagus nerve, hence the brainstem and upper cord involvement [53].

There is little information in the current literature regarding diffusion-weighted imaging of the spinal cord in EV-71 infections. The authors recently encountered a case of EV-71-positive 6-month-old child who presented with fever, vomiting, oropharyngeal/tracheal secretions, acute on chronic respiratory failure with hypoxemia. The imaging findings included anteromedial thalamic, dorsal brainstem and anterior horn cell predominant spinal cord T2 hyperintensities and restricted diffusion spanning multiple vertebral body levels (Fig. 23.11).

23.5.2 Intramedullary Abscess

The mechanism of infection is different between children and adults. In children, spinal dysraphism or neural tube defect such as a dermal sinus tract (tract from the skin surface extending towards the spinal canal) is often present allowing for direct spread of infection. In adults, it is commonly idiopathic. However identifiable causes include hematogenous spread or direct spread from spinal infection. Intramedullary abscesses of the spinal cord are very rare. Iwasaki et al. found only 54 cases reported in the world literature between 1977 and 2009. Clinical symptoms often resemble those of a structural cord lesion rather than infection.

An intramedullary abscess arising from within the spinal cord (Fig. 23.12) should be distinguished from epidural or subdural abscesses. The evolution of an intramedullary abscess seems to roughly correspond to that of an intracerebral abscess [54, 55]. T1-weighted images may show an ill-defined low signal expansile lesion within the cord with associated high T2 signal representing local edema. With evolution of the abscess, well-defined ring enhancement should be seen. Well-formed abscesses show restriction of diffusion centrally. However, the degree of diffusion restriction is variable depending on the amount of internal inflammatory cells and viscosity of abscess fluid [56]. DWI aids in differentiating abscess from a necrotic or cystic tumor, or cystic demyelinating disease as the latter will show increased rather than restricted diffusion.

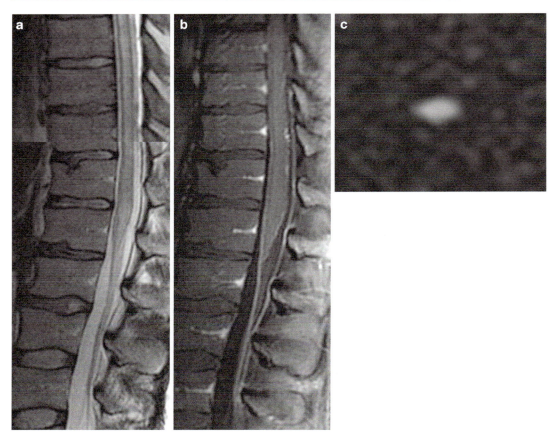

Fig. 23.10 (**a–c**) West Nile meningomyelitis in a 38-year-old male with 3-day history of worsening lower extremity paralysis. T2-weighted sagittal image shows (**a**) extensive longitudinal high T2 cord signal. Sagittal T1-weighted postcontrast image (**b**) showing dural and leptomeningeal enhancement. Diffusion is restricted in the thoracic spine (**c**) with decreased ADC (0.67×10^{-3} mm^2/s) (not shown) which represents acute demyelination process

23.6 Mechanical Cord Injury
(Table 23.3)

23.6.1 Compressive Myelopathy

Although not completely understood, the pathophysiology of compressive myelopathy is secondary to spinal stenosis from bulging or herniated disks, osseous spurs, or other form of mass effect on the cord leading to decreased perfusion, infarct, and necrosis [57, 58]. Clinical symptoms include neck or back pain, neurogenic claudication, and radiculopathy and may progress in severity to myelopathy with a combination of upper and lower motor neuron symptoms and signs plus sensory and autonomic deficits.

Beyond any obvious mass effect on the cord such as from a recent trauma or severe degenerative disease, subtle diagnosis of compressive myelopathy has typically relied on high T2 cord signal and atrophy (Fig. 23.2). Unfortunately, studies have shown that high T2 signal was only observed in 15–65% of symptomatic patients [57, 58]. Various contrast enhancement patterns have been described including peripheral, central, scattered, diffuse, and "snake eyes." Compressive myelopathy will typically be slightly hyperintense on DWI and have increased

23 Spinal Cord Lesions

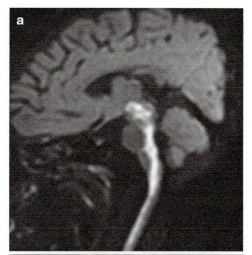
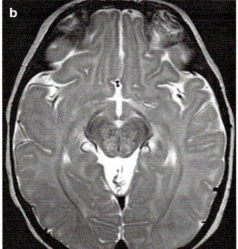
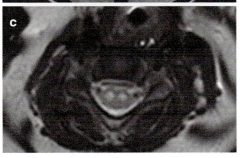

Fig. 23.11 (**a–c**) EV-71 infection. 6-month-old male who presented with fever, vomiting, and respiratory failure. Sagittal diffusion-weighted imaging demonstrated restricted diffusion involving the midbrain, dorsal pons, dorsal medulla, and anterior spinal cord (**a**). The areas of restricted diffusion within the brainstem and anterior horn cells also demonstrated T2 hyperintensities (**b** and **c**)

ADC values, representing facilitated diffusion due to chronic hypoperfusion and changes in the arrangement of axons of the spinal cord [57, 58]. Some studies have suggested that ADC maps have sensitivity as high as 80% compared to T2 sensitivity of 61% and were able to show statistically significant changes in ADC values between normal patients and those suffering from cervical myelopathy before cord compression is even appreciated on conventional MR [59, 60].

23.6.2 Spinal Cord Contusion

The most common etiology of spinal cord contusion is high velocity trauma, which tends to happen most commonly in young adults during motor vehicle accidents. Cord contusion in middle aged and older adults is typically the result of a fall. Cord contusion is most easily described as a "bruise" of the spinal cord with intramedullary hemorrhage and a variable amount of adjacent edema depending on the acuity of the injury.

Diffusion can be especially useful for spinal cord contusion (Fig. 23.13). In the acute stage, cytotoxic edema due to severe cord injury will restrict water diffusion, while adjacent vasogenic edema shows up slightly hyperintense on DWI and increased ADC helping to delineate the different types of edema [61].

23.6.3 Syrinx and Pre-syrinx State

Syringomyelia consists of a cystic cavity within the spinal cord that is not lined with ependyma. It occurs in many conditions, including posttraumatic states, Chiari malformations, arachnoiditis, spine and spinal cord tumors, and spondylosis. Although the pathophysiology is not certain, it is hypothesized that mechanical impairment of normal CSF circulation drives CSF into the cord via perivascular spaces, partially due to CSF pulsation, resulting in a syrinx cavity. Pre-syrinx states can be thought of as intramedullary interstitial edema and enlargement due to CSF flow into the cord at presumed areas of an under-

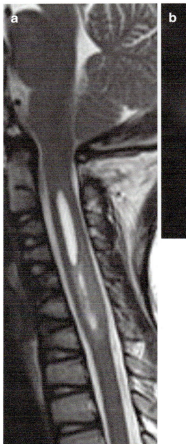
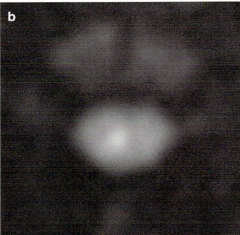

Fig. 23.12 (**a, b**) Intramedullary spinal cord abscess in a pediatric patient with Chiari I malformation and associated syrinx. Sagittal T2-weighted (**a**) image shows a syrinx in the cervical cord and abscess in the lower portion of the syrinx. Diffusion images (**b**) show high signal in the abscess with reduced ADC (0.54×10^{-3} mm^2/s) (not shown)

developed central canal, which pathologically represents interstitial edema, gliosis, and slight loss of gray matter [62]. Pre-syrinx states are of special importance because they are reversible after surgical treatment of the offending cause.

Clinical symptoms are varied and depend on size and location of the syrinx. Typically, patients present with some degree of pain and thermal sensory loss.

Syringomyelia will appear as a central tubular intramedullary cystic lesion that is high on T2-, but low on T1-weighted images along the trajectory of the central canal [62–65]. Pre-syrinx states typically present with isointense T1 and high intramedullary T2 signal (Fig. 23.3). Diffusion is typically low in signal intensity with high ADC values, reflecting interstitial edema.

23.7 Neoplasm

Ependymoma is the most common in adults and astrocytoma is the most common spinal cord tumor in children. DWI signal and ADC value of neoplasms depend on the cellularity and extracellular matrix. Low-grade astrocytoma usually shows high ADC values due to the abundant extracellular matrix which contains more free water. Ependymoma shows intermediate ADC values and often contains hemorrhage. Hypercellular tumors such as high-grade glioma,

23 Spinal Cord Lesions

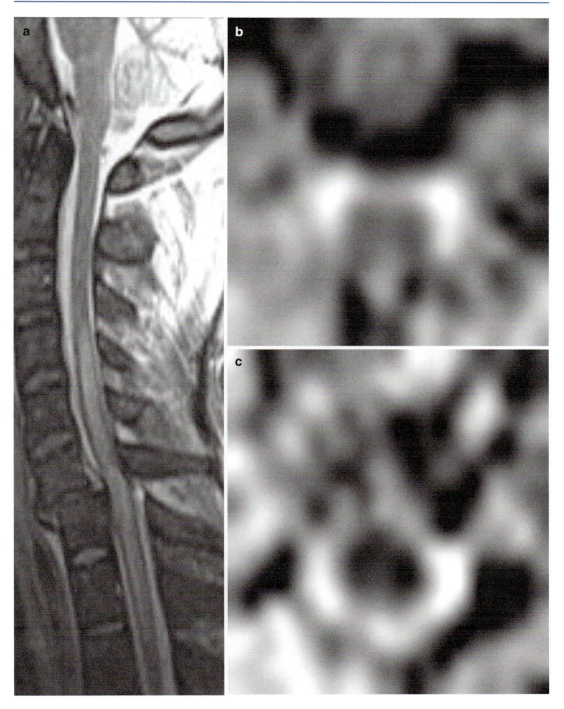

Fig. 23.13 (**a–c**) Acute cord contusion in a 39-year-old male status post motor vehicle accident. Sagittal T2-weighted images (**a**) show extensive high signal associated with a fracture dislocation. The upper region of edema (**b**) shows hyperintense diffusion signal with increased ADC (1.20×10^{-3} mm^2/s) that represents vasogenic edema. At the contusion site (**c**), there is restricted diffusion with decreased ADC (0.57×10^{-3} mm^2/s) at the fracture suggestive of cytotoxic edema

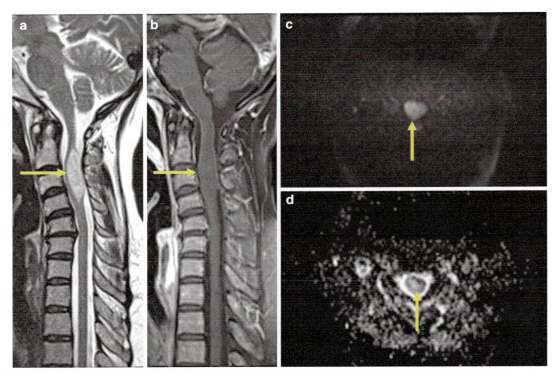

Fig. 23.14 (**a**–**d**) Astrocytoma of the cervical spinal cord. Sagittal MRI images show T2 high (**a**) and T1 low (**b**) signal mass lesion without enhancement. (**c**, **d**) DWI hyperintensity with high ADC (1.57×10^{-3} mm^2/s) which likely represents more abundant extracellular matrix seen in pilocytic astrocytoma

intramedullary metastasis, and lymphoma can show restricted diffusion with low ADC associated with less extracellular matrix.

23.7.1 Astrocytoma

A retrospective study by Yamasaki et al. found ADC values for posterior fossa pilocytic astrocytoma ranging between $1.3–1.9 \times 10^{-3}$ mm^2/s with a mean of 1.66×10^{-3} mm^2/s (Fig. 23.14). ADC values for anaplastic astrocytomas ranged between $1.04–1.57 \times 10^{-3}$ mm^2/s with a mean of 1.24×10^{-3} mm^2/s. To provide perspective, ependymomas had ADC values that ranged from $1.05–1.33 \times 10^{-3}$ mm^2/s with an average of 1.23×10^{-3} mm^2/s. Overall the authors hypothesized that higher-grade tumors roughly correlated with lower ADC values and vice versa which were corroborated in other studies [66, 67]. Similarly, Rumboldt et al. found that with a cutoff value of $>1.4 \times 10^{-3}$ mm^2/s and $<0.9 \times 10^{-3}$ mm^2/s, they were able to differentiate infratentorial juvenile pilocytic astrocytoma (WHO grade I) from medulloblastoma (WHO grade IV), respectively, with 100% specificity in posterior fossa tumors [68]. This relationship seemed to hold true in a meta-analysis for intra-axial astrocytomas, which showed that lower ADC values correlated with poor survival independent of tumor grade [69].

23.7.2 Ependymoma

A retrospective study found ADC values for intracranial ependymomas to range between $1.05–1.33 \times 10^{-3}$ mm^2/s with a mean of 1.2×10^{-3} mm^2/s [66, 70] (Fig. 23.15), which is typically lower than those seen for pilocytic

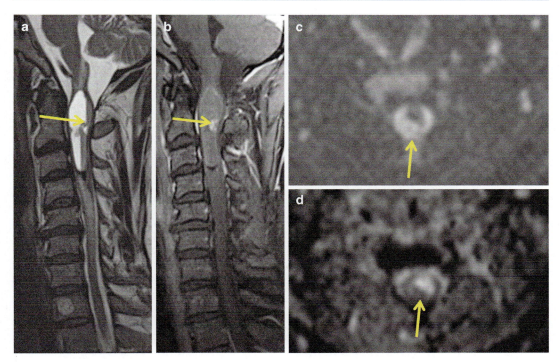

Fig. 23.15 (**a**–**d**) Cervical cord ependymoma with hemorrhage. (**a**) Sagittal T2-weighted image shows fluid-fluid levels showing hemorrhage and cystic component. (**b**) Gadolinium-enhanced T1-weighted image shows a small enhancing portion and peripheral enhancement. DWI (**c**) and ADC (**d**) of the enhancing solid portion shows intermediate ADC value (0.94×10^{-3} mm^2/s)

astrocytomas [71]. Other studies seem to confirm this trend of lower ADC values correlating with higher-grade tumors [72, 73].

23.7.3 Intramedullary Metastasis

Intramedullary metastasis is a poor prognostic indicator with a median survival of only 4 months after the time of diagnosis. Lung cancer is the most common cause, with breast cancer being the second most common. However, any primary tumor has the potential to spread to the cord either via hematogenous dissemination or through the central canal via CSF pathways (primary brain tumors). In a recent retrospective study primary malignancy was not always previously diagnosed at the time of intramedullary metastasis symptom onset or MRI imaging [74]. Patients, even those with multiple intramedullary metastases, may be asymptomatic.

With intramedullary metastasis, the cord is focally enlarged. On T2-weighted images, there is typically diffuse edema surrounding the lesion. Most metastatic lesions will show ring or homogenous enhancement (Fig. 23.16). However, if hemorrhage is present, enhancement will become heterogeneous [75]. A retrospective review of 70 intramedullary metastasis found that peri, intratumoral cysts or hemorrhage were only seen in 4% of the sample size [74]. Metastatic lesions tend to be most common in the cervical spine, followed by the thoracic and then lumbar spine. Diffusion and ADC characteristics likely depend on the cellularity of primary tumor. ADC values for intra-axial metastasis ranged between 0.89–1.58×10^{-3} mm^2/s with a mean of 1.15×10^{-3} mm^2/s [66].

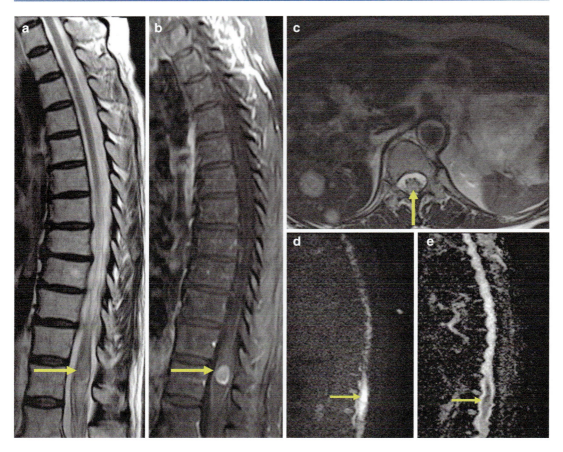

Fig. 23.16 (**a**–**e**) Intramedullary metastatic lesion from breast cancer. Sagittal T2 (**a**) and gadolinium-enhanced T1-weighted (**b**) images show an enhancing intramedullary lesion near the conus medullaris (arrow). (**c**) Axial T2-weigted image at the liver shows high signal cord lesion (arrow) and multiple liver metastases. (**d**, **e**) Sagittal DWI shows hyperintensity and corresponding low ADC (arrow)

23.7.4 Lymphoma

Most intramedullary lymphomas are highly aggressive with poor prognosis. The most common known risk factor is immunodeficiency. Immunocompetent patients tend to present older, roughly at 60 years, while immunosuppressed patients tend to present in their 30–40 years [75, 76]. The most typical presenting symptoms include back pain (30%), progressive myelopathy, and radiculopathy. More than 50% of spinal lymphomas are multifocal, which includes intracranial lesions [75, 76].

Not uncommonly, the lesion is isointense on T1-weighted images and hyperintense on T2-weighted images. Enhancement is variable and may range from patchy to diffuse to discrete. Lymphoma will typically show diffusion restriction indicative of its hypercellularity [75]. ADC values for intracranial lymphomas ranged between $0.60–1.07 \times 10^{-3}$ mm^2/s with a mean of 0.73×10^{-3} mm^2/s [66] (Fig. 23.17).

23.7.5 Waldenstrom's Macroglobulinemia and Bing-Neel Syndrome

Waldenstrom's macroglobulinemia is a rare lymphoproliferative disorder characterized by bone marrow and lymphoid tissue B cell infiltration as well as presence of IgM monoclonal gammopa-

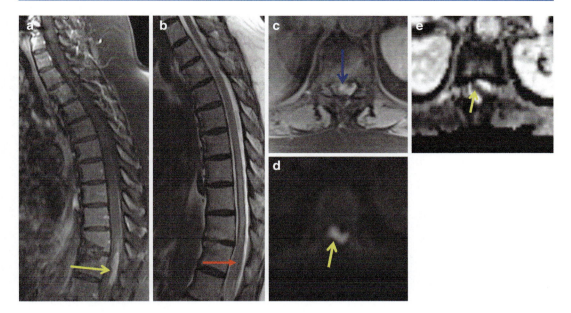

Fig. 23.17 (**a–e**) Lymphoma with invasion of the cord. (**a**) Sagittal T1 postcontrast and (**b**) sagittal T2 images demonstrate enhancing intradural lesion (arrow) with invasion of the cord better visualized on the axial T1 post- contrast image (**c**). Extensive leptomeningeal enhancement and cord edema are also present. (**d**) DWI and (**e**) ADC of the enhancing solid portion show high and low ADC (0.63×10^{-3} mm^2/s)

thy in the serum. Bing-Neel syndrome is a rare neurological complication of the already rare Waldenstrom's macroglobulinemia with central nervous system involvement by malignant cells that was first described in 1936 by Jens Bing and Axel Valdemar von Neel [77]. Diagnosis of Bing-Neel syndrome is based on cytological or histological confirmation most often via cerebrospinal fluid analysis in the setting of systemic Waldenstrom's macroglobulinemia.

Imaging plays a helpful role in diagnosis. Routine MR sequences such as FLAIR, DWI, and contrast-enhanced T1-weighted images are important in identifying Bing-Neel syndrome. The most common radiological finding is contrast enhancement of the subarachnoid space due to leptomeningeal infiltration within the brain or spine. The cranial nerves and cauda equina nerve roots may become thickened with contrast enhancement [78]. Dural thickening with enhancement is another common finding. Brain parenchymal involvement may often present with periventricular and brainstem enhancing lesions. Similar to lymphoma with hypercellular cells, lesions in Bing-Neel syndrome may sometimes show restricted diffusion (Fig. 23.18).

23.8 Conclusion

Diffusion-weighted imaging is useful in narrowing the differential diagnoses of intramedullary spinal lesions. Etiologies that cause cytotoxic edema or decreased free diffusion of water will lead to diffusion restriction, which includes spinal cord infarct, acute demyelination, intramedullary abscess, and highly cellular tumors. Conversely, lesions that have increased diffusion of water molecules will have elevated ADC values, which include subacute to chronic inflammatory and demyelinating lesions, chronic compressive myelopathy, pre-syrinx state, and low-grade primary tumors. On the other hand, technical difficulties for DWI implementation in the spine are being addressed by development of different MRI sequences that minimize magnetic homogeneity issues. Although the early data is promising in regard to the utility of DWI and

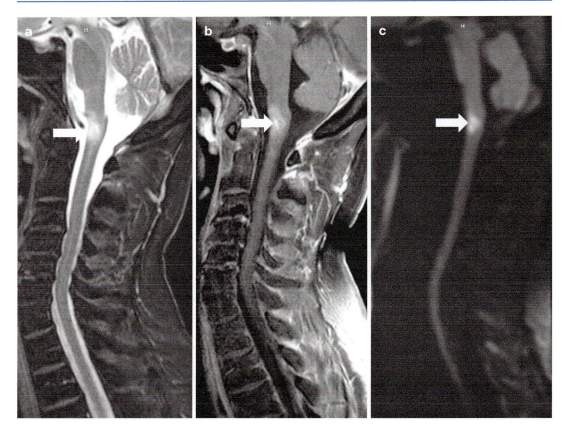

Fig. 23.18 (**a**–**c**) Bing-Neel syndrome. 67-year-old male with sensation of disequilibrium for 2 months, trouble with fine motor movements in both hands, with progressive bowel/bladder changes and radicular pain into legs. MRI of the cervical spine demonstrates T2 hyperintense (**a**), contrast-enhancing (**b**), and restricted diffusion (**c**) lesion in the cervical-medullary junction (arrows) and cauda equine enhancement (not shown) compatible with Bing-Neel syndrome. CSF cytology and flow cytometry was positive for malignant cells with elevated IgM

ADC with intramedullary lesions, more dedicated research studies will be needed in the future.

23.9 Treatment of Intramedullary Spinal Cord Tumors

Patrick W. Hitchon, Royce W. Woodroffe, Jennifer Noeller, and Kirill V. Nourski

23.9.1 Introduction

Spinal cord tumors are classified based on their anatomic location. Those originating from the spinal cord parenchyma are referred to as intramedullary, whereas those arising from the dura or elsewhere are extramedullary. Intramedullary spinal cord tumors (IMSCT) are rare lesions and constitute only 4–10% of all primary central nervous system tumors [70, 79, 80]. IMSCTs are less common in adults than in children. The most frequently involved localization was in the thoracic region (36%), followed by the cervical region (33%), the cervicothoracic region (19%), and the thoracolumbar (with conus) region (13%) [79]. The majority of IMSCTs are comprised of gliomas (80–90%), of which 60–70% are ependymomas and 30–40% are astrocytomas [80–82].

Imaging is paramount in identifying intradural from extradural spinal tumors. Diagnosis of the lesion can often be suspected or made from imaging, but confirmation of diagnosis demands surgery. In an attempt to identify radiographic features of spinal cord tumors, we reviewed our records of intramedullary spinal cord tumors for the past 10 years (IRB 201710760), including radiology reports, treatment, and outcomes.

In our experience, we encountered 30 meningiomas, 30 intramedullary gliomas, 28 nerve sheath tumors, 4 hemangioblastomas, 3 cavernomas, and 3 intramedullary metastases. Hereafter, we describe our experience and that of others in the diagnosis and management of ependymomas and astrocytomas.

23.9.2 Ependymoma

The most common intramedullary spinal cord tumor, regardless of age group, is ependymoma and accounts for 50–60% of lesions [83]. The vast majority of these lesions are WHO grade II, with WHO grade III anaplastic ependymoma being exceedingly rare. Up to 88% of patients with intramedullary spinal ependymomas present with neurologic symptoms, including motor weakness, sensory loss, or bladder dysfunction [84]. Of those who are neurologically intact, pain is the most common presenting symptom [84]. Intramedullary spinal ependymomas most commonly originate in the cervical spine, followed by the thoracic and then lumbar areas [85].

23.9.2.1 Imaging

An intramedullary tumor is radiographically recognized by focal expansion of the cord and occasionally an associated cyst. MRI shows T2-weighted (T2W) and fluid attenuated inversion recovery (FLAIR) hyperintensity, T1-weighted (T1W) hypo- or isointensity, with variable contrast enhancement [86]. Ependymomas show contrast enhancement associated with cystic changes, and hemosiderin suggestive of previous hemorrhage [87, 88] (Figs. 23.19, 23.20, and 23.21). A syrinx was present in 80% of the ependymomas [80].

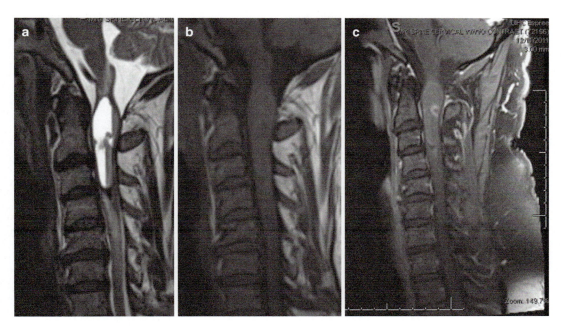

Fig. 23.19 (**a–c**) A 47-year-old male with neck pain since a fall 1 month ago endorses instability of gait. No frank weakness on exam. MRI shows a 5.6 × 1.7 × 1.2 cm intramedullary lesion in the cervical cord extending from C1 to C3 with high signal on T2 (**a**), low signal on T1 (**b**), and enhancing nodule (**c**). This is associated with fluid/fluid level (**a**) compatible with hemorrhage

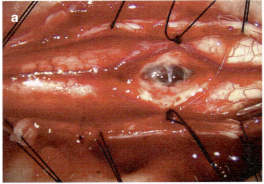
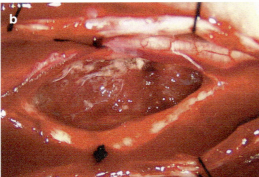
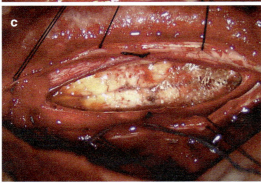

Fig. 23.20 (**a–c**) Intraoperative myelotomy (**a**), followed by total exposure of the entire ependymoma grade II (**b**). The tumor bed following excision of the tumor is seen in figure (**c**)

23.9.2.2 Treatment

The vast majority of patients with intramedullary ependymomas present with a neurologic deficit, and in that case, early excision is recommended whenever possible [89, 90]. Patients who present without neurologic deficit should be appropriately counseled on the risks of surgery. One study of such patients demonstrated worsening of preoperative complaints in 10% [84]. In general, most patients (69%) will have no changes in the neurologic status, and improvement is unlikely (20%) [91]. There is some increased risk with thoracic lesions and advanced age [90]. Depending on the plane of dissection and the infiltrative nature of the tumor, attempts should be made to achieve a gross total resection (GTR) [85]. For unresectable tumor or recurrences, radiation is recommended [85] (Figs. 23.22 and 23.23). Contrary to intramedullary astrocytomas, ependymomas yield themselves more likely to a successful GTR, which translates to a cure in the majority of patients [89]. Recurrence rates are lower as well, with one study demonstrating recurrence in only 7.3% of patients [91]. Chemotherapy is still considered investigational when other modalities have been exhausted [79].

23.9.3 Malignant Astrocytoma

Astrocytomas are the most common primary spinal cord neoplasm in the pediatric population, comprising up to 90% of all IMSCTs [92], while in the adult population they account for approximately 60% of IMSCTs [93]. Most of these lesions are low grade; however, 10–15% classify as malignant astrocytomas, including anaplastic astrocytomas (WHO grade III) and glioblastomas (WHO grade IV) [94]. Intramedullary astrocytomas most commonly originate in the cervical spine, followed by the thoracic and lumbar areas [95]. They commonly present in the third decade of life, with a range of 2–61 years found in one study [85].

23.9.3.1 Imaging

Astrocytomas appear on MRI as fusiform expansion of the cord and are less likely to be associated with cyst or syrinx. The tumor is hypo- to isointense on T1W images, hyperintense on T2W and FLAIR images, with variable contrast enhancement. Astrocytoma is more likely than ependymoma to be non-enhancing [96] (Figs. 23.24, 23.25, and 23.26).

In general, the distinction between astrocytomas and ependymomas by magnetic resonance

23 Spinal Cord Lesions

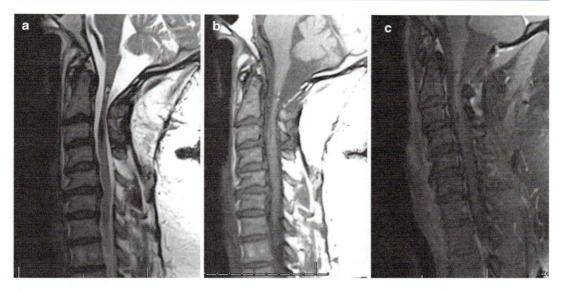

Fig. 23.21 (**a–c**) Five years following resection, there is low signal intensity on T2 (**a**), T1 (**b**), and no enhancement with Gd administration (**c**). No evidence of recurrence

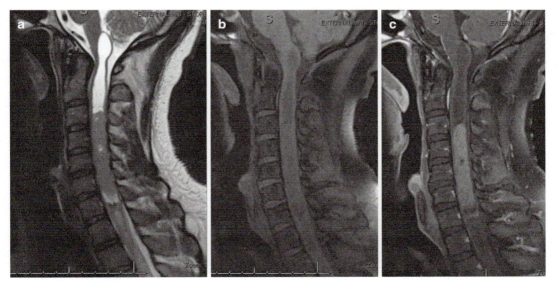

Fig. 23.22 (**a–c**) A 43-year-old male presents with neck stiffness, numbness, and weakness in his arms. MRI shows a solid isointense mass on T2 (**a**) and T1 (**b**), enhancing (**c**) from C3–7 capped with a syrinx extending to the medulla and caudally to the thoracic cord

(MR) is not possible [81], although ependymomas are generally better defined and less infiltrative than astrocytomas. A syrinx was present in 75% of the astrocytomas [80].

23.9.3.2 Treatment
Astrocytomas often lack a clear dissection plane due to their infiltrative nature, making a GTR difficult to achieve [95]. In one study that

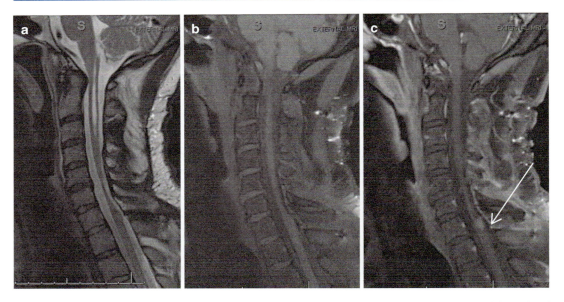

Fig. 23.23 (**a–c**) One year from surgery for excision of the grade III ependymoma in Fig. 23.23, a postoperative MRI was obtained. The study shows small residual syrinx hyperintense on T2 (**a**) and isointense on T1 (**b**). There is a small residual enhancing mass at the caudal margin of the resection cavity at C7 (**c**). As a result, the patient underwent radiation therapy and is being followed closely

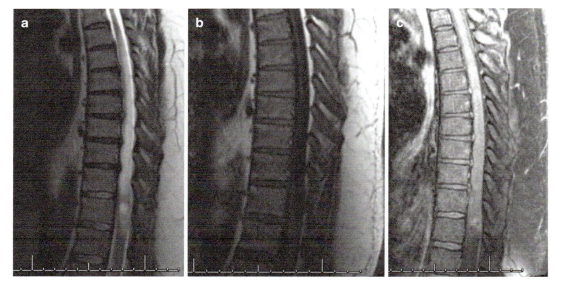

Fig. 23.24 (**a–c**) A 37-year-old male presents with shaking in his legs and stiffness in walking. He has a sensory level and clonus. MRI shows abnormal high T2 signal (**a**) and low signal on T1 (**b**) in the thoracic spinal cord. There is minimal heterogeneous enhancement compatible with astrocytoma (**c**)

23 Spinal Cord Lesions

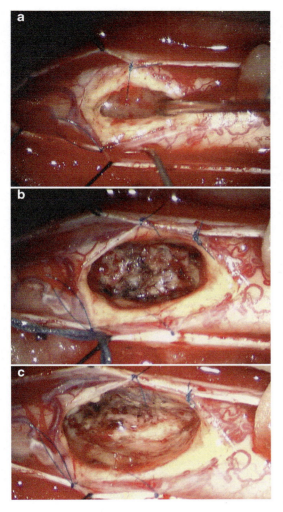

Fig. 23.25 (**a–c**) Intraoperative exposure (**a**), circumferential dissection (**b**), and following excision of infiltrating grade II astrocytoma (**c**)

included 18 patients with WHO grade III or IV astrocytomas, none achieved a GTR [87]. In fact, this is generally not advisable due to risk of damage to normal cord parenchyma [95]. This risk is evident, as 61% of those in the aforementioned study had worsened functional status postoperatively [87]. Neurologic improvement for patients postoperatively is rare, with rates as low as 5% [88]. For significant residual, recurrences, or unresectable tumor, adjuvant radiation is recommended, and the majority of patients undergo treatment and receive some benefit [95]. Subtotal resection lends to a high recurrence rate (47.6%) [88], and long-term survival is associated with a more aggressive resection [85, 91, 97]. In patients with anaplastic astrocytoma, the median overall survival is 72 months, whereas for patients with glioblastoma it is only 9 months [85]. Chemotherapy is still considered investigational when other modalities have been exhausted [79].

23.9.4 Surgical Technique

Surgery accomplishes three main goals: (1) tissue diagnosis; (2) cytoreduction; and (3) prevention of worsening of neurologic function. Timing of surgical intervention for IMSCTs is poorly studied. However, in patients with progressive neurologic decline, earlier intervention is preferred as preoperative neurologic function is strongly predictive of postoperative function [86]. Extent of tumor resection is a significant predictor of survival, as these lesions respond poorly to chemotherapy or radiation due to their low proliferation index [86]. Patient preparation is nowhere more necessary than in IMSC. The surgeon should always apprise the patient of the potential diagnosis and the risks involved. Within reason, the patient should be educated about the ease and complexity of these operations. Removal of these tumors can at times be easy, and at others quite difficult. Examples of similar cases should be presented to the patient to comprehend this potentially life-changing procedure. If the patient comprehends and the surgeon has the experience, then it is appropriate to proceed, earlier rather than later [98, 99]. If there is reluctance on the part of the patient to accept neurologic deficit in spite of malignancy, a delay in decision-making by the patient is wise.

All biopsies or resections of intramedullary tumors were accomplished with intraoperative somatosensory evoked potentials (SSEP) and motor evoked potentials (MEP). For localization, intraoperative fluoroscopy was always used. Once the levels were confirmed, laminoplasty of the levels of interest was undertaken up to one level above and below the level of the

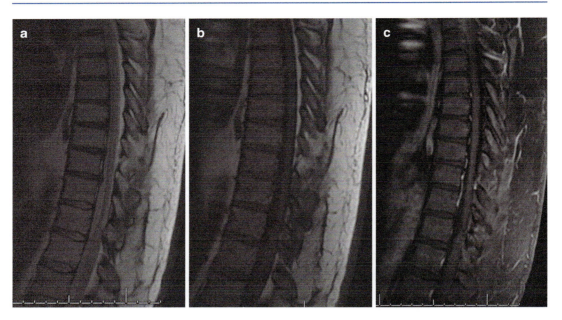

Fig. 23.26 (**a–c**) Two years postoperative, there is a stable small residual hyperintensity on T2 signal (**a**), none on T1 (**b**), and no evidence of residual tumor enhancement (**c**)

tumor, as it is unwise to undertake bony exposure once the dura is opened. Laminoplasty is commonly employed [83] and generally preferred as laminectomy can portend to the development of spinal deformity, especially in the cervical region [84]. However, in the pediatric population, laminoplasty or laminectomy of greater than four levels is still associated with the development of spinal deformity necessitating fusion [89].

Intraoperative ultrasonography is routinely used prior to dural opening. Myelotomy and dissection is always undertaken under the microscope with a suction regulator. A minimal amount of suction with a 5 French suction is necessary. The use of bipolar coagulation is minimized. Oftentimes small bleeding points can be easily controlled with Gelfoam, obviating the need for coagulation. Where a cleavage plane is identified between the tumor and spinal cord, total excision is always attempted, and oftentimes possible. The ultrasonic aspirator has provided a significant adjunct to resection of IMSCTs and has become integral to the armamentarium for resection of these lesions. SSEPs and MEPs have to be heeded, as they are extremely sensitive and specific for anticipating neurologic injury [90], and at every stage the surgeon should always reconsider the risk vs. benefit to the patient where the cleavage plane is elusive.

Intraoperative histopathologic analysis provides important information that will influence how aggressive the surgeon may be in attempting a gross total resection. Among the intramedullary tumors, ependymomas can often be entirely resected, while astrocytomas are more likely to infiltrate the spinal cord [79, 81, 98, 99]. However, it is important to keep in mind that intraoperative frozen pathology has lower diagnostic accuracy in spinal neoplasms (~70%) than with cranial neoplasms [100]. Resection of intradural but extramedullary spinal cord tumors such as meningiomas (Fig. 23.27) or nerve sheath tumors (Fig. 23.28) are by far simpler operations with far less risk of morbidity to the patient. Though hemangioblastoma tumors are also intramedullary, they are generally far simpler to remove as their borders are well delineated with significantly less trauma imparted to the cord (Fig. 23.29).

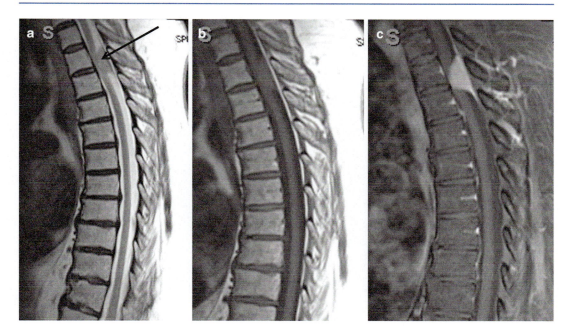

Fig. 23.27 (**a–c**) A 71-year-old female with a several-month history of progressive weakness and numbness in her legs. She failed to improve with therapy, with persistence of paraparesis, loss of sensation in her legs, and fecal incontinence. Thoracic MRI shows mild hyperintense T2 signal (**a**, arrow), low attenuation on T1 (**b**), and a homogeneously enhancing extradural extramedullary mass at T2-T3 with a dural tail effacing the right posterolateral aspect of the thecal sac and causing significant mass effect on the spinal cord (**c**). Uneventful surgery resulted in excision of the meningioma, with slow but significant improvement

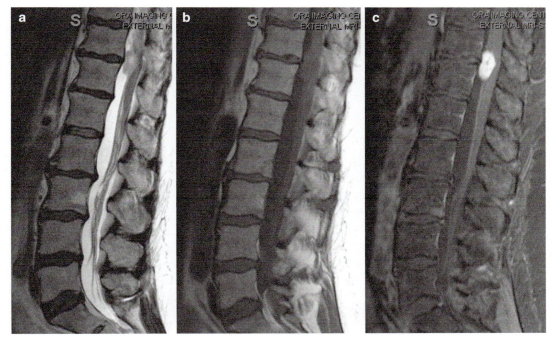

Fig. 23.28 (**a–c**) A 64-year-old lady complains of 1-year history of bilateral leg pain. MRI shows a well-defined intradural extramedullary lesion at the level of T11-T12. The lesion appears isointense on T2 (**a**) and T1 (**b**) and shows homogeneous intense contrast enhancement (**c**). Pathology revealed a benign schwannoma

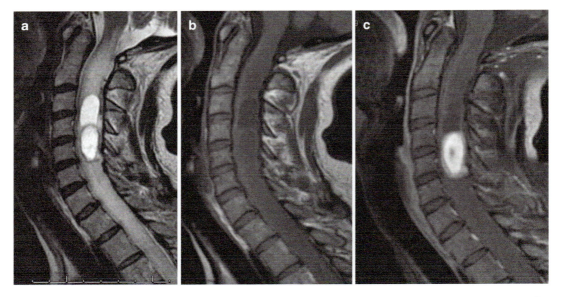

Fig. 23.29 (**a–c**) A 39-year-old lady has had problems with coordination and function on the right side of her body for the last 2–3 years. Her medical history is positive for retinoblastoma of her right eye as a child. MRI shows cord enlargement from the 4th ventricle to T3. There is hyperintensity on T2 (**a**) and decreased signal on T1 (**b**). There is intense enhancement (**c**), with a non-enhancing cyst rostral to the enhancing mass. The differential includes hemangioblastoma and ependymoma. The pathology following surgery confirmed the former

Table 23.4 Demographic and radiographic features of spinal cord tumors

Parameter	Astrocytoma	Ependymoma	P
Number	15	15	
M/F	9/6	8/7	1.0
Age	34+/−22	42+/−11	
Distribution cervical/thoracic	5/10	10/5	0.1431
Presence of syrinx	7	12	0.0253
Syrinx rostral/caudal	6/3	11/10	
MRI accuracy	13/15	15/15	

23.9.5 Our Experience

Our review yielded 54 intramedullary tumors, with 15 astrocytomas and 15 ependymomas (Table 23.4). The results suggest no gender or age predilection to one pathology over the other. The results show a prevalence of astrocytomas to the thoracic spine, whereas ependymomas were more prevalent in the cervical spine. MRI was accurate in identifying gliomas from other pathologies such as hemangioblastoma, nerve sheath tumors, or infections. However, distinguishing astrocytoma from ependymoma was not consistent, and they were listed as one or the other. A syrinx cavity was more often associated with ependymoma (12/15) compared to glioma (7/15, $p = 0.0253$).

23.9.6 Conclusion

Based on our single institution review, the differences between ependymomas and astrocytomas have meaningful clinical significance in terms of need for ancillary treatment as well as prognosis. On MRI, ependymomas were more likely to be associated with a syrinx. Distinguishing astrocytoma from ependymoma from MRI images is suspected but not always accurate.

Acknowledgement The authors acknowledge the invaluable assistance of Faith Vaughn in the editing and submission of this manuscript.

References

1. Beslow LA et al (2008) Role of diffusion MRI in diagnosis of spinal cord infarction7 in children. Neuropediatrics 39(3):188–191
2. Facon D et al (2005) MR diffusion tensor imaging and fiber tracking in spinal cord compression. AJNR Am J Neuroradiol 26(6):1587–1594
3. Kuker W et al (2004) Diffusion-weighted MRI of spinal cord infarction—high resolution imaging and time course of diffusion abnormality. J Neurol 251(7):818–824
4. Loher TJ et al (2003) Diffusion-weighted MRI in acute spinal cord ischaemia. Neuroradiology 45(8):557–561
5. Sagiuchi T et al (2002) Diffusion-weighted MRI of the cervical cord in acute spinal cord injury with type II odontoid fracture. J Comput Assist Tomogr 26(4):654–656
6. Thurnher MM, Bammer R (2006) Diffusion-weighted MR imaging (DWI) in spinal cord ischemia. Neuroradiology 48(11):795–801
7. Porter DA, Heidemann RM (2009) High resolution diffusion-weighted imaging using readout-segmented echo-planar imaging, parallel imaging and a two-dimensional navigator-based reacquisition. Magn Reson Med 62(2):468–475
8. Kumral E et al (2011) Spinal ischaemic stroke: clinical and radiological findings and short-term outcome. Eur J Neurol 18(2):232–239
9. Manara R et al (2010) Spinal cord infarction due to fibrocartilaginous embolization: the role of diffusion weighted imaging and short-tau inversion recovery sequences. J Child Neurol 25(8):1024–1028
10. Millichap JJ, Sy BT, Leacock RO (2007) Spinal cord infarction with multiple etiologic factors. J Gen Intern Med 22(1):151–154
11. Hickey R et al (1986) Autoregulation of spinal cord blood flow: is the cord a microcosm of the brain? Stroke 17(6):1183–1189
12. Marcus ML et al (1977) Regulation of total and regional spinal cord blood flow. Circ Res 41(1):128–134
13. Sandler AN, Tator CH (1976) Effect of acute spinal cord compression injury on regional spinal cord blood flow in primates. J Neurosurg 45(6):660–676

14. Weidauer S et al (2002) Spinal cord infarction: MR imaging and clinical features in 16 cases. Neuroradiology 44(10):851–857
15. Bammer MMTaR (2006) Diffusion-weighted magnetic resonance imaging of the spine and spinal cord. Semin Roentgenol 41:294–311
16. Loher TJ, Bassetti CL, Lovblad KO et al (2003) Diffusion-weighted MRI in acute spinal cord ischaemia. Neuroradiology 45:557–561
17. Wilhelm Kuker MW, Klose U et al (2004) Diffusion-weighted MRI of spinal cord infarction. High resolution imaging and time course of diffusion abnormality. J Neurol 251:818–824
18. Criscuolo GR, Oldfield EH, Doppman JL (1989) Reversible acute and subacute myelopathy in patients with dural arteriovenous fistulas. Foix-Alajouanine syndrome reconsidered. J Neurosurg 70(3):354–359
19. Heros RC (2009) Foix-Alajouanine syndrome: what is it? J Neurosurg 111(5):900–901
20. Inoue T et al (2006) Congestive myelopathy due to cervical perimedullary arteriovenous fistula evaluated by apparent diffusion coefficient values—case report. Neurol Med Chir (Tokyo) 46(11):559–562
21. Kataoka H et al (2001) Venous congestion is a major cause of neurological deterioration in spinal arteriovenous malformations. Neurosurgery 48(6):1224–1229; discussion 1229–30
22. Spetzler RF et al (2002) Modified classification of spinal cord vascular lesions. J Neurosurg 96(2 Suppl):145–156
23. Sibon I et al (2006) Diffusion MRI in spinal dural arterio-venous fistula: a case report. Spinal Cord 44(5):315–317
24. Borchers AT, Gershwin ME (2012) Transverse myelitis. Autoimmun Rev 11(3):231–248
25. Frohman EM, Wingerchuk DM (2010) Clinical practice. Transverse myelitis. N Engl J Med 363(6):564–572
26. Seifert T et al (2005) Relapsing acute transverse myelitis: a specific entity. Eur J Neurol 12(9):681–684
27. Alper G et al (2011) Idiopathic acute transverse myelitis in children: an analysis and discussion of MRI findings. Mult Scler 17(1):74–80
28. Choi KH et al (1996) Idiopathic transverse myelitis: MR characteristics. AJNR Am J Neuroradiol 17(6):1151–1160
29. Goh C, Phal PM, Desmond PM (2011) Neuroimaging in acute transverse myelitis. Neuroimaging Clin N Am 21(4):951–973
30. Renoux J et al (2006) MR diffusion tensor imaging and fiber tracking in inflammatory diseases of the spinal cord. AJNR Am J Neuroradiol 27(9):1947–1951
31. Dale RC et al (2000) Acute disseminated encephalomyelitis, multiphasic disseminated encephalomyelitis and multiple sclerosis in children. Brain 123(12):2407–2422

32. Hynson JL et al (2001) Clinical and neuroradiologic features of acute disseminated encephalomyelitis in children. Neurology 56(10):1308–1312
33. Tenembaum S, Chamoles N, Fejerman N (2002) Acute disseminated encephalomyelitis: a long-term follow-up study of 84 pediatric patients. Neurology 59(8):1224–1231
34. Marcel C et al (2010) Diffusion-weighted imaging in noncompressive myelopathies: a 33-patient prospective study. J Neurol 257(9):1438–1445
35. Balasubramanya KS et al (2007) Diffusion-weighted imaging and proton MR spectroscopy in the characterization of acute disseminated encephalomyelitis. Neuroradiology 49(2):177–183
36. Zuccoli G et al (2014) Vasogenic edema characterizes pediatric acute disseminated encephalomyelitis. Neuroradiology 56:679–684
37. Andre JB, Bammer R (2010) Advanced diffusion-weighted magnetic resonance imaging techniques of the human spinal cord. Top Magn Reson Imaging 21(6):367–378
38. Lycklama G et al (2003) Spinal-cord MRI in multiple sclerosis. Lancet Neurol 2(9):555–562
39. Clark CA, Werring DJ, Miller DH (2000) Diffusion imaging of the spinal cord in vivo: estimation of the principal diffusivities and application to multiple sclerosis. Magn Reson Med 43(1):133–138
40. McKeon A et al (2008) CNS aquaporin-4 autoimmunity in children. Neurology 71(2):93–100
41. Wingerchuk DM et al (2007) The spectrum of neuromyelitis optica. Lancet Neurol 6(9):805–815
42. Kitley J et al (2014) Neuromyelitis optica spectrum disorders with aquaporin-4 and myelin-oligodendrocyte glycoprotein antibodies: a comparative study. JAMA Neurol 71(3):276–283
43. Wingerchuk DM et al (2006) Revised diagnostic criteria for neuromyelitis optica. Neurology 66(10):1485–1489
44. Benedetti B et al (2006) Grading cervical cord damage in neuromyelitis optica and MS by diffusion tensor MRI. Neurology 67(1):161–163
45. Sohn M et al (2013) Spinal cord neurosarcoidosis. Am J Med Sci 347:195–198
46. Lee WJ, Hsu HY, Wang PY (2008) Reversible myelopathy on magnetic resonance imaging due to cobalamin deficiency. J Chin Med Assoc 71(7):368–372
47. Hirata A et al (2006) Subacute combined degeneration of the spinal cord concomitant with gastric cancer. Intern Med 45(14):875–877
48. Okada S et al (2006) Two cases of subacute combined degeneration: magnetic resonance findings. J Nippon Med Sch 73(6):328–331
49. Ravina B, Loevner LA, Bank W (2000) MR findings in subacute combined degeneration of the spinal cord: a case of reversible cervical myelopathy. AJR Am J Roentgenol 174(3):863–865
50. Tian C (2011) Hyperintense signal on spinal cord diffusion-weighted imaging in a patient with subacute combined degeneration. Neurol India 59(3):429–431
51. Kim EY et al (2013) Subacute combined degeneration revealed by diffusion-weighted imaging: a case study. Clin Neuroradiol 23(2):157–159
52. Jang S et al (2012) Enterovirus 71-related encephalomyelitis: usual and unusual magnetic resonance imaging findings. Neuroradiology 54(3):239–245
53. Li H et al (2019) MRI reveals segmental distribution of enterovirus lesions in the central nervous system: a probable clinical evidence of retrograde axonal transport of EV-A71. J Neuro-Oncol 25(3):354–362
54. Iwasaki M et al (2011) Acute onset intramedullary spinal cord abscess with spinal artery occlusion: a case report and review. Eur Spine J 20(Suppl 2):S294–S301
55. Murphy KJ et al (1998) Spinal cord infection: myelitis and abscess formation. AJNR Am J Neuroradiol 19(2):341–348
56. Dorflinger-Hejlek E et al (2010) Diffusion-weighted MR imaging of intramedullary spinal cord abscess. AJNR Am J Neuroradiol 31(9):1651–1652
57. Thurnher MM, Bammer R (2006) Diffusion-weighted magnetic resonance imaging of the spine and spinal cord. Semin Roentgenol 41(4):294–311
58. Hori M et al (2012) New diffusion metrics for spondylotic myelopathy at an early clinical stage. Eur Radiol 22(8):1797–1802
59. Demir A et al (2003) Diffusion-weighted MR imaging with apparent diffusion coefficient and apparent diffusion tensor maps in cervical spondylotic myelopathy. Radiology 229(1):37–43
60. Banaszek A et al (2014) Usefulness of diffusion tensor MR imaging in the assessment of intramedullary changes of the cervical spinal cord in different stages of degenerative spine disease. Eur Spine J 23(7):1523–1530
61. Zhang JS, Huan Y (2014) Multishot diffusion-weighted MR imaging features in acute trauma of spinal cord. Eur Radiol 24(3):685–692
62. Yurube T et al (2009) The vanishment of an intramedullary high-signal intensity lesion at the craniocervical junction after surgical treatment: a case report of the presyrinx state. Spine (Phila Pa 1976) 34(6):E235–E239
63. Eser O et al (2007) Idiopathic recurrent transverse myelitis with syringomyelia: a case report. Turk Neurosurg 17(3):228–231
64. Fischbein NJ et al (1999) The "presyrinx" state: a reversible myelopathic condition that may precede syringomyelia. AJNR Am J Neuroradiol 20(1):7–20
65. Fischbein NJ et al (2000) The "presyrinx" state: is there a reversible myelopathic condition that may precede syringomyelia? Neurosurg Focus 8(3):E4
66. Yamasaki F et al (2005) Apparent diffusion coefficient of human brain tumors at MR imaging. Radiology 235(3):985–991
67. de Fatima Vasco Aragao M et al (2014) Comparison of perfusion, diffusion, and MR spectroscopy between low-grade enhancing pilocytic astrocytomas and high-grade astrocytomas. AJNR Am J Neuroradiol 35:1495–1502

68. Rumboldt Z et al (2006) Apparent diffusion coefficients for differentiation of cerebellar tumors in children. AJNR Am J Neuroradiol 27(6):1362–1369
69. Zulfiqar M, Yousem DM, Lai H (2013) ADC values and prognosis of malignant astrocytomas: does lower ADC predict a worse prognosis independent of grade of tumor?—a meta-analysis. AJR Am J Roentgenol 200(3):624–629
70. Minehan KJ, Brown PD, Scheithauer BW, Krauss WE, Wright MP (2009) Prognosis and treatment of spinal cord astrocytoma. Int J Radiat Oncol Biol Phys 73(3):727–733
71. Brandao LA, Shiroishi MS, Law M (2013) Brain tumors: a multimodality approach with diffusion-weighted imaging, diffusion tensor imaging, magnetic resonance spectroscopy, dynamic susceptibility contrast and dynamic contrast-enhanced magnetic resonance imaging. Magn Reson Imaging Clin N Am 21(2):199–239
72. Gimi B et al (2012) Utility of apparent diffusion coefficient ratios in distinguishing common pediatric cerebellar tumors. Acad Radiol 19(7):794–800
73. Porto L et al (2013) Differentiation between high and low grade tumours in paediatric patients by using apparent diffusion coefficients. Eur J Paediatr Neurol 17(3):302–307
74. Rykken JB et al (2013) Intramedullary spinal cord metastases: MRI and relevant clinical features from a 13-year institutional case series. AJNR Am J Neuroradiol 34(10):2043–2049
75. Mechtler LL, Nandigam K (2013) Spinal cord tumors: new views and future directions. Neurol Clin 31(1):241–268
76. Flanagan EP et al (2011) Primary intramedullary spinal cord lymphoma. Neurology 77(8):784–791
77. Fitsiori A et al (2019) Imaging spectrum of Bing-Neel syndrome: how can a radiologist recognise this rare neurological complication of Waldenstrom's macroglobulinemia? Eur Radiol 29(1):102–114
78. Varettoni M et al (2017) Bing-Neel Syndrome: illustrative cases and comprehensive review of the literature. Mediterr J Hematol Infect Dis 9(1):e2017061
79. Bostrom A, Kanther NC, Grote A, Bostrom J (2014) Management and outcome in adult intramedullary spinal cord tumours: a 20-year single institution experience. BMC Res Notes 7:908
80. Manzano G, Green BA, Vanni S, Levi AD (2008) Contemporary management of adult intramedullary spinal tumors-pathology and neurological outcomes related to surgical resection. Spinal Cord 46(8):540–546
81. Chamberlain MC, Tredway TL (2011) Adult primary intradural spinal cord tumors: a review. Curr Neurol Neurosci Rep 11(3):320–328
82. Slooff JL (1964) Primary intramedullary tumors of the spinal cord and filum terminale. Saunders, Philadelphia, p 255
83. Woodroffe RW, Zanaty M, Kirby P, Dlouhy BJ, Menezes AH (2018) Resection of a pediatric intramedullary spinal cord tumor: 2-dimensional operative video. Oper Neurosurg (Hagerstown) 83. https://doi.org/10.1093/ons/opy185
84. Joaquim AF, Riew KD (2015) Management of cervical spine deformity after intradural tumor resection. Neurosurg Focus 39(2):E13
85. McGirt MJ, Goldstein IM, Chaichana KL, Tobias ME, Kothbauer KF, Jallo GI (2008) Extent of surgical resection of malignant astrocytomas of the spinal cord: outcome analysis of 35 patients. Neurosurgery 63(1):55–60; discussion -1
86. Abul-Kasim K, Thurnher MM, McKeever P, Sundgren PC (2008) Intradural spinal tumors: current classification and MRI features. Neuroradiology 50(4):301–314
87. Raco A, Esposito V, Lenzi J, Piccirilli M, Delfini R, Cantore G (2005) Long-term follow-up of intramedullary spinal cord tumors: a series of 202 cases. Neurosurgery 56(5):972–981; discussion -81
88. Karikari IO, Nimjee SM, Hodges TR, Cutrell E, Hughes BD, Powers CJ, et al (2011) Impact of tumor histology on resectability and neurological outcome in primary intramedullary spinal cord tumors: a single-center experience with 102 patients. Neurosurgery 68(1):188–197; discussion 97
89. Ahmed R, Menezes AH, Awe OO, Mahaney KB, Torner JC, Weinstein SL (2014) Long-term incidence and risk factors for development of spinal deformity following resection of pediatric intramedullary spinal cord tumors. J Neurosurg Pediatr 13(6):613–621
90. Scibilia A, Terranova C, Rizzo V, Raffa G, Morelli A, Esposito F et al (2016) Intraoperative neurophysiological mapping and monitoring in spinal tumor surgery: sirens or indispensable tools? Neurosurg Focus 41(2):E18
91. Adams H, Avendano J, Raza SM, Gokaslan ZL, Jallo GI, Quinones-Hinojosa A (2012) Prognostic factors and survival in primary malignant astrocytomas of the spinal cord: a population-based analysis from 1973 to 2007. Spine (Phila Pa 1976) 37(12):E727–E735
92. Winn HR (2017) Youmans and Winn neurological surgery. Seventh edition. ed. Elsevier, Philadelphia, PA
93. Ottenhausen M, Ntoulias G, Bodhinayake I, Ruppert FH, Schreiber S, Forschler A et al (2018) Intradural spinal tumors in adults-update on management and outcome. Neurosurg Rev 42:371–388
94. Harrop JS, Ganju A, Groff M, Bilsky M (2009) Primary intramedullary tumors of the spinal cord. Spine (Phila Pa 1976) 34(22 Suppl):S69–S77
95. Tobin MK, Geraghty JR, Engelhard HH, Linninger AA, Mehta AI (2015) Intramedullary spinal cord tumors: a review of current and future treatment strategies. Neurosurg Focus 39(2):E14
96. Kim DH, Kim JH, Choi SH, Sohn CH, Yun TJ, Kim CH et al (2014) Differentiation between intramedullary spinal ependymoma and astrocytoma: comparative MRI analysis. Clin Radiol 69(1):29–35
97. Ahmed R, Menezes AH, Awe OO, Torner JC (2014) Long-term disease and neurological outcomes in

patients with pediatric intramedullary spinal cord tumors. J Neurosurg Pediatr 13(6):600–612

98. Garces-Ambrossi GL, McGirt MJ, Mehta VA, Sciubba DM, Witham TF, Bydon A et al (2009) Factors associated with progression-free survival and long-term neurological outcome after resection of intramedullary spinal cord tumors: analysis of 101 consecutive cases. J Neurosurg Spine 11(5):591–599

99. Klekamp J (2013) Treatment of intramedullary tumors: analysis of surgical morbidity and long-term results. J Neurosurg Spine 19(1):12–26

100. Hongo HT, Takai K, Komori T, Taniguchi M (2018) Intramedullary spinal cord ependymoma and astrocytoma: intraoperative frozen-section diagnosis, extent of resection, and outcomes. J Neurosurg Spine 30:1–7

Part III

Futures of Diffusion Imaging

Future Directions for Diffusion Imaging of the Brain and Spinal Cord

24

Takayuki Obata, Jeff Kershaw, Akifumi Hagiwara, and Shigeki Aoki

The purpose of this book is to illustrate how DWI technology can be applied as an effective clinical tool. However, there are a number of DWI methods that are expected to be effective in principle, but are not yet widely used due to technological limitations and limited awareness amongst clinicians.

The biggest bottleneck in the development of DWI as a clinical tool is the strength and stability of the magnetic field gradients. Some development is required in the reduction of artifacts related to strong magnetic field gradients, in the maintenance of a reliable magnetic field environment during rapid gradient switching, and in post-acquisition correction techniques. Nevertheless, clinical applications continue to be investigated as hardware and software technology progresses. One trend in this field is to investigate new contrasts by varying the diffusion-time. The basics of diffusion-time-dependent DWI are introduced in the first two sections of this chapter. The final section discusses the extraction of microstructural information from DWI of the brain and spinal cord.

The original version of this chapter was revised. The erratum to this chapter can be found at https://doi.org/10.1007/978-3-030-62120-9_27

T. Obata (✉) · J. Kershaw
Applied MRI Research, National Institute of Radiological Sciences, QST, Chiba, Japan
e-mail: obata.takayuki@qst.go.jp; len@qst.go.jp

A. Hagiwara · S. Aoki
Department of Radiology, Juntendo University, Tokyo, Japan
e-mail: a-hagiwara@juntendo.ac.jp;
saoki@juntendo.ac.jp

24.1 Introducing the Diffusion-Time

The b-value is used in DWI as a measurement parameter that characterizes signal attenuation or decay. When DWI is performed on a liquid, the measurements agree well with a simple single-exponential signal model having an exponent equal to the product of the b-value and diffusion coefficient of the liquid. However, interpreting the signal behaviour for more complex samples like in vivo tissue is not so simple. It is sometimes found that the signal may vary between measurements even when the same b-value is applied. This phenomenon can often be attributed to changes in another parameter known as the diffusion-time. Before discussing the diffusion-time in more detail, we would first like to briefly revise the meaning of the b-value for the pulsed-gradient spin-echo (PGSE) sequence.

24.1.1 b-Value

The b-value for a standard PGSE sequence is

$$b = \left(\gamma G \delta\right)^2 \left(\Delta - \frac{\delta}{3}\right). \qquad (24.1)$$

Here, Δ represents the time between the onset of the motion-probing gradient (MPG) lobes, δ is the width of each lobe, γ is the gyro-magnetic ratio,

---

© Springer Nature Switzerland AG 2021, corrected publication 2021
T. Moritani, A. A. Capizzano (eds.), *Diffusion-Weighted MR Imaging of the Brain, Head and Neck, and Spine*, https://doi.org/10.1007/978-3-030-62120-9_24

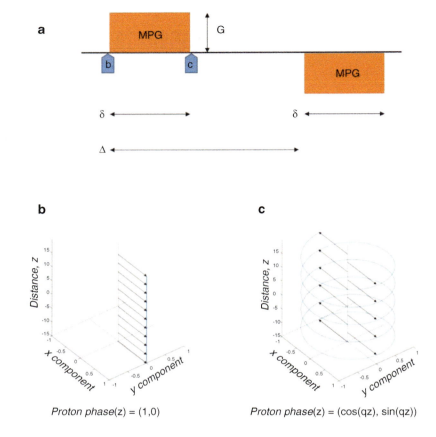

Fig. 24.1 (a) Schematic of the motion-probing gradient (MPG) for a standard PGSE sequence. Δ, the separation between the onset of each MPG; δ, represents the width of each MPG; γ, gyromagnetic ratio; G, the strength of the magnetic gradient. (b) Proton spin arrangement before and (c) after the 1st MPG. The proton spins have the same phase at all z before the 1st MPG, but after the 1st MPG the phase of the spins is dependent on z. The value of q corresponds to the spatial frequency of the proton spin rotation along the z direction

and G is the strength of the magnetic gradient (Fig. 24.1). The first factor $(\gamma G\delta)^2$ on the right side corresponds to the square of the proton-spin spatial frequency q. The frequency q characterises the distance-dependent proton spin shift generated by the 1st MPG (Fig. 24.1). The second factor, $(\Delta - \delta/3)$, is often interpreted as the period of time, called the diffusion-time t, over which water diffusion is allowed to occur before making an observation. Unlike the relaxation times T1 and T2, which are intrinsic tissue-specific parameters, the diffusion time is a measurement parameter that can be controlled by the user. Therefore, it is in the same category as TR and TE. An explanation of why the diffusion time is equal to $(\Delta - \delta/3)$ for the PGSE sequence has been omitted here. If interested, please see a reliable textbook [1]. Using the definitions of q and t, Eq. (24.1) may be rewritten as,

$$b = q^2 t. \qquad (24.2)$$

24.1.2 Gaussian or Free Diffusion

Hardware developments have made it possible to vary q and t to some extent in practice. Potentially this makes it possible to obtain more subtle information about in vivo structures. Although we will describe some cases where the signal attenuation differs depending on the specific values of t and q even if the b-value is the same, we first want to introduce the concept of Gaussian or free diffusion.

It is well known that the diffusion coefficient D is proportional to the mean square of the particle displacement ($<x^2>$) per unit time

$$D \propto \langle x^2 \rangle / t. \qquad (24.3)$$

As shown in Fig. 24.2a (blue line), if water can diffuse freely (i.e. molecular motion is unrestricted), then plotting the mean displacement against diffusion-time will produce a straight line of constant slope equal to the diffusion coefficient. In this situation a measurement will always produce the same result for the same b-value regardless of whether q and t have been varied. That is, all signal attenuation can be attributed to the b-value as a controlling parameter and the signal decays monoexponentially.

24.1.3 Restricted Diffusion

24.1.3.1 *b*-Value-Dependent Signal with Constant Diffusion Time

Free diffusion is rarely found in vivo except in the CSF, which is primarily water.

Figure 24.3 presents DWI measurements on an array of parallel cylindrical capillaries of diameter 20 μm in a glass plate sitting in water (Fig. 24.3a) [2]. This phantom can be used as a model of intracellular diffusion in an axon-like space. Here, the MPG is applied perpendicular to the axis of the cylindrical capillaries. For such a system, at long diffusion-time $<x^2>$ will asymptotically approach a constant value that is dependent on the size and shape of the water-containing space (red line, Fig. 24.2a). In this case, rather than being constant, the diffusion coefficient estimated with Eq. (24.3) will decrease with increased diffusion time. This means that plots of the logarithmic DWI signal vs. b-value will appear to be higher for longer diffusion times, with the slope of the plot reflecting the t-dependent ADC (Fig. 24.3b). It is expected that similar signal behaviour might be observed for the movement of water in cells if the cell membrane acts like a barrier.

Fig. 24.2 (a) Mean square displacement $<x^2>$ plotted against diffusion-time. Blue line, Gaussian or free diffusion case; red line, restricted diffusion. For the restricted diffusion case, as the ADC is equal to the slope of the dashed lines, it is clear that the ADC decreases at longer diffusion-time. (b) Schematic illustrating the restriction of water motion for increasing diffusion time

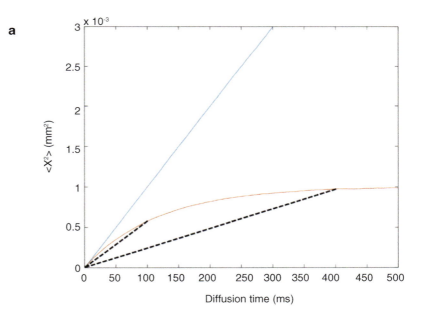

Increasing diffusion time →

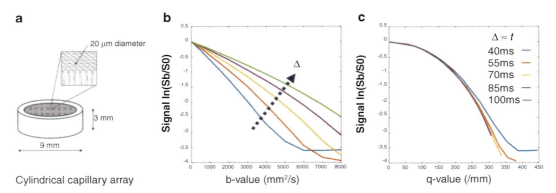

Fig. 24.3 (a) Experiment on a glass plate with an array of cylindrical capillaries drilled through it. (b) The b-value-dependent signal change was measured while varying q with constant Δ. The signal appears to be higher for longer Δ. (c) The difference between the data sets is less obvious when plotted against q alone

This phantom experiment also exhibits non-monoexponential b-value-dependent signal change. As noted in Sect. 24.1.2, free water signal attenuation is independent of diffusion time and displays single exponential behavior vs. b-value. However, in vivo signal behavior is more complicated, and requires an alternative signal description (e.g., double exponential). It is interesting that the b-value-dependent logarithmic signal change observed for the glass plate phantom is neither linear nor downwardly convex (Fig. 24.3b), which is clearly different to the signal behaviour usually observed with in vivo DWI. For more information about this phenomenon please see [3].

It should also be noted that the DWI signal at long diffusion-time is mainly determined by q. For example, when the experimental data of Fig. 24.3b is plotted against q alone, the signal curves become more and more similar with increasing diffusion-time (Fig. 24.3c). q-space imaging (QSI) is one technique that tries to utilize this phenomenon to characterize/qualify microstructure. However, QSI does not work very well for inhomogeneous structures like in vivo tissue.

24.1.3.2 b-Value-Dependent Signal with Constant q

Next, we will discuss an example where diffusion-time is varied while q is kept constant (red open circles and solid line, Fig. 24.4). As mentioned above, the DWI signal at long diffusion-time is mainly determined by q, which means that when the b-value is plotted on the horizontal axis the signal asymptotically approaches a q-dependent constant value (red dot-dashed line in Fig. 24.4). On the other hand, at low b-values, corresponding to short diffusion-times, the signal approaches the free water limit (dashed line in Fig. 24.4). This is easy to interpret. At very short diffusion-times the probability that a water molecules will collide with a barrier is very low, so the signal behaves almost like free water.

In summary, for free diffusion the logarithmic signal change is linear as a function of b-value (dashed line in Fig. 24.4). However, in an environment where water movement is limited by barriers, the b-value-dependent signal change can be quite different. This is because, the DWI signal actually depends on the individual values of q and t even if the same b-value is used. Nevertheless, this type of signal behaviour is not easily observed in clinical imaging because in vivo microstructure is far more complex than the phantom example discussed here.

24.2 In Vivo Application of Diffusion-Time-Dependent DWI

24.2.1 Shortening the Diffusion-Time

Here, we would like to talk about DWI signal attenuation when the diffusion-time is set to be shorter than the usual clinical setting. While this

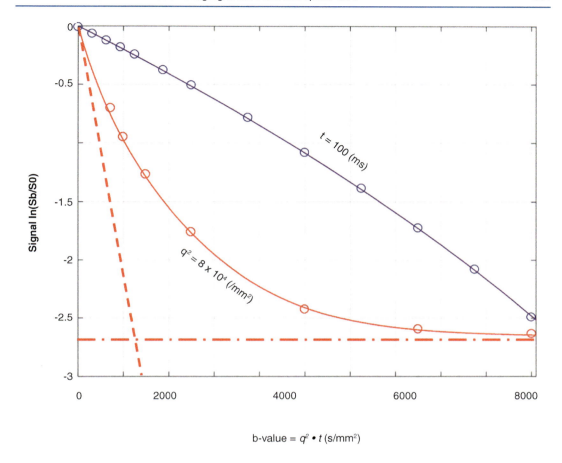

Fig. 24.4 b-Value-dependent signal change in the glass capillary plate with either q or t constant. The red open circles and corresponding solid line represent the measured and simulated signal changes, respectively, for a constant q. The red dot-dashed line is the asymptote of the red solid line as $b \to \infty$; the red dashed line is the signal for free water. The blue open circles and solid line are the measured and simulated signals, respectively, for a constant t

is a promising way to investigate complex in vivo microstructure, it also pushes the gradient hardware towards its physical limit. Since the b-value is proportional to q^2 and diffusion-time for PGSE, the maximum amplitude and slew rate of the gradient hardware will limit the minimum diffusion-time that can be reached while keeping the same b-value. One workaround for this problem is to use multiple MPG pairs with a relatively short, but practically achievable separation. When inserted into a spin-echo sequence, this multi-MPG-pair waveform provides an example of the oscillating-gradient spin-echo (OGSE) method. In using this method it is common to report the ADC as a function of the frequency of the MPG pairs instead of the diffusion-time (Fig. 24.5). Observations of in vivo tissue find that the ADC is linearly dependent on frequency, and the slope of this dependence might be used to characterise tissue microstructure. Please refer to [4] for a more comprehensive introduction to the OGSE method.

It is anticipated that biological application of the OGSE method can be used to obtain information about tissue structures. Experiments with animals have reported that the ADC in the cerebellum is frequency-dependent [5]. The granular cell layer seems to be particularly sensitive to frequency variation (Fig. 24.6), and it has been suggested that this is due to the relatively large nuclear volume of granular cells [6]. It has also been predicted that mesoscopic structural complexity can be characterized by observing the frequency dependence of the ADC [7, 8].

Fig. 24.5 The waveform (g), time integral (f), and spectra (F) corresponding to the MPGs of the pulsed-gradient spin-echo (PGSE), sine- (SOGSE) and cosine- (COGSE) oscillating-gradient spin-echo sequences. A special characteristic of the COGSE MPG is that it does not sample the central frequencies that dominate the SOGSE and PGSE spectra. Reproduced with permission from [4]

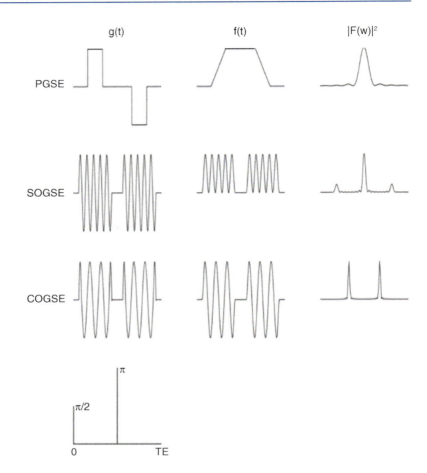

The number of neuroradiology studies using OGSE has recently been increasing. Investigations of epidermoid cyst [9] and choroid plexus cyst [10] (Fig. 24.7), revealed that the OGSE-measured ADC increased at shorter diffusion-time, indicating the spatial restriction of water diffusion inside those structures. The high DWI signal of these structures is not solely due to the T2 shine-through effect. Previous research on mouse glioblastoma models using OGSE showed that the ADC at short diffusion-time was significantly higher in tumor after radiation therapy, while PGSE failed to detect such changes [11]. This result indicates that using shorter diffusion-times increases the sensitivity of DWI to subtle changes in cellular microstructure. The utility of OGSE in the differential diagnosis of malignant and benign head and neck tumors has also been demonstrated in humans [12]. OGSE may therefore aid the diagnosis and quantitative evaluation of treatment response for tumors in the future. The clinical relevance of diffusion-time also applies to cerebral infarction. It has been demonstrated that acute cerebral infarction displays low contrast on short diffusion-time DWI (Fig. 24.8) [13–15]. Technical advances in gradient hardware that allow higher maximum gradient and slew rate may introduce an unexpected reduction in the diffusion-time and cause critical transformation of the contrast in clinical images. Hence, it is important for clinicians to understand how diffusion-time can affect DWI.

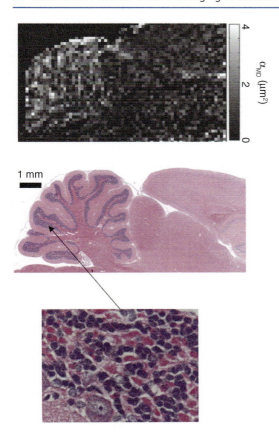

Fig. 24.6 αMD map (top), histology section (middle), and magnification of the granule cell layer (bottom) in the cerebellum. αMD is the slope of the mean diffusivity (MD) as a function of frequency. The high αMD region appears to correspond to the cerebellar granule cell layer. The histological sections have been stained with hematoxylin and eosin. Details can be found in the report by Kershaw et al. [5]

24.2.2 Increasing the Diffusion-Time

What happens if the diffusion-time is made longer than the usual clinical setting?

As shown in Fig. 24.4, if in vivo water is surrounded by impermeable barriers, the DWI signal will reach a nonzero lower limit as diffusion-time is increased (provided q is constant). As a result, when the diffusion-time increases, the measured diffusion coefficient (proportional to $<x^2>/t$) approaches zero. However, when the diffusion-time is extended in real observations, it is found that the in vivo signal is attenuated and the ADC approaches a nonzero constant value. There are two main reasons for this. One is the existence of a space that allows water to diffuse long distances through the tissue. For long diffusion-times, $<x^2>$ for the water in this space is approximately proportional to the diffusion-time, which means that the diffusion coefficient asymptotically approaches a nonzero constant value. This is sometimes called extracellular or hindered diffusion. Figure 24.9 shows experimental results from a phantom containing hydrophobic fiber bundles as a model of extracellular diffusion. The time-dependent signal changes in the experiment are small compared to those observed for the capillary phantom (Fig. 24.3), which indicates that diffusion was hindered rather than fully restricted. If in vivo DWI signal can be modelled as the sum of intracellular and extracellular signal, the b-value-dependent signal curves (each acquired with a constant t) should be either constant or increase at longer t.

In the intracellular and extracellular signal models described so far, b-value-dependent signal curves tend to increase with t for the former (Fig. 24.3), but the signal curves are less sensitive to t for the latter (Fig. 24.9). However, when measurements are taken on pathological tissue, there are certain observations that cannot be explained by the interpretations that have been discussed in this section. For example, in reports of cerebral infarction, the t-dependent signal decreases as t increases [16]. This suggests that some mechanism other than restricted or hindered diffusion must be occurring. A possible explanation for the decrease is that water exchange between the intra- and extracellular spaces makes some contribution to the DWI signal. In fact, this has been investigated in a report that compared optical one-cell imaging signals with DWI to validate the inter-compartmental water exchange-time measured for expression-controlled aquaporin-4 (AQP4) cells. It was shown that the t-dependent signal attenuation increases more for the high-permeability (AQP4 high expression) cells than for

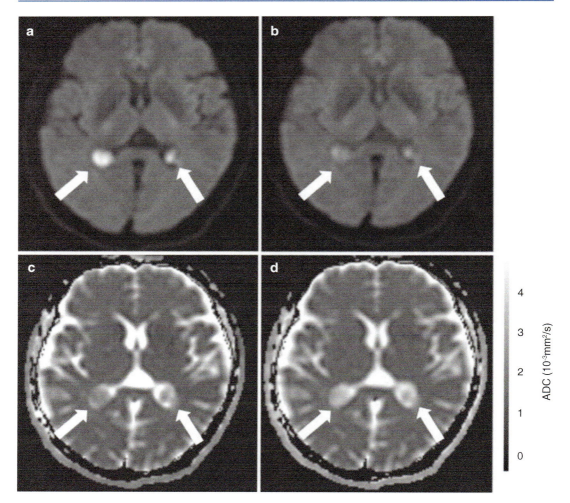

Fig. 24.7 DWI and ADC maps of choroid plexus cysts. (**a**) The choroid plexus cysts in the lateral ventricles show high intensity on pulsed-gradient spin-echo (PGSE) DWI at long diffusion-time (*t*). (**b**) On the other hand, the choroid plexus cysts showed decreased contrast on OGSE DWI at short *t*. (**c, d**) In comparison to the long *t* result, the ADCs of the choroid plexus cysts are higher at short *t*. Figure reproduced with permission from the report by Maekawa et al. [10]

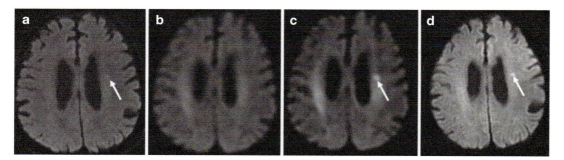

Fig. 24.8 Diffusion-weighted imaging of the brain of an 87-year-old patient showing an acute infarction (arrow). (**a**) PGSE DWI (*b*-value = 1000 s/mm^2, diffusion-time = 22.3 ms), (**b**) OGSE DWI (*b*-value = 1500 s/mm^2, diffusion-time = 8.5 ms), (**c**) PGSE DWI (*b*-value = 1500 s/mm^2, diffusion-time = 47.3 ms), (**d**) PGSE DWI (*b*-value = 1000 s/mm^2, diffusion-time = 22.3 ms) obtained 2 days after the image in Fig. **a**. Figure reproduced with permission from the report by Hori et al. [13]

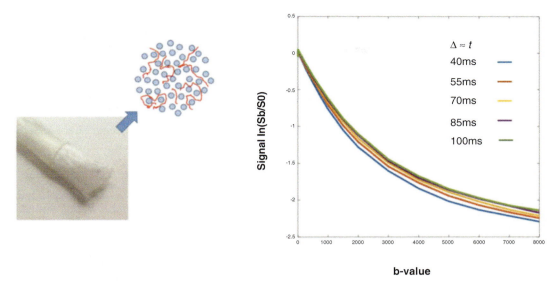

Fig. 24.9 A hydrophobic fiber bundle used as a hindered diffusion phantom (left), and the expected b-value-dependent signal curves (right). The signal is larger for longer t, but the differences are small in comparison to the restricted diffusion case (Fig. 24.3)

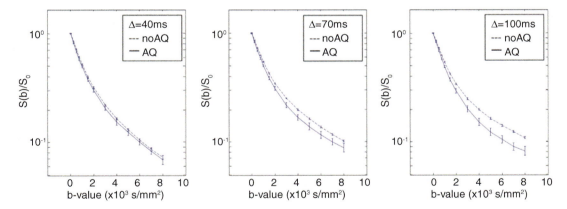

Fig. 24.10 Normalized b-value-dependent signal decay curves at different diffusion-times for in vitro AQP4-expressing (AQ) and AQP4-non-expressing (noAQ) samples. The separation between the curves corresponding to each cell type increases with diffusion-time. Also note that the AQ signal at high b-value increases from $\Delta = 40$ ms to 70 ms, but decreases from $\Delta = 70$ ms to 100 ms. This behavior cannot be explained by a simple Gaussian or restricted diffusion model. Figure reproduced from the report by Obata et al. [17]

the low-permeability (no AQP4 expression) cells (Fig. 24.10).

Many other concepts for investigating the tissue microstructure utilising the relationship between diffusion-time and DWI signal have been proposed [18–23].

24.3 Extracting Microstructural Information from DWI

The last section of this chapter is devoted to microstructural imaging of the brain and spinal cord using multi-shell DWI. A variety of DWI techniques, such as diffusion tensor imaging, diffusional kurtosis imaging, and q-space imaging, have been used to extract in vivo microstructural information. However, the metrics estimated with these techniques are not specific to microstructural features such as axon density and diameter. Hence, the relationship between observed changes in these metrics and pathology is often difficult to explain. In contrast, it is thought that DWI-based modeling of microstructural features will provide more specific information. We discuss the basics, limitations, and clinical applications of microstructural modeling for DWI.

24.3.1 Basics and Limitations

To extract microstructural information, microstructural modelling assumes at least two compartments in the brain, namely, intra-neurite and extra-neurite compartments. Some models assume an additional isotropic free water compartment, but the signal from water inside the tightly packed myelin sheath is usually ignored because the T2 is very short. The most widely used method for estimating microstructural features from DWI data is the neurite orientation dispersion and density imaging (NODDI) model. NODDI assumes 3 compartments: a restricted intracellular compartment (neurite density index, NDI), a hindered extracellular compartment, and CSF with free diffusion [24]. Neurites are composed of either an axon or a dendrite and are modelled as zero-radius sticks. NODDI provides information about the orientation of neurites through the orientation dispersion index (ODI). In contrast to DTI, which is sensitive to partial-volume averaging of fiber orientations, NODDI incorporates curving and fanning of fibers into the model so it is considered to be more robust for estimating the volume of axons [25].

The g-ratio, which is the ratio of the inner to the outer diameter of a myelinated axon, is associated with the speed of conduction [26]. Larger axons and thicker myelin sheaths give rise to faster conduction of electrochemical information, but there is always a trade-off between these dimensions because of the limited space in the nervous system. The g-ratio has a limited

dynamic range in healthy WM and depends on age and region. Combining DWI modelling and myelin imaging, we can estimate the g-ratio and axon volume fraction (AVF) in a voxel [25]. The g-ratio can differentiate between demyelination and axonal degeneration, whereas conventional T2-weighted or FLAIR images cannot.

However, modelling has some limitations. To obtain microstructural information at a scale of μm from MRI data on a scale of mm resolution in a feasible scan time, strict assumptions, which may not be true in pathological states, are required to solve complex mathematical equations. Further, modelling usually targets white matter in the brain; suitable methods for the gray matter of the brain and spinal cord still need to be developed.

24.3.2 Clinical Applications

Techniques for microstructural modelling of DWI data, especially NODDI, have been widely applied for healthy populations and patients. Two recent studies have shown that the NDI calculated using NODDI has a stronger relationship with age and is more sensitive to microstructural changes in late childhood and adolescence than DTI metrics [27, 28]. Granberg et al. [29] found that the normal-appearing white matter (NAWM) in patients with multiple sclerosis (MS) had significantly lower NDI than healthy controls. However, Hagiwara et al. [30] reported that, relative to NAWM, the myelin volume fraction estimated with synthetic MRI was more sensitive than the AVF, calculated using a combination of synthetic MRI and NODDI, to damage in plaque and peri-plaque WM (Fig. 24.11). Kamagata et al. [31] investigated the diagnostic utility of DTI and NODDI in the substantia nigra pars compacta and striatum in Parkinson's disease. Multivariate logistic analysis revealed that NDI and mean diffusivity in the contralateral substantia nigra pars compacta are independent predictors of Parkinson's disease. From ROC analysis, NDI in the contralateral substantia nigra pars compacta had the best diagnostic performance (mean cutoff, 0.62; sensitivity, 0.88; specificity, 0.83) among all DTI and NODDI metrics. In a separate study, Kamagata et al. also showed that mean kurtosis

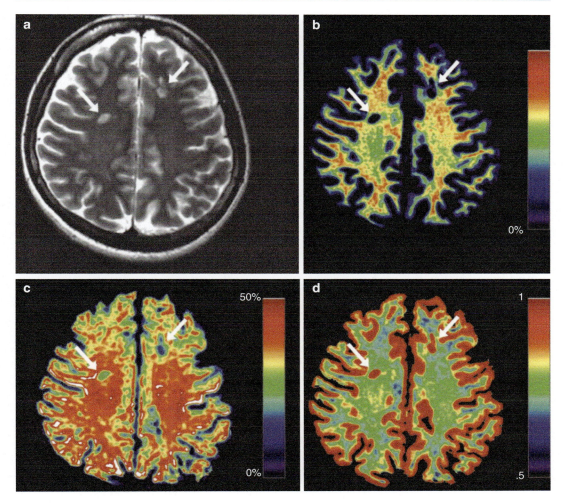

Fig. 24.11 Representative images from a patient with multiple sclerosis. T2WI (**a**) and maps of the myelin volume fraction (**b**), axon volume fraction (**c**), and g-ratio (**d**) are shown. Two plaques indicated by arrows appear in these images. Even though myelin is severely damaged in these plaques (**b**, 5.53% and 7.23%), the degrees of axon damage are milder (**c**, 31.30% and 22.95%). Because myelin is severely damaged in these plaques, the corresponding g-ratios are close to 1.00 (**d**, 0.94 and 0.91). Figures reproduced with permission from the report by Hagiwara et al. [30]

and NDI in the GM were the most accurate biomarkers of Parkinson's disease amongst all the DTI, diffusional kurtosis imaging, and NODDI metrics [32]. Kamiya et al. [33] and Irie et al. [34] investigated the utility of NODDI for patients with idiopathic normal pressure hydrocephalus and showed that ODI and NDI in the corticospinal tract were significantly lower than healthy controls, suggesting that ODI can capture the reversible straightening of nerve fibers, whereas decreased NDI may indicate irreversible microstructural damage.

Even though NODDI was originally developed for the brain, it has also been applied to and validated within the spinal cord. For example, Grussu et al. [35] characterized differences between spinal cord WM and GM using NODDI and demonstrated that NODDI is superior to DTI in terms of fitting and reproducibility. They also histologically validated the ODI measured with NODDI for characterizing MS lesions [36]. Schilling et al. [37] showed the normative values of DTI and NODDI metrics in the spinal cord, and revealed that DTI lacks specificity. However, they cautioned that NODDI indices in the spinal cord are not as strongly associated with the histology as previously reported for the brain. Hori et al. [38] investigated the utility of microstructural modelling using a combination of NODDI and myelin imaging for patients with cervical spondylotic myelopathy. They revealed that in patients the AVF of some tracts was lower than that in healthy controls, whereas myelin volume fraction showed no difference between patients and healthy controls. The g-ratio of lateral corticospinal tracts was lower in the patients than in the healthy controls. It was therefore concluded that the pathological microstructural changes in the spinal cord of patients with cervical spondylotic myelopathy may be partial axonal degenerations with preserved myelin.

24.3.3 Summary

In this chapter, some fundamental ideas related to diffusion-time-dependent DWI have been introduced. The parameter most widely used to control DWI signal attenuation is the b-value, which is calculated as the product of the spatial frequency q squared and diffusion-time t. However, in some circumstances the DWI signal may vary depending on the specific values of q and t even if the b-value is the same. Although this is not used in current clinical diagnosis, technological improvements and increased awareness within the medical field may lead to important clinical applications in the future. Also included in this chapter was a brief introduction to some of the methods used to extract microstructural information from DWI data. We are optimistic that further development will produce new and more accurate techniques for the diagnosis of pathological states in the brain and spinal cord.

References

1. Callaghan PT (2011) 5.5 Pulsed gradient spin-echo NMR: diffusion and flow. In: Translational dynamics and magnetic resonance, principles of pulsed gradient spin echo NMR. Oxford University Press, Oxford, pp 204–221

2. Tachibana A, Tachibana Y, Kershaw J, Sano H, Fukushi M, Obata T (2018) Comparison of glass capillary plates and polyethylene fiber bundles as phantoms to assess the quality of diffusion tensor imaging. Magn Reson Med Sci 17(3):251–258

3. Callaghan PT (2011) 7.1.2 diffusive diffraction in an enclosed pore. In: Translational dynamics and magnetic resonance, principles of pulsed gradient spin echo NMR. Oxford University Press, Oxford, pp 312–316

4. Gore JC, Xu J, Colvin DC, Yankeelov TE, Parsons EC, Does MD (2010) Characterization of tissue structure at varying length scales using temporal diffusion spectroscopy. NMR Biomed 23(7):745–756

5. Kershaw J, Leuze C, Aoki I, Obata T, Kanno I, Ito H, Yamaguchi Y, Handa H (2013) Systematic changes to the apparent diffusion tensor of in vivo rat brain measured with an oscillating-gradient spin-echo sequence. NeuroImage 70:10–20

6. Xu J, Does MD, Gore JC (2009) Sensitivity of MR diffusion measurements to variations in intracellular structure: effects of nuclear size. Magn Reson Med 61(4):828–833

7. Novikov DS, Jensen JH, Helpern JA, Fieremans E (2014) Revealing mesoscopic structural universality with diffusion. Proc Natl Acad Sci U S A 111(14):5088–5093

8. Novikov DS, Fieremans E, Jespersen SN, Kiselev VG (2019) Quantifying brain microstructure with diffusion MRI: Theory and parameter estimation. NMR Biomed 32(4):e3998

9. Andica C, Hori M, Kamiya K, Koshino S, Hagiwara A, Kamagata K, Fukunaga I, Hamasaki N, Suzuki M, Feiweier T, Murata K, Arakawa A, Kondo A, Akiyama O, Aoki S (2018) Spatial restriction within intracranial epidermoid cysts observed using short diffusion-time diffusion-weighted imaging. Magn Reson Med Sci 17(3):269–272

10. Maekawa T, Hori M, Murata K, Feiweier T, Andica C, Fukunaga I, Koshino S, Hagiwara A, Kamiya K, Kamagata K, Wada A, Abe O, Aoki S (2019) Choroid plexus cysts analyzed using diffusion-weighted imaging with short diffusion-time. Magn Reson Imaging 57:323–327

11. Bongers A, Hau E, Shen H (2018) Short diffusion time diffusion-weighted imaging with oscillating gradient preparation as an early magnetic resonance imaging biomarker for radiation therapy response monitoring in glioblastoma: a preclinical feasibility study. Int J Radiat Oncol Biol Phys 102(4):1014–1023

12. Iima M, Yamamoto A, Kataoka M, Yamada Y, Omori K, Feiweier T, Togashi K (2019) Time-dependent diffusion MRI to distinguish malignant from benign head and neck tumors. J Magn Reson Imaging 50(1):88–95

13. Hori M, Irie R, Suzuki M, Aoki S (2017) Teaching Neuroimages: obscured cerebral infarction on MRI. Clin Neuroradiol 27(4):519–520

14. Baron CA, Kate M, Gioia L, Butcher K, Emery D, Budde M, Beaulieu C (2015) Reduction of diffusion-weighted imaging contrast of acute ischemic stroke at short diffusion times. Stroke 46(8):2136–2141

15. Boonrod A, Hagiwara A, Hori M, Fukunaga I, Andica C, Maekawa T, Aoki S (2018) Reduced visualization of cerebral infarction on diffusion-weighted images with short diffusion times. Neuroradiology 60(9):979–982

16. Latt J, Nilsson M, van Westen D, Wirestam R, Stahlberg F, Brockstedt S (2009) Diffusion-weighted MRI measurements on stroke patients reveal water-exchange mechanisms in sub-acute ischaemic lesions. NMR Biomed 22(6):619–628

17. Obata T, Kershaw J, Tachibana Y, Miyauchi T, Abe Y, Shibata S, Kawaguchi H, Ikoma Y, Takuwa H, Aoki I, Yasui M (2018) Comparison of diffusion-weighted MRI and anti-Stokes Raman scattering (CARS) measurements of water in expression-controlled aquaporin-4 cells. Sci Rep 8(1):17954

18. Fieremans E, Novikov DS, Jensen JH, Helpern JA (2010) Monte Carlo study of a two-compartment exchange model of diffusion. NMR Biomed 23(7):711–724

19. Li H, Jiang X, Xie J, McIntyre JO, Gore JC, Xu J (2016) Time-dependent influence of cell membrane permeability on MR diffusion measurements. Magn Reson Med 75(5):1927–1934

20. Nilsson M, Latt J, van Westen D, Brockstedt S, Lasic S, Stahlberg F, Topgaard D (2013) Noninvasive mapping of water diffusional exchange in the human brain using filter-exchange imaging. Magn Reson Med 69(6):1573–1581

21. Ozarslan E, Shepherd TM, Koay CG, Blackband SJ, Basser PJ (2012) Temporal scaling characteristics of diffusion as a new MRI contrast: findings in rat hippocampus. NeuroImage 60(2):1380–1393

22. Roth Y, Ocherashvilli A, Daniels D, Ruiz-Cabello J, Maier SE, Orenstein A, Mardor Y (2008) Quantification of water compartmentation in cell suspensions by diffusion-weighted and T(2)-weighted MRI. Magn Reson Imaging 26(1):88–102

23. Thelwall PE, Shepherd TM, Stanisz GJ, Blackband SJ (2006) Effects of temperature and aldehyde fixation on tissue water diffusion properties, studied in an erythrocyte ghost tissue model. Magn Reson Med 56(2):282–289

24. Zhang H, Schneider T, Wheeler-Kingshott CA, Alexander DC (2012) NODDI: practical in vivo neurite orientation and density imaging of the human brain. NeuroImage 61(4):1000–1016

25. Stikov N, Campbell JS, Stroh T, Lavelee M, Frey S, Novek J, Nuara S, Ho MK, Bedell BJ, Dougherty RF, Leppert IR, Boudreau M, Narayanan S, Duval T, Cohen-Adad J, Picard PA, Gasecka A, Cote D, Pike GB (2015) In vivo histology of the myelin g-ratio with magnetic resonance imaging. NeuroImage 118:397–405

26. Rushton WA (1951) A theory of the effects of fibre size in medullated nerve. J Physiol 115(1):101–122

27. Genc S, Malpas CB, Holland SK, Beare R, Silk TJ (2017) Neurite density index is sensitive to age related differences in the developing brain. NeuroImage 148:373–380

28. Mah A, Geeraert B, Lebel C (2017) Detailing neuroanatomical development in late childhood and early adolescence using NODDI. PLoS One 12(8):e0182340

29. Granberg T, Fan Q, Treaba CA, Ouellette R, Herranz E, Mangeat G, Louapre C, Cohen-Adad J, Klawiter EC, Sloane JA, Mainero C (2017) In vivo characterization of cortical and white matter neuroaxonal pathology in early multiple sclerosis. Brain 140(11):2912–2926

30. Hagiwara A, Hori M, Yokoyama K, Nakazawa M, Ueda R, Horita M, Andica C, Abe O, Aoki S (2017) Analysis of white matter damage in patients with multiple sclerosis via a novel In Vivo MR method for measuring myelin, axons, and G-Ratio. AJNR Am J Neuroradiol 38(10):1934–1940

31. Kamagata K, Hatano T, Okuzumi A, Motoi Y, Abe O, Shimoji K, Kamiya K, Suzuki M, Hori M, Kumamaru KK, Hattori N, Aoki S (2016) Neurite orientation dispersion and density imaging in the substantia nigra in idiopathic Parkinson disease. Eur Radiol 26(8):2567–2577

32. Kamagata K, Zalesky A, Hatano T, Ueda R, Di Biase MA, Okuzumi A, Shimoji K, Hori M, Caeyenberghs K, Pantelis C, Hattori N, Aoki S (2017) Gray matter abnormalities in idiopathic Parkinson's disease: evaluation by diffusional kurtosis imaging and neurite orientation dispersion and density imaging. Hum Brain Mapp 38(7):3704–3722

33. Kamiya K, Hori M, Irie R, Miyajima M, Nakajima M, Kamagata K, Tsuruta K, Saito A, Nakazawa M, Suzuki Y, Mori H, Kunimatsu A, Arai H, Aoki S, Abe O (2017) Diffusion imaging of reversible and irreversible microstructural changes within the corticospinal tract in idiopathic normal pressure hydrocephalus. NeuroImage Clinical 14:663–671

34. Irie R, Tsuruta K, Hori M, Suzuki M, Kamagata K, Nakanishi A, Kamiya K, Nakajima M, Miyajima M, Arai H, Aoki S (2017) Neurite orientation dispersion and density imaging for evaluation of corticospinal tract in idiopathic normal pressure hydrocephalus. Jpn J Radiol 35(1):25–30

35. Grussu F, Schneider T, Zhang H, Alexander DC, Wheeler-Kingshott CA (2015) Neurite orientation dispersion and density imaging of the healthy cervical spinal cord in vivo. NeuroImage 111:590–601

36. Grussu F, Schneider T, Tur C, Yates RL, Tachrount M, Ianus A, Yiannakas MC, Newcombe J, Zhang H, Alexander DC, DeLuca GC, Gandini Wheeler-Kingshott CAM (2017) Neurite dispersion: a new marker of multiple sclerosis spinal cord pathology? Ann Clin Transl Neurol 4(9):663–679

37. Schilling KG, By S, Feiler HR, Box BA, O'Grady KP, Witt A, Landman BA, Smith SA (2019) Diffusion MRI microstructural models in the cervical spinal cord—application, normative values, and correlations with histological analysis. NeuroImage 201:116026

38. Hori M, Hagiwara A, Fukunaga I, Ueda R, Kamiya K, Suzuki Y, Liu W, Murata K, Takamura T, Hamasaki N, Irie R, Kamagata K, Kumamaru KK, Suzuki M, Aoki S (2018) Application of quantitative microstructural MR imaging with atlas-based analysis for the spinal cord in cervical spondylotic myelopathy. Sci Rep 8(1):5213

Diffusion Imaging of the Head and Neck in the Future

25

Ashok Srinivasan

25.1 Current State of Diffusion Imaging in the Head and Neck

While diffusion-weighted imaging (DWI) has been present in clinical practice for more than a decade, its primary use in neuroradiology has centered around its utility in brain pathologies including acute ischemic stroke, abscesses, and tumors. Multiple studies that have focused on DWI in the head and neck over the past 15 years or so have been crucial in increasing our understanding of the clinical applications of DWI in head and neck pathologies. The advent of Echo Planar Imaging (EPI) and intravoxel incoherent motion (IVIM) has allowed for the rapid acquisition necessary to collect DWI data with a significant reduction in motion artifact. With improved imaging technology and advances in MRI sequences, it has become possible to tackle the inherent challenges in applying DWI in the head and neck that include geometric contour variations, motion artifact from pulsating vessels and physiological maneuvers such as swallowing and susceptibility artifacts from air-soft tissue interfaces.

For the most part, the different applications of DWI in head and neck imaging have been attributed to its ability to serve as a surrogate marker for tissue cellularity. Apparent diffusion coefficient (ADC) derived from DWI is a quantitative metric measuring the freedom of water molecular motion and has been demonstrated to have an inverse correlation with cellularity; for example, higher ADC values for a specific voxel correlate with a lower cellularity in that voxel [1] (Figs. 25.1, 25.2, 25.3, and 25.4).

However, there are other tissue factors that determine DWI signal and ADC that could play a role in influencing the ADC and the interpretation of the images. Some non-tumor causes of reduced ADC include increased viscosity and presence of macromolecules (increased protein content of inspissated secretions). In this chapter, we will look at the current state of techniques and clinical applications of DWI in head and neck imaging, and discuss the future state.

25.2 Techniques: Current and Future

While there are a number of techniques available for acquiring DWI, routine head and neck DWI continues to employ EPI and is typically acquired as a single shot technique with 2 or 3 b values due to simplicity of operation and shorter

A. Srinivasan (✉)
Division of Neuroradiology, Department of Radiology, University of Michigan, Ann Arbor, MI, USA
e-mail: ashoks@med.umich.edu

© Springer Nature Switzerland AG 2021
T. Moritani, A. A. Capizzano (eds.), *Diffusion-Weighted MR Imaging of the Brain, Head and Neck, and Spine*, https://doi.org/10.1007/978-3-030-62120-9_25

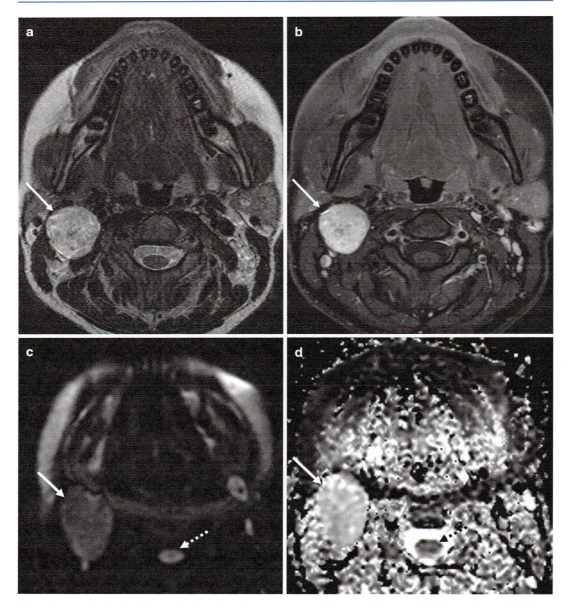

Fig. 25.1 (**a–d**) Axial T2-weighted (**a**) and post-gadolinum T1-weighted (**b**) images in a 42-year-old female demonstrate a T2 hyperintense, enhancing lesion in the right carotid sheath that was proven to be a schwannoma. Corresponding trace DWI image (**c**) and ADC map (**d**) show the DWI signal intensity to be lower than the spinal cord and the ADC higher, seen typically with benign lesions in the head and neck

acquisition time. Non-EPI techniques that take longer to acquire are usually employed in regions such as skull base and temporal bone where significant susceptibility artifacts can degrade image quality [2].

25.2.1 EPI Diffusion

The main advantages of EPI diffusion are its short acquisition time and relative insensitivity to motion. This makes it attractive for its applica-

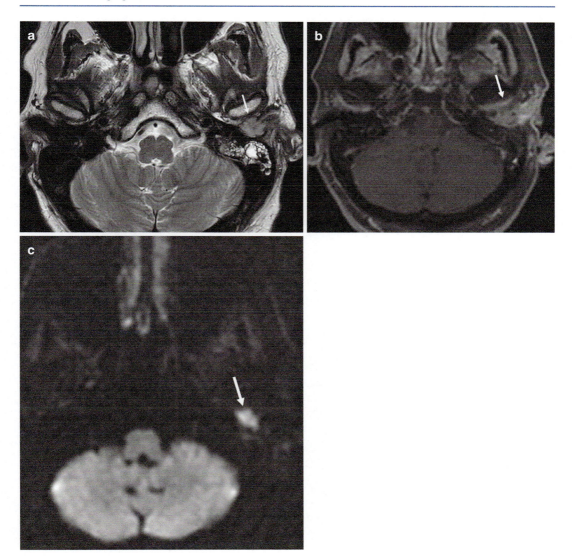

Fig. 25.2 (**a–c**) Axial T2-weighted (**a**) and post-gadolinum T1-weighted (**b**) images in a 74-year-old male demonstrate a heterogeneous enhancing lesion in the left external auditory canal that was proven to be squamous cell carcinoma. Corresponding trace DWI image (**c**) shows high signal intensity similar to that observed in the brainstem, seen typically in hypercellular lesions such as malignancies

tion in routine head and neck imaging. This can be performed either as a single-shot technique where the entire K-space is filled with one TR or multi-shot where multiple TRs are used. The latter technique, while longer in acquisition compared to single-shot technique, has the benefit of reduced susceptibility effects and geometric distortion and improved spatial resolution.

25.2.2 Non-EPI Diffusion (TSE Diffusion)

While multi-shot EPI diffusion can reduce the susceptibility artifacts associated with EPI diffusion, non-EPI techniques can provide a further reduction in artifacts, increase spatial resolution, thereby providing an overall improvement in

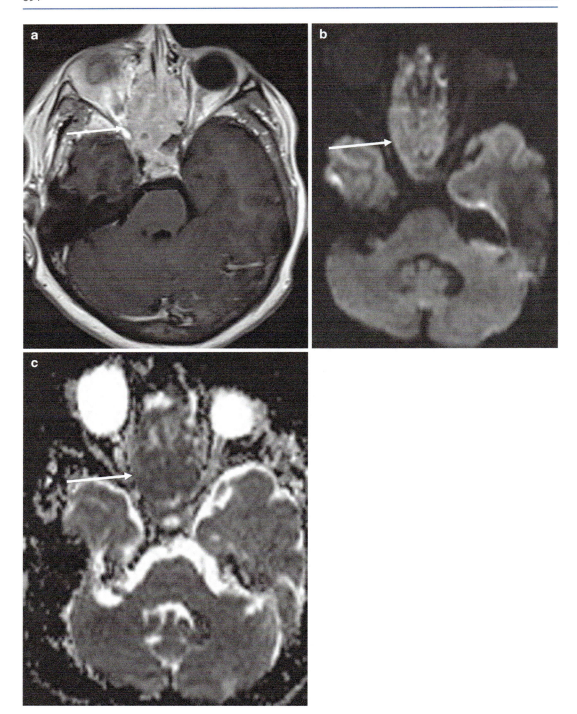

Fig. 25.3 (**a–c**) Axial post-gadolinum T1-weighted (**a**) image in a 63-year-old male with a history of previously treated adenocarcinoma in the nasal cavities demonstrates an enhancing posttreatment mass at the site of the treated primary cancer. Corresponding trace DWI image (**b**) and ADC map (**c**) show high DWI signal intensity and low ADC, suggesting hypercellularity. Final pathology was recurrent adenocarcinoma

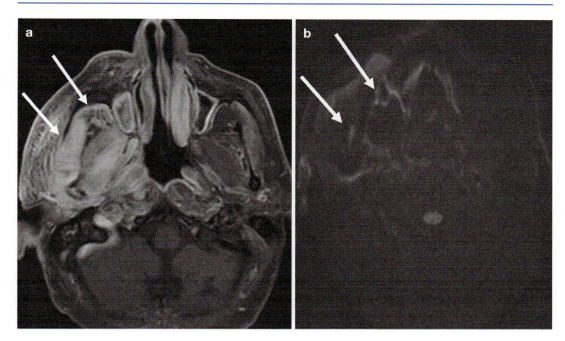

Fig. 25.4 (**a**, **b**) Axial post-gadolinum T1-weighted (**a**) image in a 50-year-old male with treated squamous cell carcinoma of the mandibular gingiva (oral cavity) demonstrates asymmetric mass-like enhancement within the right masticator space. Corresponding trace DWI image (**b**) shows no areas of high signal intensity that would be suggestive of a hypercellular process. Multiple biopsies revealed only benign granulation tissue with no evidence of recurrent malignancy

image quality. They do have a relatively lower signal-to-noise ratio (SNR) that necessitates multiple averages for better SNR and prolongs scanning time.

25.2.3 Intravoxel Incoherent Motion

It is important to realize that ADC values are influenced by the choice of b values, a phenomenon partly explained in the work by Le Bihan et al. that demonstrated that the water molecular motion contributing to DWI signal arose from different compartments: extracellular space diffusion, intracellular space diffusion, and intravascular space diffusion (or perfusion) [3]. Intravoxel incoherent motion (IVIM) imaging enables separation of water molecular diffusion from perfusion in the microcirculation from that due to diffusion in the extravascular space. Using this technique, multiple parameters can be generated including "f" representing the perfusion fraction (or the contribution of water moving in capillaries), "D" representing the tissue diffusion coefficient, and "D^*" representing the pseudodiffusion coefficient (or diffusion within the microcirculation). Above b values of 200 s/mm^2, the contribution of D^* is negligible since it is greater than D by several orders of magnitude [3–5].

25.2.4 Reproducibility of ADC Values

In a study by Kolff-Gart et al., the authors evaluated the reproducibility of ADC values in the head and neck region in healthy subjects and attempted to identify the most suitable reference tissue [6]. They studied 7 subjects with both EPI and TSE sequences on 5 different MR imaging systems at 3 time points in 2 institutions. Mean ADC values for different tissues (submandibular gland, sternocleidomastoid muscle, spinal cord, subdigastric lymph node, and tonsil) were evaluated for intra- and intersubject, intersystem, and intersequence variability. Their results showed that the ADC values derived from EPI-DWI with 2 b-values and calculated EPI-DWI with 2 b-values extracted from EPI-DWI with 6 b-values did not differ significantly with the least standard error of measurement seen in the tonsil and spinal cord. They also noted that the intersystem difference for mean ADC values and the influence of the MR imaging system on ADC values among the subjects were statistically significant. Based on their results, they concluded that the spinal cord was the most appropriate reference tissue and that EPI-DWI with 6 b-values was the most reproducible sequence [6]. This study shows that quantitative ADC measurements performed as part of clinical care would be more accurate if the patients were scanned on the same MR imaging system and with the same sequence. ADC values differed significantly between MR imaging systems and sequences. If this is not possible for various reasons, the next best option would be to use the spinal cord as an internal standard. This was also corroborated in another study by Koontz et al. who were able to successfully use ADC ratios between tumor tissue and spinal cord to differentiate benign and malignant head and neck lesions [7].

25.2.5 Enhanced Dual-Stage Correlated Diffusion Imaging

Correlated diffusion imaging (CDI) is a new form of diffusion imaging which accounts for the joint correlation of diffusion signal attenuation across multiple gradient pulse strengths and timings in order to improve the separability of cancerous and healthy tissues [8]. However, CDI does not capture anatomical information. Dual-stage CDI (D-CDI) is a recent version of CDI where an additional signal mixing stage between the correlated diffusion signal from the first signal mixing stage (CDI) and an auxiliary diffusion signal is performed to incorporate anatomical context. This technique has been evaluated so far in prostate cancer and found to

be beneficial over T2-weighted images and DWI used in the form of ADC maps; future studies in the head and neck may prove its utility too since the basic principles of cancer detection and characterization would be similar across different tissues [8].

25.3 Clinical Applications

25.3.1 Benign Versus Malignant Lesions

While pathological confirmation using tissue biopsy is the gold standard for differentiating benign and malignant lesions in the head and neck, there are deeper anatomical locations that may not be accessible for a biopsy. Furthermore, biopsies themselves are not zero risk procedures, suggesting the need for robust noninvasive techniques to predict presence of malignancy.

Multiple studies have demonstrated the ability and reliability of DWI in characterizing the malignant potential of a head and neck lesion. Based on the hypothesis that malignant tumors demonstrate lower ADC values compared to benign tumors due to their relatively higher cellularity, Wang et al. demonstrated that benign and malignant lesions yielded significantly different ADC values, and using an ADC value of 1.22×10^{-3} mm^2/s, the authors were able to categorize lesions as benign (above the cutoff) or malignant (below), with an accuracy of 86%, sensitivity of 84%, and specificity of 91% [9]. Other authors have also shown this utility using different MRI systems and magnet strengths. Razek et al. demonstrated an apparent diffusion coefficient cutoff value of 1.15×10^{-3} mm^2/s yielded a sensitivity of 95%, a specificity of 91%, and an accuracy of 93% [10]. Similarly, Srinivasan et al. compared 33 patients with head and neck masses on a 3T magnet and found that there was a statistically significant difference between benign and malignant lesions with the latter showing lower ADC values than the former. In their study, the threshold value of 1.3×10^{-3} mm^2/s provided the best differentiation [11].

Since absolute ADC values vary based on the magnet strength, manufacturer, and number of b values, it would be better to use an internal reference standard such as the adjacent brainstem or spinal cord to determine whether a lesion may be benign or malignant. If the clinical workflow does not permit quantitative ROI measurements, a qualitative assessment may suffice in most instances; lesions that appear darker on the ADC map than the brainstem/spinal cord can be expected to have higher cellularity and hence more likely in the malignant spectrum. Exceptions to this rule of thumb would be the presence of high protein content within inspissated secretions and benign lesions with high cellularity such as paragangliomas.

In a few scenarios, DWI can help distinguish different malignant tumors from one another. Dreissen et al. demonstrated that positive HPV status correlates with low mean ADC when compared with non-HPV squamous cell cancers of the oropharynx [12]. Given the significant differences in treatment response of HPV+ and HPV− oropharyngeal cancers, this differentiation may lead to more patient focused treatment options based on MRI findings.

25.3.2 Prediction and Monitoring of Treatment Response

Predicting a tumor's response to treatment using noninvasive imaging based biomarkers can be helpful to tailor individualized management options. To this effect, many DWI based biomarkers have been studied by different investigators with variable results. Guo et al. found a notably lower pretreatment ADC value, and D value (IVIM derived bi-exponential diffusion coefficient) in responders compared to non-responders as well as a higher posttreatment ADC, and concluded that lower pretreatment ADC value correlated with therapy response [4]. In another study by Kim et al., the authors showed that complete responders had significantly lower pretreatment ADC values than partial responders; furthermore, pretreatment ADC value achieved 65% sensitivity and 86% speci-

ficity in predicting response [13]. This was also corroborated in a separate study by Srinivasan et al. who showed that a histographic analysis of ADC values may be of benefit as well; in their study, lesions with lower pretreatment ADC and more than 45% of their volume below a threshold of 1.15×10^{-3} mm^2/s had better response to chemoradiation 2 years after treatment [14].

Other metrics apart from ADC may also have utility in predicting response. Using IVIM in metastatic lymph nodes, Hauser et al. showed that an elevated perfusion fraction (or f-value) at baseline examination may predict locoregional failure after treatment [5].

However, the clinical applicability of DWI in this field is not settled yet. Contrasting results have been reported in other studies; King et al. failed to demonstrate a significant correlation between pretreatment ADC and treatment response [15].

Having a reliable way to assess treatment response during early stages and at the end of therapy is important for making management decisions on continuing therapy and for prognostication. ADC has been investigated as a potential biomarker for evaluating early therapy response. In a study by Paudyal et al., the authors used IVIM technique and found a significant difference in change in D (bi-exponential diffusion coefficient) between complete responders and incomplete responders, and suggested that with more research, MRI may not only be able to assess response, but also characterize its magnitude to allow for individualized treatment options [16].

Other authors have also shown similar results, thereby suggesting that ADC can be a valuable metric for this application.

25.3.3 Recurrence Versus Posttreatment Changes

Based on the hypothesis that recurrent malignancies would demonstrate higher cellularity and therefore lower ADC compared to benign posttreatment masses, multiple authors have shown the utility of ADC for this differentiation.

Vaid et al. examined 80 treated head and neck cancer patients and were able to show that recurrent malignancy demonstrated decreased ADC values when compared to posttreatment changes [17]. Using a threshold ADC value of 1.2×10^{-3} mm^2/s, they achieved 90.13% sensitivity and 82.5% specificity for this differentiation. In a study of 50 laryngeal cancer patients who underwent either surgery or chemoradiation, Desouky et al. compared DWI and dynamic contrast enhanced imaging and demonstrated that an ADC threshold value of 0.9667×10^{-3} mm^2/s differentiated benign and malignant lesions with 100% sensitivity, and 74.2% specificity [18].

Vandacaveye et al. evaluated 26 patients with recurrent head and neck squamous cell cancer and showed that the signal was significantly higher for HNSCC than for nontumoral tissue on native b-1000 images, with a 71.6% sensitivity and 71.3% specificity [19]. In this study, differentiation based on ADC values (lower for HNSCC than for benign tissue) achieved a 94.6% sensitivity and 95.9% specificity. In addition, DWI detected nodal metastases smaller than 1 cm, and gave fewer false positive results in both the original tumor bed and in residual adenopathies, when compared with CT, TSE-MRI, and FDG-PET. While ADC is often utilized in clinical practice for differentiating recurrence from posttreatment changes, the lack of a consensus on well-defined ADC values and thresholds makes it difficult to compare results across institutions.

25.4 What the Future Holds

While DWI has shown utility in multiple head and neck applications, the major obstacle in its routine integration in day-to-day clinical practice has been the lack of standardization of protocols and well-defined threshold values for quantitative analysis. This can be overcome to some extent if ADC values can be standardized against an internal structure such as the brain/spinal cord or by using qualitative analysis. In addition, there are issues with susceptibility artifacts and image distortion that can prevent appropriate assessment of head and neck tissues but this can be overcome to a large degree by utilizing parallel imaging, reducing echo train length and by adopting technical improvements such as reduced field of view diffusion imaging [20]. However, it is important to remember that DWI alone may not be the answer to the problem in many instances and hence the proper integration of DWI with conventional imaging information and other advanced techniques such as perfusion are key to a better understanding of pathologies in the head and neck.

References

1. Chen L, Liu M, Bao J, Xia Y, Zhang J, Zhang L et al (2013) The correlation between apparent diffusion coefficient and tumor cellularity in patients: a meta-analysis. PLoS One 8(11):e79008
2. Schakel T, Hoogduin JM, Terhaard CH, Philippens ME (2013) Diffusion weighted MRI in head-and-neck cancer: geometrical accuracy. Radiother Oncol 109(3):394–397
3. Le Bihan D, Breton E, Lallemand D, Grenier P, Cabanis E, Laval-Jeantet M (1986) MR imaging of intravoxel incoherent motions: application to diffusion and perfusion in neurologic disorders. Radiology 161(2):401–407
4. Guo W, Luo D, Lin M, Wu B, Li L, Zhao Y et al (2016) Pretreatment intra-voxel incoherent motion diffusion-weighted imaging (IVIM-DWI) in predicting induction chemotherapy response in locally advanced hypopharyngeal carcinoma. Medicine 95(10):e3039
5. Hauser T, Essig M, Jensen A, Laun FB, Munter M, Maier-Hein KH et al (2014) Prediction of treatment response in head and neck carcinomas using IVIM-DWI: evaluation of lymph node metastasis. Eur J Radiol 83(5):783–787
6. Kolff-Gart AS, Pouwels PJW, Noij DP, Ljumanovic R, Vandecaveye V, de Keyzer F, de Bree R, de Graaf P, Knol DL, Castelijns JA (2015) Diffusion-weighted imaging of the head and neck in healthy subjects: reproducibility of ADC values in different MRI systems and repeat sessions. AJNR 36(2):384–390
7. Koontz NA, Wiggins RH 3rd (2017) Differentiation of Benign and Malignant head and neck lesions with diffusion tensor imaging and DWI. AJR 208(5):1110–1115
8. Khalvati F, Zhang J, Haider MA, Wong A (2016) Enhanced dual-stage correlated diffusion imaging. Conf Proc IEEE Eng Med Biol Soc 2016:5537–5540
9. Wang J, Takashima S, Takayama F, Kawakami S, Saito A, Matsushita T et al (2001) Head and neck lesions: characterization with diffusion-weighted echo-planar MR imaging. Radiology 220(3):621–630

10. Razek AA, Elkhamary S, Mousa A (2011) Differentiation between benign and malignant orbital tumors at 3-T diffusion MR-imaging. Neuroradiology 53(7):517–522
11. Srinivasan A, Dvorak R, Perni K, Rohrer S, Mukherji SK (2008) Differentiation of benign and malignant pathology in the head and neck using 3T apparent diffusion coefficient values: early experience. AJNR 29(1):40–44
12. Driessen JP, van Bemmel AJ, van Kempen PM, Janssen LM, Terhaard CH, Pameijer FA et al (2016) Correlation of human papillomavirus status with apparent diffusion coefficient of diffusion-weighted MRI in head and neck squamous cell carcinomas. Head Neck 38(Suppl 1):E613–E618
13. Kim S, Loevner L, Quon H, Sherman E, Weinstein G, Kilger A et al (2009) Diffusion-weighted magnetic resonance imaging for predicting and detecting early response to chemoradiation therapy of squamous cell carcinomas of the head and neck. Clin Cancer Res 15(3):986–994
14. Srinivasan A, Chenevert TL, Dwamena BA, Eisbruch A, Watcharotone K, Myles JD, Mukherji SK (2012) Utility of pretreatment mean apparent diffusion coefficient and apparent diffusion coefficient histograms in prediction of outcome to chemoradiation in head and neck squamous cell carcinoma. J Comput Assist Tomogr 36(1):131–137
15. King AD, Mo FK, Yu KH, Yeung DK, Zhou H, Bhatia KS et al (2010) Squamous cell carcinoma of the head and neck: diffusion-weighted MR imaging for prediction and monitoring of treatment response. Eur Radiol 20(9):2213–2220
16. Paudyal R, Oh JH, Riaz N, Venigalla P, Li J, Hatzoglou V et al (2017) Intravoxel incoherent motion diffusion-weighted MRI during chemoradiation therapy to characterize and monitor treatment response in human papillomavirus head and neck squamous cell carcinoma. JMRI 45(4):1013–1023
17. Vaid S, Chandorkar A, Atre A, Shah D, Vaid N (2017) Differentiating recurrent tumours from post-treatment changes in head and neck cancers: does diffusion-weighted MRI solve the eternal dilemma? Clin Radiol 72(1):74–83
18. Desouky SE, Paudyal R, OH JH (2015) Role of dynamic contrast enhanced and diffusion weighted MRI in the differentiation between post treatment changes and recurrent laryngeal cancers. Egypt J Radiol Nucl Med 46:379–389
19. Vandecaveye V, De Keyzer F, Nuyts S, Deraedt K, Dirix P, Hamaekers P et al (2007) Detection of head and neck squamous cell carcinoma with diffusion weighted MRI after (chemo)radiotherapy: correlation between radiologic and histopathologic findings. Int J Radiat Oncol Biol Phys 67(4):960–971
20. Vidiri A, Minosse S, Piludu F, Curione D, Pichi B, Spriano G et al (2017) Feasibility study of reduced field of view diffusion-weighted magnetic resonance imaging in head and neck tumors. Acta Radiol 58(3):292–300

Part IV

How to use this book

How to Use This Book

26

Toshio Moritani and Per-Lennart A. Westesson

The aim of this chapter is to help the reader understand major topics and various cases of DWI in this book visually.

In Table 26.1, we demonstrated the most important 33 images of color schemas, tables, and pathologies from each chapter with the figure numbers, so that the reader can go back to the text and learn more detailed information.

In Tables 26.2–26.8 we demonstrated DWI signal characteristics and the corresponding ADC and T2 characteristics. Each table is essentially a list of differential diagnoses. When combined with the knowledge of patient symptomatology and demographic criteria, the radiologist will be able to narrow the differential diagnosis to a few conditions. These tables take into account that the same condition may have variable imaging characteristics. This chapter makes direct reference to other chapters of the book, where a full description is then provided.

T. Moritani (✉)
Division of Neuroradiology, University of Michigan,
Ann Arbor, MI, USA
e-mail: tmoritan@med.umich.edu

P.-L. A. Westesson
University of Rochester Medical Center,
Rochester, NY, USA
e-mail: perlennart_westesson@urmc.rochester.edu

© Springer Nature Switzerland AG 2021
T. Moritani, A. A. Capizzano (eds.), *Diffusion-Weighted MR Imaging of the Brain, Head and Neck, and Spine*, https://doi.org/10.1007/978-3-030-62120-9_26

Table 26.1 The list of 33 important schemas, tables and pathologies

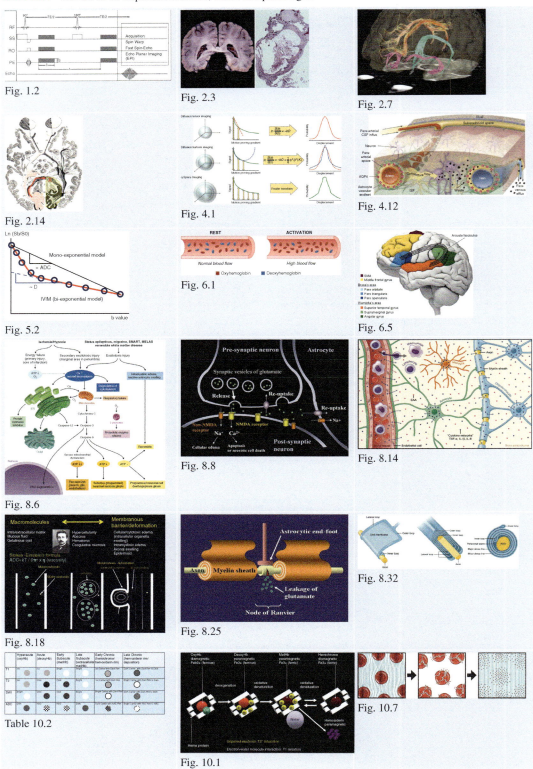

26 How to Use This Book

Table 26.1 (continued)

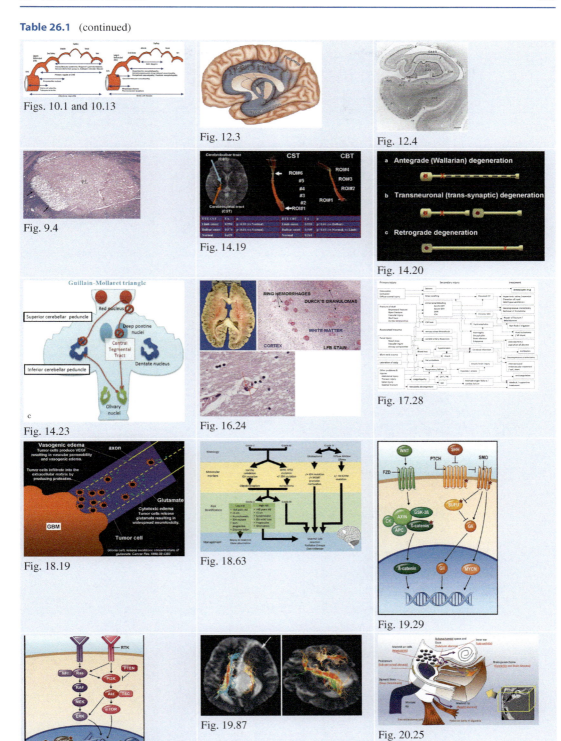

Figs. 10.1 and 10.13

Fig. 12.3

Fig. 12.4

Fig. 9.4

Fig. 14.19

Fig. 14.20

Fig. 14.23

Fig. 16.24

Fig. 17.28

Fig. 18.19

Fig. 18.63

Fig. 19.29

Fig. 19.39

Fig. 19.87

Fig. 20.25

Table 26.2 Differential diagnoses for lesions with a **high diffusion** signal associated with **low ADC** and **isointense** T2 signal

Diagnoses	Reference images		
	DWI high	ADC low	T2WI iso
Infarction/hypoxia/trauma			
Nonaccidental head injury	Fig. 19.15d	Fig. 19.15e	Fig. 19.15b
Hyperacute infarction	Fig. 9.1b	Fig. 9.1c	Fig. 9.1a
Hypoxic ischemic encephalopathy	Fig. 19.10c	Fig. 19.10d	Fig. 19.10a
Toxic/metabolic			
Methotrexate leukoencephalopathy	Fig. 15.2b	Fig. 15.2c	Fig. 15.2a

26 How to Use This Book

Table 26.3 Differential diagnoses for lesions with a **high diffusion** signal associated with **iso-high ADC** and a **high intense T2** signal

Diagnoses	Reference images		
	DWI high	ADC iso-high	T2 high
Degeneration			
Amyotrophic lateral sclerosis	Fig.14.18b	Fig. 14.18c	Fig. 14.18a
Demyelination			
Acute disseminated encephalomyelitis (ADEM)	Fig. 13.12c	Fig. 13.12d	Fig. 13.12a
Multiple sclerosis (MS)	Fig. 13.3c	Fig. 13.3d	Fig. 13.3a
Progressive multiple leukoencephalopathy (PML)	Fig. 13.21b	Fig. 13.21c	Fig. 13.21a

(continued)

Table 26.3 (continued)

Diagnoses	Reference images		
	DWI high	ADC iso-high	T2 high
Epilepsy Postictal encephalopathy	Fig. 12.16d	Fig. 12.16e	Fig. 12.16a
Infarction Venous infarction	Fig. 9.7c	Fig. 9.7d	Fig. 9.7b
Infection Subdural empyema	Fig. 16.12b	Fig. 16.12c	Fig. 16.12a
Toxic/metabolic Marchiafava-Bignami disease	Fig. 15.8c	Fig. 15.8d	Fig. 15.8a

26 How to Use This Book

Table 26.3 (continued)

Diagnoses	Reference images		
	DWI high	ADC iso-high	T2 high
Tumor			
Epidermoid	Fig. 16.16c	Fig. 16.16d	Fig. 16.16a
Brain stem glioma	Fig. 18.7d	Fig. 18.7e	Fig. 18.7a
Anaplastic astrocytoma	Fig. 3.2c	Fig. 3.2d	Fig. 3.2a
Low-grade oligoastrocytoma	Fig. 18.8c	Fig. 18.8d	Fig. 18.8a

(continued)

Table 26.3 (continued)

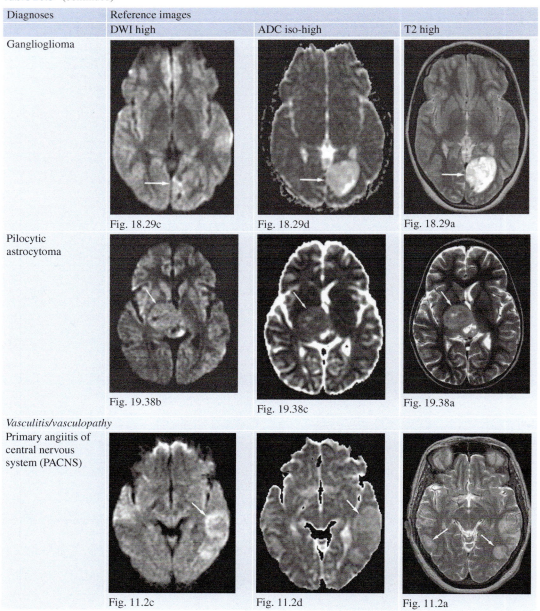

26 How to Use This Book

Table 26.3 (continued)

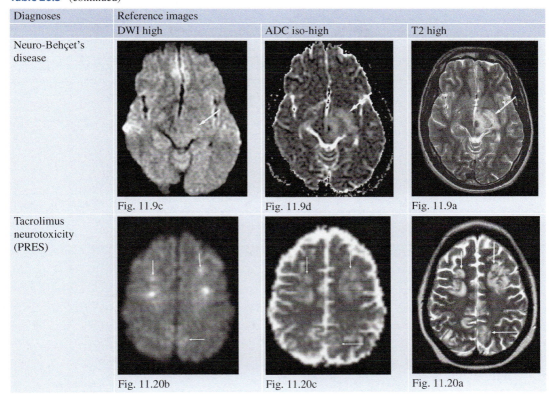

Table 26.4 Differential diagnoses for lesions with a **high diffusion** signal associated with a **low ADC** and **high intense T2** signal

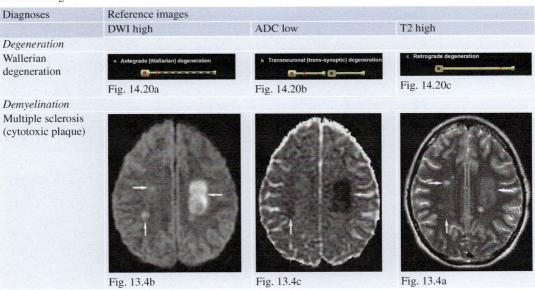

(continued)

Table 26.4 (continued)

Diagnoses	Reference images		
	DWI high	ADC low	T2 high
Epilepsy Status epileptics	Fig. 8.20b	Fig. 8.20c	Fig. 8.20a
Postictal encephalopathy	Fig. 12.17d	Fig. 12.17e	Fig. 12.17a
Hematoma Late subacute hematoma (Extracellular methemoglobin)	Fig. 10.6c	Fig. 10.6e	Fig. 10.6a
Subdural hematoma (SDH)	Fig. 10.8c	Fig. 10.8e	Fig. 10.8d

26 How to Use This Book

Table 26.4 (continued)

Diagnoses	Reference images		
	DWI high	ADC low	T2 high
Infarction/Ischemia			
Hyperacute reversible ischemia (2 h)	 Fig. 9.5b	 Fig. 9.5c	 Fig. 9.5a
Acute infarction (24 h)	 Fig. 3.3d	 Fig. 3.3e	 Fig. 3.3c
Subacute infarction (10 day)	 Fig. 9.3c	 Fig. 9.3d	 Fig. 9.3a
Infection			
Abscess	 Fig. 16.1c	 Fig. 16.1d	 Fig. 16.1a

(continued)

Table 26.4 (continued)

Diagnoses	Reference images		
	DWI high	ADC low	T2 high
Septic emboli	Fig. 16.4b	Fig. 16.4c	Fig. 16.4a
Ventriculitis	Fig. 16.14c	Fig. 16.14d	Fig. 16.14b
Acquired immunodeficiency syndrome (AIDS)	Fig. 16.47b	Fig. 16.47c	Fig. 16.47a
Aspergillosis (disseminated)	Fig. 16.23b	Fig. 16.23c	Fig. 16.23a

26 How to Use This Book

Table 26.4 (continued)

Diagnoses	Reference images		
	DWI high	ADC low	T2 high
Creutzfeldt-Jakob disease (CJD)	Fig. 14.13b	Fig. 14.13c	Fig. 14.13a
Group B Streptococcus meningitis	Fig. 16.17b	Fig. 16.17c	Fig. 16.17a
Herpes simplex virus encephalitis	Fig. 19.19b	Fig. 19.19c	Fig. 19.19a
Toxoplasmosis (exceptional case)	Fig. 16.20c	Fig. 16.20d	Fig. 16.20a

(continued)

Table 26.4 (continued)

Diagnoses	Reference images		
	DWI high	ADC low	T2 high
Toxic/metabolic			
Carmofur leukoencephalopathy	Fig. 15.3b	Fig. 15.3c	Fig. 15.3a
Heroin-induced leukoencephalopathy	Fig. 15.5b	Fig. 15.5c	Fig. 15.5a
Central pontine myelinolysis (CPM)	Fig. 15.17b	Fig. 15.17c	Fig. 15.17a
Extrapontine myelinolysis (EPM)	Fig. 15.18b	Fig. 15.18c	Fig. 15.18a

26 How to Use This Book

Table 26.4 (continued)

Diagnoses	Reference images		
	DWI high	ADC low	T2 high
L-2-hydroxyglutaric aciduria	Fig. 19.75b	Fig. 19.75c	Fig. 19.75a
Mitochondrial encephalopathy, lactic acidosis, and stroke-like episodes (MELAS)	Fig. 15.24f	Fig. 15.24e	Fig. 15.24g
Phenylketonuria (PKU)	Fig. 19.72b	Fig. 19.72c	Fig. 19.72a
Trauma Nonaccidental head injury	Fig. 19.16b	Fig. 19.16d	Fig. 19.16a

(continued)

Table 26.4 (continued)

Diagnoses	Reference images		
	DWI high	ADC low	T2 high
Contusion	Fig. 17.20b	Fig. 17.20c	Fig. 17.20a
Diffuse axonal injury (DAI)	Fig. 17.2c	Fig. 17.2d	Fig. 17.2a
Tumor Glioblastoma (solid)	Fig. 18.13d	Fig. 18.13e	Fig. 18.13a
Lymphoma	Fig. 18.47d	Fig. 18.47e	Fig. 18.47a

26 How to Use This Book

Table 26.4 (continued)

Diagnoses	Reference images		
	DWI high	ADC low	T2 high
Meningioma (meningothelial)	Fig. 18.38c	Fig. 18.38d	Fig. 18.38a
Meningioma (atypical)	Fig. 18.43c	Fig. 18.43d	Fig. 18.43a
Metastasis (lung)	Fig. 16.9c	Fig. 16.9d	Fig. 16.9a
Primitive neuroectodermal tumor (PNET)	Fig. 18.34c	Fig. 18.34d	Fig. 18.34a

(continued)

Table 26.4 (continued)

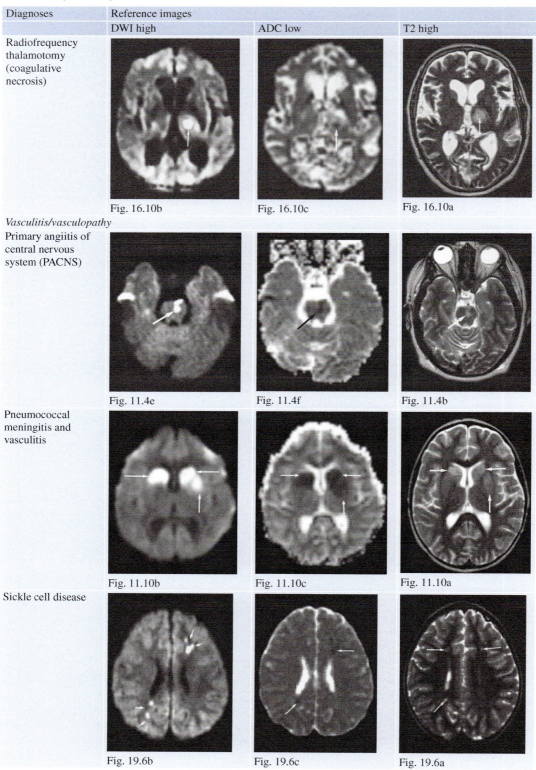

Table 26.4 (continued)

Diagnoses	Reference images		
	DWI high	ADC low	T2 high
Hemolytic uremic syndrome (HUS)	Fig. 11.25b	Fig. 11.25c	Fig. 11.25a

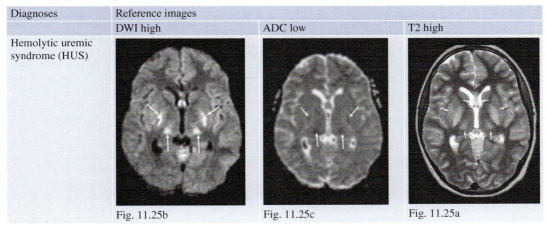

Table 26.5 Differential diagnoses for lesions with an **iso diffusion** signal associated with a **high ADC** and **high intense T2** signal

Diagnoses	Reference images		
	DWI iso	ADC high	T2 high
Vasculitis/Vasculopathy			
Posterior reversible encephalopathy syndrome (PRES)	Fig. 3.4c	Fig. 3.4d	Fig. 3.4b
Vasogenic edema (metastasis)	Fig. 3.5e	Fig. 3.5d	Fig. 3.5a

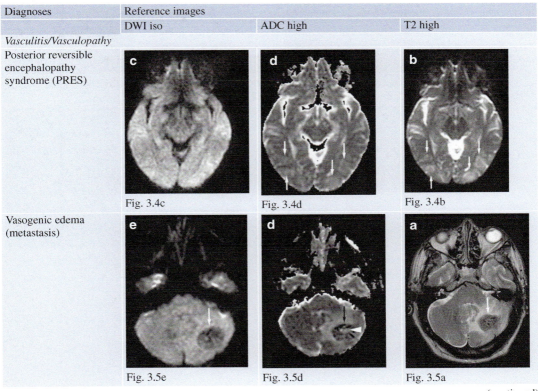

(continued)

Table 26.5 (continued)

Diagnoses	Reference images		
	DWI iso	ADC high	T2 high
Tacrolimus neurotoxicity	Fig. 11.20b	Fig. 11.20c	Fig. 11.20a
Postictal encephalopathy	Fig. 12.14d	Fig. 12.14e	Fig. 12.14a
Metabolic disease Wernicke encephalopathy	Fig. 15.21b	Fig. 15.21c	Fig. 15.21a

26 How to Use This Book

Table 26.6 Differential diagnoses for lesions with a **low diffusion** signal associated with a **high ADC** and **high intense T2** signal

Diagnoses	Reference images		
	DWI low	ADC high	T2 high
Infarction			
Chronic infarction (10 months)	Fig. 9.4c	Fig. 9.4d	Fig. 9.4b
Tumor			
Glioblastoma (necrosis)	Fig. 16.8c	Fig. 16.8d	Fig. 16.8a
Craniopharyngioma	Fig. 18.55c	Fig. 18.55b	Fig. 18.55a
Metastasis (lung)	Fig. 18.60c	Fig. 18.60d	Fig. 18.60a

(continued)

Table 26.6 (continued)

Diagnoses	Reference images		
	DWI low	ADC high	T2 high
Arachnoid cyst	Fig. 18.54c	Fig. 18.54d	Fig. 18.54a
Vanishing white matter disease	Fig. 19.83b	Fig. 19.83c	Fig. 19.83a
Van der Knaap disease	Fig. 19.80b	Fig. 19.80c	Fig. 19.80a
Vasogenic edema (toxoplasmosis)	Fig. 8.35b	Fig. 8.35c	Fig. 8.35a

Table 26.7 Differential diagnoses for lesions with a **low diffusion** signal associated with a **high ADC**

Diagnoses	Reference images		
	DWI low	ADC high	T2 iso
Normal			
Neonate			

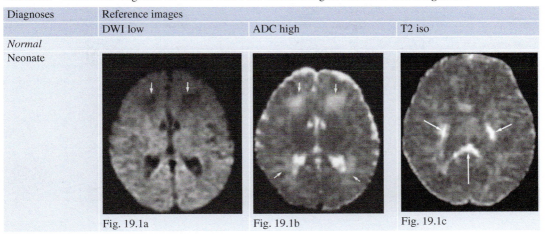

Fig. 19.1a   Fig. 19.1b   Fig. 19.1c

Table 26.8 Differential diagnoses for lesions with **artifacts**

Diagnoses	Reference images		
	DWI	ADC	T2
Susceptibility artifacts			
Physiological iron deposition			
Oxy/deoxy hemoglobin			

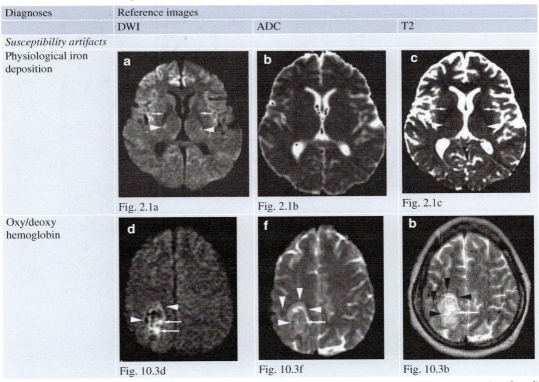

Fig. 2.1a   Fig. 2.1b   Fig. 2.1c

Fig. 10.3d   Fig. 10.3f   Fig. 10.3b

(continued)

Table 26.8 (continued)

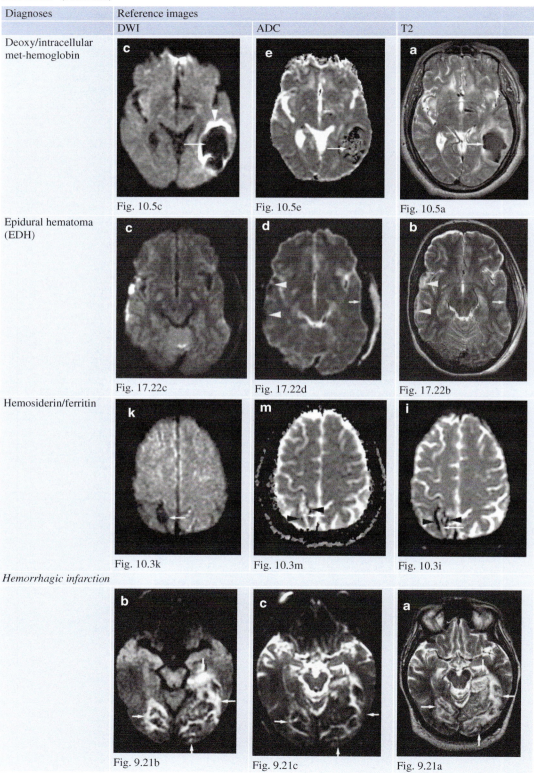

26 How to Use This Book

Table 26.8 (continued)

Diagnoses	Reference images		
	DWI	ADC	T2
Disseminated aspergillosis	Fig. 11.11c	Fig. 11.11d	Fig. 11.11a
Metastasis (melanoma)	Fig. 18.61d	Fig. 18.61e	Fig. 18.61b
Contusion	Fig. 17.19c	Fig. 17.19d	Fig. 17.19b

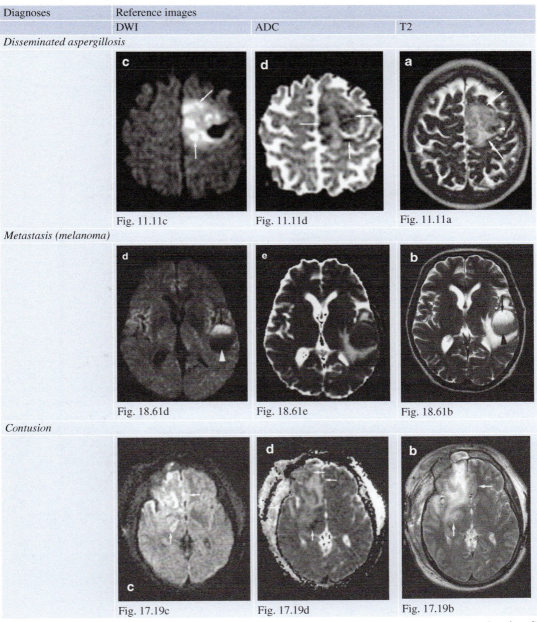

(continued)

Table 26.8 (continued)

Diagnoses	Reference images		
	DWI	ADC	T2
Eddy current artifacts			
N/2 ghosting artifacts			
Motion artifacts			

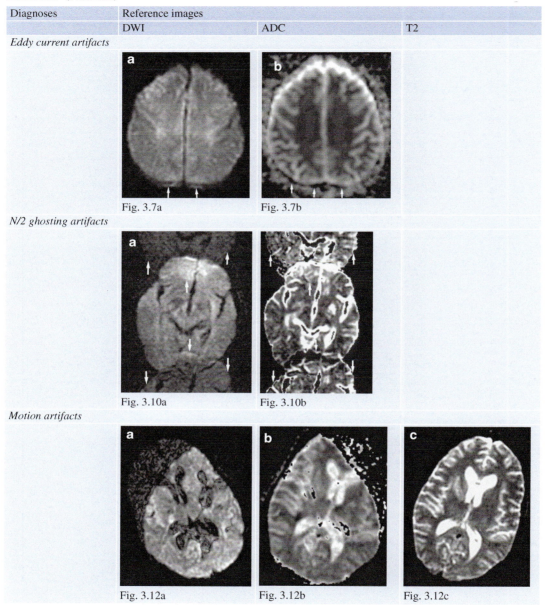

Fig. 3.7a   Fig. 3.7b

Fig. 3.10a   Fig. 3.10b

Fig. 3.12a   Fig. 3.12b   Fig. 3.12c

Correction to: Future Directions for Diffusion Imaging of the Brain and Spinal Cord

Takayuki Obata, Jeff Kershaw, Akifumi Hagiwara, and Shigeki Aoki

---

Correction to:
T. Moritani, A. A. Capizzano (eds.), *Diffusion-Weighted MR Imaging of the Brain, Head and Neck, and Spine*,
https://doi.org/10.1007/978-3-030-62120-9

The texts "Permission not yet received" and "Permission from the Journal is not yet received, but it is open access and I am 1st and corresponding author" in the figure captions of the following figures 24.5, 24.7, 24.8, 24.10, 24.11 have been removed. The chapter has been updated.

The updated online version of this chapter can be found at
https://doi.org/10.1007/978-3-030-62120-9_24

© Springer Nature Switzerland AG 2021
T. Moritani, A. A. Capizzano (eds.), *Diffusion-Weighted MR Imaging of the Brain, Head and Neck, and Spine*, https://doi.org/10.1007/978-3-030-62120-9_27

Printed in the United States
by Baker & Taylor Publisher Services